D1504646

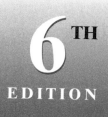

MODERN
PHARMACOLOGY
with Clinical Applications

MODERN
PHARMACOLOGY
with Clinical Applications

6TH
EDITION

Charles R. Craig, PhD
PROFESSOR OF NEUROBIOLOGY AND ANATOMY
West Virginia University School of Medicine
Morgantown, West Virginia

Robert E. Stitzel, PhD
PROFESSOR AND ASSOCIATE CHAIRMAN OF BIOCHEMISTRY AND MOLECULAR PHARMACOLOGY
West Virginia University School of Medicine
Morgantown, West Virginia

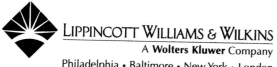

LIPPINCOTT WILLIAMS & WILKINS
A **Wolters Kluwer** Company
Philadelphia • Baltimore • New York • London
Buenos Aires • Hong Kong • Sydney • Tokyo

Editor: Betty Sun
Managing Editor: Rebecca Kerins
Marketing Manager: Joseph Schott
Production Editor: Jennifer Ajello
Designer: Doug Smock
Compositor: Graphic World
Printer: Quebecor World-Dubuque

Copyright © 2004 Lippincott Williams & Wilkins

351 West Camden Street
Baltimore, MD 21201

530 Walnut Street
Philadelphia, PA 19106

All rights reserved. This book is protected by copyright. No part of
this book may be reproduced in any form or by any means, including
photocopying, or utilized by any information storage and retrieval
system without written permission from the copyright owner.

The publisher is not responsible (as a matter of product liability,
negligence, or otherwise) for any injury resulting from any material
contained herein. This publication contains information relating to
general principles of medical care that should not be construed as
specific instructions for individual patients. Manufacturers' product
information and package inserts should be reviewed for current information, including contraindications, dosages, and precautions.

04 05 06 07 08
1 2 3 4 5 6 7 8 9 10
Printed in the United States of America

Library of Congress Cataloging-in-Publication Data

Modern pharmacology with clinical applications / edited by Charles
   R. Craig, Robert E. Stitzel.—6th ed.
         p. ; cm.
      Includes index.
      ISBN 0-7817-3762-1
      1. Clinical pharmacology.   I. Craig, Charles R. II. Stitzel,
      Robert E.
      [DNLM: 1. Pharmacology. 2. Drug Therapy. QV 4 M6898
      2003]
   RM301.28.M63 2003
   615′.1—dc21

The publishers have made every effort to trace the copyright holders
for borrowed material. If they have inadvertently overlooked any, they
will be pleased to make the necessary arrangements at the first oppor-
tunity.

To purchase additional copies of this book, call our customer service
department at **(800) 638-3030** or fax orders to **(301) 824-7390.**
International customers should call **(301) 714-2324.**

Visit Lippincott Williams & Wilkins on the Internet:
http://www.LWW.com. Lippincott Williams & Wilkins customer
service representatives are available from 8:30 am to 6:00 pm, EST.

PREFACE

The sixth edition of *Modern Pharmacology With Clinical Applications* continues our commitment to enlisting experts in pharmacology to provide a textbook that is up-to-date and comprehensive. Designed to be used during a single semester, the book focuses on the clinical application of drugs within a context of the major principles of pharmacology. It is meant to serve students in medicine, osteopathy, dentistry, pharmacy, and advanced nursing, as well as undergraduate students.

SUMMARY OF FEATURES

This edition includes a number of new or updated features that further enhance the appeal of the text.

Study Questions: Each chapter includes five to seven examination questions (following the United States Medical Licensing Examination guidelines) with detailed answers to help students test their knowledge of the covered material.

Case Studies: Appearing at the end of each chapter, case studies present students with real-life examples of clinical scenarios and require them to apply their knowledge to solve the problem.

Refined Focus: In this edition, we chose to focus more on drug classes rather than on individual drugs, eliminate unnecessary detail such as chemical structures, and maintain emphasis on structure–activity relationships in drug action and development.

Updated Information: This edition also includes new information from the clinic and the laboratory. Emerging information has been added within chapters and when appropriate (as in the case of herbal drugs and erectile dysfunction), through the addition of new chapters.

With these revisions, we hope we have provided a book that is readable, up-to-date, comprehensive but not exhaustive, and accurate—a text that supplies both students and faculty with a clear introduction to modern pharmacotherapeutics.

Charles R. Craig
Robert E. Stitzel

ACKNOWLEDGMENT

The editors began working together on *Modern Pharmacology* almost 25 years ago. We are grateful to be working together still as colleagues and friends and are very pleased to dedicate this sixth edition to a new generation of students, and to our grandchildren, Kaya Seneca Stitzhal and Andrew, Megan, and Taylor Craig.

CONTRIBUTING AUTHORS

Albert J. Azzaro, PhD
Chief Scientific Officer, Clinical Development
Somerset Pharmaceuticals
2202 North West Shore Blvd., Suite 450
Tampa, FL 33607

Suzanne Barone, PhD
9710 Bellevue Drive
Bethesda, MD 20814

Steven M. Belknap, MD
Associate Professor
Department of Biomedical & Therapeutic Sciences
University of Illinois College of Medicine at Peoria
PO Box 1649
Peoria, Ill 61656

William O. Berndt, PhD
Vice Chancellor, Academic Affairs
Dean, Graduate Studies and Research
Professor of Pharmacology
University of Nebraska Medical Center
986810 Nebraska Medical Center
Omaha, NE 68198-6810

David R. Bickers, MD
Carl Truman Nelson Professor and Chairman
Department of Dermatology
College of Physicians & Surgeons of Columbia
University
New York, NY 10032

Leo R. Brancazio, PhD
Instructor, Division of Maternal/Fetal Medicine
4010 Hospital South
Duke University Medical Center
Durham, NC 27710-3967

Eric L. Carter, MD
Assistant Clinical Professor of Dermatology
Columbia University College of Physicians and
Surgeons
151 Ft. Washington Avenue
New York, NY 10032

Lisa A. Cassis, PhD
Professor, Division of Pharmaceutical Sciences
University of Kentucky, College of Pharmacy
Lexington, KY 40536-0082

Richard J. Cenedella, PhD
Professor and Chairman, Department of Biochemistry
Kirksville College of Osteopathic Medicine
800 West Jefferson Street
Kirksville, MO 63501

Mary-Margaret Chren, MD
Associate Professor in Residence
University of California at San Francisco
San Francisco VAMC 190
4150 Clement Street
San Francisco, CA 94121

John M. Connors, PhD
Associate Professor
Department of Physiology and Pharmacology
West Virginia University School of Medicine
Morgantown, WV 26506-9229

Charles R. Craig, PhD
*Director of West Virginia University Research
Compliance*
Professor of Neurobiology and Anatomy
West Virginia University School of Medicine
Morgantown, WV 26506-9142

John W. Dailey, PhD
Professor Emeritus
Department of Basic Science
University of Illinois College of Medicine
PO Box 1649
Peoria, IL 61656

Priscilla S. Dannies, PhD
Professor of Pharmacology
Department of Pharmacology School of Medicine
Yale University
333 Cedar Street
New Haven, CT 06510

Mary E. Davis, PhD
Professor of Physiology and Pharmacology
West Virginia University School of Medicine
Morgantown, WV 26506-9229

William L. Dewey, PhD
Professor of Pharmacology and Toxicology
Virginia Commonwealth University
310 N. 12th Street
PO Box 980613
Richmond, VA 23219-0613

Jeffrey S. Fedan, PhD
Professor of Physiology and Pharmacology
West Virginia University School of Medicine
Research Pharmacologist
National Institute for Occupational Safety and Health
Morgantown, WV 26506

Mitchell S. Finkel, MD
Professor of Medicine and Biochemistry and Molecular Pharmacology
West Virginia University School of Medicine
Morgantown, WV 26506-9157

Peter S. Fischbach, MD
Department of Pediatric & Communicable Diseases
Division of Pediatric Cardiology
F1310 Mott Children's Hospital
Ann Arbor, MI 48109-0204

Janet Fleetwood, PhD
Director, Medical Humanities Program
Medical College of Pennsylvania
3300 Henry Avenue
Philadelphia, PA 19129

Peter A. Friedman, PhD
Professor of Pharmacology
University of Pittsburgh School of Medicine
Pittsburgh, PA 15261

William W. Fleming, PhD
Professor Emeritus
Department of Physiology and Pharmacology
West Virginia University School of Medicine
Morgantown, WV 26506-9229

Lisa M. Gangarosa, MD
Assistant Professor
Section of Gastroenterology
C.B. 7080
University of North Carolina
Burnett-Womack Bldg., Room 724
Chapel Hill, NC 27599

Jennifer Rubin Grandis, M.D
Associate Professor of Otolaryngology
University of Pittsburgh School of Medicine
Pittsburgh, PA 15261

James F. Graumlich, MD
Assistant Professor of Biomedical & Therapeutic Sciences
University of Illinois College of Medicine
One Illini Drive, Box 1649
Peoria, IL 61656-1649

Garrett J. Gross, PhD
Professor of Pharmacology & Toxicology
Medical College of Wisconsin
8701 Watertown Plank Road
Milwaukee, WI 53226

David Haddox, D.D.S., MD, F.A.C.P.M.
Medical Director, Internal Analgesics
Purdue Pharmaceuticals
100 Connecticut Avenue
Norwalk, CT 06850-3590

Douglas W. P. Hay, PhD
Associate Fellow, Department of Pulmonary Pharmacology
SmithKline Beecham Pharmaceuticals
King of Prussia, PA 19406-0639

Arthur F. Hefti, D.MD, P.D.
Associate Dean
Research and Graduate Studies
Ohio State University College of Medicine and Dentistry
305 W. 12th Ave.
Columbus, OH 43210

J. Thomas Hjelle, PhD
Associate Professor of Pharmacology
Department of Biomedical and Therapeutic Sciences
University of Illinois College of Medicine at Peoria
One Illini Drive
Peoria, IL 61605

Michael B. Howie, MD
Professor of Anesthesia
The Ohio State University College of Medicine
Columbus, OH 43210

Mir Abid Husain, MD
Saint Francis Medical Center
530 NE Glen Oak Avenue
Peoria, IL 61637

Gregory Juckett, MD
Professor of Family Medicine
West Virginia University Health Sciences Center
Morgantown, WV 26506-9247

Stephen M. Lasley, PhD
Department of Biomedical & Therapeutic Sciences
University of Illinois College of Medicine
PO Box 1649
Peoria, IL 61656-1649

John S. Lazo, PhD
Professor and Chair, Department of Pharmacology
University of Pittsburgh School of Medicine
E1340 Biomedical Sciences Tower
Pittsburgh, PA 15261-0001

Tony J.-F. Lee
Professor of Pharmacology
Southern Illinois University
School of Medicine
Springfield, IL 62794-9629

Benedict R. Lucchesi, MD, PhD
Professor of Pharmacology
Department of Pharmacology
University of Michigan Medical School
1301 MSRB III
Ann Arbor, MI 48109-0632

Angelo Mariotti, D.D.S., PhD
Chair, Department of Periodontology
Ohio State University College of Medicine and
Dentistry
305 W. 12th Ave.
Columbus, OH 43210

Billy R. Martin, PhD
Professor and Chair
Department of Pharmacology & Toxicology
Virginia Commonwealth University
410 N. 12th St., 7th floor, Room 760
PO Box 980613
Richmond, VA 23298-0377

Jeane McCarthy, MD
Clinical Professor of Pediatrics
University of South Florida
All Children's Hospital
St. Petersburg, FL 33701

Joseph J. McPhillips, PhD
Retired, formerly Director of Clinical Research
Boehringer Mannheim Pharmaceuticals Corp.
Current address: 20611 Highland Hall Drive
Montgomery Village, MD 20886-4024

Marcia A. Miller-Hjelle, PhD
*Chief, Section of Medical Microbiology and Infectious
Diseases*
Department of Biomedical and Therapeutic Sciences
University of Illinois College of Medicine
One Illini Drive, Box 1649
Peoria, IL 61656-1649

Roman J. Miller, PhD
Professor of Biology
Eastern Mennonite College
Harrisonburg, VA 22801

Humayun Mirza, MD
Interventional Fellow
Section of Cardiology, Department of Medicine
West Virginia University School of Medicine
Morgantown, WV 26506-9157

Michael D. Miyamoto, PhD
Professor of Pharmacology
East Tennessee State University College of Medicine
Johnson City, TN 37614-0577

Richard P. O'Connor, MD
C/o Caterpillar Corporate Medical
Caterpillar Inc.
PO Box 600
Mossville, IL 61552-0600

Mark Reasor, PhD
Professor of Physiology and Pharmacology
West Virginia University School of Medicine
Morgantown, WV 26506-9229

Ronald P. Rubin, PhD
Professor and Chair
Department of Pharmacology and Toxicology
State University of New York at Buffalo
School of Medicine
102 Farber Hall
Buffalo, NY 14214-3000

Leonard J. Sauers, PhD, D.A.B.T.
*Director, Product Safety, Regulatory Affairs, &
Analytical Sciences*
The Procter & Gamble Company
Ivorydale Technical Center
5299 Spring Grove Avenue
Cincinnati, OH 45217

Leonard William Scheibel, MD
Chief, Section of Clinical Pharmacology
University of Illinois College of Medicine
Department of Biomedical & Therapeutic Sciences
PO Box 1649
Peoria, IL 61656-1649

Frank L. Schwartz, MD
Associate Professor of Medicine
West Virginia University School of Medicine
Morgantown, WV 26506
Medical Director, Diabetes Center
Camden Clark Memorial Hospital
Parkersburg, WV 26101

Donald G. Seibert, MD
Gastroenterology Associates of Southwest Virginia
2012 Stephenson Ave SW
Roanoke, VA 24014

Branimir I. Sikic, MD, PhD
*Professor of Medicine (Oncology) and Clinical
Pharmacology*
Stanford University Medical Center
Stanford, CA 94305-5151

David C. Slagle, MD
Saint Francis Medical Center
530 N. E. Glen Oak Avenue
Peoria, IL 61637

David J. Smith, PhD
*Professor of Biochemistry and Molecular
Pharmacology*
West Virginia University School of Medicine
Morgantown, WV 26506-9142

Vijaya Somaraju, MD
Saint Francis Medical Center
530 N. E. Glen Oak Avenue
Peoria, IL 61637

Patricia K. Sonsalla, PhD
Associate Professor of Neurology
UMDNJ-RW Johnson Medical School
675 Hoes Lane
Piscataway, NJ 08854-5635

Robert E. Stitzel, PhD
Director of University Graduate Education
Professor and Associate Chair
Department of Biochemistry and Molecular
Pharmacology
West Virginia University School of Medicine
Morgantown, WV 26506-9142

Jeannine Strobl, PhD
*Professor of Biochemistry and Molecular
Pharmacology*
West Virginia University School of Medicine
Morgantown, WV 26506-9142

V. C. Swamy, PhD
Chair, Biomedical Pharmacology
School of Pharmacy
State University of New York at Buffalo
313 Hochstetter Hall
Buffalo, NY 14260

David A. Taylor, PhD
Professor and Chair of Pharmacology
East Carolina University School of Medicine
Greenville, NC 27858-4353

John A. Thomas, PhD
219 Wood Shadow
San Antonio, TX 78216-1633

Michael J. Thomas, MD, PhD
*Associate Professor of Medicine, Division of
Endocrinology*
University of North Carolina School of Medicine
6101 Thurston Bowles, CB #7170
Chapel Hill, NC 27599-7170

Theodore J. Torphy, PhD
Vice President and Director of Pharmacology
Centocor, Inc.
200 Great Valley Parkway
Malvern, PA 19355

Timothy S. Tracy, PhD
Associate Professor of Basic Pharmaceutical Sciences
West Virginia University School of Pharmacy
Morgantown, WV 26506-9530

David Triggle, PhD
Dean, State University of New York at Buffalo
School of Pharmacy
126 Cooke
Buffalo, NY 14260-0001

Knox Van Dyke, PhD
*Professor of Biochemistry and Molecular
Pharmacology*
West Virginia University School of Medicine
Morgantown, WV 26506-9142

Herbert E. Ward, MD
Department of Psychiatry
University of Florida
PO Box 100256
Gainesville, FL 32610-0256

Sandra P. Welch, PhD
Professor of Pharmacology & Toxicology
Virginia Commonwealth University
PO Box 980613
Richmond, VA 23298-0613

David P. Westfall, PhD
Professor of Pharmacology
University of Nevada-Reno, MS318
Reno, NV 89557-0046

Thomas C. Westfall, PhD
Professor and Chair
Department of Pharmacology and Physiological
Sciences
St. Louis University School of Medicine
1402 S. Grand Blvd.
St. Louis, MO 63104-1083

William F. Wonderlin, PhD
*Associate Professor of Biochemistry and Molecular
Pharmacology*
West Virginia University School of Medicine
Morgantown, WV 26506-9142

Karen A. Woodfork, PhD
*Adjunct Associate Professor in Biochemistry and
Molecular Pharmacology*
West Virginia University School of Medicine
Morgantown, WV 26506-9142

TABLE OF CONTENTS

I

GENERAL PRINCIPLES OF PHARMACOLOGY

1 | Progress in Therapeutics

Robert E. Stitzel and Joseph J. McPhillips

Early in human history a natural bond formed between religion and the use of drugs. Those who became most proficient in the use of drugs to treat disease were the "mediators" between this world and the spirit world, namely, the priests, shamans, holy persons, witches, and soothsayers. Much of their power within the community was derived from the cures that they could effect with drugs. It was believed that the sick were possessed by demons and that health could be restored by identifying the demon and finding a way to cast it out.

Originally, religion dominated its partnership with *therapeutics,* and divine intervention was called upon for every treatment. However, the use of drugs to effect cures led to a profound change in both religious thought and structure. As more became known about the effects of drugs, the importance of divine intervention began to recede, and the treatment of patients effectively became a province of the priest rather than the gods whom the priest served. This process lead to a growing understanding of the curative powers of natural products and a decreasing reliance on supernatural intervention and forever altered the relationship between humanity and its gods. Furthermore, when the priests began to apply the information learned from treating one patient to the treatment of other patients, there was a recognition that a regularity prevailed in the natural world independent of supernatural whim or will. Therapeutics thus evolved from its roots in magic to a foundation in experience. This was the cornerstone for the formation of a science-based practice of medicine.

CONTRIBUTIONS OF MANY CULTURES

The ancient Chinese wrote extensively on medical subjects. The *Pen Tsao,* for instance, was written about 2700 B.C. and contained classifications of individual medicinal plants as well as compilations of plant mixtures to be used for medical purposes. The Chinese *doctrine of signatures* (like used to treat like) enables us to understand why medicines of animal origin were of such great importance in the Chinese pharmacopoeia.

Ancient Egyptian medical papyri contain numerous prescriptions. The largest and perhaps the most important of these, the *Ebers papyrus* (1550 B.C.), contains about 800 prescriptions quite similar to those written today in that they have one or more active substances as well as vehicles (animal fat for ointments; and water, milk, wine, beer, or honey for liquids) for suspending or dissolving the active drug. These prescriptions also commonly offer a brief statement of how the preparation is to be prepared (mixed, pounded, boiled, strained, left overnight in the dew) and how it is to be used (swallowed, inhaled, gargled, applied externally, given as an enema). Cathartics and purgatives were particularly in vogue, since both patient and physician could tell almost immediately whether a result had been achieved. It was reasoned that in causing the contents of the gastrointestinal tract to be forcibly ejected, one simultaneously drove out the disease-producing evil spirits that had taken hold of the unfortunate patient.

The level of drug usage achieved by the Egyptians undoubtedly had a great influence on Greek medicine and literature. Observations on the medical effects of various natural substances are found in both the *Iliad* and the *Odyssey*. Battle wounds frequently were covered with powdered plant leaves or bark; their astringent and pain-reducing actions were derived from the tannins they contained. It may have been mandrake root (containing atropinelike substances that induce a twilight sleep) that protected Ulysses from Circe. The oriental hellebore, which contains the cardiotoxic *Veratrum* alkaloids, was smeared on arrow tips to increase their killing power. The fascination of the Greeks with the toxic effects of various plant extracts led to an increasing body of knowledge concerned primarily with the poisonous aspects of drugs (the science of *toxicology*). Plato's description of the death of Socrates is an accurate description of the toxicological properties of the juice of the hemlock fruit. His description of the paralysis of sensory and motor nerves, followed eventually by central nervous system depression and respiratory paralysis, precisely matches the known actions of the potent hemlock alkaloid, coniine.

The Indian cultures of Central and South America, although totally isolated from the Old World, developed drug lore and usage in a fashion almost parallel with that of the older civilization. The use of drugs played an intimate part in the rites, religions, history, and knowledge of the South American Indians. New World medicine also was closely tied to religious thought, and Indian cultures treated their patients with a blend of religious rituals and herbal remedies. Incantations, charms, and appeals to various deities were as important as the appropriate application of poultices, decoctions, and infusions.

Early drug practitioners, both in Europe and South America, gathered herbs, plants, animals, and minerals and often blended them into a variety of foul-smelling and ill-flavored concoctions. The fact that many of these preparations were so distasteful led to an attempt to improve on the "cosmetic" properties of these mixtures to ensure that patients would actually use them. Individuals who searched for improved product formulations were largely responsible for the founding of the disciplines of *pharmacy* (the science of preparing, compounding, and dispensing medicines) and *pharmacognosy* (the identification and preparation of crude drugs from natural sources).

There has long been a tendency of some physicians to prescribe large numbers of drugs where one or two would be sufficient. We can trace the history of this polypharmaceutical approach to Galen (A.D. 131–201), who was considered the greatest European physician after Hippocrates. Galen believed that drugs had certain essential properties, such as warmth, coldness, dryness, or humidity, and that by using several drugs he could combine these properties to adjust for deficiencies in the patient. Unfortunately, he often formulated general rules and laws before sufficient factual information was available to justify their formulations.

By the first century A.D. it was clear to both physician and protopharmacologist alike that there was much variation to be found from one biological extract to another, even when these were prepared by the same individual. It was reasoned that to fashion a rational and reproducible system of therapeutics and to study pharmacological activity one had to obtain standardized and uniform medicinal agents.

At the turn of the nineteenth century, methods became available for the isolation of active principles from crude drugs. The development of chemistry made it possible to isolate and synthesize chemically pure compounds that would give reproducible biological results. In 1806, Serturner (1783–1841) isolated the first pure active principle when he purified morphine from the opium poppy. Many other chemically pure active compounds were soon obtained from crude drug preparations, including emetine by Pelletier (1788–1844) from ipecacuanha root; quinine by Carentou (1795–1877) from cinchona bark; strychnine by Magendie (1783–1855) from nux vomica; and, in 1856, cocaine by Wohler (1800–1882) from coca.

The isolation and use of pure substances allowed for an analysis of what was to become one of the basic concerns of pharmacology, that is, the quantitative study of drug action. It was soon realized that drug action is produced along a continuum of effects, with low doses producing a less but essentially similar effect on organs and tissues as high doses. It also was noted that the appearance of toxic effects of drugs was frequently a function of the dose–response relationship.

Until the nineteenth century, the rapid development of pharmacology as a distinct discipline was hindered by the lack of sophisticated chemical methodology and by limited knowledge of physiological mechanisms. The significant advances made through laboratory studies of animal physiology accomplished by early investigators such as Françoise Magendie and Claude Bernard provided an environment conducive to the creation of similar laboratories for the study of pharmacological phenomena.

One of the first laboratories devoted almost exclusively to drug research was established in Dorpat, Estonia, in the late 1840s by Rudolph Bucheim (1820–1879) (Fig. 1.1). The laboratory, built in Bucheim's home, was devoted to studying the actions of agents such as cathartics, alcohol, chloroform, anthelmintics, and heavy metals. Bucheim believed that "the investigation of drugs . . . is a task for a pharmacologist and not for a chemist or pharmacist, who until now have been expected to do this."

Although the availability of a laboratory devoted to pharmacological investigations was important, much more was required to raise this discipline to the same prominent position occupied by other basic sciences; this included the creation of chairs in pharmacology at other

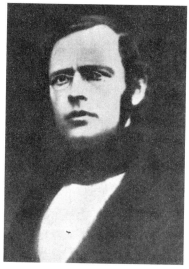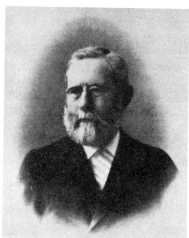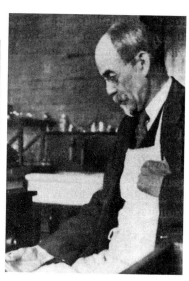

FIGURE 1.1

The three important figures in the early history of pharmacology are (left to right) Rudolf Bucheim, Oswald Schmiedeberg, and John Jacob Abel. They not only created new laboratories devoted to the laboratory investigation of drugs but also firmly established the new discipline through the training of future faculty, the writing of textbooks, and the founding of scientific journals and societies.

academic institutions and the training of a sufficient number of talented investigators to occupy these positions. The latter task was accomplished largely by Bucheim's pupil and successor at Dorpat, Oswald Schmiedeberg (1838–1921), undoubtedly the most prominent pharmacologist of the nineteenth century (Fig. 1.1). In addition to conducting his own outstanding research on the pharmacology of diuretics, emetics, cardiac glycosides, and so forth, Schmiedeberg wrote an important medical textbook and trained approximately 120 pupils from more than 20 countries. Many of these new investigators either started or developed laboratories devoted to experimental pharmacology in their own countries.

One of Schmiedeberg's most outstanding students was John Jacob Abel, who has been called the founder of American pharmacology (Fig 1.1). Abel occupied the chair of pharmacology first at the University of Michigan and then at Johns Hopkins University. Among his most important research accomplishments is an examination of the chemistry and isolation of the active principles from the adrenal medulla (a monobenzyl derivative of epinephrine) and the pancreas (crystallization of insulin). He also examined mushroom poisons, investigated the chemotherapeutic actions of the arsenicals and antimonials, conducted studies on tetanus toxin, and designed a model for an artificial kidney. In addition, Abel founded the *Journal of Experimental Medicine,* the *Journal of Biological Chemistry,* and the *Journal of Pharmacology and Experimental Therapeutics.* His devotion to pharmacological research, his enthusiasm for the training of students in this new discipline, and his establishment of journals and scientific societies proved critical to the rise of experimental pharmacology in the United States.

Pharmacology, as a separate and vital discipline, has interests that distinguish it from the other basic sciences and pharmacy. Its primary concern is not the cataloguing of the biological effects that result from the administration of chemical substances but rather the dual aims of (1) providing an understanding of normal and abnormal human physiology and biochemistry through the application of drugs as experimental tools and (2) applying to clinical medicine the information gained from fundamental investigation and observation.

A report in the *Status of Research in Pharmacology* has described some of the founding principles on which the discipline is based and that distinguish pharmacology from other fields of study. These principles include the study of the following:

- The relationship between drug concentration and biological response
- Drug action over time
- Factors affecting absorption, distribution, binding, metabolism, and elimination of chemicals
- Structure-activity relationships
- Biological changes that result from repeated drug use: tolerance, addiction, adverse reactions, altered rates of drug metabolism, and so forth
- Antagonism of the effects of one drug by another
- The process of drug interaction with cellular macromolecules (receptors) to alter physiological function (i.e., receptor theory)

In the past 100 years there has been extraordinary growth in medical knowledge. This expansion of information has come about largely through the contributions of the biological sciences to medicine by a systematic approach to the understanding and treatment of disease. The experimental method and technological advances are the foundations upon which modern medicine is built.

DRUG CONTROL AND DEVELOPMENT

Before the twentieth century, most government controls were concerned not with drugs but with impure and adulterated foods. Medicines were thought to pose problems similar to those presented by foods. Efficacy was questioned in two respects: adulteration of active medicines by addition of inert fillers and false claims made for the so-called patent (secret) medicines or nostrums. Indeed, much of the development of the science of pharmacy in the nineteenth century was standardizing and improving prescription drugs.

A landmark in the control of drugs was the 1906 Pure Food and Drug Act. Food abuses, however, were the primary target. Less than one quarter of the first thousand decisions dealt with drugs, and of these, the majority were concerned with patent medicines.

The 1906 law defined *drug* broadly and governed the labeling but not the advertising of any substance used to affect disease. This law gave the *Pharmacopoeia* and the *National Formulary* equal recognition as authorities for drug specifications. In the first contested criminal prosecution under the law, action was taken against the maker of a headache mixture bearing the beguiling name of *Cuforhedake-Brane-Fude*. In 1912, Congress passed an amendment to the Pure Food and Drug Act that banned false and fraudulent therapeutic claims for patent medicines.

Prescription drugs also were subject to control under the 1906 law. In fact, until 1953 there was no fixed legal boundary between prescription and nonprescription medications. Prescription medications received a lower priority, since food and patent medicine abuses were judged to be the more urgent problems.

For the next 30 years, drug control was viewed primarily as a problem of prohibiting the sale of dangerous drugs and tightening regulations against misbranding. Until the 1930s, new drugs posed little problem because there were few of them.

MODERN DRUG LEGISLATION

The modern history of United States drug regulation began with the Food, Drug and Cosmetic Act of 1938, which superseded the 1906 Pure Food and Drug Act. The 1938 act was viewed as a means of preventing the marketing of untested, potentially harmful drugs. An obscure provision of the 1938 act was destined to be the starting point for some of the most potent controls the Food and Drug Administration (FDA) now exercises in the drug field. This provision allowed the prescription drug to come under special control by requiring that it carry the legend "Caution—to be used only by or on the prescription of a physician."

A major defect of the generally strong 1938 law was its inadequate control of advertising. Regulations now require that the "labeling on or within the package from which the drug is to be dispensed" contain adequate information for the drug's use; this requirement explains the existence of the package insert. If the pharmaceutical manufacturer makes claims for its product beyond those contained in an approved package insert, the FDA may institute legal action against the deviations in advertising.

The 1938 act required manufacturers to submit a New Drug Application (NDA) to the FDA for its approval before the company was permitted to market a new drug. *Efficacy* (proof of effectiveness) became a requirement in 1962 with the Kefauver-Harris drug amendments. These amendments established a requirement that drugs show "substantial evidence" of efficacy before receiving NDA approval. Substantial evidence was defined in the amendments as evidence consisting of adequate and well-controlled investigations, including clinical investigations, by experts qualified by scientific training and experience to evaluate the effectiveness of the drug, on the basis of which such experts could fairly and responsibly conclude that the drug would have the claimed effect under the conditions of use named on the label.

Drug regulation in the United States is continuing to evolve rapidly, both in promulgation of specific regulations and in the way regulations are implemented (Table 1.1). The abolition of patent medicines is an outstanding example, as is control over the accuracy of claims made for drugs. Since the 1962 amendments, the advertising of prescription drugs in the United States has been increasingly controlled—to a greater extent than in most other countries. All new drugs introduced since 1962 have some proof of efficacy. This is not to say that misleading drug advertisements no longer exist; manufacturers still occasionally make unsubstantiated claims.

TABLE 1.1   **Phases of Clinical Investigation**

Phase	Purpose
I	Establish safety
II	Establish efficacy and dose
III	Verify efficacy and detect adverse affects
IV	Obtain additional data following approval

CLINICAL TESTING OF DRUGS

Experiments conducted on animals are essential to the development of new chemicals for the management of disease. The safety and efficacy of new drugs, however, can be established only by adequate and well-controlled studies on human subjects. Since findings in animals do not always accurately predict the human response to drugs, subjects who participate in clinical trials are put at some degree of risk. The risk comes not only from the potential toxicity of the new drug but also from possible lack of efficacy, with the result that the condition under treatment becomes worse. Since risk is involved, the primary consideration in any clinical trial should be the welfare of the subject. As a consequence of unethical or questionably ethical practices committed in the past, most countries have established safeguards to protect the rights and welfare of persons who participate in clinical trials. Two of the safeguards that have been established are the *institutional review board* (IRB) and the requirement for *informed consent.*

The IRB, also known as the ethics committee or human subjects committee, originally was established to protect people confined to hospitals, mental institutions, nursing homes, and prisons who may be used as subjects in clinical research. In the United States any institution conducting clinical studies supported by federal funds is required to have proposed studies reviewed and approved by an IRB.

People who volunteer to be subjects in a drug study have a right to know what can and will happen to them if they participate (informed consent). The investigator is responsible for ensuring that each subject receives a full explanation, in easily understood terms, of the purpose of the study, the procedures to be employed, the nature of the substances being tested, and the potential risks, benefits, and discomforts.

PHASES OF CLINICAL INVESTIGATION

The clinical development of new drugs usually takes place in steps or phases conventionally described as clinical pharmacology (*phase I*), clinical investigation (*phase II*), clinical trials (*phase III*), and postmarketing studies (*phase IV*). Table 1.1 summarizes the four phases of clinical evaluation.

Phase I

When a drug is administered to humans for the first time, the studies generally have been conducted in healthy *men* between 18 and 45 years of age; this practice is coming under increasing scrutiny and criticism. For certain types of drugs, such as antineoplastic agents, it is not appropriate to use healthy subjects because the risk of injury is too high. *The purpose of phase I studies is to establish the dose level at which signs of toxicity first appear.* The initial studies consist of administering a single dose of the test drug and closely observing the subject in a hospital or clinical pharmacology unit with emergency facilities. If no adverse reactions occur, the dose is increased progressively until a predetermined dose or serum level is reached or toxicity supervenes. Phase I studies are usually confined to a group of 20 to 80 subjects. If no untoward effects result from single doses, short-term multiple-dose studies are initiated.

Phase II

If the results of phase I studies show that it is reasonably safe to continue, *the new drug is administered to patients for the first time.* Ideally, these individuals should have no medical problems other than the condition for which the new drug is intended. Efforts are concentrated on evaluating efficacy and on establishing an optimal dose range. Therefore, dose–response studies are a critical part of phase II studies. Monitoring subjects for adverse effects is also an integral part of phase II trials. The number of subjects in phase II studies is usually between 80 and 100.

Phase III

When an effective dose range has been established and no serious adverse reactions have occurred, large numbers of subjects can be exposed to the drug. In phase III studies the number of subjects may range from several hundred to several thousand, depending on the drug. *The purpose of phase III studies is to verify the efficacy of the drug* and to detect effects that may not have surfaced in the phase I and II trials, during which exposure to the drug was limited. A new drug application is submitted at the end of phase III. However, for drugs intended to treat patients with life-threatening or severely debilitating illnesses, especially when no satisfactory therapy exists, the FDA has established procedures designed to expedite development, evaluation, and marketing of new therapies. In the majority of cases, the procedure applies to drugs being developed for the treatment of cancer and acquired immunodeficiency syndrome (AIDS). Under this procedure, drugs can be approved on the basis of phase II studies conducted in a limited number of patients.

Phase IV

Controlled and uncontrolled studies often are conducted after a drug is approved and marketed. Such studies are intended to broaden the experience with the drug and compare it with other drugs.

SPECIAL POPULATIONS

One of the goals of drug development is to provide sufficient data to permit the safe and effective use of the drug.

Therefore, the patient population that participates in clinical trials should be representative of the patient population that will receive the drug when it is marketed. To a varying extent, however, *women, children, and patients over 65 years of age have been underrepresented in clinical trials of new drugs.* The reasons for exclusion vary, but the consequence is that prescribing information for these patient populations is often deficient.

ADVERSE REACTION SURVEILLANCE

Almost all drugs have adverse effects associated with their use; these range in severity from mild inconveniences to severe morbidity and death. Some adverse effects are extensions of the drug's pharmacological effect and are predictable, for example, orthostatic hypotension with some antihypertensive agents, arrhythmias with certain cardioactive drugs, and electrolyte imbalance with diuretics. Other adverse effects are not predictable and may occur rarely or be delayed for months or years before the association is recognized. Examples of such reactions are aplastic anemia associated with chloramphenicol and clear cell carcinoma of the uterus in offspring of women treated with diethylstilbestrol during pregnancy. Postmarketing surveillance programs and adverse reaction reporting systems may detect such events. The best defense against devastating adverse actions is still the vigilance and suspicion of the physician.

Study QUESTIONS

1. The primary consideration in all clinical trials is to
   (A) Determine the safety of the drug
   (B) Determine the efficacy of the drug
   (C) Ensure that there is no risk to the subject
   (D) Provide for the welfare of the subject
2. To conduct reliable clinical trials with a potential new drug, it is necessary to establish a dose level that toxicity first appears. This is commonly determined in
   (A) Phase I Studies
   (B) Phase II Studies
   (C) Phase III Studies
   (D) Phase IV Studies
3. The history of pharmacology includes a long list of heroes. The person considered to be the founder of American pharmacology is
   (A) Claude Bernard
   (B) Rudolph Bucheim
   (C) John Jacob Abel
   (D) Oswald Schmeideberg

ANSWERS

1. **D.** There is always some degree of risk in clinical trials; the object is to minimize the risk to the patient. The primary consideration in any clinical trial is the welfare of the subject. The safety of the drug is one objective for certain clinical trials as is the efficacy of the drug in other trials.
2. **A.** Phase I studies are carried out in normal volunteers. The object of phase I studies is to determine the dose level at which signs of toxicity first appear. Phase II studies are carried out in patients in which the drug is designed to be effective in. It is conducted to determine efficacy and optimal dosage. Phase III studies are a continuation of phase II, but many more patients are involved. The purpose of phase III studies is to verify efficacy established earlier in phase II studies and to detect adverse effects that may not have surfaced in earlier studies. Phase IV studies are conducted when the drug has been approved and is being marketed. The purpose of these studies is to broaden the experience with the drug and to compare the new drug with other agents that are being used clinically.
3. **C.** John Jacob Abel occupied the first chair of a department of pharmacology in the United States. This was at the University of Michigan. Abel subsequently left Michigan to chair the first department of pharmacology at Johns Hopkins University. Claude Bernard was an early French physiologist and pharmacologist. Rudolph Bucheim established one of the first pharmacology laboratories at the University of Dorpat (Estonia). Oswald Schmiedeberg is considered the founder of pharmacology. He trained approximately 120 pupils from around the world, including the father of American pharmacology, John Jacob Abel.

SUPPLEMENTAL READING

Burks TF. Two hundred years of pharmacology: A midpoint assessment. Proc West Pharmacol Soc 2000;43:95–103.

Guarino RA. (ed). New Drug Approval Process. New York: Dekker, 1992.

Holmstead B and Liljestrand G. (eds.). Readings in Pharmacology. New York: Macmillan, 1963.

Huang KC. The Pharmacology of Chinese Herbs. Boca Raton, FL: CRC, 1993.

Lemberger L. Of mice and men: The extension of animal models to the clinical evaluation of new drugs. Clin Pharmacol Ther 1986;40:599–603.

Muscholl E. The evolution of experimental pharmacology as a biological science: The pioneering work of Bucheim and Schmiedeberg. Brit J Pharmacol 1995;116:2155–2159.

O'Grady J and Joubert PH (eds.). Handbook of Phase I/II Clinical Drug Trials. Boca Raton, FL: CRC, 1997.

Parascandola J. John J. Abel and the emergence of U.S. pharmacology. Pharmaceut News 1995;2:911.

Spilker, B. Guide to Clinical Trials. New York: Raven, 1991.

2 Mechanisms of Drug Action

William W. Fleming

RECEPTORS

A fundamental concept of pharmacology is that to initiate an effect in a cell, most drugs combine with some molecular structure on the surface of or within the cell. This molecular structure is called a *receptor*. The combination of the drug and the receptor results in a molecular change in the receptor, such as an altered configuration or charge distribution, and thereby triggers a chain of events leading to a *response*. This concept applies not only to the action of drugs but also to the action of naturally occurring substances, such as hormones and neurotransmitters. Indeed, many drugs mimic the effects of hormones or transmitters because they combine with the same receptors as do these endogenous substances.

It is generally assumed that all receptors with which drugs combine are receptors for neurotransmitters, hormones, or other physiological substances. Thus, the discovery of a specific receptor for a group of drugs can lead to a search for previously unknown endogenous substances that combine with those same receptors. For example, evidence was found for the existence of endogenous peptides with morphinelike activity. A series of these peptides have since been identified and are collectively termed *endorphins* and *enkephalins* (see Chapter 26). It is now clear that drugs such as morphine merely mimic endorphins or enkephalins by combining with the same receptors.

DRUG RECEPTORS AND BIOLOGICAL RESPONSES

Although the term *receptor* is convenient, one should never lose sight of the fact that *receptors are in actuality molecular substances or macromolecules in tissues that combine chemically with the drug.* Since most drugs have a considerable degree of *selectivity* in their actions, it follows that the receptors with which they interact must be equally unique. Thus, *receptors will interact with only a limited number of structurally related or complementary compounds.*

The drug–receptor interaction can be better appreciated through a specific example. The end-plate region of a skeletal muscle fiber contains large numbers of receptors having a high affinity for the transmitter acetylcholine. Each of these receptors, known as nicotinic receptors, is an integral part of a channel in the postsynaptic membrane that controls the inward movement of sodium ions (see Chapter 28). At rest, the postsynaptic membrane is relatively impermeable to sodium. Stimulation of the nerve leading to the muscle results in the release of acetylcholine from the nerve fiber in the region of the end plate. The acetylcholine combines with the receptors and changes them so that channels are opened and sodium flows inward. The more acetylcholine the end-plate region contains, the more receptors are occupied and the more channels are open. When the number of open channels reaches a critical value, sodium enters rapidly enough to disturb the ionic balance of the membrane, resulting in local depolarization. The local depolarization (end-plate potential) triggers the activation of large numbers of voltage-dependent sodium channels, causing the conducted depolarization known as an action potential. The action potential leads to the release of calcium from intracellular binding sites. The calcium then interacts with the contractile proteins, resulting in shortening of the muscle cell. The sequence of events can be shown diagrammatically as follows:

$$\text{Ach} + \text{receptor} \rightarrow \text{Na}^+ \text{ influx} \rightarrow \text{action potential}$$
$$\rightarrow \text{increased free Ca}^{++} \rightarrow \text{contraction}$$

where Ach = acetylcholine. The precise chain of events following drug–receptor interaction depends on the particular receptor and the particular type of cell. The important concept at this stage of the discussion is that *specific receptive substances serve as triggers of cellular reactions.*

If we consider the sequence of events by which acetylcholine brings about muscle contraction through receptors, we can easily appreciate that foreign chemicals (drugs) can be designed to interact with the same process. Thus, such a drug would *mimic* the actions of acetylcholine at the motor end plate; nicotine and carbamylcholine are two drugs that have such an effect. *Chemicals that interact with a receptor and thereby initiate a cellular reaction are termed* agonists. Thus, acetylcholine itself, as well as the drugs nicotine and carbamylcholine, are agonists for the receptors in the skeletal muscle end plate.

On the other hand, if a chemical is somewhat less similar to acetylcholine, it may interact with the receptor but be unable to induce the exact molecular change necessary to allow the inward movement of sodium. In this instance the chemical does not cause contraction, but because it occupies the receptor site, it prevents the interaction of acetylcholine with its receptor. Such a drug is termed an *antagonist.* An example of such a compound is *d*-tubocurarine, an antagonist of acetylcholine at the end-plate receptors. Since it competes with acetylcholine for its receptor and prevents acetylcholine from producing its characteristic effects, administration of *d*-tubocurarine results in muscle relaxation by interfering with acetylcholine's ability to induce and maintain the contractile state of the muscle cells.

Historically, receptors have been identified through recognition of the relative selectivity by which certain exogenously administered drugs, neurotransmitters, or hormones exert their pharmacological effects. By applying mathematical principles to *dose–response relationships*, it became possible to estimate dissociation constants for the interaction between specific receptors and individual agonists or antagonists. Subsequently, methods were developed to measure the specific binding of radioactively labeled drugs to receptor sites in tissues and thereby determine not only the *affinity* of a drug for its receptor, but also the *density of receptors* per cell.

In recent years much has been learned about the chemical structure of certain receptors. The nicotinic receptor on skeletal muscle, for example, is known to be composed of five subunits, each a glycoprotein weighing 40,000 to 65,000 daltons. These subunits are arranged as interacting helices that penetrate the cell membrane completely and surround a central pit that is a sodium ion channel. The binding sites for acetylcholine (see Chapter 12) and other agonists that mimic it are on one of the subunits that project extracellularly from the cell membrane. The binding of an agonist to these sites changes the conformation of the glycoprotein so that the side chains move away from the center of the channel, allowing sodium ions to enter the cell through the channel. The glycoproteins that make up the nicotinic receptor for acetylcholine serve as both the walls and the gate of the ion channel. This arrangement represents one of the simpler mechanisms by which a receptor may be coupled to a biological response.

SECOND-MESSENGER SYSTEMS

Many receptors are capable of initiating a chain of events involving second messengers. Key factors in many of these second-messenger systems are proteins termed G *proteins,* short for guanine nucleotide–binding proteins. G proteins have the capacity to bind guanosine triphosphate (GTP) and hydrolyze it to guanosine diphosphate (GDP).

G proteins couple the activation of several different receptors to the next step in a chain of events. In a number of instances, the next step involves the enzyme adenylyl cyclase. Many neurotransmitters, hormones, and drugs can either stimulate or inhibit adenylyl cyclase through their interaction with different receptors; these receptors are coupled to adenylate cyclase through either a stimulatory (G_s) or an inhibitory (G_i) G protein. During the coupling process, the binding and subsequent hydrolysis of GTP to GDP provides the energy needed to terminate the coupling process.

The activation of adenylyl cyclase enables it to catalyze the conversion of adenosine triphosphate (ATP) to 3′5′-cyclic adenosine monophosphate (cAMP), which in turn can activate a number of enzymes known as *kinases.* Each kinase phosphorylates a specific protein or proteins. Such phosphorylation reactions are known to be involved in the opening of some calcium channels as well as in the activation of other enzymes. In this system, the receptor is in the membrane with its binding site on the outer surface. The G protein is totally within the membrane while the adenylyl cyclase is within the membrane but projects into the interior of the cell. The cAMP is generated within the cell (see Figure 10.4).

Whether or not a particular agonist has any effect on a particular cell depends initially on the presence or absence of the appropriate receptor. However, the *nature* of the response depends on these factors:

- Which G protein couples with the receptor
- Which kinase is activated
- Which proteins are accessible for the kinase to phosphorylate

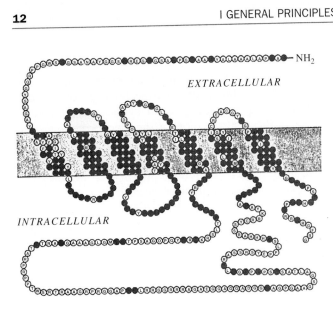

FIGURE 2.1

Primary structure of the human kidney α_2-adrenoceptor. The amino acid sequence is represented by the one-letter code. (Reprinted with permission from Regan JW et al. Cloning and expression of a human kidney cDNA. Proc Natl Acad Sci USA 85:6301, 1988.)

The variety of possible responses is further increased by the fact that receptor-coupled G proteins can either activate enzymes other than adenylate cyclase or can directly influence ion channel functions.

Many different receptor types are coupled to G proteins, including receptors for norepinephrine and epinephrine (α- and β-adrenoceptors), 5-hydroxytryptamine (serotonin or 5-HT receptors), and muscarinic acetylcholine receptors. Figure 2.1 presents the structure of one of these, the α_2-adrenoceptor from the human kidney. All members of this family of G protein–coupled receptors are characterized by having seven membrane-enclosed domains plus extracellular and intracellular loops. *The specific binding sites for agonists occur at the extracellular surface, while the interaction with G proteins occurs with the intracellular portions of the receptor.* The general term for any chain of events initiated by receptor activation is *signal transduction.*

THE CHEMISTRY OF DRUG–RECEPTOR BINDING

Biological receptors are capable of combining with drugs in a number of ways, and the forces that attract the drug to its receptor must be sufficiently strong and long-lasting to permit the initiation of the sequence of events that ends with the biological response. Those forces are *chemical bonds,* and a number of types of bonds participate in the formation of the initial drug–receptor complex.

The bond formed when two atoms share a pair of electrons is called a *covalent bond.* It possesses a bond energy of approximately 100 kcal/mole and therefore is strong and stable; that is, it is essentially irreversible at body temperature. Covalent bonds are responsible for the stability of most organic molecules and can be broken only if sufficient energy is added or if a catalytic agent that can facilitate bond disruption, such as an enzyme, is present. Since bonds of this type are so stable at physiological temperatures, the binding of a drug to a receptor through covalent bond formation would result in the formation of a long-lasting complex.

Although most drug–receptor interactions are readily reversible, some compounds, such as the anticancer nitrogen mustards (see Chapter 56) and other alkylating agents form relatively irreversible complexes. Covalent bond formation is a desirable feature of an antineoplastic or antibiotic drug, since long-lasting inhibition of cell replication is needed. However, covalent bond formation between environmental pollutants and cellular constituents may result in mutagenesis or carcinogenesis in normal, healthy cells.

The formation of an *ionic bond* results from the electrostatic attraction that occurs between oppositely charged ions. The strength of this bond is considerably less (5 kcal/mole) than that of the covalent bond and diminishes in proportion to the square of the distance between the ionic species. Most macromolecular receptors have a number of ionizable groups at physiological pH (e.g., carboxyl, hydroxyl, phosphoryl, amino) that are available for interaction with an ionizable drug.

The hydrogen atom, with its strongly electropositive nucleus and single electron, can be bound to one strongly electronegative atom and still accept an electron from another electronegative donor atom, such as nitrogen or oxygen, and thereby form a bridge (*hydrogen bond*) between these two donor atoms. The formation of several such bonds between two molecules (e.g., drug and receptor) can result in a relatively stable but reversible interaction. Such bonds serve to maintain the tertiary structure of proteins and nucleic acids and are thought to play a significant role in establishing the selectivity and specificity of drug–receptor interactions.

Van der Waals bonds are quite weak (0.5 kcal/mole) and become biologically important only when two atoms are brought into sufficiently close contact. Van der Waals forces play a significant part in determining drug–receptor specificity. Like the hydrogen bonds, several van der Waals bonds may be established between two molecules, especially if the drug molecule and a receptor have complementary three-dimensional conformations and thus fit closely together. The closer the drug comes to the receptor, the stronger the possible binding forces that can be established. Slight differences in three-dimensional shape among a group of agonists and therefore slight differences in fit or strength of bonding forces that can be established between agonists and receptor form the basis for the *structure–activity relationships* among related agonists.

DYNAMICS OF DRUG–RECEPTOR BINDING

The drug molecule, following its administration and passage to the area immediately adjacent to the receptor surface (sometimes called the *biophase*), must bond with the receptor before it can initiate a response. Resisting this bond formation is a random thermal agitation that is inherent in every molecule and tends to keep the molecule in constant motion. Under normal circumstances, the electrostatic attraction of the ionic bond, which can be exerted over longer distances than can the attraction of either the hydrogen or van der Waals bond, is the first force that draws the ionized molecule toward the oppositely charged receptor surface. This is a reasonably strong bond and will lend some stability to the drug–receptor complex.

Generally, the ionic bond must be reinforced by a hydrogen or van der Waals bond or both before significant receptor activation can occur. This is true because unreinforced bonds are too easily and quickly broken by the energy of thermal agitation to permit sufficient time for adequate drug–receptor interaction to take place. The better the structural congruity (i.e., fit) between drug and its receptor, the more secondary (i.e., hydrogen and van der Waals) bonds can form.

Even if extensive binding has taken place, unless covalent bond formation has occurred, the drug–receptor complex can still dissociate. Once dissociation has occurred, drug action is terminated. For most drug–receptor interactions, there is a continual random association and dissociation. The frequencies of association and dissociation are a function of the affinity between the drug and the receptor, the density of receptors, and the concentration of drug in the biophase. *The magnitude of the response is generally considered to be a function of the concentration of the drug–receptor complexes formed at any moment in time.*

DOSE–RESPONSE RELATIONSHIP

To understand drug–receptor interactions, it is necessary to quantify the relationship between the drug and the biological effect it produces. Since the degree of effect produced by a drug is generally a function of the amount administered, we can express this relationship in terms of a *dose–response curve.* Because we cannot always quantify the concentration of drug in the biophase in the intact individual, it is customary to correlate effect with dose administered.

In general, biological responses to drugs are *graded;* that is, the response continuously increases (up to the maximal responding capacity of the given responding system) as the administered dose continuously increases. Expressed in receptor theory terminology, this means that *when a graded dose–response relationship exists, the response to the drug is directly related to the number of receptors with which the drug effectively interacts.* This is one of the tenets of pharmacology.

The principles derived from dose–response curves are the same in animals and humans. However, obtaining the data for complete dose–response curves in humans is generally difficult or dangerous. We shall therefore use animal data to illustrate these principles.

Quantal Relationships

In addition to the responsiveness of a given patient, one may be interested in the relationship between dose and some specified quantum of response among *all* individuals taking that drug. Such information is obtained by evaluating data obtained from a *quantal dose–response curve.*

Anticonvulsants can be suitably studied by use of quantal dose–response curves. For example, to assess the potential of new anticonvulsants to control epileptic seizures in humans, these drugs are initially tested for their ability to protect animals against experimentally induced seizures. In the presence of a given dose of the drug, the animal either has the seizure or does not; that is, it either is or is not protected. Thus, in the design of this experiment, the effect of the drug (protection) is *all or none.* This type of response, *in contrast to a graded response,* must be described in a noncontinuous manner.

The construction of a quantal dose–response curve requires that data be obtained from many individuals. Although any given patient (or animal) either will or will not respond to a given dose, a comparison of individuals within a population shows that members of that population are not identical in their ability to respond to a particular dose. This variability can be expressed as a type of dose–response curve, sometimes termed a *quantal dose–response curve,* in which the dose (plotted on the horizontal axis) is evaluated against the percentage of animals in the experimental population that is protected by each dose (vertical axis). Such a dose–response curve for the anticonvulsant phenobarbital is illustrated in Figure 2.2*A.* Five groups of 10 rats per group were used. The animals in any one group received a particular dose of phenobarbital of 2, 3, 5, 7, or 10 mg/kg body weight. The percentage of animals in each group protected against convulsions was plotted against the dose of phenobarbital. As Figure 2.2*A* shows, the lowest dose protected none of the 10 rats to which it was given, whereas 10mg/kg protected 10 of 10. With the intermediate doses, some rats were protected and some

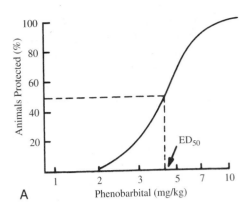
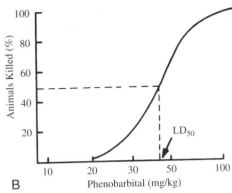

A

B

FIGURE 2.2
Quantal dose–response curves based on all-or-none responses. **A.** Relationship between the dose of phenobarbital and the protection of groups of rats against convulsions. **B.** Relationship between the dose of phenobarbital and the drug's lethal effects in groups of rats. ED_{50}, effective dose, 50%; LD_{50}, lethal dose, 50%.

were not; this indicates that the rats differ in their sensitivity to phenobarbital.

The quantal dose–response curve is actually a *cumulative plot* of the normal frequency distribution curve. The frequency distribution curve, in this case relating the minimum protective dose to the frequency with which it occurs in the population, generally is bell shaped. If one graphs the cumulative frequency versus dose, one obtains the sigmoid-shaped curve of Figure 2.2*A*. *The sigmoid shape is a characteristic of most dose–response curves when the dose is plotted on a geometric, or log, scale.*

Therapeutic Index
Effective Dose

The quantal dose–response curve represents estimates of the *frequency* with which each dose elicits the desired response in the population. In addition to this information, it also would be useful to have some way to express the average sensitivity of the entire population to phenobarbital. This is done through the calculation of an ED_{50} (effective dose, 50%; i.e., the dose that would protect 50% of the animals). This value can be obtained from the dose–response curve in Figure 2.2*A*, as shown by the broken lines. The ED_{50} for phenobarbital in this population is approximately 4mg/kg.

Lethal Dose

Another important characteristic of a drug's activity is its *toxic effect.* Obviously, the ultimate toxic effect is death. A curve similar to that already discussed can be constructed by plotting percent of animals killed by phenobarbital against dose (Fig. 2.2*B*). From this curve, one can calculate the LD_{50} (lethal dose, 50%). Since *the degree of safety associated with drug administration depends on an adequate separation between doses producing a therapeutic effect* (e.g., ED_{50}) *and doses producing toxic effects* (e.g., LD_{50}), one can use a comparison of

these two doses to estimate drug safety. Thus, one estimate of a drug's margin of safety is the ratio LD_{50}/ED_{50}; this is the *therapeutic index.* The therapeutic index for phenobarbital used as an anticonvulsant is approximately 40/4, or 10.

As a general rule, a drug should have a high therapeutic index; however, some important therapeutic agents have low indices. For example, although the therapeutic index of the cardiac glycosides is only about 2 for the treatment and control of cardiac failure, these drugs are important for many cases of cardiac failure. Therefore, in spite of a low margin of safety, they are often used for this condition. The identification of a low margin of safety, however, dictates particular caution in its use; the appropriate dose for each individual must be determined separately.

It has been suggested that a more realistic estimate of drug safety would include a comparison of the lowest dose that produces toxicity (e.g., LD_1) and the highest dose that produces a maximal therapeutic response (e.g., ED_{99}). A ratio less than unity would indicate that a dose effective in 99% of the population will be lethal in more than 1% of the individuals taking that dose. Figure 2.2 indicates that Phenobarbital's ratio LD_1/ED_{99} is approximately 2.

Protective Index

The margin of safety is only *one* of several criteria to be used in determining a drug's clinical merit. Clearly, *the therapeutic index is a very rough measure of safety and generally represents only the starting point* in determining whether a drug is safe enough for human use. Usually, undesirable side effects occur in doses lower than the lethal doses. For example, phenobarbital induces drowsiness and an associated temporary neurological impairment. Since anticonvulsant drugs are intended to allow people with epilepsy to live normal seizure-free lives, sedation is unacceptable. Thus, an important measure of safety for an anticonvulsant would be the ratio ED_{50} (neurological impairment)/ED_{50} (seizure protection). This ratio is called a *protective index*. The protective index for phenobarbital is approximately 3. It is easy to see that data derived from dose–response curves can be used in a variety of ways to compare the clinical usefulness of drugs. For instance, a drug with a protective index of 1 is useless as an anticonvulsant, since the dose that protects against convulsion causes an unacceptable degree of drowsiness. A drug with a protective index of 5 would be a more promising anticonvulsant than one with an index of 2.

Graded Responses

More common than the quantal dose–response relationship is the situation in which a single animal (or patient) gives graded responses to graded doses; that is, as the dose is increased, the response increases. *With graded responses, one can obtain a complete dose-response curve in a single animal.* A good example is the effect of the drug levarterenol (L-norepinephrine) on heart rate.

Results of experiments with levarterenol in guinea pigs are shown in Figure 2.3. The data are typical of what one might obtain from constructing complete dose–response curves in each of five different guinea pigs (*a–e*). In animal *a*, a small increase in heart rate occurs at a dose of 0.001 µg/kg body weight. As the dose is increased, the response increases until at 1 µg/kg, the maximum increase of 80 beats per minute occurs. Further increases in dose do not produce greater responses. At the other extreme, in guinea pig *e*, doses below 0.3 µg/kg have no effect at all, and the maximum response occurs only at about 100 µg/kg.

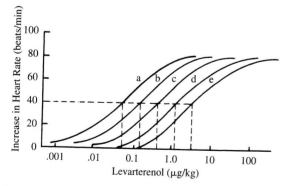

FIGURE 2.3
Dose-response curves illustrating the graded responses of five guinea pigs (a-e) to increasing doses of levarterenol. The responses are increases in heart rate above the rate measured before the administration of the drug. Broken lines indicate 50% of maximum response (horizontal) and individual ED_{50} values (vertical).

Since an entire dose–response relationship is determined from one animal, the curve cannot tell us about the degree of biological variation inherent in a population of such animals. Rather, variability is reflected by a *family* of dose–response curves, such as those given in Figure 2.3. The ED_{50} in this type of dose–response curve is the dose that produced 50% of the maximum response in one animal. In guinea pig *e*, the maximum response is an increase in heart rate of 80 beats per minute. Thus, 50% of the maximum is 40 beats per minute. From Figure 2.3, it can be seen that the dose causing this effect in guinea pig *e* is about 3 µg/kg. The average sensitivity of all of the animals to levarterenol can be estimated by combining the separate dose-response curves into a mean (average) dose–response curve and then calculating the mean ED_{50}. An estimate of the variation within the population can be indicated by calculating a statistical parameter, such as a confidence interval.

It is also possible to construct quantal dose–response curves for drugs that produce graded responses. To do so, one chooses a quantum of effect, for example, an increase in heart rate of 20 to 30 beats per minute above the control, or resting, rate. Doses of the drug are then plotted against the frequency with which each dose produces this amount of effect. The resulting graph has the same characteristics as the graph for the anticonvulsant activity of phenobarbital.

The doses in Figures 2.2 and 2.3 are on not an arithmetic but a logarithmic, or geometric, scale (i.e., the doses are displayed as multiples). This is more apparent in Figure 2.3 because of the greater range of doses. There are many reasons for the common practice of using geometric scales, some of which will become apparent later in this book. One important reason is that in most instances significant increases in response generally occur only when doses are increased in multiples. For example, in Figure 2.3, curve *e*, if one increased the dose from 10 to 11 or 12 µg/kg, the change in response would hardly be measurable. However, if one increased it 3 times or 10 times (i.e., to 30 or 100 µg/kg), one could easily discern increased responses.

The concept of the therapeutic index as a measure of the margin of safety has already been discussed. In the ratio LD_{50}/ED_{50}, the ED_{50} can be obtained from either quantal (Fig. 2.2*A*) or graded (Fig. 2.3) dose–response curves. In the latter case, it must be a *mean* ED_{50}, that is, the average ED_{50} obtained from several individuals.

Potency and Intrinsic Activity

Another drug characteristic that can be compared by use of ED_{50} values is *potency*. Figure 2.4 illustrates the mean dose–response curves of three hypothetical drugs that increase heart rate. Drugs *a* and *b* produce the same maximum response (an increase in heart rate of

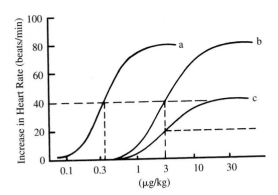

FIGURE 2.4

Idealized dose–response curves of three agonists (a, b, c) that increase heart rate but differ in potency, maximum effect, or both. Broken lines indicate 50% of maximum response (horizontal) and individual ED_{50} values (vertical).

80 beats per minute). However, the fact that the dose–response curve for drug *a* lies to the left of the curve for drug *b* indicates that drug *a* is more potent, that is, *less of drug a is needed to produce a given response*. The difference in potency is quantified by the ratio $ED_{50}b/ED_{50}a$: $3/0.3 = 10$. Thus, drug *a* is 10 times as potent as drug *b*. In contrast, drug *c* has less maximum effect than either drug *a* or drug *b*. Drug *c* is said to have a lower *intrinsic activity* than the other two. Drugs *a* and *b* are full agonists with an intrinsic activity of 1; drug *c* is called a *partial agonist* and has an intrinsic activity of 0.5 because its maximum effect is half the maximum effect of *a* or *b*. The potency of drug *c*, however, is the same as that of drug *b*, because both drugs have the same ED_{50} (3 µg /kg). The ED_{50} is the dose producing a response that is one-half of the maximal response to that *same* drug.

It is important not to equate greater potency of a drug with therapeutic superiority, since one might simply increase the dose of a less potent drug and thereby obtain an identical therapeutic response. Such factors as the severity and frequency of undesirable effects associated with each drug and their cost to the patient are more relevant factors in the choice between two similar drugs.

EQUATIONS DERIVED FROM DRUG–RECEPTOR INTERACTIONS

It is important not to confuse the term *potency* with *affinity* or the term *intrinsic activity* with *efficacy*. The constants that relate an agonist A and its receptor R to the response may be represented as follows:

$$A + R \underset{k_2}{\overset{k_1}{\rightleftharpoons}} AR \overset{k_3}{\rightarrow} \text{response}$$

Affinity is k_1/k_2, and efficacy is represented by k_3. Thus, affinity and efficacy represent kinetic constants that relate the drug, the receptor, and the response at the molecular level. Affinity is the measure of the net molecular attraction between a drug (or neurotransmitter or hormone) and its receptor. Efficacy is a measure of the efficiency of the drug–receptor complex in initiating the signal transduction process. In contrast, potency and intrinsic activity are simple measurements, respectively, of the relative positions of dose–response curves on their horizontal axes and of their relative maxima. Affinity is *one* of the determinants of potency; efficacy contributes *both* to potency and to the maximum effect of the agonist. Figure 2.4 shows that drug *c* has less efficacy (and less intrinsic activity) than either drug *a* or drug *b*. However, in contrast to intrinsic activity, no numerical value of efficacy can be calculated from the data presented. Unfortunately, the terms *potency* and *efficacy* are frequently used in a loose and misleading manner.

The mathematical relationship of response to efficacy and affinity is the following:

$$\frac{E_A}{E_m} = f\left\{ \frac{e[A]}{K_A + [A]} \right\}$$

This equation states that the ratio of the response (E_A) to a given concentration of an agonist to the maximum response (E_m) of the test system, such as an isolated strip of muscle, is a function (f) of efficacy (e) times the concentration of the agonist ([A]) divided by the dissociation constant (K_A) plus the concentration of the agonist. K_A is the reciprocal of the affinity constant and, under equilibrium conditions,

$$K_A = \frac{[R][A]}{[RA]}$$

[R] is the concentration of free receptors and [RA] is the concentration of receptors bound to agonist. Although the details are beyond the scope of this textbook, it should be noted that by the use of combinations of agonists and antagonists, dose–response curves, and mathematical relationships, it is possible to estimate the dissociation constants of agonists and antagonists for a given receptor and to estimate the relative efficacy of two agonists acting on the same receptor.

DRUG ANTAGONISM

The terms *agonist* and *antagonist* have already been introduced. The several types of antagonism can be classified as follows:

1. Chemical antagonism
2. Functional antagonism

3. Competitive antagonism
    a. Equilibrium competitive
    b. Nonequilibrium competitive
4. Noncompetitive antagonism

Chemical Antagonism

Chemical antagonism involves a *direct chemical interaction between the agonist and antagonist* in such a way as to render the agonist pharmacologically inactive. A good example is the use of chelating agents to assist in the biological inactivation and removal from the body of toxic metals. *Chelation* involves a particular type of two-pronged attachment of the antagonist to a metal (the agonist). One chemical chelator, dimercaprol, is used in the treatment of toxicity from mercury, arsenic, and gold. After complexing with the dimercaprol, mercury is biologically inactive and the complex is excreted in the urine.

Functional Antagonism

Functional antagonism is a term used to represent the interaction of two agonists that act independently of each other but happen to cause opposite effects. Thus, indirectly, each tends to cancel out or reduce the effect of the other. A classic example is acetylcholine and epinephrine. These agonists have opposite effects on several body functions. Acetylcholine slows the heart, and epinephrine accelerates it. Acetylcholine stimulates intestinal movement, and epinephrine inhibits it. Acetylcholine constricts the pupil, and epinephrine dilates it; and so on.

Competitive Antagonism

Competitive antagonism is the most frequently encountered type of drug antagonism in clinical practice. *The antagonist combines with the same site on the receptor as does the agonist, but unlike the agonist, does not induce a response;* that is, the antagonist has little or no *efficacy.* The antagonist competes with the agonist for its binding site on the receptor. Competitive antagonists can fall into either of two subtypes, depending on the type of bond formed between the antagonist and the receptor. If the bond is a loose one, the antagonism is called *equilibrium competitive* or *reversibly competitive.* If the bond is covalent, however, the combination of the antagonist with the receptor is not readily reversible, and the antagonism is termed *nonequilibrium competitive or irreversibly competitive.*

If the antagonism is of the equilibrium type, the antagonism increases as the concentration of the antagonist increases. Conversely, the antagonism can be overcome (surmounted) if the concentration of the agonist in the *biophase* (the region of the receptors) is in-

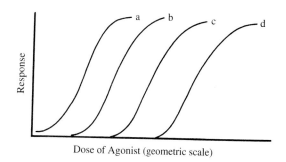

Dose of Agonist (geometric scale)

FIGURE 2.5
Idealized dose–response curves of an agonist in the absence (a) and the presence (b, c, d) of increasing doses of an equilibrium-competitive antagonist.

creased. This relationship can best be appreciated by examining dose–response curves, as in Figure 2.5. Curve *a* is obtained in the absence of the antagonist. Curve *b* is obtained in the presence of a modest amount of the antagonist. The curves are parallel, and the maximum effects are equal. The antagonist has shifted the dose–response curve of the agonist to the right. Any level of response is still possible, but greater amounts of the agonist are required. If the amount of the antagonist is increased, the dose–response curve is shifted farther to the right (curve *c),* still with no decrease in the maximum effect of the agonist. However, the amount of agonist required to achieve maximum response is greater with each increase in the amount of antagonist. Examples of equilibrium-competitive antagonists are atropine, *d*-tubocurarine phentolamine, and naloxone.

Of course, this continual shift of the curve to the right with no change in maximum as the dose of antagonist is increased assumes that very large amounts of the agonist can be achieved in the biophase. This is generally true when the agonist is a drug being added from outside the biological system. However, if the agonist is a naturally occurring substance released from within the biological system (e.g., a neurotransmitter), the supply of the agonist may be quite limited. In that case, increasing the amount of antagonist ultimately abolishes all response.

The effect of a nonequilibrium antagonist on the dose–response curve of an agonist is quite different from the effect of an equilibrium antagonist, as illustrated in Figure 2.6. As the dose of nonequilibrium antagonist is increased, the slope of the agonist curve and the maximum response achieved are progressively depressed. When the amount of antagonist is adequate (curve *d),* no amount of agonist can produce any response. The haloalkylamines, such as phenoxybenzamine, which form covalent bonds with receptors, are examples of nonequilibrium-competitive antagonists (see Chapter 11).

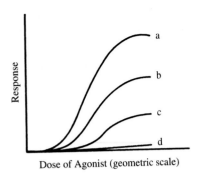

FIGURE 2.6
Idealized dose–response curves of an agonist in the
absence (a) and the presence (b, c, d) of increasing doses
of a non–equilibrium-competitive antagonist.

Noncompetitive Antagonism

*In noncompetitive antagonism, the antagonist acts at a
site beyond the receptor for the agonist.* The difference
between a competitive and a noncompetitive antagonist
can be appreciated from the following scheme, in which
two agonists, A and B, interact with totally different receptor systems, R_A and R_B, to initiate a chain of events
leading to contraction of a vascular smooth muscle cell.
X is a competitive antagonist, and Y is a noncompetitive
antagonist.

$$A + R_A \searrow$$
$$\text{Depolarization} \rightarrow \text{increased}$$
$$\nearrow \qquad \text{free}$$
$$B + R_B \qquad\qquad \text{calcium} \rightarrow \text{contraction}$$
$$\uparrow \qquad\qquad\qquad\qquad \uparrow$$
$$X \qquad\qquad\qquad\qquad Y$$

Antagonist X (competitive) has an affinity for R_B but
not R_A. Thus, it specifically antagonizes agonist B. It
does not antagonize agonist A. Antagonist Y acts on a
receptor associated with the cellular translocation of
calcium and inhibits the increase in intracellular free
calcium. It will therefore antagonize the effects of both
A and B, since they both ultimately depend on calcium
movement to cause contraction.

The effect of a noncompetitive antagonist on the
dose–response curve for an agonist would be the same as
the effect of a non–equilibrium-competitive antagonist
(Fig. 2.6). The practical difference between a noncompetitive antagonist and a nonequilibrium-competitive antagonist is *specificity*. The noncompetitive antagonist
antagonizes agonists acting through more than one receptor system; the nonequilibrium-competitive antagonist antagonizes only agonists acting through one receptor system. The antihypertensive drug diazoxide is one of
the few examples of therapeutically useful noncompetitive antagonists (see Chapter 20).

Study QUESTIONS

1. Receptors are macromolecules that
   (A) Are designed to attract drugs
   (B) Are resistant to antagonists
   (C) Exist as targets for physiological neurotrans-
   mitters and hormones
   (D) Are only on the outer surface of cells
   (E) Are only inside of cells
2. All of the following are capable of initiating a signal
   transduction process EXCEPT
   (A) Combination of an agonist with its receptor
   (B) Combination of an antagonist with its receptor
   (C) Combination of a neurotransmitter with its
   receptor
   (D) Combination of a hormone with its receptor

3. Which of the following chemical bonds would cre-
   ate an irreversible combination of an antagonist
   with its receptor?
   (A) Ionic bond
   (B) Hydrogen bond
   (C) Van der Waals bond
   (D) Covalent bond
4. Potency is determined by
   (A) Affinity alone
   (B) Efficacy alone
   (C) Affinity and efficacy
   (D) Affinity and intrinsic activity
   (E) Efficacy and intrinsic activity

ANSWERS

1. **C.** There are a large number of receptors in the
   body. Although many drugs are attracted to receptors, the receptors are not designed for that purpose. Antagonists also are attracted to receptors.
   Some receptors are on the cell surface, while others
   are found inside the cell.

2. **B.** An antagonist binds to a receptor and prevents
   the action of an agonist. Choice A is wrong because
   this combination does initiate a signal transduction
   process. C and D are incorrect because both neurotransmitters and hormones work through their appropriate receptor to initiate signal transduction.

3. D. A covalent bond is a strong and stable bond that is essentially irreversibly formed at normal body temperature. The other bonds are much weaker.

4. C. Potency is a useful measure of the comparison between two or more drugs. It does not equate to therapeutic superiority but rather is a measure of the size of the dose required to produce a particular level of response.

SUPPLEMENTAL READING

Brown BL and Dobson PRM (eds.). Cell Signaling: Biology and Medicine of Signal Transduction. New York: Raven, 1993.

Foreman JC and Johansen T. (eds). Textbook of Receptor Pharmacology. Boca Raton, FL: CRC, 1995.

Kenakin TP. Pharmacological Analysis of Drug–receptor Interaction. New York: Lippincott-Raven, 1993.

Kenakin TP, Bond RA, and Bonner TI. Definition of pharmacological receptors. Pharmacol Rev 1992; 44:351–362.

Ruffolo RR and Hollinger MA (eds.). G-Protein Coupled Transmembrane Signaling Mechanisms. Boca Raton, FL: CRC, 1995.

Ruffolo RR et al. Structure and function of α-adreno-ceptors. Pharmacol Rev 1991;43:475–505.

3

Drug Absorption and Distribution

Timothy S. Tracy

Unless a drug acts topically (i.e., at its site of application), it first must enter the bloodstream and then be distributed to its site of action. The mere presence of a drug in the blood, however, does not lead to a pharmacological response. To be effective, the drug must leave the vascular space and enter the intercellular or intracellular spaces or both. The rate at which a drug reaches its site of action depends on two rates: absorption and distribution. *Absorption* is the passage of the drug from its site of administration into the blood; *distribution* is the delivery of the drug to the tissues. To reach its site of action, a drug must cross a number of biological barriers and membranes, predominantly lipid. Competing processes, such as binding to plasma proteins, tissue storage, metabolism, and excretion (Fig. 3.1), determine the amount of drug finally available for interaction with specific receptors.

PROPERTIES OF BIOLOGICAL MEMBRANES THAT INFLUENCE DRUG PASSAGE

Although some substances are translocated by specialized transport mechanisms and small polar compounds may filter through membrane pores, most foreign compounds penetrate cells by diffusing through lipid membranes. A model of membrane structure, shown in Figure 3.2, envisions the membrane as a mosaic structure composed of a discontinuous *bimolecular* lipid layer with fluidlike properties. A smaller component consists of glycoproteins or lipoproteins that are embedded in the lipid matrix and have ionic and polar groups protruding from one or both sides of the membrane. This membrane is thought to be capable of undergoing rapid local shifts, whereby the relative geometry of specific adjacent proteins may change to form channels, or pores. The pores permit the membrane to be less restrictive to the passage of low-molecular-weight hydrophilic substances into cells. In addition to its role as a barrier to solutes, the cell membrane has an important function in providing a structural matrix for a variety of enzymes and drug receptors. The model depicted is *not* thought to apply to capillaries.

Physicochemical Properties of Drugs and the Influence of pH

The ability of a drug to diffuse across membranes is frequently expressed in terms of its lipid–water partition coefficient rather than its lipid solubility per se. This coefficient is defined as the ratio of the concentration of the drug in two immiscible phases: a nonpolar liquid or organic solvent (frequently octanol), representing the membrane; and an aqueous buffer, usually at pH 7.4, representing the plasma. The partition coefficient is a measure of the relative affinity of a drug for the lipid and aqueous phases. Increasing the polarity of a drug, either by increasing its degree of ionization or by adding a carboxyl, hydroxyl, or amino group to the molecule, decreases the lipid–water partition coefficient. Alternatively, reducing drug polarity through suppression of ionization or adding lipophilic (e.g., phenyl or t-butyl) groups results in an increase in the lipid–water partition coefficient.

Drugs, like most organic electrolytes, generally do not completely dissociate (i.e., form ions) in aqueous solution. Only a certain proportion of an organic drug molecule will ionize at a given pH. The smaller the fraction of total drug molecules ionized, the weaker the electrolyte. Since most drugs are either weak organic acids or bases (i.e., weak electrolytes), their degree of

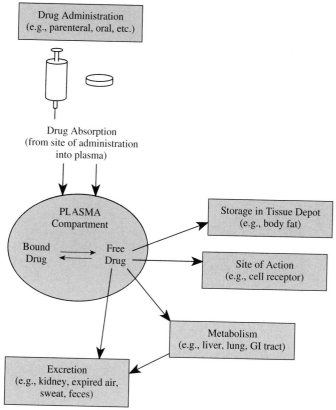

FIGURE 3.1

Factors that affect drug concentration at its site of action. Once a drug has been absorbed into the blood, it may be subjected to varying degrees of metabolism, storage in nontarget tissues, and excretion. The quantitative importance of each of these processes for a given drug determines the ultimate drug concentration achieved at the site of action.

ionization will influence their lipid–water partition coefficient and hence their ability to diffuse through membranes.

The proportion of the total drug concentration that is present in either ionized or un-ionized form is dictated by the drug's dissociation or ionization constant (K) and the local pH of the solution in which the drug is dissolved.

The dissociation of a weak acid, RH, and a weak base, B, is described by the following equations:

$$RH \rightleftharpoons H^+ + R^- \text{ (acid)}$$
$$B + H^+ \rightleftharpoons BH^+ \text{ (base)}$$

If these equations are rewritten in terms of their dissociation constants (using K_a for both weak acids and weak bases), we obtain

$$K_a = \frac{[R^-][H^+]}{[RH]} \text{ (acid)}$$

$$K_a = \frac{[H^+][B]}{[BH^+]} \text{ (base)}$$

By taking logarithms and then substituting the terms pK and pH for the negative logarithms of K_a and [H$^+$], respectively, we arrive at the Henderson-Hasselbach equations:

$$pH = pK_a + \log\frac{[R^-]}{[RH]} \text{ (acid)}$$

and

$$pH = pK_a + \log\frac{[B]}{[BH^+]} \text{ (base)}$$

It is customary to describe the dissociation constants of *both* acids and bases in terms of pK_a values. This is possible in aqueous biological systems because a simple mathematical relationship exists between pK_a, pK_b, and the dissociation constant of water pK_w.

$$pK_a + pK_b = pK_w = 14$$
$$pK_a = 14 - pK_b$$

The use of only pK_a values to describe the relative strengths of either weak bases or weak acids makes comparisons between drugs simpler. The lower the pK_a value ($pK_a < 6$) of an acidic drug, the stronger the acid (i.e., the larger the proportion of ionized molecules). The higher the pK_a value ($pK_a > 8$) of a basic drug, the stronger the base. Thus, knowing the pH of the aqueous medium in which the drug is dissolved and the pK_a of the drug, one can, using the Henderson-Hasselbach equation, calculate the relative proportions of ionized and un-ionized drug present in solution. For example, when the pK_a of the drug (e.g., 7) is the same as the pH (e.g., 7) of the surrounding medium, there will be equal proportions of ionized [R$^-$] and un-ionized [RH] molecules; that is, 50% of the drug is ionized.

The effect of pH on drug ionization is shown in Figure 3.3. The relationship between pH and degree of drug ionization is not linear but sigmoidal; that is, small changes in pH may greatly influence the degree of drug ionization, especially when pH and pK_a values are initially similar.

MECHANISMS OF SOLUTE TRANSPORT ACROSS MEMBRANES

Except for intravenous administration, all routes of drug administration require that the drug be transported from the site of administration into the systemic circulation. A drug is said to be absorbed only when it has entered the blood or lymph capillaries. The transport of drugs across membranes entails one or more of

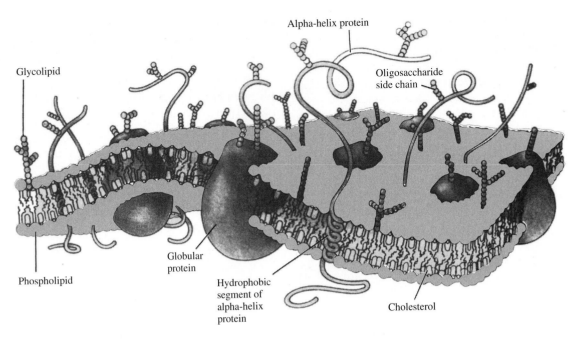

FIGURE 3.2
The plasma membrane, a phospholipid bilayer in which cholesterol and protein molecules are embedded. The bottom layer, which faces the cytoplasm, has a slightly different phospholipid composition from that of the top layer, which faces the external medium. While phospholipid molecules can readily exchange laterally within their own layer, random exchange across the bilayer is rare. Both globular and helical kinds of protein traverse the bilayer. Cholesterol molecules tend to keep the tails of the phospholipids relatively fixed and orderly in the regions closest to the hydrophilic heads; the parts of the tails closer to the core of the membrane move about freely. This model is not believed to apply to blood or lymph capillaries. (Reprinted with permission from Bretscher MS. The molecules of the cell membrane. Sci Am 1985;253:104. Copyright 1985 by Scientific American, Inc. All rights reserved.)

Drug	Intestinal lumen pH 5.0		Membrane barriers		
			Plasma pH 7.4		Stomach pH 1.4
Weak acid— acetaminophen (pK_a 9.5)	[U] $\downarrow\uparrow$ [I] [Total]	= 100 = 0.003 = 100.003	[U] $\downarrow\uparrow$ [I] [Total] = 100 = 0.79 = 100.79		[U] $\downarrow\uparrow$ [I] [Total] = 100 = 0.0 = 100.0
Weak base— diazepam (pK_a 3.3)	[U] $\downarrow\uparrow$ [I] [Total]	= 100 = 2.0 = 102.0	[U] $\downarrow\uparrow$ [I] [Total] = 100 = 0.008 = 100.008		[U] $\downarrow\uparrow$ [I] [Total] = 100 = 7940.0 = 8040.0

FIGURE 3.3
Relative concentrations of the weak acid acetaminophen (pK_a 9.5) and a weak base, diazepam (pK_a 3.3), in some body fluid compartments. [ ], concentration; U, un-ionized drug; I, ionized drug.

the following processes: (1) passive diffusion, (2) filtration, (3) bulk flow, (4) active transport, (5) facilitated transport, (6) ion pair transport, (7) endocytosis, and (8) exocytosis (Fig. 3.4). These processes also participate in the transport of substances necessary for cellular maintenance and growth.

Passive Diffusion

Most drugs pass through membranes by passive diffusion (down their concentration gradient) of the *unionized* moiety. The rate of diffusion depends mainly on the lipid–water partition coefficient rather than on lipid solubility per se. For example, the central nervous system depressant barbital is almost completely un-ionized at physiological pH and therefore should be able to cross membranes easily. However, barbital's lipid–water partition coefficient is sufficiently low that diffusion across membranes proceeds at an extremely slow rate. This slow rate of passage across central nervous system (CNS) membranes largely explains why the time of onset (*latent period*) of drug action after barbital administration is delayed.

A drug will accumulate in the membrane until the ratio of its concentration in the membrane and its concentration in the extracellular fluid equal its partition coefficient. A concentration gradient is thereby established between the membrane and the intracellular space; this gradient is the driving force for the *passive transfer* of the drug into the cell. Thus, a drug that has a very high lipid–water partition coefficient will have a large concentration gradient, and this favors its rapid diffusion across the membrane and into the cell.

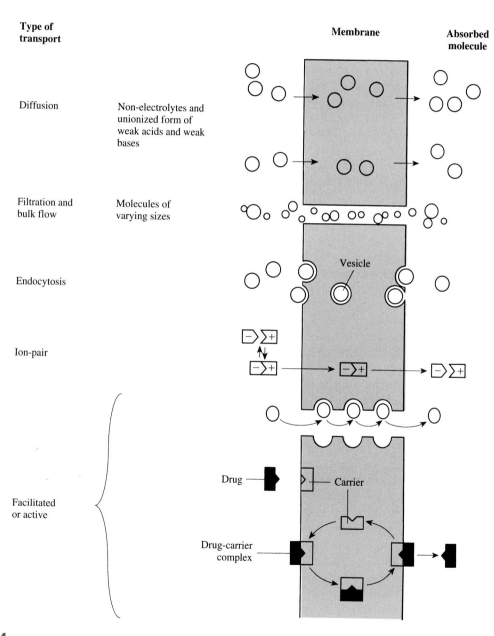

FIGURE 3.4

Mechanisms involved in the passage of drugs across membranes. (Adapted with permission from Smyth DH. Absorption and Distribution of Drugs. Baltimore: Williams & Wilkins, 1964; and Forth W and Rummel W (eds.). Pharmacology of Intestinal Absorption: Gastrointestinal Absorption of Drugs. Vols. 1 and 2. Oxford, UK: Pergammon, 1975).

Filtration

The rate of filtration depends both on the existence of a pressure gradient as a driving force and on the size of the compound relative to the size of the pore through which it is to be filtered. In biological systems, the passage of many small water-soluble solutes through aqueous channels in the membrane is accomplished by filtration. The hypothetical diameter of these pores is about 7 Å, a size that generally limits passage to compounds of molecular weight less than 100 (e.g., urea, ethylene glycol).

Bulk Flow

Most substances, lipid soluble or not, cross the capillary wall at rates that are extremely rapid in comparison with their rates of passage across other body membranes. In fact, the supply of most drugs to the various tissues is limited by blood flow rather than by restraint imposed by the capillary wall. This *bulk flow* of liquid occurs through intercellular pores and is the major mechanism of passage of drugs across most capillary endothelial membranes, with the exception of those in the CNS.

Active Transport

The energy-dependent movement of compounds across membranes, most often against their concentration gradient, is referred to as *active transport*. In general, drugs will not be actively transported unless they sufficiently resemble the endogenous substances (such as sugars, amino acids, nucleic acid precursors) that are the normal substrates for the particular carrier system. This transport involves the reversible binding of the molecule to be transferred to a membrane component (a carrier) of complementary configuration.

Several mechanisms of active transport have been postulated. One transport model proposes that the drug molecule combines with a specific mobile carrier (Fig. 3.4), probably a protein, on one side of the membrane. The complex formed diffuses across the membrane to the opposite side, where the complex dissociates, thus releasing the drug into the aqueous compartment bordering the opposite membrane surface. The carrier protein can then return to its initial side to bind more drug. Another model involves a chainlike arrangement of sites in transport channels to which the drug can bind. The drug would be transferred from one site to another until it had traversed the membrane.

Active transport of a particular substance occurs in one direction only. The number of molecules transported per unit of time will reach a maximum (T_m) once the binding capacity of the carrier becomes saturated. Drugs such as levodopa (for parkinsonism) and α-methyldopa (for hypertension) are actively transported.

Since active transport often requires energy in the form of adenosine triphosphate (ATP), compounds or conditions that inhibit energy production (e.g., iodoacetate, fluoride, cyanide, anaerobiosis) will impair active transport. The transport of a given compound also can be inhibited competitively by the coadministration of other compounds of sufficient structural similarity that they can compete with the first substance for sites on the carrier protein.

Facilitated Diffusion

The transfer of drugs by facilitated diffusion has many of the characteristics associated with active transport, including being a protein carrier–mediated transport system that shows saturability and selectivity. It differs from active transport, however, in that no energy input is required beyond that necessary to maintain normal cellular function. In facilitated transport the movement of the transported molecule is from regions of higher to regions of lower concentrations, so *the driving force for facilitated transport is the concentration gradient*. Although the initial rate of drug transfer will be proportional to the magnitude of the concentration gradient, at some point further increases in drug concentration no longer increase the transport rate; that is, T_m has been reached, since the binding sites on the carrier are now completely saturated.

Ion Pair Transport

Absorption of some highly ionized compounds (e.g., sulfonic acids and quaternary ammonium compounds) from the gastrointestinal tract cannot be explained in terms of the transport mechanisms discussed earlier. These compounds are known to penetrate the lipid membrane despite their low lipid–water partition coefficients. It is postulated that these highly lipophobic drugs combine reversibly with such endogenous compounds as mucin in the gastrointestinal lumen, forming neutral ion pair complexes; it is this neutral complex that penetrates the lipid membrane by passive diffusion.

Endocytosis

Endocytosis involves the cellular uptake of exogenous molecules or complexes inside plasma membrane–derived vesicles. This process can be divided into two major categories: (1) adsorptive or phagocytic uptake of particles that have been bound to the membrane surface and (2) fluid or pinocytotic uptake, in which the particle enters the cell as part of the fluid phase. The solute within the vesicle is released intracellularly, possibly through lysosomal digestion of the vesicle membrane or by intermembrane fusion (Fig. 3.4).

ABSORPTION OF DRUGS FROM THE ALIMENTARY TRACT

Oral Cavity and Sublingual Absorption

In contrast to absorption from the stomach and intestine, drugs absorbed from the oral cavity enter the general circulation directly. Although the surface area of the oral cavity is small, absorption can be rapid if the drug has a high lipid–water partition coefficient and therefore can readily diffuse through lipid membranes. Since the diffusion process is very rapid for un-ionized drugs, pK_a will be a major determinant of the lipid–water partition coefficient for a particular therapeutic agent. For instance, the weak base nicotine (pK_a 8.5) reaches peak blood levels four times faster when absorbed from the mouth (pH 6), where 40 to 50% of the drug is in the un-ionized form, than from the gastrointestinal tract (pH 1–5), where the drug exists mainly in its ionized (protonated) form.

Although the oral mucosa is highly vascularized and its epithelial lining is quite thin, drug absorption from the oral cavity is limited. This is due in part to the relatively slow dissolution rate of most solid dosage forms and in part to the difficulty in keeping dissolved drug in contact with the oral mucosa for a sufficient length of time. These difficulties may be overcome if the drug is placed under the tongue (sublingual administration) or between the cheek and gum (buccal cavity) in a formulation that allows rapid tablet dissolution in salivary secretions. The extensive network of blood vessels facilitates rapid drug absorption. Sublingual administration is the route of choice for a drug like nitroglycerin (glyceryl trinitrate), whose coronary vasodilator effects are required quickly in cases of angina. Furthermore, if swallowed, the drug would be absorbed from the gastrointestinal tract and carried to the liver, where nitroglycerin is subject to rapid metabolism and inactivation.

Absorption from the Stomach

Although *the primary function of the stomach is not absorption,* its rich blood supply and the contact of its contents with the epithelial lining of the gastric mucosa provide a potential site for drug absorption. However, since stomach emptying time can be altered by many variables (e.g., volume of ingested material, type and viscosity of the ingested meal, body position, psychological state), the extent of gastric absorption will vary from patient to patient as well as at different times within a single individual.

The low pH of the gastric contents (pH 1–2) may have consequences for absorption because it can dramatically affect the degree of drug ionization. For example, the weak base diazepam (pK_a 3.3) will be highly protonated in the gastric juice, and consequently, ab-

sorption across lipid membranes of the stomach will be particularly slow. On the other hand, the weak acid acetaminophen (pK_a 9.5) will exist mainly in its un-ionized form and can more readily diffuse from the stomach into the systemic circulation (Fig. 3.3).

Because of the influence of pH on ionization of weak bases, basic drugs may be trapped in the stomach even if they are administered intravenously. Since basic compounds exist primarily in their un-ionized form in the blood (pH 7.4), they readily diffuse from the blood into the gastric juice. Once in contact with the gastric contents (pH 1–2), they will ionize rapidly, which restricts their diffusibility. At equilibrium, the concentration of the un-ionized lipid-soluble fraction will be identical on both sides of the gastric membranes, but there will be more *total* basic drug on the side where ionization is greatest (i.e., in gastric contents). This means of drug accumulation is called *ion trapping.*

Absorption from the Small Intestine

The epithelial lining of the small intestine is composed of a single layer of cells called enterocytes. It consists of many villi and microvilli and has a complex supply of blood and lymphatic vessels into which digested food and drugs are absorbed. The small intestine, with its large surface area and high blood perfusion rate, has a greater capacity for absorption than does the stomach. *Most drug absorption occurs in the proximal jejunum* (first 1–2 m in humans).

Although transfer of drugs across the intestinal wall can occur by facilitated transport, active transport, endocytosis, and filtration, the predominant process for most drugs is diffusion. Thus, the pK_a of the drug and the pH of the intestinal fluid (pH 5) will strongly influence the rate of drug absorption. While weak acids like phenobarbital (pK_a 7.4) can be absorbed from the stomach, they are more readily absorbed from the small intestine because of the latter's extensive surface area.

Conditions that shorten intestinal transit time (e.g., diarrhea) decrease intestinal drug absorption, while increases in transit time will enhance intestinal absorption by permitting drugs to remain in contact with the intestinal mucosa longer. Although delays in gastric emptying time will increase gastric drug absorption, in general, *total* drug absorption may actually decrease, since material will not be transferred to the large absorptive surface of the small intestine.

Absorption from the Large Intestine

The large intestine has a considerably smaller absorptive surface area than the small intestine, but it may still serve as a site of drug absorption, especially for compounds that have not been completely absorbed from the small intestine. However, little absorption occurs from this site, since the relatively solid nature of the intestinal contents impedes diffusion of the *drug* from the contents to the mucosa.

The most distal portion of the large intestine, the rectum, can be used directly as a site of drug administration. This route is especially useful where the drug may cause gastric irritation, after gastrointestinal surgery, during protracted vomiting, and in uncooperative patients (e.g., children) or unconscious ones. Dosage forms include solutions and suppositories. The processes involved in rectal absorption are similar to those described for other sites.

Although the surface area available for absorption is not large, absorption can still occur, owing to the extensive vascularity of the rectal mucosa. Drugs absorbed from the rectum largely escape the biotransformation to which orally administered drugs are subject, because *a portion of the blood that perfuses the rectum is not delivered directly to the liver, and therefore, rectally administered drug, at least in part, escapes hepatic first-pass metabolism.*

FACTORS AFFECTING RATE OF GASTROINTESTINAL ABSORPTION

In addition to the lipid–water partition coefficient of drugs, local blood flow, and intestinal surface area, other factors may affect absorption from the gastrointestinal tract.

Gastric Emptying Time

The rate of gastric emptying markedly influences the rate at which drugs are absorbed, whether they are acids, bases, or neutral substances. In general, factors that accelerate gastric emptying time, thus permitting drugs to reach the large absorptive surface of the small intestine sooner, will increase drug absorption unless the drug is slow to dissolve. A list of physiological, pathological, and pharmacological factors that in-

fluence the rate of gastric emptying is provided in Table 3.1.

Intestinal Motility

Increased gastrointestinal motility may facilitate drug absorption by thoroughly mixing intestinal contents and thereby bringing the drug into more intimate contact with the mucosal surface. However, the opposite may also occur in that an increase in motility may reduce contact time in the upper portion of the intestine where most of drug absorption occurs. Conversely, a decrease in gastrointestinal motility may promote absorption by increasing contact time. Thus, the effect depends on the drug and change in motility. Serious intestinal diseases, particularly those associated with intestinal sloughing, can be expected to alter drug absorption dramatically.

Food

Absorption of most drugs from the gastrointestinal tract is reduced or delayed by the presence of food in the gut. Drugs such as the tetracyclines, which are highly ionized, can complex with Ca^{++} ions in membranes, food, or milk, leading to a reduction in their rate of absorption. For drugs that are ionized in the stomach and un-ionized in the intestine, overall absorption will be delayed by any factor that delays gastric emptying. Finally, increased splanchnic blood flow, as occurs during eating, will increase the rate of drug absorption.

Formulation Factors

The ability of solid drug forms to dissolve and the solubility of the individual drug in the highly acidic gastric juice must be considered. For example, although the anticoagulant dicumarol has a very high lipid–water partition coefficient, it precipitates at the low pH of gastric juice, and the rate of its absorption is

TABLE 3.1   **Some Factors Influencing Gastric Emptying Time**

Factor	Increased gastric emptying rate	Decreased gastric emptying rate
Physiological	Liquids, gastric distention	Solids, acids, fat
Pathological	Duodenal ulcers, gastroenterostomy, chronic pancreatitis	Acute abdominal trauma and pain, labor of child birth, gastric juices, intestinal obstruction, pneumonia, diabetes mellitus
Pharmacological	Reserpine, anticholinesterases, guanethidine, cholinergic agents	Anticholinergic drugs, ganglionic blocking drugs, narcotic analgesics

Reprinted with permission from W. S. Nimmo. Drugs, disease and altered gastric emptying. Clin Pharmacokinet 1976; 1:189.

thereby reduced. This may be overcome by covering the tablets with an enteric coating that dissolves only in the relatively alkaline secretions in the small intestine. Drugs administered in aqueous solution are absorbed faster and more completely than tablet or suspension forms. Suspensions of fine particles (microcrystalline) are better absorbed than are those of larger particles.

Metabolism and Efflux Transporters

Drugs may be inactivated in the gastrointestinal tract before they are absorbed. Until recently, only gut microflora were implicated in the metabolism of drugs in the gastrointestinal system, affecting drug absorption. However, it has now become apparent that drug-metabolizing enzymes, such as the cytochrome P450 enzymes, play a major role in determining the extent of drug absorption of some drugs. Significant expression of cytochrome P450 3A4 and 3A5 occurs in the enterocytes lining the small intestine. These drug-metabolizing enzymes are responsible for approximately 50% of the cytochrome P450–mediated drug metabolism (see Chapter 4) and thus can be expected to play a major role in the presystemic metabolism of a number of drugs. For example, less than 20% of a dose of the immunosuppressant cyclosporine reaches the systemic circulation intact. In fact, most of the metabolism of cyclosporine prior to reaching the systemic circulation takes place in the gut via cytochrome P450 3A4 and 3A5, not in the liver, as might be expected. Thus, gut metabolism is the major factor responsible for the low percentage of an oral dose of cyclosporine reaching the systemic circulation. Cytochrome P450 2C9 and 2C19 are also expressed in measurable quantities in the human intestine. With any of these four cytochrome P450 enzymes, the variation in expression between individuals is substantial, and so their relative contribution to presystemic metabolism of drugs will vary from person to person.

Recently, it has also been discovered that efflux transporters (transporters that pump drug or substrate out of a cell) are also present in human intestinal enterocytes on the apical side nearest the lumen of the intestine. The predominant transporter protein identified to date is P glycoprotein (Pgp), which is a product of the MDR1 gene. This transporter was originally identified as being overexpressed in tumor cells and responsible in part for multidrug resistance because of its role in the efflux of drugs out of tumor cells; thus the name multidrug resistance (MDR) gene. It has become apparent that many of the drugs that are substrates for cytochrome P450 3A4 are also substrates for Pgp. As a substrate for Pgp, a drug will enter the cell, usually via passive diffusion, but then be picked up by the Pgp transporter and carried back to the gut lumen (efflux). As this continually occurs along the intestine, some of the drug molecules are prevented from being absorbed, which decreases overall absorption. Taken together, the Pgp transporter and the cytochrome P450 enzymes form a mechanism to reduce the amount of drug reaching the systemic circulation.

ABSORPTION OF DRUGS FROM THE LUNG

The lungs serve as a major site of administration for a number of agents given for both local and systemic effects. Such drugs can be inhaled as gases (e.g., volatile anesthetics) or as aerosols (suspended liquid droplets or solid particles). Absorption of agents from the lung is facilitated by the large surface area of the pulmonary alveolar membranes (50–100 m²), the limited thickness of these membranes (approximately 0.2 μ), and the high blood flow to the alveolar region.

Pulmonary absorption of volatile anesthetics across the alveolar–capillary barrier is very rapid because of the relatively high lipid–water partition coefficients and small molecular radii of such agents. The driving force for diffusion is a combination of the blood–air partition coefficient (which is a measure of the capacity of blood to dissolve drug) and the difference in partial pressure between the alveoli and the arterial and venous blood. Agents with high blood–air partition coefficients require more drug to be dissolved in the blood for equilibrium to be reached.

ABSORPTION OF DRUGS THROUGH THE SKIN

Most drugs that have been incorporated into creams or ointments are applied to the skin for their local effect. The diffusion rate of a drug through the skin is largely determined by the compound's lipid–water partition coefficient. However, the stratum corneum, or outer layer of the epidermis, forms a barrier against the rapid penetration of most drugs. This is due in large part to the relatively close-packed cellular arrangement and decreased amount of lipid in these cells. Thus, even highly lipid-soluble compounds will be absorbed much more slowly through the skin than from other sites. The dermis, on the other hand, is well supplied with blood and lymph capillaries and therefore is permeable to both lipid-soluble and water-soluble compounds. If penetration of the skin by lipid-insoluble compounds does occur, it is probably accomplished by diffusion through the hair follicles, sweat glands, or sebaceous glands.

ABSORPTION OF DRUGS AFTER PARENTERAL ADMINISTRATION

Intramuscular and Subcutaneous Administration

Intramuscular and subcutaneous injections are by far the most common means of parenteral drug administration. Because of the high tissue blood flow and the ability of the injected solution to diffuse laterally, drug absorption generally is more rapid after intramuscular than after subcutaneous injection. Drug absorption from intramuscular and subcutaneous sites depends on the quantity and composition of the connective tissue, the capillary density, and the rate of vascular perfusion of the area. These factors can be influenced by the coinjection of agents that alter local blood flow (e.g., vasoconstrictors or vasodilators) or by substances that decrease tissue resistance to lateral diffusion (e.g., hyaluronidase).

Advantages of the intramuscular and subcutaneous routes include an increased reliability and precision in the drug blood level finally achieved and reasonably rapid absorption and onset of drug action. There are, however, serious disadvantages as well. Pain, tenderness, local tissue necrosis (primarily with highly alkaline injections), microbial contamination, and nerve damage may be associated with these forms of parenteral administration.

Intravenous Administration

Intravenous drug administration ensures immediate pharmacological response; problems of absorption are circumvented because the entire quantity of drug enters the vasculature directly. This route is also useful for compounds that are poorly or erratically absorbed, are extremely irritating to tissues, or are rapidly metabolized before or during their absorption from other sites. The rate of injection should be slow enough, however, to prevent excessively high local drug concentrations and to allow for termination of the injection if undesired effects appear.

A serious disadvantage of intravenous drug administration becomes clearly apparent when an overdose is inadvertently given: Neither can the drug be removed nor its absorption retarded. Other disadvantages include the possibilities of embolism (particularly if an insoluble drug is given), introduction of bacteria, and when this route is used for prolonged periods, subcutaneous tissue infiltration. The possible introduction of the human immunodeficiency virus (HIV) is a well-known consequence of intravenous drug administration in addicts who use contaminated needles.

FACTORS INFLUENCING DRUG DISTRIBUTION

Distribution is the delivery of drug from the systemic circulation to tissues. Once a drug has entered the blood compartment, the *rate* at which it penetrates tissues and other body fluids depends on several factors. These include (1) capillary permeability, (2) blood flow–tissue mass ratio (i.e., perfusion rate), (3) extent of plasma protein and specific organ binding, (4) regional differences in pH, (5) transport mechanisms available, and (6) the permeability characteristics of specific tissue membranes.

Drug delivery and eventual drug equilibration with intercellular tissue spaces are largely determined by the extent of organ blood flow. The composition of the capillary bed is usually not a limiting factor except with the capillaries of the CNS. The renal and hepatic capillaries are especially permeable to the movement of most molecules, except those of particularly large size. The rate of passage of drugs across capillary walls can be influenced by agents that affect capillary permeability (e.g., histamine) or capillary blood flow rate (e.g., norepinephrine).

AVAILABLE DISTRIBUTION VOLUME

The total volume of the fluid compartments of the body into which drugs may be distributed is approximately 40 L in a 70-kg adult. These compartments include plasma water (approximately 10 L), interstitial fluid (10 L), and the intracellular fluid (20 L). Total extracellular water is the sum of the plasma and the interstitial water. Factors such as sex, age, edema, pregnancy, and body fat can influence the volume of these various compartments.

The rate at which an equilibrium concentration of a drug is reached in the extracellular fluid of a particular tissue will depend on the tissue's perfusion rate; the greater the blood flow the more rapid the distribution of the drug from the plasma into the interstitial fluid. Thus, a drug will appear in the interstitial fluid of liver, kidney, and brain more rapidly than it will in muscle and skin (Table 3.2). The pharmacokinetic concept of volume of distribution (a derived parameter that relates the amount of drug in the body to the plasma concentration) is discussed more fully in Chapter 5.

BINDING OF DRUGS TO PLASMA PROTEINS

Most drugs found in the vascular compartment are bound reversibly with one or more of the macromolecules in plasma. Although some drugs simply dissolve in plasma water, most are associated with plasma compo-

TABLE 3.2 Blood Perfusion Rates in Adult Humans

Tissue	Percent of cardiac output	Blood flow (L/min)	Percent of body weight	Perfusion rate (mL/min/100 g tissue)
Kidney	20	1.23	0.5	350
Brain	12	0.75	2.0	55
Lung	100	5.40	1.5	400
Liver	24	1.55	2.8	85
Heart	4	0.25	0.5	84
Muscle	23	0.80	40.0	5
Skin	6	0.40	10.0	5
Adipose tissue	10	0.25	19.0	3

nents such as albumin, globulins, transferrin, ceruloplasmin, glycoproteins, and α- and β-lipoproteins. While many acidic drugs bind principally to albumin, basic drugs frequently bind to other plasma proteins, such as lipoproteins and α_1-acid glycoprotein (α_1-AGP), in addition to albumin. The extent of this binding will influence the drug's distribution and rate of elimination because *only the unbound drug can diffuse through the capillary wall, produce its systemic effects, be metabolized, and be excreted.*

Drugs ordinarily bind to protein in a reversible fashion and in dynamic equilibrium, according to the law of mass action. Since only the unbound (or free) drug diffuses through the capillary walls, extensive binding may decrease the intensity of drug action. The magnitude of this decrease is directly proportional to the fraction of drug bound to plasma protein. At low drug concentrations, the stronger the affinity between the drug and protein, the smaller the fraction that is free. As drug dosage increases, eventually the binding capacity of the protein becomes saturated and any additional drug will remain unbound.

The binding of a drug to plasma proteins will decrease its effective plasma to tissue concentration gradient, that is, the force that drives the drug out of the circulation, thereby slowing the rate of transfer across the capillary. As the free drug leaves the circulation, the protein–drug complex begins to dissociate and more free drug becomes available for diffusion. Thus, binding does not prevent the drug from reaching its site of action but only retards the rate at which this occurs. Extensive plasma protein binding may prolong drug availability and duration of action.

Protein binding also plays a role in the distribution of drugs and thus the volume of distribution. Drugs that are highly bound to plasma proteins may distribute less widely because they remain trapped in the peripheral vasculature, since the plasma proteins themselves cannot tra-

verse into the extravascular space. However, if the affinity of a drug for tissues (e.g., fat, muscle) is greater than the affinity for plasma proteins, widespread distribution can occur despite a high degree of plasma protein binding.

Albumin

Of the plasma proteins, the most important contributor to drug binding is albumin. Although albumin has a *net* negative charge at serum pH, it can interact with both positive and negative charges on drugs. Many highly albumin-bound drugs are poorly soluble in water, and for such drugs, binding to hydrophobic sites on albumin is often important. In general, only one or two molecules of an acidic drug are bound per albumin molecule, whereas basic, positively charged drugs are more weakly bound to a larger number of binding sites.

The binding of drugs to plasma proteins is usually nonspecific; that is, many drugs may interact with the same binding site. A drug with a higher affinity may displace a drug with weaker affinity. Increases in the non–protein-bound drug fraction (i.e., free drug) can theoretically result in an increase in the drug's intensity of pharmacological response, side effects, and potential toxicity. However, in practice, changes in protein binding result in clinically significant effects for only a limited number of drugs.

Some disease states (e.g., hyperalbuminemia, hypoalbuminemia, uremia, hyperbilirubinemia) have been associated with changes in plasma protein binding of drugs. For example, in uremic patients the plasma protein binding of certain acidic drugs (e.g., penicillin, sulfonamides, salicylates, and barbiturates) is reduced.

Lipoproteins

Drugs that bind to lipoproteins do so by dissolving in the lipid portion of the lipoprotein core. The binding capacity of individual lipoproteins generally depends on their lipid content. It is also possible that the lipid and protein fractions cooperate in the binding process, the drug first binding to a number of sites on the protein moiety and then dissolving in the lipid phase.

α_1-Acid Glycoprotein

The importance of α_1-AGP as a determinant of the plasma protein binding of basic drugs, including the psychotherapeutic drugs chlorpromazine, imipramine, spiroperidol, and nortriptyline, is becoming apparent. There is evidence of increased plasma α_1-AGP levels in certain physiological and pathological conditions, such as injury, stress, surgery, trauma, rheumatoid arthritis, and celiac disease.

SELECTIVE ACCUMULATION OF DRUGS

Drugs will not always be uniformly distributed to and retained by body tissues. The concentrations of some drugs will be either considerably higher or considerably lower in particular tissues than could be predicted on the basis of simple distribution assumptions. This observation is demonstrated in the following examples:

1. *Kidney.* Since the kidneys receive 20 to 25% of the cardiac output, they will be exposed to a relatively large amount of any systemically administered drug. The kidney also contains a protein, metallothionein, that has a high affinity for metals. This protein is responsible for the renal accumulation of cadmium, lead, and mercury.
2. *Eye.* Several drugs have an affinity for the retinal pigment melanin and thus may accumulate in the eye. Chlorpromazine and other phenothiazines bind to melanin and accumulate in the uveal tract, where they may cause retinotoxicity. Chloroquine concentration in the eye can be approximately 100 times that found in the liver.
3. *Fat.* Drugs with extremely high lipid–water partition coefficients have a tendency to accumulate in body fat. However, since blood flow to adipose tissue is low (about 3 mL/100 g/minute), distribution into body fat occurs slowly. Drug accumulation in body fat may result either in decreased therapeutic activity owing to the drug's removal from the circulation or in prolonged activity when only low levels of the drug are needed to produce therapeutic effects. In the latter instance, fat depots provide a slow, sustained release of the active drug. Should body fat be seriously reduced, as during starvation, stored compounds (e.g., DDT and chlordane) may be mobilized, and toxic symptoms may ensue.
4. *Lung.* The lung receives the entire cardiac output; therefore, drug distribution into it is very rapid. Most compounds that accumulate in the lung are basic amines (e.g., antihistamines, imipramine, amphetamine, methadone, phentermine, chlorphentermine, and chlorpromazine) with large lipophilic groups and pK values greater than 8. However, some nonbasic amines, such as the herbicide paraquat, also can accumulate in the lung.
5. *Bone.* Although bone is a relatively inert tissue, it can accumulate such substances as tetracyclines, lead, strontium, and the antitumor agent cisplatin. These substances may accumulate in bone by absorption onto the bone crystal surface and eventually be incorporated into the crystal lattice. Tetracycline deposition during odontogenesis may lead to a permanent yellow-brown discoloration of teeth, dysplasia, and poor bone development. Lead can substitute for calcium in the bone crystal lattice, resulting in bone brittleness. Bone may become a reservoir for the slow release of toxic substances, such as lead and cisplatin.

PHYSIOLOGICAL BARRIERS TO DRUG DISTRIBUTION

Blood-Brain Barrier

The capillary membrane between the plasma and brain cells is much less permeable to water-soluble drugs than is the membrane between plasma and other tissues. Thus, the transfer of drugs into the brain is regulated by the *blood-brain barrier*. To gain access to the brain from the capillary circulation, drugs must pass through cells rather than between them. Only drugs that have a high lipid–water partition coefficient can penetrate the tightly apposed capillary endothelial cells.

Drugs that are partially ionized and only moderately lipid soluble will penetrate at considerably slower rates. Lipid-insoluble or highly ionized drugs will fail to enter the brain in significant amounts. Because the pH of the cerebrospinal fluid is about 7.35, there is some tendency for weak organic bases to concentrate in the cerebrospinal fluid and for weak organic acids to be excluded. In addition, because only the unbound form of a drug is available for diffusion, extensive plasma protein binding also can have dramatic effects on the extent of drug transfer into the brain.

Inflammation, such as occurs in bacterial meningitis or encephalitis, may increase the permeability of the blood-brain barrier, permitting the passage of ionized lipid-insoluble compounds (e.g., penicillin and ampicillin) that would otherwise be restricted from penetrating into the brain extracellular fluid.

The flow of cerebrospinal fluid is essentially unidirectional; that is, it flows from its site of formation in the choroid plexus through the ventricles to its site of exit at the arachnoid villi. Drugs in this fluid can either enter the brain tissue or be returned to the venous circulation in the *bulk flow* of cerebrospinal fluid carried through the arachnoid villi. Some drugs, such as penicillin, will not leave the cerebrospinal fluid compartment by bulk flow but will be actively transported by the choroid plexus out of the fluid and back into the blood. Finally, drugs may diffuse from brain tissue directly into blood capillaries.

Though drugs appear to cross the blood-brain barrier by passive diffusion, transporter systems in the blood-brain barrier pump drugs back *out* into the systemic circulation. As in the gut, the Pgp transporter system is the primary active transporter in the blood-brain barrier identified to date. This ATP-dependent transporter system picks up substrates that have crossed the capillary endothelial cells and transports them back to the systemic circulation, limiting their penetration into the CNS. Thus, not only are the physicochemical properties of the drug a determinant for penetration into the CNS but penetration also depends on whether the drug is a substrate for the Pgp transporter system.

An important consequence of the existence of a variety of routes of drug removal from the brain is that drugs that slowly penetrate the CNS may never achieve adequate therapeutic brain concentrations. Penicillin, for example, is a less effective antibiotic centrally than it is peripherally.

Placental Barrier

The blood vessels of the fetus and mother are separated by a number of tissue layers that collectively constitute the *placental barrier*. Drugs that traverse this barrier will reach the fetal circulation. The placental barrier, like the blood-brain barrier, does not prevent transport of all drugs but is selective, and factors that regulate passage of drugs through any membrane (e.g., pK_a, lipid solubility, protein binding) are applicable here.

In general, substances that are lipid soluble cross the placenta with relative ease in accordance with their lipid–water partition coefficient and degree of ionization. Highly polar or ionized drugs do not cross the placenta readily. However, most drugs used in labor and delivery are not highly ionized and will cross. They are generally weak bases with pK_a values of about 8 and tend to be more ionized in the fetal bloodstream, since the pH of fetal blood is around 7.3 as compared with the maternal blood pH of 7.44. Differences in maternal and fetal blood pH can give rise to unequal concentrations of ionizable drugs in the mother and the fetus.

Active efflux transporters also exist in the placenta, analogous to the gut and blood-brain barrier. These are Pgp, multidrug resistance–associated protein (MRP), and breast cancer resistance protein (BCRP). These transport proteins are located in many tissues but also appear to be expressed in the placenta. Though the substrate specificities of these proteins have not been completely described, they appear to function as efflux transporters, moving endogenous and exogenous chemicals from the placental cells back to the systemic circulation. In this way, they serve as a mechanism to protect the fetus from exposure to unintended chemicals.

Blood-Testis Barrier

The existence of a barrier between the blood and testes is indicated by the absence of staining in testicular tissue after the intravascular injection of dyes. Morphological studies indicate that the barrier lies beyond the capillary endothelial cells and is most likely to be found at the specialized Sertoli–Sertoli cell junction. It appears that Pgp, the efflux transporter protein, also plays a role in forming this blood-testis barrier. This protein probably plays a role in preventing certain chemotherapeutic agents from reaching specific areas of the testis and thus hinders treatment of the neoplasm.

Study QUESTIONS

1. Following oral administration, a drug is absorbed into the body, wherein it can exert its action. For a drug given orally, the primary site of drug absorption is:
   (A) The esophagus
   (B) The stomach
   (C) The upper portion of the small intestine
   (D) The large intestine

2. Patients can exhibit alterations in the rate and extent of drug absorption because of various factors. All of the following factors might affect the rate and/or extent of drug absorption EXCEPT:
   (A) Gastric emptying time
   (B) Intestinal motility
   (C) The presence of food
   (D) The formulation of the drug
   (E) A generic form of the drug

3. The body has developed defense mechanisms that reduce the amount of foreign chemicals, such as drugs, that enter the body. One of the more prominent of these mechanisms is an efflux transport system that pumps some drugs back into the intestinal lumen following absorption into the enterocytes and that is responsible for the lack of complete absorption of some drugs. This efflux transport system is:
   (A) Facilitated diffusion
   (B) P glycoprotein
   (C) Cytochrome P450 3A
   (D) Pinocytosis

4. All of the following statements concerning the blood-brain barrier and the passage of drugs from the systemic circulation into the cerebrospinal fluid are TRUE EXCEPT:
   (A) Ionized drugs are more likely to cross into the CSF than un-ionized drugs.
   (B) The higher the lipid solubility of a drug, the more likely it will cross into the CSF.
   (C) Inflammation of the meninges improves the likelihood that drugs will cross the blood-brain barrier as compared to the uninflamed state (i.e., normal condition).
   (D) P glycoprotein serves to pump drugs back into the systemic circulation from endothelial cells lining the blood-brain barrier.

5. Which of the following organs or tissues is a potential site for drug accumulation of lead that has been ingested?
   (A) Eyes
   (B) Fat
   (C) Bone
   (D) Lungs
   (E) Blood

ANSWERS

1. **C.** The primary site of absorption is the small intestine. Because of its large surface area and high blood perfusion rate, the small intestine is optimal for absorbing drugs. Some drug absorption occurs in the stomach and large intestine, but because of their reduced surface area in relative terms and for some drugs less than optimal physicochemical conditions, these tissues play a lesser role in drug absorption. Because of the tissue type, very little drug absorption occurs through the esophagus.

2. **E.** To be approved, generic formulations must exhibit the same rate and extent of absorption as the trademark compound. All of the other choices can affect drug absorption. For example, slowing gastric emptying time may increase the absorption of a drug absorbed in the stomach. Alterations in gastric motility may affect the amount of time a drug spends in the region of the gastrointestinal tract, where it undergoes the most extensive absorption. The presence of food may cause decreased absorption through binding to the drug or may increase absorption through making a better local environment for absorption of particular drugs. Finally, changes in drug formulation can alter absorption by changing dissolution rates.

3. **B.** P-glycoprotein transporters in the intestinal lumen serve as an efflux transporter for many drugs. This transporter pumps drugs out of the enterocytes into which they were absorbed and back into the intestinal lumen, reducing absorption. Facilitated diffusion and pinocytosis generally result in drug influx (absorption). The cytochrome P450 3A enzymes metabolize drugs; therefore, even though they may reduce the amount of drug absorbed, the reduction is due to drug metabolism, not efflux transport back into the intestinal lumen.

4. **A.** Un-ionized drugs cross into the cerebrospinal fluid more readily than ionized drugs. All of the other choices are correct.

5. **C.** Lead can substitute for calcium in the bone crystal lattice, resulting in bone brittleness. Bone may become a reservoir for other substances as well. Several drugs, such as chlorpromazine, may accumulate in the eye. Drugs with extremely high lipid–water partition coefficients tend to accumulate in fat, while basic amines tend to accumulate in the lungs. Many agents bind avidly to albumin in the blood.

SUPPLEMENTAL READING

Amidon G, Lee P, and Topp E (eds.). Transport Processes in Pharmaceutical Systems. New York: Decker, 2000.

Blackmore CG, McNaughton PA, and van Veen HW. Multidrug transporters in prokaryotic and eukaryotic cells: physiological functions and transport mechanisms. Mol Membr Biol 2001;18:97–103.

Oie S. Drug distribution and binding. J Clin Pharmacol 1986;26:583–586. Potts RO and Guy RH (eds.). Mechanisms of Transdermal Drug Delivery. New York: Decker, 1997.

Segal MB. The Barriers and Fluids of the Eye and Brain. Boca Raton, FL: CRC, 1989.

Tillement J-P and Lindenlaub E (eds). Protein Binding and Drug Transport. New York: Liss, 1987.

Zhang Y and Benet LZ. The gut as a barrier to drug absorption: combined role of cytochrome P4503A and p-glycoprotein. Clin Pharmacokinet 2001;40:159–168.

CASE Study   Improving Drug Absorption

A 47-year-old man recently received a heart transplant and is being discharged home with oral medications, including cyclosporine. The physician also prescribed diltiazem, a calcium channel blocker used for the treatment of hypertension. Since he did not have hypertension, the patient wondered why this additional drug was being prescribed.

ANSWER: Cyclosporine is an immunosuppressant drug used to prevent transplant rejections. Though an oral formulation is available, it has low bioavailability (very little reaches the systemic circulation as intact drug). Diltiazem will inhibit cytochrome P450 3A4 in the gut. CYP3A4 is the primary enzyme responsible for the presystemic metabolism of cyclosporine and has been implicated as the primary cause for the low amounts of orally administered cyclosporine reaching the systemic circulation. Coadministration of diltiazem greatly increases the bioavailability of cyclosporine, reducing the dose of drug needed. Furthermore, because cyclosporine is relatively expensive, a substantial cost savings is realized. Finally, a common adverse effect of cyclosporine therapy is the development of hypertension, and the diltiazem somewhat protects the patient from this adverse effect.

4 | Metabolism and Excretion of Drugs

Timothy S. Tracy

Both metabolism and excretion can be viewed as processes responsible for elimination of drug (parent and metabolite) from the body. Drug metabolism changes the chemical structure of a drug to produce a drug *metabolite,* which is frequently but not universally less pharmacologically active. Metabolism also renders the drug compound more water soluble and therefore more easily excreted.

Drug metabolism reactions are carried out by enzyme systems that evolved over time to protect the body from exogenous chemicals. The enzyme systems for this purpose for the most part can be grouped into two categories: phase I oxidative or reductive enzymes and phase II conjugative enzymes. Enzymes within these categories exhibit some limited specificity in relation to the substrates acted upon; a given enzyme may interact with only a limited number of drugs. Some nonspecific hydrolytic enzymes, such as esterases and amidases, have not received much research attention. The focus of this discussion therefore is on phase I and phase II reactions and the enzymes that carry out these processes.

OXIDATIVE AND REDUCTIVE ENZYMES: PHASE I REACTIONS

Phase I enzymes act by causing the drug molecule to undergo oxidation or more rarely, reduction. Examples of oxidation reactions carried out by phase I enzymes are listed in Table 4.1 and encompass a broad range of drugs with varying chemical structures. However, as discussed later, there is still a great deal of substrate specificity within a given enzyme family.

Cytochrome P450 Enzymes

The cytochrome P450 (CYP450) enzyme superfamily is the primary phase I enzyme system involved in the oxidative metabolism of drugs and other chemicals. These enzymes also are responsible for all or part of the metabolism and synthesis of a number of endogenous compounds, such as steroid hormones and prostaglandins.

Though it was originally described as the CYP450 enzyme, it is now apparent that it is a group of related enzymes, each with its own substrate specificity. To date, 12 unique isoforms (e.g., CYP3A4, CYP2D6) have been identified as playing a role in human drug metabolism, and others may be discovered. These isoforms, along with examples of compounds for which each isoform plays a substantial role in their metabolism, are listed in Table 4.2. More than one CYP isoform may be involved in the metabolism of a particular drug. For example, the calcium channel blocking drug verapamil is primarily metabolized by CYP3A4, but CYPs 2C9, 2C8 and 2D6 participate to some degree, particularly in the secondary metabolism of the verapamil metabolites. Thus, the degree to which a drug interaction involving competition for a CYP isoform may occur will depend on the extent of metabolism of each compound that can be attributed to that isoform. The more isoforms involved in the metabolism of a drug, the less likely is a clinically significant drug interaction.

Substrate Specificity of the CYP Enzymes

CYP3A4 is thought to be the most predominant CYP isoform involved in human drug metabolism, both in terms of the amount of enzyme in the liver and the variety of drugs that are substrates for this enzyme isoform.

TABLE 4.1 Types of Oxidation Reactions Involved in Enzymatic Drug Metabolism

Reaction	Examples
Aliphatic and aromatic hydroxylation	Ibuprofen, flurbiprofen
N-demethylation	Morphine
O-demethylation	Codeine
Epoxidation	Carbamazepine
N-Oxidation	Morphine
S-oxidation	Sulindac
Deamination	Amphetamine

This isoform may account for more than 50% of all CYP-mediated drug oxidation reactions, and CYP3A4 is likely to be involved in the greatest number of drug–drug interactions. The active site of CYP3A4 is thought to be large relative to other isoforms, as evidenced by its ability to accept substrates up to a molecular weight of 1200 (e.g., cyclosporine). This active site size allows drugs with substantial variation in molecular structure to bind within the active site. However, the fact that two drugs are metabolized predominantly by CYP3A4 does not mean that coadministration will result in a drug–drug interaction, since drugs can bind in different regions of the CYP3A4 active site, and these binding regions may be distinct. In fact, it is believed that two drugs (substrates) can occupy the active site simultaneously, with both available for metabolism by the enzyme. This finding helps account for a number of absent interactions that would have been predicted to occur based on strict substrate specificity rules.

CYP3A5, whose amino acid sequence is similar to that of CYP3A4, appears to possess roughly the same substrate specificity characteristics as CYP3A4. However, it differs in that it is not present in all individuals. Thus, patients expressing both CYP3A4 and CYP3A5 have the potential to exhibit increased metabolism of CYP3A substrates as compared to individuals expressing only the CYP3A4 isoform.

Levels of CYP enzyme expression of any isoform can vary substantially among individuals. The other identified human CYP3A isoform is CYP3A7, which appears to be expressed only in the fetus and rapidly disappears following birth, to be replaced by CYP3A4 and CYP3A5. It is becoming increasingly clear that different enzyme expression patterns, and thus different drug metabolism capabilities, are observed throughout the various stages of life. Neonates are different from 6-month-old infants, who differ from year-old infants, who differ from preadolescents, who differ from adolescents, who differ from adults, who differ from the elderly. Thus, consideration must be given to the person's age when assessing drug metabolism capacity.

The second most common CYP isoform involved in human drug metabolism is CYP2D6. It may account for 30% of the CYP-mediated oxidation reactions involving drugs, including the metabolism of drugs in such diverse therapeutic categories as antipsychotic agents, tricyclic antidepressants, β-blocking agents, and opioid analgesics. Though this isoform accepts a number of drugs as substrates, its relative abundance in the liver is quite low. CYP2D6 is most known for its propensity to exhibit genetic polymorphisms (see Pharmacogenetics, later in the chapter).

The other isoform responsible for a substantial portion (about 10%) of the CYP-mediated drug oxidation

TABLE 4.2 Representative Drugs Metabolized by Each of the CYP Isoforms in Human Drug Metabolism

CYP Isoform	Examples of Substrates	Comments
CYP1A1	Essentially same as CYP1A2	
CYP1A2	Polycyclic aromatic hydrocarbons, caffeine, theophylline	
CYP2A6	Nicotine, 5-fluorouracil, coumarin	
CYP2B6	Bupropion, cyclophosphamide, propofol	
CYP2C8	Paclitaxel	
CYP2C9	Phenytoin, warfarin, nonsteroidal antiinflammatory drugs	Polymorphic
CYP2C19	Omeprazole	Polymorphic
CYP2D6	Tricyclic antidepressants, codeine, dextromethorphan, some β-blockers, some antipsychotics, some antiarrhythmics	Polymorphic
CYP2E1	Acetaminophen, chlorzoxazone	
CYP3A4	Midazolam, triazolam, cyclosporine, erythromycin, HIV protease inhibitors, calcium channel blockers	Polymorphic
CYP3A5	Essentially same as CYP3A4	
CYP3A7	Unclear but may be similar to CYP3A4	Polymorphic Present only in the fetus

CYP, cytochrome P450.

reactions is CYP2C9. This isoform metabolizes several clinically important drugs with narrow therapeutic indices. Two of these drugs are the antiepileptic agent phenytoin and the anticoagulant warfarin. Any change in the metabolism of these two drugs, either increased or decreased, can have profound adverse effects. CYP2C9 appears to prefer weakly acidic drugs as substrates, which limits the number of drugs metabolized by this isoform, since most drugs are weak bases).

The remaining CYP isoforms involved in human drug metabolism (Table 4.2) are present in the liver in varying amounts, and each is thought to contribute 2–3% or less of the CYP-mediated drug oxidation reactions. Though they may not be involved in the metabolism of a broad range or significant number of drugs, if they are the primary enzyme responsible for the metabolism of the drug of interest, then their importance in that instance is obviously increased.

Regulation of the CYP Enzymes

CYP450 enzymes can be regulated by the presence of other drugs or by disease states. This regulation can either decrease or increase enzyme function, depending on the modulating agent. These phenomena are commonly referred to as enzyme inhibition and enzyme induction, respectively.

Enzyme Inhibition

Enzyme inhibition is the most frequently observed result of CYP modulation and is the primary mechanism for drug–drug pharmacokinetic interactions. The most common type of inhibition is simple competitive inhibition, wherein two drugs are vying for the same active site and the drug with the highest affinity for the site wins out. In this scenario, addition of a second drug with greater affinity for the enzyme inhibits metabolism of the primary drug, and an elevated primary drug blood or tissue concentration is the result. In the simplest case, each drug has its own unique degree of affinity for the CYP enzyme active site, and the degree of inhibition depends on how avidly the secondary (or effector) drug binds to the enzyme active site. For example, ketoconazole and triazolam compete for binding to the CYP3A4 active site and thus exhibit their own unique rate of metabolism. However, when given concomitantly, the metabolism of triazolam by the CYP3A4 enzyme (essentially the only enzyme that metabolizes triazolam) is decreased to such a degree that the patient is exposed to 17 times as much of parent triazolam as when ketoconazole is not present. Table 4.3 lists the common CYP isoforms and representative inhibitory agents.

A second type of CYP enzyme inhibition is mechanism-based inactivation (or suicide inactivation). In this type of inhibition, the effector compound (i.e., the in-

TABLE 4.3 Representative Inhibitors for Each of the CYP Isoforms Involved in Human Drug Metabolism

CYP Isoform	Examples of Inhibitors
CYP1A1	Thought to be same as CYP1A2
CYP1A2	Amiodarone, fluoroquinolone antibiotics, fluvoxamine
CYP2A6	Tranylcypromine, methoxsalen
CYP2B6	Efavirenz, nelfinavir, ritonavir
CYP2C8	Probably similar to CYP2C9
CYP2C9	Amiodarone, fluconazole, fluvastatin, lovastatin, zafirlukast
CYP2C19	Cimetidine, ketoconazole, omeprazole, ticlopidine[a]
CYP2D6	Amiodarone, cimetidine, fluoxetine, paroxetine, quinidine
CYP2E1	Disulfiram[a]
CYP3A4	HIV antivirals (e.g., Ritonavir), amiodarone, cimetidine, diltiazem, erythromycin[a], grapefruit juice, ketoconazole
CYP3A5	Thought to be same as CYP3A4
CYP3A7	Unclear at this time but may be similar to CYP3A4

[a]Mechanism-based inactivator.
CYP, cytochrome P450.

hibitor) is itself metabolized by the enzyme to form a reactive species that binds irreversibly to the enzyme and prevents any further metabolism by the enzyme. This mechanism-based inactivation lasts for the life of the enzyme molecule and thus can be overcome only by the proteolytic degradation of that particular enzyme molecule and subsequent synthesis of new enzyme protein. A drug that is commonly used in clinical practice and yet is known to be a mechanism-based inactivator of CYP3A4 is the antibiotic erythromycin.

Enzyme Induction

Induction of drug-metabolizing activity can be due either to synthesis of new enzyme protein or to a decrease in the proteolytic degradation of the enzyme. Increased enzyme synthesis is the result of an increase in messenger RNA (mRNA) production (transcription) or in the translation of mRNA into protein. Regardless of the mechanism, the net result of enzyme induction is the increased turnover (metabolism) of substrate. Whereas one frequently associates enzyme inhibition with an increase in potential for toxicity, enzyme induction is most commonly associated with therapeutic failure due to inability to achieve required drug concentrations.

Table 4.4 lists representative inducers of each of the CYP isoforms. No inducers of CYP2D6 have been identified.

TABLE 4.4	Representative Inducers for Each of the CYP Isoforms Involved in Human Drug Metabolism
CYP Isoform	**Examples of Inducers**
CYP1A1	Smoking (polycyclic aromatic hydrocarbons), char-grilled meat, omeprazole
CYP1A2	Same as CYP1A1
CYP2A6	Phenobarbital, dexamethasone
CYP2B6	Phenobarbital, dexamethasone, rifampin
CYP2C8	Same as CYP2C9
CYP2C9	Rifampin, dexamethasone, phenobarbital
CYP2C19	Rifampin
CYP2D6	None known
CYP2E1	Ethanol, isoniazid
CYP3A4	Efavirenz, nevirapine, barbiturates, carbamazepine, glucocorticoids, phenytoin, pioglitazone, rifampin, St. John's wort
CYP3A5	Thought to be same as CYP3A4
CYP3A7	Unclear but may be similar to CYP3A4

The time course of enzyme induction is important, since it may play a prominent role in the duration of the effect and therefore the potential onset and offset of the drug interaction. Both time required for synthesis of new enzyme protein (transcription and translation) and the half-life of the inducing drug affect the time course of induction. An enzyme with a slower turnover rate will require a longer time before induction reaches equilibrium (steady state), and conversely, a faster turnover rate will result in a more rapid induction. With respect to the drug inducer, drugs with a shorter half-life will reach equilibrium concentrations sooner (less time to steady state) and thus result in a more rapid maximal induction, with the opposite being true for drugs with a longer half-life.

Flavin Monooxygenases

The flavin monooxygenases (FMOs) are a family of five enzymes (FMO 1–5) that operate in a manner analogous to the cytochrome P450 enzymes in that they oxidize the drug compound in an effort to increase its elimination. Though they possess broad substrate specificity, in general they do not play a major role in the metabolism of drugs but appear to be more involved in the metabolism of environmental chemicals and toxins.

CONJUGATIVE ENZYMES: PHASE II REACTIONS

Phase II conjugative enzymes metabolize drugs by attaching (conjugating) a more polar molecule to the original drug molecule to increase water solubility, thereby permitting more rapid drug excretion. This conjugation can occur following a phase I reaction involving the molecule, but prior metabolism is not required. The phase II enzymes typically consist of multiple isoforms, analogous to the CYPs, but to date are less well defined.

Glucuronosyl Transferases

Glucuronosyl transferases (UGTs) conjugate the drug molecule with a glucuronic acid moiety, usually through establishment of an ether, ester, or amide bond. Examples of each of these types of conjugates are presented in Figure 4.1. The glucuronic acid moiety, being very water soluble, generally renders the new conjugate more water soluble and thus more easily eliminated. Typically this conjugate is inactive, but sometimes it is active. For example, UGT-mediated conjugation of morphine at the 6- position results in the formation of morphine-6-glucuronide, which is 50 times as potent an analgesic as morphine.

It is now apparent that UGTs are also a superfamily of enzyme isoforms, each with differing substrate specificities and regulation characteristics. Of the potential products of the UGT1 gene family, only expression of UGT1A1, 3, 4, 5, 6, 9 and 10 occurs in humans. Depending on the isoform, these enzymes have varying reactivity toward a number of pharmacologically active compounds, such as opioids, androgens, estrogens, progestins, and nonsteroidal antiinflammatory drugs; UGT1A1 is the only physiologically significant enzyme involved in the conjugation of bilirubin. UGT1A4 appears to be inducible by phenobarbital administration, and UGT1A7 is induced by the chemopreventive agent oltipraz.

UGT2B7 is probably the most important of the UGT2 isoforms and possibly of all of the UGTs. It exhibits broad substrate specificity encompassing a variety of pharmacological agents, including many already mentioned as substrates for the UGT1A family. Little is known about the substrate specificities of the other UGT2B isoforms or the inducibility of this enzyme family.

N-Acetyltransferases

As their name implies, the *N*-acetyltransferase (NAT) enzymes catalyze to a drug molecule the conjugation of an acetyl moiety derived from acetyl coenzyme A. Examples of this type of reaction are depicted in Figure 4.1. The net result of this conjugation is an increase in water solubility and increased elimination of the compound. The NATs identified to date and involved in human drug metabolism include NAT-1 and NAT-2. Little overlap in substrate specificities of the two isoforms appears to exist. NAT-2 is a polymorphic enzyme, a

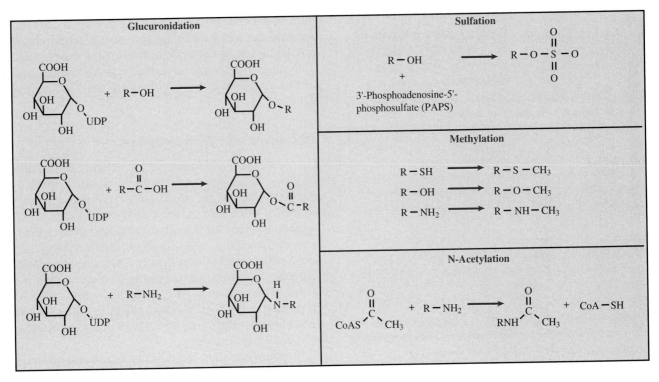

FIGURE 4.1

Examples of phase II conjugation reactions in drug metabolism.

property found to have important pharmacological consequences (discussed later). To date, little information exists on the regulation of the NAT enzymes, such as whether they can be induced by chemicals. However, reports have suggested that disease states such as acquired immunodeficiency syndrome (AIDS) may down-regulate NAT-2, particularly during active disease.

Sulfotransferases and Methyltransferases

Sulfotransferases (SULTs) are important for the metabolism of a number of drugs, neurotransmitters, and hormones, especially the steroid hormones. The cosubstrate for these reactions is 3'-phosphoadenosine 5'-phosphosulfate (PAPS) (Fig. 4.1). Like the aforementioned enzymes, sulfate conjugation typically renders the compound inactive and more water soluble. However, this process can also result in the activation of certain compounds, such as the antihypertensive minoxidil and several of the steroid hormones. Seven SULT isoforms identified in humans, including SULTs 1A1 to 1A3, possess activity toward phenolic substrates such as dopamine, estradiol, and acetaminophen. SULT1B1 possesses activity toward such endogenous substrates as dopamine and triiodothyronine. SULT1E1 has substantial activity toward steroid hormones, especially estradiol and dehydroepiandrosterone, and toward the anti-

hypertensive minoxidil. SULT2A1 also is active against steroid hormones. Little is known about the substrate specificity of SULT1C1. Regulation of the SULT enzymes appears to be controlled by levels of the available sulfate pool in the body or that of PAPS. Patients who consume a low-sulfate diet or have ingested multiple SULT substrates may be susceptible to inadequate metabolism by this enzyme and thus drug toxicity.

The methyltransferases (MTs) catalyze the methyl conjugation of a number of small molecules, such as drugs, hormones, and neurotransmitters, but they are also responsible for the methylation of such macromolecules as proteins, RNA, and DNA. A representative reaction of this type is shown in Figure 4.1. Most of the MTs use S-adenosyl-L-methionine (SAM) as the methyl donor, and this compound is now being used as a dietary supplement for the treatment of various conditions. Methylations typically occur at oxygen, nitrogen, or sulfur atoms on a molecule. For example, catechol-O-methyltransferase (COMT) is responsible for the biotransformation of catecholamine neurotransmitters such as dopamine and norepinephrine. N-methylation is a well established pathway for the metabolism of neurotransmitters, such as conversion of norepinephrine to epinephrine and methylation of nicotinamide and histamine. Possibly the most clinically relevant example of MT activity involves S-methylation by the enzyme thiopurine methyltransferase (TPMT). Patients who are low or lacking in TPMT (i.e., are polymorphic) are at high risk for development of severe bone marrow suppression when given normal doses of the chemotherapeutic agent 6-mercaptopurine. Patients are now studied for TPMT activity prior to administration of 6-mercaptopurine so that the dose may be adjusted downward if they are found to be deficient in this enzyme.

TISSUE SPECIFICITY OF HUMAN DRUG METABOLISM ENZYMES

Though most drug metabolism enzymes reside in the liver, other organs may also play an important role. All of the enzymes previously mentioned are found in the human liver, but other tissues and organs may have some complement of these enzymes. CYP3A4 and CYP3A5 have been found in the human gut and can contribute to substantial metabolism of orally administered drugs, even before the compound reaches the liver. For example, CYP3A4 may play a substantial role in the low bioavailability of cyclosporine. Drug-metabolizing enzymes have also been found in measurable quantities in the kidney, brain, placenta, skin, and lungs.

PHARMACOGENETICS OF DRUG-METABOLIZING ENZYMES

One of the most interesting and heavily researched areas of drug metabolism today is genetic polymorphism of drug-metabolizing enzymes (pharmacogenetics). As early as the late 1950s it was recognized that individuals might differ in whether they could acetylate certain drugs, such as isoniazid (see Chapter 49). In this case, the individuals studied appeared to segregate into two distinct groups, rapid acetylators and slow acetylators.

It was later discovered that this polymorphism existed in the *N*-acetyltransferase-2 gene and thus the NAT-2 enzyme. More important, it has become clear that slow acetylators (about 50% of the caucasian population) are more prone to adverse effects following administration of certain drugs than fast acetylators. For example, it is well established that slow acetylators receiving the antiarrhythmic drug procainamide are much more likely to develop the systemic lupus erythematosus–like syndrome that has been described as a characteristic and therapy-limiting event associated with this drug. In fact, this adverse event is rare in fast acetylators. Fortunately, the number of drugs that depend on NAT-2 for their primary metabolic fate is small, so this polymorphism is clinically relevant only in certain situations.

Possibly the most studied genetic polymorphism is that associated with CYP2D6. At least 17 variant alleles of this enzyme have been identified, most being associated with a deficiency in the ability to carry out CYP2D6-mediated oxidation reactions. Approximately 7% of the caucasian population is CYP2D6 deficient, whereas only 1–3% of African Americans and Asians are deficient in this enzyme. CYP2D6 is responsible for about 30% of the CYP-mediated reactions (Table 4.2) and exhibits this polymorphism. Likelihood of adverse events, such as the dyskinesias associated with certain antipsychotic agents, have been linked to this polymorphism, since individuals who are CYP2D6 deficient have a higher incidence of these side effects. To minimize adverse events and toxicity, care should be exercised when prescribing drugs that depend on CYP2D6 metabolism.

Recently, variant alleles (and thus polymorphisms) have been elucidated for most of the CYP isoforms. For example, six alleles of CYP2C9 have been discovered, and several of them profoundly affect therapy. The variant allele CYP2C9*3 occurs in fewer than 1% of the population, but affected individuals generally require doses of the anticoagulant warfarin that are 10–25% of those required by unaffected individuals. A CYP2C19 polymorphism also has been identified in 2–3% of caucasians and 20–30% of Asians. In this case, individuals who are CYP2C19 deficient are more likely to have complete ulcer healing after therapy with omeprazole (a proton pump inhibitor that reduces gastric acid) than are extensive metabolizers, a positive benefit.

EXCRETION OF DRUGS

Despite the reduction in activity that occurs as a drug leaves its site of action, it may remain in the body for a considerable period, especially if it is strongly bound to tissue components. Thus, reduction in pharmacological activity and drug elimination are to be seen as related but separate phenomena.

Excretion, along with metabolism and tissue redistribution, is important in determining both the duration of drug action and the rate of drug elimination. Excretion is a process whereby drugs are transferred from the internal to the external environment, and the principal organs involved in this activity are the kidneys, lungs, biliary system, and intestines.

The physicochemical considerations discussed in Chapter 3 that govern the passage of drugs across biological barriers are applicable to both excretory and absorptive phenomena.

RENAL EXCRETION

Although some drugs are excreted through extrarenal pathways, the kidney is the primary organ of removal for most drugs (Figure 4.2), especially for those that are water soluble and not volatile. *The three principal processes that determine the urinary excretion of a drug are glomerular filtration, tubular secretion, and tubular reabsorption (mostly passive back-diffusion).* Active

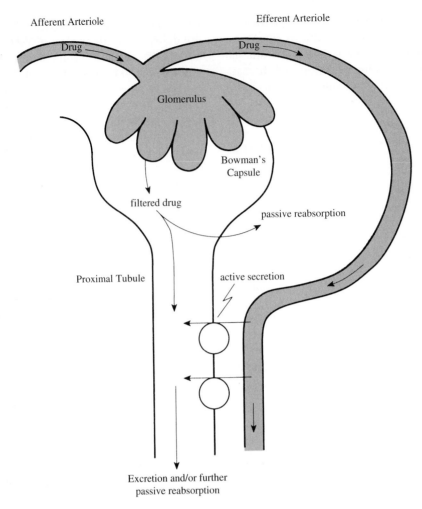

Afferent Arteriole

Efferent Arteriole

Drug

Drug

Glomerulus

Bowman's
Capsule

filtered drug

passive reabsorption

Proximal Tubule

active secretion

Excretion and/or further
passive reabsorption

FIGURE 4.2

Renal excretion of drugs. Filtration of small non–protein-bound drugs occurs through glomerular capillary pores. Lipid-soluble and un-ionized drugs are passively reabsorbed throughout the nephron. Active secretion of organic acids and bases occurs only in the proximal tubular segment.

tubular reabsorption also may have some influence on the rate of excretion for a limited number of compounds.

Glomerular Filtration

The ultrastructure of the glomerular capillary wall is such that it permits a high degree of fluid filtration while restricting the passage of compounds having relatively large molecular weights. This selective filtration is important in that it prevents the filtration of plasma proteins (e.g., albumin) that are important for maintaining an osmotic gradient in the vasculature and thus plasma volume.

Several factors, including molecular size, charge, and shape, influence the glomerular filtration of large molecules. The restricted passage of macromolecules can be thought of as a consequence of the presence of a glomerular capillary wall barrier with uniform pores.

Since approximately 130 mL of plasma water is filtered across the porous glomerular capillary membranes each minute (190 L/day), the kidney is admirably suited for its role in drug excretion. As the ultrafiltrate is formed, any drug that is free in the plasma water, that is, not bound to plasma proteins or the formed elements in the blood (e.g., red blood cells), will be filtered as a result of the driving force provided by cardiac pumping.

All unbound drugs will be filtered as long as their molecular size, charge, and shape are not excessively large. Compounds with an effective radius above 20 Å may have their rate of glomerular filtration restricted; hindrance to passage increases progressively as the molecular radius increases, and passage approaches zero when the compound radius becomes greater than about 42Å.

Charged substances (e.g., sulfated dextrans) are usually filtered at slower rates than neutral compounds (e.g., neutral dextrans), even when their molecular sizes are comparable. The greater restriction to filtration of charged molecules, particularly anions, is probably due to an electrostatic interaction between the filtered molecule and the fixed negative charges within the glomerular capillary wall. These highly anionic structural components of the wall contribute to an electrostatic barrier and are most likely in the endothelial or glomerular basement membrane regions.

Molecular configuration also may influence the rate of glomerular filtration of drugs. Differences in the three-dimensional shape of macromolecules result in a restriction of glomerular passage of globular molecules (e.g., proteins) to a greater extent than of random coil or extended molecules (e.g., dextrans). Thus, the efficient retention of proteins within the circulation is attributed to a combination of factors, including their globular structure, their large molecular size, and the magnitude of their negative charge.

Factors that affect the glomerular filtration rate (GFR) also can influence the rate of drug clearance. For instance, inflammation of the glomerular capillaries may increase GFR and hence drug filtration. Most drugs are at least partially bound to plasma proteins, and therefore their actual filtration rates are less than the theoretical GFR. Anything that alters drug–protein binding, however, will change the drug filtration rate. The usual range of half-lives seen for most drugs that are cleared solely by glomerular filtration is 1 to 4 hours. However, considerably longer half-lives will be seen if extensive protein binding occurs.

Also, since water constitutes a larger percentage of the total body weight of the newborn than of individuals in other age groups, the apparent volume of distribution of water-soluble drugs is greater in neonates. This results in a lower concentration of drug in the blood coming to the kidneys per unit of time and hence a decreased rate of drug clearance. The lower renal plasma flow in the newborn also may decrease the glomerular filtration of drugs.

Passive Diffusion

An important determinant of the urinary excretion of drugs (i.e., weak electrolytes) is the extent to which substances diffuse back across the tubular membranes and reenter the circulation. In general, the movement of drugs is favored from the tubular lumen to blood, partly because of the reabsorption of water that occurs throughout most portions of the nephron, which results in an increased concentration of drug in the luminal fluid. The concentration gradient thus established will facilitate movement of the drug out of the tubular lumen, given that the lipid solubility and ionization of the drug are appropriate.

The pH of the urine (usually between 4.5 and 8) can markedly affect the rate of passive back-diffusion. The

back-diffusion occurs primarily in the distal tubules and collecting ducts, where most of the urine acidification takes place. Since it is the un-ionized form of the drug that diffuses from the tubular fluid across the tubular cells into the blood, it follows that acidification increases reabsorption (or decreases elimination) of weak acids, such as salicylates, and decreases reabsorption (or promotes elimination) of weak bases, such as amphetamines. However, should the un-ionized form of the drug not have sufficient lipid solubility, urinary pH changes will have little influence on urinary drug excretion.

Effects of pH on urinary drug elimination may have important applications in medical practice, especially in cases of overdose. For example, one can enhance the elimination of a barbiturate (a weak acid) by administering bicarbonate to the patient. This procedure alkalinizes the urine and thus promotes the excretion of the now more completely ionized drug. The excretion of bases can be increased by making the urine more acidic through the use of an acidifying salt, such as ammonium chloride.

Active Tubular Secretion

A number of drugs can serve as substrates for the two active secretory systems in the proximal tubule cells. These transport systems, which actively transfer drugs from blood to luminal fluid, are independent of each other; one secretes organic anions (Figure 4.3), and the other secretes organic cations. One drug substrate can compete for transport with a simultaneously administered or endogenous similarly charged compound; this competition will decrease the overall rate of excretion of each substance. The secretory capacity of both the organic anion and organic cation secretory systems can be saturated at high drug concentrations. Each drug will

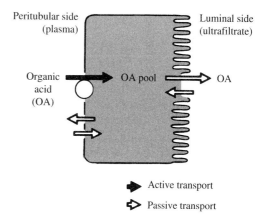

FIGURE 4.3

Active renal elimination of an organic anion. The transport mechanism is in the peritubular portion of the membrane of the proximal tubular cell.

have its own characteristic maximum rate of secretion (transport maximum, T_m).

Some drugs that are not candidates for active tubular secretion may be metabolized to compounds that are. This is often true for metabolites that are formed as a result of conjugative reactions. Because the conjugates are generally not pharmacologically active, increases in their rate of elimination through active secretion usually have little effect on the drug's overall duration of action.

These active secretory systems are important in drug excretion because *charged anions and cations are often strongly bound to plasma proteins* and therefore are not readily available for excretion by filtration. However, since the protein binding is usually reversible, the active secretory systems can rapidly and efficiently remove many protein-bound drugs from the blood and transport them into tubular fluid.

Any drug known to be largely excreted by the kidney that has a body half-life of less than 2 hours is probably eliminated, at least in part, by tubular secretion. Some drugs can be secreted and have long half-lives, however, because of extensive passive reabsorption in distal segments of the nephron (see Passive Diffusion, earlier in the chapter). Several pharmacologically active drugs, both anions and cations, known to be secreted are listed in Table 4.5.

It is important to appreciate that these tubular transport mechanisms are not as well developed in the neonate as in the adult. In addition, their functional capacity may be diminished in the elderly. Thus, *compounds normally eliminated by tubular secretion will be excreted more slowly in the very young and in the older adult.* This age dependence of the rate of renal drug secretion may have important therapeutic implications and must be considered by the physician who prescribes drugs for these age groups.

Finally, compounds that undergo active tubular secretion also are filtered at the glomerulus (assuming protein binding is minimal). Hence, a reduction in secretory activity does not reduce the excretory process to zero but rather to a level that approximates the glomerular filtration rate.

Active Tubular Reabsorption

Some substances filtered at the glomerulus are reabsorbed by active transport systems found primarily in the proximal tubules. Active reabsorption is particularly important for endogenous substances, such as ions, glucose, and amino acids (Fig. 4.4), although a small number of drugs also may be actively reabsorbed. The probable location of the active transport system is on the luminal side of the proximal cell membrane. *Bidirectional* active transport across the proximal tubule also occurs for some compounds; that is, a drug may be both actively reabsorbed and secreted. The occurrence of such bidirectional active transport mechanisms across the proximal tubule has been described for several organic anions, including the naturally occurring uric acid (see Chapter 37). The major portion of *filtered* urate is probably reabsorbed, whereas that eventually found in the urine is mostly derived from active tubular secretion.

Most drugs act by reducing active transport rather than by enhancing it. Thus, drugs that promote uric acid loss (uricosuric agents, such as probenecid and sulfinpyrazone) probably inhibit active urate reabsorption, while pyrazinamide, which reduces urate excretion, may block the active tubular secretion of uric acid. A complicating observation is that a drug may primarily inhibit active reabsorption at one dose and active secretion at another, frequently lower, dose. For example, small amounts of salicylate will decrease total urate ex-

TABLE 4.5	Compounds Secreted by Renal Tubular Transport Systems
Organic Anion Transport	**Organic Cation Transport**
Acetazolamide	Acetylcholine
Bile salts	Atropine
Hydrochlorothiazide	Cimetidine
Furosemide	Dopamine
Indomethacin	Epinephrine
Penicillin G	Morphine
Prostaglandins	Neostigmine
Salicylate	Quinine

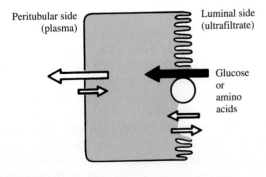

FIGURE 4.4
Active reabsorption of important substances that have been filtered at the glomerular membranes. The transport mechanism is in the luminal portion of the membrane of the proximal tubular cell. *Solid arrow* indicates active transport.

cretion, while high doses have a uricosuric effect. This is offered as an explanation for the apparently paradoxical effects of low and high doses of drugs on the total excretory pattern of compounds that are handled by renal active transport.

Clinical Implications of Renal Excretion

The rate of urinary drug excretion will depend on the drug's volume of distribution, its degree of protein binding, and the following renal factors:

1. Glomerular filtration rate
2. Tubular fluid pH
3. Extent of back-diffusion of the unionized form
4. Extent of active tubular secretion of the compound
5. Possibly, extent of active tubular reabsorption

Changes in any of these factors may result in clinically important alterations in drug action. In the final analysis, the amount of drug that finally appears in the urine will represent a balance of filtered, reabsorbed (passively and actively), and secreted drug. For many drugs, the duration and intensity of pharmacological effect will be influenced by the status of renal function, because of the major role played by the kidneys in drug and metabolite elimination. Ultimately, whether or not dosage adjustment (e.g., prolongation of dosing interval, reduction in the maintenance dose, or both) becomes necessary will depend on an assessment of the degree of renal dysfunction, the percentage of drug cleared by the kidney, and the potential for drug toxicity, especially if renal function is reduced.

Biliary Excretion

The liver secretes about 1 L of bile daily. Bile flow and composition depend on the secretory activity of the hepatic cells that line the biliary canaliculi. As the bile flows through the biliary system of ducts, its composition can be modified in the ductules and ducts by the processes of reabsorption and secretion, especially of electrolytes and water. For example, osmotically active compounds, including bile acids, transported into the bile promote the passive movement of fluid into the duct lumen. In the gallbladder, composition of the bile is modified further through reabsorptive processes.

The passage of most foreign compounds from the blood into the liver normally is not restricted because the endothelium of the hepatic blood sinusoids behaves as a porous membrane. Hence, drugs with molecular weights lower than those of most protein molecules readily reach the hepatic extracellular fluid from the plasma. A number of compounds are taken up into the liver by carrier-mediated systems, while more lipophilic

drugs pass through the hepatocyte membrane by diffusion. The subsequent passage of substances into the bile, however, is much more selective.

At least three groups of compounds enter the bile. Compounds of group A are those whose concentration in bile and plasma are almost identical (bile–plasma ratio of 1). These include glucose, and ions such as $Na+$, K^+, and Cl^-. Group B contains the bile salts, bilirubin glucuronide, sulfobromophthalein, procainamide, and others, whose ratio of bile to blood is much greater than 1, usually 10 to 1,000. Group C is reserved for compounds for which the ratio of bile to blood is less than 1, for example, insulin, sucrose, and proteins. Drugs can belong to any of these three categories. Only small amounts of most drugs reach the bile by diffusion. However, biliary excretion plays a major role (5–95% of the administered dose) in drug removal for some anions, cations, and certain un-ionized molecules, such as cardiac glycosides. In addition, biliary elimination may be important for the excretion of some heavy metals.

Cardiac glycosides, anions, and cations are transported from the liver into the bile by three distinct and independent carrier-mediated active transport systems, the last two closely resembling those in the renal proximal tubules that secrete anions and cations into tubular urine. As is true for renal tubular secretion, protein-bound drug is completely available for biliary active transport. In contrast to the bile acids, the *actively secreted drugs* generally do not recycle, because they are not substrates for the intestinal bile acid transport system, and they are generally too highly charged to back-diffuse across the intestinal epithelium. Thus, the ability of certain compounds to be actively secreted into bile accounts for the large quantity of these drugs removed from the body by way of the feces.

On the other hand, most drugs that are secreted by the liver into the bile and then into the small intestine are not eliminated through the feces. The physicochemical properties of most drugs are sufficiently favorable for passive intestinal absorption that the compound will reenter the blood that perfuses the intestine and again be carried to the liver. Such recycling may continue (*enterohepatic cycle* or *circulation*) until the drug either undergoes metabolic changes in the liver, is excreted by the kidneys, or both. This process permits the conservation of such important endogenous substances as the bile acids, vitamins D_3 and B_{12}, folic acid, and estrogens (Table 4.6).

Extensive enterohepatic cycling may be partly responsible for a drug's long persistence in the body. Orally administered activated charcoal and/or anion exchange resins have been used clinically to interrupt enterohepatic cycling and trap drugs in the gastrointestinal tract.

As stated earlier, many foreign compounds are either partially or extensively metabolized in the liver.

TABLE 4.6 Drugs that Undergo Enterohepatic Recirculation

Adriamycin	Methadone
Amphetamine	Metronidazole
Chlordecone	Morphine
1,25-Dihydroxyvitamin D_3	Phenytoin
Estradiol	Polar Glucuronic Acid Conjugates
Indomethacin	Polar Sulfate Conjugates
Mestranol	Sulindac

Conjugation of a compound or its metabolites is especially important in determining whether the drug will undergo biliary excretion. Frequently, when a compound is secreted into the intestine through the bile, it is in the form of a conjugate. *Conjugation generally enhances biliary excretion,* since it both introduces a strong polar (i.e., anionic) center into the molecule and increases its molecular weight. Molecular weight may, however, be less important in the biliary excretion of organic cations. Conjugated drugs will not be reabsorbed readily from the gastrointestinal tract unless the conjugate is hydrolyzed by gut enzymes such as β-glucuronidase. Chloramphenicol glucuronide, for example, is secreted into the bile, where it is hydrolyzed by gastrointestinal flora and largely reabsorbed. Such a continuous recirculation may lead to the appearance of drug-induced toxicity.

The kidney and liver are, in general, capable of actively transporting the same organic anion substrates. However, the two organs have certain quantitative differences in drug affinity for the transporters. It has been suggested that several subsystems of organic anion transport may exist and that the binding specificities of the transporters involved are not absolute but overlapping.

Liver disease or injury may impair bile secretion and thereby lead to accumulation of certain drugs, for example probenecid, digoxin, and diethylstilbestrol. Impairment of liver function can lead to decreased rates of both drug metabolism and secretion of drugs into bile. These two processes, of course, are frequently interrelated, since many drugs are candidates for biliary secretion only after appropriate metabolism has occurred.

Decreases in biliary excretion have been demonstrated at both ends of the age continuum. For example, ouabain, an unmetabolized cardiac glycoside that is secreted into the bile, is particularly toxic in the newborn. This is largely due to a reduced ability of biliary secretion to remove ouabain from the plasma.

Increases in hepatic excretory function also may take place. After the chronic administration of either phenobarbital or the potassium-sparing diuretic spirono-lactone, the rate of bile flow is augmented. Such an increase in bile secretion can reduce blood levels of drugs that depend on biliary elimination.

Finally, the administration of one drug may influence the rate of biliary excretion of a second coadministered compound. These effects may be brought about through an alteration in one or more of the following factors: hepatic blood flow, uptake into hepatocytes, rate of biotransformation, transport into bile, or rate of bile formation. In addition, antibiotics may alter the intestinal flora in such a manner as to diminish the presence of sulfatase and glucuronidase-containing bacteria. This would result in a persistence of the conjugated form of the drug and hence a decrease in its enterohepatic recirculation.

PULMONARY EXCRETION

Any volatile material, irrespective of its route of administration, has the potential for pulmonary excretion. Certainly, gases and other volatile substances that enter the body primarily through the respiratory tract can be expected to be excreted by this route. *No specialized transport systems are involved in the loss of substances in expired air; simple diffusion across cell membranes is predominant.* The rate of loss of gases is not constant; it depends on the rate of respiration and pulmonary blood flow.

The degree of solubility of a gas in blood also will affect the rate of gas loss. Gases such as nitrous oxide, which are not very soluble in blood, will be excreted rapidly, that is, almost at the rate at which the blood delivers the drug to the lungs. *Increasing cardiac output has the greatest effect on the removal of poorly soluble gases;* for example, doubling the cardiac output nearly doubles the rates of loss. Agents with high blood and tissue solubility, on the other hand, are only slowly transferred from pulmonary capillary blood to the alveoli. Ethanol, which has a relatively high blood gas solubility, is excreted very slowly by the lungs. *The arterial concentration of a highly soluble gas falls much more slowly, and its rate of loss depends more on respiratory rate than on cardiac output.*

A more detailed discussion of the uptake, distribution, and elimination of compounds administered by inhalation can be found in Chapter 25.

EXCRETION IN OTHER BODY FLUIDS

Sweat and Saliva

Excretion of drugs into sweat and saliva occurs but has only minor importance for most drugs. The mechanisms involved in drug excretion are similar for sweat and saliva. Excretion mainly depends on the diffusion of the un-ionized lipid-soluble form of the drug across the epithelial cells of the glands. Thus, the pK_a of the drug and the pH of the individual secretion formed in the glands are important determinants of the total quantity of drug appearing in the particular body fluid. It is not definitely established whether active drug transport occurs across the ducts of the glands.

Lipid-insoluble compounds, such as urea and glycerol, enter saliva and sweat at rates proportional to their molecular weight, presumably because of filtration through the aqueous channels in the secretory cell membrane. Drugs or their metabolites that are excreted into sweat may be at least partially responsible for the dermatitis and other skin reactions caused by some therapeutic agents. Substances excreted into saliva are usually swallowed, and therefore their fate is the same as that of orally administered drugs (unless expectoration is a major characteristic of a person's habits). The excretion of a drug into saliva accounts for the drug taste patients sometimes report after certain compounds are given intravenously.

Milk

Many drugs in a nursing mother's blood are detectable in her milk (Table 4.7). The ultimate concentration of the individual compound in milk will depend on many factors, including the amount of drug in the maternal blood, its lipid solubility, its degree of ionization, and the extent of its active excretion. Thus, the physicochemical properties that govern the excretion of drugs into saliva and sweat also apply to the passage of drugs into milk.

Since milk is more acidic (pH 6.5) than plasma, basic compounds (e.g., alkaloids, such as morphine and codeine) may be somewhat more concentrated in this fluid. In contrast, the levels of weak organic acids will probably be lower than those in plasma. In general, a high maternal plasma protein binding of drug will be associated with a low milk concentration. A highly lipid-soluble drug should accumulate in milk fat. Low-molecular-weight un-ionized water-soluble drugs will diffuse passively across the mammary epithelium and transfer into milk. There they may reside in association with one or more milk components, for example, bound to protein such as lactalbumin, dissolved within fat globules, or free in the aqueous compartment. Substances that are not electrolytes, such as ethanol, urea, and antipyrine, readily enter milk and reach approximately the same concentration as in plasma. Compounds used in agriculture also may be passed from cows to humans by this route. Finally, antibiotics such as the tetracyclines, which can function as chelating agents and bind calcium, have a higher milk than plasma concentration.

Both maternal and infant factors determine the final amount of drug present in the nursing child's body at any particular time. Variations in the daily amount of milk formed within the breast (e.g., changes in blood flow to the breast) as well as alterations in breast milk pH will affect the total amount of drug found in milk. In addition, composition of the milk will be affected by the maternal diet; for example, a high-carbohydrate diet will increase the content of saturated fatty acids in milk.

The greatest drug exposure occurs when feeding begins shortly after maternal drug dosing. Additional factors determining exposure of the infant include milk volume consumed (about 150 mL/kg/day) and milk composition at the time of feeding. Fat content is highest in the morning and then gradually decreases until about 10 P.M. A longer feed usually results in exposure of the infant to more of a fat-soluble drug, since milk fat content increases somewhat during a given nursing period.

Whether or not a drug accumulates in a nursing child is affected in part by the infant's ability to eliminate via metabolism and excretion the ingested compound. In general, the ability to oxidize and conjugate drugs is low in the neonate and does not approach full adult rates until approximately age 6. It follows, therefore, that drug accumulation should be less in an older infant who breast-feeds than in a suckling neonate.

Although abnormalities in fetal organ structure and function can result from the presence of certain drugs in breast milk, it would be quite inappropriate to deny the breast-feeding woman appropriate and necessary drug therapy. A pragmatic approach on the part of both the physician and patient is necessary. *Breast-feeding should be discouraged when inherent drug toxicity is known or when adverse pharmacological actions of the drug on the infant are likely.* Infant drug exposure can be minimized, however, through short intermittent maternal drug use and by drug dosing immediately after breast-feeding.

TABLE 4.7 **Examples of Drugs That Appear in Breast Milk**

Acetylsalicylic acid
Antithyroid uracil compounds
Barbiturates
Caffeine
Ethanol
Glutethimide
Morphine
Nicotine

Study QUESTIONS

1. Concerning regulation of CYP-mediated drug metabolism, all of the following statements are true EXCEPT
   (A) Drugs that competitively inhibit CYP enzymes cause a decrease in concentrations of the object (original) drug.
   (B) Induction of drug-metabolizing enzymes results in a decrease in concentrations of the object (original) drug, thus potentially reducing efficacy.
   (C) Induction of drug-metabolizing enzymes frequently requires the synthesis of new enzyme protein and thus may not occur immediately upon introduction of the inducing agent.
   (D) Mechanism-based inactivation results in irreversible inactivation of the enzyme that lasts for the duration of the enzyme molecule.

2. Which of the following CYP enzymes is associated with metabolism of the greatest number of drugs and thus most likely to be involved in drug–drug interactions?
   (A) CYP3A4
   (B) CYP2C9
   (C) CYP2D6
   (D) CYP2E1
   (E) CYP1A2

3. Conjugation of a drug with glucuronic acid via the glucuronosyl transferases will result in all of the following EXCEPT
   (A) Production of a more water-soluble moiety that is more easily excreted
   (B) A new compound that may also possess pharmacological activity
   (C) A drug molecule that may be more susceptible to biliary elimination
   (D) A drug molecule that may undergo enterohepatic recirculation and reintroduction into the bloodstream
   (E) A drug with a different pharmacological mechanism of action

4. Concerning the renal excretion of drugs:
   (A) Drugs that are ionized in the renal tubule are more likely to undergo passive reabsorption than those that are unionized
   (B) Low-molecular-weight drugs are much more likely to be actively secreted than filtered.
   (C) Only drug that is not bound to plasma proteins (i.e., free drug) is filtered by the glomerulus.
   (D) Decreasing renal tubular fluid pH will increase elimination of weakly acidic drugs.

5. Drug presence in breast milk is most likely for:
   (A) Drugs highly bound to plasma proteins
   (B) Lipid-soluble molecules

   (C) Large ionized water-soluble molecules
   (D) Acidic compounds

ANSWERS

1. **A.** When one inhibits the action of a drug-metabolizing enzyme (A), one would expect an increase instead of a decrease in drug concentrations, since less is being metabolized. Induction of an enzyme (B) would have the opposite effect, since there would be more enzyme available to metabolize the drug. C is correct, since the most common mechanism of enzyme induction is through synthesis of new enzyme protein, which does not occur immediately. Finally, mechanism-based inactivation (D) is also correct, since this is irreversible, leaving the enzyme inactive and eventually it is degraded by the body.

2. **A.** CYP3A4 is the predominant cytochrome P450 drug-metabolizing enzyme in the body, both in terms of amount of enzyme and the number of drugs that it metabolizes. It has been estimated to carry out approximately 50% of the cytochrome P450–mediated reactions observed. The other enzymes have been reported to carry out 30% (CYP2D6), 15–20% (CYP2C9) and 1–2% (both CYP2E1 and CYP1A2).

3. **E.** Most glucuronic acid conjugates are less effective than the parent drug. The conjugate, however, usually maintains the same pharmacological mechanism of action, although frequently of a lesser magnitude. Conjugation with glucuronic acid makes a drug molecule more water soluble (A), and glucuronic acid conjugates are more likely to be eliminated by secretion into the bile (C) than are unconjugated compounds. These glucuronide conjugates, once secreted into the bile, may be cleaved by β-glucuronidases to liberate the parent compound, which can then be reabsorbed (D). Several glucuronic acid conjugates of drugs (e.g., morphine 6-glucuronide) possess pharmacological activity (B).

4. **C.** Plasma proteins are too large to be filtered by the glomerulus, so that any drug molecules bound to these plasma proteins will not undergo filtration. A is not correct: ionized drugs are *less* likely to undergo reabsorption, since this is generally thought to be a passive process. B is also not correct: low-molecular-weight drugs are more likely to be filtered, since they can easily pass through the glomerulus filter. Finally, weakly acidic drugs will be un-ionized at a low (acidic) pH, hence more likely to undergo reabsorption, thus *reducing* the net elimination (D).

5. B. Lipid-soluble molecules are more likely to be excreted in breast milk because it is primarily a passive diffusion process. A, C, and D are not correct because they are opposite of the typical characteristics of drugs excreted into breast milk.

SUPPLEMENTAL READING

Bennett PN (ed). Drugs and Human Lactation. Amsterdam: Elsevier, 1988.

Boyer JL, Graf J, and Meier PJ. Hepatic transport systems regulating pH, cell volume, and bile secretion. Ann Rev Physiol 1992;54:415–438.

Cutler RE, Forland SC, Hammond, P, and Evans, JR. Extracorporeal removal of drugs and poisons by hemodialysis and hemoperfusion. Annu Rev Pharmacol Toxicol 1987;27:169–191.

Goldstein RS. Biochemical heterogeneity and site-specific tubular injury. In Hook JB and Goldstein RS (eds.). Toxicology of the Kidney (2nd ed.). New York: Raven, 1993.

Grantham JJ and Chonko AM. Renal handling of organic anions and cations: Excretion of uric acid. In Brenner BM and Rector FC (eds.).7 The Kidney (4th ed). Philadelphia: Saunders, 1991.

Levy RH et al. (eds.) Metabolic Drug Interactions. Philadelphia: Lippincott, Williams & Wilkins, 2000.

Roberts RJ. Drug Therapy in Infants. Philadelphia: Saunders, 1984.

Walker RI and Duggin GG. Drug nephrotoxicity. Annu Rev Pharmacol Toxicol 1988;28:331–345.

CASE Study Why am I not getting pain relief?

A 37-year-old woman visited her dentist for removal of her wisdom teeth. The teeth were found to be impacted, and removal necessitated extensive surgery. Following completion of the procedure on one side of the mouth, the patient was given a prescription for acetaminophen 300 mg with codeine 30 mg (combination product) for the relief of pain. The patient took the prescription as prescribed for approximately 2 days, but little pain relief was achieved. She called the dentist to get a prescription for another analgesic. What is a possible explanation for this lack of efficacy?

ANSWER: Codeine itself is a very weak analgesic but is metabolized to morphine, which produces most of the analgesic effect following codeine administration. The metabolism of codeine to morphine is carried out by cytochrome P450 2D6, an enzyme that exhibits genetic polymorphism. The patient may be deficient in CYP2D6 and thus unable to convert codeine into its active metabolite, morphine; hence analgesic efficacy is lacking.

5 | Pharmacokinetics

Timothy S. Tracy

Pharmacokinetics is the description of the time course of a drug in the body, encompassing absorption, distribution, metabolism, and excretion. In simplest terms, it can be described as what the body does to the drug. Pharmacokinetic concepts are used during drug development to determine the optimal formulation of a drug, dose (along with effect data), and dosing frequency. For drugs with a wide therapeutic index (difference between the minimum effective dose and the minimum toxic dose), knowledge of the drug's pharmacokinetic properties in that individual patient may not be particularly important. For example, nonsteroidal antiinflammatory drugs, such as ibuprofen, have a wide therapeutic index, and thus knowledge of the pharmacokinetic parameters in a given individual is relatively unimportant, since normal doses can vary from 400 to 3200 mg per day with no substantial difference in acute toxicity or effect. However, for drugs with a narrow therapeutic index, knowledge of that drug's pharmacokinetic profile in an individual patient has paramount importance.

If there is little difference between the minimum effective dose and the toxic dose, slight changes in a drug's pharmacokinetic profile, or even simply interindividual differences, may require dosage adjustments to minimize toxicity or maximize efficacy. For example, the blood concentrations of the antiasthmatic drug theophylline must usually be maintained within the range of 10–20 μg/mL. At concentrations below this, patients may not obtain relief of symptoms, while concentrations above 20 μg/mL can result in serious toxicities, such as seizures, arrhythmias, and even death. Thus, a drug's pharmacokinetic profile may have important clinical significance beyond its use in drug development.

DRUG CONCENTRATION–TIME PROFILES AND BASIC PHARMACOKINETIC PARAMETERS

The time course of a drug in the body is frequently represented as a concentration–time profile in which the concentrations of a drug in the body are measured analytically and the results plotted in semilogarithmic form against time. A representative profile of a drug given intravenously is presented in Figure 5.1. Drug concentrations are measured in samples typically taken from the brachial vein, since this vein is readily accessible, since sampling results in minimal patient discomfort and since obtained values reflect the concentrations of drug in the bloodstream. Concentrations in the blood may not be identical to concentrations at the site of action, such as a receptor, but one hopes they serve as a surrogate that correlates in a proportional manner.

Figure 5.1 shows that for a drug given intravenously, maximum concentrations are achieved almost instantaneously, since absorption across membranes is not required, though distributive processes may also occur (not depicted for the sake of simplicity). The concentrations of drug in the blood decline over time according to the elimination rate of that particular drug. More commonly, drug is given via extravascular routes (e.g., orally), so absorption and distribution must occur, and therefore it will take some time before maximum concentrations are achieved.

The blood concentration–time profile for a theoretical drug given extravascularly (e.g., orally) is shown in Figure 5.2. Some pharmacokinetic parameters, such as C_{max}, T_{max}, *area under the curve*, and *half-life*, can be estimated by visual inspection or computation from a con-

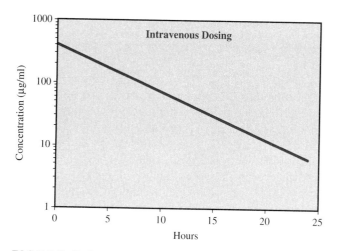

FIGURE 5.1

Concentration–time profile for a hypothetical drug administered intravenously. Following intravenous dosing of a drug, blood concentrations of the drug reach a maximum almost immediately. Y-axis is logarithmic scale.

centration–time profile. C_{max} is defined as the maximum concentration achieved in the blood. In Figure 5.2, C_{max} can be estimated to be approximately 225 µg/mL. The other pharmacokinetic parameter that can be easily estimated from a concentration–time profile is T_{max}, or the time needed to reach maximum concentration. In Figure 5.2, the T_{max} is estimated by visual inspection to be approximately 2 hours. The same drug in a formulation that permits a faster rate of absorption would have a shorter T_{max} and generally a higher C_{max} than the formulation with slower absorptive properties. Likewise, all other things being equal, a drug with a slower elimi-

nation rate will generally exhibit a longer T_{max} and higher C_{max}. Once administered, a drug begins undergoing absorption, distribution, metabolism, and excretion all at once, not in a sequential fashion, such that all of these processes are involved in determining the shape of a concentration–time profile.

One indicator of the overall exposure of a person to a drug is through the calculation of the *area under the curve (AUC)*. As the name implies, AUC is the mathematically integrated area under the concentration–time curve and is most commonly calculated using the trapezoidal rule of mathematics. In Figure 5.2, the AUC is represented by the shaded area. Though the shape of the concentration–time profile may affect the AUC for a drug, two drugs with entirely different concentration–time profile shapes may have the same AUC. It is, in fact, this property that makes calculating the AUC useful, because it can be used to assess the person's overall exposure to a drug, even though the individual may have reached different T_{max} and C_{max} values from those of other individuals. Furthermore, as will be discussed shortly, AUC is also useful for calculating another pharmacokinetic parameter, clearance.

An additional parameter that can be determined from a concentration–time profile is the half-life of the drug, that is, the time it takes for half of the drug to be eliminated from the body. Half-life determination is very useful, since it can readily be used to evaluate how long a drug is expected to remain in the body after termination of dosing, the time required for a drug to reach steady state (when the rate of drug entering the body is equal to the rate of drug leaving the body), and often the frequency of dosing. The following equation is used to calculate the half-life of a drug:

$$t_{1/2} = \frac{0.693}{k_e}$$

where $t_{1/2}$ is the half-life and k_e is the elimination rate constant calculated from the slope of the declining portion of the concentration–time profile (Fig. 5.3). By definition, half-life denotes that 50% of the drug in the body at a given time will be eliminated over the calculated period. However, this does not mean that the same *amount* of drug is eliminated each half-life. For example, Figure 5.3 shows that during the first half-life period (0–5 hours) the drug concentration is reduced from 100 µg/mL to 50 µg/mL. However, during the second half-life period (5–10 hours), even though the amount in the body is reduced by 50%, the concentration falls only from 50 µg/mL to 25 µg/mL (a reduction in concentration of 25 µg/mL). This concept is also illustrated in Table 5.1. It takes approximately five half-lives for 97% of the drug to be eliminated from the body (regardless of the duration of the half-life). Thus, if one wished to switch a patient from one drug to another but not have both drugs present in substantial quantities,

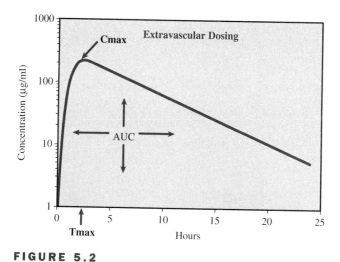

FIGURE 5.2

Concentration–time profile for a hypothetical drug administered extravascularly. C_{max}, maximum concentration achieved. T_{max}, time required to achieve maximum concentration. AUC = Area under the curve. Y-axis is on logarithmic scale.

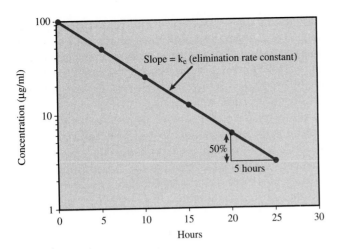

FIGURE 5.3

Elimination of a hypothetical drug with a half-life of 5 hours. The drug concentration decreases by 50% every 5 hours (i.e., $t_{1/2}$ = 5 hours). The slope of the line is the elimination rate (k_e).

the clinician must wait five half-lives (in this case, 25 hours) before administering the second drug. It will also require five half-lives for a drug to reach steady state (see Pharmacokinetics of Single Versus Multiple Dosing, later in the chapter), again, independent of the duration of the half-life. Steady state is when the amount of drug entering the body is equal to the amount of drug being eliminated in a given period. Finally, it is a rule of thumb (though certainly not absolute) that drugs are generally dosed every half-life (with allowance for rounding to convenient intervals). Thus, the concept of half-life has considerable importance for determining dosing frequency or adjusting doses in a patient.

ADDITIONAL PHARMACOKINETIC PARAMETERS

Bioavailability

Bioavailability (designated as F) is defined as the fraction of the administered drug reaching the systemic circulation as intact drug. Bioavailability is highly dependent on both the route of administration and the drug formulation. For example, drugs that are given intravenously exhibit a bioavailability of 1, since the entire dose reaches the systemic circulation as intact drug. However, for other routes of administration, this is not necessarily the case.

Subcutaneous, intramuscular, oral, rectal, and other extravascular routes of administration require that the drug be absorbed first, which can reduce bioavailability. The drug also may be subject to metabolism prior to reaching the systemic circulation, again potentially reducing bioavailability. For example, when the β-blocking agent propranolol is given intravenously, F = 1, but when it is given orally, F = ~0.2, suggesting that only approximately 20% of the administered dose reaches the systemic circulation as intact drug.

With respect to the effect of drug formulation on bioavailability, the drug digoxin provides a good example. Given orally as a solution, the bioavailability of digoxin approaches F = 1, suggesting essentially complete bioavailability and one that approaches that of the intravenous formulation. Digoxin liquid capsules also exhibit F = ~1 when given orally and thus are also completely available. However, for digoxin tablets, F = ~0.7, suggesting incomplete bioavailability, probably because of lack of absorption.

Two types of bioavailability can be calculated, depending on the formulations available and the information required. The gold standard is a calculation of the *absolute* bioavailability of a given product compared to

---

TABLE 5.1   Elimination Characteristics of a Drug with a 5-Hour Half-life

Concentration at Beginning of Period[a]	Concentration at End of Period[a]	Period (hours)	Percent of Original Concentration
100.00	50.000	0–5	50.000
50.00	25.000	5–10	25.000
25.00	12.500	10–15	12.500
12.50	6.250	15–20	6.250
6.25	3.125	20–25	3.125

Half of the concentration at the beginning of any period is eliminated during the period. Thus, each successive half-life removes less drug, but the concentration at the beginning of the period is reduced by 50% during the period.
[a]Micrograms per milliliter.

the intravenous formulation (F = 1). The absolute bioavailability of a drug can be calculated as:

$$F = \frac{Dose_{iv} \cdot (AUC_{0-\infty})_{other}}{Dose_{other} \cdot (AUC_{0-\infty})_{iv}}$$

where the route of administration is other than intravenous (e.g., oral, rectal). For calculation of absolute bioavailability, complete concentration-time profiles are needed for both the intravenous and other routes of administration.

The other computation is that of *relative* bioavailability. This calculation is determined when two products are compared to each other, not to an intravenous standard. This is commonly calculated in the generic drug industry to determine that the generic formulation (e.g., a tablet) is bioequivalent to the original formulation (e.g., another tablet). Thus, bioavailability is not routinely calculated in an individual patient but reserved for product development by a drug manufacturer. However, it is important to have an idea of how formulations or routes of administration differ with respect to bioavailability so as to allow proper dosage adjustment when changing formulations or routes of administration.

Clearance

Clearance is a pharmacokinetic parameter used to describe the efficiency of irreversible elimination of drug from the body. More specifically, clearance is defined as the volume of blood from which drug can be completely removed per unit of time (e.g., 100 mL/minute). Clearance can involve both metabolism of drug to a metabolite and excretion of drug from the body. For example, a molecule that has undergone glucuronidation is described as having been cleared, even though the molecule itself may not have left the body. Clearance of drug can be accomplished by excretion of drug into the urine, gut contents, expired air, sweat, and saliva as well as metabolic conversion to another form. However, uptake of drug into tissues does not constitute clearance.

In the broadest sense, total (systemic) clearance is the clearance of drug by all routes. Total (systemic) clearance (Cl) can be calculated by either of the equations given below:

$$Cl = Vd \cdot k_e$$

or

$$Cl = \frac{Dose}{AUC}$$

where Vd is the volume of distribution (see below) and the remainder of the parameters are as defined previously. One must give the drug intravenously to assure 100% bioavailability, because lack of 100% bioavail-

ability can change the dose numerator, which is required to calculate total clearance. Frequently, however, one wishes to calculate drug clearance but intravenous administration is not feasible. In this situation, the apparent clearance (also called oral clearance) can be estimated by the following equation:

$$Cl_{app} = \frac{Dose \cdot F}{AUC}$$

and can be rearranged to give

$$\frac{Cl_{app}}{F} = \frac{Dose}{AUC}$$

The term *apparent clearance* is used because the bioavailability of the compound is unknown. Thus, estimations of apparent clearance will always be higher than the true systemic clearance because of this unknown bioavailability.

The final clearance value that is frequently calculated is that of renal clearance, or that portion of clearance that is due to renal elimination. Renal clearance is calculated as:

$$Clr = \frac{Ae}{AUC}$$

where Ae is the total amount of drug excreted unchanged into the urine. Calculation of renal clearance is especially useful for drugs that are eliminated primarily by the kidney.

Because clearance estimates the efficiency of the body in eliminating drug, the calculation of clearance can be especially useful in optimizing dosing of patients. Since this parameter includes both the volume of distribution and the elimination rate, it adjusts for differences in distribution characteristics and elimination rates among people, thus permitting more accurate comparisons among individuals. However, as stated earlier, by far the easiest clearance parameter to estimate is that of apparent (oral) clearance, since it does not require intravenous administration, yet this parameter can be profoundly affected by bioavailability of the drug.

Volume of Distribution

Vd relates a concentration of drug measured in the blood to the total amount of drug in the body. This mathematically determined value gives a rough indication of the overall distribution of a drug in the body. For example, a drug with a Vd of approximately 12 L (i.e., interstitial fluid plus plasma water) is probably distributed throughout extracellular fluid but is unable to penetrate cells. In general, the greater the Vd, the greater the diffusibility of the drug.

The volume of distribution is not an actual volume, since its estimation may result in a volume greater than the volume available in the body (~40 L in a 70-kg adult). Such a value will result if the compound is bound or sequestered at some *extravascular* site. For example, a highly lipid-soluble drug, such as thiopental, that can be extensively stored in fat depots may have a Vd considerably in excess of the entire fluid volume of the body. Thus, because of their physicochemical characteristics, different drugs can have quite different volumes of distribution in the same person.

The antiinflammatory drug ibuprofen, for example, typically exhibits a volume of distribution of 0.14 L/kg such that for a 70-kg person, the Vd would be 10.8 L. This volume (10.8 L) is approximately equal to the plasma volume of a person that size, suggesting that this drug does not distribute widely into tissues (though it does reach tissues to some degree to exert its action). In contrast, the antiarrhythmic amiodarone has a Vd of 60 L/kg, giving a total Vd of 4200 L for this same 70-kg person. This large Vd suggests that amiodarone distributes widely throughout the body; in fact, it does distribute to various tissues, such as the liver, lungs, eyes, and adipose tissue. Since the total volume of the body does not equal 4200 L, it can clearly be seen that this is not a "real" volume but one that relates the blood concentration to the amount of drug in the body.

Protein Binding

Most drugs bind to plasma proteins such as albumin and α_1-acid glycoprotein (AGP) to some degree. This becomes clinically important as it is assumed that only unbound (free) drug is available for binding to receptors, being metabolized by enzymes, and eliminated from the body. Thus, the free fraction of drug is important. For example, phenytoin is approximately 90% bound to plasma proteins, leaving 10% of the concentration in the blood as free drug and available for pharmacological action and metabolism. If the presence of renal disease or a drug interaction were to alter the degree of protein binding to only 80%, this change could have substantial clinical consequences. Even though the total percent bound changes relatively little, the net result is to double the amount of free drug. In fact, for phenytoin, this can have clinical consequences. However, for most drugs, displacement from protein binding sites results in only a transient increase in free drug concentration, since the drug is rapidly redistributed into other body water compartments. Thus, interactions or changes in protein binding in most cases have little clinical effect despite these theoretical considerations.

PHARMACOKINETICS OF SINGLE VERSUS MULTIPLE DOSING

Administration of single doses of a drug are occasionally encountered in clinical practice, but it is more common to use single doses to determine the pharmacokinetic profile of a drug. Figures 5.1 and 5.2 illustrate such a use of single doses. Following a single dose, concentrations can be monitored until no longer analytically detectable and a complete pharmacokinetic profile is described.

In clinical practice, drugs are more commonly administered in multiple doses, with the second dose usually given before the first dose is completely eliminated. Figure 5.4 shows a representative time–concentration profile for multiple dosing of a drug with a $t_{1/2}$ of 8 hours. With each successive dose up to approximately five doses, the concentration of drug keeps increasing, a phenomenon known as accumulation. The final concentrations of drug reached depend on the elimination rate of the drug, the dosing frequency, and the actual dose. Thus, for a given drug, *concentrations* will reach higher steady-state values if the drug is given more frequently or in greater doses. In contrast, the *time* to reach steady state is affected by neither the dose amount nor dosing frequency. The time to reach steady state is solely affected by the elimination rate (which is reflected in the $t_{1/2}$). Giving a larger dose or giving the dose more often will not change the time needed to reach steady state (except in the case of a bolus dose, as discussed later).

Just as it takes approximately five half-lives for a drug to be essentially (97%) eliminated, it also requires five half-lives for a drug to reach steady state. This is exemplified in the concentration–time profiles of Figure 5.4. The hypothetical drug in this example has a half-life of 8 hours and is dosed every 8 hours. The graph shows that at about 40 hours (five half-lives), the maximum and minimum concentrations become consistent, indi-

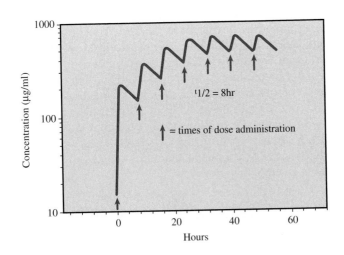

FIGURE 5.4
Concentration–time profile for a hypothetical drug administered orally in multiple doses. The drug is administered once every half-life (i.e., every 8 hours). Drug continues to accumulate (i.e., concentrations rise) until steady state (rate in = rate out) is reached at approximately 5 half-lives (about 40 hours).

cating achievement of a steady state of concentration (drug input = drug elimination).

The only practical method for achieving steady-state concentrations prior to five half-lives is to administer a bolus dose of drug (a dose much higher than normal and designed to bring concentrations up to steady state immediately) followed by standard dosing (Figure 5.5). In this way, the "accumulation" of drug occurs rapidly because of the large amount of drug given initially. However, bolus doses must be calculated in accordance with both the drug's pharmacokinetic parameters and the physiological characteristics of the individual to avoid potential toxicities.

NONLINEAR PHARMACOKINETICS

The underlying assumption in the discussion of these concepts is that the drug of interest follows linear pharmacokinetic principles; that is, the concentrations achieved are proportional to the dose given. For example, a doubling of the dose will produce a doubling of the blood concentration. For some drugs, however, this is not the case: an increase in dose may produce a concentration much greater than expected. For example, increases in dosage of the antiepileptic agent phenytoin above approximately 300 mg daily usually produce a greater than expected increase in blood concentrations. This is illustrated in the graph of Figure 5.6, which shows that for a hypothetical patient, phenytoin blood concentrations are plotted against dose of phenytoin. The graph demonstrates that as one approaches doses that result in therapeutic concentrations of phenytoin, the rise in concentrations becomes nonlinear such that an increase in dose from 300 to 400 mg (33% increase) produces a 300% increase in phenytoin concentration. Thus, it is easy to see how toxicity may arise quickly following what was seemingly a small increase in dose; under linear circumstances such a small increase in dose would have resulted in concentrations still within the therapeutic range. This nonlinearity often occurs because the drug-metabolizing enzymes for the drug become saturated at typical blood concentrations, such that despite increases in dose, drug is still metabolized at the same rate and blood concentrations go up unexpectedly. In this case, following Michaelis-Menten enzyme kinetics, the maximum velocity (V_{max}) has been reached and the rate of drug metabolism remains constant.

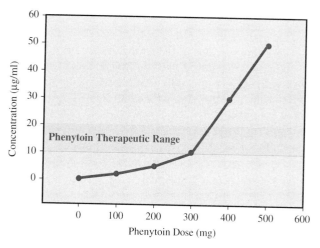

FIGURE 5.6
Theoretical depiction of phenytoin concentrations achieved following various doses of the antiepileptic phenytoin. Shaded area indicates the therapeutic range of phenytoin concentrations: below 10 µg/mL, results in subtherapeutic effect; above 20 µg/mL, results in toxicity. Within the therapeutic range, a relatively small increase in dose results in a greater than proportional increase in concentration, suggesting nonlinear pharmacokinetics.

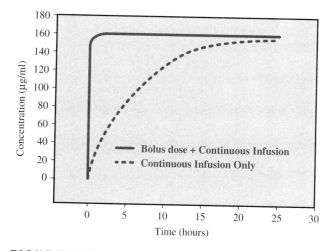

FIGURE 5.5
Theoretical depiction of plasma concentrations following either an intravenous bolus dose immediately followed by initiation of a continuous intravenous infusion or initiation of a continuous intravenous infusion only.

Study QUESTIONS

1. Frequently it is useful to consider the overall exposure of a person to a drug during the dosing interval. Which of the following pharmacokinetic parameters defines the exposure of a person to a drug?
   (A) C_{max}
   (B) T_{max}
   (C) AUC (area under the curve)
   (D) Half-life
   (E) Clearance

2. Organs such as the liver remove exogenous chemicals, such as drugs, from the body. For drugs such as phenytoin, for which the difference between the minimum effective concentration and the minimum toxic concentration is small, clinicians must calculate the rate at which a given individual removes drug from the body. The volume of fluid from which drug can be completely removed per unit of time (rate of drug removal) is termed:
   (A) Distribution
   (B) Clearance
   (C) Metabolism
   (D) Excretion

3. For a drug such as piroxicam with a 40-hour half-life and being dosed once daily (i.e., every 24 hours), steady state will be reached *shortly following* which DOSE (not which half-life)?
   (A) 1st dose
   (B) 3rd dose
   (C) 5th dose
   (D) 8th dose
   (E) 12th dose

4. Volume of distribution (Vd), though not a physiological volume, helps a clinician to estimate drug distribution in the body. Drugs distribute throughout the body to differing degrees depending on a number of factors. Which of the following factors is TRUE concerning drug distribution?
   (A) In general, a drug with a higher degree of plasma protein binding will have a lower volume of distribution.
   (B) All drugs distribute to the same degree in all tissues.
   (C) The binding of drugs to tissues has no relationship to the distribution of drug in the body.
   (D) In general, lipophilic drugs distribute to a lesser extent than hydrophilic drugs.

5. A clinician must be concerned with the amount of a drug dose that reaches the systemic circulation, since this will affect the plasma concentration and therapeutic effects observed. The fraction of a dose reaching the systemic circulation as unchanged drug (i.e., intact) is defined as:

   (A) Theoretical dose
   (B) C_{max}
   (C) Bioavailability
   (D) Ideal dose

ANSWERS

1. **C.** The AUC (area under the curve) best describes the overall exposure of a person to a given drug over the course of the dosing interval. It describes the concentration of drug integrated over the period assessed, usually the dosing interval. A (C_{max}) is not correct, as C_{max} gives the maximum concentration achieved but does not reveal how long measurable concentrations of the drug were present or how long until this concentration was achieved. B (T_{max}) only refers to the time until the maximum concentration is achieved, again not giving a reference to overall exposure over time. D (half-life) simply describes how much time is required for the concentration to decrease by one-half. Finally, clearance (E) is the volume of fluid (usually plasma) from which drug can be removed per unit of time and as such does not define exposure.

2. **B.** Clearance is defined as the volume of fluid from which drug is completely removed per unit of time and as such is a measure of the body's ability to remove drug by whatever manner (e.g., elimination, metabolism, excretion). Distribution is the theoretical volume to which the drug distributes and metabolism and excretion are simply methods of clearing drug.

3. **D.** Approximately five half-lives are required for a drug to reach steady-state concentrations. Since piroxicam has a half-life of 40 hours, it will require approximately 200 hours before steady state is reached. If given every 24 hours, shortly after the 8th dose (192 hours at exactly the 8th dose) steady state will be reached.

4. **A.** Drugs with a higher degree of plasma protein binding in general have a lower volume of distribution, since the plasma proteins (and thus the drug bound to the plasma protein) tend to stay in the plasma and not distribute to the extravascular tissues. Different drugs can have widely disparate volumes of distribution, so B is incorrect. Tissue binding of drugs is extremely important to drug distribution and can override plasma protein binding, so C is incorrect. Finally, D is incorrect, since in general the more lipophilic a drug is, the greater volume of distribution it has.

5. **C.** Bioavailability describes the portion of the drug that reaches the systemic circulation without being

metabolized or eliminated. Bioavailability is highly dependent on the drug and the route of administration. C_{max} (B) is incorrect, since this is only the maximum concentration reached following a dose and gives no measure of the amount reaching the circulation. The other terms (ideal dose and theoretical dose) are fabricated.

SUPPLEMENTAL READING

Birkett DJ. Pharmacokinetics Made Easy. Sydney: McGraw-Hill, 1998.

Rowland M and Tozer TN. Clinical Pharmacokinetics (3rd ed.). Baltimore: Williams & Wilkins, 1995.

Schumacher GE. Therapeutic Drug Monitoring. Norwalk, CT: Appleton & Lange, 1995.

CASE Study   How Long Until My Warfarin Dose Stabilizes?

A 67-year-old woman with atrial arrhythmia has been treated for 3 years with the antiarrhythmic amiodarone 200 mg and the anticoagulant warfarin 10 mg, both daily. The patient began having liver and ocular toxicity due to amiodarone. The physician decided to discontinue amiodarone therapy because of these adverse effects. Upon checkup, a month after discontinuation of amiodarone, the patient's international normalized ratio (INR), a measure of blood clotting, was greatly elevated, placing the patient at risk for bleeding. The physician reduced the dose of warfarin to 7.5 mg daily. The half-life of amiodarone is approximately 35 days. For how long should the physician continue to monitor the INR?

ANSWER: The half-life of amiodarone is 35 days. Approximately five half-lives are required for functionally complete drug elimination. Thus, it will take approximately 6 months (5 half-lives) before the amiodarone is eliminated from the body. Since amiodarone strongly inhibits metabolism of S-warfarin (active enantiomer), it will continue to affect warfarin metabolism for 6 months following discontinuation of amiodarone. Thus, the dose of warfarin will have to be monitored approximately every month and adjusted if necessary. This monthly monitoring should be continued for at least 6 months, until the metabolism of warfarin stabilizes and a constant dose of warfarin can again be maintained.

6

Drug Metabolism and Disposition in Pediatric and Gerontological Stages of Life

Jeane McCarthy

The clinical responses to drug administration can be greatly influenced both by the chronological age of the patient and by the relative maturity of the particular organ system that is being targeted. Human development follows a continuum of time-related events. There are unique therapeutic differences and concerns associated with the treatment of the very young and the elderly patient. Age-dependent changes in body function are known to alter the pharmacokinetic parameters that determine each compound's duration of action, extent of drug–receptor interaction, and the drug's rates of absorption, distribution, metabolism, and excretion. This chapter discusses some of these principles and the cautions that must be considered when treating these particular patient populations.

DRUG DISPOSITION IN PEDIATRIC PATIENTS

In spite of recent advances in this area, knowledge of the disposition and actions of drugs in children is limited. This lack of information has made drug therapy for them difficult and dangerous. There are two major obstacles to clinical drug studies in children. One is an ethical issue, the inability to obtain true informed consent. The second obstacle is inherent to children; they grow and change rapidly. Drug studies must be performed on children at each stage of their development to determine appropriate usage for all patients.

To study drug disposition in children it is most informative to divide them into five age groups: preterm infants, term infants from birth through the first month of life, children 1 month to 2 years of age, children 2 to 12 years of age, and children 12 to 18 years of age. Tanner staging of sexual maturation may more appropriately break down this latter group. Children that are Tanner stages I, II, and III are appropriately considered children; those who are Tanner stages IV and V are considered adults.

Preterm infants, especially those near the limits of viability (24 weeks' gestation), have glomerular filtration rates approximately one-tenth that of a term newborn. Because of limitations on tubular reabsorption, they have increased urinary loss of filtered substances. Glucuronidation pathways appear after 20 weeks of gestation and so are limited in extremely premature infants.

Recent advances have made it possible for drug therapy to begin prior to birth. Many mothers and therefore their infants are receiving corticosteroids to induce maturation of the lungs. Some fetal cardiac arrhythmias, such as supraventricular tachycardia, are successfully managed by treating the mother during pregnancy. Since most drugs cross the placenta, the infant has the potential to be affected by drugs that the mother takes. Metabolism and excretion are not the responsibility of the fetus, as the placenta and the maternal liver and kidneys contribute significantly to drug elimination.

At birth, term infants can metabolize and eliminate drugs. For most patients these systems did not function during fetal life and therefore even at birth are not very efficient. Table 6.1 outlines the time required for maturation of some of the systems used in drug absorption and elimination. Table 6.2 lists other factors that alter drug disposition in newborns. The ability to absorb and eliminate drugs increases slowly over the first month of life.

<table>
<tr><td colspan="2">TABLE 6.1 Age-related Maturation of Selected Systems</td></tr>
</table>

System	Age Adult Level Attained
Gastric acid production	3 mo
Gastric emptying	6–8 mo
Hepatic metabolism	
Phase I enzyme reactions	5 mo–5 yr
Phase II enzyme reactions	3–6 mo
Excretion	
Glomerular filtration	3–5 mo
Tubular secretion	6–9 mo
Renal blood flow	5–12 mo

TABLE 6.3 Age-dependent $t_{1/2}$ of Trimethoprim

Age	$t_{1/2}$ (hr)
Newborn	10.8
1–3 yr	3.7
8–10 yr	5.4
Young adult	11.2

Maternally administered drugs also may affect infants who are breast-fed. Most drugs are present in breast milk in small quantities. However, several drugs can reach concentrations sufficient to adversely affect the newborn. Drugs that are contraindicated during breast-feeding include cocaine, ergotamine, and cimetidine. Unfortunately, for many drugs the information regarding risks to the infant from drug in breast milk is not available.

The period from 1 month to 2 years of age is a time of rapid growth and maturation. By the end of this period, most systems function at adult levels. Paradoxically, between 2 and 12 years of age drug clearance greatly increases and often exceeds adult levels. Half-lives are shorter and dosing requirements are frequently greater than for adults (Table 6.3).

From 12 to 18 years of age sex differences start to appear. These differences are often associated with a decreased drug absorption and elimination in the female as opposed to the male. Females have less gastric acidity and an increased gastric emptying time. Estrogens decrease hepatic cytochrome P450 content and therefore may decrease metabolism of some drugs via phase I pathways. Cyclic changes in glomerular filtration are noted during the menstrual cycle.

Absorption

Oral absorption of drugs is influenced by gastric acidity and emptying time. Gastric acid is rarely found in the

TABLE 6.2 Other Factors Affecting Newborn Drug Disposition

Increased body water
Decreased body fat
Decreased exocrine pancreatic function
Decreased albumin concentration and binding
Decreased total plasma protein

stomach of infants at less than 32 weeks' gestation. Acid initially is secreted within the first few hours after birth, reaching peak levels within the first 10 days of life. It decreases during the next 20 days of extrauterine life. Gastric acid secretion approaches the lower limits of adult values by 3 months of age. The initiation of acid secretion is often delayed in infants with delayed initiation of oral feedings, such as extreme preemies and those with anomalies of the gastrointestinal tract.

Gastric emptying time in infants is related to their age and to the type of formula they receive. Formulas containing long-chain fatty acids will delay gastric emptying. Both gastric emptying time and small-intestine peristalsis tend to be slow until the later part of the first year of life. In children aged 2 to 12 years gastric emptying time dramatically increases, as does splanchnic blood flow. These physiological changes result in faster drug absorption and increased peak blood concentrations of drug. The decreased small intestine transit time during this period may result in decreased absorption of some drugs. Because of low blood flow through muscles in the neonatal period, drugs administered intramuscularly are absorbed erratically.

Percutaneous drug absorption can present special problems in newborns, especially in preterm infants. While the skin of a newborn term infant may have the same protective capacity as the skin of an adult, a preterm infant will not have this protective barrier until after 2 to 3 weeks of life. Excessive percutaneous absorption has caused significant toxicity to preterm babies. Absorption of hexachlorophene soap used to bathe newborns has resulted in brain damage and death. Aniline dyes on hospital linen have caused cyanosis secondary to methemoglobinemia, and EMLA (lidocaine/prilocaine) cream may cause methemoglobinemia when administered to infants less than 3 months of age.

Distribution

The total body water of prematures, newborns, and infants is significantly greater than it is for older children and adults. This increased total body water increases the volume of drug distribution for water-soluble compounds. As a consequence, there is a need to administer loading doses of some drugs. Differences in total body water are basically insignificant after the first year of life. Newborns have decreased body fat and therefore less storage ability for fat-soluble drugs.

Newborns, especially prematures, have decreased plasma albumin and total plasma protein concentrations. In addition, albumin from these patients shows a decreased drug-binding affinity. This may result in increased plasma levels of free drug and the potential for toxicity. In the past, concerns were raised that certain drugs, such as sulfonamides, could displace endogenous substances, like bilirubin, from albumin-binding sites. Theoretically, such an interaction would increase the risk for kernicterus. Although this belief has been challenged recently, reluctance to treat newborns with sulfonamides persists.

Metabolism

As with adults, the primary organ responsible for drug metabolism in children is the liver. Although the cytochrome P450 system is fully developed at birth, it functions more slowly than in adults. Phase I oxidation reactions and demethylation enzyme systems are significantly reduced at birth. However, the reductive enzyme systems approach adult levels and the methylation pathways are enhanced at birth. This often contributes to the production of different metabolites in newborns from those in adults. For example, newborns metabolize approximately 30% of theophylline to caffeine rather than to uric acid derivatives, as occurs in adults. While most phase I enzymes have reached adult levels by 6 months of age, alcohol dehydrogenase activity appears around 2 months of age and approaches adult levels only by age 5 years.

Phase II synthetic enzyme reactions are responsible for the elimination of endogenous compounds, such as bilirubin, and many exogenous substances. The immaturity of the glucuronidation pathway was responsible for the development of gray baby syndrome (see Chapter 47) in newborns receiving chloramphenicol. Preterm and newborn infants dying of this syndrome developed anemia and cardiovascular collapse because of high blood concentrations of unconjugated chloramphenicol. The plasma half-life was found to be 26 hours in these patients compared with 4 hours in older children.

Infants and children have a greater capacity to carry out sulfate conjugation than do adults. For example, acetaminophen is excreted predominantly as a sulfate conjugate in children as opposed to a glucuronide conjugate in adults. This enhanced sulfation of acetaminophen, along with decreased metabolism via cytochrome P450 pathways and increased glutathione turnover, are thought to explain the decreased hepatotoxicity caused by this analgesic in children under 6 years of age. Phase II enzyme systems reach adult levels between 3 and 6 months of age.

Excretion

Renal blood flow, glomerular filtration rate, and tubular function are reduced in both preterm and term neonates. Therefore, newborns, especially those less than 34 weeks' gestation, require less frequent dosing intervals for many drugs. Aminoglycosides are administered every 8 hours in older children, every 12 hours in newborns, and every 24 hours in extremely premature infants. The glomerular filtration rate of the term newborn is approximately 50% less than the adult level but reaches adult values by 1 year of age. Renal blood flow approaches adult values between ages 5 and 12 months. Tubular secretory functions mature at a slower rate than does glomerular filtration. Renal excretion of organic anions, such as penicillin, furosemide, and indomethacin, is very low in the newborn. Tubular secretion and reabsorption reach adult levels by 7 months of age. Renal elimination of drugs appears to play a greater role than does metabolism in newborns. Over the first year of life the infant develops a more adult-type excretory pattern.

Drug Action

Most drugs are administered to infants and children for the same therapeutic indications as for adults. However, a few drugs have found unique uses in children. Among these are theophylline and caffeine, which are used to treat apnea of prematurity; indomethacin, which closes a patent ductus arteriosus; and prostaglandin E_1, which maintains the patency of the ductus arteriosus. Paradoxically, drugs such as phenobarbital, which have a sedating action on adults, may produce hyperactivity in children, and some adult stimulant drugs, such as methylphenidate, are used to treat children with hyperactivity.

Adverse Reactions

Children may display adverse reactions different from those noted in adult patients. Table 6.4 lists a number of drugs that demonstrate unique actions in children.

Special Considerations

Several problems unique to pediatric drug therapy deserve special mention. For example, most medications are commercially available only in adult dose forms. Preparing pediatric doses from adult tablets or capsules can be very difficult and may require special skill on the part of the pharmacist. For some drugs it is simpler to administer the intravenous (IV) preparation orally than to develop a preparation from the oral medication.

IV drug administration is most effective in children when given via a pump infusion system close to the site of IV insertion. Because of the small size of many pediatric doses and the fact that some drugs adhere to IV tubing, a significant percentage of the drug can be lost if

TABLE 6.4   Pediatric Specific Adverse Drug Reactions

Drug	Reaction
Furosemide (*Lasix*)	Nephrocalcinosis
Indomethacin (*Indocin*)	Renal Failure, bowel perforation
Adrenocorticoids	Delayed development, growth suppression
Tetracyclines	Discolored teeth
Phenobarbital	Hyperactivity, impaired intellectual development
Phenytoin (*Dilantin*)	Thickened skull, coarse features
Chloramphenicol	Gray baby syndrome
Phenothiazines	Extrapyramidal reaction
Valproic acid (*Depakene*)	Hepatotoxicity ($<$2 yr)
Aspirin	Reye's syndrome in patients with chickenpox or influenza

Compiled from Outslander JG. Drug therapy in the Elderly. Ann Intern Med 1981;95:711; and Richey DP and Bender AD. Pharmacokinetic consequences of aging. Annu Rev Pharmacol Toxicol 1977;17:49; and references therein.

it is given using techniques usually reserved for adults. For many prematures and newborns, the volume of administration is also critical and therefore much more easily managed by IV infusion pumps.

Most adult drugs must be diluted to achieve appropriate pediatric dosages. Some drugs must be diluted several times. This introduces the potential for significant error in dilution. Some drugs such as NPH (Neutral Protamine Hagedorn) insulin may lose their effectiveness if diluted.

Children with chronic illnesses require special consideration. For example, patients with cystic fibrosis have increased hepatic metabolism and therefore increased drug clearance. This may necessitate the administration of increased drug dosages.

Calculation of pediatric dosages is usually done on the basis of weight (e.g., milligrams per kilogram) for infants and toddlers and on the basis of weight or body surface area (milligrams per square meter) for older children. Repeated increases in drug dosage are required to accommodate for growth in children receiving chronic drug therapy.

In summary, children, especially those in the first year of life, present significant pharmacological challenges. Drug administration must be tailored to meet the unique needs of children at their varied stages of development. Special attention must be given to unexpected drug actions and adverse reactions in these patients, who are maturing at variable rates. When planning drug therapy for children, it is important to remember:

- Children are not small adults.
- Infants are not small children.
- Newborns are not small infants.
- Preemies are not small newborns.

DRUG DISPOSITION IN GERIATRIC PATIENTS

The elderly (individuals over 65 years of age) constitute more than 13% of the population. This figure is increasing steadily and is expected to reach 50 million by the year 2020. This segment of our society is the most highly drug-treated and accounts for about 25% of prescription drugs dispensed. The average Medicare patient in an acute-care hospital receives approximately 10 different drugs daily, and this translates into a higher incidence of adverse drug reactions in geriatric patients than in the general population.

Chronological aging may not necessarily be an accurate index of biological aging, which is the result of many genetic and environmental factors. While most 20-year-olds have a similar response to a given drug, it is difficult to predict the response among 80-year-olds. A clear relationship between the appearance of untoward effects to drugs and aging has been demonstrated only for about 10 drugs. For some 90 other drugs in common clinical use, age alone was not a major determinant of clinical toxicity. It is apparent that an increase in life span is accompanied by an increase in chronic illnesses such as hypertension, congestive heart failure, arthritis, and diabetes. The pharmacological management of these conditions, especially when the same person has several diseases, becomes increasingly complex.

Age-related alterations in pharmacokinetics (absorption, distribution, metabolism, and excretion) have received considerable attention. Thus, physiological changes in elderly patients, when taken together, may contribute to impairments in drug clearance in this segment of the population (Table 6.5).

Absorption

Elderly patients may absorb drugs less completely or more slowly because of decreased splanchnic blood flow or delayed gastric emptying. Reduced gastric acidity may decrease the absorption of drugs that require high acidity.

Distribution

Drug distribution in elderly patients may be altered by hypoalbuminemia, qualitative changes in drug-binding sites, reductions in relative muscle mass, increases in the proportion of body fat, and decreases in total body water. The plasma level of free, active drug is often a direct function of the extent of drug binding to plasma proteins. There is a well-documented age-dependent decline (about 20%) in plasma albumin concentration in humans due to a reduced rate of hepatic albumin

TABLE 6.5 Plasma Half-lives of Several Drugs in Young Adult and Elderly Patients

	Plasma or serum $t_{1/2}$	
Drug	Young (20–30 yr)	Elderly (65–80 yr)
Penicillin G	20.7 min	39.1 min
Dihydrostreptomycin	5.2 hr	8.4 hr
Tetracycline	3.5 hr	4.5 hr
Kanamycin	107.0 min	282.0 min
Digoxin	52.0 hr	73.0 hr
Aminopyrine	3.0 hr	10.0 hr
Phenobarbital	71.0 hr	107.0 hr
Diazepam	20.0 hr	80.0 hr
Lidocaine	80.6 min	139.6 min
Chlordiazepoxide	8.9 hr	16.7 hr
Antipyrine	12.0 hr	17.4 hr
Phenylbutazone	81.2 hr	104.6 hr
Isoniazid	1.4 hr	1.5 hr
Warfarin	37.0 hr	44.0 hr

Source: Compiled from J.G. Ouslander, Drug therapy in the elderly. *Ann. Intern. Med.* 95:711, 1981; and D.P. Richey and A.D. Bender, Pharmacokinetic consequences of aging. *Annu. Rev. Pharmacol. Toxicol.* 17:49, 1977, and references therein.

synthesis. These changes in serum albumin may affect the free drug concentration for a number of highly bound drugs, such as phenytoin, warfarin, and meperidine.

Metabolism

In addition to changes in metabolism that occur as a result of reduced hepatic enzyme activity, metabolism may be impaired by a reduction in hepatic mass, volume, and blood flow (Fig. 6.1). Phase I oxidative pathways are decreased with age, while phase II conjugation pathways are unchanged.

In a carefully controlled clinical study, the plasma half-life of diazepam (Valium), a widely used antianxiety agent, exhibited a striking age dependency. In patients aged 20 years, the $t_{1/2}$ was about 20 hours, and this increased linearly with age to about 90 hours at 80 years. Half-lives of other drugs in young and old patients are presented in Table 6.5. These data demonstrate changes in drug half-life with increasing age, suggesting that at least for some drugs, elderly patients have reduced metabolism, drug clearance, or both.

Excretion

Renal elimination of foreign compounds may change dramatically with increasing age by factors such as reduced renal blood flow, reduced glomerular filtration rate, reduced tubular secretory activity, and a reduction in the number of functional nephrons. It has been estimated that in humans, beginning at age 20 years, renal function declines by about 10% for each decade of life. This decline in renal excretion is particularly important for drugs such as penicillin and digoxin, which are eliminated primarily by the kidney.

Adverse Drug Effects

The incidence of iatrogenic complications is three to five times greater in the elderly than in the general population. Adverse drug reactions account for 20 to 40% of these complications. Inappropriate drug use has been noted in almost half of hospitalized elderly patients. One-fourth of these patients were receiving contraindicated drugs, and three-fourths were receiving unneces-

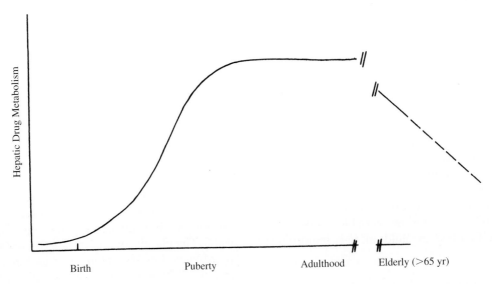

FIGURE 6.1
The ontogeny of hepatic drug metabolic activity.

sary drugs. Half of adverse drug reactions occur in patients receiving inappropriate drugs.

Delirium and cognitive impairment are common adverse reactions in the elderly. While almost every class of drugs has the potential to produce delirium in the elderly, it is most frequent with psychoactive drugs. The risk increases with the number of drugs the patient is receiving, reaching a 14-fold increase in risk for patients taking more than 6 drugs.

Special Considerations

The following should be considered when prescribing drugs for elderly patients.

Drugs should be prescribed only if nonpharmacological techniques are ineffective, such as for problems like sleeplessness and anxiety. When drugs are prescribed for these conditions, they should be given for a limited time and the patient closely monitored for adverse effects. Dosage should start at or below the lowest recommended levels.

Keep it simple. Prescribe drugs only if you have available extensive experience and prescribing information for that drug in elderly patients. Use the least number of drugs and doses per day.

Reevaluate the continued use of all medications the patient is receiving, including over-the-counter medications, on a regular basis.

Noncompliance is a significant problem, with almost 50% of elderly patients failing to take their medications as prescribed. Some of the reasons for noncompliance are inability to pay for the drug, side effects, mental impairment, and inability to understand complex instructions.

SUMMARY

Physicians should exercise caution when prescribing drugs for pediatric and geriatric patients. This is virtually axiomatic in premature infants, whose severely restricted ability to metabolize drugs is well documented. Caution also must be exerted in prescribing for the elderly population, since these individuals may be taking 10 to 15 different drugs daily. Problems associated with drug interaction and declining physiological function are very real. It is simply inadequate to administer drugs to very young and very old patients strictly on a body mass basis. Dose adjustments often must be made empirically, depending upon the changing pharmacokinetic characteristics of the drug in question, the nature of the disease, and the physiological status of the major organs and tissues involved in drug absorption, distribution, metabolism, and excretion.

Study QUESTIONS

1. It is well established that most drugs taken by pregnant women are capable of crossing the placenta and reaching the developing fetus. The placenta itself can aid in the protection of the fetus from excessive exposure to drugs in the maternal circulation by
   (A) Impairing diffusion of lipid soluble drugs
   (B) Preventing the passage of drugs having a molecular weight under 250
   (C) Playing a role as a site of drug metabolism
   (D) Secreting drugs from the fetal circulation to the maternal circulation

2. Neonates having a patent ductus arteriosus can be treated with which agent to induce a relatively rapid closure and thus often avoid surgical intervention?
   (A) Phenobarbital
   (B) Indomethacin
   (C) Hydrochlorothiazide
   (D) Prostaglandin E_1
   (E) Epinephrine

3. Which of the following is an accurate description of changes taking place in elderly individuals compared to younger adults?
   (A) Increased lean body mass
   (B) Diminished body fat as a relative percentage of total body mass

   (C) Increase in the levels of plasma proteins
   (D) General increase in hepatic drug metabolizing capacity
   (E) Decrease in renal clearance of many drugs

4. A neonate is given drug A, a compound with a high affinity for plasma proteins, in a dose that does not exceed the binding capacity of albumin. Later, a second drug, B, that also binds strongly to albumin, is given in amounts that greatly exceed albumin's binding capacity. Which of the following statements is most likely to be true?
   (A) The free plasma concentration of drug A is decreased.
   (B) The relative free drug concentration of both compounds is unchanged.
   (C) The concentration of drug A in tissues is likely to be increased.
   (D) The concentration of drug A in tissues is likely to be decreased.
   (E) The free plasma concentration of drug B would likely be markedly increased if drug A were given second rather than first.

5. Mr. Johnson, a 70-year-old, has come into a physician's office complaining of not being able to sleep well at night because of residual pain associated

with a recent hip replacement. He is taking a thiazide diuretic (A) for mild hypertension, digitalis (B) for congestive heart failure, and an oral hypoglycemic agent (C) for mild type 2 diabetes. An opioid analgesic (D) that gave him considerable pain relief when he broke his arm 30 years ago is prescribed. About a week later Mr. Johnson is seen in the emergency department complaining of shortness of breath and a feeling of suffocation. Which of the drugs he is receiving is a likely possible cause of this particular symptom?

ANSWERS

1. **C.** The placenta can serve as a site of metabolism for some drugs passing through it. The placenta can carry out a number of drug metabolizing reactions, including dealkylation and hydroxylation. Lipophilic drugs readily diffuse across the placenta and enter the fetal circulation; drugs with a molecular weight of under 500 generally can easily cross the placenta; and no known active transport systems play any important role in drug secretion in the placenta.

2. **B.** Indomethacin's action as a potent nonselective COX inhibitor appears to be important in speeding up ductus closure. The other drugs do not have such an action, and prostaglandin E_1 given by infusion would cause the ductus to remain open.

3. **E.** The kidney, the most important organ involved in drug clearance, especially of highly water-soluble drugs, shows an age-related decline in function. Lean body mass decreases, percentage of body fat increases, production of plasma proteins decrease, and drug metabolism decreases for most drugs as patients reach their seventh and eighth decade.

4. **C.** The large amounts of drug B that are given can displace the almost completely bound drug A from its albumin binding site and lead to an increase in free drug. The latter is then available to be distributed outside the blood compartment and reach tissues where its concentrations will increase.

5. **D.** The elderly are frequently sensitive to the pulmonary depressing actions of opioid analgesics. These agents should be used with caution in the elderly until an adequate dosage has been determined for a particular patient. This does not mean that the older patient should not be given opioid analgesics for pain, however, since appropriate pain management should always be part of any total clinical treatment plan.

SUPPLEMENTAL READING

Avorn J and Gurwitz JH. Drug use in the nursing home. Ann Intern Med 1995;123:195–204.

Briggs GG, Freeman RK, and Yaffe SJ. Drugs in Pregnancy and Lactation (5th ed.). Baltimore: Williams & Wilkins, 1998.

Hazzard WR et al. Principles of Geriatric Medicine and Gerontology (4th ed.). New York: McGraw-Hill, 1999.

Medical Letter. Some drugs that cause psychiatric symptoms. 1998;40:21–24.

Nahata MC. Variability in clinical pharmacology of drugs in children. J Clin Pharmacol Ther 1992; 17:365–368.

Rochon P and Gurwitz JH. Drug therapy. Lancet 1995;346:32–36.

Rylace GW. Pharmacology. In Rennie JM and Roberton NRC (eds.). Textbook of Neonatology. Edinburgh: Churchill Livingstone, 1999.

Sastry BVR (ed). Placental Toxicology. Boca Baton, FL: CRC, 1995.

CASE Study   A Choice of Sedative

Mrs. Jones celebrated her 71st birthday by taking her grandchildren to the park. She fell while pushing the merry-go-round and broke her wrist. She has no pain now but is too uncomfortable with the cast to sleep well. She has tried soothing music, reading, and relaxing techniques but is still unable to sleep. She has requested a sleeping pill. Based on knowledge of psychotropic drugs in elderly patients, what medication would be an appropriate choice?

ANSWER: Benzodiazepines are effective for short-term use as sedative–hypnotics. Long-acting types with active metabolites, such as diazepam, would normally be expected to have a prolonged half-life. The half-life would be even more prolonged in Mrs. Jones because of the increase in body fat and decreased renal excretion that are typical for persons of her age. After several weeks of administration, daytime confusion may occur in this patient and may put her at risk for a fall and another serious injury. A short-acting benzodiazepine with inactive metabolites, such as oxazepam, could provide the desired effect with minimal adverse effects.

7

Principles of Toxicology

Mary E. Davis and Mark J. Reasor

The discipline of toxicology considers the adverse effects of chemicals, including drugs, and other agents, such as biological toxins and radiation, on biological systems. Toxicity associated with drug action can generally be characterized as either an extension of the therapeutic effect, such as the fatal central nervous system (CNS) depression that may follow a barbiturate overdose, or as an effect that is unrelated to the therapeutic effect, such as the liver damage that may result from an acetaminophen overdose. This chapter focuses on the tissue response associated with the latter type of drug toxicity and on the toxicities associated with several important classes of nontherapeutic agents.

The target organ for the expression of xenobiotic toxicity is not necessarily the tissue or organ in which the drug produces its therapeutic effect, nor is it necessarily the tissue that has the highest concentration of the agent. For example, lead accumulates in bone but produces no toxicity there; certain chlorinated pesticides accumulate in adipose tissue but produce no local adverse effects. Drugs such as acetaminophen cause necrosis in the centrilobular portion of the liver at a site of the monooxygenase enzymes that bioactivate the analgesic.

It is necessary to distinguish between the intrinsic toxicity of a chemical and the hazard it poses. While a chemical may have high intrinsic toxicity, it may pose little or no hazard if exposure is low. In contrast, a relatively nontoxic chemical may be quite hazardous if exposure is large or the route of exposure is not physiological.

MANIFESTATIONS OF TOXICITY

Organ Toxicity

The events that initiate cell death are not completely understood. The common final stages of necrotic cell death are disruption of normal metabolic processes and ensuing inability to maintain intracellular electrolyte homeostasis. If the insult is severe or prolonged enough, the cell will not regain normal function. At the same time, other cells show apoptotic cell death, characterized by cell shrinkage, cleavage of DNA between nucleosomes, and formation of apoptotic bodies. Some chemicals are metabolized to reactive products that bind to cellular macromolecules. If such binding impairs the function of crucial macromolecules, cell viability is lost. How severely organ function will be impaired depends on the reserve capacity of that organ. The ultimate outcome will depend on the affected organ's regenerative capacity and response to damage.

Pulmonary Toxicity

Inhaled gases, solid particles, or liquid aerosols may deposit throughout the respiratory system, depending on their chemical and physical properties. The large surface area of the respiratory passages and alveolar region and the large volume of air delivered to that area (approximately 6–7 L/minute in a young man) provide great opportunity for interaction between inhaled materials and lung tissue. Examples of inhaled xenobiotics that cause lung damage and those that have entered the body by ingestion, injection, or dermal absorption are presented in Figure 7.1.

Exposure of the lungs to xenobiotics may result in a number of disease conditions including bronchitis, emphysema, asthma, hypersensitivity pneumonitis, pneumoconiosis, and cancer. During repair, damaged lung alveolar epithelium may be replaced by fibrous tissue that does not allow for gas exchange, which intensifies the damage caused by the initial lesion.

Hepatotoxicity

The blood draining the stomach and small intestine is delivered directly to the liver via the hepatic portal vein, thus exposing the liver to relatively large concentrations of ingested drugs or toxicants (e.g., Fig. 7.1). Hepatic exposure to agents that undergo bioactivation to toxic species can be significant.

Hepatic necrosis can be classified by the zone of the liver tissue affected. Xenobiotics, such as acetaminophen or chloroform, that undergo bioactivation to toxic intermediates cause necrosis of the cells surrounding the central veins (*centrilobular*) because the components of the cytochrome P450 system are found in those cells in abundance. At higher doses or in the presence of agents that increase the synthesis of cytochrome P450 (inducers), the area of necrosis may incorporate the

midzonal area (midway between the portal triad and central vein). Cells around the portal triad are exposed to the highest concentrations; necrosis occurs with direct-acting agents. A single large dose of a hepatotoxin may cause liver necrosis yet resolve with little or no tissue scarring. Continued exposure to the toxic agent, however, can result in hepatic cirrhosis and permanent scarring.

Allergic reactions to drugs produce foci of necrosis that are scattered throughout the liver. Other agents cause severe (chlorpromazine) or mild (estrogens) cholestatic liver damage, including cholestasis and inflammation of the portal triad and hepatocellular necrosis.

Nephrotoxicity

The kidneys are susceptible to toxicity from xenobiotics (Fig. 7.1) because they too have a high blood flow. Cells of the tubular nephron face double-sided exposure, to agents in the blood on the basolateral side and in the filtered urine on the luminal side. Proximal tubule cells are generally the site of nephrotoxicity, since these cells have an abundance of cytochrome P450 and can transport organic anions and cations from the blood into the cells, thereby concentrating these chemicals manyfold.

Chemically induced kidney damage is typically seen as acute tubular necrosis (ATN). The cells in the proximal tubule are affected. Reabsorption of water, elec-

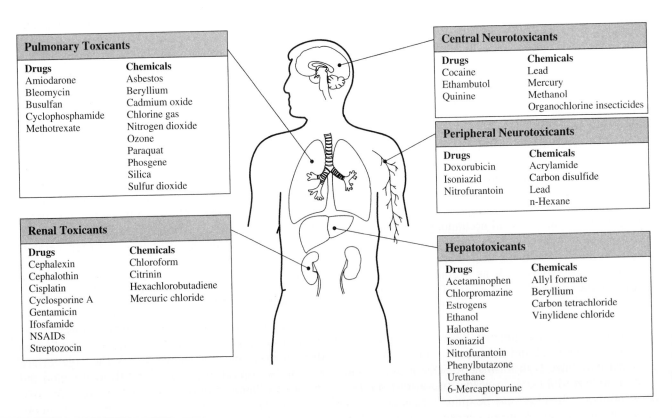

FIGURE 7.1
Organ toxicity of selected chemicals.

trolytes, glucose, and amino acids is impaired. Feedback mechanisms decrease glomerular filtration and thus prevent delivery of large volumes of water to nephron segments. Urine output may be increased, decreased, or unchanged. Markers of glomerular filtration, *blood urea nitrogen (BUN)* and *creatinine,* are increased only if filtration falls by 80%. The urine may contain glucose and protein, including proteinaceous casts formed in the nephron of tubular debris.

Neurotoxicity

Although the CNS is protected from a number of xenobiotics by the blood-brain barrier, the barrier is not effective against lipophilic compounds, such as solvents or insecticides (Fig. 7.1). Similarly, the peripheral nervous system is protected by a blood-neural barrier. The barriers are less well developed in the immature nervous system, rendering the fetus and neonate even more susceptible to neurotoxicants. Neural tissue susceptibility is due in large part to its high metabolic rate, high lipid content, and for the CNS, high rate of blood flow.

Since damaged neural tissue cannot easily replicate, glial and other nonconducting cells may proliferate and occupy the space of the dead neurons, and the damage may be expressed as deficits of sensory and motor functions and behavior. Alternatively, other neurons may take on the functions of the damaged neurons such that there is little or no perceptible damage.

Immunotoxicity

A number of drugs and environmentally and occupationally important chemicals can impair the activity of one or more components of the immune system. Immunodeficiency may result in increased susceptibility to infection, decreased surveillance against precancerous or cancerous cells, or tissue-damaging reactions (Table 7.1). Allergic and autoimmune reactions are examples of this form of toxicity.

Clinical expressions of cutaneous allergic reactions include eczematous, indurate–inflammatory, and urticarial eruptions. Irritant responses causing direct damage to the skin may be confused with allergic responses involving immune mechanisms. An important difference is that allergic reactions require an initial exposure to sensitize the individual; dermatitis is then elicited by minimal subsequent exposure to the agent.

Toxic Effects on Genetic Material and Cell Replication

Mutagenesis, teratogenesis, and carcinogenesis are different manifestations of damage to genetic material (*genotoxicity*). Chemically induced genotoxicity occurs in several steps, and at each step there is opportunity for repair. Generally, xenobiotics are not themselves muta-

TABLE 7.1	Chemicals that Suppress the Immune System in Humans and Animals
Drugs	**Chemicals**
Azathioprine	Arsenic
Corticosteroids	Benzene
Cyclophosphamide	Dibenzodioxins (TCDD)
Cyclosporine A	Lead
Methotrexate	Organophosphate and organochlorine insecticides
	Ozone
	Polybrominated and polychlorinated biphenyls

genic, but rather they must be bioactivated to metabolites that are sufficiently reactive to bind to DNA and disrupt its coding. The reactive intermediates must be formed close enough to the DNA to interact with it before interacting with other less important macromolecules or before being further metabolized to inactive forms. Nongenotoxic carcinogens act by altering cell replication control.

Reproductive Toxicity

Most drugs and chemicals pose a threat to the developing fetus. An estimated 4 to 5% of developmental defects in humans result from prenatal exposure to drugs or environmental chemicals. This is particularly important, since women with irregular menstrual cycles may be exposed to teratogens and enter the sensitive period of *organogenesis* before pregnancy is suspected.

Gestation is generally considered to consist of three periods of development, each with differing sensitivities to chemicals. During the *preimplantation* or predifferentiation phase, expression of toxicity is an all-or-none phenomenon; damage to the embryo results in either death or no effect. *Organogenesis* occurs during the embryonic period (the first 3 months of pregnancy), and therefore, susceptibility to teratogenesis is high; the embryo is particularly vulnerable to teratogens on days 25 through 40. The *fetal period* consists of the last 6 months of gestation and is a time of reduced susceptibility to teratogenic alterations. Certain organs, such as the genitals and the nervous system, however, are still undergoing differentiation during this period. Functional impairment in tissues without marked structural damage and growth retardation is the most common effect of chemical exposure during the fetal period.

Chemicals such as 1,2-dibromo-3-chloropropane can disrupt spermatogenesis, leading to impaired reproductive function, including sterility. Men and women undergoing cancer chemotherapy with alkylating drugs are at increased risk for sterility.

TREATMENT OF POISONINGS

Specific antidotes are available for only a few toxic agents (Table 7.2). Even these are not always effective, particularly if the poisoning is severe. The best treatment begins with supportive care. This includes resuscitation (if necessary) and maintenance of respiratory and cardiovascular functions. Imbalances in fluid and electrolytes may have to be corrected. An approach to the treatment of victims of poisoning is presented in Table 7.3.

EXPOSURE TO NONTHERAPEUTIC TOXICANTS

Worldwide production of chemicals has increased dramatically in recent decades, resulting in increased human exposure. This applies not only to workers who manufacture the chemicals and final products but also to those who use the products or are exposed through contamination of surface and ground water and air.

Air Pollution

Industrial activity has polluted the outdoor air with a number of chemicals known to be hazardous to human health. These include a variety of gases, such as carbon monoxide, ozone, and the oxides of sulfur and nitrogen. Unacceptable levels of air pollutants can occur indoors as well. While some of these pollutants may be the same as for the outdoor air, they also include biological

agents (e.g., fungal spores, viruses, bacteria, actinomycetes), volatile organic compounds, carbon dioxide, and formaldehyde.

Gases

Carbon monoxide arises from the incomplete combustion of organic material. Of principal concern is its generation by the internal combustion engine and by home heating units, particularly in poorly ventilated areas. Carbon monoxide emission by automobiles in closed garages and by unvented space heaters results in numerous deaths each year. Following inhalation, carbon monoxide binds to hemoglobin, displacing oxygen and forming carboxyhemoglobin. This decreases the oxygen-carrying capacity of the blood and impairs the blood cells' ability to release bound oxygen. The resulting hypoxia is the principal mechanism of carbon monoxide toxicity.

Nitrogen oxides, principally nitrogen dioxide, and ozone are classified as oxidizing pollutants. The major source of nitrogen dioxide is the internal combustion engine. Photolysis of nitrogen dioxide by ultraviolet radiation liberates oxygen atoms, which can then combine with molecular oxygen to form ozone. Both gases cause irritation of the deep lung and can result in increased susceptibility to respiratory infection, pulmonary edema, and impaired lung function.

Oxides of sulfur (principally sulfur dioxide) are generated during the burning of fossil fuels, most notably coal, and are classified as reducing pollutants because of

TABLE 7.2   Some Specific Antidotes for Toxic Drugs and Chemicals

Agent	Antidote	Mechanism of Action
Drugs		
Heparin	Protamine	Ionically neutralizes heparin
Acetaminophen	*N*-acetylcysteine	Inactivates toxic metabolite
Narcotics and opioids	Naloxone	Displaces drugs from receptors
Insulin, oral hypoglycemics	Glucose	Reverses glucose depletion
Chemicals		
Methanol	Ethanol	Blocks metabolism to toxic metabolite
Ethylene glycol	Ethanol	Blocks metabolism to toxic metabolite
Botulinum toxin	Antiserum	Immunologically neutralizes toxicant
Cyanide	Sodium nitrate	Forms methemoglobin, which binds cyanide, thus removing it from active pool
	Sodium thiosulfate	Provides a source of sulfur to detoxify cyanide
Organophosphates	Atropine	Displaces acetylcholine from its receptor
	Pralidoxime	Reactivates acetylcholinesterase
Carbon monoxide	Oxygen	Displaces toxicant from hemoglobin
Nitrites	Methylene blue	Reduces methemoglobin to hemoglobin
Arsenic	Dimercaprol	Forms inactive complex with metal
Iron	Deferoxamine	Forms inactive complex with metal
Lead	Calcium disodium edetate	Forms inactive complete with metal
Warfarin	Vitamin K_1	Stimulates coagulation factor synthesis

TABLE 7.3 A General Approach to the Treatment of Acute Poisoning

Provide emergency management
  Perform cardiopulmonary resuscitation if necessary
  If victim is in a coma, administer naloxone hydrochloride (in narcotic or opioid overdose) and 50% glucose (in case of insulin shock)
Evaluation
  Identify the toxic agent and dose if possible
  Assess vital signs and level of consciousness
  Conduct laboratory tests
Reduce absorption and enhance removal of poison
  Irrigate eyes and skin if involved
  Induce emesis with syrup of ipecac if victim is conscious and has not ingested acids, alkali, hydrocarbons, or petroleum distillates
  Perform gastric lavage if victim is unconscious or in some instances when conscious
  Administer activated charcoal to bind poison
  Administer milk or water if alkali, acid, hydrocarbon, or petroleum distillates have been ingested
  Administer antidote, if one exists, that is specific for the poison
  Consider forced diuresis, urine acidification, or alkalinization if specific antidotes are not available
  Hemodialysis or charcoal hemoperfusion may be appropriate for rapid elimination if antidotes are not available

the types of reactions they undergo. Particulate matter associated with most emissions promotes the conversion of sulfur dioxide to the more toxic sulfuric acid and facilitates deposition in the deep lungs. The acid can cause bronchospasm and lung damage, including alveolitis. Asthmatic episodes can be exacerbated by sulfur dioxide and sulfuric acid.

Particulates

Industrial processes, such as milling and mining, construction work, and the burning of wood or fossil fuel, generate particulates that can be directly toxic or can serve as vectors for the transfer of bound material, such as sulfuric acid, metals, and hydrocarbons, into the lungs. Natural products such as pollen, anthrax spores, and animal dander can elicit toxic reactions on inhalation or skin contact. The inhalation of asbestos, silica, or coal dust can cause pneumoconiosis, which may develop into serious lung disease. The size of the particle, ventilatory rate, and depth of breathing will determine the extent of pulmonary deposition.

Food Additives and Contaminants

Thousands of substances are added to foods to enhance their marketability (appearance, taste, texture, etc.), storage properties, or nutritive value, any of which may cause toxicity in susceptible individuals (Table 7.4). Microbial or fungal contamination of food, either during processing or storage, can introduce potent toxins into food.

Metals

Characteristics of toxicity for a number of metals are presented in Table 7.5. While the exact tissue and molecular site of the toxic action of each metal is different, toxicity generally results from interaction of the metal with specific functional groups on macromolecules in the cell. These groups include sulfhydryl, carboxyl, amino, phosphoryl, and phenolic moieties. Interactions of such groups with metals can lead to disruption of enzyme activities and transport processes and eventually

TABLE 7.4 Examples of Toxic Food Additives and Contaminants

Agent	Type	Source and Effects
Nitrate, nitrite	Preservative	Present in vegetables; form carcinogenic nitrosamines
Sulfites	Preservative	Antioxidants used to reduce spoilage; can produce allergic reactions, especially in asthmatics
Tartrazine	Food color	Can cause urticaria in sensitive individuals
Botulinum toxin	Contaminant	Produced by *Clostridium botulinum* in improperly canned vegetables; nausea, vomiting, diarrhea, paralysis
Salmonella	Contaminant	Improper processing of food allows *Salmonella* from intestinal tract to survive; the most common cause of gastroenteritis
Aflatoxins	Contaminant (mycotoxin)	Produced by *Aspergillus flavus*, especially grains, corn, and peanuts; carcinogenic and hepatotoxic
Ochratoxin, citrinin	Contaminant (mycotoxin)	Produced by *Penicillium* strains; nephropathy (endemic Balkan nephropathy)
Polybrominated biphenyls (PBBs)	Contaminant	Fire retardant inadvertently substituted for feed supplement in Michigan; livestock loss, undetermined effect on human health

TABLE 7.5 Characteristics of Toxicity of Selected Metals*

Metal	Selected features of toxicity
Arsenic	
Inorganic	Diarrhea, hyperkeratosis, garlic breath, Mees' lines on fingernails
Arsine gas	Hemolysis
Beryllium	Pneumonitis, chronic granulomatous disease, contact dermatitis
Cadmium	Pneumonitis, emphysema, kidney damage
Iron	Gastric irritation, liver damage
Lead	Peripheral and central neurotoxicity, kidney damage, anemia
Mercury	
Elemental	Pneumonitis, neuropsychiatric toxicity (excitability, emotional instability, depression, insomnia), motor dysfunction (tremors)
Organic	Sensory neuropathy (dysarthia, paresthesia, constriction of visual field, loss of taste, hearing, smell), motor dysfunction (tremors)
Inorganic	Kidney damage, irritation of oral cavity and gastrointestinal tract

*Representative toxicities are presented; for most metals, other symptoms of toxicity may be demonstrated. Nature of the toxicities is dependent on level of exposure, whether the exposure is acute or chronic, and the route of exposure.

to loss of such cellular functions as energy production and ion regulation. In general, toxicity is related to the form of the metal (inorganic, organic, or elemental), the route of exposure, and the route of excretion.

Solvents

Solvents are generally classified as aliphatic or aromatic, and either type may be halogenated, most commonly with chlorine. The toxicity of representative solvents is summarized in Table 7.6. Occupational exposure to solvents occurs in cleaning, degreasing, painting, and gluing. Exposure to solvents is generally through inhalation of vapors, although direct skin contact also occurs. The concentration of solvent in air is determined by the vapor pressure of the solvent, the ambient temperature, and the effectiveness of ventilation systems. These factors and the rate of pulmonary air exchange will affect the extent of exposure. Sniffing glue fumes is one form of substance abuse.

Solvents are generally lipid-soluble, and therefore they are readily absorbed across the skin. Once absorbed, they tend to concentrate in the brain, and CNS dysfunction is common at high exposures. Symptoms can range from confusion to unconsciousness. Solvents often undergo bioactivation and may cause systemic toxicity as a result of the formation of reactive intermediates.

Pesticides

Pesticides are chemicals used to eliminate unwanted organisms. Common targets for pesticides include insects, weeds (herbicides), fungi, and rodents. Poisoning from pesticides often affects professional exterminators, agricultural workers, and consumers (Table 7.7). More than half of the poisonings due to agricultural pesticides affect children.

Insecticides

The prototypical *organochlorine insecticide* is DDT. It was first used in World War II for vector control of malaria. The organochlorine insecticides are very stable in the environment. This persistence allows toxic concentrations to build up in nontarget organisms.

Organophosphate insecticides (e.g., malathion, parathion, diazinon) undergo metabolic activation to

TABLE 7.6 Toxicity of Selected Solvents

Solvent	Uses	Effect and Mechanism
Aliphatic solvents		
Chloroform	Drug purification	Hepatic centrilobular necrosis, likely from reactive metabolites
Trichloroethylene	Degreasing, dry cleaning	Sensitizes the myocardium to epinephrine, interferes with alcohol metabolism
Methylene chloride	Degreasing, paint stripping, aerosol propellant	Metabolized to CO, resulting in formation of carboxyhemoglobin
Hexane, methyl n-butyl ketone	Wood glue, plastics manufacturing	Polyneuropathy from their metabolite, 2,5-hexanedione
Aromatic solvents		
Benzene	Petroleum product, adhesives and coatings	Leukemia, aplastic anemia, likely from reactive intermediates
Toluene	Adhesives	Cerebellar degeneration with repeated high-dose exposure (glue sniffing)

TABLE 7.7 Toxicity of Selected Pesticides

Class and Examples	Effect and Mechanism
Organochlorine insecticides	Neuronal hyperactivity; convulsions; impaired vision, concentration, and memory
DDT, chlordane, aldrin, heptachlor	Altered membrane permeability to Na^+, K^+
	Block repolarization by inhibiting Na^+, K^+-ATPase
	Block GABA-stimulated chloride uptake
Organophosphate insecticides	Bronchoconstriction and secretion, muscular weakness or paralysis, CNS depression, including respiratory centers
Bromophos, chlorpyrifos, parathion, malathion, diazinon	Inhibition of acetylcholinesterase (reversible or irreversible)
Carbamate insecticides	Same as organophosphate insecticides
Carbaryl	Inhibition of acetylcholinesterase (reversible)
Pyrethrin and pyrethroid insecticides	Neuronal hyperactivity, incoordination, tremors with hyperthermia, seizures
Pyrethrin I, II; fenvalerate, permethrin	Delayed inactivation of channels in excitable tissues, causing repetitive firing and at high doses, depolarization
	Block GABA-stimulated chloride uptake
Chlorophenoxy herbicides	Muscle weakness, aching, and tenderness; hypotonia
2,4-D; 2,4,5-T	
Bipyridyl herbicides	Delayed respiratory distress, fibrosis, and atelectasis
Paraquat, diquat	Gastrointestinal, liver, and kidney toxicity
	Formation of reactive oxygen species
Rodenticides	Block tricarboxylic acid cycle (fluoroacetates)
Compound 1080, warfarin, strychnine	Prevent blood clotting
	Induce seizures

ATPase, adenosine triphosphatase; GABA, γ-aminobutyric acid; 2,4-D, 2,4-dichlorophenoxyacetic acid; 2,4,5-T, 2,4,5-trichlorophenoxyacetic acid.

yield an oxygenated metabolite that will react with the active site of acetylcholinesterase (AChE), resulting in irreversible enzyme inhibition. Symptoms of poisoning are due to excessive stimulation of cholinergic receptors. In cases of lethal poisoning in humans, death is from respiratory failure. Distal neuropathy of the lower limbs also has been seen.

The *carbamate insecticides* also inhibit AChE. The mechanism of inhibition is similar, but the reaction is reversible.

Herbicides and Rodenticides

Herbicidal activity generally consists of interference with plant-specific biochemical reactions. Thus, mammalian toxicity is generally low and not predictable from the mechanism of herbicidal action. In contrast, rodenticide target selectivity is not based on differences in biochemistry between humans and rodents but rather on differences in physiology or behavior, especially feeding behavior. For example, an emetic may be included in a rodenticide formulation to promote vomiting in humans who accidentally consume the product; rodents do not have a vomit reflex.

The *chlorophenoxy herbicides,* 2,4-dichlorophenoxyacetic acid (2,4-D) and 2,4,5-trichlorophenoxyacetic acid (2,4,5-T), were used in defoliating operations in Vietnam, and the adverse health effects of the contaminant 2,3,7,8-tetrachlorodibenzodioxin (dioxin) continue to be controversial.

The *bipyridyl herbicides* paraquat and diquat are broad-spectrum herbicides. As little as 10 mL of paraquat concentrate is lethal in adults. Paraquat damages the lungs and may result in the appearance of a respiratory distress syndrome appearing 1 or 2 weeks after poisoning. In contrast, diquat causes minimal lung damage because it does not selectively accumulate in the lung. Acute renal failure, liver toxicity, and gastrointestinal damage are sequelae to diquat poisoning.

Warfarin, a coumarin anticoagulant, is incorporated into cornmeal for use as a rat poison. Repeated exposure results in sufficient inhibition of prothrombin synthesis to cause fatal internal hemorrhage.

APPLICATIONS OF TOXICOLOGICAL PRINCIPLES

Health professionals may be asked to provide an opinion of the cause and effect relationship between exposure to a xenobiotic and an adverse health effect ranging from symptoms of toxicity to death. Certain principles, including an assessment of temporality, should be considered in such an evaluation. Do the symptoms or disease follow the exposure within a proper time frame? In addition, an evaluation of the toxicological properties of the substance should be included. Does the xenobiotic possess properties that can logically be expected to cause the damage or disease in question? For many chemicals, the qualitative consideration of the types of symptoms, injury, or disease that may occur after exposure can be predicted based on the available toxicological data or known biological activity of the chemicals. If the toxicity or disease does not fit into this known profile, a causal relationship between the chemical and the problem should be questioned further. If the xenobiotic has the appropriate toxicological

properties, quantitative consideration of the total dose received must be carefully evaluated. Was the dose high enough to produce health effects? Finally, the possibility of alternate causes of the health problems must be investigated carefully. Are there other more logical explanations for the symptoms? If appropriate, drug side effects should be considered as a possible cause of the adverse health effects. Lifestyle and avocations also must be evaluated. Alternate causation is ideally evaluated by a thorough and frequently tedious review of complete medical, occupational, and social records of the patient.

Study QUESTIONS

1. A dental technician begins to display symptoms, including tremors, depression, and insomnia. Which of the following chemicals present in the workplace may be responsible for the symptoms?
   (A) Solvents used in dental adhesives
   (B) Fluoride used in oral rinses
   (C) Mercury used in the preparation of amalgams
   (D) Lidocaine used as an anesthetic

2. A patient learned recently that she is about 5 weeks pregnant, but because she has been suffering from depression, she asks her physician for a prescription for a drug to treat this problem. Her physician refuses to prescribe a drug at this time because he is concerned that the fetus is at risk for toxicity from in utero exposure to the drug. What is the most likely adverse outcome if the woman began taking the drug at this time?
   (A) The fetus would die.
   (B) A teratogenic response would occur in the fetus.
   (C) The growth of the fetus would be retarded.

3. Exposure to air pollutants can have adverse effects on human health. Exposure to one such pollutant, carbon monoxide, can result in which of the following conditions?
   (A) Irritation of the deep lungs because of damage to the epithelium
   (B) An increased susceptibility to respiratory infection due to impairment in phagocyte function
   (C) Exacerbation of asthmatic episodes because of bronchoconstriction
   (D) Hypoxia due to displacing oxygen from hemoglobin

4. A 4-year-old boy is taken to the emergency department by his parents in the afternoon the first Saturday in June. The family is moving into a house. They found the boy almost unconscious in a corner

in the garage, having difficulty breathing. He was surrounded by chemical containers left by the previous owners. The labels had deteriorated and couldn't be read. On examination you noted bronchoconstriction and profuse airway secretion, weakness of the muscles, difficulty breathing, and CNS depression. Which of the following chemicals do you suspect was involved?
   (A) Compound 1080
   (B) Pyrethrin
   (C) Parathion
   (D) Diquat

5. You are a staff physician at a major chemical manufacturing company. A worker on the maintenance crew has complained of being light-headed and tired occasionally at work and that if it occurs, it clears up after he leaves for the day. He was asked to write down where he had worked on the days this occurred; these are listed below. In which of these areas is he most likely to have exposures that would cause these symptoms?
   (A) Herbicide production area
   (B) Insecticide packaging area
   (C) Label printing area
   (D) Kitchen area of the cafeteria

6. You have been told there has been a large spill at the chemical company but in the confusion you weren't told where it occurred. The exposed workers were agitated and irritable and said to be having difficulty walking in a coordinated manner. Some feel quite hot as if they are burning up, and one had a seizure. Which area do you suspect had the spill?
   (A) Herbicide production area
   (B) Insecticide packaging area
   (C) Label printing area
   (D) Kitchen area of the cafeteria

ANSWERS

1. **C.** The symptoms are characteristic of a person chronically exposed to vapors released from elemental mercury. Since the dental technician may handle elemental mercury, including mishandling, the symptoms presented may occur. While the technician may be exposed to solvent vapors released from dental adhesives, the symptoms are not characteristic of this type of exposure. Fluoride toxicity would not be expected because these are not symptoms associated with fluoride ingestion, and the patient and not the technician would be most likely exposed to quantities high enough to cause any symptoms. The technician has little exposure to lidocaine, and the symptoms are not typical of lidocaine toxicity.

2. **B.** The fetus is particularly vulnerable to teratogens between days 25 and 40 of gestation, and this patient is within this window of time. The fetus is at much greater risk for death if exposure occurs during the first 2 weeks of gestation. Growth retardation of the fetus is the principal outcome if exposure to drugs occurs during the last 6 months of gestation.

3. **D.** Carbon monoxide can cause hypoxia because it reduces the oxygen carrying capacity of the blood by displacing oxygen from hemoglobin as well as impairing the erythrocyte's ability to release oxygen. Particulate air pollutants and reactive air pollutant gases, such as ozone and nitrogen dioxide, can damage the lungs, including increasing susceptibility to respiratory infection and irritation of the deep lungs, while exposure to sulfur dioxide can exacerbate asthmatic episodes.

4. **C.** Bronchoconstriction and secretion and muscular weaknesses occur from acetylcholine accumulation after inhibition of acetylcholinesterase. Parathion is an organophosphate insecticide that inhibits acetylcholinesterase, and it is readily available. Poisoning with compound 1080 (fluorocitrate) inhibits mitochondrial respiration and causes seizures and cardiac arrhythmias. Pyrethrin and pyrethroids are generally low in toxicity and few poisonings have been reported; however, seizures are a symptom. Diquat causes gastrointestinal disturbances.

5. **C.** Symptoms that occur during the work day and clear up after work are often due to inhalation exposure of volatile or aerosol materials. The solvents used in printing inks cause light-headedness and sedation. The symptoms are not those of herbicide exposure and insecticide exposure.

6. **B.** Spills cause acute high-dose exposures. The symptoms are referable to an acute high exposure to an organochlorine or pyrethroid insecticide. While organochlorine pesticides are not used in this country, they are manufactured for export. An acute high exposure to herbicide would be primarily irritation of skin and mucous membranes. The solvents in printing ink would cause CNS depression.

SUPPLEMENTAL READING

Ellenhorn MJ. Ellenhorn's Medical Toxicology: Diagnosis and Treatment of Human Poisoning (2nd ed.). Baltimore: Williams & Wilkins, 1997.

Gosselin RE, Smith RP, and Hodge HC. Clinical Toxicology of Commercial Products (5th ed.). Baltimore: Williams & Wilkins, 1984.

Haddad LM, Shannon MW, and Winchester JF. Clinical Management of Poisoning and Drug Overdose (3rd ed.). Philadelphia: Saunders, 1998.

Hayes AW (ed.). Principles and Methods of Toxicology (4th ed.). Philadelphia: Taylor & Francis, 2001.

Klaassen CD (ed.). Casarett and Doull's Toxicology, the Basic Science of Poisons (6th ed.). New York: McGraw Professional, 2001.

Rom WM (ed.). Environmental and Occupational Medicine (3rd ed.). Philadelphia: Lippincott-Raven, 1998.

Sullivan JB, Jr. and Krieger GR (eds.). Hazardous Materials Toxicology: Clinical Principles of Environmental Health. Baltimore: Williams & Wilkins, 1992.

CASE **Study**   **A Case of Poisoning**

A 5-year-old girl is taken to the doctor's office by her mother following a conference with her kindergarten teacher. The teacher is concerned because compared to her kindergarten classmates, she is hyperactive, restless, and easily distracted. Recent testing revealed that the child's vision was normal but hearing acuity was below normal. Recently the child has complained of abdominal pain and has had occasional constipation. About 3 years ago the parents moved into a 75-year-old house in the inner city and have been renovating it extensively. Within the past year, the parents separated and the father moved out of the house.

1. What is the most likely cause of the child's problems?
2. What tests should be run to help in the diagnosis?
3. What is the best treatment option?

ANSWERS:

1. These symptoms are consistent with childhood lead poisoning. The paint used originally in older homes usually contains lead. Since the parents have been renovating this older home, it is likely that they have removed some of the older paint, generating lead-containing dust and paint chips. Small children may exhibit pica, which is the compulsive eating of nonfood items, and this can occur during times of stress, such as the separation of parents. If the parents have not cleaned up adequately after removing the paint, it is probable that the child has had the opportunity to consume substantial quantities of lead.

2. Measuring the child's blood lead level will be very useful in assessing the possibility of lead poisoning. There is evidence that at blood lead levels of about 10 μg/dL, children are at risk for developmental impairment. Other tests that may be useful include examination for microcytic anemia and erythrocyte stippling and radiographic examination of the long bones for lead lines.

3. Several chelators can effectively lower the child's blood lead level. These include dimercaprol, edetate calcium disodium ($CaNa_2EDTA$) and succimer. Protocols are available for using the chelators depending upon the severity of symptoms.

8 | Contemporary Bioethical Issues in Pharmacology and Pharmaceutical Research

Janet Fleetwood

BIOMEDICAL ETHICS IN PHARMACOLOGY: AN INTRODUCTION AND FRAMEWORK

The relationship between physicians, scientists, and the pharmaceutical industry is a mutually advantageous one that is fraught with ethical complexity. Seemingly straightforward questions, such as whether a physician ought to enroll patients in a drug trial, which drug to prescribe when any one of several may be effective, and how to stay abreast of new drugs while remaining objective, become difficult when examined closely. This chapter provides a conceptual framework for bioethical analysis, presents some cases that illustrate ethical problems, and delineates some guidelines for consideration.

Bioethics is the study of ethical issues associated with providing health care or pursuing biomedical research. Most approaches to bioethics in the United States are secular in nature and presuppose no particular religious or theological perspective. While one's religious beliefs may play an important role in determining personal morality, the broader endeavor of bioethical analysis attempts to be devoid of any particular religious perspective. Similarly, bioethical analysis stands independent of legal analysis. Although the law is often a consideration in bioethical decision making, laws in themselves do not determine the morality of an action. Laws are supposed to reflect a societal consensus on issues and are established to set a minimum standard of behavior.

Thus, while religion and law provide guidelines for acceptable actions, religious beliefs, and knowledge of the law are frequently insufficient to guide moral action, in the realm of health care. Solving problems that arise in the scientific and clinical contexts requires knowledge of ethical principles and the methodology for applying them. While bioethical analysis is multifactorial, four moral principles play key roles in establish-

ing a basic framework. These principles were developed from a pluralistic, albeit North American, framework. Although not every problem will involve all four principles of bioethics, an understanding of the principles of autonomy, beneficence, nonmaleficence, and justice will build a solid framework for critical analysis.

The *principle of autonomy* entails that persons should be treated as inherently valuable individuals with the moral right to make decisions about their own lives. To the extent that one's actions and choices do not negatively affect others, individuals with the capacity to make their own decisions should be free to do as they wish, even if their choices are risky or harmful to themselves. The principle also entails that persons with diminished autonomy, such as those who are illiterate or retarded, deserve to have their interests protected. Many moral obligations for professionals engaged in scientific research or health care are derived from the principle of autonomy, such as the physician–researcher's obligation to fully inform potential research subjects and respect the individual's informed consent or informed refusal. This obligation is founded on the principle that individuals are the appropriate decision makers for choices that do not harm others.

The *principle of beneficence* entails helping people to further their interests. As the primary moral principle quoted in medical codes and oaths, the principle of beneficence is fundamental to the practice of medicine and clinical research. For example, concerns about beneficence motivate physicians, pharmacologists, pharmacists, and clinical investigators, all of whom share the goal of conducting studies that will ultimately benefit society by producing or refining effective treatments.

The *principle of nonmaleficence* asserts that professionals have an obligation to prevent harm or if harm is unavoidable, minimize that harm. This principle plays an important role in clinical research, as it entails an obligation to minimize risks to each participant. Moreover, drug approval procedures, such as those implemented by the Food and Drug Administration (FDA), are designed to protect patients from harm while ultimately facilitating the marketing of drugs that have maximal therapeutic benefits. Thus the principles of beneficence and nonmaleficence dictate that the overall goal of scientific advancement cannot trump the duty to protect human subjects of clinical research from harm.

The *principle of justice* states that individuals should be given what they deserve, be that benefit or burden. Cases that are alike should be treated similarly, and relevant distinctions should be drawn consistently. The principle of justice does not specifically state what distinctions are fair or which criteria are reasonable; it simply requires that, once criteria are determined, they be applied fairly. Justice is important in many areas, such as recruitment of research subjects for pharmaceutical studies. For example, researchers must guard against distributing the burdens of participation disproportionately among populations that are poorly equipped to give informed consent, such as children or the mentally incompetent.

The principles of autonomy, beneficence, nonmaleficence, and justice form a foundation for analysis of ethical quandaries. In addition, a comprehensive ethical analysis will include considerations of cultural and religious diversity of patient–subjects, health care providers and interpersonal relationships; an assessment of the profession-based duties and obligations of the health care professionals, including an examination of relevant professional oaths and codes; and an analysis of relevantly similar previous bioethical dilemmas.

BIOMEDICAL ETHICS AND CLINICAL RESEARCH

For more than 50 years, scientists, physicians, bioethicists, and the media have focused on a variety of issues in research with human subjects, or clinical research. In 1948, in response to the atrocities perpetrated by Nazi experimentation, the Nuremberg Code was developed to set forth guidelines for the acceptable conduct of scientific research. In 1964 the World Medical Association adopted the Declaration of Helsinki, which specifically guides physicians in biomedical research. These documents specify basic moral guidelines ultimately founded on concerns for autonomy, beneficence, and justice. The guidelines require the following:

- Subjects must give voluntary consent before being enrolled in any study after being fully advised of the study's aims, methods, benefits, risks, and discomforts.

- Proposed studies must have sufficient scientific merit to warrant their risks.
- Studies must be designed to avoid all unnecessary physical and mental suffering.
- Potential benefits to subjects must outweigh risks to subjects.
- Researchers must ensure subjects' privacy and confidentiality.
- Subjects must have the right to withdraw from the study at any time.
- Researchers are obligated to stop the study if continuation is likely to result in injury to subjects.

The guidelines further require that research on human subjects be conducted by qualified individuals and that most clinical research be reviewed by an independent committee, which is generally an institutional review board.

In addition to the Nuremberg Code and Declaration of Helsinki, The International Ethical Guidelines for Biomedical Research Involving Human Subjects was issued in 1982 and revised in 1993 by the Council for the International Organization of Medical Sciences (CIOMS). Those guidelines define national policies for biomedical research, apply ethical standards to the circumstances often present in research in economically developing nations, and define mechanisms for ethical review of human subjects research.

In drug studies, specific ethical concerns focus on balancing benefits and burdens to subjects, on the need for investigators to use noninvasive and minimally painful means of determining drug disposition, on minimizing the frequency of bodily fluid sampling, and on choosing study subjects who are representative of the target population whenever possible rather than exposing healthy volunteer subjects. Placebo-controlled studies create special obligations pertaining to the potential deception of subjects and raise difficult questions about subjects' informed consent.

Recently, attention has focused on the issue of international medical research, especially that done with patients in economically developing nations. For example, one controversy focused on a highly publicized placebo-controlled study in Africa examining the prevention of perinatal transmission of HIV using azidothymidine (AZT). Since such a study in an economically developed nation would probably not have a placebo arm, critics argue that this reflects a double standard for research. They assert that one standard for ethical research should prevail, regardless of the social and economic conditions of the subjects. Bioethicists and those directly involved in research are reconsidering whether subjects who are already suffering under impoverished conditions might suffer further exploitation at the hands of medical researchers.

Those who designed the study point out that placebo-controlled studies are the most rigorous available and that AZT would not otherwise be available to this population. Enrollment in the study offered a benefit over and above the status quo, they assert, and did not deprive subjects of anything they could otherwise obtain. Yet such "studies in nature" pose complex ethical issues. If the research relies on the continuation of undesirable social conditions, such as the general lack of prenatal care, critics assert that there is a fundamental obligation to improve those background conditions rather than take advantage of access to the perfect "laboratory." While the clinical study has certainly not made the underlying conditions worse, the study has done little to correct the underlying deprivations. Even so, is that the role of pharmaceutical research or a broader social role that goes beyond what researchers should have to provide? While it would be foolhardy to insist that the only ethically acceptable research is done on patients with full access to comprehensive health care, we do not want to make those who are already deprived and in poverty into "lab rats" who participate in research that ultimately benefits primarily those in the developed world.

Clinical research can target the needs of those in economically developing nations and those who are medically underserved in the United States. Yet we must be cautious in the design and implementation of research studies to ensure that those who are the most vulnerable, whether locally or abroad, are offered the most protections and stand to gain proportionately from the studies in which they participate. Research must satisfy the needs of the population in which it is undertaken, and the products developed during the course of the research must subsequently be made reasonably available.

CONFLICTS OF INTEREST AND THE PHARMACEUTICAL INDUSTRY

A *conflict of interest* occurs when an individual's private goals are inconsistent with that person's official responsibilities. The interrelationship between scientists, physicians, and researchers and the pharmaceutical industry has given rise to a variety of well-publicized cases raising concerns about conflicts of interest.

Researchers and drug companies are interdependent. The pharmaceutical industry depends on scientists and clinicians for research, development, and marketing. Conversely, the medical profession depends on research that is largely financed by the pharmaceutical industry. While this interdependence often benefits industry, research, and patient care, conflicts of interest may arise in two main areas: (1) drug research and development and (2) clinical education and product marketing.

Drug Research and Development

Pharmacology, unlike some other basic science disciplines, has a unique status when it comes to potential conflicts of interest. The pharmaceutical industry combines a desire for discovery and development with profit-motivated marketing and sales goals. Although scientists and physicians share the desire for drug discovery and development and are motivated by the desire to contribute to scientific advancement and improved patient care, pharmaceutical companies are simultaneously under strong commercial pressures. Pharmaceutical companies are therefore willing to offer financial incentives to physician–researchers who conduct studies, recruit patients, or are helpful in product development and testing. In some cases, this financial support may compromise professional judgment in conducting, analyzing, or reporting research.

For example, often a pharmaceutical company will contract with a private physician to recruit patients into a drug study. While this arrangement frequently offers patients access to treatment that might otherwise be unavailable, the potential conflict may ultimately result in lack of objectivity in study design, data interpretation, and dissemination of research results. For example, a 1986 study in the *Journal of General Internal Medicine* found a statistically significant relationship between drug company funding and outcomes favoring a new therapy.

In addition, this kind of arrangement places the physician in a dual role as a clinician–researcher, with sometimes competing obligations to the drug company and the patient. The doctor assumes a position of responsibility to the company while simultaneously maintaining the usual duties to protect and benefit his or her patients. The physician's role as patient advocate can easily be compromised, since physicians also have a potentially competing interest in enrolling patients in the trial. In fact, patients may mistakenly believe that when their personal family physician suggests they enroll as a subject in a study, the doctor is suggesting enrollment because it is in that specific patient's interest to participate. However, the enrollment offer probably has little to do with that particular patient's care and more to do with the physician's desire to enroll subjects.

At minimum, the principles of autonomy and beneficence require that patients be told the source of funding for sponsored studies in which they are invited to enroll and advised of any potential conflicts between the physician's research interests and treatment recommendations.

Although disclosure to patients is important, patients are generally ill suited to assess how a potential conflict of interest actually affects their treatment. In addition to disclosure to patients, we need rigorous reporting requirements for those engaged in drug studies.

Institutions should implement clear policies, and professional guidelines should be developed, to prohibit relationships that place patient care secondary to financial gain.

Clinical Education and Product Marketing

The second area for ethical concern is clinical education and product marketing. The line between "education" and marketing is frequently a blurry one, and it is often difficult to separate a company's desire to educate physicians about products that may genuinely enhance patient care from the company's desire to increase profits. As the gatekeepers for all prescription drugs, physicians have the power to determine which drugs will compete successfully in the marketplace, making doctors the logical targets for marketing efforts by pharmaceutical firms. In fact, pharmaceutical companies spend more than $11 billion each year on promotion and marketing. Between $8,000 and $13,000 is spent annually on each physician. However, many company-sponsored arrangements may conflict with the physician's responsibility to act in the best interest of the patient. A voluntary code has recently been adopted by the Pharmaceutical Research and Manufacturers of America which establishes guidelines for relationships between the pharmaceutical industry and health care professionals.

Ultimately, prescribing practices are the main source of concern, as physicians may be induced to prescribe some products rather than others based on factors other than therapeutic effectiveness or cost. Many drug companies have generous programs for providing their products free of charge to those who cannot afford them. However, free samples provided by drug companies directly to physicians' offices should be used cautiously, and the choice of drugs should be made on the basis of medical indications, not sample availability. While samples supplied to physicians' offices to be given to patients may enable a patient to try a drug for a few weeks to be sure it is tolerated, they also serve to get patients started on a particular product which presumably will have to be continued and paid for by the patient or a third-party payer. The patient, as a health care consumer, is not in a position to assess the need for a certain drug or decide whether it is prescribed appropriately and sometimes cannot accurately determine whether it is therapeutically effective. Thus, the patient is entitled to be protected by the physician, whose primary role is that of patient advocate as dictated by the principles of beneficence and nonmaleficence.

Product marketing presents other ethical issues as well. In addition to direct product advertising in medical journals and direct to consumer advertising in the popular media, pharmaceutical company sales representatives frequently visit physicians. Although the salesperson's goal is clearly to promote sales, often these visits take the form of "education" for busy clinicians. Company representatives present "educational" information, provide meals, and may give gifts or incentives to the doctor. Although such visits may keep clinicians informed about current products, they may also precipitate conflicts of interest. Gifts of more than token value, trips to resort areas for "educational" programs with little scientific merit, and cash incentives for prescribing a drug or having it added to a hospital formulary all are cause for concern. The line between a gift and a bribe is not a sharp one, and clinicians and drug company employees should strive to avoid any impropriety. The American Medical Association has stated in its Current Opinions that gifts should primarily benefit patients and should not be of substantial value. While textbooks, modest meals, and educational or work-related gifts, such as notepads or textbooks, may be appropriate, cash payments are not appropriate. Physicians should not accept gifts from companies if the gift might compromise or appear to compromise the physician's objectivity. A helpful criterion suggested by the American College of Physicians when considering the ethical appropriateness of a particular interaction between a physician and drug company is to ask whether one would be willing to have the arrangement generally known. If not, the action falls outside the realm of ethical acceptability and should be avoided.

Medical students and residents are not exempt from the influence of drug companies. Many students and residents are offered gifts of educational books or equipment or are invited to attend company-sponsored events. Young professionals need to be extremely careful to avoid impropriety and should receive specific instruction about the ethically appropriate scope and limits of interactions with drug company representatives.

The area of continuing medical education is similarly mired with controversy, as "educational" meetings may be simply soft sells at company expense to encourage physicians to prescribe one company's product over a competitor's. While some industry-sponsored education provides a good opportunity for unbiased scientific exchange, such as when a drug company underwrites the cost of an educational program but places no restrictions on topics discussed or speakers chosen, too often "education" is a euphemism for marketing. To be considered legitimate, a conference or meeting must be primarily dedicated to scientific and educational activities, and the main incentive for bringing attendees together must be to further broad knowledge.

In addition, physicians may be invited to serve as a drug company "consultant." These "consultants" are invited to a company-sponsored symposium, which is sometimes nothing more than a sales pitch for that company's products with little real interaction or consultancy. While consultants who provide genuine services may receive reasonable compensation and accept reimbursement for travel expenses, token consulting or advisory arrangements cannot be used to justify compensating physicians.

Speakers at company-sponsored events who are drawn from the professional community should subject their presentation to the same level of scientific rigor as they would apply to a presentation at a professional meeting. In particular, they should refrain from allowing the pharmaceutical company to influence the data they present, the means of presenting it, or the outcomes drawn. When companies financially support conferences or lectures other than their own, the organizers of the conference should maintain control over the topics and speakers selected. If a speaker wishes to mention a specific product, he or she should be sure to avoid any appearance of impropriety by comparing it fairly and completely with competing products. Researchers and clinicians who are invited to conduct studies supported by drug companies and present their data at company-sponsored educational events should take special care to conduct the study meticulously, analyze the data rigorously, and present the data as objectively as possible. Speakers should avoid accepting lecture invitations to events at which the drug company pays the audience to attend and should object if the company's marketing representatives conduct sales activities, such as distributing samples or brochures about a specific product, when an event has been promoted as educational. In addition, industry sponsorship should be noted in any publication reporting study results. Finally, both attendees and speakers should demand that financial sponsorship be revealed before registration and that financial relationships between speakers and the promoter be plainly stated. In short, to ensure objectivity and eliminate any appearance of conflict of interest, doctors should get their information primarily from professional peer-reviewed journals and not rely solely on material provided by drug companies.

In addition to these general guidelines, three questions are useful to assess the ethics of an arrangement between pharmaceutical company and researcher–clinician. First, would it be embarrassing for the clinician if the public knew about the financial arrangement? Arrangements that would cause embarrassment or lead others to suspect a conflict of interest should be avoided. Second, can the physician reveal the financial arrangements to patients whom the clinician invites to participate in the study? If the physician feels uncomfortable discussing the remuneration with patient recruits because of the appearance of a conflict of interest, the physician should not participate. Third, would the clinician pursue the same treatment strategy if there were no financial incentive? If the physician would likely choose another treatment were it not for the financial rewards from the drug company, the physician should reconsider offering enrollment for the patient. Finally, do any professional codes, institutional policies, or other guidelines preclude participation?

FINAL CONSIDERATIONS

The principles of autonomy, beneficence, nonmaleficence, and justice provide a conceptual framework for analyzing issues pertaining to clinical research and the complex relationship between science, industry, and patient care. To develop a broad understanding of these issues, that basic framework should be filled in with an understanding of cultural considerations, profession-based duties and obligations, and an analysis of previous bioethical issues. Continual scrutiny of bioethical issues in pharmacology is warranted as we develop better insight into the moral dilemmas of the field.

Study QUESTIONS

1. Joel Martin, a pediatrician at a residential facility for mentally retarded children, has been approached by the Modern Pharmaceutical Company. The company would like Dr. Martin to enroll children aged 4 to 7 in one of their clinical trials for a new drug to treat conjunctivitis (pinkeye). Dr. Martin recognizes that the children's parents would be able to give informed consent or refusal on behalf of their children, that risks have been minimized, and that overall, the study drug is likely to help the participants. He is concerned, however, about the drug companies' decision to enroll retarded children before healthy children in the community. Modern's representative points out that the incidence of conjunctivitis in the facility is very high and so provides an excellent setting for the study to be completed quickly. Dr. Martin considers the population of the facility extremely vulnerable. The ethical principle that underlies Dr. Martin's concerns is:
(A) Autonomy
(B) Beneficence
(C) Nonmaleficence
(D) Justice
(E) Medical neediness

2. The main ethical problem with medical research in economically developing nations in which subjects are medically underserved is that:
(A) Subjects are frequently not compliant, as they do not understand the importance of the study, raising ethical issues about risks and benefits for the subjects that complete the study.
(B) Researchers cannot generalize from the outcome with a medically underserved population to draw conclusions that would be applicable in the United States because of the numerous other variables that affect the outcome of the study.
(C) Subjects are not asked to give informed consent, as they cannot understand the complexities of a research study.
(D) Subjects are included in studies of treatments that are not available in underserved countries but are available in the United States, raising issues of equity and fairness toward disadvantaged populations.
(E) Subjects are deprived access to medical treatments that would be available in their country were they not part of a randomized, placebo-controlled study.

3. When does a conflict of interest occur?
(A) When an individual's private goals are inconsistent with that person's official responsibilities
(B) When an individual's research interests are in conflict with the research of an individual in another institution or corporation
(C) When two researchers want to do research in the same area but there is only enough available funding for one researcher to do the research adequately
(D) When an individual has a conflict between his or her research interests and the requirements set forth by the Nuremberg Code

4. Susan Brown, a community-based internist in Little Town, U. S. A., has received a letter inviting her to become a consultant to the Modern Pharmaceutical Company. Modern would like Dr. Brown to attend a medical consultants' meeting at the Golden Sunset Resort, an elegant resort about an hour away from Little Town. The agenda includes a Saturday morning presentation by representatives from Modern, with time over lunch for the medical consultants to give feedback to the company representative about the company's products. The rest of the weekend is unscheduled time for Dr. Brown to enjoy the resort. Dr. Brown will be paid $1000 for her consulting services. When considering whether or not to attend Dr. Brown should:
(A) Decide whether she thinks she would be biased toward Modern products by the company's generosity; if she believes she can remain objective, it is acceptable to attend.
(B) Determine whether she feels favorably toward Modern's product line; if she already prescribes Modern products and prefers them to the competition's, she cannot be biased by their presentations, so there is no ethical issue in attending.
(C) Consider how important it is for drug companies to be able to get feedback on their products from physicians and attend to ensure that the company gets accurate information.
(D) Consider that her time is valuable, so she deserves to be compensated by Modern.
(E) Consider the guidelines by the American Medical Association and choose not to attend under the stated conditions.

5. A helpful criterion suggested by the American College of Physicians when considering the ethical appropriateness of a particular interaction between a physician and industry is to:
(A) Determine whether the interaction violates any laws or statutes; if not, the action is acceptable.
(B) Determine whether one would be willing to have the arrangement generally known; if not, the action should be avoided.
(C) Determine whether the action compromises the profit margin of the pharmaceutical company and therefore is not in the interest of the shareholders; if so, the action should be avoided.
(D) Determine whether patient care is negatively affected; if not, the action is ethically acceptable.

ANSWERS

1. **D.** The principle of justice is a relevant consideration when subjects are selected for clinical research. It requires that members of a vulnerable population, such as institutionalized patients with mental retardation, not be exploited. The principle of autonomy would be most relevant to the parents' ability to consent or refuse on the child's behalf, something Dr. Martin thinks is handled satisfactorily. Dr. Martin believes risks have been minimized and the overall study drug is likely to help the participants, so the study has satisfied the principles of nonmaleficence and beneficence. The principle of medical priority is not mentioned in the chapter and pertains to treating the most medically needy patients first, which is not at issue here.

2. **D.** An ethical issue arises when one includes medically underserved patients in a study without providing them with the level of care available to others. Problems with noncompliance, while potentially damaging to a study, do not pose ethical problems in medically underserved populations not encountered elsewhere. Effective study design can overcome problems with generalizing from one population to the next. Subjects everywhere should be

provided with information at a level the subject can comprehend and asked to give informed consent. Subjects in medically underserved populations are not deprived of access to medical treatments that are available in their own country, only those that are available only elsewhere.

3. **A.** A conflict of interest occurs when an individual's personal interests conflict with official responsibilities, such as those required by one's profession. So, for example, a physician who owns shares in a drug company that is sponsoring a clinical trial in which the doctor enrolls patients may have a conflict of interest. Conflicts of interest do not generally pertain to conflicts between researchers or the requirements set forth by the Nuremberg Code.

4. **E.** The American Medical Association guidelines suggest that Dr. Brown should not attend. Clearly, the educational nature of the meeting is dubious. Even if we consider it a consultancy rather than an educational meeting, Dr. Brown's role as a "consultant" is not well specified, and the compensation for her consultancy may be seen as excessive. Although she may believe that she can remain objective despite the company's generosity, numerous studies show that prescribing patterns change in response to pharmaceutical company largesse. Similarly, the fact that she often prescribes their products does not mean that her objectivity cannot be compromised. For example, she may not consider new products from other companies as carefully because of her preference to keep prescribing Modern's products. While admittedly her time is valuable, the amount this company will spend on her expenses and honoraria far exceed what is reasonable.

5. **B.** Considering whether one would be willing to have an arrangement generally known is a quick test of the ethical appropriateness of an action. While some individuals may have a relatively low standard for what they would be willing to have publicly known, for most people this test can provide a useful guideline. The simple fact that an action falls within the law does not make it morally acceptable. Considerations of the profit margin for the pharmaceutical company shareholders is impor-

tant for company employees but bears little relevance on physician–pharmaceutical company interactions, in which the physician is supposed to be primarily a patient advocate. Finally, although patient care may not be directly affected by an action, the action may be ethically problematic if it gives the impression that the physician is under undue influence of the pharmaceutical company and thereby willing to put patient care behind company profit.

SUPPLEMENTAL READING

Council on Ethical and Judicial Affairs, American Medical Association. Gifts to physicians from industry. JAMA 1991;265:501. Updated June 1996 and June 1998. Available online at http://www.ama-assn.org (E-8.061 Gifts to Physicians from Industry.)

Davidson R. Source of funding and outcome of clinical trials. J Gen Intern Med 1986:1:155–158.

Emanuel E, Wendler D, and Grady C. What Makes Clinical Research Ethical? JAMA 2000;283(20):2701–2711.

Executive Committee of the Pharmaceutical Research and Manufacturers of American (PhRMA), PhRMA Code on Interactions with Healthcare Professionals, July 1, 2002. Available online at http://www.phrma.org

Fletcher J et al. Introduction to Clinical Ethics (2nd ed.). Frederick, MD: University Publishing, 1997.

Kessler DA. Drug promotion and scientific exchanges: The role of the clinical investigator. N Engl J Med 1991;325:201–203.

Levine RJ. Some recent developments in the international guidelines on the ethics of research involving human subjects. Annu N Y Acad Sci 2000;918:10–8.

Svensson C. Ethical considerations in the conduct of clinical pharmacokinetic studies. Clin Pharmacokinet 1989;17:217–222.

Wazana A. Physicians and the Pharmaceutical Industry: Is A Gift Ever Just a Gift? JAMA 2000;283(3):373–380.

Wolfe SM. Why do American drug companies spend more than $12 billion a year pushing drugs? J Gen Intern Med 1996;11:637–639.

CASE Study   Dr. Drew and the Hypertension Drug Trial

Lee Drew, MD, has been invited by Modern Pharmaceutical Company to participate in a new drug trial for hypertension. For every patient Dr. Drew recruits through his small private practice, he will receive $1,000 to help defray the costs of quarterly blood draws and the additional paperwork required by the study. In addition, Modern Pharmaceuticals will replace Dr. Drew's computer system to enable better patient tracking. Given the declining reimbursement rates from third-party payers, Dr. Drew could really use the financial support but wonders what benefits this drug offers to patients. Is it simply a me-too or copycat drug, designed primarily to make money for the drug company? And, if so, can Dr. Drew be justified in asking patients to enroll in the study? Still, Dr. Drew finds the financial incentives tempting and knows the risk to patients is low. How should Dr. Drew resolve the ethical dilemma?

ANSWER: Dr. Drew faces many ethical questions in deciding whether or not to participate in the drug trial for hypertension sponsored by the Modern Pharmaceutical Company. In analyzing whether to participate, Dr. Drew should focus on the primacy of the role of *physician*, with the attendant duty to protect patients from harm, and recognize that the role of *investigator* must remain secondary. Having established the priority of Dr. Drew's obligations to provide good patient care and protect patients from harm, Dr. Drew should assess the study's value. Assessing value entails analyzing whether the data generated will change the course of patient care or otherwise provide a valuable scientific benefit, over and above profit for the pharmaceutical company.

Further, Dr. Drew should examine the scientific validity of the study and assess whether the study is well designed and positioned to answer the question at hand while minimizing risks and maximizing benefits to subjects. Dr. Drew should consider whether subjects will be selected fairly, and whether subjects will be well informed. Dr. Drew should consider the quality of the ethical and scientific review that the protocol has undergone by the Institutional Review Board, and see if the protocol raises ethical issues that have not been addressed. Finally, Dr. Drew should consider whether the payment offered is commensurate with the time, effort, and actual expenditures to enroll patients and implement the trial. The offer of a computer system to enable better patient tracking is especially troubling, since it is debatable whether such a system really serves the needs of patients or primarily serves the needs of the drug company. In any case, PhRMA guidelines recommend that physicians not accept gifts over $100 in value even if they offer benefit to patients, so Dr. Drew should not accept the computer system even if its absence makes it impossible to participate in the study. Finally, if Dr. Drew feels that the study is valuable, well designed, and meets ethical standards, before enrolling any patient Dr. Drew should consider whether that patient is doing well on current therapy. Enrollment is most easily justifiable for a patient who is not doing well on standard therapy and most ethically problematic for patients whose current therapy is effective. These issues, although complex, must be considered and resolved before Dr. Drew can determine the ethical justifiability of participating.

DRUGS AFFECTING THE AUTONOMIC NERVOUS SYSTEM

General Organization and Functions of the Nervous System

William W. Fleming

GENERAL ORGANIZATION AND FUNCTIONS OF THE NERVOUS SYSTEM

The nervous system is divided into two parts: the central nervous system (CNS) and the peripheral nervous system (PNS). The CNS consists of the brain and spinal cord. The PNS consists of all *afferent* (sensory) neurons, which carry nerve impulses into the CNS from sensory end organs in peripheral tissues, and all *efferent* (motor) neurons, which carry nerve impulses from the CNS to effector cells in peripheral tissues. The peripheral efferent system is further divided into the *somatic nervous system* and the *autonomic nervous system*. The effector cells innervated by the somatic nervous system are skeletal muscle cells. The autonomic nervous system innervates three types of effector cells: (1) smooth muscle, (2) cardiac muscle, and (3) exocrine glands. While the somatic nervous system can function on a reflex basis, voluntary control of skeletal muscle is of primary importance. In contrast, in the autonomic nervous system voluntary control can be exerted, but reflex control is paramount.

Both somatic and autonomic effectors may be reflexly excited by nerve impulses arising from the same sensory end organs. For example, when the body is exposed to cold, heat loss is minimized by vasoconstriction of blood vessels in the skin and by the curling up of the body. At the same time, heat production is increased by an increase in skeletal muscle tone and shivering and by an increase in metabolism owing in part to secretion of epinephrine.

In general terms, the function of the autonomic nervous system is to maintain the constancy of the internal environment (*homeostasis*). This includes the regulation of the cardiovascular system, digestion, body temperature, metabolism, and the secretion of the exocrine glands.

ANATOMIC DIFFERENCES BETWEEN THE SOMATIC AND AUTONOMIC NERVOUS SYSTEMS

Anatomical differences between the peripheral somatic and autonomic nervous systems have led to their classification as separate divisions of the nervous system. These differences are shown in Figure 9.1. The axon of a somatic motor neuron leaves the CNS and travels without interruption to the innervated effector cell. In contrast, two neurons are required to connect the CNS and a visceral effector cell of the autonomic nervous system. The first neuron in this sequence is called the *preganglionic* neuron. The second neuron, whose cell body is within the ganglion, travels to the visceral effector cell; it is called the *postganglionic* neuron.

AUTONOMIC NERVOUS SYSTEM

The preganglionic neurons of the *sympathetic* nervous system have their cell bodies in the thoracic and lumbar regions of the spinal cord, termed the thoracolumbar division. The preganglionic neurons of the *parasympathetic* division have their cell bodies in the brainstem and in the sacral region of the spinal cord, termed the craniosacral division. The cranial part of the parasympathetic nervous system innervates structures in the head, neck, thorax, and abdomen (e.g., the stomach, part of the intestines, and pancreas). The cranial parasympathetic fibers leave the CNS in the oculomotor, facial, glos-

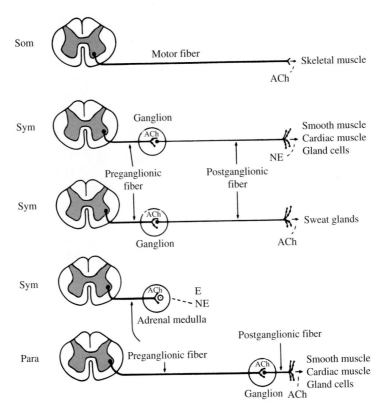

FIGURE 9.1

Anatomical characteristics and neurotransmitters of the somatic (Som), sympathetic (Sym), and parasympathetic (Para) divisions of the PNS. ACh, acetylcholine; E, epinephrine; NE, norepinephrine

sopharyngeal, and vagal cranial nerves. The sacral division of the parasympathetic nervous system innervates the remainder of the intestines and the pelvic viscera.

Location of the Autonomic Ganglia

The sympathetic ganglia consist of two chains of 22 segmentally arranged ganglia lateral to the vertebral column. The preganglionic fibers leave the spinal cord in adjacent ventral roots and enter neighboring ganglia, where they make synaptic connections with postganglionic neurons. Some preganglionic fibers pass through the vertebral ganglia without making synaptic connections and travel by way of splanchnic nerves to paired prevertebral ganglia in front of the vertebral column, where they make synaptic connections with postganglionic neurons. In addition, some sympathetic preganglionic fibers pass through the splanchnic nerves into the adrenal glands and make synaptic connections on the chromaffin cells of the adrenal medulla.

Because sympathetic ganglia lie close to the vertebral column, sympathetic preganglionic fibers are generally short. Postganglionic fibers are generally long, since they arise in vertebral ganglia and must travel to the innervated effector cells. There are exceptions to

this generalization. A few sympathetic ganglia lie near the organs innervated (e.g., urinary bladder and rectum); thus, these preganglionic fibers are long and the postganglionic fibers are short. In contrast, the parasympathetic ganglia lie very close to or actually within the organs innervated by the parasympathetic postganglionic neurons.

Ratio of Preganglionic to Postganglionic Neurons

A single sympathetic preganglionic fiber branches a number of times after entering a ganglion and makes synaptic connection with a number of postganglionic neurons. Furthermore, some branches of this preganglionic fiber may ascend or descend to adjacent vertebral ganglia and terminate on an additional number of postganglionic neurons in these ganglia as well. Therefore, activity in a single sympathetic preganglionic neuron may result in the activation of a number of effector cells in widely separated regions of the body. Anatomically, *the sympathetic nervous system is designed to produce widespread physiological activity.* The sympathetic nervous system prepares the body for strenuous muscular activity, stress, and emergencies.

By contrast, parasympathetic preganglionic neurons are extremely limited in their distribution. In general, a single parasympathetic preganglionic fiber makes a synaptic connection with only one or two postganglionic neurons. For this reason, along with the fact that the ganglia are near or are embedded in the organs innervated, individual *parasympathetic preganglionic neurons influence only a small region of the body or affect only specific organs.* The parasympathetic nervous system is involved with the accumulation, storage, and preservation of body resources.

When the sympathetic integrative centers in the brain are activated (by anger, stress, or emergency), the body's resources are mobilized for combat or for flight. Stimulation of the sympathetic nervous system results in acceleration of the heart rate and an increase in the contractile force of the heart muscle. There is increased blood flow (*vasodilation*) through skeletal muscle and decreased blood flow (*vasoconstriction*) through the skin and visceral organs. Activity of the gastrointestinal tract, such as peristaltic and secretory activity, is decreased, and intestinal sphincters are contracted. The pupils are dilated. The increased breakdown of glycogen (*glycogenolysis*) in the liver produces an increase in blood sugar, while the breakdown of lipids (*lipolysis*) in adipose tissue produces an increase in blood fatty acids; these biochemical reactions make energy available for active tissues. In addition to generalized activation of the sympathetic system in response to stress, there can be more discrete homeostatic activation of the sympathetic system. For example, a selective reflex-associated alteration in the sympathetic outflow to the cardiovascular system can occur.

The parasympathetic system is designed to function more or less on an organ system basis, usually under conditions of minimal stress. For example, the activation of the gastrointestinal tract takes place during digestion of a meal; constriction of the pupil and accommodation for near vision are essential for reading.

AUTONOMIC NEUROTRANSMITTERS

Two PNS neurotransmitters, acetylcholine and norepinephrine, have particular clinical importance. Both are synthesized and stored primarily in the nerve terminals until released by a nerve impulse. It should be noted, to avoid confusion, that in the United States the transmitter in the sympathetic nervous system is referred to as *norepinephrine* and the major adrenal medullary hormone is referred to as *epinephrine.* In Europe and most of the world these two substances are called *noradrenaline* and *adrenaline,* respectively.

Neurotransmission in the PNS occurs at three major sites: (1) preganglionic synapses in both parasympathetic and sympathetic ganglia, (2) parasympathetic and

sympathetic postganglionic neuroeffector junctions, and (3) all somatic motor end plates on skeletal muscle. Acetylcholine is the transmitter released at all of these sites except for the majority of sympathetic neuroeffector junctions. Neurons that release acetylcholine are called *cholinergic* neurons.

Norepinephrine is the transmitter released at most sympathetic postganglionic neuroeffector junctions. Neurons that release this substance are called *adrenergic* or *noradrenergic* neurons. Not all sympathetic postganglionic neurons are noradrenergic. The sympathetic postganglionic neurons that innervate the sweat glands and some of the blood vessels in skeletal muscle are cholinergic; that is, they release acetylcholine rather than norepinephrine, even though anatomically they are sympathetic neurons (Fig. 9.1).

Drugs that mimic the actions of acetylcholine are termed *cholinomimetic,* and those that mimic epinephrine and/or norepinephrine are *adrenomimetic.* The cholinomimetic drugs are also called parasympathomimetic drugs. The adrenomimetic drugs are often called sympathomimetic.

The receptors with which acetylcholine and other cholinomimetic drugs interact are called *cholinoreceptors,* while the receptors with which norepinephrine, epinephrine, or other adrenomimetic drugs combine are called *adrenoceptors.* It is common both in textbooks and the scientific literature to see these receptors referred to as cholinergic or adrenergic receptors. This is improper usage of the terms *cholinergic* and *adrenergic,* since these terms should be applied only to nerves.

Drugs that antagonize the actions of acetylcholine are known as *cholinoreceptor antagonists;* those that antagonize norepinephrine are known as *adrenoceptor antagonists.*

A number of other substances are released by sympathetic and parasympathetic neurons, often the same neurons that release norepinephrine or acetylcholine. These substances include adenosine triphosphate (ATP), neuropeptide Y, and substance P.

INNERVATION OF VARIOUS ORGANS BY THE SYMPATHETIC AND PARASYMPATHETIC NERVOUS SYSTEMS

Many visceral organs are innervated by both divisions of the autonomic nervous system. In most instances, when an organ receives dual innervation, the two systems work in opposition to one another. In some tissues and organs, the two innervations exert an opposing influence on the same effector cells (e.g., the sinoatrial node in the heart), while in other tissues opposing actions come about because different effector cells are activated (e.g., the circular and radial muscles in the iris).

Some organs are innervated by only one division of the autonomic nervous system.

Many neurons of both divisions of the autonomic nervous system are tonically active; that is, they are continually carrying some impulse traffic. The moment-to-moment activity of an organ such as the heart, which receives a dual innervation by sympathetic (noradrenergic) and parasympathetic (cholinergic) neurons, is controlled by the level of tonic activity of the two systems.

Blood Vessels

Most vascular smooth muscle is innervated solely by the sympathetic (noradrenergic) nervous system, but there are exceptions. Some blood vessels in the face, tongue, and urogenital tract (especially the penis) are innervated by parasympathetic (cholinergic) as well as sympathetic (noradrenergic) neurons. The parasympathetic innervation of blood vessels has only regional importance, for example, in salivary glands, where increased parasympathetic activity causes vasodilation that supports salivation.

The primary neural control of total peripheral resistance is through sympathetic nerves. The diameter of blood vessels is controlled by the tonic activity of noradrenergic neurons. There is a continuous outflow of noradrenergic impulses to the vascular smooth muscle, and therefore some degree of constant vascular constriction is maintained. An increase in impulse outflow causes further contraction of the smooth muscle, resulting in greater vasoconstriction. A decrease in impulse outflow permits the smooth muscle to relax, leading to vasodilation.

The Heart

The heart is innervated by both sympathetic and parasympathetic neurons; however, their distribution in the heart is quite different. Postganglionic noradrenergic fibers from the stellate and inferior cervical ganglia innervate the sinoatrial (S-A) node and myocardial tissues of the atria and ventricles. Activation of the sympathetic outflow to the heart results in an increase in rate (*positive chronotropic effect*), in force of contraction (*positive inotropic effect*), and in conductivity of the atrioventricular (A-V) conduction tissue (*positive dromotropic effect*).

The postganglionic cholinergic fibers of the parasympathetic nervous system terminate in the S-A node, atria, and A-V conduction tissue. Cholinergic fibers do not innervate the ventricular muscle to any significant degree. Activation of the parasympathetic outflow to the heart results in a decrease in rate (*negative chronotropic effect*) and prolongation of A-V conduction time (*negative dromotropic effect*). There is a decrease in the contractile force of the atria but little effect on ventricular contractile force.

The effect of a drug on the heart depends on the balance of sympathetic and parasympathetic activity at the time the drug is administered. An example is the effect of the ganglionic blocking agents (see Chapter 14), which nonselectively inhibit transmission in both sympathetic and parasympathetic ganglia. Normally, during rest or mild activity, the heart is predominantly under the influence of the vagal parasympathetic system. Blockade of the autonomic innervation of the heart by the administration of a ganglionic blocking agent accelerates the heart rate. Conversely, if sympathetic activity is dominant, as in exercise, ganglionic blockade will decrease the heart rate and also reduce ventricular contractility. Likewise, the magnitude of effect of a drug antagonist of sympathetic activity will depend upon how much sympathetic activity exists at the time it is given. A similar relationship exists between parasympathetic antagonists and the level of parasympathetic activity.

Cardiovascular Reflexes

Any sudden alteration in the mean arterial blood pressure tends to produce compensatory reflex changes in heart rate, contractility, and vascular tone, which will oppose the initial pressure change and restore the homeostatic balance. The primary sensory mechanisms that detect changes in the mean arterial blood pressure are stretch receptors (*baroreceptors*) in the carotid sinus and aortic arch.

The injection of a vasoconstrictor, which causes an increase in mean arterial blood pressure, results in activation of the baroreceptors and increased neural input to the cardiovascular centers in the medulla oblongata. The reflex compensation for the drug-induced hypertension includes an increase in parasympathetic nerve activity and a decrease in sympathetic nerve activity. This combined alteration in neural firing reduces cardiac rate and force and the tone of vascular smooth muscle. As a consequence of the altered neural control of both the heart and the blood vessels, the rise in blood pressure induced by the drug is opposed and blunted.

Injection of a drug that causes a fall in the mean arterial blood pressure triggers diametrically opposite reflex changes. There is decreased impulse traffic from the cardiac inhibitory center, stimulation of the cardiac accelerator center, and augmented vasomotor center activity. These changes in cardiac and vasomotor center activity accelerate the heart and increase sympathetic transmission to the vasculature; thus, the drug-induced fall in blood pressure is opposed and blunted.

The Eye

Two sets of smooth muscle in the iris control the diameter of the pupil. One set of muscles, which is arranged radially (dilator pupillae), is innervated by sympathetic (noradrenergic) fibers that arise from cells in the superior cervical ganglion. Stimulation of them causes contraction of the radial smooth muscle cells, leading to dilation of the pupil (*mydriasis*). The other set of smooth muscle cells in the iris (constrictor pupillae) is circular and is innervated by parasympathetic neurons arising from cells in the ciliary ganglion. Stimulation of these cholinergic neurons causes contraction of the circular smooth muscle of the iris and constriction of the pupil (*miosis*).

The lens, which aids in visual accommodation, is attached at its lateral edge to the ciliary body by suspensory ligaments. When the smooth muscles of the ciliary body are relaxed, the ciliary body exerts tension on the lens, causing it to flatten. Thus, the eye is accommodated for far vision. Stimulation of parasympathetic cholinergic neurons, which arise in the ciliary ganglion, causes contraction of the smooth muscle of the ciliary body; this decreases the lateral tension on the lens. Naturally elastic, the lens thickens, and the eye accommodates for near vision. Drugs that block accommodation are called *cycloplegic*. Since the parasympathetic system is dominant in the eye, blockade of this system by atropine or of both autonomic systems by a ganglionic blocking agent will result in pupillary dilation and a loss of accommodative capacity.

Pulmonary Smooth Muscle

The bronchial tree is innervated by both divisions of the autonomic nervous system. Postganglionic parasympathetic neurons innervate bronchial smooth muscle directly and produce bronchoconstriction when stimulated. Sympathetic noradrenergic neurons appear to innervate vascular smooth muscle and parasympathetic ganglion cells. The effect of noradrenergic fibers on ganglion cells is to inhibit their firing. There is some controversy concerning the role of noradrenergic fibers in the regulation of airway smooth muscle tone. There is no doubt, however, that adrenoceptors are present on bronchial smooth muscle and that epinephrine from the adrenal gland and drugs such as epinephrine and isoproterenol produce bronchodilation of the airway.

Gastrointestinal Tract

The innervation of the gastrointestinal tract is complex. The myenteric and submucosal plexuses contain many interneurons. These possess a number of neurotransmitters and neuromodulators, including several peptides, such as enkephalins, substance P, and vasoactive intestinal peptide. Reflex activity within the plexuses regulates peristalsis and secretion locally. The effects of sympathetic and parasympathetic nerve stimulation are superimposed on this local neural regulation.

The myenteric and submucosal plexuses contain ganglion cells giving rise to excitatory cholinergic fibers that directly innervate the smooth muscle and gland cells of the gut. The sympathetic fibers that enter the gastrointestinal tract are postganglionic noradrenergic fibers, stimulation of which inhibits gut motility and gland secretion and contracts sphincters. Most of the noradrenergic fibers terminate either in blood vessels or on the cholinergic ganglionic cells of the intramural plexuses. These fibers alter gut motility by inhibiting acetylcholine release from the intramural nerves. Direct noradrenergic innervation of smooth muscle of the nonsphincter portion of the gut is sparse.

Salivary Glands

One exception to the generalization that the two systems work in opposition to each other is secretion by the salivary glands; both sympathetic (noradrenergic) and parasympathetic (cholinergic) activation of these glands leads to an increase in the flow of saliva. However, the nature of the saliva produced by the two systems is qualitatively different. The saliva produced by activation of the sympathetic system is a sparse, thick, mucinous secretion, whereas that produced by parasympathetic activation is a profuse, watery secretion.

THE ADRENAL MEDULLA

The cells of the adrenal medulla, called *chromaffin* cells, are homologous with sympathetic postganglionic neurons. The adrenal medulla may in fact be considered a modified sympathetic ganglion. The adrenal medulla secretes two hormones. One is norepinephrine, which is also the primary neurotransmitter of sympathetic postganglionic neurons. The other medullary hormone is epinephrine.

General activation of the sympathetic system during stress, fear, or anxiety is accompanied by increased secretion of adrenal medullary hormones, which consist primarily of epinephrine in the human. The secretory activity of the adrenal medulla is regulated by the CNS.

Some blood-borne substances of endogenous origin, such as histamine, angiotensin, and bradykinin, can directly stimulate the chromaffin cells to secrete epinephrine and norepinephrine. A variety of exogenously administered drugs, such as cholinomimetic agents and caffeine, can directly stimulate the secretion of adrenal medullary hormones. The neuronally induced secretion of medullary hormones is antagonized by ganglionic blocking agents.

TRANSMISSION OF THE NERVE IMPULSE

Microscopic studies of the structure of the terminal axons of the autonomic nerves have shown that the axons branch many times on entering the effector tissue, forming a plexus among the innervated cells. "Swollen" areas found at intervals along the terminal axons are referred to as *varicosities* (Figs. 9.2 and 9.3). Within each varicosity are mitochondria and numerous *vesicles* containing neurotransmitters.

The vesicles are intimately involved in the release of the transmitter into the *synaptic* or *neuroeffector cleft* in response to an action potential. Following release, the transmitter must diffuse to the effector cells, where it interacts with receptors on these cells to produce a response. The distance between the varicosities and the effector cells varies considerably from tissue to tissue. Smooth muscle, cardiac muscle, and exocrine gland cells do not contain morphologically specialized regions comparable to the end plate of skeletal muscle.

In the autonomic ganglia, the varicosities in the terminal branches of the preganglionic axons come into close contact primarily with the dendrites of the ganglionic cells and make synaptic connection with them.

STEPS IN NEUROCHEMICAL TRANSMISSION

Regardless of the type of neuron under consideration, the fundamental steps in chemical transmission are the same. Each of these steps is a potential site for pharmacological intervention in the normal transmission process:

1. Synthesis of the transmitter
2. Storage of the transmitter
3. Release of the transmitter by a nerve action potential
4. Interaction of the released transmitter with receptors on the effector cell membrane and the associated change in the effector cell
5. Rapid removal of the transmitter from the vicinity of the receptors
6. Recovery of the effector cell to the state that preceded transmitter action

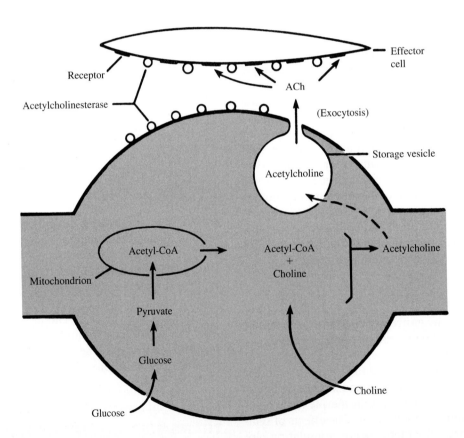

FIGURE 9.2
Varicosity showing processes of synthesis and storage of acetylcholine within a cholinergic neuron. Also shown are the release of acetylcholine (exocytosis) and the location of acetylcholinesterase, which inactivates acetylcholine.

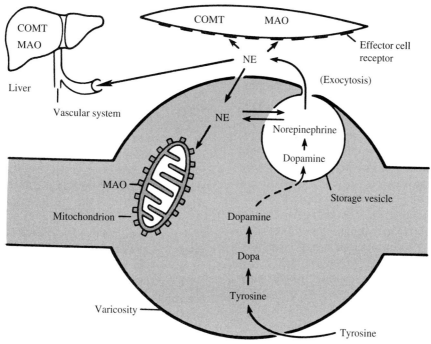

FIGURE 9.3

Varicosity of a noradrenergic neuron showing synthesis and storage of norepinephrine. Also shown is the release of norepinephrine (NE) and multiple routes for degradation. COMT, catechol-O-methyltransferase; MAO, monoamine oxidase.

Synthesis, Storage, Release, and Removal of Acetylcholine

The processes involved in neurochemical transmission in a cholinergic neuron are shown in Figure 9.2. The initial substrates for the synthesis of acetylcholine are *glucose* and *choline*. Glucose enters the neuron by means of facilitated transport. There is some disagreement as to whether choline enters cells by active or facilitated transport. Pyruvate derived from glucose is transported into mitochondria and converted to *acetylcoenzyme A* (*acetyl-CoA*). The acetyl-CoA is transported back into the cytosol. With the aid of the enzyme choline acetyltransferase, acetylcholine is synthesized from acetyl-CoA and choline. The acetylcholine is then transported into and stored within the storage vesicles by as yet unknown mechanisms.

Conduction of an action potential through the terminal branches of an axon causes depolarization of the varicosity membrane, resulting in the release of transmitter molecules via *exocytosis*. Once in the junctional extracellular space (biophase), acetylcholine interacts with cholinoreceptors.

A key factor in the process of exocytosis is the entry of extracellular calcium ions during the depolarization.

Modification of extracellular calcium concentration or of calcium entry therefore can markedly affect neurotransmission.

The interactions between transmitters and their receptors are readily reversible, and the number of transmitter–receptor complexes formed is a direct function of the amount of transmitter in the biophase. The length of time that intact molecules of acetylcholine remain in the biophase is short because *acetylcholinesterase*, an enzyme that rapidly hydrolyzes acetylcholine, is highly concentrated on the outer surfaces of both the prejunctional (neuronal) and postjunctional (effector cell) membranes. A rapid hydrolysis of acetylcholine by the enzyme results in a lowering of the concentration of free transmitter and a rapid dissociation of the transmitter from its receptors; little or no acetylcholine escapes into the circulation. Any acetylcholine that does reach the circulation is immediately inactivated by plasma esterases.

The rapid removal of transmitter is essential to the exquisite control of neurotransmission. As a consequence of rapid removal, the magnitude and duration of effect produced by acetylcholine are directly related to the frequency of transmitter release, that is, to the frequency of action potentials generated in the neuron.

Synthesis, Storage, Release, and Removal of Norepinephrine

Transmission in noradrenergic neurons is somewhat more complex, particularly in regard to the mechanisms by which the transmitter is removed from the biophase subsequent to its release. Noradrenergic transmission is represented diagrammatically in Figure 9.3.

Synthesis of norepinephrine begins with the amino acid *tyrosine*, which enters the neuron by active transport, perhaps facilitated by a permease. In the neuronal cytosol, tyrosine is converted by the enzyme *tyrosine hydroxylase* to *dihydroxyphenylalanine* (*dopa*), which is converted to *dopamine* by the enzyme *aromatic L–amino acid decarboxylase*, sometimes termed *dopa-decarboxylase*. The dopamine is actively transported into storage vesicles, where it is converted to norepinephrine (the transmitter) by *dopamine β-hydroxylase*, an enzyme within the storage vesicle.

In noradrenergic neurons, the end product is norepinephrine. In the adrenal medulla, the synthesis is carried one step further by the enzyme *phenylethanolamine N-methyltransferase*, which converts norepinephrine to epinephrine. The human adrenal medulla contains approximately four times as much epinephrine as norepinephrine. The absence of this enzyme in noradrenergic neurons accounts for the absence of significant amounts of epinephrine in noradrenergic neurons. The structures of these compounds are shown in Figure 9.4.

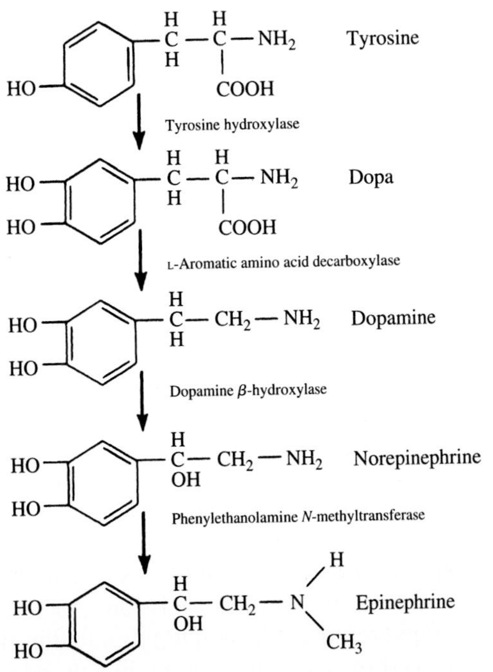

Since the enzyme that converts dopamine to norepinephrine (dopamine β-hydroxylase) is located only within the vesicles, the transport of dopamine into the vesicle is an essential step in the synthesis of norepinephrine. This same transport system is essential for the storage of norepinephrine. There is a tendency for norepinephrine to leak from the vesicles into the cytosol. If norepinephrine remains in the cytosol, much of it will be destroyed by a mitochondrial enzyme, *monoamine oxidase (MAO)*. However, most of the norepinephrine that leaks out of the vesicle is rapidly returned to the storage vesicles by the same transport system that carries dopamine into the storage vesicles. *It is important for a proper understanding of drug action to remember that this single transport system, called vesicular transport, is an essential element of both synthesis and storage of norepinephrine.*

Like the cholinergic transmitter, the noradrenergic transmitter is released by action potentials through exocytosis, the contents of entire vesicles being emptied into the biophase (synaptic or junctional region). Similarly, the formation of transmitter–receptor complexes is a direct function of the concentration of transmitter in the biophase and is readily reversible. In this instance, the receptors are adrenoceptors.

Three processes contribute to the removal of norepinephrine from the biophase:

1. Transport back into the noradrenergic neuron (*reuptake*), followed by either vesicular storage or by enzymatic inactivation by mitochondrial MAO. The transport of norepinephrine into the neurons is a sodium-facilitated process similar to that for choline transport.
2. Diffusion from the synapse into the circulation and ultimate enzymatic destruction in the liver and renal excretion.
3. Active transport of the released transmitter into effector cells (*extraneuronal uptake*) followed by enzymatic inactivation by catechol-*O*-methyltransferase.

The neuronal transport system is the most important mechanism for removing norepinephrine. Any norepinephrine or epinephrine in the circulation will equilibrate with the junctional extracellular fluid and thus become accessible both to the receptors and to neuronal transport. Thus, neuronal transport is also an important mechanism for limiting the effect and duration of action of norepinephrine or epinephrine, whether these are released from the adrenal medulla or are administered as drugs. *Neuronal uptake is primarily a mechanism for removing norepinephrine rather than conserving it.* Under most circumstances, synthesis of new norepinephrine is quite capable of keeping up with the needs of transmission, even in the complete absence of neuronal reuptake.

FIGURE 9.4
Steps in the synthetic pathway of epinephrine and norepinephrine.

It is important to make a clear distinction between neuronal and vesicular transport. *Neuronal transport* occurs from the junctional extracellular fluid (biophase) across the cell membrane of the neuron and into the neuronal cytosol. *Vesicular transport* is from the neuronal cytosol across the membrane of the vesicle and into the vesicle. Although these two systems readily transport both norepinephrine and epinephrine, certain drugs will selectively inhibit one or the other transport system.

The second most important mechanism for removing norepinephrine from the synapse is the escape of neuronally released norepinephrine into the general circulation and its metabolism in the liver. The liver has two enzymes that perform this function: *catechol-O-methyltransferase (COMT)* and *MAO*.

COMT is a specific enzyme, accepting only catechols as substrates. A catechol is a substance with two adjacent hydroxyl groups on an unsaturated six-member ring. The end result of the action of COMT is the *O*-methylation of the meta-hydroxyl group on the catechol nucleus. Figure 9.5 illustrates the action of COMT on norepinephrine or epinephrine. This reaction reduces the biological activity of norepinephrine or epinephrine at least 100-fold.

MAO is a much less discriminating enzyme in that it will catalyze the removal of an amine group from a variety of substrates. The action of MAO on norepinephrine and epinephrine also is indicated in Figure 9.5. The list of its substrates is very large, including endogenous substances (norepinephrine, epinephrine, dopamine, tyramine, 5-hydroxy-tryptamine) and many drugs that are amines. At least in the brain, two separate forms of MAO have been described: MAO type A and MAO type B. The two types are differentiated on the basis of substrate and inhibitor specificity.

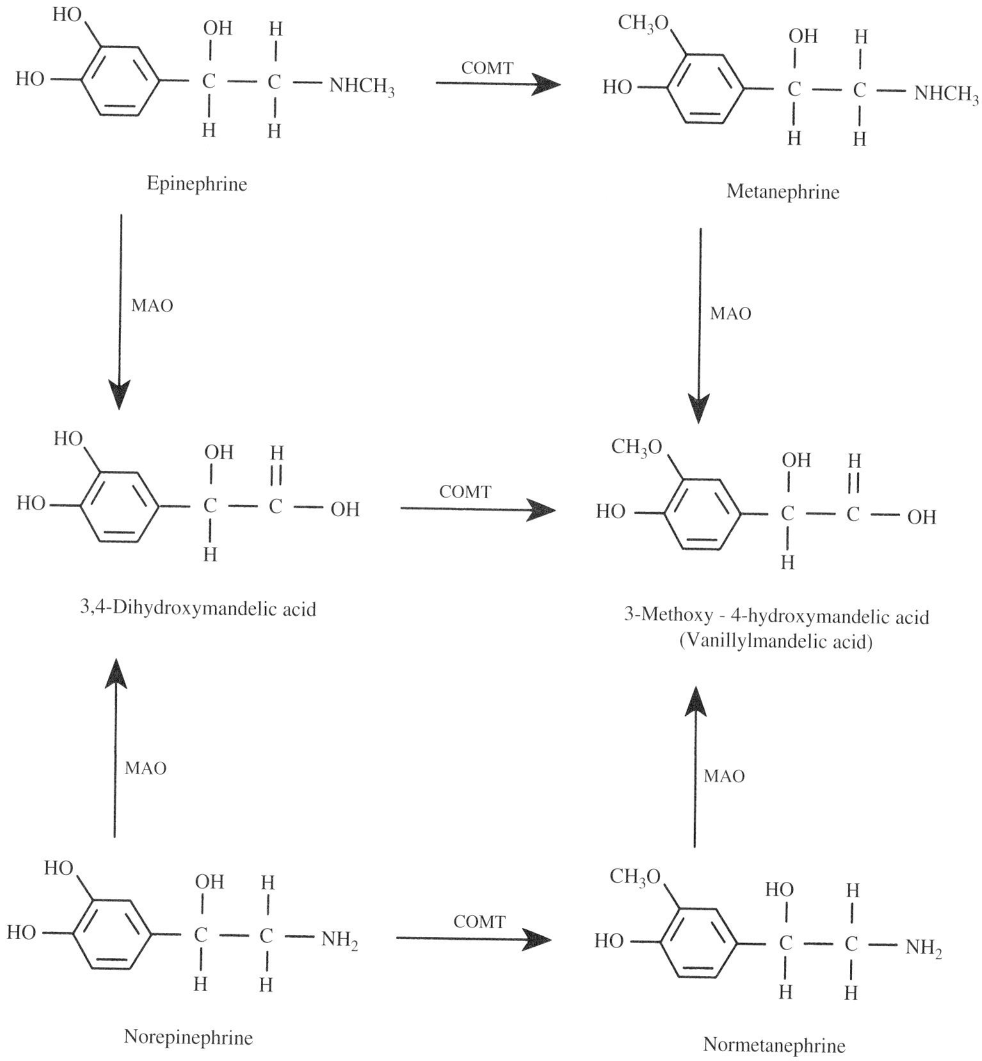

FIGURE 9.5

Primary route of metabolism of norepinephrine and epinephrine. COMT, catechol-*O*-methyltransferase; MAO, monoamine oxidase.

Although either COMT or MAO may act first on circulating norepinephrine or epinephrine, COMT is the more rapidly acting enzyme, and therefore more molecules are O-methylated and then deaminated than the reverse. Some norepinephrine and epinephrine appear unchanged in the urine. The larger portion, however, is metabolized and the products of metabolism excreted in the urine, often as conjugates.

Measurements of norepinephrine, epinephrine, and their metabolites in the urine constitute valuable diagnostic aids, particularly in the detection of tumors that synthesize and secrete norepinephrine and epinephrine (e.g., pheochromocytoma).

Catecholamines can be transported into effector cells (extraneuronal uptake). These cells generally contain both COMT and MAO. The combined processes of extraneuronal uptake and O-methylation are believed to be a minor but functionally significant, site of irreversible loss of catecholamines. The precise role of extraneuronal MAO in transmitter inactivation remains unknown.

RECEPTORS ON THE AUTONOMIC EFFECTOR CELLS

The receptors for acetylcholine and related drugs (cholinoreceptors) and for norepinephrine and related drugs (adrenoceptors) are different. Acetylcholine will not interact with receptors for norepinephrine, and norepinephrine will not interact with cholinoreceptors. These receptors are selective not only for their respective agonists but also for their respective antagonist drugs; that is, drugs that antagonize or block acetylcholine at cholinoreceptors will not antagonize norepinephrine at adrenoceptors and vice versa.

Cholinoceptors

The action of administered acetylcholine on effector systems innervated by parasympathetic postganglionic neurons (smooth muscle cells, cardiac muscle cells, and exocrine gland cells) resembled the actions produced by the naturally occurring plant alkaloid muscarine. The actions of both acetylcholine and muscarine on the visceral effectors are similar to those produced by parasympathetic nerve stimulation. Furthermore, the effects of acetylcholine, muscarine, and parasympathetic nerve stimulation on visceral effectors are antagonized by atropine, another plant alkaloid.

The administration of acetylcholine mimics the stimulatory effect of nicotine, the alkaloid from the tobacco plant, on autonomic ganglia and the adrenal medulla. It has become common practice to refer to the effects of acetylcholine on visceral effectors as the muscarinic action of acetylcholine and to its effects on the autonomic ganglia and adrenal medulla as the nicotinic action of acetylcholine. The respective receptors are called the muscarinic and nicotinic cholinoreceptors or the muscarinic and nicotinic receptors of acetylcholine.

The action of acetylcholine at the skeletal muscle motor end plate resembles that produced by nicotine. Thus, the cholinoreceptor on skeletal muscle is a nicotinic receptor. Based on antagonist selectivity, however, the autonomic and somatic nicotinic receptors are not pharmacologically identical (see Chapter 14).

Acetylcholine can stimulate a whole family of receptors. However, these receptors are sufficiently chemically diverse that different exogenous agonists and antagonists can distinguish among them. Great therapeutic benefit has been obtained from this diversity because it allows the development of therapeutic agents that can selectively mimic or antagonize actions of acetylcholine. Such a diversity of receptor subtypes exists for other neurotransmitters in addition to acetylcholine.

Adrenoceptors

Adrenoceptors interact not only with norepinephrine but also with the adrenal medullary hormone epinephrine and a number of chemically related drugs. However, the responses produced by the drugs in different autonomic structures differ quantitatively or qualitatively from one another.

On the basis of the observed selectivity of action among agonists and antagonists, it was proposed that two types of adrenoceptors exist. These were designated as α- and β-adrenoceptors. Subsequently, it has become necessary to classify the adrenoceptors further into α_1-, α_2-, β_1-, and β_2-receptor subtypes. Table 9.1 indicates present knowledge of the distribution of the subtypes of adrenoceptors in various tissues.

The α_1-adrenoceptors are located at postjunctional (postsynaptic) sites on tissues innervated by adrenergic neurons. α_2-Adrenoceptors having a presynaptic (i.e., neuronal) location are involved in the feedback inhibition of norepinephrine release from nerve terminals (discussed later). α_2-Receptors also can occur postjunctionally. The β_1-adrenoceptors are found chiefly in the heart and adipose tissue, while β_2-adrenoceptors are located in a number of sites, including bronchial smooth muscle and skeletal muscle blood vessels, and are associated with smooth muscle relaxation.

Activation of α_1-adrenoceptors in smooth muscle of blood vessels leads to vasoconstriction, while activation of β_2-adrenoceptors in blood vessels of skeletal muscle produces vasodilation. Activation of β_1-adrenoceptors on cardiac tissue produces an increase in the heart rate and contractile force.

Norepinephrine and epinephrine are potent α-adrenoceptor agonists, while isoproterenol, a synthetic

TABLE 9.1   Responses to Adrenergic and Cholinergic Nerve Stimulation

Organ or Tissue Function	Predominant Adrenoceptor Type	Adrenergic Response	Cholinergic Response[a]
Heart[b]			
Rate (chronotropic effect)	β_1	Increase	Decrease
Contractile force (inotropic effect)	β_1	Increase	None
Conduction velocity (dromotropic effect)	β_1	Increase	Decrease
Eye			
Pupil size	α_1	Constriction of radial muscle causing dilation (mydriasis)	Contraction of circular muscle (miosis)
Accommodation		No innervation	Contraction of ciliary muscle producing accommodation for near vision
Bronchial smooth muscle	β_2	Relaxation	Contraction
Blood vessels (arteries and arterioles)[c]			
Cutaneous	α_1	Constriction	No innervation[e]
Visceral	α_1	Constriction	No innervation[e]
Pulmonary	α_1	Constriction	No innervation[e]
Skeletal muscle	α_1, β_2	Constriction[d]	No innervation[e]
Coronary	α_1, β	Constriction, dilation[f]	No innervation[e]
Cerebral	α_1	Constriction	
Veins	α_1	Constriction	No innervation
Gastrointestinal tract (tone, motility, and secretory activity)	α_2, β_2	Decrease[g]	Increase
Sphincters	α	Contraction	Relaxation
Splenic capsule	α_1	Contraction	No innervation
Urinary bladder			
Detrusor muscle	β	Relaxation	Contraction
Trigone-sphincter muscle	α_1	Contraction	Relaxation
Uterus	α_1, β_2	Contraction-relaxation[h]	Contraction-relaxation
Glycogenolysis			
Skeletal muscle	β_2	Increase	None
Liver	α_1, β_2	Increase	None
Lipolysis	β_1	Increase	None
Renin secretion	β_1	Increase	None
Insulin secretion	α_2	Decrease	Increase

[a]Muscarinic cholinoceptors. See Chapter 12 for a discussion of subtypes.
[b]There are some β_2-receptors in the heart. The ratio of β_1 to β_2 varies with the region and the species. In the human heart, the ratio of β_1 to β_2 is about 3:2 in atria and 4:1 in ventricles.
[c]There are some α_2-receptors in some vascular smooth muscle.
[d]Low doses of epinephrine of endogenous or exogenous origin plus other β_2-receptor agonists dilate these blood vessels.
[e]Exogenously administered cholinergic drugs dilate these blood vessels.
[f]Dilation is the dominant in vivo response, owing to indirect effects.
[g]α_2-Adrenoceptors may be involved in hypersecretory responses.
[h]Responses depend on hormonal state.

adrenomimetic, is selective for β_1- and β_2-adrenoceptors. Norepinephrine and epinephrine are thus potent vasoconstrictors of vascular beds that contain predominantly α-adrenoceptors, while isoproterenol has little effect in these vessels.

Isoproterenol and epinephrine are potent β_2-adrenoceptor agonists; norepinephrine is a relatively weak β_2-adrenoceptor agonist. Isoproterenol and epinephrine produce vasodilation in skeletal muscle, but norepinephrine does not; rather it produces vasoconstriction through the α_1-adrenoceptors. Isoproterenol,

epinephrine, and norepinephrine are potent β_1-adrenoceptor agonists; thus, all three can stimulate the heart (Table 9.1).

The existence of a β_3-adrenoceptor has recently been demonstrated in human adipose tissue along with the β_1-adrenoceptor. This observation raises the possibility that eventually therapeutic drugs may selectively alter lipid metabolism and therefore provide therapeutic management of obesity. The β_3-receptor and the recently identified subtypes within the α_1- and α_2-receptor groups (α_{1A}, α_{1B}, etc.) also have not been included in the table, since as yet few therapeutic drugs distinguish among these further subtypes. One exception is tamsulosin, an antagonist with some selectivity for α_{1A}-receptors in the urinary tract.

Presynaptic Receptors

Presynaptic or *prejunctional receptors* are located on the presynaptic nerve endings and function to control the amount of transmitter released per nerve impulse and in some instances to affect the rate of transmitter synthesis through some as yet undetermined feedback mechanism. For instance, during repetitive nerve stimulation, when the concentration of transmitter released into the synaptic or junctional cleft is relatively high, the released transmitter may activate presynaptic receptors and thereby reduce the further release of transmitter. Such an action may prevent excessive and prolonged stimulation of the postsynaptic cell. In this case, the activation of the presynaptic receptor would be part of a *negative feedback mechanism.*

The presynaptic receptors may have pharmacological significance, since several drugs may act in part either by preventing the transmitter from reaching the presynaptic receptor, thus causing excessive transmitter release, or by directly stimulating presynaptic receptors and thereby diminishing the amount of transmitter released per impulse.

The inhibitory presynaptic α-adrenoceptors found on noradrenergic neurons are of the α_2-subtype. Adrenoceptors of the β_2 subclass also occur presynaptically, and activation of these receptors leads to enhanced norepinephrine release. The physiological and pharmacological importance of these presynaptic β_2-receptors is less certain than it is for presynaptic α_2-receptors.

Presynaptic receptors for nonadrenomimetic substances (e.g., acetylcholine, adenosine) also have been found on the sympathetic presynaptic nerve ending. Their importance and role in the modulation of neurotransmission have not been definitively established.

PHARMACOLOGICAL INTERVENTION IN NEUROTRANSMISSION

The drugs listed in Table 9.2 affect specific steps in cholinergic or adrenergic transmission. These and many other drugs that alter transmission are discussed in subsequent chapters.

TABLE 9.2 Drugs that interfere with Specific Steps in Chemical Transmission

Transmission Step	Adrenergic Nerves	Cholinergic Nerves
Synthesis of transmitter	α-Methyldopa	Hemicholinium
Storage of transmitter	Reserpine	None known
Release of transmitter	Guanethidine	Botulinum toxin
Combination of transmitter with receptor	Prazosin (α-receptors)	Atropine (muscarinic receptors)
	Propranolol (β-receptors)	d-Tubocurarine (nicotinic receptors)
Destruction or removal of transmitter from site of action	Tolcapone (COMT inhibitor)	Physostigmine (cholinesterase inhibitor)
	Phenelzine (MAO inhibitor)	
	Tricyclic antidepressants (inhibit neuronal transport)	
Recovery of postsynaptic cell from the effects of the transmitter	None known	Succinylcholine

COMT, catechol-*O*-methyltransferase; MAO, monoamine oxidase.

Study QUESTIONS

1. All of the following types of cells are innervated by the autonomic nervous system EXCEPT:
   (A) Smooth muscle of blood vessels
   (B) Skeletal muscle
   (C) Sinoatrial node
   (D) Salivary glands
   (E) Intestinal smooth muscle

2. All of the following structures have a significant cholinergic innervation EXCEPT:
   (A) Ventricular wall
   (B) Sinoatrial node
   (C) Atrioventricular node
   (D) Bladder
   (E) Ileum

3. The radial smooth muscle of the iris is innervated by:
   (A) Primarily sympathetic noradrenergic neurons
   (B) Primarily sympathetic cholinergic neurons
   (C) Primarily parasympathetic noradrenergic neurons
   (D) Primarily parasympathetic cholinergic neurons
   (E) Equally by sympathetic and parasympathetic neurons
4. The receptors on the skeletal muscle end plate respond to:
   (A) Acetylcholine and muscarine
   (B) Acetylcholine and nicotine
   (C) Acetylcholine, muscarine, and nicotine
   (D) Only muscarine of the three choices in C
   (E) Only nicotine of the three choices in C
5. α_1-Adrenoceptors are prominently involved in which one of the following?
   (A) Cardiac acceleration
   (B) Intestinal relaxation
   (C) Cardiac contractility
   (D) Presynaptic inhibition
   (E) Vasoconstriction
6. Smooth muscle relaxation is most associated with which one of the following adrenoceptors?
   (A) β_1
   (B) β_2
   (C) β_3
   (D) α_1
   (E) α_2

ANSWERS

1. **B.** Skeletal muscle is innervated by the somatic nervous system. All other choices are tissues that are innervated by the autonomic nervous system.
2. **A.** Cholinergic fibers do not innervate the ventricular muscles, although there is significant cholinergic innervation to the SA node (B) and the AV node (C). The gastrointestinal tract, including the ileum (E), is extensively innervated by cholinergic fibers, as is the bladder (D).
3. **A.** Stimulation of the sympathetic noradrenergic neurons to the iris causes contraction of the radial smooth muscle and dilation of the pupil (mydriasis).

4. **B.** The receptor on skeletal muscle end plate is characterized as a nicotinic receptor. It responds to both nicotine and to acetylcholine. It does not respond to muscarine; that is, it is not a muscarinic receptor.
5. **E.** α_1-Receptors are prominent in smooth muscle of blood vessels; activation of these receptors leads to vasoconstriction. Cardiac acceleration (A) and cardiac contraction (C) are primarily due to β_1-receptor stimulation. Intestinal relaxation occurs as a result of stimulation of α_1- and β_1-receptor stimulation.
6. **B.** Smooth muscle relaxation is primarily under the influence of the sympathetic nervous system. This control is primarily through β_2-receptors. β_1-Receptors are found chiefly in the heart and adipose tissue. α_1-Receptors are at postjuctional sites on tissues innervated by adrenergic neurons. α_2-Receptors are usually presynaptic, while β_3-adrenoceptors appear to be primarily in adipose tissue.

SUPPLEMENTAL READING

Appenzeller O. The Autonomic Nervous System (4th ed.). Amsterdam: Elsevier, 1990.
Ciriello J et al. Organization of the Autonomic Nervous System: Central and Peripheral Mechanisms. New York: Liss, 1987.
Furness JB and Costa M. The Enteric Nervous System. New York: Churchill Livingstone, 1987.
Hieble JR et al. Recommendation for nomenclature of α_1-adrenoceptors: Consensus update. Pharmacol Rev1995;47:267–270.
International Union of Pharmacology. The IUPHAR Compendium of Receptor Characterization and Classification (2nd ed.) London: IUPHAR Media, 2000.
Limbird, LE (ed). The Alpha-2 Adrenergic Receptors. Clifton, NJ: Humana, 1988.
Perkins, JD (ed). The Beta-Adrenergic Receptors. Clifton, NJ: Humana, 1991.

10 | Adrenomimetic Drugs

Tony J.-F. Lee and Robert E. Stitzel

 DRUG LIST

GENERIC NAME	PAGE	GENERIC NAME	PAGE
Albuterol	105	Isoproterenol	102
Amphetamine	106	Metaraminol	105
Dobutamine	105	Methoxamine	105
Dopamine	103	Norepinephrine	101
Ephedrine	105	Phenylephrine	105
Epinephrine	101	Terbutaline	105

The *adrenomimetic drugs* mimic the effects of adrenergic sympathetic nerve stimulation on sympathetic effectors; these drugs are also referred to as *sympathomimetic agents*. The adrenergic transmitter norepinephrine and the adrenal medullary hormone epinephrine also are included under this broad heading. The adrenomimetic drugs are an important group of therapeutic agents that can be used to maintain blood pressure or to relieve a life-threatening attack of acute bronchial asthma. They are also present in many over-the-counter cold preparations because they constrict mucosal blood vessels and thus relieve nasal congestion.

CHEMISTRY

The adrenomimetic drugs can be divided into two major groups on the basis of their chemical structure: the catecholamines and the noncatecholamines. The catecholamines include norepinephrine, epinephrine, and dopamine, all of which are naturally occurring, and several synthetic substances, the most important of which is isoproterenol (isopropyl norepinephrine). The skele-

tal structure of the catecholamines is shown in Figure 10.1.

The L-isomers are the naturally occurring forms of epinephrine and norepinephrine and possess considerably greater pharmacological effects than do the D-isomers. Throughout most of the world, epinephrine and norepinephrine are known as *adrenaline* and *noradrenaline,* respectively.

Noncatecholamine adrenomimetic drugs differ from the basic catecholamine structure primarily by having substitutions on their benzene ring.

MECHANISM OF ACTION

Many adrenomimetic drugs produce responses by interacting with the adrenoceptors on sympathetic effector cells. An examination of Table 9.1 reveals that sympathetic effectors have activity at α_1-, α_2-, β_1-, or β_2-adrenoreceptors or in some cases, combinations of these adrenoceptors. Adrenomimetic drugs vary in their affinities for each subgroup of adrenoceptors. Some, like epinephrine, have a high affinity for all of the adrenocep-

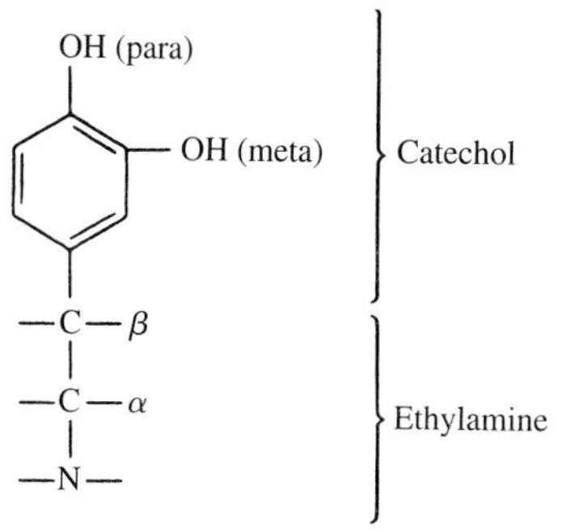

OH (para)

—— OH (meta) } Catechol

—C—β
—C—α } Ethylamine
—N—

FIGURE 10.1
Skeletal structure of catecholamines.

tors. Others are relatively selective. For example, isoproterenol has a high affinity for β_1- and β_2-adrenoceptors but a very low affinity for α-adrenoceptors; isoproterenol is considered a nearly pure β-agonist. Norepinephrine has a high affinity for α- and β_1-adrenoceptors but a relatively low affinity for β_2-receptors.

The effect of a given adrenomimetic drug on a particular type of effector cell depends on the receptor selectivity of the drug, the response characteristics of the effector cells, and the predominant type of adrenoceptor found on the cells. For example, the smooth muscle cells of many blood vessels have only or predominantly α-adrenoceptors. The interaction of compounds with these adrenoceptors initiates a chain of events in the vascular smooth muscle cells that leads to activation of the contractile process. Thus, norepinephrine and epinephrine, which have high affinities for α-adrenoceptors, cause the vascular muscle to contract and the blood vessels to constrict. Since bronchial smooth muscle contains β_2-adrenoceptors, the response in this tissue elicited by the action of β_2-adrenoceptor agonists is relaxation of smooth muscle cells. Epinephrine and isoproterenol, which have high affinities for β_2-adrenoceptors, cause relaxation of bronchial smooth muscle. Norepinephrine has a lower affinity for β_2-adrenoceptors and has relatively weak bronchiolar relaxing properties.

Adrenomimetic drugs can be divided into two major groups on the basis of their mechanism of action. Norepinephrine, epinephrine, and some closely related adrenomimetics produce responses in effector cells by directly stimulating α- or β-adrenoceptors and are referred to as *directly acting* adrenomimetic drugs.

Many other adrenomimetic drugs, such as amphetamine, do not themselves interact with adrenoceptors, yet they produce sympathetic effects by releasing norepinephrine from neuronal storage sites (vesicles). The norepinephrine that is released by these compounds interacts with the receptors on the effector cells. These adrenomimetics are called *indirectly acting* adrenomimetic drugs. *The effects elicited by indirectly acting drugs resemble those produced by norepinephrine.*

An important characteristic of indirectly acting adrenomimetic drugs is that repeated injections or prolonged infusion can lead to *tachyphylaxis* (gradually diminished responses to repeated administration). This is a result of a gradually diminishing availability of releasable norepinephrine stores on repeated drug administration. The time frame of the tachyphylaxis will vary with individual agents.

The actions of many indirectly acting adrenomimetic drugs are reduced or abolished by the prior administration of either cocaine or tricyclic antidepressant drugs (e.g., imipramine). These compounds can block the adrenergic neuronal transport system and thereby prevent the indirectly acting drug from being taken up into the nerve and reaching the norepinephrine storage vesicles. Lipophilic drugs (e.g., amphetamine), however, can enter nerves by diffusion and do not need membrane transport systems.

Destruction or surgical interruption of the adrenergic nerves leading to an effector tissue renders indirectly acting adrenomimetic drugs ineffective because neuronal norepinephrine is no longer available for release since the nerves have degenerated. Also, patients being treated for hypertension with reserpine or guanethidine, which deplete the norepinephrine stores in adrenergic neurons (see Chapter 20), respond poorly to administration of indirectly acting adrenomimetic drugs.

Some adrenomimetic drugs act both directly and indirectly; that is, they release some norepinephrine from storage sites and also directly activate tissue receptors. Such drugs are called *mixed-action* adrenomimetics. However, most therapeutically important adrenomimetic drugs in humans act either directly or indirectly.

Structure–Activity Relationships Among Adrenomimetic Drugs

The nature of the substitutions made on the basic phenylethylamine skeleton at the para and meta positions of the benzene ring or on the β-carbon of the side chain determine whether an adrenomimetic drug will act directly or indirectly. Directly acting adrenomimetic drugs, which have two or more carbon atoms (e.g., isoproterenol) added to their amino group, are virtually pure β-adrenoceptor agonists. Directly acting drugs, which have only small substitutions on their amino groups (e.g., norepinephrine and epinephrine), are usually α-adrenoceptor agonists, but may be β-adrenoceptor agonists as well. Norepinephrine has very weak actions on β_2-adrenoceptors but strong β_1-adrenoceptor actions. Epinephrine has a high affinity for both β_1- and β_2-adrenoceptors.

Adrenomimetic drugs with no substitutions on their benzene ring (e.g., amphetamine and ephedrine) are generally quite lipid soluble, readily cross the blood-brain barrier, and can cause central nervous system (CNS) stimulation.

The structure of a particular adrenomimetic drug will influence its susceptibility to metabolism by catechol-*O*-methyltransferase (COMT) and monoamine oxidase (MAO). The actions of COMT are specific for the catechol structure. If either the meta or para hydroxyl group is absent, COMT will not metabolize the drug. The presence of a substitution, such as a methyl group, on the α-carbon of the side chain reduces the affinity of the adrenomimetic drug for MAO. Also, drugs with a large substitution on the terminal nitrogen will not be degraded by MAO. A noncatecholamine that has a methyl group attached to its α-carbon will not be metabolized by either enzyme and will have a greatly prolonged duration of action (e.g., amphetamine).

The Role of Second Messengers in Receptor-mediated Responses

The adrenomimetic drugs, including the naturally occurring catecholamines, initiate their responses by combining with α-, β-, or dopamine adrenoceptors. This interaction triggers a series of biochemical events starting within the effector cell membrane that eventually culminates in the production of a physiological response,

for example contraction, secretion, relaxation, or altered metabolism. The total process of converting the action of an external signal (e.g., norepinephrine interacting with its receptor) to a physiological response (e.g., vascular smooth muscle contraction) is called *signal transduction.*

Following the binding of the agonist (the first *messenger*) to its appropriate receptor on the external surface of the effector cell, a *second messenger* is generated (or synthesized) and participates in a particular series of biochemical reactions that ultimately result in the generation of a specific physiological response by that cell (Figs. 10.2 and 10.3). For both α- and β-adrenoceptors, the signal transduction process seems to involve the participation of G proteins (see Chapter 2).

The specific second-messenger pathways constitute a highly versatile signaling system that can modify (stimulate or inhibit) numerous cellular processes including secretion, contraction and relaxation, metabolism, neuronal excitability, cell growth, and apoptosis. The second messengers that participate in signal transduction include *cyclic adenosine monophosphate (cAMP), diacylglycerol,* and *inositol triphosphate.* Once liberated within the cell, second messengers will activate specific

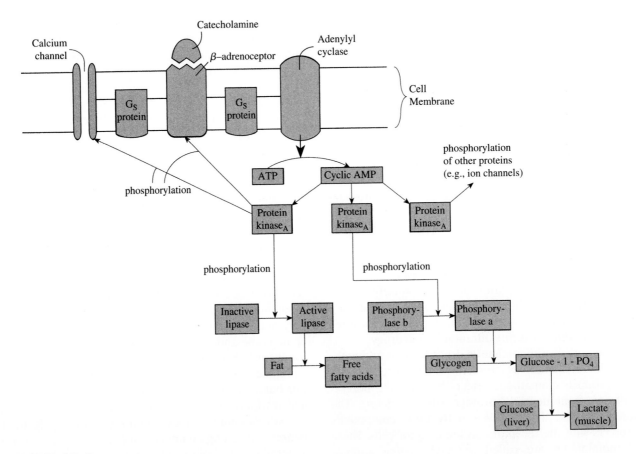

FIGURE 10.2
The role of cyclic 3′,5′-adenosine monophosphate (cAMP) as a second messenger in the actions of catecholamines acting on β-receptors. ATP, adenosine triphosphate.

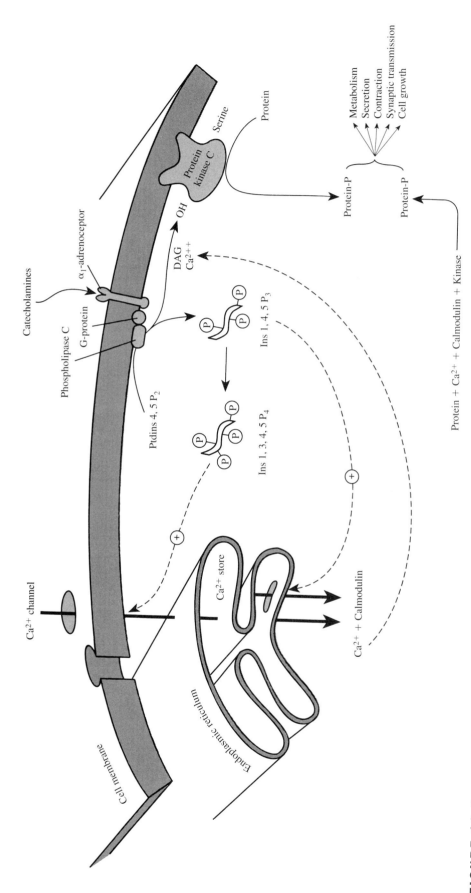

FIGURE 10.3

The role of diacylglycerol (DAG) and inositol triphosphate (Ins 1,4,5 P$_3$) as second messengers linked to agonist-receptor (α_1-adrenoceptor) interactions. Ptdins 4,5 P$_2$ is a phosphatidylinositol precursor in cell membranes that is hydrolyzed following receptor activation to form the two second messengers, Ins 1,4,5 P$_3$ and DAG. Once liberated within the cell, these second messengers activate separate but interacting pathways. Ins 1,4,5 P$_3$ releases Ca^{++} stored in cells and can be phosphorylated to form a tetraphosphate (Ins 1,3,4,5 P$_4$), which can open Ca^{++} channels in the membrane. DAG triggers protein phosphorylation through the activation of protein kinase C. Ca^{++}-induced activation of the enzyme calmodulin also phosphorylates protein. Adenylyl cyclase traverses the membrane. Cyclic AMP–dependent protein kinase can phosphorylate and inactivate the β-adrenoceptors. This kinase may have a role in homologous desensitization of G$_s$-protein–coupled β-adrenoceptors. β-Receptor stimulation can (1) activate Ca^{++} channels through an action of G$_s$ proteins without the participation of cAMP and (2) affect other ion channels through phosphorylation via kinases. (Modified from Berridge MJ. Inositol triphosphate and diacylglycerol: Two interacting second messengers. ISI Atlas of Science: Pharmacology, 1:91, 1987.)

signal pathways. For example, inositol triphosphate functions by mobilizing calcium from intracellular stores or opening channels; the calcium can be used to initiate vascular smooth muscle contraction, probably through a protein phosphorylation pathway (Fig. 10.3). Diacylglycerol is known to stimulate an enzyme, protein kinase C, that phosphorylates specific intracellular proteins, some of which regulate ionic mechanisms such as the Na^+/H^+ exchanger and potassium channels.

The basic features of the signaling system found in different cells are remarkably similar. It appears that protein phosphorylation is a final common pathway in the molecular mechanisms through which neurotransmitters, hormones, and the nerve impulse produce many of their biological effects in target cells.

PHARMACODYNAMIC ACTIONS OF NOREPINEPHRINE, EPINEPHRINE, AND ISOPROTERENOL

Vascular Effects

The cardiovascular effects of norepinephrine, epinephrine, and isoproterenol are shown in Table 10.1. Differences in the action of these three catecholamines on various vascular beds are due both to the different affinities possessed by the catecholamines for α- and β-adrenoceptors and to differences in the relative distribution of the receptors in a particular vascular bed. The hemodynamic responses of the major vascular beds to these amines are shown in Table 10.2.

The blood vessels of the skin and mucous membranes predominantly contain α-adrenoceptors. Both epinephrine and norepinephrine produce a powerful constriction in these tissues, substantially reducing blood flow through them. Isoproterenol, which is almost a pure β-adrenoceptor agonist, has little effect on the vasculature of the skin and mucous membranes. The blood vessels in visceral organs, including the kidneys, contain predominantly α-adrenoceptors, although some β$_2$-adrenoceptors are also present. Consequently, epinephrine and norepinephrine cause vasoconstriction and reduced blood flow through the kidneys and other visceral organs. Isoproterenol produces either no effect or weak vasodilation.

The blood vessels in skeletal muscle contain both α- and β$_2$-adrenoceptors. Norepinephrine constricts these blood vessels and reduces blood flow through an interaction with α-adrenoceptors. Isoproterenol dilates the vessels in skeletal muscle and consequently increases blood flow through the tissue by interaction with the β$_2$-adrenoceptors. Epinephrine has a more complex ac-

TABLE 10.1   Cardiovascular Effects of Catecholamines in Humans (in therapeutic doses of 0.1-0.4 μg/kg/min IV or 0.5–1.0 mg SC)

Cardiovascular function	Epinephrine	Norepinephrine	Isoproterenol
Systolic blood pressure	+ +	+ + +	0+
Diastolic blood pressure	−	+ +	− −
Mean blood pressure	+0−	+ +	− −
Total peripheral resistance	− −	+ + +	− − −
Heart rate (chronotropic effect)	+	−	+ +
Stroke output (inotropic effect)	+ +	+	+ +
Cardiac output	+ + +	−0	+ + +

Key: 0 = no effect; + = increased; − = decreased. The number of symbols indicates the approximate magnitude of the response.

TABLE 10.2   Response of the Major Vascular Beds to Usual Doses of the Catecholamines

Vascular bed	Receptor type*	Norepinephrine	Epinephrine	Isoproterenol
Cutaneous blood vessels	α	Constriction	Constriction	None
Visceral blood vessels	α	Constriction	Constriction	None (weak dilation)
Renal blood vessels	α	Constriction	Constriction	None (weak dilation)
Coronary blood vessels	α, β	Dilation	Dilation	Dilation
Skeletal muscle blood vessels	α, β$_2$	Constriction	Dilation	Dilation
Pial blood vessels	α, β$_1$	Constriction/dilation	Constriction/dilation	Dilation

*While virtually all blood vessels have α$_1$-receptors, some also have α$_2$-receptors. Stimulation of either subtype generally results in vasoconstriction.

tion on these blood vessels because of its high affinity for both α- and β$_2$-adrenoceptors. Whether epinephrine produces vasodilation or vasoconstriction in skeletal muscle depends on the dose administered. Low doses of epinephrine will dilate the blood vessels; larger doses will constrict them.

Although several factors can influence the flow of blood through the coronary vessels, the most important of these is the local production of vasodilator metabolites that results from stimulation-induced increased work by the heart. α-Adrenoreceptors and β-adrenoceptors in the coronary vascular beds do not play a major role in determining the vasodilator effects of the administration of epinephrine or norepinephrine.

Effects on the Intact Cardiovascular System

An increase in sympathetic neuronal activity causes an increase in heart rate (positive chronotropic effect, or tachycardia) and an increase in cardiac contractile force (positive inotropic effect) such that the stroke output is increased. Cardiac output, which is a function of rate and stroke output, is thus increased. *A physiological increase in sympathetic tone is almost always accompanied by a diminution of parasympathetic vagal tone;* this allows full expression of the effects of increased sympathetic tone on the activity of the heart.

An increase in sympathetic tone constricts blood vessels in most vascular beds and therefore causes a net increase in total peripheral resistance. Increased sympathetic tone increases neural release of norepinephrine and its interaction both with β-adrenoceptors on cardiac cells and with α-adrenoceptors on vascular smooth muscle cells. As a consequence, the systolic and diastolic blood pressures are elevated. It follows that the mean arterial blood pressure must also be increased.

Norepinephrine

Norepinephrine, administered to a normotensive adult either subcutaneously or by slow intravenous injection, constricts most blood vessels. Venules as well as arterioles are constricted. As a consequence, there is a net increase in the total peripheral resistance.

The effects of norepinephrine on cardiac function are complex because of the dynamic interaction of the direct effects of norepinephrine on the heart and the initiation of powerful cardiac reflexes. The baroreceptor reflexes are discussed in detail in Chapter 9.

Important considerations are as follows: (1) *The direct effect of norepinephrine on the heart is stimulatory.* (2) *The reflex initiated is inhibitory,* that is, opposite to the direct effect. (3) The reflex varies with the level of sympathetic and parasympathetic activity just before the initiation of the reflex. (4) The distribution of sympathetic and parasympathetic nerves is not uniform in the heart.

The net effect of norepinephrine administration on heart rate and ventricular contractile force therefore varies with the dose of norepinephrine, the physical activity of the subject, any prior cardiovascular and baroreceptor pathology, and the presence of other drugs that may alter reflexes.

In a normal resting subject who is receiving no drugs, there is a moderate parasympathetic tone to the heart, and sympathetic activity is relatively low. *The ventricular muscle receives little, if any, parasympathetic innervation.* As the blood pressure rises in response to norepinephrine, the baroreceptor reflex is activated, parasympathetic impulses (which are inhibitory) to the heart increase in frequency, and what little sympathetic outflow there is may be reduced. Heart rate is slowed so much that the direct effect of norepinephrine to increase the rate is masked and there is a *net* decrease in rate. Under the conditions described, however, the impact of the reflex on the ventricles is very slight because there is no parasympathetic innervation and the preexisting level of sympathetic activity is already low. A further decrease in sympathetic activity therefore would have little further effect on contractility in this subject. Thus, a decrease in heart rate and an increase in stroke volume will occur, and cardiac output will change very little.

The reflex nature of the bradycardia induced by parenterally administered norepinephrine can readily be demonstrated by administration of atropine, a cholinoreceptor antagonist. Atropine abolishes the compensatory vagal reflexes. Under conditions of vagal blockade, the direct cardiac stimulatory effects of norepinephrine are unmasked. There is marked tachycardia, an increase in stroke volume, and as a consequence, a marked increase in cardiac output (Fig. 10.4).

Epinephrine

A small dose of epinephrine causes a fall in mean and diastolic pressure with little or no effect on systolic pressure. This is due to the net decrease in total peripheral resistance that results from the predominance of vasodilation in the skeletal muscle vascular bed. The intravenous infusion or subcutaneous administration of epinephrine in the range of doses used in humans generally increases the systolic pressure, but the diastolic pressure is decreased. Therefore, the mean pressure may decrease, remain unchanged, or increase slightly, depending on the balance between the rise in systolic and fall in diastolic blood pressures (Fig. 10.4).

The cardiac effects of epinephrine are due to its action on β-adrenoceptors in the heart. The rate and contractile force of the heart are increased; consequently, cardiac output is markedly increased. Because total peripheral resistance is decreased, the increase in cardiac output is largely responsible for the increase in systolic pressure. Since epinephrine causes little change in the

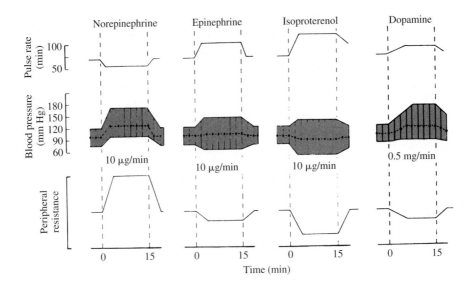

FIGURE 10.4

Cardiovascular effects of infusion of norepinephrine, epinephrine, isoproterenol, and dopamine in humans. Infusions were made intravenously during the time indicated by the broken lines. Heart rate is given in beats per minute, blood pressure in millimeters of mercury, and peripheral resistance in arterial blood pressure. (Reprinted with permission from Allwood MJ, Cobbald AF, and Ginsburg J. Peripheral vascular effects of noradrenaline, isopropyl-noradrenaline, and dopamine. Br Med Bull 19:132, 1963. Reproduced by permission of the Medical Department, The British Council.

mean arterial blood pressure, reflex slowing of the heart is usually not seen in humans.

Isoproterenol

Slow intravenous infusion of therapeutic doses of isoproterenol in humans produces a marked decrease in total peripheral resistance, owing to the predominance of vasodilation in skeletal muscle vascular beds. As a consequence, diastolic and mean blood pressures fall (Fig. 10.4). The depressor action of isoproterenol is more pronounced than that of epinephrine because isoproterenol causes no vasoconstriction, whereas epinephrine does in some vascular beds. Systolic blood pressure may remain unchanged or may increase. When an increase in systolic blood pressure is seen, it is due to the marked increase in cardiac output produced by isoproterenol.

Isoproterenol usually increases the heart rate and stroke volume more than does epinephrine. This is partly due to its ability to decrease mean blood pressure, which then reflexively diminishes vagal activity, and partly to its action on the heart.

Effects on Vascular Smooth Muscle

Postjunctional α_1-adrenoceptors are always found in veins, arteries, and arterioles. Activation of these receptors results in the entry of extracellular calcium through receptor-operated channels and in the release of intracellularly stored calcium; this is brought about through the participation of the inositol triphosphate second-

messenger system. This system plays an important role in the regulation of blood pressure and vascular tone.

Vascular endothelium also plays an important role in maintaining vascular tone. The endothelium can modulate both vasodilation and vasoconstriction through its ability to locally synthesize and release vasodilators such as nitric oxide, endothelium-derived hyperpolarizing factor, and PGI_2, and vasoconstrictors such as endothelin, which in turn directly affect vascular smooth muscle activity. Stimulation of α_2-adrenoceptors located on the endothelial cells in certain vascular beds (such as the coronary artery) results in the release of nitric oxide and vasodilation.

In any blood vessel, the final integrated response to either neuronally released norepinephrine or to circulating epinephrine probably depends on the relative participation of at least four populations of α-adrenoceptors: postjunctional α_1- and α_2-adrenoceptors mediate constriction of vascular smooth muscle, while prejunctional and endothelial α_2-adrenoceptors mediate vasodilation. An understanding of the vessel vascular response to adrenomimetic drugs also must include the effects of drugs on adventitial innervation, smooth muscle, and other vascular factors that may be present.

Effects on Nonvascular Smooth Muscle

In general, the responses to administered catecholamines are similar to those seen after sympathetic nerve stimulation and depend on the type of adrenoceptor in the muscle.

Bronchial smooth muscle is relaxed by epinephrine and isoproterenol through their interaction with β_2-adrenoceptors. Epinephrine and isoproterenol are potent bronchodilators, while norepinephrine has a relatively weak action in this regard (see Chapter 39).

Smooth muscle of the gastrointestinal tract is generally relaxed by catecholamines, but this may depend on the existing state of muscle tone. Usually motility of the gut is reduced by catecholamines while the gastrointestinal sphincters are contracted. Catecholamines appear to produce relaxation of the gut through an action on α_2-adrenoceptors on ganglionic cells. Activation of these receptors reduces acetylcholine release from cholinergic neurons. Catecholamines also may produce gastrointestinal relaxation through an action on β_2-adrenoceptors on smooth muscle cells. Contraction of the sphincters occurs through an action on α_1-adrenoceptors. These effects are quite transient in humans and therefore have no therapeutic value.

The *radial (dilator) muscle of the iris* contains α-adrenoceptors. Epinephrine and norepinephrine cause dilation of the pupil (*mydriasis*) by contracting the dilator muscle.

Uterine muscle contains both α- and β-adrenoceptors, which mediate contraction and relaxation, respectively. The response of the human uterus to catecholamines is variable and depends on the endocrine balance of the individual at the time of amine administration (see Chapter 62). During the last stage of pregnancy and during parturition, epinephrine inhibits the uterine muscle, as does isoproterenol; norepinephrine contracts the uterus.

The *detrusor muscle* (which contains β_2-adrenoceptors) in the body of the urinary bladder is relaxed by epinephrine and isoproterenol. On the other hand, the trigone and sphincter (which contain α_1-receptors) are contracted by norepinephrine and epinephrine; this action inhibits the voiding of urine.

Central Nervous System Effects

Epinephrine, in therapeutic doses, mildly stimulates the CNS. The most noticeable features of this stimulation are apprehension, restlessness, and increased respiration. In therapeutic doses both isoproterenol and norepinephrine also have minor CNS stimulant properties. Since these compounds do not easily cross the blood-brain barrier, the mechanism of their stimulatory effects is not clear. It is likely that the stimulating effects are primarily, if not entirely, due to actions in the periphery that alter the neural input to the CNS.

Metabolic Effects

The catecholamines, primarily epinephrine and isoproterenol, exert a number of important effects on metabolic processes. Most of these are mediated through an interaction with β-adrenoceptors. Norepinephrine is usually effective only in large doses. Epinephrine and isoproterenol in therapeutic doses increase oxygen consumption by 20 to 30%. Endogenous epinephrine secreted by the adrenal medulla in response to stress such as exercise increases blood levels of glucose, lactic acid, and free fatty acids.

Epinephrine, the most potent stimulant of hepatic glycogenolysis, gives rise to glucose, which readily enters the circulation; isoproterenol produces relatively weak hyperglycemia. Administration of both α- and β-adrenoceptor blocking agents is necessary for complete antagonism of glycogenolysis in this tissue.

Isoproterenol is the most potent stimulant of skeletal muscle glycogenolysis, followed by epinephrine and norepinephrine. β_2-Adrenoceptors mediate muscle glycogenolysis. Stimulation of skeletal muscle glycogenolysis will raise blood lactic acid levels rather than blood glucose levels because skeletal muscle lacks the enzyme glucose-6-phosphatase, which catalyzes the conversion of glucose-6-phosphate to glucose.

The release of free fatty acids from adipose tissue (lipolysis) is mediated through β_3-adrenoceptors. Isoproterenol is the most potent agonist, followed by epinephrine and norepinephrine.

Potassium Homeostasis

The catecholamines can play an important role in the short-term regulation of plasma potassium levels. Stimulation of hepatic α-adrenoceptors will result in the release of potassium from the liver. In contrast, stimulation of β_2-adrenoceptors, particularly in skeletal muscle, will lead to the uptake of potassium into this tissue. The β_2-adrenoceptors are linked to the enzyme Na$^+$, K$^+$ adenosine triphosphatase (ATPase). Excessive stimulation of these β_2-adrenoceptors may produce hypokalemia, which in turn can be a cause of cardiac arrhythmias.

PHARMACOLOGICAL ACTIONS OF DOPAMINE

Dopamine is a naturally occurring catecholamine; it is the immediate biochemical precursor of the norepinephrine found in adrenergic neurons and the adrenal medulla. It is also a neurotransmitter in the CNS, where it is released from dopaminergic neurons to act on specific dopamine receptors (see Chapter 31).

Dopamine is a unique adrenomimetic drug in that it exerts its cardiovascular actions by (1) releasing norepinephrine from adrenergic neurons, (2) interacting with α-and β_1-adrenoceptors, and (3) interacting with specific dopamine receptors.

The cardiovascular response to dopamine in humans depends on the concentration infused. Low rates of dopamine infusion can produce vasodilation in the renal, mesenteric, coronary, and intercerebral vascular beds with little effect on other blood vessels or on the heart. The vasodilation produced by dopamine is not antagonized by the β-adrenoceptor blocking agent propranolol but is antagonized by haloperidol and other dopamine receptor–blocking agents.

Dopamine can exert pronounced cardiovascular and renal effects through the activation of both D_1- and D_2-receptor subtypes. Stimulation of the D_1-receptor, which is present on blood vessels and certain other peripheral sites, will result in vasodilation, natriuresis, and diuresis. D_2-receptors are found on ganglia, on sympathetic nerve terminals, on the adrenal cortex, and within the cardiovascular centers of the CNS; their activation produces hypotension, bradycardia, and regional vasodilation (e.g., renal vasodilation). The kidney appears to be a particularly rich source for endogenous dopamine in the periphery.

The infusion of moderately higher concentrations of dopamine increases the rate and contractile force of the heart and augments the cardiac output. This action is mediated by β_1-adrenoceptors and norepinephrine release and is antagonized by propranolol. In contrast to isoproterenol, which has a marked effect on both the rate and the contractile force of the heart, dopamine has a greater effect on the force than on cardiac rate. The advantage of this greater inotropic than chronotropic effect of dopamine is that it produces a smaller increase in oxygen demand by the heart than does isoproterenol. Systolic blood pressure is increased by dopamine, whereas diastolic pressure is usually not changed significantly. Total peripheral resistance is decreased because of the vasodilator effect of dopamine (Fig. 10.4).

At still higher concentrations, dopamine causes α-adrenoceptor-mediated vasoconstriction in most vascular beds and stimulates the heart. Total peripheral resistance may be increased. If the concentration of dopamine reaching the tissue is high enough, vasoconstriction of the renal and mesenteric beds also occurs. The vasoconstrictive action of dopamine is antagonized by α-adrenoceptor blocking agents such as phentolamine.

CLINICAL USES OF CATECHOLAMINES

The clinical uses of catecholamines are based on their actions on bronchial smooth muscle, blood vessels, and the heart. Epinephrine is also useful for the treatment of allergic reactions that are due to liberation of histamine in the body, because it produces certain physiological effects opposite to those produced by histamine. It is the primary treatment for anaphylactic shock and is useful in the therapy of urticaria, angioneurotic edema, and serum sickness.

Epinephrine also has been used to lower intraocular pressure in open-angle glaucoma. Its use promotes an increase in the outflow of aqueous humor. Because epinephrine administration will decrease the filtration angle formed by the cornea and the iris, its use is contraindicated in angle-closure glaucoma; under these conditions the outflow of aqueous humor via the filtration angle and into the venous system is hindered, and intraocular pressure may rise abruptly.

The vasoconstrictor actions of epinephrine and norepinephrine have been used to prolong the action of local anesthetics by reducing local blood flow in the region of the injection. Epinephrine has been used as a topical hemostatic agent for the control of local hemorrhage. Norepinephrine is infused intravenously to combat systemic hypotension during spinal anesthesia or other hypotensive conditions in which peripheral resistance is low, but it is not used to combat the hypotension due to most types of shock. In shock, marked sympathetic activity is already present, and perfusion of organs, such as the kidneys, may be jeopardized by norepinephrine administration.

Dopamine is used in the treatment of shock owing to inadequate cardiac output (cardiogenic shock), which may be due to myocardial infarction or congestive heart failure. It is also used in the treatment of septic shock, since renal circulation is frequently compromised in this condition. An advantage of using dopamine in the treatment of shock is that its inotropic action increases cardiac output while dilating renal blood vessels and thereby increasing renal blood flow.

Adverse Effects

Because they increase the force of the heartbeat, all three catecholamines may produce an excessively rapid heart rate. Palpitations produced by epinephrine and isoproterenol are accompanied by tachycardia, whereas those produced by norepinephrine usually are accompanied by bradycardia owing to reflex slowing of the heart. Headache and tremor are also common. Epinephrine is especially likely to produce anxiety, fear, and nervousness.

The greatest hazards of accidental overdosage with epinephrine and norepinephrine are cardiac arrhythmias, excessive hypertension, and acute pulmonary edema. Large doses of isoproterenol can produce such excessive cardiac stimulation, combined with a decrease in diastolic blood pressure, that coronary insufficiency may result. It also may cause arrhythmias and ventricular fibrillation. Tissue sloughing and necrosis due to severe local ischemia may follow extravasation of norepinephrine at its injection site.

OTHER ADRENOMIMETIC AGENTS

A number of adrenomimetic amines are not catecholamines. Some of these are directly acting amines that must interact with adrenoceptors to produce a response in effector tissues. Some directly acting compounds, such as phenylephrine and methoxamine, activate α-adrenoceptors almost exclusively, whereas others, like albuterol and terbutaline, are nearly pure β-adrenoceptor agonists. Drugs that exert their pharmacological actions by releasing norepinephrine from its neuronal stores (indirectly acting) produce effects that are similar to those of norepinephrine. They tend to exert strong α-adrenoceptor activity, but β_1-adrenoceptor activity typical of norepinephrine, such as myocardial stimulation, also occurs.

Some of the indirectly acting adrenomimetic amines are used primarily for their vasoconstrictive properties. They are applied locally to the nasal mucosa or to the eye. Other amines are used as bronchodilators, while still others are used exclusively for their ability to stimulate the CNS. Many noncatecholamine adrenomimetic amines resist enzymatic destruction, have prolonged actions, and are orally effective. The indirectly acting drugs are effective only when given in large doses, and they often produce tachyphylaxis.

Directly Acting Adrenomimetic Drugs
Phenylephrine, Metaraminol, and Methoxamine

These drugs are directly acting adrenomimetic amines that exert their effects primarily through an action on α-adrenoceptors. Consequently, these agents have little or no direct action on the heart. All three drugs increase both systolic and diastolic blood pressures through their vasoconstrictor action. The pressor response is accompanied by reflex bradycardia, no change in the contractile force of the heart, and little change in cardiac output. They do not precipitate cardiac arrhythmias and do not stimulate the CNS.

Phenylephrine is not a substrate for COMT, while metaraminol and methoxamine are not metabolized by either COMT or MAO. Consequently, their duration of action is considerably longer than that of norepinephrine. Following intravenous injection, pressor responses to phenylephrine may persist for 20 minutes, while pressor responses to metaraminol and methoxamine may last for more than 60 minutes.

The clinical uses of these drugs are associated with their potent vasoconstrictor action. They are used to restore or maintain blood pressure during spinal anesthesia and certain other hypotensive states. The reflex bradycardia induced by their rapid intravenous injection has been used to terminate attacks of paroxysmal atrial tachycardia. Phenylephrine is commonly used as a nasal decongestant, although occasional nasal mucosal

damage has occurred from injudicious use of the nasal spray. It is also employed in ophthalmology as a mydriatic agent. Phenylephrine, however, should not be given to patients with closed-angle glaucoma before iridectomy, since further increases in intraocular pressure may result. In dentistry, phenylephrine is used to prolong the effectiveness of a local anesthetic.

Dobutamine

Dobutamine (*Dobutrex*), in contrast to dopamine, does not produce a significant proportion of its cardiac effects through the release of norepinephrine from adrenergic nerves; dobutamine acts directly on β_1-adrenoceptors in the heart. Dobutamine exerts a greater effect on the contractile force of the heart relative to its effect on the heart rate than does dopamine. Dobutamine increases the oxygen demands on the heart to a lesser extent than does dopamine. Like dopamine, although at higher doses, it produces vasodilation of renal and mesenteric blood vessels. Dobutamine may be more useful than dopamine in the treatment of cardiogenic shock.

Terbutaline and Albuterol

Terbutaline and albuterol are relatively selective β_2-adrenoceptor agonists. Both have a longer duration of action than isoproterenol because they are not metabolized by COMT. Like isoproterenol, they are not metabolized by MAO and are not transported into adrenergic neurons. Terbutaline and albuterol are effectively administered either orally or subcutaneously. Because of their selectivity for β_2-adrenoceptors, they produce less cardiac stimulation than does isoproterenol but are not completely without effects on the heart.

Therapeutically, terbutaline and albuterol are used to treat bronchial asthma and bronchospasm associated with bronchitis and emphysema (see Chapter 39).

Side effects include nervousness, tremor, tachycardia, palpitations, headache, nausea, vomiting, and sweating. The frequency of appearance of these adverse effects is minimized, however, when the drugs are given by inhalation.

Indirectly Acting Adrenomimetic Drugs
Ephedrine

Ephedrine is a naturally occurring alkaloid that can cross the blood-brain barrier and thus exert a strong CNS-stimulating effect in addition to its peripheral actions. The latter effects are primarily due to its indirect actions and depend largely on the release of norepinephrine. However, ephedrine may cause some direct receptor stimulation, particularly in its bronchodilating effects. Because it resists metabolism by both COMT and MAO, its duration of action is longer than that of norepinephrine. As is the case with all indirectly acting adrenomimetic amines, ephedrine is much less potent than norepinephrine; in addition, tachyphylaxis develops to its peripheral actions. Unlike epinephrine or norepinephrine, however, ephedrine is effective when administered orally.

Pharmacological Actions

Ephedrine increases systolic and diastolic blood pressure; heart rate is generally not increased. Contractile force of the heart and cardiac output are both increased. Ephedrine produces bronchial smooth muscle relaxation of prolonged duration when administered orally. Aside from pupillary dilation, ephedrine has little effect on the eye.

Clinical Uses

Ephedrine is useful in relieving bronchoconstriction and mucosal congestion associated with bronchial asthma, asthmatic bronchitis, chronic bronchitis, and bronchial spasms. It is often used prophylactically to prevent asthmatic attacks and is used as a nasal decongestant, as a mydriatic, and in certain allergic disorders. Although its bronchodilator action is weaker than that of isoproterenol, its oral effectiveness and prolonged duration of action make it valuable in the treatment of these conditions. *Because of their oral effectiveness and greater bronchiolar selectivity, terbutaline and albuterol are replacing ephedrine for bronchodilation.*

Adverse Effects

Symptoms of overdose are related primarily to cardiac and CNS effects. Tachycardia, premature systoles, insomnia, nervousness, nausea, vomiting, and emotional disturbances may develop. Ephedrine should not be used in patients with cardiac disease, hypertension, or hyperthyroidism.

Amphetamine

Amphetamine is an indirectly acting adrenomimetic amine that depends for its action on the release of norepinephrine from noradrenergic nerves. Its pharmacological effects are similar to those of ephedrine; however, its CNS stimulant activity is somewhat greater. Both systolic and diastolic blood pressures are increased by oral dosing with amphetamine. The heart rate is frequently slowed reflexively. Cardiac output may remain unchanged in the low- and moderate-dose range.

The therapeutic uses of amphetamine are based on its ability to stimulate the CNS. The D-isomer (dextroamphetamine) is three to four times as potent as the L-isomer in producing CNS effects. It has been used in the treatment of obesity because of its anorexic effect, although tolerance to this effect develops rapidly. It prevents or overcomes fatigue and has been used as a CNS stimulant. *Amphetamine is no longer recommended for these uses because of its potential for abuse.* Amphetamine is useful in certain cases of narcolepsy or minimal brain dysfunction.

Further discussion of amphetamine can be found in Chapters 29 and 35.

Study QUESTIONS

1. Selective β_2-agonists, such as terbutaline
   (A) Have shorter durations of action than catecholamines when taken orally
   (B) Have stronger cardiac stimulant effects than epinephrine
   (C) Can be taken orally because these agents are not degraded by COMT
   (D) Are definitely no better than methylxanthines for asthmatic patients who are hypertensive.
2. Which drug does not induce mydriasis?
   (A) Phenylephrine
   (B) Cocaine
   (C) Phentolamine
   (D) Norepinephrine
   (E) Ephedrine
3. Epinephrine given in small therapeutic doses
   (A) Increases systolic blood pressure through β_2 receptor stimulation in the left ventricle
   (B) Decreases heart rate reflexively.
   (C) Decreases peripheral resistance through stimulation of β_1-receptors on the vascular smooth muscle cells.
   (D) Decreases peripheral resistance through β_2-adrenoceptor stimulation predominantly in skeletal muscle vascular beds.
4. The pressor response to amphetamine is
   (A) Decreased in the presence of a monoamine oxidase (MAO) inhibitor.
   (B) Potentiated by a reuptake inhibitor, such as cocaine
   (C) Associated with marked tolerance (tachyphylaxis)
   (D) Potentiated by pretreatment with reserpine
5. When phenylephrine is administered by slow infusion of the therapeutic dose, which is the most likely effect illustrated in the following table: increase ($\uparrow$); decrease ($\downarrow$); no change (0)?

	Blood Pressure (total peripheral resistance)	Heart Rate Effect		
		Reflex (via baroreceptor)	Direct	Reflex and Direct
(A)	↑	↓	↑	↑ or ↓
(B)	↑	↓	0	↓
(C)	↓	↑	↑	↑ or ↓

ANSWERS

1. **C.** Structural modification by placing the hydroxy groups at positions 3 and 5 of the phenyl ring has resulted in compounds that are not substrates for COMT, resulting in lower rates of metabolism and enhanced oral bioavailability compared to catecholamines.

2. **C.** α-Adrenoceptors mediate contraction of the radial muscle of the iris. The shortening of the radial muscle cells opens the pupil. Phentolamine blocks α-adrenoceptors, allowing parasympathetic nerves innervating the sphincter muscle to take over. This leads to a less opposed contraction of the sphincter muscle induced by transmitter acetylcholine and a constriction of the pupil or miosis.

3. **D.** A small dose of epinephrine (0.1 μg/kg) given by intravenous route may cause the blood pressure to fall, decreasing peripheral resistance. The depressor effect of small doses is due to greater sensitivity to epinephrine of vasodilator β_2-adrenoceptors than of constrictor α-adrenoceptors and a dominant action on β_2-adrenoceptors of vessels in skeletal muscle. Consequently, diastolic blood pressure usually falls. The mean blood pressure in general, however, is not greatly elevated. The compensatory baroreceptor reflexes do not appreciably antagonize the direct cardiac actions.

4. **C.** Amphetamine is an indirectly acting adrenomimetic amine that depends on the release of norepinephrine from noradrenergic nerves for its action. Thus, its effect depends on neuronal uptake (blocked by cocaine) to displace norepinephrine from the vesicles and the availability of norepinephrine (depleted by reserpine). The substitution on the α-carbon atom blocks oxidation by monoamine oxidase. With no substitution on its benzene ring, amphetamine resists metabolism by COMT.

5. **B.** Phenylephrine is an α_1-selective agonist. It causes an increase in peripheral vascular resistance. The major cardiovascular response to this drug is a rise in blood pressure associated with reflex bradycardia. The slowing of the heart rate is blocked by atropine.

SUPPLEMENTAL READING

Burnstock G and Griffith SG. Nonadrenergic Innervation of Blood Vessels. Boca Raton, FL: CRC, 1988.

Gootman PM (ed.). Developmental Neurobiology of the Autonomic Nervous System. Clifton, NJ: Humana, 1986.

Insel PA and Feldman RD. β-Adrenergic Receptors in Health and Disease. Boca Raton, FL: CRC, 1994.

Lee TJF. Endothelial messengers and cerebral vascular tone regulation. In: Olesen J and Edvinsson L (eds.). Headache Pathogenesis: Monoamines, Neuropeptides, Purines, and Nitric Oxide. Philadelphia: Lippincott-Raven, 1997:61–72.

Limbird E (ed.). The Alpha-2 Adrenergic Receptors. Clifton, NJ: Humana, 1988.

Missale C et al. Dopamine receptors: From structure to function. Physiol Rev 1998;78:189–225.

Moncada SR, Palmer MJ, and Higgs EA. Nitric oxide: Physiology, pathophysiology, and pharmacology. Pharmacol Rev 1991;43:109–142.

Patel TB et al. Molecular biological approaches to unravel adenylyl cyclase signaling and function. Gene 2001;16:13–25.

Post SR, Hammond HR, and Insel PA. Beta-adrenergic receptors and receptor signaling in heart failure. Annu Rev Pharmacol Toxicol 1999;39:343–360.

CASE Study   Help for the Heart

T. L. is a highly successful scientist who spends long hours in the laboratory and is constantly in demand as a speaker and reviewer for scientific papers and grants. He has a family history of cardiovascular disease, having lost both his father and grandfather before either reached age 60. He has recently noticed decreased energy, especially during exercise, and had symptoms (difficulty in breathing, chest pain) that took him to the emergency department. The examining physician thought the best treatment would be short-term therapy with a directly acting inotropic agent, especially one that would not markedly increase an already elevated heart rate. Based on a knowledge of the distribution of cardiovascular autonomic receptors, which of the following agents—epinephrine, norepinephrine, amphetamine, or dobutamine—would be a logical choice to use in this initial short-term treatment?

ANSWER: Dobutamine injection would provide particular benefit in meeting the therapeutic needs of this patient. Dobutamine augments ventricular contractility and thus enhances cardiac output, especially stroke volume, in patients with depressed cardiac function. It does this by stimulating β-adrenoceptors in the heart while producing relatively little increase in chronotropic activity or any significant elevation in systemic blood pressure since it lacks α-adrenoceptor stimulating effects. Thus, in contrast to a nonselective β-adrenoceptor stimulant such as isoproterenol, which increases cardiac output primarily by increasing heart rate, dobutamine's actions increase cardiac output without being accompanied by either a marked increase in heart rate or a significant increase in systemic vascular resistance.

11 Adrenoceptor Antagonists

David P. Westfall

 DRUG LIST

GENERIC NAME	PAGE	GENERIC NAME	PAGE
Acebutolol	114	Nadolol	114
Atenolol	114	Phenoxybenzamine	113
Betaxolol	114	Phentolamine	113
Bucindolol	117	Pindolol	114
Carteolol	114	Prazosin	112
Carvedilol	117	Propranolol	113
Doxazosin	111	Terazosin	112
Esmolol	112	Timolol	114
Labetalol	116	Tolazoline	112
Medroxalol	117	Trimazosin	112
Metoprolol	113		

ADRENOCEPTORS

Drugs that produce responses by interacting with adrenoceptors are referred to as *adrenoceptor agonists* or *adrenergic agonists*. Norepinephrine and isoproterenol are examples of such compounds. Agents that inhibit responses mediated by adrenoceptor activation are known as *adrenoceptor antagonists, adrenergic antagonists,* or *adrenergic blocking agents*. Prazosin and propranolol are examples of receptor-blocking drugs. The pharmacology of the adrenoceptor antagonists is described in this chapter.

Norepinephrine is released from the varicosities of the postganglionic sympathetic nerves during neural activity and interacts with the adrenoceptors of the effector organ, producing the characteristic response of the effector. This occurs because norepinephrine has an *affinity* for the receptors and possesses *intrinsic activity;* that is, it has the capacity to activate the receptors. Circulating catecholamines and other directly acting adrenomimetic drugs also interact with these receptors.

The adrenergic blocking agents also have an affinity for the adrenoceptors. The antagonists, however, have only limited or no capacity to activate the receptors; that is, they have little or negligible intrinsic activity. The blocking drugs compete with adrenomimetic substances for access to the receptors. Thus, *these agents reduce the effects produced by both sympathetic nerve stimulation and by exogenously administered adrenomimetics*. This action forms the basis for their therapeutic and investigational use.

109

Competition for receptors, hence receptor antagonism, is governed by the *law of mass action;* that is, the interaction between drug and receptor depends on the concentration of drug in the vicinity of the receptor and the number of receptors present. Because agonist and antagonist have an affinity for the same receptors, the two substances compete for binding to the receptors.

For most adrenoceptor antagonists (and agonists), the attachment of the blocking agent to the adrenoceptor is by relatively weak forces, such as hydrophobic, hydrogen, or van der Waals bonding. Because the drug easily dissociates from the receptor, the antagonism exhibited by these compounds is readily reversible on removal of the antagonists from the biophase. This type of antagonism is referred to as *reversibly competitive* or *equilibrium competitive* (see Chapter 2). However, one group of antagonists, the haloalkylamines, is highly chemically reactive. These compounds are capable of forming covalent bonds with various chemical groupings on receptors. Removal of these antagonists from the biophase is not sufficient to restore the responsiveness of the effector to agonists. Full tissue responsiveness may not occur for several days. Because of the apparently irreversible nature of this drug antagonism, it is termed *irreversibly competitive* or *non–equilibrium competitive* (see Chapter 2).

Adrenoceptor-blocking agents do not prevent the release of transmitters from adrenergic nerves as do the neuron-blocking agents, such as guanethidine, and they are not catecholamine-depleting agents, such as reserpine (see Chapter 20). *They prevent the agonist from interacting with its receptor.*

CLASSIFICATION OF BLOCKING DRUGS

An α-receptor is one that mediates responses for which the adrenomimetic order of potency is epinephrine greater than or equal to norepinephrine greater than isoproterenol, and that is susceptible to blockade by phentolamine and phenoxybenzamine. It follows from this definition that phentolamine and phenoxybenzamine are called α-adrenoceptor antagonists or α-blocking agents. A β-receptor mediates responses for which the adrenomimetic order of potency is isoproterenol greater than epinephrine greater than or equal to norepinephrine, and this receptor is susceptible to blockade by propranolol. Propranolol is, therefore, called a β-adrenoceptor antagonist or β-blocking agent.

β-Receptor Subtypes

The two main types of β-receptors have been given the designations β_1 and β_2. Among the responses mediated by β_1-receptors is cardiac stimulation, whereas β_2-receptor stimulation mediates bronchodilation and re-

laxation of vascular and uterine smooth muscle (see Chapters 9 and 62). These findings are significant, since a number of both agonists and antagonists have some degree of selectivity for either β_1- or β_2-receptors.

A comparison of the effects produced by propranolol, a nonselective β-receptor blocking agent, with those of metoprolol, a relatively selective β_1-receptor blocker, illustrates the clinical utility of such drugs. For example, a patient who is a candidate for β-blocker therapy (angina, hypertension), but who also has obstructive airway disease probably should not receive a nonselective β-blocking agent such as propranolol because of the possibility of aggravating bronchospasm. In this instance, metoprolol would be advantageous, since β-receptors of the respiratory system are β_2, hence less affected by metoprolol than by propranolol. However, metoprolol's selectivity is only relative, and at high concentrations the drug will also antagonize β_2 responses.

Absolute selectivity of drug action does not exist. Any given effector tissue probably contains more than one receptor subtype, and it is likely that the proportion of receptor subtypes varies within that effector. Nevertheless, the designation of a drug as a selective agent for either a β_1-receptor or a β_2-receptor seems both useful and justified if one keeps in mind that the designation represents a shorthand notation for what is only a predominance of activities.

Molecular genetic techniques have confirmed the existence of multiple subtypes of β-adrenoceptors. β_1-Receptors and β_2-receptors have been cloned, and recent molecular biological evidence indicates the existence of at least one additional β-receptor subtype, called the β_3-receptor. It is suggested that the β_3-receptor may mediate some of the metabolic effects of catecholamines, although no available β-blocker has been shown to rely on β_3-receptor antagonism for its therapeutic effectiveness.

α-Receptor Subtypes

There are differences between the receptors on nerves (*presynaptic* receptors) and those on effector cells (*postsynaptic* receptors). Furthermore, some α-agonists and antagonists exhibit selectivity for one of these receptor types. Terminology classifies receptors as either α_1 or α_2. α_1-Receptors are those whose stimulation has traditionally been associated with the postsynaptic α-receptors of smooth muscle, while α_2-receptors are those originally associated with the presynaptic α-receptors of peripheral nerves. However, the designation of receptors as either α_1 or α_2 cannot be categorized strictly by anatomical location (i.e., presynaptic or postsynaptic), since evidence now indicates that α_2-receptors occupy, in addition to peripheral nerves, a variety of sites including smooth muscle, adrenal medullary cells, the brain, and melanocytes.

The existence of α-receptor subclasses and the receptor selectivity exhibited by certain α-blocking agents have therapeutic implications. Phentolamine is a disappointing antihypertensive drug because its administration results in a reflex increase in both heart rate and contractile force; these effects tend to negate the reduction in blood pressure that it produces. In contrast, prazosin is an effective antihypertensive drug because the reflex cardiac stimulation it induces is much less. The differing hemodynamic effects produced by phentolamine and prazosin appear to be related to their relative degree of selectivity for α_1- and α_2- receptors. Phentolamine is a relatively nonselective receptor blocking agent, since in addition to blocking postsynaptic α_1-receptors, it will block presynaptic α_2-receptors; the latter action enhances release of norepinephrine, hence augments cardiac rate and contractile force. Blockade of α_2-receptors may actually potentiate the cardiac effects of sympathetic nerve stimulation. Prazosin, in contrast to phentolamine, is relatively selective for α_1-receptors; that is, it preferentially blocks responses mediated by the postsynaptic α_1-receptors in the blood vessels without having a substantial effect on presynaptic α_2-receptors. Thus, prazosin stimulates the heart less than does phentolamine.

Absolute selectivity of action for α_1- or α_2-receptors does not exist for any available α-agonists and antagonists. Furthermore, as is the case with β-receptors, a given effector tissue may contain more than one α-receptor subtype. Recent evidence suggests that in addition to α_1-receptors, vascular smooth muscle may possess α_2-receptors. Although the functional importance of α_2-receptors in blood vessels seems to be less than that of α_1-receptors, this can account for certain clinical observations, as for example the pressor response that occurs upon initiation of treatment with the α_2-agonist clonidine.

It is becoming increasingly clear that neither α_1- nor α_2-receptors are homogeneous. There seem to be at least three subtypes of both α_1- and α_2-receptors, that is, α_{1A}, α_{1B}, α_{1D}, α_{2A}, α_{2B} and α_{2C}. At this point, the pharmacology and therapeutic usefulness of the major α-antagonists can be reasonably well explained by considering their relative selectivity for the two main classes of α-receptors, α_1 and α_2. This is beginning to change, however. For example, tamsulosin (*Flomax*), a recently introduced α-antagonist, reportedly exhibits some selectivity for α_{1A}-receptors, which are rich in the prostate, as compared to α_{1B}-receptors, which are more plentiful in vascular smooth muscle. This may provide some advantage to tamsulosin as an agent for treatment of patients with benign prostate hypertrophy (discussed later).

α-RECEPTOR BLOCKING AGENTS

The clinically important α-blockers fall primarily into three chemical groups: the *haloalkylamines* (e.g., phe-noxybenzamine), the *imidazolines* (e.g., phentolamine), and the *quinazoline derivatives* (e.g., prazosin). Of these three classes of α-adrenoceptor antagonists, the quinazoline compounds are of greatest clinical utility and are emphasized in this chapter. The use of the haloalkylamines and imidazolines has diminished in recent years because they lack selectivity for α_1- and α_2-receptors. Comparative information concerning the three chemical classes of antagonists is presented in Table 11.1

Quinazoline Derivatives

The chief use of these drugs is in the management of primary hypertension. Examples of quinazoline α-blockers include prazosin (*Minipress*), trimazosin (*Cardovar*), terazosin (*Hytrin*), and doxazosin (*Cardura*).

Mechanism of Action

The α-antagonism produced by prazosin and the other quinazoline derivatives is of the *equilibrium-competitive* type. The drugs are selective for α_1-adrenoceptors, so that at usual therapeutic concentrations there is little or negligible antagonism of α_2-adrenoceptors. However, selectivity is only relative and can be lost with high drug concentrations. While most of the pharmacological effects of prazosin are directly attributable to α_1-antagonism, at high doses the drug can cause vasodilation by a direct effect on smooth muscle independent of α-receptors. This action appears to be related to an inhibition of phosphodiesterases that results in an enhancement of intracellular levels of cyclic nucleotides.

Absorption, Metabolism, Excretion

Prazosin is readily absorbed after oral administration, peak serum levels occur approximately 2 hours after a single oral dose, and the antihypertensive effect of prazosin persists for up to 10 hours. Its half-life in plasma ranges from 2.5 to 4 hours, and elimination from plasma appears to follow first-order kinetics. The drug is extensively (perhaps as high as 97%) bound to plasma proteins; this observation partially explains the lack of correlation between plasma drug levels and persistence of antihypertensive effect.

Hepatic *O*-dealkylation and glucuronide formation appear to be major pathways of biotransformation. Only about 10% of orally administered prazosin is excreted in the urine. Plasma levels of prazosin are increased in patients with renal failure; the nature of this interaction is unknown.

Pharmacological Actions

The most important pharmacological effect of prazosin is its ability to antagonize vascular smooth muscle contraction that is caused by either sympathetic nervous activity

TABLE 11.1   Comparative Information About the Three Classes of α-Adrenoceptor Antagonists

	Haloalkylamines	Imidazolines	Quinazolines
Prototype	Phenoxybenzamine (*Dibenzyline*)	Phentolamine (*Regitine*)	Prazosin (*Minipress*)
Others		Tolazoline (*Priscoline*)	Terazosin (*Hytrin*) Doxazosin (*Cardura*) Trimazosin (*Cardovar*)
Antagonism	Irreversible (non-equilibrium) competitive	Equilibrium competitive	Equilibrium competitive
Selectivity Hemodynamic effects	Somewhat selective for α_1 Decreased peripheral vascular resistance and blood pressure Venodilation is prominent Cardiac stimulation occurs because of cardiovascular reflexes and enhanced release of norepinephrine	Nonselective Similar to phenoxybenzamine	Selective for α_1 Decreased peripheral vascular resistance and blood pressure Veins seem to be less susceptible to antagonism than arteries; thus, postural hypotension is less of a problem Cardiac stimulation is less because release of norepinephrine is not enhanced
Actions other than α-blockade	Some antagonism of responses to ACh, 5-HT, and histamine Blockade of neuronal and extraneuronal uptake	Cholinomimetic, adrenomimetic, and histaminelike actions Antagonism of responses to 5-HT	At high doses some direct vasodilator action, probably due to phosphodiesterase inhibition
Routes	Intravenous and oral Oral absorption incomplete and erratic	Similar to phenoxybenzamine	Oral
Adverse reactions	Postural hypotension, tachycardia, miosis, nasal stuffiness, failure of ejaculation	Same as phenoxybenzamine and in addition gastrointestinal disturbances	Some postural hypotension, especially with the first dose; less of a problem overall than with phenoxybenzamine or phentolamine
Therapeutic uses	Conditions of catecholamine excess such as pheochromocytoma Peripheral vascular disease Benign prostatic hypertrophy	Same as phenoxybenzamine	Primary hypertension Benign prostatic hypertrophy

ACh, acetylcholine; 5-HT, 5-hydroxytryptamine.

or the action of adrenomimetics. Hemodynamically, the effects of prazosin differ from those of phenoxybenzamine and phentolamine in that venous smooth muscle is not as much affected by prazosin. Postural hypotension during chronic treatment is also less of a problem. Also, increases in heart rate, contractile force, and plasma renin activity, which normally occur after the use of vasodilators and α-blockers, are much less prominent following chronic treatment with prazosin.

Phenoxybenzamine and phentolamine, in addition to blocking postsynaptic α-receptors, also block α_2-receptors on nerves and therefore can enhance the release of norepinephrine. When norepinephrine exerts a postsynaptic action by means of β-adrenoceptors (e.g., cardiac stimulation, renin release), blockade of presynaptic α_2-receptors by phenoxybenzamine and phentolamine may actually potentiate the responses. *Prazosin blocks responses mediated by postsynaptic α_1-receptors but has no effect on the presynaptic α_2-receptors.* Thus,

stimulation of the heart and renin release is less prominent with this drug.

Clinical Uses

Prazosin is effective in reducing all grades of hypertension. The drug can be administered alone in mild and (in some instances) moderate hypertension. When the hypertension is moderate or severe, prazosin generally is given in combination with a thiazide diuretic and a β-blocker. The antihypertensive actions of prazosin are considerably potentiated by coadministration of thiazides or other types of antihypertensive drugs.

Prazosin may be particularly useful when patients cannot tolerate other classes of antihypertensive drugs or when blood pressure is not well controlled by other drugs. Since prazosin does not significantly influence blood uric acid or glucose levels, it can be used in hypertensive patients whose condition is complicated by diabetes mellitus or gout.

Prazosin and other α-antagonists find use in the management of benign prostatic obstruction, especially in patients who are not candidates for surgery. Blockade of α-adrenoceptors in the base of the bladder and in the prostate apparently reduces the symptoms of obstruction and the urinary urgency that occurs at night.

Adverse Effects

Although less of a problem than with phenoxybenzamine or phentolamine, symptoms of postural hypotension, such as dizziness and light-headedness, are the most commonly reported side effects associated with prazosin therapy. These effects occur most frequently during initial treatment and when the dosage is sharply increased. Postural hypotension seems to be more pronounced during Na^+ deficiency, as may occur in patients on a low-salt diet or being treated with diuretics, β-blockers, or both.

β-ADRENOCEPTOR BLOCKING AGENTS

A large number of β-blockers are on the market in the United States. Of these, propranolol, a nonselective β-antagonist, was the first to be introduced and is the prototypical drug with which the others are compared. Metoprolol was the first β_1-selective drug and timolol the first β-blocker approved for ophthalmic use.

As a class, β-blocking agents have greater structural similarity to their corresponding agonists than do the α-blockers. This structural similarity also accounts for the greater specificity of action exhibited by the β-receptor blocking drugs than by the α-adrenoceptor blocking drugs.

The similarity in structure to β-agonists is most certainly responsible for the finding that some β-blockers activate β-receptors; that is, they have some intrinsic sympathomimetic activity. The intrinsic activity of these compounds is generally modest in comparison with an agonist, such as isoproterenol, and they are generally referred to as *partial agonists* (see Chapter 2).

Mechanism of Action

All of the β-blockers exert equilibrium-competitive antagonism of the actions of catecholamines and other adrenomimetics at β-receptors. Probably the best-recognized action of these compounds that is not mediated by a β-receptor is depression of cellular membrane excitability. This effect has been described as a membrane-stabilizing action, a quinidinelike effect, or a local anesthetic effect. This action is not too surprising in view of the structural similarities between β-blockers and local anesthetics. *However, with the usual therapeutic doses, the actions of the β-receptor blocking agents appear to be almost entirely accounted for by their β-receptor antagonism.*

Because the β-receptors of the heart are primarily of the β_1 type and those in the pulmonary and vascular smooth muscle are β_2 receptors, β_1-selective antagonists are frequently referred to as *cardioselective blockers.* The intrinsic activity, cardioselectivity, and membrane-stabilizing actions of a number of β-blockers are summarized in Table 11.2

Absorption, Metabolism, and Excretion

Propranolol (*Inderal*) is suitable for both parental and oral administration. Absorption from the gastrointestinal tract is extensive. The peak therapeutic effect after oral administration occurs in 1 to 1.5 hours. The plasma half-life of propranolol is approximately 3 hours. The drug is concentrated in the lungs and to a lesser extent in the liver, brain, kidneys, and heart. Binding to plasma proteins is extensive (90%). The liver is the chief organ involved in the metabolism of propranolol, and the drug is subject to a significant degree of first-pass metabolism. At least eight metabolites have been recovered from the urine, the major excretory route.

The pharmacokinetic profile of metoprolol (*Lopressor*) is similar to that of propranolol. Metoprolol is readily and rapidly absorbed after oral administration and is subject to a significant amount of first-pass metabolism by the liver. Curiously, the duration of metoprolol's action is longer than one would predict from its plasma half-life, which ranges from 0.5 to 2.5 hours. The degree of binding of metoprolol to plasma proteins is modest (10%). The extensive distribution of metoprolol to the lungs and kidney is typical of a moderately lipophilic drug. Metoprolol undergoes considerable metabolism;

TABLE 11.2	Characteristics and Preparations of β-Blockers		
β-Blocker	Cardio-selective	Partial Agonist Activity	Membrane Stabilizing Activity
Propranolol	No	None	Yes
Acebutolol	Yes	Slight	None
Atenolol	Yes	None	None
Betaxolol	Yes	None	Slight
Carteolol	No	Slight	None
Esmolol	Yes	None	None
Levobunolol	No	None	None
Metoprolol	Yes	None	Slight
Nadolol	No	None	None
Penbutolol	No	Slight	None
Pindolol	No	Yes	Slight
Timolol	No	Slight	None

only 3 to 10% of an administered dose is recovered as unchanged drug. The metabolites are essentially inactive as β-receptor blocking agents and are eliminated primarily by renal excretion. Small amounts of the drug are present in the feces.

Timolol (*Timoptic*) is almost completely absorbed from the gastrointestinal tract. Peak plasma levels occur 2 to 4 hours after oral administration; the plasma half-life of timolol is approximately 5.5 hours. The extensive tissue distribution of timolol into lung, liver, and kidney is similar to that of other β-blockers. Approximately 70% of the drug is excreted in the urine within 24 hours, mostly as highly polar unconjugated metabolites. Only 6% of an administered dose is recovered in the feces. Although timolol is approved for the *topical* treatment of elevated intraocular pressure, there is limited information about its pharmacokinetics following administration by this route. The drug apparently can reach the systemic circulation after intraocular instillation, but plasma levels are only about 7% of those achieved in the aqueous humor.

About half of an orally administered dose of acebutolol (*Sectral*) is absorbed. Approximately 25% of the drug is bound to plasma proteins, and its plasma half-life is about 4 hours. Metabolism of acebutolol produces a metabolite with β-blocking activity whose half-life is 10 hours.

Roughly half of an orally administered dose of atenolol (*Tenormin*) is absorbed. The drug is eliminated primarily by the kidney and unlike propranolol, undergoes little hepatic metabolism. Its plasma half-life is approximately 6 hours, although if it is administered to a patient with impaired renal function, its half-life can be considerably prolonged.

Absorption of an oral dose of betaxolol (*Kerlone, Betoptic*) is almost complete. The drug is subject to a slight first-pass effect such that the absolute bioavailability of the drug is about 90%. Approximately 50% of administered betaxolol binds to plasma proteins, and its plasma half-life is about 20 hours; it is suitable for dosing once per day. The primary route of elimination is by liver metabolism, with only 15% of unchanged drug being excreted.

Carteolol (*Cartrol*) is a long-acting β-blocker that is suitable for dosing once per day. It is almost completely absorbed and exhibits about 30% binding to plasma proteins. Unlike many β-blockers, carteolol is not extensively metabolized. Up to 70% of an administered dose is excreted unchanged.

The β-blocker esmolol (*Brevibloc*) is unusual in that it is very rapidly metabolized; its plasma half-life is only 9 minutes. It is subject to hydrolysis by cytosolic esterases in red blood cells to yield methanol and an acid metabolite, the latter having an elimination half-life of about 4 hours. Only 2% of the administered esmolol is excreted unchanged. Because of its rapid onset and short duration of action, esmolol is used by the intravenous route for the control of ventricular arrhythmias in emergencies.

Nadolol (*Corgard*) is slowly and incompletely absorbed from the gastrointestinal tract, and only 30% of an orally administered dose is absorbed. Appreciable metabolism does not seem to occur; nadolol is excreted primarily unchanged in the urine and feces. The plasma half-life is quite long, approaching 24 hours, which permits dosing once per day.

Pindolol (*Visken*) is extensively absorbed from the gastrointestinal tract. First-pass metabolism is estimated at about 15%, and its plasma half-life is on the order of 3 to 4 hours. The binding of pindolol to plasma proteins is approximately 50%. The metabolic fate of pindolol is not completely understood, although 50% of an administered dose is recovered, primarily in the urine, as unchanged drug.

Pharmacological Actions

The most important actions of the β-blocking drugs are on the cardiovascular system. *β-Blockers decrease heart rate, myocardial contractility, cardiac output, and conduction velocity within the heart.* These effects are most pronounced when sympathetic activity is high or when the heart is stimulated by circulating agonists.

The actions of β-blockers on blood pressure are complex. After acute administration, blood pressure is only slightly altered. This is because of the compensatory reflex increase in peripheral vascular resistance that results from a β-blocker–induced decrease in cardiac output. Vasoconstriction is mediated by α-receptors, and α-receptors are not antagonized by β-receptor blocking agents. Chronic administration of β-blockers, however, results in a reduction of blood pressure, and this is the reason for their use in primary hypertension (see Chapter 20). The mechanism of this effect is not well understood, but it may include such actions as a reduction in renin release, antagonism of β-receptors in the central nervous system, or antagonism of presynaptic facilitatory β-receptors on sympathetic nerves.

Total coronary blood flow is reduced by the β-blockers. This effect may be due in part to the unopposed α-receptor–mediated vasoconstriction that follows β-receptor blockade in the coronary arteries. Additional contributing factors to the decrease in coronary blood flow are the negative chronotropic and inotropic effects produced by the β-blockers; these actions result in a decrease in the amount of blood available for the coronary system. The decrease in mean blood pressure may also contribute to the reduced coronary blood flow.

In view of the effects of the β-receptor blocking agents on coronary blood flow, it seems paradoxical that these drugs are useful for the prophylactic treatment of *angina pectoris,* a condition characterized by inadequate myocardial perfusion. The chief benefit of the β-blockers in this condition derives from their ability to decrease cardiac work and oxygen demand. The use of the β-blockers in angina is considered in Chapter 17. The ability of β-blockers to decrease cardiac work and oxygen demand may also be responsible for the favorable effects of these agents in the long-term management of congestive heart failure.

The release of renin from the juxtaglomerular cells of the kidney is believed to be regulated in part by β-receptors; most β-blockers decrease renin release. While the drug-induced decrease in renin release may contribute to their hypotensive actions, it is probably not the only factor (see Chapter 20). Nevertheless, β-blockers are useful and logical agents to use when treating hypertension that is accompanied by high plasma renin activity, although angiotensin converting enzyme inhibitors are also widely used in this situation.

The glycogenolytic and lipolytic actions of endogenous catecholamines are mediated by β-receptors and are subject to blockade by β-blockers. This metabolic antagonism exerted by the β-blockers is particularly pronounced if the levels of circulating catecholamines have been increased reflexively in response to hypoglycemia. Other physiological changes induced by hypoglycemia, such as tachycardia, may be blunted by β-blockers. These agents therefore must be used with caution in patients susceptible to hypoglycemia (e.g., diabetics treated with insulin). Because the metabolic responses to catecholamines are mediated by β_2-receptors and possibly by β_3-receptors, β_1-selective antagonists such as metoprolol and atenolol may be better choices whenever β-blocker therapy is indicated for a patient who has hypoglycemia.

Propranolol increases airway resistance by antagonizing β_2-receptor–mediated bronchodilation. Although the resulting bronchoconstriction is not a great concern in patients with normal lung function, it can be quite serious in the asthmatic. *The cardioselective β-blockers produce less bronchoconstriction than do the nonselective antagonists.*

β-Blockers can reduce intraocular pressure in glaucoma and ocular hypertension. The mechanism is believed to be related to a decreased production of aqueous humor.

Clinical Uses

The β-receptor blocking agents have widespread and important uses in the management of cardiac arrhythmias, angina pectoris, and hypertension. Their uses in these conditions are reviewed in Chapters 16, 17, and 20, respectively. Even though acute administration of β-blockers can precipitate congestive heart failure in patients who are largely dependent on enhanced sym-

pathetic nerve activity to maintain sufficient cardiac output, the β-blockers have been shown to be quite useful in the long-term management of patients with mild to moderate heart failure. The β-blockers also offer proven benefit in preventing the recurrence of a myocardial infarction (MI). For this purpose, it is best if β-blocker therapy is instituted soon after the MI and continued for the long term. Other therapeutic applications of the β-blockers are discussed later in the chapter.

Hyperthyroidism

The β-blockers significantly reduce the peripheral manifestations of hyperthyroidism, particularly elevated heart rate, increased cardiac output, and muscle tremors. Although the β-blockers can improve the clinical status of the hyperthyroid patient, the patient remains biochemically hyperthyroid. The β-blockers should not be used as the sole form of therapy in hyperthyroidism. They are most logically employed in the management of hyperthyroid crisis, in the preoperative preparation for thyroidectomy, and during the initial period of administration of specific antithyroid drugs (see Chapter 65).

Glaucoma

β-Blockers can be used topically to reduce intraocular pressure in patients with chronic open-angle glaucoma and ocular hypertension. The mechanism by which ocular pressure is reduced appears to depend on decreased production of aqueous humor. Timolol has a somewhat greater ocular hypotensive effect than do the available cholinomimetic or adrenomimetic drugs. The β-blockers also are beneficial in the treatment of acute angle-closure glaucoma.

Anxiety States

Patients with anxiety have a variety of psychic and somatic symptoms. The peripheral manifestations of anxiety may include a number of symptoms (e.g., palpitations) that are due in part to overactivity of the sympathetic nervous system. The β-blocking agents may offer some benefit in the treatment of anxiety.

Migraine

The β-blockers may offer some value in the prophylaxis of migraine headache, possibly because a blockade of craniovascular β-receptors results in reduced vasodilation. The painful phase of a migraine attack is believed to be produced by vasodilation.

Adverse Effects and Contraindications

The most prominent side effects associated with the administration of the β-blockers are those directly attributable to their ability to block β-receptors. Although β-blockers prevent an increase in heart rate and cardiac output resulting from an activation of the autonomic nervous system, these effects may not be troublesome in patients with adequate or marginal cardiac reserve. However, they can be life threatening for a patient with congestive heart failure. Also, because conduction of impulses in the heart may be slowed by β-blockers, patients with conduction disturbances, particularly through the atrioventricular node, should not be treated with β-blockers.

Caution must be exercised in the use of β-blockers in obstructive airway disease, since these drugs promote further bronchoconstriction. Cardioselective β-blockers have less propensity to aggravate bronchoconstriction than do nonselective β-blockers.

β-Blockers potentiate hypoglycemia by antagonizing the catecholamine-induced mobilization of glycogen. The use of β-blockers in hypoglycemic patients is therefore dangerous and must be undertaken with caution. If β-blocker therapy is required, a cardioselective β-blocker is preferred.

Whenever β-blocker therapy is employed, the period of greatest danger for asthmatics or insulin-dependent diabetics is during the initial period of drug administration, since the greatest disruption of the autonomic balance will occur at this time. If marked toxicity does not occur during this period, further doses are less likely to cause problems.

Although the β-blockers produce a number of central effects, it is not clear whether these effects are due to blockade of central β-receptors. After high doses, patients may have hallucinations, nightmares, insomnia, and depression.

Topical application of timolol to the eye is well tolerated, and the incidence of side effects, which consist of burning or dryness of the eyes, is reported to be 5 to 10%.

In spite of the potential seriousness of some of their side effects, β-blockers as a class are well tolerated and patient compliance is good.

DRUGS WITH COMBINED β- AND α-BLOCKING ACTIVITY

Labetalol

Labetalol (*Normodyne, Trandate*) possesses both β-blocking and α-blocking activity and is approximately one-third as potent as propranolol as a β-blocker and one-tenth as potent as phentolamine as an α-blocker. The ratio of β- to α-activity is about 3:1 when labetalol is administered orally and about 7:1 when it is administered intravenously. Thus the drug can be most conveniently thought of as a β-blocker with some α-blocking properties.

Mechanism of Action

Labetalol produces *equilibrium-competitive antagonism* at β-receptors but does not exhibit selectivity for β₁- or β₂-receptors. Like certain other β-blockers (e.g., pindolol and timolol), labetalol possesses some degree of intrinsic activity. This intrinsic activity, or partial agonism, especially at β₂-receptors in the vasculature, has been suggested to contribute to the vasodilator effect of the drug. The membrane-stabilizing effect, or local anesthetic action, of propranolol and several other β-blockers, is also possessed by labetalol, and in fact the drug is a reasonably potent local anesthetic.

The α-blockade produced by labetalol is also of the equilibrium-competitive type. In a manner similar to prazosin, labetalol exhibits selectivity for α₁-receptors. Presynaptic α-receptors, which are of the α₂ subclass, are not antagonized by labetalol. The drug also has some intrinsic activity at α-receptors, although this action is less than its intrinsic β-receptor–stimulating effects.

Labetalol appears to produce relaxation of vascular smooth muscle not only by α-blockade but also by a partial agonist effect at β₂-receptors. In addition, labetalol may produce vascular relaxation by a direct non–receptor-mediated effect.

Labetalol can block the neuronal uptake of norepinephrine and other catecholamines. This action, plus its slight intrinsic activity at α-receptors, may account for the seemingly paradoxical, although infrequent, increase in blood pressure seen on its initial administration.

Absorption, Metabolism, and Excretion

Labetalol is almost completely absorbed from the gastrointestinal tract. However, it is subject to considerable first-pass metabolism, which occurs in both the gastrointestinal tract and the liver, so that only about 25% of an administered dose reaches the systemic circulation. While traces of unchanged labetalol are recovered in the urine, most of the drug is metabolized to inactive glucuronide conjugates. The plasma half-life of labetalol is 6 to 8 hours, and the elimination kinetics are essentially unchanged in patients with impaired renal failure.

Pharmacological Actions

Although capable of antagonizing a variety of responses in a number of effectors that are mediated by both β- and α-receptors, *the most important actions of labetalol are on the cardiovascular system.* These effects vary from individual to individual and depend on the sympathetic and parasympathetic tone at the time of drug administration.

The most common hemodynamic effect of acutely administered labetalol in humans is a *decrease in peripheral vascular resistance and blood pressure without an appreciable alteration in heart rate or cardiac output.*

This pattern differs from that seen following administration with either a conventional β- or α-blocker. Acute administration of a β-blocker produces a decrease in heart rate and cardiac output with little effect on blood pressure, while acute administration of an α-blocker leads to a decrease in peripheral vascular resistance and a reflexively initiated increase in cardiac rate and output. Thus, the pattern of cardiovascular responses observed after labetalol administration combines the features of β- and α-blockade, that is, a decrease in peripheral vascular resistance (due to α-blockade and direct vascular effects) without an increase in cardiac rate and output (due to β-blockade).

Prolonged oral therapy with labetalol results in cardiovascular responses similar to those obtained following conventional β-blocker administration, that is, decreases in peripheral vascular resistance, blood pressure, and heart rate. Generally, however, the decrease in heart rate is less pronounced than after administration of propranolol or other β-blockers.

Clinical Uses

Labetalol is useful for the chronic treatment of primary hypertension. It can be used alone but is more often employed in combination with other antihypertensive agents. Labetalol also has been used intravenously for the treatment of hypertensive emergencies. Like conventional β-blockers, labetalol may be useful for patients with coexisting hypertension and anginal pain due to ischemia. It is also being investigated as a possible therapeutic modality for ischemic heart disease, even in the absence of hypertension. The benefit derives from its β-blocking activity, which decreases cardiac work, and from its ability to decrease afterload by virtue of its α-blocking activity.

Labetalol, because it possesses both α- and β-blocking activity, is useful for the preoperative management of patients with a pheochromocytoma.

Adverse Effects

There have been reports of excessive hypotension and paradoxical pressor effects following intravenous administration of labetalol. These latter effects may be due to a labetalol-induced blockade of neuronal amine uptake, which increases the concentrations of norepinephrine in the vicinity of its receptors.

Approximately 5% of the patients who receive labetalol complain of side effects typical of noradrenergic nervous system suppression. These include postural hypotension, gastrointestinal distress, tiredness, sexual dysfunction, and tingling of the scalp. Most of these effects are related to α-blockade, although the tingling of the scalp may be due to the drug's intrinsic activity at α-receptors. Side effects associated with β-blockade, such as induction of bronchospasm and congestive heart failure, may also occur, but generally at a lower frequency than α-receptor–associated effects.

Skin rashes have been reported, as has an increase in the titer of antinuclear antibodies. Despite the latter observation, the appearance of a systemic lupus syndrome is rare. Labetalol also has been reported to interfere with chemical measurements of catecholamines and metabolites.

Other Compounds

Several other β-adrenoceptor antagonists, similar to labetalol, exhibit some degree of α-receptor antagonism. These include bucindolol, carvedilol, and medroxalol.

S t u d y Q U E S T I O N S

1. Which of the following actions of epinephrine would be antagonized by prazosin but not by propranolol?
   (A) Increase in heart rate
   (B) Mydriasis
   (C) Release of renin
   (D) Bronchiolar dilation
   (E) Glycogenolysis

2. Which of the following adrenoceptor antagonists will reduce responses mediated by both α- and β-receptors?
   (A) Propranolol
   (B) Prazosin
   (C) Phenoxybenzamine
   (D) Labetalol
   (E) Metoprolol

3. This question is based on the information provided in the accompanying diagram. Shown is the effect of applying norepinephrine on the arterial pressure of an isolated (in vitro) segment of artery from an experimental animal before and after adding drug X to the tissue. Drug X is present during the second application of norepinephrine. Drug X is most likely:

(A) Guanethidine
(B) Propranolol
(C) Cocaine
(D) Prazosin
(E) Atropine

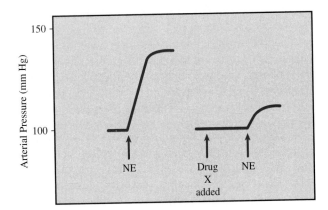

5. This question refers to the accompanying graphs. Shown are dose–response curves for isoproterenol (control) both alone and in the presence of one or the other of two β-receptor antagonists, drugs X and Y. The responses being measured are an increase in heart rate of a human subject and relaxation of an in vitro strip of human bronchiolar smooth muscle. Drug X is most likely:

(A) Metoprolol
(B) Propranolol
(C) Pindolol
(D) Timolol
(E) Nadolol

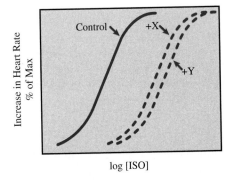

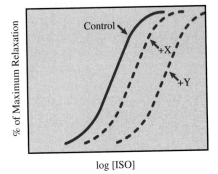

4. This question is based on the information provided in the accompanying diagram. The experimental set up is the same as in the previous question. Drug Y is administered before and after timolol. Drug Y is most likely:

(A) Bradykinin
(B) Histamine
(C) Isoproterenol
(D) Acetylcholine
(E) Phenylephrine

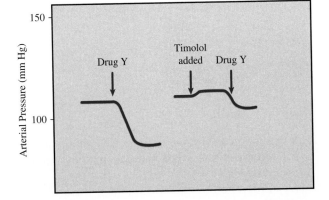

ANSWERS

1. **B.** The adrenoceptors that epinephrine acts on to affect heart rate, renin release, bronchiolar tone, and glycogenolysis are β-receptors. Prazosin is an α-antagonist so would not antagonize epinephrine at those receptors. The radial smooth muscle in the iris has α-receptors that when activated, contract the radial muscle which dilates the pupil. This action is antagonized by prazosin.

2. **D.** Propranolol and metoprolol are selective for β-receptors, whereas prazosin and phenoxybenzamine are selective for α-receptors. Labetalol is the only antagonist in this list that has the ability to reduce responses mediated by both α- and β-receptors.

3. **D.** What is shown is an increase in pressure caused by norepinephrine and the reduction of the effect by drug X. Therefore, drug X is an antagonist of norepinephrine. Two of the choices are adrenoceptor antagonists, prazosin and propranolol, which are α- and β-receptor antagonists, respectively. The adrenoceptors that mediate vasoconstriction are α-receptors. Therefore, prazosin, the α-blocker, is the correct choice. Cocaine, because it blocks neuronal uptake of norepinephrine, would actually enhance the response to this catecholamine, as would guanethidine, because it also blocks neuronal uptake of norepinephrine. Atropine is a muscarinic receptor antagonist and would not affect responses to norepinephrine.

4. **C.** The vasodilation produced by drug Y is antagonized by timolol, a β-receptor antagonist. Although bradykinin, histamine, acetylcholine, and isoproterenol will all cause vasodilation, only isoproterenol does so by activating β-receptors. Phenylephrine is a sympathomimetic that is selective for α-receptors and would be expected to increase, rather than decrease, perfusion pressure.

5. **A.** Both sets of responses to isoproterenol are mediated by β-adrenoceptors, and all the choices are β-antagonists. However, drug X is more effective in antagonizing cardiac responses to isoproterenol than it is the bronchiolar responses. Drug X is therefore a cardioselective β-blocker, that is, selective for β_1 over β_2 receptors. Metoprolol is the only β_1-selective antagonist among the choices.

SUPPLEMENTAL READING

Brodde O-E. β_1- and β_2-adrenoceptors in the human heart: Properties, function, and alterations in chronic heart failure. Pharmacol Rev 1991;43:203–242.

Brooks AM and Gillies WE. Ocular beta blockers in glaucoma management: Clinical pharmacology aspects. Drugs Aging 1992;2:208–221.

Bylund DB et al. Nomenclature of adrenoceptors. Pharmacol Rev 1994;46:1211–1236.

Cruickshank JM and Prichard BNC. Beta-Blockers in Clinical Practice (2nd ed). London: Churchill Livingstone, 1994.

Harrison JK et al. Molecular characterization of α_1- and α_2- adrenoceptors. Trends Pharmacol Sci 1991;12:62–67.

Lonnqvist F et al. Evidence for a functional β_3-adrenoceptor in man. Br J Pharmacol 1993;110:929–936.

Piascik MT and Perez DM. Alpha 1-adrenergic receptors: New insights and directions. J Pharmacol Exp Ther 2001;298:403–410.

Ruffolo RR Jr. et al. Structure and function of α-adrenoceptors. Pharmacol Rev 1991;43:475–505.

CASE **Study**   **Cardiopulmonary Complications of Eyedrops**

A 61-year-old man with congenital heart disease and a history of chronic congestive heart failure was seen by an ophthalmologist for a routine eye examination. In general, the patient's health was reasonable and cardiac output was well compensated. During the examination, the physician found that the patient had open-angle glaucoma that required treatment to reduce the pressure in the eye. The ophthalmologist prescribed one eyedrop twice daily in each eye. Several months later the patient began to gain weight, became dyspneic and complained of "asthmatic attacks." An examination showed bronchospasm and severe congestive heart failure with a slow ventricular rate. Gastrointestinal function was normal. The eyedrops were stopped and the patient's condition stabilized. Is it possible that the eyedrops were responsible for the development of cardiopulmonary complications, and if so, what is a likely offending drug?

ANSWER: The finding that the patient's symptoms subsided after terminating the treatment certainly implicates the eyedrops in precipitating the congestive heart failure. Although it is unusual to absorb enough drug through the eye to produce systemic effects, it does happen and physicians should be aware of it. The usual classes of drugs used to treat open-angle glaucoma include the carbonic anhydrase inhibitors (e.g., acetazolamide), cholinergic miotic agents (e.g., pilocarpine), β-adrenoceptor antagonists (e.g., timolol), and epinephrinelike drugs. Acetazolamide is unlikely to be the offending agent because it is usually administered orally. The clinical symptoms in this patient, including the bronchoconstriction and slow heart rate, are not consistent with the actions of epinephrine, which would be expected to cause bronchodilation and an increase in heart rate.

Pilocarpine, a naturally occurring cholinomimetic, and timolol, a β-blocking agent, both should be considered. Pilocarpine, because of its agonistic effect at muscarinic receptors, can cause bronchoconstriction and precipitate an asthmatic attack; β-blockers, such as timolol, should always be used with caution in an asthmatic patient and are known to worsen symptoms in some individuals with congestive heart failure. The weight gain in this patient, due to edema, and the dyspnea, due to pulmonary congestion, are classic signs of congestive heart failure and can be caused in a susceptible individual by a β-blocker. The slow heart rate is also consistent with either a β-blocker or use of pilocarpine. One might have expected gastrointestinal disturbances if the reaction to the glaucoma medication was due to the systemic accumulation of pilocarpine. All in all, the most likely choice is a β-blocker, and a different class of drug should be used to treat the glaucoma in this patient.

12

Directly and Indirectly Acting Cholinomimetics

William F. Wonderlin

 DRUG LIST

GENERIC NAME	PAGE	GENERIC NAME	PAGE
Acetylcholine	122	Isofluorophate	127
Ambenonium	126	Methacholine	123
Bethanechol	123	Neostigmine	130
Carbachol	123	Physostigmine	130
Demecarium	130	Pilocarpine	123
Donepezil	128	Pralidoxime	131
Echothiophate	130	Pyridostigmine	127
Edrophonium	126	Rivastigmine	127
Galanthamine	128	Tacrine	128

Cholinomimetic drugs can elicit some or all of the effects that acetylcholine (ACh) produces. This class of drugs includes agents that act directly as agonists at cholinoreceptors and agents that act indirectly by inhibiting the enzymatic destruction of endogenous ACh (i.e., cholinesterase inhibitors). The directly acting cholinomimetics can be subdivided into agents that exert their effects primarily through stimulation of muscarinic receptors at parasympathetic neuroeffector junctions (parasympathomimetic drugs) and agents that stimulate nicotinic receptors in autonomic ganglia and at the neuromuscular junction (see Chapter 9). This chapter focuses on the parasympathomimetic drugs and cholinesterase inhibitors. Drugs acting at nicotinic receptors are presented in Chapters 14 and 28.

Muscarinic Receptors and Signal Transduction

Classical studies by Sir Henry Dale demonstrated that the receptors activated by *muscarine*, an alkaloid isolated from the mushroom *Amanita muscaria*, are the same receptors activated by ACh released from parasympathetic nerve endings, from which the general notion that muscarinic agonists have parasympathomimetic properties was born. This conclusion is true but incomplete, and we now know that muscarinic receptors have a broader distribution and many functional roles. To understand the actions of cholinomimetic drugs it is essential to recognize that muscarinic receptors: (1) mediate the activation of effectors by ACh released from parasympathetic nerve endings; (2) mediate the activation of sweat glands by ACh released from sympathetic fibers; (3) are found on vascular endothelial cells that receive no cholinergic innervation; (4) are widely distributed in the central nervous system (CNS), from basal ganglia to neocortex; and (5) are present on presynaptic nerve terminals, including terminals that release ACh and terminals associated with other neurotransmitter systems, such as the catecholamines. Therefore, the activation of muscarinic receptors may influence most of the organ systems along with CNS pathways involved in regulating voluntary motor activity, memory, and cognition. Activation of presynaptic muscarinic receptors can inhibit the release of endogenous neurotransmitters, and may account for some paradoxical effects of cholinomimetic stimulation.

Binding studies with high-affinity receptor antagonists revealed four subtypes of muscarinic receptors that can be distinguished on the basis of (1) the rank order of potency of specific antagonists in functional experiments and (2) the affinity of these antagonists for muscarinic receptors in the same tissues. More recently, molecular studies have revealed five genetically distinct receptor subtypes, named M1 through M5, the first four of which correspond to functionally defined receptors. The different subtypes of muscarinic receptors are heterogeneously distributed: (1) M1 receptors are present in brain, exocrine glands, and autonomic ganglia. (2) M2 receptors are found in the heart, brain, autonomic ganglia, and smooth muscle. (3) M3 receptors are present in smooth muscle, exocrine glands, brain, and endothelial cells. (4) M4 receptors are present in brain and autonomic ganglia. (5) M5 receptors are found in the CNS.

All muscarinic receptors are members of the seven transmembrane domain, G protein–coupled receptors, and they are structurally and functionally unrelated to nicotinic ACh receptors. Activation of muscarinic receptors by an agonist triggers the release of an intracellular G-protein complex that can specifically activate one or more signal transduction pathways. Fortunately, the cellular responses elicited by odd- versus even-numbered receptor subtypes can be conveniently distinguished. Activation of M1, M3, and M5 receptors produces an inosine triphosphate (IP3) mediated release of intracellular calcium, the release of diacylglycerol (which can activate protein kinase C), and stimulation of adenylyl cyclase. These receptors are primarily responsible for activating calcium-dependent responses, such as secretion by glands and the contraction of smooth muscle.

Activation of M2 and M4 receptors inhibits adenylyl cyclase, and activation of M2 receptors opens potassium channels. The opening of potassium channels hyperpolarizes the membrane potential and decreases the excitability of cells in the sinoatrial (SA) and atrioventricular (A-V) nodes in the heart. The inhibition of adenylyl cyclase decreases cellular cyclic adenosine monophosphate (cAMP) levels, which can override the opposing stimulation of adenylyl cyclase by β-adrenoceptor agonists.

Although muscarinic receptors as a class can be selectively activated and they demonstrate strong stereoselectivity among both agonists and antagonists (see Chapter 13), the therapeutic use of cholinomimetics is limited by the paucity of drugs selective for specific *subtypes* of muscarinic receptors. This lack of specificity combined with the broad-ranging effects of muscarinic stimulation on different organ systems makes the therapeutic use of cholinomimetic drugs a challenge, and the careful consideration of the pharmacokinetic properties of the drugs plays an especially important role in making therapeutic decisions.

DIRECT-ACTING PARASYMPATHOMIMETIC DRUGS

Acetylcholine

Acetylcholine is an ester of choline and acetic acid, the prototype for a small family of choline ester compounds. The choline moiety of ACh contains a quaternary ammonium group that gives ACh a permanent positive charge, making it very hydrophilic and membrane impermeant.

ACh is degraded by a group of enzymes called cholinesterases. These enzymes catalyze the hydrolysis of ACh to choline and acetic acid (Fig. 12.1). The active center of cholinesterase has two areas that interact with ACh: the anionic site and the esteratic site. The anionic site contains a negatively charged amino acid that binds the positively charged quaternary ammonium group of ACh through coulombic forces. This probably serves to bring the ester linkage of ACh close to the esteratic site of the enzyme. The esteratic site contains a serine residue, which is made more reactive by hydrogen bonding to a nearby histidine residue. The nucleophilic oxygen of the serine reacts with the carbonyl carbon of ACh, thereby breaking the ester linkage. During this reaction, choline is liberated and an acetylated enzyme is formed. The latter intermediate is rapidly hydrolyzed to release acetic acid and regenerate the active enzyme. The entire process takes about 150 microseconds, one of the fastest enzymatic reactions known.

There are two major types of cholinesterases: acetylcholinesterase (AChE) and pseudocholinesterase (pseudo-ChE). AChE (also known as true, specific, or erythrocyte cholinesterase) is found at a number of sites in the body, the most important being the cholinergic neuroeffector junction. Here it is localized to the prejunctional and postjunctional membranes, where it rapidly terminates the action of synaptically released ACh. It is essential to recognize that *the action of ACh is ter-*

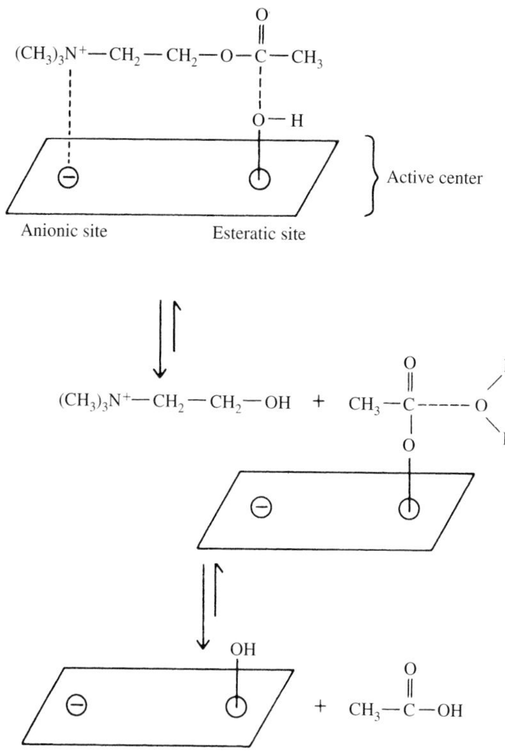

FIGURE 12.1
Simplified scheme of ACh hydrolysis at the active center of ACh. Rectangular area represents the active center of the enzyme with its anionic and esteratic sites. *Top*, the initial bonding of ACh at the active center. The broken line at left represents electrostatic forces. The broken line at right represents the initial interaction between the serine oxygen of the enzyme and the carbonyl carbon of ACh. The ester linkage is broken, choline is liberated, and an acetylated enzyme intermediate is formed (*middle*). Finally, the acetylated intermediate undergoes hydrolysis to free the enzyme and generate acetic acid (*bottom*).

minated only by its hydrolysis. There is no reuptake system in cholinergic nerve terminals to reduce the concentration of ACh in a synaptic cleft, unlike the reuptake systems for other neurotransmitters such as dopamine, serotonin, and norepinephrine. Therefore, inhibition of AChE can greatly prolong the activation of cholinoreceptors by ACh released at a synapse.

Pseudo-ChE (also known as butyryl-, plasma, and nonspecific cholinesterase) has a widespread distribution, with enzyme especially abundant in the liver, where it is synthesized, and in the plasma. In spite of the abundance of pseudo-ChE, its physiological function has not been definitively identified. It does, however, play an important role in the metabolism of such clinically important compounds as succinylcholine, procaine, and numerous other esters.

Derivatives of ACh: Methacholine, Carbachol, and Bethanechol

The therapeutic usefulness of ACh is limited by (1) its lack of selectivity as an agonist for different types of cholinoreceptors and (2) its rapid degradation by cholinesterases. These limitations have been circumvented in part by the development of three *choline ester* derivatives of ACh: methacholine (*Provocholine*), carbachol (*Isopto Carbachol, Miostat*) and bethanechol (*Urecholine*). Methacholine differs from ACh only in the addition of a methyl group at the β-carbon of ACh. This modification greatly increases its selectivity for muscarinic receptors relative to nicotinic receptors, and it renders methacholine resistant to the pseudo-ChE in the plasma and decreases its susceptibility to AChE, thereby increasing its potency and duration of action compared to those of ACh. Carbachol differs from ACh only in the substitution of a carbamoyl group for the terminal methyl group of ACh. This substitution makes carbachol completely resistant to degradation by cholinesterases but does not improve its selectivity for muscarinic versus nicotinic receptors. Bethanechol combines the addition of the methyl group and the substitution of the terminal carbamoyl group, producing a drug that is a selective agonist of muscarinic receptors and is resistant to degradation by cholinesterases.

All of these drugs are very hydrophilic and membrane impermeant because they retain the quaternary ammonium group of the choline moiety of ACh.

Pilocarpine is a naturally occurring cholinomimetic alkaloid that is structurally distinct from the choline esters. It is a tertiary amine that crosses membranes relatively easily. Therefore, it is rapidly absorbed by the cornea of the eye, and it can cross the blood-brain barrier. Pilocarpine is a pure muscarinic receptor agonist, and it is unaffected by cholinesterases. *Muscarine* is an alkaloid with no therapeutic use, but it can produce dangerous cholinomimetic stimulation following ingestion of some types of mushrooms (e.g., *Inocybes*).

Basic Pharmacology of the Directly Acting Parasympathomimetic Drugs

Methacholine, bethanechol, and pilocarpine are selective agonists of muscarinic receptors, whereas carbachol and ACh can activate both muscarinic and nicotinic receptors. However, at usual therapeutic doses, the effects of carbachol and ACh are entirely due to the activation of muscarinic receptors. This apparent preference for muscarinic receptors can be attributed to the greater accessibility and abundance of these cholinoreceptors compared with the nicotinic receptors.

Cardiovascular Effects

Low doses of muscarinic agonists given intravenously relax arterial smooth muscle and produce a fall in blood pressure. These responses result from the stimulation of muscarinic receptors on vascular endothelial cells (Fig. 12.2). Activation of these receptors causes the endothelial cells to synthesize and release nitric oxide. Nitric oxide can diffuse into neighboring vascular smooth muscle cells, where it activates soluble guanylyl cyclase, thereby increasing the synthesis of cyclic guanosine monophosphate (cGMP) and relaxing the muscle fibers. Most of the resistance vasculature is not innervated by cholinergic neurons, and the physiological function of the endothelial muscarinic receptors is not known. However, activation of these receptors by directly acting cholinomimetic drugs has major pharmacological significance, as the potentially dangerous hypotension produced by their activation is an important limitation to the systemic administration of muscarinic agonists.

Although the release of ACh onto the heart by the vagus nerve slows the heart rate, a low dose of a muscarinic agonist can sometimes increase the heart rate. This paradoxical effect is produced when the decrease in blood pressure produced by stimulation of endothelial muscarinic receptors, as described earlier, triggers the activation of a compensatory sympathetic reflex stimulation of the heart. Sympathetic stimulation increases heart rate and vasomotor tone, partially counteracting the direct vasodilator response. Therefore, the tachycardia produced by muscarinic agonists is indirect. At higher concentrations of a muscarinic agonist, the direct effects on cardiac muscarinic (M2) receptors in the

SA node and A-V fibers become dominant. Activation of M2 receptors increases the potassium permeability and reduces cAMP levels, slowing the rate of depolarization and decreasing the excitability of SA node and A-V fiber cells. This results in marked bradycardia and a slowing of A-V conduction that can override the stimulation of the heart by catecholamines released during sympathetic stimulation. In fact, very high doses of a muscarinic agonist can produce lethal bradycardia and A-V block. Choline esters have relatively minor direct effects on ventricular function, but they can produce negative inotropy of the atria.

The Eye

When solutions of directly acting cholinomimetics are applied to the eye (i.e., conjunctival sac), they cause contraction of the smooth muscle in two important structures, the iris sphincter and the ciliary muscles (Fig. 12.3). Contraction of the iris sphincter decreases the diameter of the pupil (miosis). Contraction of the circular fibers of the ciliary muscle, which encircles the lens, reduces the tension on the suspensory ligaments that normally stretch and flatten the lens, allowing the highly elastic lens to spontaneously round up and focus for near vision (accommodation to near vision).

Other Organ Systems

Prominent effects within the digestive tract include stimulation of salivation and acid secretion, increased intestinal tone and peristaltic activity, and relaxation of most sphincters. Bronchoconstriction and stimulation of secretions are prominent effects in the respiratory system. Muscarinic agonists can also evoke secretion from nasopharyngeal glands. Urination is promoted by stimulation of the detrusor muscle of the bladder and is facilitated by relaxation of the trigone and external sphincter muscles.

Clinical Uses
Glaucoma

Cholinomimetic drugs are useful for treating glaucoma because they can decrease the resistance to the movement of fluid (aqueous humor) out of the eye (Fig. 12.3), thereby reducing the intraocular pressure. It is useful to distinguish between open-angle glaucoma, a chronic condition in which the porosity of the trabecular meshwork is insufficient to permit the movement of fluid into the canal of Schlemm, and angle-closure glaucoma, an emergency condition in which an abnormal position of the peripheral iris blocks the access of fluid to the trabecular meshwork. Open-angle glaucoma can be effectively treated with cholinomimetics such as pilocarpine and carbachol, because contraction of the ciliary muscle stretches the trabecular network, increasing its porosity

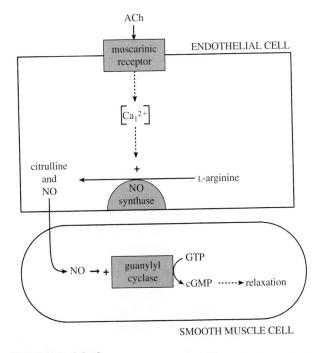

FIGURE 12.2

Mechanism for vasodilation produced by ACh. Arrows with broken tail indicate multiple steps or that other factors are involved. NO, nitric oxide.

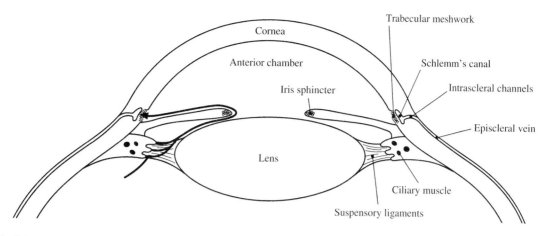

FIGURE 12.3

Diagram of eye depicting major pathway for outflow of aqueous humor (*arrow*) and ocular smooth muscles, which contract in response to parasympathomimetics or cholinesterase inhibitors (i.e., iris sphincter and ciliary muscle).

and permeability to the outflow of fluid. This beneficial effect, however, comes at the price of a spasm of accommodation and miosis, which seriously disturb vision. Cholinomimetics, therefore, have been replaced by β-blockers and carbonic anhydrase inhibitors, both of which decrease the formation of aqueous humor without affecting vision. However, some patients simply do not respond to these treatments or do not tolerate the cardiovascular side effects of the β-blockers, and cholinomimetics (most notably pilocarpine) remain as important treatment alternatives.

Contraction of the iris sphincter (miosis) by cholinomimetic stimulation is less important than contraction of the ciliary muscle for treating angle-closure glaucoma, but it may be essential as emergency therapy for acute-angle glaucoma to reduce intraocular pressure prior to surgery (iridectomy). Contraction of the iris sphincter by pilocarpine pulls the peripheral iris away from the trabecular meshwork, thereby opening the path for aqueous outflow.

Pilocarpine is the first choice among cholinomimetics for the treatment of glaucoma. Pilocarpine can be applied to the eye as a gel (Pilopine HS Gel) or time-release system (Ocusert) for the chronic treatment of open-angle glaucoma, or as drops (Pilocar) for an acute reduction of intraocular pressure, as in the emergency management of angle-closure glaucoma. Carbachol is sometimes effective in treating cases of open-angle glaucoma that are resistant to pilocarpine.

Surgery of the Eye

Because ACh is rapidly inactivated by cholinesterases, its use is best suited for clinical applications requiring only a brief duration of action, such as when it is employed to cause miosis during cataract surgery. ACh

(Miochol) can produce a brief (10 minutes) miosis, and carbachol is used during eye surgery necessitating miosis of a longer duration.

Urinary Retention

Bethanechol is used to treat postsurgical bladder dysfunction associated with the retention of urine. It is most commonly given orally for this purpose, although the subcutaneous route is also used. Effects are more rapid and intense after subcutaneous administration, but the duration of action is shorter.

Diagnosis of Bronchial Hyperreactivity

Methacholine is used to identify bronchial hyperreactivity in patients without clinically apparent asthma. For this indication, the drug is administered by inhalation, and patients who may be developing asthma usually produce an exaggerated airway contraction. Upon completion of the test, a rapid-acting bronchodilator (e.g., inhaled β-adrenoceptor agonist) can be given to counter the bronchoconstrictor effect of methacholine and relieve the patient's discomfort.

Adverse Effects

Potentially severe adverse effects can result from systemic administration of cholinomimetic drugs, and none should be administered by intramuscular or intravenous injection. If significant amounts of these drugs enter the circulation, nausea, abdominal cramps, diarrhea, salivation, hypotension with reflex tachycardia, cutaneous vasodilation, sweating, and bronchoconstriction can result. Pilocarpine can cross the blood-brain barrier and affect cognitive function. Even the topical application of cholinomimetics to the eyes can present some risk, and the escape of cholinomimetics into the circulatory system following topical application to the eye can be minimized by pressure applied to the lacrimal duct. Within the eye, cholinomimetics elicit miosis and spasm of accommodation, both of which disturb vision.

Bethanechol is relatively selective in activating cholinoreceptors in the gastrointestinal and urinary tracts when taken orally, but it is less selective when given subcutaneously, and it is very dangerous when given intramuscularly or intravenously, having the potential to produce circulatory collapse and cardiac arrest. Systemic poisoning with cholinomimetics can be treated with the muscarinic receptor antagonist atropine.

Bethanechol should not be used in patients with possible mechanical obstruction of the bladder or gastrointestinal tract or when contraction of smooth muscles in these tissues may be harmful (e.g., recent intestinal resection). It is also contraindicated in patients with bronchial asthma, peptic ulcer disease, coronary artery disease, gastrointestinal hypermotility or inflammatory disease, hypotension or marked bradycardia, hyperthyroidism, parkinsonism, or epilepsy. Care should be exercised in administering pilocarpine to elderly patients because it can enter the CNS and affect memory and cognition, even when applied topically to the eye.

CHOLINESTERASE INHIBITORS

Inhibition of AChE slows or prevents the degradation of ACh released at synapses, and this can greatly prolong the activation of cholinoreceptors produced by synaptically released ACh. In a functional sense, the indirect cholinomimetic effect of AChE inhibitors is more selective than the effect of directly acting cholinomimetics, because the inhibitors of AChE increase the activation of cholinoreceptors only at active cholinergic synapses. This permits strengthening of the phasic stimulation of synaptically activated cholinoreceptors rather than the persistent activation by directly acting cholinomimetics. At therapeutic concentrations, inhibitors of AChE do not activate cholinoreceptors at sites that do not receive cholinergic synaptic input, such as endothelial muscarinic receptors, and therefore do not present the same risk of eliciting large vasodilator responses.

Acetylcholinesterase can be inhibited by two general mechanisms. In the first mechanism, positively charged quaternary ammonium compounds bind to the anionic site and prevent ACh from binding—a simple competitive inhibition. In the second mechanism, the agents act either as a false substrate for the cholinesterase or directly attack the esteratic site; in both cases they covalently modify the esteratic site and noncompetitively prevent further hydrolytic activity. Either mechanism can be effective in preventing the hydroly-

sis of ACh, but they differ markedly in their pharmacokinetic properties.

Inhibition of AChE can increase the stimulation of both muscarinic and nicotinic receptors produced by synaptically released ACh. Nicotinic receptors can also be stimulated directly by AChE inhibitors with a quaternary ammonium group, and this can potentiate their cholinomimetic effect. Finally, although inhibition of true AChE is most important for potentiating the synaptic activity of ACh, several AChE inhibitors also inhibit the pseudo-ChE in plasma. This can permit plasma concentrations of ACh to rise markedly and activate endothelial muscarinic receptors.

Quaternary Ammonium Agents

Edrophonium (*Enlon, Tensilon*) and ambenonium (*Mytelase*) are monoquaternary and bisquaternary ammonium alcohols, respectively. Their positive charge allows them to bind to the anionic site at the reactive center, competitively displacing ACh from the active site without covalent modification of the site. Edrophonium has a very short duration of action, lasting only 5 to 10 minutes, whereas inhibition by ambenonium can last 4 to 8 hours. These drugs have direct agonist activity at nicotinic receptors.

Carbamates

Carbamate anticholinesterase agents are carbamic acid esters that are hydrolyzed by AChE in a manner similar to that of ACh. Carbamates have this general structure:

$$R_2 - N - C - O - R_3$$

with R_1 on the nitrogen and O double-bonded to the carbon.

The clinically useful carbamates generally contain a tertiary or quaternary amine group that can bind noncovalently to the anionic site of the enzyme. The inhibition of AChE by *neostigmine* (Prostigmin) illustrates the general mechanism. The quaternary ammonium group of neostigmine binds electrostatically to the anionic site of the enzyme, thereby orienting the drug. The serine oxygen at the esteratic site of the enzyme then reacts with the carbonyl carbon of neostigmine, just as it did with ACh (Fig. 12.1). However, a carbamylated intermediate is formed instead of an acetylated one, and this carbamylated enzyme undergoes hydrolysis much more slowly. Whereas the acetylated enzyme is hydrolyzed nearly instantly, the half-life for hydrolysis of this particular carbamylated intermediate is about an hour. The carbamates generally inhibit pseudo-ChE as well as true AChE, and their suicidal degradation by cholinesterases contributes importantly to terminating their duration of effect. Physostigmine (also called eserine) (*Antilirium*) is a tertiary amine that can inhibit

AChE in the CNS, and it can be used in life-threatening cases to treat antimuscarinic poisoning.

Pyridostigmine (*Mestinon*) is a quaternary ammonium carbamate. Neostigmine and pyridostigmine also have direct agonist activity at nicotinic receptors on skeletal muscle. Rivastigmine (*Exelon*) is a carbamate cholinesterase inhibitor with good penetration into the brain.

Organophosphates

The organophosphate compounds also react at the esteratic site of AChE (Fig. 12.4). In general, however, they are much less selective than are the carbamates, inhibiting many enzymes that contain a serine molecule at an active center. The organophosphate compounds have this general structure:

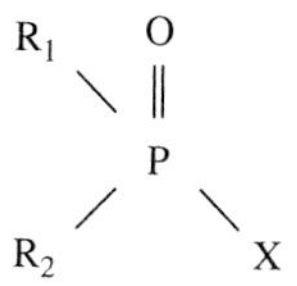

$$\begin{array}{c} R_1 \quad O \\ \diagdown \quad \| \\ P \\ \diagup \quad \diagdown \\ R_2 \qquad X \end{array}$$

Examples of X groups are fluorine in isoflurophate (*Floropryl*, no longer available in the United States or Canada) and echothiophate (*Phospholine*). Parathion and malathion (insecticides) are thiophosphates

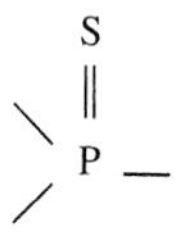

$$\begin{array}{c} S \\ \| \\ \diagdown \quad P \\ \diagup \quad \diagdown \end{array}$$

that must be converted to oxyanalogues to become active. The organophosphates, except for echothiophate, are very lipid soluble.

In the interaction of isoflurophate with AChE, a phosphorylated intermediate is formed and fluoride is released. An important characteristic of the organophosphate-induced inhibition is that the bond between the phosphate and the enzyme is very stable. While the regeneration of most carbamylated enzymes occurs with a half-life of minutes or hours, the recovery of a phosphorylated enzyme is generally measured in days. These agents are referred to, therefore, as irreversible inhibitors.

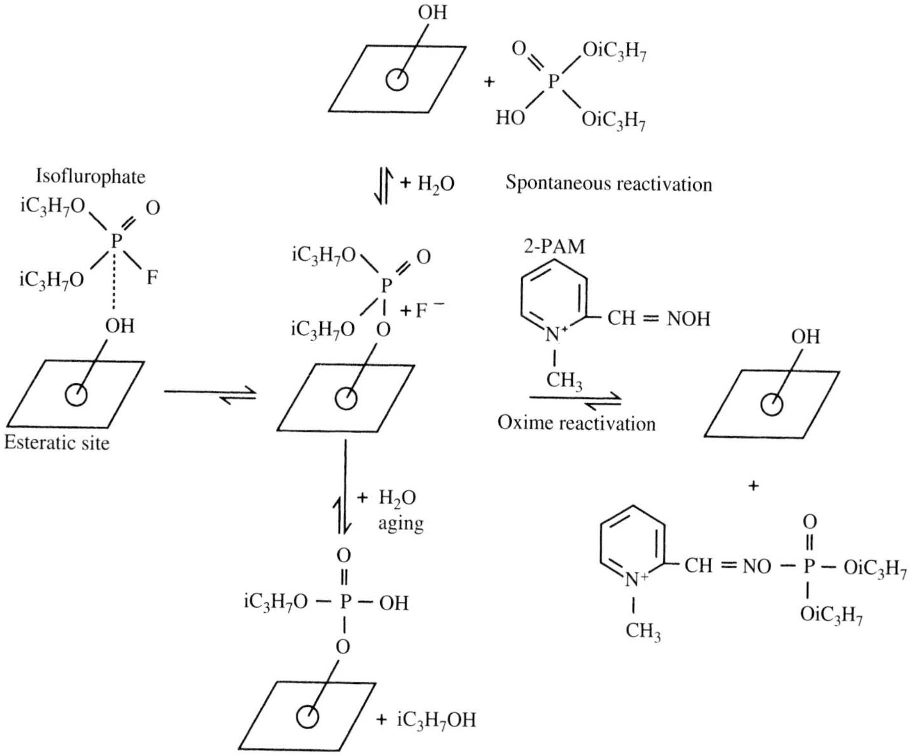

FIGURE 12.4

Isofluorophate reaction at AChE esteratic site, aging, spontaneous reactivation, and oxime reactivation. *Left,* the nucleophilic attack on the phosphorus of isofluorophate by the serine oxygen. This results in a stable phosphorylated enzyme intermediate, which undergoes dephosphorylation at a negligible rate (*top*). A more favorable reaction is the loss of an isopropoxy group, a process termed aging (*bottom*). This renders the phosphorylated enzyme resistant to dephosphorylation by an oxime. The original phosphorylated intermediate (*center*) will react with the nucleophilic oxygen of pralidoxime (2-PAM), resulting in dephosphorylation of the enzyme and formation of an oxime phosphonate (*lower right*).

Although the spontaneous hydrolysis of a phosphorylated enzyme is generally very slow, compounds called oximes can cause dephosphorylation (Fig. 12.4). Pralidoxime chloride (2-PAM) (Protopam chloride) is an oxime used therapeutically to reactivate phosphorylated AChE. It has the additional feature that its quaternary ammonium group binds to the anionic site of the enzyme and thereby promotes dephosphorylation. If the oxime is not administered soon enough (minutes to hours) after AChE has been inhibited, an alkoxy group may be lost from the phosphorylated enzyme. This reaction is called aging. Once aging has occurred, oximes can no longer regenerate free enzymes. The rate of aging appears to depend both on the nature of the enzyme (AChE or pseudo-ChE) and on the particular inhibitor employed. Since pralidoxime is a quaternary amine, it does not cross the blood-brain barrier, and it is not useful for reactivating cholinesterases in the CNS.

Inhibitors targeted at AChE in the CNS

Several inhibitors of AChE have been developed for use in treating Alzheimer's disease, which requires that the drugs readily enter the CNS. These inhibitors are structurally unrelated and vary in their mechanism of inhibition, although all are reversible inhibitors. Tacrine (*Cognex*) is a monoamine acridine. Donepezil (*Aricept*) is a piperidine derivative that is a relatively specific inhibitor of AChE in the brain, with little effect on pseudo-ChE in the periphery. Galanthamine (*Reminyl*) is a tertiary alkaloid and phenanthrene derivative extracted from daffodil bulbs that is a reversible competitive inhibitor of AChE; it also acts on nicotinic receptors.

Absorption, Metabolism, and Excretion

Physostigmine and rivastigmine are tertiary amines that are rapidly absorbed from the gastrointestinal tract, as are tacrine, donepezil, and galanthamine, whereas quaternary ammonium compounds are poorly absorbed after oral administration. Nevertheless, quaternary ammonium compounds like neostigmine and pyridostigmine are orally active if larger doses are employed. Only the quaternary ammonium inhibitors do not readily enter the CNS. Because of their high lipid solubility and low molecular weight, most of the organophosphates are absorbed by all routes of administration; even percutaneous exposure can result in the absorption of sufficient drug to permit the accumulation of toxic levels of these compounds.

Edrophonium is partially metabolized to a glucuronide conjugate in the liver. Some of this metabolite is excreted in bile. Carbamates undergo both nonenzymatic and enzymatic hydrolysis, with enzymatic hydrolysis generally resulting from an interaction of the drug with the pseudo-ChE in plasma and liver. Organophosphates are metabolized to inactive products by hydrolytic enzymes in the plasma, kidney, liver, and lungs. In contrast, the organophosphate insecticide parathion requires metabolism (oxidative desulfuration) to become an effective insecticide.

Metabolites of the cholinesterase inhibitors and in some instances significant amounts of the parent compound are eliminated in the urine. Renal excretion is very important in the clearance of agents such as neostigmine, pyridostigmine, and edrophonium. This is demonstrated by a twofold to threefold increase in elimination half-lives for these drugs in anephric patients. Renal elimination is largely the result of glomerular filtration but probably also involves, at least in the case of quaternary amines, secretion via the renal cationic transport system.

Basic Pharmacology

Inhibition of AChE potentiates and prolongs the stimulation of cholinoreceptors resulting from ACh released at cholinergic synapses (Fig. 12.5). These synapses include those found at the skeletal neuromuscular junction, adrenal medulla, autonomic ganglia, cholinergic neuroeffector junctions of the autonomic nervous system, and cholinergic synapses in the CNS. The degree and range of effects observed depend on the inhibitor chosen, the dose employed, and the route of exposure or administration.

Neuromuscular transmission in skeletal muscle is enhanced by low concentrations of anticholinesterase agents, whereas high concentrations result in cholinergic blockade. This blockade is initially due to a persistent membrane depolarization and inactivation of voltage-gated sodium channels, but if ACh levels remain high, the nicotinic cholinergic receptors can quickly become desensitized. Although anticholinesterase agents will facilitate cholinergic transmission at autonomic ganglia, their action at these sites is less marked than at the neuromuscular junction. See Chapter 28 for further discussion of this topic. Muscarinic receptors do not exhibit comparable desensitization.

Anticholinesterase agents of all classes can initiate antidromic firing of action potentials in motor neurons, possibly due to an activation of prejunctional ACh receptors that are activated by the elevated synaptic ACh. Quaternary ammonium inhibitors can also act as agonists at these receptors. The initiation of antidromic firing may be a mechanism by which cholinesterase inhibitors produce fasciculation of skeletal muscle.

The actions of anticholinesterase agents on the cardiovascular system are complex. The primary effect produced by potentiation of vagal stimulation is bradycardia with a consequent decrease in cardiac output and blood pressure. However, potentiation of both parasympathetic and sympathetic ganglionic transmis-

A No Drug   B AChE Inhibitor (—||→)

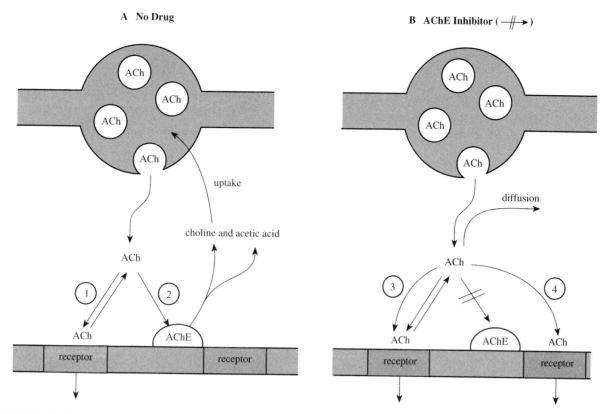

FIGURE 12.5

Action of AChE at a cholinergic neuroeffector function and effects of AChE inhibition. **A.** Key features of cholinergic neurotransmission in the absence of drugs. After release from a cholinergic nerve terminal or varicosity, ACh can (1) bind reversibly to cholinergic receptors in the postsynaptic membrane and elicit a response or (2) bind to AChE and undergo hydrolysis to choline and acetic acid (inactive metabolites). The survival time of released ACh is quite brief because of the abundance and effectiveness of AChE. **B.** The consequences of inhibiting AChE. Since ACh no longer has access to the active site of AChE, the concentration of ACh in the synaptic cleft increases. This can result in enhanced transmission due to (3) repeated activation of receptors and (4) activation of additional cholinergic receptors.

sion, including that in the adrenal medulla, can produce complicated effects on the cardiovascular system, including vasoconstrictor responses. The activation of reflexes can also complicate the total cardiovascular response to cholinesterase inhibitors.

Clinical Uses
Myasthenia Gravis

Myasthenia gravis is an autoimmune disease in which antibodies recognize nicotinic cholinoreceptors on skeletal muscle. This decreases the number of functional receptors and consequently decreases the sensitivity of the muscle to ACh. Muscle weakness and rapid fatigue of muscles during use are characteristics of the disease. Anticholinesterase agents help to alleviate the weakness by elevating and prolonging the concentration of ACh in the synaptic cleft, producing a greater activation

of the remaining nicotinic receptors. By contrast, thymectomy, plasmapheresis, and corticosteroid administration are treatments directed at decreasing the autoimmune response.

Anticholinesterase agents play a key role in the diagnosis and therapy of myasthenia gravis, because they increase muscle strength. During diagnosis, the patient's muscle strength is examined before and immediately after the intravenous injection of edrophonium chloride. In myasthenics, an increase in muscle strength is obtained for a few minutes.

The pronounced weakness that may result from inadequate therapy of myasthenia gravis (myasthenic crisis) can be distinguished from that due to anticholinesterase overdose (cholinergic crisis) by the use of edrophonium. In cholinergic crisis, edrophonium will briefly cause a further weakening of muscles, whereas improvement in muscle strength is seen in the myasthenic patient whose anticholinesterase therapy is inadequate. Means for artificial respiration should be available when patients are being tested for cholinergic crisis.

Pyridostigmine and neostigmine are the major anticholinesterase agents used in the therapy of myasthenia gravis, but ambenonium can be used when these drugs are unsuitable. When it is feasible, these agents are given orally. Pyridostigmine has a slightly longer duration of action than neostigmine, with smoother dosing, and it causes fewer muscarinic side effects. Ambenonium may act somewhat longer than pyridostigmine, but it produces more side effects and tends to accumulate.

Smooth Muscle Atony

Anticholinesterase agents can be employed in the treatment of adynamic ileus and atony of the urinary bladder, both of which may result from surgery. Neostigmine is most commonly used, and it can be administered subcutaneously or intramuscularly in these conditions. Cholinesterase inhibitors are, of course, contraindicated if mechanical obstruction of the intestine or urinary tract is known to be present.

Antimuscarinic Toxicity

A number of drugs in addition to atropine and scopolamine have antimuscarinic properties. These include tricyclic antidepressants, phenothiazines, and antihistamines. Physostigmine has been used in the treatment of acute toxicity produced by these compounds. However, physostigmine can produce cardiac arrhythmias and other serious toxic effects of its own, and therefore, it should be considered as an antidote only in life-threatening cases of anticholinergic drug overdose.

Alzheimer's Disease

Alzheimer's disease is a slowly developing neurodegenerative disease that produces a progress loss of memory and cognitive function, that is, dementia. These functional changes appear to result primarily from the loss of cholinergic transmission in the neocortex. The four cholinesterase inhibitors that have been approved for use in the palliative treatment of Alzheimer's disease are tacrine, donepezil, rivastigmine, and galanthamine. These agents can cross the blood-brain barrier to produce a reversible inhibition of AChE in the CNS. These compounds produce modest but significant improvement in the cognitive function of patients with mild to moderate Alzheimer's disease, but they do not delay progression of the disease. Donepezil, rivastigmine, and galanthamine are as effective as tacrine in increasing cognitive performance but do not share tacrine's hepatotoxic effects.

Glaucoma

Long-lasting AChE inhibitors, such as demecarium (*Humorsol*), echothiophate, and physostigmine are also effective in treating open-angle glaucoma, although they have now been largely replaced by less toxic drugs. Topical application of long-acting cholinesterase inhibitors to the eye not only presents the risk of systemic effects, but they can cause cataracts; this is a primary reason for reluctance to use these drugs even in resistant cases of glaucoma. Pilocarpine should be used rather than AChE inhibitors for treating angle-closure glaucoma.

Strabismus

Drug treatment of *strabismus* (turning of one or both eyes from the normal position) is largely limited to certain cases of accommodative *esotropia* (inward deviation). Long-acting anticholinesterase agents, such as echothiophate or demecarium, are employed to potentiate accommodation by blocking ACh hydrolysis at the ciliary muscle and decreasing the activity of extraocular muscles of convergence. This results in reduced accommodative convergence. The same side effects and precautions mentioned for the use of these drugs in glaucoma apply to the therapy of strabismus.

Reversal of Neuromuscular Blockade

Anticholinesterase agents are widely used in anesthesiology to reverse the neuromuscular blockade caused by nondepolarizing muscle relaxants (see Chapter 28). The blockade by these drugs is competitive and can be overcome by increasing the concentration of ACh available to stimulate nicotinic cholinoreceptors at the neuromuscular junction. Neostigmine, pyridostigmine, and edrophonium are anticholinesterase agents that are used for this purpose. Atropine or glycopyrrolate is administered in conjunction with the anticholinesterase agents to prevent the bradycardia and other side effects that result from excessive stimulation of muscarinic receptors.

Adverse Effects

Accidental poisoning by cholinesterase inhibitors can arise in many settings, since these agents are not only used clinically but also widely used as agricultural and household insecticides, and accidental poisoning sometimes occurs during their manufacture and use. In addition, a number of cholinesterase inhibitors, including the nerve gases *sarin* and *soman,* have been used in chemical warfare. The acute toxicity of all of these agents results from the accumulation of ACh at cholinergic synapses. With increasing inhibition of AChE and accumulation of ACh, the first signs are muscarinic stimulation, followed by nicotinic receptor stimulation and then desensitization of nicotinic receptors. Excessive inhibition can ultimately lead to a *cholinergic crisis* that includes gastrointestinal distress (nausea, vomiting, diarrhea, excessive salivation), respiratory distress (bronchospasm and increased bronchial secretions), cardiovascular distress (bradycardia or tachycardia, A-V block, hypotension), visual disturbance (miosis, blurred vision), sweating, and loss of skeletal motor function (progressing through incoordination, muscle cramps, weakness, fasciculation, and paralysis). CNS symptoms include agitation, dizziness, and mental confusion. Death usually results from paralysis of skeletal muscles required for respiration but may also result from cardiac arrest. The progression through the adverse effects can be rapid.

Although anticholinesterase agents can be used in the treatment of atony of the bladder and adynamic ileus, they are contraindicated in cases of mechanical obstruction of the intestine or urinary tract. Caution should also be used in giving these drugs to a patient with bronchial asthma or other respiratory disorders, since they will further constrict the smooth muscle of the bronchioles and stimulate respiratory secretions.

Because anticholinesterase agents also inhibit plasma pseudo-ChE, they will potentiate the effects of succinylcholine by inhibiting its breakdown. This is important, for example, when succinylcholine is to be employed in patients who have previously received cholinesterase inhibitors for the treatment of myasthenia gravis or glaucoma.

Adverse effects unrelated to inhibition of AChE can also occur. Tacrine presents a high risk of hepatotoxicity, which limits its use. Some organophosphorous compounds produce delayed neurotoxicity unrelated to inhibition of any cholinesterase. Clinically, this syndrome is characterized by muscle weakness that begins a few weeks after acute poisoning and may progress to flaccid paralysis and eventually to spastic paralysis. This syndrome appears to result from changes in axonal transport. There is no specific therapy for organophosphate-induced neuropathy, and clinical recovery occurs only in the mildest cases.

Treatment of Anticholinesterase Poisoning

The first step in treatment of anticholinesterase poisoning should be injection of increasing doses of atropine sulfate to block all adverse effects resulting from stimulation of muscarinic receptors. Since atropine will not alleviate skeletal and respiratory muscle paralysis, mechanical respiratory support may be required.

If the poisoning is due to an organophosphate, prompt administration of pralidoxime chloride will result in dephosphorylation of cholinesterases in the periphery and a decrease in the degree of the blockade at the skeletal neuromuscular junction. Since pralidoxime is a quaternary amine, it will not enter the CNS and therefore cannot reactivate central cholinesterases. In addition, pralidoxime is effective only if there has been no aging of the phosphorylated enzyme. Pralidoxime has a greater effect at the skeletal neuromuscular junction than at autonomic effector sites.

Study QUESTIONS

1. A young patient is being treated for myasthenia gravis, which requires frequent adjustment of the optimal dose of neostigmine. The patient is challenged with edrophonium to evaluate the effectiveness of the cholinesterase inhibition. Optimal dosing will be indicated by
   (A) An increase in muscle strength
   (B) A decrease in muscle strength
   (C) No change in muscle strength

2. A young man broke his leg in a skiing accident, causing severe muscular spasm that necessitated relaxation of the muscle with a competitive nicotinic receptor antagonist before the fracture could be set. At the end of the orthopaedic procedure, the doctor restored neuromuscular transmission by administering:

   (A) Succinylcholine
   (B) Carbachol
   (C) Physostigmine
   (D) Neostigmine

3. A patient has developed glaucoma that is refractory to noncholinergic therapies. You decide to prescribe eyedrops containing pilocarpine, but you are concerned about the patient's ability to self-administer the drops. The most sensitive indicator of excessive administration of pilocarpine is
   (A) An increased heart rate
   (B) A decreased heart rate
   (C) Mental confusion
   (D) Constriction of the pupil

4. An 80-year-old man is increasingly forgetful, and his wife is afraid he is developing Alzheimer's disease. You are considering prescribing an anti-AChE drug to see if this will decrease his forgetfulness. Before making this prescription, you want to be sure that these drugs are suitable given the patient's medical history. Of the possible preexisting conditions listed below, you should be least concerned about
    (A) Asthma
    (B) Weak atrioventricular conduction
    (C) Glaucoma
    (D) Obstruction of the GI tract

5. The choice of route of administration plays an important role in the actions of directly acting cholinomimetics. An adverse effect of choline esters that may be avoided by selection of an appropriate route of administration is:
    (A) Bradycardia
    (B) Hypotension
    (C) Delirium
    (D) Sweating

ANSWERS

1. **C.** At an optimal dose of neostigmine, there should be no change in muscle strength with administration of edrophonium. If edrophonium increases muscle strength, the inhibition of AChE is insufficient and the maximum therapeutic benefit is not being achieved. If edrophonium decreases muscle strength, the dose of neostigmine is too high, bordering on the production of a depolarizing block of neuromuscular transmission.

2. **D.** Neostigmine will inhibit AChE and increase the ACh available to compete with the antagonist at the neuromuscular junction, overcoming the block of neurotransmission. Succinylcholine, a nicotinic agonist, will only very transiently increase the strength of the muscle, after which it will produce a depolarizing block. Carbachol is a nonselective cholinoreceptor agonist that will stimulate nicotinic and muscarinic receptors without therapeutic benefit. Physostigmine will increase the strength of the muscle by the same mechanism as neostigmine, but it will also enter the CNS, producing undesirable side effects.

3. **A.** Excessive administration of pilocarpine can cause it to enter the circulatory system, activate endothelial muscarinic receptors, and produce a fall in blood pressure. This will activate sympathetic re-

flexes that increase the heart rate. Higher levels of pilocarpine would be required to stimulate muscarinic receptors on the heart that can decrease the heart rate. Although pilocarpine can enter the CNS and produce confusion in older patients, this also requires higher doses. Pilocarpine will constrict the pupil at therapeutically appropriate doses.

4. **C.** Glaucoma as a preexisting condition does not contraindicate an AChE inhibitor. The other preexisting conditions preclude the administration of AChE inhibitors. Potentiation of parasympathetic stimulation can constrict airway smooth muscle and aggravate asthma, further weaken A-V conduction, and risk perforation of the bowel if an obstruction is present.

5. **B.** Hypotension, which can be life threatening, can be avoided by preventing the entry of directly acting cholinomimetics into the circulatory system. Bradycardia and sweating are also avoided by the same precaution, but they are less significant. Delirium is not an issue for choline esters, since they do not enter the CNS.

SUPPLEMENTAL READING

Abou-Donia M and Lapadula DM. Mechanisms of organophosphorus ester-induced delayed neurotoxicity: Type I and type II. Annu Rev Pharmacol Toxicol 1990;30:405–440.

Evoli A, Batocchi AP, and Tonali P. A practical guide to the recognition and management of myasthenia gravis. Drugs 1996;52:662–670.

Farlow MR. Pharmacokinetic profiles of current therapies for Alzheimer's disease: implications for switching to galanthamine. Clin Ther 2001;23:A13–A24.

Felder C. Muscarinic acetylcholine receptors: Signal transduction through multiple effectors. FASEB J 1995;9:619–625.

Hoyng PF and van Beek LM. Pharmacological therapy for glaucoma: a review. Drugs 2000;411–34.

Millard CB and Broomfield CA. Anticholinesterases: Medical applications of neurochemical principles. J Neurochem 1995 64:1909–1918.

Schneider LS. Treatment of Alzheimer's disease with cholinesterase inhibitors. Clin Geriatr Med 2001;17:337–358.

Treatment of nerve gas poisoning. Med Lett 1995;37:43–44.

CASE Study   Will you give 2-PAM to Pam?

A young woman named Pam has been brought to the emergency department. She is sweating profusely, vomiting, and having difficulty breathing. She cannot walk without assistance, and she has a pulse of 30. She is delirious and unable to explain her condition. The friend who brought her in said that the woman had threatened suicide 2 hours earlier. What should you do?

ANSWER: It is very likely that Pam has ingested an AChE inhibitor, most likely an insecticide. An additional diagnostic test would be to examine the size of the pupils and test for pupillary reflexes. If it is an anti-AChE overdose, the pupils will be constricted, and they will open only slightly (if at all) when the eye is darkened. The easy decision is to administer atropine, a treatment that typically presents relatively little risk. This will reduce or eliminate many symptoms, including the bradycardia, nausea, hypotension, sweating, and the component of the respiratory difficulty resulting from bronchoconstriction. A more difficult decision is whether to give an oxime (2-pralidoxime) to reactivate the AChE. It appears that the ingestion occurred in the past 2 hours, so reactivation by an oxime is still possible. The more difficult question is whether oxime treatment is necessary. Insecticides can include reversible carbamate AChE inhibitors or irreversible phosphorylating compounds. Unfortunately, you don't know which she has ingested. Certainly a quick inquiry to see if the product can be identified would be worth the effort. Oximes are effective in reactivating AChE inhibited by carbamates as well as phosphorylating inhibitors. However, oxime treatment does present some risk of its own, and it is not typically used for carbamate poisoning, since the life-threatening stage should pass within a few hours. You should immediately prepare for ventilatory support, as paralysis of the muscles of respiration is the primary cause of death. So there is no definitive answer to whether to administer an oxime. If there is reason to suspect a phosphorylating inhibitor was ingested or the patient is descending further into severe respiratory distress, treatment with an oxime might be warranted. However, if the patient's condition appears to be stable and adequate ventilatory support is available, it might be better to treat the patient symptomatically.

13 Muscarinic Blocking Drugs

William F. Wonderlin

 DRUG LIST

GENERIC NAME	PAGE	GENERIC NAME	PAGE
Atropine	136	Oxybutynin	137
Cyclopentolate	137	Propantheline	137
Dicyclomine	137	Scopolamine	136
Glycopyrrolate	137	Tolterodine	137
Ipratropium	138	Tropicamide	137

Muscarinic blocking drugs are compounds that selectively antagonize the responses to acetylcholine (ACh) and other parasympathomimetics that are mediated by activation of muscarinic receptors. These agents are also referred to as *muscarinic antagonists, antimuscarinic drugs,* and *anticholinergics.* The belladonna alkaloids, such as atropine, are the oldest known muscarinic blocking compounds, and their medicinal use preceded the concept of neurochemical transmission.

CHEMISTRY

The best known of the muscarinic blocking drugs are the belladonna alkaloids, atropine (*Atropine*) and scopolamine (*Scopolamine*). They are tertiary amines that contain an ester linkage. Atropine is a racemic mixture of DL-hyoscyamine, of which only the levorotatory isomer is pharmacologically active. Atropine and scopolamine are parent compounds for several semisynthetic derivatives, and some synthetic compounds with little structural similarity to the belladonna alkaloids are also in use. All of the antimuscarinic compounds are amino alcohol esters with a tertiary amine or quaternary ammonium group.

The control of access to muscarinic receptors in the central nervous system (CNS) by a tertiary amine versus quaternary ammonium group is fundamentally important in selecting among antimuscarinic agents.

MECHANISM OF ACTION

Antimuscarinic drugs are competitive antagonists of the binding of ACh to muscarinic receptors. The seven transmembrane helices of these receptors have a ringlike organization in the cell membrane that forms a narrow central cleft where ACh binds. At least seven amino acids from four transmembrane helices have been implicated in agonist binding to the muscarinic receptors. Some of these residues, particularly a negatively charged aspartate, interact electrostatically with the positively charged quaternary ammonium moiety of ACh, whereas other residues are required for binding to the ester moiety. Although the tertiary amine and quaternary ammonium groups of antimuscarinic drugs bind to the same anionic site on the receptor that agonists occupy, these drugs do not fit into the narrow cleft and consequently cannot activate the receptor.

134

Dicyclomine (*Bentyl*), oxybutynin (*Ditropan*), and tolterodine (*Detrol*) are nonselective smooth muscle relaxants that produce relatively little antagonism of muscarinic receptors at therapeutic concentrations. The mechanism of relaxation is not known. Finally, some other classes of drugs can act in part as muscarinic antagonists. For example, the antipsychotics and antidepressants produce antimuscarinic side effects (e.g., dry mouth).

PHARMACOLOGICAL ACTIONS

Muscarinic antagonists have no intrinsic activity, and they can produce effects only by blocking the activation of muscarinic receptors by muscarinic agonists or by neuronally released ACh. Therefore, the magnitude of the response produced by muscarinic antagonists depends on the existing level of cholinergic activity or on the presence of muscarinic agonists. Also, the nature of the response of an organ to the administration of a muscarinic antagonist will depend on the organ's pattern of innervation; for example, some organs receive dual innervation from adrenergic and cholinergic pathways. At these locations, block of the activation of muscarinic receptors can increase the tone provided by the adrenergic input.

The effects of muscarinic blocking drugs on various human organ systems are summarized in Table 13.1. The tissues or systems affected will depend on the dose administered, the drug's pharmacokinetic properties (e.g., increased entry into the CNS at higher concentrations), and the differential sensitivity of muscarinic receptors in various organs to individual blocking agents. Although muscarinic *agonists* typically do not exhibit selectivity among muscarinic receptors (see Chapter 12), some muscarinic *antagonists* are selective in their ability to block subtypes of muscarinic receptors.

Heart

Intravenous administration of low doses of atropine or scopolamine often produces slight bradycardia, whereas higher doses produce tachycardia by directly blocking the parasympathetic input to the sinoatrial node. Although it has been suggested that the bradycardia results from an effect of the drugs on the CNS (thought to be central vagal stimulation), this appears unlikely, since methylatropine (a quaternary ammonium derivative of atropine) produces a similar response. One plausible explanation for the *paradoxical bradycardia* produced by low doses of muscarinic blockers is that they block presynaptic muscarinic receptors that normally provide feedback inhibition of the release of ACh. Antagonism of these presynaptic muscarinic receptors prevents feedback inhibition and increases the release

TABLE **13.1**	Effects of Muscarinic Blocking Drugs in Humans
Tissue or system	**Effects**
Skin	Inhibition of sweating (hyperpyrexia may result); flushing
Visual	Cycloplegia (relaxation of ciliary muscle); mydriasis (relaxation of sphincter pupillae muscle); increase in aqueous outflow resistance (increases intraocular pressure in many cases of glaucoma)
Digestive	Decreased salivation; reduced tone and motility in the gastrointestinal tract; decrease in vagus-stimulated gastric, pancreatic, intestinal, and biliary secretions
Urinary	Urinary retention (relaxation of the detrusor muscle); relaxation of ureter
Respiratory	Bronchial dilation and decreased secretions
Cardiovascular	Bradycardia at low doses (may be a CNS effect) and tachycardia at higher doses (peripheral effect); increased cardiac output if patient is recumbent
Central nervous system	Decreased concentration and memory; drowsiness; sedation; excitation; ataxia; asynergia; decrease in alpha EEG and increase in low-voltage slow waves (as in drowsy state); hallucinations; coma

of ACh, and this effect may dominate postsynaptic muscarinic receptor blockade produced by low doses of antagonist. Atropine can also facilitate atrioventricular (A-V) conduction and block parasympathetic effects on the cardiac conduction system and on myocardial contractility.

Blood Vessels

Atropine and other muscarinic antagonists produce minimal effects on the circulation in the absence of circulating muscarinic agonists. This reflects the relatively minor role of cholinergic innervation in determining vascular smooth muscle tone. Atropine can produce flushing in the blush area owing to vasodilation. It is not known whether this is a direct effect or a response to the hyperthermia induced by the drug's ability to inhibit sweating.

Gastrointestinal Tract

Muscarinic antagonists have numerous effects on the digestive system (see Chapter 40). The inhibition of salivation by low doses of atropine results in a dry mouth and difficulty in swallowing. Antimuscarinic drugs also inhibit gastric acid secretion and gastrointestinal motility, because both processes are partly under the control of the vagus nerve. Relatively large doses of atropine are required to inhibit acid secretion, and side effects such as dry mouth, tachycardia, ocular disturbances, and urinary retention are drawbacks to the use of muscarinic antagonists in the treatment of peptic ulcers.

Bladder

Muscarinic antagonists can cause urinary retention by blocking the excitatory effect of ACh on the detrusor muscle of the bladder. During urination, cholinergic input to this smooth muscle is activated by a stretch reflex.

Central Nervous System

Although atropine and scopolamine share many properties, an important difference is the easier entry of scopolamine into the CNS. Typical doses of atropine (0.2–2 mg) have minimal central effects, while larger doses can produce a constellation of responses collectively termed the *central anticholinergic syndrome*. At intermediate doses (2–10 mg), memory and concentration may be impaired, and the patient may be drowsy. If doses of 10 mg or more are used, the patient may exhibit confusion, excitement, hallucinations, ataxia, asynergia, and possibly coma.

Even low doses of scopolamine have central effects. Sedation, amnesia, and drowsiness are common during the clinical use of this drug. Large doses of scopolamine can produce all of the responses seen with atropine. Other tertiary amine compounds with muscarinic receptor blocking activity have similar central effects.

Eye

Antimuscarinic drugs block contraction of the iris sphincter and ciliary muscles of the eye produced by ACh. This results in dilation of the pupil (*mydriasis*) and paralysis of accommodation (*cycloplegia*), responses that cause photophobia and inability to focus on nearby objects. Ocular effects are produced only after higher parenteral doses. Atropine and scopolamine produce responses lasting several days when applied directly to the eyes.

Lung

Muscarinic antagonists inhibit secretions and relax smooth muscle in the respiratory system. The parasympathetic innervation of respiratory smooth muscle is most abundant in large airways, where it exerts a dominant constrictor action. In agreement with this innervation pattern, muscarinic antagonists produce their greatest bronchodilator effect at large-caliber airways.

By this mechanism they can block reflex laryngospasm during surgery. In addition, these drugs are potent inhibitors of secretions throughout the respiratory system, from the nose to the bronchioles.

Nicotinic Receptors

Although the antimuscarinic drugs are normally selective for muscarinic cholinergic receptors, high concentrations of agents with a quaternary ammonium group (e.g., propantheline) can block nicotinic receptors on autonomic ganglia and skeletal muscles. However, these effects are generally not clinically important at usual therapeutic doses.

ABSORPTION, METABOLISM, AND EXCRETION

Both atropine and scopolamine are tertiary amines that cross biological membranes readily. They are well absorbed from the gastrointestinal tract and conjunctiva and can cross the blood-brain barrier. After the intravenous injection of atropine (DL-hyoscyamine), the biologically inactive isomer, D-hyoscyamine, is excreted unchanged in the urine. The active isomer, however, can undergo dealkylation, oxidation, and hydrolysis.

The quaternary ammonium derivatives of the belladonna alkaloids, as well as the synthetic quaternary ammonium compounds, are incompletely absorbed from the gastrointestinal tract. Consequently, greater amounts of these compounds are eliminated in the feces following oral administration. The blood-brain barrier prevents quaternary ammonium muscarinic blockers from gaining significant access to the CNS.

CLINICAL USES

Cardiovascular Uses

Atropine can be useful in patients with *carotid sinus syncope*. This condition results from excessive activity of afferent neurons whose stretch receptors are in the carotid sinus. By reflex mechanisms, this excessive afferent input to the medulla oblongata causes pronounced bradycardia, which is reversible by atropine.

Atropine can be used in the differential diagnosis of S-A node dysfunction. If sinus bradycardia is due to extracardiac causes, atropine can generally elicit a tachycardic response, whereas it cannot elicit tachycardia if the bradycardia results from intrinsic causes. Under certain conditions, atropine may be useful in the treatment of acute myocardial infarction. Bradycardia frequently occurs after acute myocardial infarction, especially in the first few hours, and this probably results from excessive vagal tone. The increased tone and bradycardia facilitate the development of ventricular ectopy. Although atropine sulfate has proved beneficial in patients whose bradycardia is accompanied by hypotension or ventricular ectopy, it *is generally not otherwise recommended in this condition*. Use of atropine is not without hazard, because cardiac work can be increased without improved perfusion, and ventricular arrhythmias may occur. Atropine can also be used to induce positive chronotropy during cardiopulmonary resuscitation.

Uses in Anesthesiology

At one time, atropine or scopolamine was routinely administered before the induction of general anesthesia to block excessive salivary and respiratory secretions induced by certain inhalation anesthetics (e.g., diethyl ether). With the newer, less irritating anesthetics, antimuscarinic premedication is not routinely required as an *antisialagogue* (i.e., to counteract the formation of saliva). Sedation can occur following scopolamine administration, and preanesthetic or postoperative agitation has been observed in some patients. High serum levels of drugs with antimuscarinic activity can produce postoperative delirium. Glycopyrrolate bromide (*Robinul*) has also been given intramuscularly as a preanesthetic medication with satisfactory results. This agent is a quaternary ammonium compound and therefore produces no central effects.

Use With Cholinesterase Inhibitors

During reversal of competitive neuromuscular blockade with neostigmine or other anticholinesterase agents and in the management of myasthenia gravis with cholinesterase inhibitors, atropine or another muscarinic antagonist should be given to prevent the stimulation of muscarinic receptors that accompanies excessive inhibition of AChE. However, extra care must be exercised because the prevention of muscarinic receptor stimulation eliminates an important early sign of cholinergic crisis (see Chapter 12).

Uses in Ophthalmology

Antimuscarinic drugs are widely used in ophthalmology to produce mydriasis and cycloplegia. These actions permit an accurate determination of the refractive state of the eye, and the antimuscarinics are also useful in treating specific ocular diseases and for the treatment of patients following iridectomy.

Atropine, scopolamine, cyclopentolate (*Cyclogyl, AK-Pentolate,* and others) and tropicamide (*Mydriacyl, Tropicacyl,* and others) are among the antimuscarinic drugs used in ophthalmology. All of these agents are tertiary amines that reach the iris and ciliary body after topical application to the eye. Systemic absorption of these drugs from the conjunctival sac is minimal, but significant absorption and toxicity can occur if the antimuscarinic drugs come into contact with the nasal and pharyngeal mucosa via the nasolacrimal duct. To minimize this possibility, pressure should be applied to the lacrimal sac for a few minutes after topical application of muscarinic blockers.

The mydriatic and cycloplegic actions of atropine and scopolamine can persist for a week after topical application to the eye. Shorter-acting drugs, such as cyclopentolate and tropicamide, are now favored for this application because complete recovery of accommodation occurs within 6 to 24 hours and 2 to 6 hours, respectively.

Uses in Disorders of the Digestive System

Nonselective antimuscarinic drugs have been employed in the therapy of peptic ulcers (see Chapter 40) because they can reduce gastric acid secretion; they also have been used as adjunctive therapy in the treatment of *irritable bowel syndrome*. Antimuscarinic drugs can decrease the pain associated with postprandial spasm of intestinal smooth muscle by blocking contractile responses to ACh. Some of the agents used for this disorder have only antimuscarinic activity (e.g., propantheline), while other drugs have additional properties that contribute to their antispasmodic action. Dicyclomine (*Bentyl*) and oxybutynin (*Ditropan*) at therapeutic concentrations primarily have a direct smooth muscle relaxant effect with little antimuscarinic action.

Uses in Urology

Propantheline (*Pro-Banthine*), oxybutynin, dicyclomine, and several other agents have been used for uninhibited bladder syndrome, bladder spasm, enuresis, and urge incontinence. Tolterodine (*Detrol*), a nonselective muscarinic antagonist, exhibits functional specificity for blocking muscarinic receptors in the bladder, with fewer side effects than oxybutynin. However, total prevention of involuntary bladder contractions is difficult to achieve. The participation of noncholinergic, nonadrenergic nerves in bladder contraction may explain this apparent resistance to muscarinic blocking agents.

Uses in Respiratory Disorders

For a long time, muscarinic receptor–blocking drugs occupied a major place in the therapy of asthma, but they have been largely displaced by the adrenergic drugs (see Chapter 41). The problems associated with the use of antimuscarinic alkaloids in respiratory disorders are low therapeutic index and impaired expectoration. The latter is a consequence of their inhibition of mucous secretion, ciliary activity, and mucous transport.

Ipratropium bromide (*Atrovent*), in contrast, is a synthetic muscarinic blocking drug that has gained widespread use in recent years for the treatment of respiratory disorders. The drug is a quaternary ammonium compound, and it is applied topically to the airways through the use of a metered-dose inhaler. A substantial portion of the dose is swallowed, but absorption from the airways and gastrointestinal tract is negligible and most of the drug is eliminated in the feces. Consequently, systemic antimuscarinic effects are not observed with ipratropium. Dryness of the mouth, cough, and a bad taste have been reported by some patients, but the drug appears to have no other significant adverse effects. Ipratropium does not affect mucociliary transport or the volume and viscosity of sputum.

Clinical studies have demonstrated the effectiveness of ipratropium in chronic obstructive lung disease, for which it is equal or better in effectiveness than β2-adrenergic agonists. Maximum bronchodilator responses to ipratropium develop in 1.5 to 2 hours. Consequently, it would be less suitable than a rapidly acting β-adrenergic agonist in emergencies. Ipratropium is less effective than the β2-receptor agonists in asthma, but it may be useful when combined with other bronchodilators.

Uses in Parkinsonism

Antimuscarinic agents can have beneficial effects in the treatment of parkinsonism, since there is an apparent excess of cholinergic activity in the striatum of patients suffering from this disorder. Although therapy of Parkinson's disease is directed toward replacement of the dopaminergic deficiency rather than blocking the cholinergic excess, antimuscarinics are sometimes employed for mild cases and in combination with other agents (e.g., levodopa) for treatment of advanced cases. Side effects due to peripheral muscarinic blockade are common, and CNS side effects (e.g., confusion and hallucinations) can occasionally limit their use (see Chapter 31 for a more detailed discussion of the use of antimuscarinic drugs in extrapyramidal disorders).

Uses in Motion Sickness

Scopolamine is useful for prevention of motion sickness when the motion is very stressful and of short duration. A transdermal preparation (*Transderm-Scop*) with a 72-hour duration of action has been marketed for this purpose. Blockade of cholinergic sites in the vestibular nuclei and reticular formation may account for the effectiveness of this agent. When the motion is less stressful and lasts longer, the antihistamines (H1-antagonists) are probably preferable to the antimus-

carinic drugs, especially for the prophylactic treatment of motion sickness.

Uses as Antidotes for Cholinomimetic Poisoning

Atropine is used as an antidote in poisoning by an overdose of a cholinesterase inhibitor (see Chapter 14). It also is used in cases of poisoning from species of mushroom that contain high concentrations of muscarine and related alkaloids (e.g., *Clitocybe dealbata*).

ANTIMUSCARINIC POISONING

Antimuscarinic poisoning can result from the intake of excessive doses of belladonna alkaloids, synthetic antimuscarinic drugs, and drugs from other pharmacological groups that have significant antimuscarinic activity (Table 13.2).

Signs of peripheral muscarinic blockade (e.g., speech disturbances, swallowing difficulties, cardioacceleration, and pupillary dilation) are most common at lower doses, whereas CNS effects (e.g., headache, restlessness, ataxia, and hallucinations) are more apparent after large doses. Antimuscarinic drugs can produce atrial arrhythmias, A-V dissociation, and ventricular tachycardia and fibrillation. Many cases of antimuscarinic poisoning can be managed by removing unab-

TABLE 13.2 Sources of Anticholinergic Poisoning

Group	Examples
Antihistamines (H1-receptor antagonists)	Diphenhydramine, Chlorpheniramine, Dimenhydrinate
Antiparkinsonian drugs	Benztropine, Trihexyphenidyl
Antipsychotics	Chlorpromazine, Thioridazine, Loxapine
Antispasmodics	Dicyclomine, Propantheline
Belladonna alkaloids and related drugs	Atropine, Scopolamine
Belladonna alkaloid-containing plants	Deadly nightshade, Angel's trumpet, Jimsonweed
Cyclic antidepressants	Amitriptyline, Doxepin, Fluoxetine
Cycloplegics and mydriatics	Cyclopentolate, Tropicamide
Muscle relaxants	Orphenadrine, Cyclobenzaprine

Source: Modified from L. Goldfrank, *Goldfrank's Toxicologic Emergencies.* East Norwalk, CT: Appleton & Lange, 1990.

sorbed drug, treating symptoms, and providing supportive therapy. However, any life-threatening effects (i.e., seizures, severe hypertension, hallucinations, or life-threatening arrhythmias) would justify the use of specific antidotal therapy with the cholinesterase-inhibiting compound physostigmine. Special caution should be employed if the patient has any disorder that might be aggravated by the cholinergic stimulation resulting from the use of physostigmine.

CONTRAINDICATIONS AND CAUTIONS

Muscarinic blocking agents are contraindicated in angle-closure glaucoma. Caution also should be used in individuals with untreated open-angle glaucoma, cardiac disease, hyperthyroidism, or prostatic hypertrophy. Muscarinic antagonists can aggravate reflux esophagitis by decreasing the tone of the lower esophageal sphincter. Infants and children are especially sensitive to the hyperthermic action of muscarinic blockers. Elderly patients are especially sensitive to antimuscarinic effects in the CNS, such as impairment of memory. Phenothiazines and tricyclic antidepressants have antimuscarinic activity and can produce effects that are additive to those of the muscarinic blocking drugs. Antimuscarinics should not be given to patients with gastrointestinal infections because the drug will slow gastric motility and cause the patient to retain the infectious organisms in the gastrointestinal tract.

Study QUESTIONS

1. Which of the responses to atropine listed below is most likely to be different in an elderly versus a young patient?
   (A) Inhibition of sweating
   (B) Tachycardia
   (C) Mydriasis
   (D) Drowsiness
2. You have successfully prescribed neostigmine to a young patient with myasthenia gravis, and her muscle strength has improved markedly. However, she also exhibits cardiovascular and gastrointestinal signs of excessive vagal tone, which you would like to block with atropine. Which of the following risk factors in prescribing atropine is most important to you?
   (A) Dry mouth
   (B) Ocular disturbances
   (C) Paralysis of the respiratory muscles
   (D) Tachycardia
3. Antimuscarinic mydriatics, such as tropicamide, are useful in ophthalmological examinations. Prior to administering tropicamide, it would be most important to know
   (A) If the patient has angle-closure glaucoma
   (B) If the patient has open-angle glaucoma
   (C) If the patient is taking a cholinomimetic miotic drug
4. In which of the following conditions would atropine be the *least* likely to increase blood pressure?
   (A) A healthy young medical student
   (B) A patient being treated with an AChE inhibitor
   (C) A patient being treated with bethanechol
5. A patient has come to you complaining of feeling drowsy and finding it hard to concentrate. The patient tells you that he is taking a medication, but he cannot remember the name of the medication. You proceed to ask questions that might provide a clue to the source of his problems. Which of the following questions would be *least* likely to be helpful?
   (A) Has the patient had problems with hay fever and stuffiness?
   (B) Is the patient being treated for glaucoma?
   (C) Has the patient had back spasms?
   (D) Is the patient being treated for mood disorders?

ANSWERS

1. **B.** The resting level of vagal stimulation of the heart decreases with age, which is typically accompanied by a gradual increase in heart rate with age. Therefore, the tachycardia produced by atropine is greater in young patients with strong vagal tone, and the response decreases with age in parallel with the decrease in vagal tone.
2. **C.** Atropine will not directly paralyze the respiratory muscles. However, it can prevent the detection of early signs of an overdose of neostigmine, which can quickly progress to a depolarizing block of skeletal muscle and paralysis of the respiratory muscles. Dry mouth, ocular disturbances, and tachycardia are common side effects of atropine given alone, but these effects are less likely to occur with competition between atropine and the increase in the synaptic ACh produced by inhibition of AChE by neostigmine.
3. **A.** Application of tropicamide to the eye of a patient with narrow-angle (angle-closure) glaucoma is a very serious risk, because the peripheral movement of the relaxed iris can block the outflow of fluid and trigger a rapid rise in intraocular pressure. Open-angle glaucoma does not present the same

risk for the application of a short-acting mydriatic such as tropicamide. If the patient is taking a cholinomimetic miotic for open-angle glaucoma, there is even less risk of applying tropicamide, although potential competition between the miotic and the antagonist may have to be considered.

4 A. Atropine has little effect on blood pressure in the absence of a circulating muscarinic agonist because the muscarinic receptors on endothelial cells do not receive synaptic input. Therefore, the blood pressure of a healthy patient will not change with treatment with atropine. In contrast, patients being treated with an AChE inhibitor may have slightly elevated plasma ACh levels, and patients being treated with bethanechol may be hypotensive because of its direct actions on the muscarinic receptors on endothelial cells.

5 B. The symptoms are suggestive of central antimuscarinic effects of a drug. Glaucoma is treated with muscarinic agonists or noncholinergic drugs. Although the entry of pilocarpine into the CNS can disturb CNS function, it is not as likely as an antimuscarinic drug to produce drowsiness and loss of concentration. The other questions would all be useful. A patient who has hay fever or stuffiness may be taking an antihistamine. A patient with back spasms may be taking a muscle relaxant, such as cyclobenzaprine. One who is being treated for mood disorders may be taking antipsychotic medication.

All of these treatments can produce significant central antimuscarinic side effects.

SUPPLEMENTAL READING

Barnes PJ. Modulation of neurotransmission in airways. Physiol Rev 1992;72:699–729.

Campbell SC. Clinical aspects of inhaled anticholinergic therapy. Respir Care 2000;45:864–867.

Eglen RM, Choppin A, and Watson N. Therapeutic opportunities from muscarinic receptor research. Trends Pharmacol Sci 2001;22:409–414.

Friedman C. Treatment of the irritable bowel syndrome. Gastroenterol Clin North Am1991;20:325–333.

Gross NJ. Ipratropium bromide. N Engl J Med 1988;319:486–494.

Jacoby DB and Fryer AD. Anticholinergic therapy for airway diseases. Life Sci 2001;68:2565–2572.

Mirakhur RK. Anticholinergic drugs in anesthesia. Br J Hosp Med 1991;46:409–411.

Ouslander JG, Shih YT, Malone-Lee J, and Luber K. Overactive bladder: Special considerations in the geriatric population. Am J Manag Care 2000;6:S599–S606.

Pickford EJ et al. Infants and atropine: A dangerous mixture. J Paediatr Child Health 1991;27:55–56.

Ruckenstein MJ and Harrison RV. Motion sickness: Helping patients tolerate the ups and downs. Postgrad Med 1991;89:139–144.

CASE Study   The Risks of Treating Peptic Ulcers with Antimuscarinic Drugs

A 55-year-old man who works in the furnace room at a steel foundry has developed chronic peptic ulcer disease that has not responded to treatment with antibiotics and H_2 receptor blockers. You are considering giving him an antimuscarinic drug to block gastric acid secretion as adjunctive therapy. What are your concerns regarding the suitability of this treatment for this worker?

ANSWER: Antimuscarinics are not frequently used for peptic ulcer disease today because of their many side effects, but they still can play a useful role as adjunctive therapy. Unfortunately, high concentrations are required to block gastric acid secretion, which means that many side effects are difficult to avoid. This man works in a dangerous environment, and his concentration cannot be compromised. Although CNS depression and loss of concentration is a concern with tertiary amine muscarinic antagonists, quaternary ammonium muscarinic antagonists that do not enter the CNS, such as glycopyrrolate, can be prescribed for blocking gastric acid secretion, thereby avoiding central side effects. Probably the most important risk factor for this worker is his exposure to a hot workplace. Antimuscarinics prevent sweating, which can impair temperature regulation and produce hyperthermia. Hyperthermia alone is a health risk, and it is aggravated by the fact that heart rate increases steeply in proportion to increased body temperature. This worker is probably required to do heavy physical labor, which will add to the hyperthermia and cardiac stimulation. Compensatory feedback via the vagus nerve to slow the heart rate will be blocked by a peripherally acting muscarinic antagonist, and this could lead to very dangerous tachycardia and arrhythmia. Overall, antimuscarinic therapy would not be a good choice for this worker unless he can be moved to a safer work environment.

14 | Ganglionic Blocking Drugs and Nicotine

Thomas C. Westfall

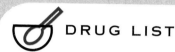

DRUG LIST

GANGLIONIC TRANSMISSION

Transmission through autonomic ganglia is more complex than neurotransmission at the neuromuscular and postganglionic neuroeffector junctions and is subject to numerous pharmacological and physiological influences. In some ganglionic synapses, especially at parasympathetic ganglia, there is a simple presynaptic to postsynaptic cell relationship; in others, the presynaptic to postsynaptic cell relationship may involve neurons interposed between the presynaptic and postsynaptic elements (interneurons).

In a variety of sympathetic and certain parasympathetic ganglion cells (e.g., vagal ganglia in the sinoatrial node), cells exhibiting the characteristic catecholamine fluorescence spectrum have been found. These cells are referred to as small intensely fluorescent (SIF) cells. At some autonomic ganglia, the SIF cell is a true interneuron, receiving afferent innervation from preganglionic cholinergic neurons and forming efferent synapses with postganglionic neurons. At other autonomic ganglia, its function is not completely understood, but the SIF cell is believed to play a role in the modulation of ganglionic transmission. Many SIF cells are thought to contain dopamine or norepinephrine as their neurotransmitter.

Unlike the receptors at postganglionic neuroeffector junctions or at skeletal neuromuscular junctions, both types of cholinergic receptors, that is, nicotinic and mus-

carinic, are present on the cell bodies of the postganglionic neurons. Stimulation of the preganglionic neuron results in the release of acetylcholine (ACh) from the preganglionic nerve terminal, which in turn activates postganglionic cholinergic receptors and leads ultimately to the formation of a propagated action potential down the postganglionic axon. At the more complicated synapses, the release of ACh from preganglionic neurons results in the appearance of complex postsynaptic potential changes consisting of several temporally arranged components. There is an initial fast excitatory postsynaptic potential (EPSP) followed by a succession of much slower postsynaptic potential changes, including a slow EPSP that lasts for 2 to 5 seconds, a slow inhibitory postsynaptic potential (IPSP) lasting about 10 seconds, and a late slow EPSP lasting for 1 to 2 minutes.

There is considerable diversity among nicotinic acetylcholine receptors, and at least one source of this diversity is the multiplicity of acetylcholine receptor genes. Cholinergic–nicotinic receptors in skeletal muscle are different from those in autonomic ganglia and the central nervous system.

Excitatory and Inhibitory Potentials

The interaction of ACh with the postsynaptic nicotinic receptor results in depolarization of the membrane, an influx of Na$^+$ and Ca^{++} through a neuronal nicotinic receptor channel, and the generation of the fast EPSP. This change in postsynaptic potential is principally responsible for the generation of the propagated action potential in the postganglionic neuron. Generally, several presynaptic terminals innervate a single ganglion cell, and several preganglionic axon terminals must fire simultaneously for transmission to take place. Ganglionic blocking agents prevent transmission by interfering with the postsynaptic action of ACh. The drugs either interact with the nicotinic–cholinergic receptor itself or with the associated ionic channel complex.

Interaction of ACh with the postsynaptic ganglionic cell muscarinic receptor is responsible for slowly developing depolarization, the slow EPSP, which has a longer latency than the fast EPSP and a duration of 30 to 60 seconds. The slow EPSP is due to inhibition of a voltage-dependent K$^+$ current called the M current, and inhibition of the M current involves activation of G proteins. At least five types of muscarinic receptors (M$_1$, M$_2$, M$_3$, M$_4$ and M$_5$) have been identified using functional studies and at least five subtypes (m$_1$, m$_2$, m$_3$, m$_4$, and m$_5$) identified by molecular cloning techniques. The M$_1$ receptor, which appears responsible for inhibiting the M current, can be blocked by atropine.

Release of ACh may activate SIF cells between preganglionic and postganglionic neurons. In this case, activation of a muscarinic receptor on the SIF cells results in the release of a catecholamine; this in turn activates a receptor on the postganglionic cell, leading to the slow IPSP. The catecholamine most frequently released from SIF cells appears to be dopamine. Finally, a late slow EPSP, lasting for 1 to 2 minutes, can be seen at some ganglionic synapses. The mediator is unclear, but it is now well established that there are a large number of peptides in the ganglia, including luteinizing hormone–releasing hormone (LHRH), substance P, angiotensin, calcitonin gene related peptide, vasoactive intestinal polypeptide, neuropeptide Y, and enkephalin.

In addition to the cholinergic and adrenergic receptors on autonomic ganglion cells, there also appear to be receptors for a variety of excitatory and inhibitory substances, including angiotensin, bradykinin, histamine, 5-hydroxytryptaimine (serotonin), and substance P. The existence of these receptors provides a wide variety of options to modulate ganglionic transmission. Agonists for these receptors most likely reach the ganglia through the circulation. A composite picture of the status of ganglionic transmission is shown in Figure 14.1. For simplicity, the figure has been divided into a type A synapse, which includes SIF cells, and a type B synapse, which lacks SIF cells. Table 14.1 summarizes the type of ganglionic action potential generated at various synapses, the type of receptor mediating the response, and the primary transmitter or mediator that activates the receptor.

GANGLIONIC STIMULANTS

A variety of agents, including nicotine, lobeline, and dimethylphenyl piperazinium (DMPP), can stimulate ganglionic nicotinic receptors. Although these drugs have little or no therapeutic use, they offer considerable interest for several reasons. First, drugs such as nicotine that both stimulate and block ganglionic receptors have proved valuable as an aid in identifying and localizing postganglionic fibers. Second, nicotine's use as a potent insecticide and rodenticide and its presence in tobacco smoke have endowed it with considerable toxicological interest.

Mechanism of Ganglionic Stimulation

Nicotine, lobeline, trimethylammonium, and DMPP stimulate all autonomic ganglia by simple combination with ganglionic nicotinic receptors on the postsynaptic membrane. This leads to membrane depolarization, an influx of sodium and calcium ions, and the generation of a fast EPSP. These agents produce general stimulation of autonomic ganglia and a complex pattern of mixed sympathetic and parasympathetic responses.

In addition to autonomic ganglia, nicotinic receptors are found in a variety of organs, and their stimulation will produce quite different results in these different tissues. Activation of nicotinic receptors on the plasma membrane of the cells of the adrenal medulla leads to the exocytotic release of epinephrine and norepinephrine; stimulation of nicotinic receptors at the neuromuscular junction results in the contraction of skeletal muscle (see

TABLE 14.1 Type of Ganglionic Action Potential per Synapse Type

Neurotransmitter/Neuromodulator	Ganglionic Receptor	Ganglionic Action Potential
Acetylcholine (from preganglionic neuron)	Nicotinic cholinergic	Fast EPSP
Acetylcholine (from preganglionic neuron)	Muscarinic cholinergic	Slow EPSP
Acetylcholine (from preganglionic neuron)	Muscarinic cholinergic or interneuron	Slow IPSP
Norepinephrine, epinephrine, dopamine (from interneuron)	Adrenergic/dopaminergic	Slow IPSP
Autacoid (angiotensin, etc.) or peptide (LHRH, etc.)	Autacoid or peptide receptor	Late slow EPSP

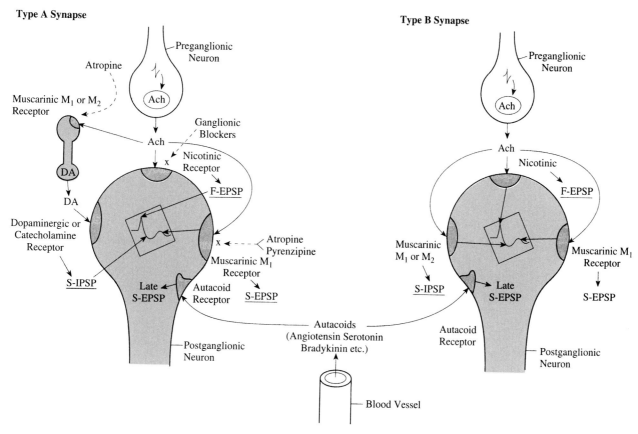

FIGURE 14.1

Composite drawing of ganglionic neurotransmission. For simplicity, it has been divided into a type A synapse containing interneurons or small intensely fluorescent (SIF) cells and a type B synapse lacking interneurons. In the type A synapse, ACh is released from the preganglionic neuron and activates nicotinic and muscarinic receptors on the SIF cells (when present), leading to the release of a catecholamine, presumably dopamine. Dopamine subsequently activates a receptor on the postganglionic nerve. The insert depicts the temporal postganglionic action potential, consisting of a fast excitatory postsynaptic potential (EPSP) due to activation of nicotinic receptors by ACh, a slow inhibitory postsynaptic potential (IPSP) due to dopamine or another catecholamine activating the appropriate receptor, and a slow EPSP due to activation by ACh of an M_1 muscarinic cholinergic receptor on the postganglionic nerve cell body. The muscarinic receptor on the SIF cell is either an M_1 or M_2 cholinergic receptor. The postganglionic nerve cell body also contains autacoid receptors that generate a late slow EPSP. The broken line and X represent the appropriate receptor antagonists. The type B synapse is similar to type A but lacks interneurons and SIF cells. In this case, ACh activates both nicotinic receptors leading to the fast EPSP and muscarinic receptors leading to the slow IPSP and slow EPSP. The receptor type leading to the slow IPSP is either M_1 or M_2; that leading to the slow EPSP is M_1. ACh, acetylcholine; DA, dopamine.

Chapter 28). Stimulation of nicotinic receptors in adrenergic nerve terminals leads to the release of norepinephrine; and activation of nicotinic chemoreceptors in the aortic arch and carotid bodies causes nausea and vomiting. Nicotinic receptors in the central nervous system mediate a complex range of excitatory and inhibitory effects.

Mechanism of Ganglionic Blockade

Large doses of nicotine produce a prolonged blockade of ganglionic nicotinic receptors. Unlike the blockade of ganglionic transmission produced by most ganglionic blocking agents, that is, a nondepolarizing competitive antagonism, the blockade produced by nicotine consists of two phases. Phase 1 can be described as persistent depolarization of the ganglion cell. The initial application of nicotine to the ganglion cells depolarizes the cell, which initiates an action potential. After a few seconds, however, this discharge stops and transmission is blocked. At this time, antidromic stimuli fail to induce an action potential. In fact, during this phase, the ganglia fail to respond to the administration of any ganglionic stimulant, regardless of the type of receptor it activates. The main reason for the loss of electrical or receptor-mediated excitability during a period of maintained depolarization is that the voltage-sensitive sodium channel is inactivated and no longer opens in response to a brief depolarizing stimulus. During the latter part of phase 1, all ganglionic stimulants that are not nicotinic, such as histamine, angiotensin, bradykinin, and serotonin, become effective.

Phase 1 is followed by a postdepolarization phase (phase 2) during which only the actions of nicotinic receptor agonists are blocked. This phase takes place after nicotine has acted for several minutes. At this time, the cell partially repolarizes, and its electrical excitability returns. The main factor responsible for phase 2 block appears to be desensitization of the receptor to ACh, which causes transmission failure.

Pharmacological Actions of Nicotine

Nicotine is present in varying amounts in all forms of tobacco smoke. Following its absorption from the lungs, the blood nicotine levels are sufficient to cause stimulation but not blockade of nicotinic receptors. In addition to stimulating receptors on autonomic ganglia, all other nicotinic receptors mentioned earlier can be activated. Thus, tobacco smoking stimulates the cardiovascular, respiratory, and nervous systems.

Cardiovascular System

The effects of nicotine on the cardiovascular system mimic those seen after activation of the sympathoadrenal system, and they are principally the result of a release of epinephrine and norepinephrine from the adrenal medulla and adrenergic nerve terminals. These effects include a positive inotropic and chronotropic effect on the myocardium as well as an increase in cardiac output. In addition, both systolic and diastolic blood pressures are increased secondary to stimulation of the sympathoadrenal system. These effects are the end result of a summation of adrenergic and cholinergic stimulation.

Respiratory System

Low doses of nicotine stimulate respiration through activation of chemoreceptors in the aortic arch and carotid bodies, while high doses directly stimulate the respiratory centers. In toxic doses, nicotine depresses respiration by inhibiting the respiratory centers in the brainstem and by a complex action at the receptors at the neuromuscular junction of the respiratory muscles. At these neuromuscular receptors, nicotine appears to occupy the receptors, and the end plate is depolarized. After this, the muscle accommodates and relaxes. These central and peripheral effects paralyze the respiratory muscles.

Central Nervous System

The actions of nicotine on the central nervous system are the result of a composite of stimulatory and depressant effects. These can include tremors, convulsions, respiratory stimulation or depression, and release of antidiuretic hormone from the pituitary. Nausea and emesis are frequently observed after the initial use of nicotine in the form of tobacco smoke. However, tolerance to these effects rapidly develops. This is in contrast to the effects of nicotine on the cardiovascular system, where tolerance develops much more slowly.

Other Systems

Additional effects of nicotine include an increase in gastric acid secretion and an increase in the tone and motility of the gastrointestinal tract. These effects are produced because of the predominance of cholinergic input to these effector systems.

Absorption, Distribution, and Excretion of Nicotine

Nicotine is well absorbed from the mucous membranes in the oral cavity, gastrointestinal tract, and respiratory system. If tobacco smoke is held in the mouth for 2 seconds, 66 to 77% of the nicotine in the smoke will be absorbed across the oral mucosa. If tobacco smoke is inhaled, approximately 90 to 98% of the nicotine will be absorbed. Nicotine is distributed throughout the body, readily crossing the blood-brain and placental barriers. The liver, kidney, and lung metabolize approximately 80 to 90% of the alkaloid. The kidney rapidly eliminates nicotine and its metabolites.

GANGLIONIC BLOCKING DRUGS

Although a number of drugs possessing ganglionic blocking properties have been developed, at the present time they are rarely used clinically. Other drugs, such as curare, are not employed as ganglionic blocking agents, although they block ganglionic nicotinic receptors, especially at high doses. The ganglionic blockers are still important in pharmacological and physiological research because of their ability to block autonomic ganglia.

Mechanism of Action

Drugs can block autonomic ganglia by any one of several mechanisms. They may act presynaptically by affecting nerve conduction or neurotransmitter synthesis, release, or reuptake. Acting postjunctionally, drugs may affect the interaction between ACh and its receptor, or they may affect depolarization of the ganglion cell or initiation of a propagated action potential.

Ganglionic nicotinic blockers can be divided into two groups. The first group, characterized by nicotine and related drugs (e.g., lobeline, tetraethylammonium), initially stimulates the ganglia and then blocks them (discussed earlier). These agents are not therapeutically useful. The second group of drugs, which have some therapeutic usefulness but are rarely used, inhibit the postsynaptic action of ACh and do not themselves produce depolarization, thereby blocking transmission without causing initial stimulation.

The site of action of many blocking drugs has been shown to be at the associated ionic channel rather than at the receptor. Prolonged administration of ganglionic blocking drugs leads to the development of tolerance to their pharmacological effects.

Pharmacological Actions

In any given tissue, the magnitude of the response produced by ganglionic blocking drugs depends largely on the quantity and relative proportion of the total autonomic input coming from sympathetic and parasympathetic nerves at the time of drug administration (Table 14.2). For example, if cardiac vagal tone is high at the time ganglion blockade is induced, tachycardia results. If heart rate is high, a decrease in rate may be seen.

The extent of the hypotension, especially postural hypotension, produced by a ganglionic blocking agent also depends on the degree of sympathetic tone at the time of drug administration. For instance, patients with normal cardiac function may have their cardiac output diminished after ganglionic blockade, while patients in cardiac failure often respond to ganglionic blockade with an increase in cardiac output. To date, it has not been possible to develop ganglionic blocking drugs that have a high degree of selectivity for either sympathetic or parasympathetic ganglia. However, since these drugs do not affect all of the various ganglia equally, and since the time at which their peak effect occurs will vary among the various types of ganglia, some degree of selectivity of action does in fact exist.

Clinical Uses
Hypertensive Cardiovascular Disease

Ganglionic blockers were once widely used in the management of essential hypertension, and they constituted an important advance in the treatment of that disease. Unfortunately, the development of tolerance to these drugs and their numerous undesirable side effects resulting from their nonselective ganglion-blocking properties led to a decline in their use. They have now been completely replaced by more effective and less toxic drugs. They do, however, retain some usefulness in the emergency treatment of hypertensive crisis.

TABLE 14.2 Predominant Autonomic Tone at Various Neuroeffector Junctions and the Effect Produced by Ganglionic Blockade

Site	Effect of Ganglionic Blockade
Tissues predominantly under parasympathetic (cholinergic) tone	
Myocardium	
Atrium; S-A node	Tachycardia
Eye	
Iris	Mydriasis
Ciliary muscle	Cycloplegia
GI tract	Decrease in tone and motility; constipation
Urinary bladder	Urinary retention
Salivary gland	Dry mouth
Tissues predominantly under sympathetic (adrenergic) tone	
Myocardium	
Ventricles	Decrease in contractile force
Blood vessels	
Arterioles	Vasodilation; increase in peripheral blood flow; hypotension
Veins	Vasodilation; pooling of blood; decrease in venous return; decrease in cardiac output
Sweat glands[a]	Decrease in secretion

[a]Anatomically sympathetic; transmitter is ACh.

Controlled Hypotension

Ganglionic blocking agents have been used to achieve controlled hypotension in plastic, neurological, and ophthalmological surgery. They are most commonly used in surgical procedures involving extensive skin dissection.

Adverse Effects

All of the responses summarized in Table 14.2 can be produced by administration of ganglionic blocking agents. Many of these responses are undesirable effects that limit the therapeutic usefulness of these agents. Mild untoward responses include mydriasis, difficulty in vision accommodation, dry mouth, urinary hesitancy, constipation, diarrhea, abdominal discomfort, anorexia, and syncope. More serious but less frequent disturbances include marked hypotension, constipation, paralytic ileus, urinary retention, and anginal pain.

INDIVIDUAL AGENTS

Trimethaphan

Trimethaphan camsylate (*Arfonad*) is an extremely short-acting agent whose major therapeutic use is in the production of controlled hypotension in certain surgical procedures and in the emergency treatment of hypertensive crisis. Continuous infusion may be employed to maintain its antihypertensive effect, especially in patients with an acute dissecting aortic aneurysm. Much of the decrease in blood pressure following trimethaphan administration is thought to be due to its direct vasodilating properties.

Trimethaphan can produce prolonged neuromuscular blockade in some patients, and therefore, it should be used with caution as a hypotensive agent during surgery. It also has been reported to potentiate the neuromuscular blocking action of tubocurarine, and because of its histamine-releasing properties, trimethaphan should be used with caution in patients with allergies.

Mecamylamine

Mecamylamine hydrochloride (*Inversine*) is a secondary amine and can therefore easily penetrate cell membranes. Its absorption from the gastrointestinal tract is more complete than that of the quaternary ammonium compounds. Mecamylamine is well absorbed orally and crosses both the blood-brain and placental barriers; its distribution is not confined to the extracellular space. High concentrations of the drug accumulate in the liver and kidney, and it is excreted unchanged by the kidney. In contrast to most of the highly ionized ganglionic blocking agents, mecamylamine can produce central nervous system effects, including tremors, mental confusion, seizures, mania, and depression. The mechanism by which these central effects are produced is unclear. Mecamylamine is rarely used today as an antihypertensive drug because it blocks both parasympathetic and sympathetic ganglia.

Study QUESTIONS

During a laboratory demonstration to depict the complexity of neurotransmission in autonomic ganglia, Professor Smith sets up an anesthetized mammalian preparation in which she is recording postsynaptic events following the electrical stimulation of preganglionic sympathetic nerves. This demonstrates a complex action potential that consists of a fast EPSP followed by a slow IPSP followed by a slow EPSP and finally by a late very slow EPSP.

1. In Professor Smith's demonstration, the mediator of the fast EPSP is
   (A) Dopamine
   (B) Neuropeptide Y
   (C) Serotonin
   (D) Angiotensin
   (E) Acetylcholine
2. In Professor Smith's demonstration, the slow EPSP and slow IPSP can both be blocked by prior administration of
   (A) Prazosin
   (B) Sumatriptan
   (C) Atropine
   (D) Losartan
   (E) Chlorpromazine
3. In Professor Smith's demonstration, the receptor most likely mediating the slow EPSP is
   (A) Nicotinic cholinergic
   (B) Muscarinic cholinergic
   (C) α-Adrenergic
   (D) P_{2x} Purinergic
   (E) β-Adrenergic

4. A patient you are treating in the hospital has a hypertensive emergency, with blood pressure of 210/140 mm Hg. Of the following drugs, which would be most effective intravenously?
   (A) Hydralazine
   (B) Hydrochlorothiazide
   (C) Trimethaphan
   (D) Methyldopa
   (E) Spironolactone
5. Ganglionic blocking agents are rarely used because of the numerous side effects they may produce. One such side effect is
   (A) Increased stimulation of the genital tract
   (B) Urinary hesitation or urgency
   (C) Vasoconstriction
   (D) Increased cardiac output
   (E) Mydriasis

ANSWERS
1. **E.** The principal neurotransmitter released from preganglionic nerve terminals in all autonomic ganglia is acetylcholine. It acts on the postganglionic cell body to activate a nicotinic–cholinergic receptor resulting in a fast EPSP. Dopamine or norepinephrine or both are the mediators released from SIF cells or interneurons. Neuropeptide Y is a peptide neurotransmitter. Angiotensin and serotonin are modulatory mediators. These last three contribute to the late very slow EPSP.
2. **C.** The slow EPSP results from activation of muscarinic–cholinergic receptors on SIF cells or in-

terneurons, which release norepinephrine or dopamine from their terminals. These catecholamines then cause a slow IPSP in the ganglionic cell body. Therefore, both the slow EPSP and subsequent slow IPSP would be prevented by the muscarinic antagonist atropine. Prazosin is an α_1-adrenergic antagonist; sumatriptan is a serotonin $5HT_{1D}$ agonist; losartan is an angiotensin receptor antagonist; and chlorpromazine is a dopamine antagonist. Only atropine would block both the slow EPSP and the slow IPSP.

3. **B.** The receptor contributing to the slow EPSP is a muscarinic–cholinergic receptor and is activated by ACh. The nicotinic–cholinergic receptor mediates the fast EPSP, an α-receptor may mediate the slow IPSP, and a P_{2X} receptor and a β-adrenergic receptor do not appear to be involved in the complex action potentials seen at autonomic ganglia.

4. **C.** Trimethaphan is a ganglionic blocking agent that will lower blood pressure very rapidly. Hydralazine is a vasodilator; hydrochlorothiazide and spironolactone are diuretics; and methyldopa is a sympatholytic acting in the central nervous system. All of these drugs are used clinically as antihypertensive agents. None work as rapidly as trimethaphan. Clinically, however, either nitroprusside or clonidine is used much more commonly than trimethaphan in this situation.

5. **E.** The effect of ganglionic blockade depends upon the predominant autonomic tone exerted within various organ systems. Since the activity of the parasympathetic nervous system predominates in the eye, the effect of ganglionic blockade is mydriasis, not miosis. Similarly, stimulation of the genital tract and urinary retention would be decreased. Since sympathetic nervous system activity predominates in blood vessels and the ventricles, vasodilation and a decreased cardiac output would follow ganglionic blockade.

SUPPLEMENTAL READING

Benowitz NL (ed). Nicotine Safety and Toxicity. New York: Oxford University Press, 1998.

Clementi F, Fornasari D, and Gotti C. (eds). Neuronal Nicotinic Receptors. Berlin: Springer Verlag, 2000.

Elfvin L-G, Lindh B and Höokfelt T. The chemical neuroanatomy of sympathetic ganglia. Annu Rev Neurosci 1993;16:471–507.

Fant RV, Owen CC, and Henningfield JE. Nicotine replacement therapy. Prim. Care 1999;26:633–652.

Lee EW and D'Alonzo GE. Cigarette smoking, nicotine addiction and its pharmacological treatment. Arch Intern Med 1993;153:34–48.

Sargent PB. The diversity of neuronal nicotine acetylcholine receptors. Annu Rev Neurosci 1993;16:403–443.

CASE Study Smoking Cessation

A patient who has been a heavy smoker (2 packs of cigarettes per day for 30 years) comes to you for advice to quit smoking. You inform your patient that sudden cessation of smoking will result in withdrawal symptoms that may include restlessness, irritability, anxiety, tension, stress, intolerance, drowsiness, frequent awakenings from sleep, fatigue, depression, impotence, confusion, impaired concentration, gastrointestinal disturbances, decreased heart rate, and impaired reaction times. You advise your patient that successful cessation of tobacco use requires attention to both the positive and negative (withdrawal) reinforcement properties of nicotine and tobacco use. You plan, therefore, to combine both psychological and pharmacological treatment. What are some therapeutic approaches you can suggest?

ANSWER: Several options are available for the pharmacological approach, including nicotine replacement and antidepressant drugs (e.g., bupropion).

You explain that nicotine replacement can be carried out with chewing gum (nicotine polacrilex), transdermal patches (e.g., *Nicoderm, Habitrol*), nasal spray (*Nicotrol NS*), or vapor inhaler (*Nicotrol Inhaler*). The objective of the nicotine replacement is to obtain a sustained plasma nicotine concentration that is lower than the venous blood concentrations after smoking. It is known that arterial blood concentrations immediately following cigarette smoke inhalation can be as much as 10 times the venous concentration. You decide on a nicotine patch and combine this strategy with counseling and motivational therapy from a professional trained in such methods. It is quite likely that the combination of the patch plus counseling will ultimately result in a successful cessation of smoking in your patient after a couple of relapses. During a second relapse period, you may wish to consider combining the antidepressant drug bupropion with the other forms of treatment.

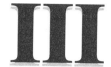

DRUGS AFFECTING THE CARDIOVASCULAR SYSTEM

15 Pharmacological Management of Chronic Heart Failure

Mitchell S. Finkel and Humayun Mirza

DRUG LIST

GENERIC NAME	PAGE	GENERIC NAME	PAGE
Amrinone	157	Hydralazine	155
Captopril	158	Losartan	156
Carvedilol	156	Metoprolol	156
Digitoxin	152	Milrinone	157
Dobutamine	157	Spironolactone	155
Digoxin	152	Valsartan	156
Furosemide	155		

CHRONIC (CONGESTIVE) HEART FAILURE

Patients who have a significant loss of cardiac pump function develop progressively severe symptoms of fatigue, dyspnea (shortness of breath), chest pain, syncope (loss of consciousness), and death. The management of these patients requires an understanding that it is an ongoing process in which the response to the initial injury causes damage beyond the insult alone. The challenge of the clinician is to keep the congestive heart failure (CHF) patient out of the hospital while reducing morbidity and mortality in this high-risk population.

Chronic CHF may be defined as the clinical condition in which an individual expels less than 40% of the blood from the left ventricle per heartbeat (ejection fraction [EF] < 40%). A normal individual expels about 55 to 65% of the blood from the left ventricle per heartbeat (EF = 55–65%). The rationale for choosing the 40% EF is based on clinical findings demonstrating pro-gressive deterioration and early mortality in individuals who have an EF below 40%.

It is remarkable that the therapeutic approach to a decreased EF is the same regardless of the etiology. The principles that guide the pharmacological management of CHF is the same for patients who had damage from a myocardial infarction (MI), viral infection, valvular disease, alcohol, and so on. This chapter reviews the recommended approach to the pharmacological management of systolic dysfunction. An historic perspective will be followed to provide an appreciation of the evolution in our understanding of the pathophysiology of this condition.

The management of heart failure in the presence of normal systolic function is not reviewed. This form of heart failure commonly occurs in the elderly with chronic hypertension and left ventricular hypertrophy. The failure of the left ventricle to relax during diastole (diastolic dysfunction) results in elevated end diastolic pressures and volumes. The shortness of breath (dyspnea), chest pain, and fatigue that result from elevated pulmonary venous pressures are similar in both systolic and diastolic dysfunction. Also excluded from discussion are nondrug therapies for CHF, such as coronary artery bypass, percutaneous coronary interventions, electronic pacemakers, and cardiac transplantation.

A considerable body of literature supports abnormalities in myocardial excitation–contraction coupling in CHF. An appreciation of the principles involved in this cell signaling process is crucial to understand current and future pharmacotherapies for CHF. A brief overview of myocardial excitation–contraction coupling will be provided.

MYOCARDIAL EXCITATION–CONTRACTION COUPLING

The physiological processes that begin with cardiac sarcolemmal membrane depolarization and culminate in contraction are collectively defined as *myocardial excitation–contraction coupling*. Depolarization of the cardiac myocyte sarcolemmal membrane during the action potential results in the intracellular entry of extracellular calcium. The major regulators of the transsarcolemmal entry of calcium include L-type calcium channels and autonomic receptors (Fig. 15.1). These membrane-bound proteins all contribute to the influx of a minute quantity of calcium from outside the cell into the myocyte. The entry of this small quantity of calcium causes the release of the large reservoir of calcium stored in the sarcoplasmic reticulum (SR) through the SR calcium release channel (ryanodine receptor). This large reservoir of calcium interacts with tropomyosin to allow the actin and myosin filaments to overlap, resulting in systolic myocardial contraction. Diastolic relaxation results from the resequestration of this large reservoir of calcium back into the sarcoplasmic reticulum through the SR calcium adenosine triphosphatase (ATPase). Calcium exits the cell through the $Na^+–Ca^{++}$ exchanger and sarcolemmal Ca^{++}ATPase.

Autonomic receptors further regulate calcium influx through the sarcolemma (Fig. 15.1). β-Adrenergic stimulation results in the association of a catalytic subunit of a G protein coupled to the β-receptor. This stimulates the enzyme adenylyl cyclase to convert ATP to cyclic adenosine monophosphate (cAMP). Increasing cAMP production results in a cAMP-dependent phosphorylation of the L-type calcium channel and a subsequent increase in the probability of the open state of the channel. This translates to an increase in transsarcolemmal calcium influx during phase 2 (the plateau phase) of the cardiac muscle action potential. The effects of transient increases in intracellular levels of cAMP are tightly controlled by phosphodiesterases and phosphatases that prevent indefinite phosphorylation and activation of regulatory proteins. α-Adrenoceptor stimulation results in the phospholipase C–mediated breakdown of phosphatidylcholine to inositol triphosphate and diacyl glycerol; these second messengers further enhance mobilization of both transsarcolemmal calcium influx and SR calcium efflux.

Binding of angiotensin II to its cardiac myocyte receptor acutely increases Ca^{++} influx through sarcolemmal L-type calcium channels. The long-term effects of chronic angiotensin II receptor stimulation include cardiac myocyte hypertrophy through enhanced expression of growth factor genes.

The maintenance of a resting membrane potential in cardiac myocytes, as well as all cells, depends on metabolic energy (ATP) that is used by the $Na^+–K^+$ ATPase to drive the gradients for Na^+ and K^+ between the intracellular and extracellular spaces. Cardiac glycosides are known to bind to this protein.

CARDIAC GLYCOSIDES

Historical Background

In "An Account of the Foxglove" William Withering related his experiences while in private practice more than 200 years ago. He traveled between two towns where he took care of the wealthy patients on a fee-for-service basis in one town and the poor people for free in the other. He encountered during one of his commutes a practitioner of the healing arts who was referred to as a witch. She provided care for people with obvious signs and symptoms of fluid overload who were diagnosed with dropsy (later called CHF). She gave these patients a group of herbs that contained digitalis, and it was Withering who identified *Digitalis purpura* as the active plant in this mixture. Unfortunately, he lacked any insight into potential mechanisms of action. Although Withering thought that digitalis worked by inducing emesis, he was actually describing digitalis toxicity and not the mechanism of action at all.

Digitalization

Digitalis remains notorious today for its very narrow dosage window for therapeutic efficacy without toxicity. A unique process, *digitalization*, for dosing digitalis (digoxin [*Lanoxin*]; digitoxin [*Crystodigin*]) has been widely accepted over the years as a means of minimizing toxicity. This process is to start patients on several repeated doses of digitalis over 24 to 36 hours before establishing a lower daily maintenance dose. Digitalis has become the mainstay of therapy for CHF despite its

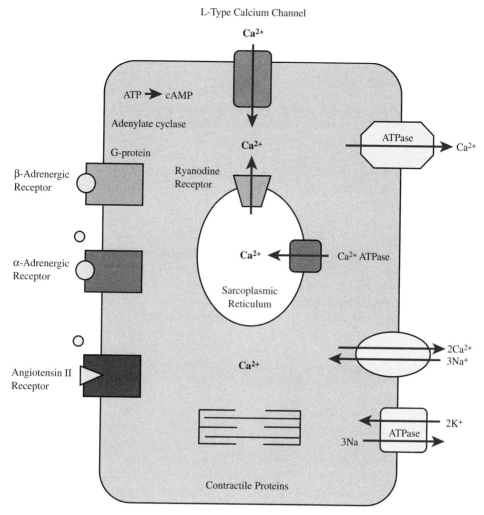

FIGURE 15.1

Principles of excitation-contraction coupling in the cardiac myocyte. Calcium enters the myocyte through L-type calcium channels that are modulated by α- and β-adrenergic receptors. This small quantity of calcium triggers release of the large reservoir of intracellular calcium stored in the SR by activation of the SR calcium release channel (ryanodine receptor). Calcium is resequestered in the SR by the SR calcium–ATPase. Calcium is extruded from the cell largely through the Na^+–Ca^{++} exchanger and the sarcolemmal calcium ATPase. β-Adrenergic agonists (e.g., dobutamine) bind to the β-adrenoceptor and activate a stimulatory G protein to couple with adenylyl cyclase to convert ATP to cAMP. Phosphodiesterase inhibitors (e.g., milrinone) increase intracellular cAMP levels by blocking the degradation of cAMP by phosphodiesterases. β-Adrenergic antagonists (e.g., metoprolol, carvedilol) bind to the same site and prevent endogenous catecholamines (e.g., norepinephrine) from binding to that site and activating a stimulatory G protein. α-Adrenergic antagonists (e.g., prazosin) and angiotensin II receptor blockers (e.g., valsartan, losartan) similarly prevent the endogenous mediators (i.e., norepinephrine, angiotensin II, respectively) from increasing intracellular ionized free calcium levels in the cardiac myocyte. ACE inhibitors (e.g., captopril, fosinopril, lisinopril) block conversion of inert angiotensin I to active angiotensin II by ACE. Digitalis glycosides initially increase intracellular Na^+ levels by binding to the Na^+–K^+ ATPase. The increase in intracellular Na^+ causes the Na^+–Ca^{++} exchanger to extrude Na^+ from the myocyte in exchange for extracellular Ca^{++}. This increases intracellular ionized free calcium levels sufficiently to enhance contractility.

toxicity, the lack of understanding of its mode of action, and the lack of any definitive evidence describing its safety and efficacy.

Toxicity

Digitalis toxicity includes nausea, vomiting, anorexia, fatigue, and a characteristic visual disturbance (green-yellow halos around bright objects). Cardiac toxicities have included tachyarrhythmias and bradyarrhythmias, including supraventricular and ventricular tachycardia and atrioventricular (A-V) block. The most classic (but not most frequent) manifestations of digitalis toxicity include atrial tachycardia with A-V block. Treatment for digitalis toxicity ranges from mild cases that respond to simply stopping the drug to the use of antidigitalis antibodies in life-threatening situations. The availability of a radioimmunoassay for digitalis levels and antidigitalis antibodies, useful in reversing digitalis's actions, have minimized the frequency of fatal toxicity.

Clinical Use

Randomized clinical trials have been conducted to explore the safety and efficacy of digitalis in the management of CHF. The first major trial showed an improvement in quality of life but no mortality benefit. A second major clinical trial revealed that treatment with digitalis diminished the combined end points of death and hospitalizations but did not specifically improve overall survival. Thus, no studies have demonstrated that digitalis therapy improves survival in CHF patients. However, digitalis does decrease morbidity by diminishing the number of admissions to the hospital for symptoms such as dyspnea (shortness of breath) and fatigue. Current guidelines for the treatment of CHF indicate that physicians must at least consider including digitalis in the regimen. The consensus now is to prescribe a dose that achieves a digitalis blood level of 0.8 to 1.2 ng/dL. This lower dose reduces the incidence of side effects while optimizing the benefit.

Mechanism of Action

Digitalis has the unique characteristic of increasing contractility (positive inotropy) while decreasing heart rate (negative chronotropy). This pharmacological profile results from indirect as well as direct effects of digitalis glycosides on the heart. Digitalis is a fat-soluble steroid that crosses the blood-brain barrier and enhances vagal tone. The slowing and/or conversion of a patient with supraventricular arrhythmia (e.g., atrial fibrillation, supraventricular tachycardia) with digitalis results from enhancement of vagal tone. This increased vagal activity increases acetylcholine release, which in turn is coupled to the opening of a K^+ channel. Opening of this K^+

channel results in closing of the L-type sarcolemmal Ca^{++} channel. Ca^{++} channel inhibition slows the heart rate and/or converts the rhythm to a sinus mechanism.

Digitalis works directly on the heart through an action on the sodium–potassium (Na^+–K^+) ATPase. Since all living cells have a resting membrane potential, there is an electrochemical gradient across the cell membrane that is not at a steady state electrically. There is an imbalance in that all cells are intracellularly negative compared to the outside of the cell. The maintenance of this gradient requires metabolic energy to maintain this difference in ions. This electrochemical gradient is lost after death. The activity of the Na^+–K^+ ATPase results in serum sodium levels of roughly 140 to 145 mmol and serum potassium around 5 mmol. Inside cells the Na^+ concentration is low and the K^+ concentration is high. The reason for this difference between the intracellular and extracellular sodium and potassium is the action of the Na^+–K^+ ATPase enzyme. Digitalis binds to this enzyme and inhibits its activity. This results in an elevation in intracellular Na^+ that leads to an increase in extrusion of Na^+ through the Na^+–Ca^{++} exchanger, which functions to maintain a relatively constant level of both Na^+ and Ca^{++} in the cell. The Na^+–Ca^{++} exchanger normally extrudes Ca^{++} in exchange for Na^+. However, in the presence of increased intracellular Na^+, it will extrude Na^+ by exchanging it for extracellular Ca^{++}. This reversal in the activity of the Na^+–Ca^{++} exchanger results in an increase in intracellular ionized free Ca^{++} that enhances myocardial contractility.

The current hypothesis regarding the cellular basis for the positive inotropic effect of digitalis helps to explain some of the wide individual variability in the dosage required to develop digitalis toxicity. Differences in pH, ischemia, Na^+, K^+, and Ca^{++} can each alter the likelihood of developing toxicity within the same patient and between individuals.

DIURETICS

One cannot discuss the management of heart failure without including comments about the kidney. The relationship between the heart and the kidney makes intuitive sense when one considers the importance of the kidney in maintaining an appropriate volume status throughout the body. An analogy that may be useful to consider is the situation in which an individual turns on the faucet at home to find that little water is flowing. The first assumption is that a leak somewhere in the system is responsible for the lower water pressure. An appropriate response is to turn off the water to the house. In an analogous manner, the kidney perceives low cardiac output from a failing heart as a leak. The kidney begins to elaborate hormones designed to retain fluid. Many of the problems in CHF result from an inappropriate neurohumoral activation by the kidney in response to perceived volume depletion from hemorrhage. Mechanisms that result in vasoconstriction are normally compensatory in the short term for acute bleeding. These same adaptive mechanisms become damaging in chronic heart failure.

The usefulness of diuretics in the management of CHF cannot be overstated. Before diuretics were available, rotating tourniquets were used to diminish venous return by ligating the lower extremities. Less venous blood returned to the right side of the heart and pooled in the legs. This procedure diminished the effective intravascular volume that would otherwise have accumulated in the lungs. The availability of loop diuretics (particularly furosemide) has resulted in the virtual elimination of this practice.

Loop Diuretics

Diuretics and their mechanisms of action will be discussed in detail in Chapter 21. Loop diuretics, such as furosemide (*Lasix*), block the Na^+–K^+–$2Cl^-$ symporter in the ascending limb of the loop of Henle. The resultant effect is delivery of more Na^+ to the distal tubule and enhanced urinary loss of Na^+ and water. Unfortunately, the resultant increase in urinary excretion of H^+ and K^+ can lead to arrhythmias. The potential for arrhythmias is exacerbated by the loss of Mg^{++} and Ca^{++} and an underlying vulnerability of the myocardium in CHF. However, loop diuretics are still part of the mainstay of therapy for CHF despite these potential problems and the absence of well-controlled multicenter clinical trials. The rationale for their use is so compelling that placebo-controlled studies appear unethical. Moreover, furosemide was accepted as the standard of care in all of the clinical trials that form the basis for recommended therapy for CHF. The use of the potassium-sparing diuretic spironolactone has been shown to improve survival and is discussed below.

Spironolactone

Spironolactone (*Aldactone*) is the only diuretic that has been shown in a double-blind multicenter prospective clinical trial to improve survival in CHF. The addition of spironolactone to digitalis and an angiotensin-converting enzyme (ACE) inhibitor significantly improved survival among patients with chronic severe heart failure. This study was conducted with patients who were not taking a β-adrenoceptor blocking agent. It is unclear at present whether the addition of spironolactone to a combination of digitalis, ACE inhibitor, and a β-blocker will also confer additional benefit.

Spironolactone competitively inhibits the binding of aldosterone to cytosolic mineralocorticoid receptors in the epithelial cells in the late distal tubule and collect-ing duct of the kidney. Aldosterone enhances salt and water retention at the expense of enhanced renal K^+ and H^+ excretion. Spironolactone enhances diuresis by blocking sodium and water retention while retaining potassium. An obvious potential side effect is hyperkalemia, which is aggravated by the potassium-retaining properties of the ACE inhibitors. The likely concomitant use of the loop diuretic furosemide, which depletes K^+, dictates careful monitoring of serum potassium to avoid life-threatening rhythm disturbances.

There is also evidence for the existence of mineralocorticoid receptors on cardiac myocytes. This raises the intriguing possibility that spironolactone could mediate important direct effects on the myocardium in CHF.

HYDRALAZINE AND NITRATES

A major advance in the pharmacological management of CHF has been the demonstration that afterload reduction improved survival. The concept of afterload reduction was developed for the treatment of mitral regurgitation. It was noted that a decrease in systemic vascular resistance, as reflected in lower arterial blood pressure, resulted in an increase in the percentage of blood that flowed from the left ventricle to the aorta as opposed to the left atrium (decreased regurgitant fraction). The decrease in backup of blood into the lungs provided considerable symptomatic relief from dyspnea, fatigue, and chest pain. It was reasoned that patients with CHF often also have mitral regurgitation and might similarly benefit from more forward (left ventricle to aorta), as opposed to backward (left ventricle to left atrium), blood flow. A VA Cooperative Study in which vasodilators were added to digitalis and furosemide was the first to demonstrate a significant improvement in survival in CHF. Patients were given either prazosin as an α-adrenoceptor blocking agent or the combination of the direct vasodilator hydralazine and a nitric oxide–mediated vasodilator, that is, one of the nitrates. There were fewer deaths among the patients on the combination of hydralazine and nitrates. Patients taking prazosin did not benefit, probably because chronic therapy with prazosin results in tachyphylaxis. The mechanisms of action of prazosin, hydralazine, and organic nitrates are discussed in more detail elsewhere.

ANGIOTENSIN-CONVERTING ENZYME INHIBITORS

The relative ease of administration and superior efficacy of angiotensin-converting enzyme inhibitors and angiotensin II receptor blockers (ARB) have largely relegated hydralazine and nitrate therapy to second-line therapies for CHF. The demonstration of the survival benefit conferred by vasodilator therapy resulted in a paradigm shift in the approach to CHF. It was recognized that the way to improve survival in heart failure was not by directly addressing the weakened heart pump but rather by reversing the inappropriate peripheral vasoconstriction that results from neurohumoral activation.

Captopril (*Capoten*) was the original prototype product, and it was administered three times a day. A once-a-day preparation was subsequently patented and marketed. Prospective multicenter double-blind placebo-controlled clinical trials have repeatedly demonstrated an early and persistent survival benefit with ACE inhibitors in CHF patients. ACE inhibitors were found superior to hydralazine and nitrates in a direct comparison. *ACE inhibitors are now clearly the agents of first choice in the pharmacological management of CHF.* There are also a number of additional reasons to use ACE inhibitors. The HOPE trial and other studies demonstrated additional survival and renal protective benefits of ACE inhibition in diabetic and/or hypertensive patients long before they develop CHF.

Our understanding of the mechanism of action of ACE inhibitors has evolved along with our growing appreciation of the physiological and pathophysiological role of angiotensin II. Initially, angiotensin II was shown to be elaborated in response to low blood flow to the kidney in animal models of hypertension. Low flow to the kidney occurs when damage to the heart results in a low cardiac output. The low EF criterion for CHF noted previously is a noninvasively determined surrogate marker for a low cardiac output. The low flow to the kidney is perceived as bleeding. The appropriate response by the kidney to low flow is to elaborate renin. Renin circulates to the liver. Renin in the liver converts angiotensinogen to angiotensin I. Angiotensin I travels to the lung, where it is converted to angiotensin II by *ACE*.

Angiotensin II binds to its receptor and increases intracellular ionized free calcium. This increase in intracellular ionized free calcium causes vasoconstriction by vascular smooth muscle cells, aldosterone secretion by adrenal glomerulosa cells, increased central sympathetic outflow, and enhanced thirst. This system is activated as part of the normal host response to stressful injury, such as bleeding or trauma. The systemic angiotensin II levels rise acutely to retain fluid and improve short-term survival following injury. Unfortunately, these short-term adaptive mechanisms are not designed to protect against the long-term consequences of chronic low blood flow from CHF. The extraordinary success of ACE inhibitors in CHF clearly demonstrates the harmful effects of chronic angiotensin II activation.

Further refinement of this basic understanding followed. First of all, ACE inhibitors not only block the conversion of angiotensin I to angiotensin II; they also block the breakdown of bradykinin. Kinins are vasodilators and serve as part of the yin–yang of the vas-

cular system (i.e., vasoconstrictors vs. vasodilators). The use of an ACE inhibitor results in the elaboration of more kinins and less angiotensin II. Thus, the benefits of ACE inhibitors may derive from their elaboration of more kinins in addition to their inhibition of angiotensin II formation.

Efforts to elucidate the mechanisms responsible for the pharmacological efficacy of ACE inhibitors have been further complicated by the discovery of alternative pathways for forming angiotensin II independent of the conversion of angiotensin I to angiotensin II. Other cellular enzymes, such as chymases and trypsin, can also elaborate angiotensin II. And finally, at least two distinct angiotensin II receptors have been cloned and sequenced; they are confusingly named the type 1 and type 2 angiotensin II (AT-1;AT-2) receptors.

Elaboration of angiotensin II can result in either of two effects on an individual cell, depending on the relative numbers of AT-1 and AT-2 receptors. Relatively selective AT-1 receptor blockers have been developed in an effort to achieve superior efficacy with enhanced selectivity. Thus far, clinical studies indicate that ARBs may be as effective as ACE inhibitors and have fewer side effects. The consensus in their use is to try an ACE inhibitor as the first-line therapy before using an ARB, such as valsartan or losartan. However, ACE inhibitors can induce a very troubling cough in susceptible individuals as a result of the increase in kinins. ARBs serve as a very good substitute for such patients.

β-ADRENOCEPTOR BLOCKING DRUGS

For many years the prevailing view was that β-blockers are contraindicated in CHF. The physiological rationale for not using β-blockers in heart failure was certainly well founded. Heart failure patients have a decrease in cardiac output. Since cardiac output is a function of stroke volume times heart rate (CO = SV ×HR), an increased heart rate would be necessary to maintain an adequate cardiac output in the presence of the relatively fixed decrease in stroke volume observed in CHF. A rapid increase in heart rate does play an important role in the physiological response to acute hemorrhage. Thus, a decrease in heart rate, along with a depression in contractility produced by β-blockers, would be expected to precipitate catastrophic decompensation; and this certainly can happen in the acute setting.

Several subsequent studies have led to the incorporation of β-blocker therapy, using either carvedilol or metoprolol, into the standard of care for CHF. Patients already taking digitalis, furosemide, and an ACE inhibitor were prescribed a β-blocker in these studies. Surprisingly, the long-term use of β-blockers in CHF improved ventricular function and prolonged survival. The assumption that an increased heart rate is necessary to maintain an adequate cardiac output in the face of a reduced stroke volume is clearly not true in CHF.

The benefits of the use of β-blockade appear to exceed by far the risks of bronchospasm in patients diagnosed with chronic obstructive pulmonary disease (COPD) and/or suppression of hypoglycemic responses in diabetics. COPD is very different from bronchospastic asthma. Young people with asthma have highly reactive airways and can die within hours of a bronchospasm in response to an exposure to an external agent. This highly reversible dynamic condition contrasts sharply with the destruction of connective tissue in lung parenchyma and dead airway sacs that are not very reactive. This is a very different phenomenon.

β-Blockers are adrenoceptor antagonists that bind to the β-receptor at the same site as do endogenous β-adrenergic agonists, such as norepinephrine. Norepinephrine binds to the adrenergic receptor, which activates a G protein, which participates in the conversion of ATP to cAMP via adenylyl cyclase. cAMP activates protein kinase A (protein kinase A, or PKA) to phosphorylate proteins, such as the sarcolemmal L-type Ca^{++} channel, that subsequently increase calcium, increase heart rate, conduction, and contraction. β-Blockers bind to the same receptor as does norepinephrine but do not facilitate G protein coupling. Occupation of the binding site by the β-blocker prevents norepinephrine from binding to it and stimulating cAMP formation.

Circulating plasma norepinephrine levels correlate inversely with survival in CHF; that is, higher levels of norepinephrine are associated with a decrease in survival. It appears that norepinephrine levels are more than just markers of disease severity: norepinephrine is actually directly toxic to cardiac myocytes, at least in culture. The addition of either an α- or β-blocker confers partial protection from norepinephrine damage. Combined α- and β-blockade confers additive protection. These data from animal studies may be relevant to human heart failure, since they suggest that both α- and β- adrenoceptor blockade may be beneficial in the man-

agement of CHF. This rationale favors the use of the combined nonselective β- and α-blocker carvedilol over the relatively selective β1-antagonist metoprolol. In addition, in CHF the number of β1-receptors decreases while the number of β2-receptors increases, and the ratio of β1- to β2-receptors changes. Thus, the β1-selectivity of metoprolol may not confer any advantage over the less specific β-blocker carvedilol. It is clear from clinical trial data that β-adrenoceptor blockers are not all the same. Use of some has produced improvements in survival, and others have produced no improvements at all. The mechanisms responsible for these benefits are not yet established. Speculation includes up-regulation of β-adrenoceptors, improved G-protein coupling, altered regulation of nitric oxide, and so on.

cAMP-ELEVATING AGENTS

The immediate effect of increasing intracellular cAMP levels is an increase in contractility. This has been observed repeatedly in acutely ill patients in the intensive care unit with the intravenous infusion of either β-adrenergic agonists (e.g., dobutamine) or the phosphodiesterase inhibitors milrinone (*Corotrope*) and amrinone (*Inocor*). Binding of dobutamine to cardiac myocyte adrenoceptors results in G-protein coupling, activation of adenylyl cyclase, and the conversion of ATP to cAMP.

Administration of either milrinone or amrinone increases cAMP levels by preventing its degradation by cardiac myocyte phosphodiesterases. Both classes of cAMP-elevating agents have been shown to be helpful for the acute short-term management of the decompensated patient. Unfortunately, the long-term continuous use of either of these classes of agents in the outpatient setting has been associated with an increase in mortality in CHF. However, the use of these drugs in appropriately selected patients is highly effective for symptomatic relief.

Study QUESTIONS

1. A 40-year-old man goes to the emergency department because of an intractable cough for the past few days. No one else in his household has any cough, fever, upper respiratory infection, and so on. He was released from the hospital a week ago with the diagnosis of idiopathic dilated cardiomyopathy following an extensive evaluation that revealed normal coronary anatomy and a left ventricular EF of 38%. He was discharged with prescriptions for digitalis, furosemide, captopril, and carvedilol. He has

been more active and has noted improvement in his dyspnea and fatigue that prompted his initial presentation 10 days ago. He appreciates all of the care that he received and apologizes for making a fuss over the cough. He states that his wife made him come in because she was concerned that it might be his heart. He states that the cough is different from the congested feeling he had 10 days ago. On examination, he was afebrile; his heart rate was 60 beats per minute; blood pressure, 100/60. Neck veins were flat; carotid upstrokes were normal. Chest and lungs were clear. Heart revealed a regular rate and rhythm without murmurs, gallops, or rubs. Abdomen was soft and not tender. Bowel sounds were present without organomegaly. Extremities revealed no cyanosis, clubbing, or edema. Chest radiograph and electrocardiogram revealed no acute changes and no active disease. The physician was satisfied that he was hemodynamically stable and the cough was not resulting from worsening heart failure. What is a reasonable next step?

(A) Admit to the hospital to exclude (rule out) a myocardial infarction

(B) Apply a PPD skin test to exclude tuberculosis

(C) Substitute an angiotensin II receptor blocker for the ACE inhibitor

(D) Provide reassurance and continue with current medications

(E) Immediately stop the β-adrenergic blocker, carvedilol

2. A 67 year old woman has had fatigue and shortness of breath over the past few months. She has diabetes and hypertension for which she has been treated for 25 years with appropriate medications. She is status post three myocardial infarctions (MI ×3) and has known inoperable coronary artery disease and CHF. She has been very compliant with her complicated medical regimen, which includes digitalis, an ACE inhibitor (fosinopril), loop diuretic (furosemide), β-adrenergic receptor blocker (carvedilol) and aldosterone antagonist (spironolactone). On examination she was noted to be in acute respiratory distress with a respiratory rate of 24, a heart rate of 60, and blood pressure of 110/60. She was anxious and uncomfortable but polite and cooperative. Neck veins were elevated to 8 cm with the patient partially supine. Lungs revealed rales to the angles of the scapulae bilaterally. Heart revealed a third heart sound and a high pitched holosystolic murmur at the apex consistent with mitral regurgitation. Abdomen was protuberant with a fluid shift consistent with ascites. Extremities revealed 2 to 3 + pretibial pitting edema bilaterally. What can the physician offer this woman?

(A) Intravenous (cAMP elevating) positive inotropic agents

(B) Vasodilator therapy with hydralazine

(C) α-Adrenergic blockade with prazosin

(D) Stop the diuretic, furosemide

(E) Stop the ACE inhibitor, fosinopril

3. Digitalis functions to improve congestive heart failure by

(A) Induction of emesis

(B) Activation of α-adrenergic receptors

(C) Improving survival in patients of heart failure

(D) Binding to and inhibiting the Na–K ATPase enzyme in cardiac myocytes

(E) Deactivation of the angiotensin receptor

4. The combination of hydralazine and nitrates has been shown to improve survival in patients of heart failure. All of the following statements about this combination are true except:

(A) The combination serves to decrease both afterload and preload.

(B) Prazosin is as effective as the combination in treatment of congestive heart failure.

(C) The concept of afterload reduction is principally derived from patients of significant mitral regurgitation.

(D) The VA cooperative study was a landmark trial demonstrating the beneficial effect of hydralazine and nitrate combination in patients of heart failure.

5. β-Blockers have been effective in the treatment of heart failure. They primarily exert their effect by

(A) Binding to the receptor that binds norepinephrine

(B) Inducing a prominent diuretic effect

(C) Increasing contractility

(D) Improving asthma control

(E) Increasing heart rate to meet the additional demands placed upon the heart in CHF

ANSWERS

1. **C.** The most likely diagnosis is ACE inhibitor–induced cough. A reasonable approach is to substitute an ARB (angiotensin II receptor blocker) such as valsartan or losartan for the ACE inhibitor, captopril. Reassure and encourage the patient and spouse that you think the cough will resolve a few days after stopping the ACE inhibitor. There is generally no benefit to trying any other ACE inhibitor, as the side effect is a class effect resulting from enhanced kinin activity from ACE inhibition. Myocardial infarction is extremely unlikely in this patient based on the catheterization data showing normal coronary anatomy. Abrupt withdrawal of a β-blocker may precipitate tachycardia and hypertension and should be avoided.

2. **A.** This woman with CHF has obviously decompensated despite compliance with standard care. She is symptomatic and may benefit from a short course of high-intensity intravenous therapy with a cAMP-elevating agent (e.g., dobutamine, milrinone, amrinone). This may be a reversible event or part of the inevitable decline of the disease process. Approximately 45% of CHF patients die suddenly of a presumed electrical event (e.g., ventricular tachycardia, asystole). The others die slowly of progressive deterioration. Many patients at the end stages of CHF prefer to try repeated outpatient inotropic (cAMP elevating) therapy for symptomatic

relief even though it may be associated with a higher incidence of sudden death.

3. **D.** Inhibition of Na–K ATPase leads to an elevation of intracellular Na^+. This results in an increase in intracellular Ca^{++} and an enhanced myocardial contractibility. There is no definitive evidence that digitalis improves survival of patients in heart failure, but it clearly improves the symptoms of this condition.

4. **B.** Prazosin has been shown not to be as effective as the combination of hydralazine and nitrates.

5. **A.** The salutary effect of β-blockers appears to be due solely to its binding to the β-receptor, which prevents norepinephrine binding and stimulates cAMP formation. The other choices do not occur.

SUPPLEMENTAL READING

Brophy JM, Joseph L, and Rouleau JL. Beta-blockers in congestive heart failure: A Bayesian meta-analysis. Ann Intern Med 2001;134:550–560.

Digitalis Investigation Group. The effects of digoxin on mortality and morbidity in patients with heart failure. N Engl J Med 1997;336:525–533.

Cohn JN et al. Effect of vasodilator therapy on mortality in chronic congestive heart failure: Results of a Veterans Administration Cooperative Study. N Engl J Med 1986;314:1547–1552.

CONSENSUS Trial Study Group. Effects of enalapril on mortality in severe congestive heart failure: Results of the Cooperative North Scandinavian Enalapril Survival Study (CONSENSUS). N Engl J Med 1987;316:1429–1435.

Hunt SA et al. ACC/AAAHA guidelines for the evaluation and management of CHF in the adult: Executive summary: A report of the American College of Cardiology/American Heart Association Task Force on Practice Guidelines. Circulation 2001;104:2996–3007.

Packer M et al. Effect of carvedilol on survival in severe chronic heart failure. N Engl J Med 2001;344:1651–1658.

Pitt B et al. The effect of spironolactone on morbidity and mortality in patients with severe heart failure. N Engl J Med 1999;341:709–717.

CASE Study   Therapy for Inoperable Coronary Artery Disease

A 75-year-old man has inoperable coronary artery disease with an EF of 31%. He is receiving digoxin, furosemide, and an ACE inhibitor. He is unable to walk more than 50 feet on flat ground before getting short of breath (dyspnea on exertion at 50 feet). His heart rate at rest is 85 beats per minute and his blood pressure while seated is 130/85. His neck veins are flat; carotid upstrokes are normal; lungs are clear; and heart examination reveals no murmurs, gallops, or rubs. His extremities reveal no cyanosis, clubbing, or edema. The remainder of the physical examination is unremarkable. What is your next therapeutic option?

ANSWER: Start a low-dose β-adrenergic blocker. Presently the choices are either the β1-selective adrenergic blocker, metoprolol, or the combined nonselective β- and α-adrenergic blocker carvedilol. The target heart rate at rest should be in the range of 50 to 60 beats per minute. The target blood pressure should be in the range of 90 to 110 systolic, or orthostatic symptoms of light-headedness develop.

16 Antiarrhythmic Drugs

Peter S. Fischbach and Benedict R. Lucchesi

DRUG LIST

GENERIC NAME	PAGE	GENERIC NAME	PAGE
Acebutolol	184	Lidocaine	176
Adenosine	192	Mexiletine	179
Amiodarone	186	Moricizine	175
Bretylium	185	Phenytoin	177
Digoxin	192	Procainamide	173
Diltiazem	192	Propafenone	180
Disopyramide	174	Propranolol	182
Dofetilide	189	Quinidine	170
Esmolol	185	Sotalol	188
Flecainide	180	Tocainide	178
Ibutilide	190	Verapamil	191

Cardiac arrhythmias result from alterations in the orderly sequence of depolarization followed by repolarization in the heart. Cardiac arrhythmias may result in alterations in heart rate or rhythm and arise from alterations in impulse generation or conduction. The clinical implications of disordered cardiac activation range from asymptomatic palpitations to lethal arrhythmia.

Pharmacological management of arrhythmias uses drugs that exert effects directly on cardiac cells by inhibiting the function of specific ion channels or by altering the autonomic input into the heart. Recent technological advances have lead to an increase in nondrug strategies, including transcatheter radiofrequency ablation, intraoperative cryoablation, implanted pacemakers, and defibrillation. Physicians caring for patients with arrhythmias therefore must understand and appreciate the benefits and risks provided by each therapeutic modality, what the indication for each is, and how these modalities may interact.

Successful antiarrhythmic drug therapy requires a combination of understanding the pathophysiology of the arrhythmia, identification of a drug that can influence the relevant electrophysiological parameters, and careful titration of the drug's dose to correct the abnormal electrophysiological events giving rise to the arrhythmia. This is accomplished while avoiding the omnipresent risk of side effects such as proarrhythmia.

This chapter first provides a brief overview of the cellular events that underlie the cardiac action potential and lead to the formation and propagation of the normal cardiac impulse. Basic mechanisms of arrhythmias are reviewed, and the pharmacology of specific antiarrhythmic agents is discussed.

CARDIAC ELECTROPHYSIOLOGY

Transmembrane Potential

Figure 16.1 shows the phases of the cardiac action potential recorded with an intracellular microelectrode. The characteristic action potential is the result of activation and inactivation of multiple ion channels, which allows the flow of charged ions across the sarcolemmal membrane. The ion channels are transmembrane proteins possessing two important features: an ion selective pore that allows the passage of a specific cation or anion and regulatory components that respond to chemical stimulation or changes in the transmembrane potential by opening or closing. The ions flow through open channels according to the electrochemical driving forces at any given moment.

Like all other electrically active cells, the interior of the cardiac muscle cell is electrically negative with respect to the surrounding medium. This difference between the exterior and interior of a myocardial cell results from the action of several energy-requiring pumps, such as the Na^+–K^+–ATPase, which pumps Na^+ out of and K^+ into the cell in a ratio of $3Na^+$ to $2K^+$, and the presence of large negatively charged intracellular proteins that do not diffuse freely across the sarcolemmal membrane. The normal resting $[K^+]_i$ is 140 mM, whereas the extracellular K^+ concentration, $[K^+]_o$, is 4 mM. The resting myocardial cell tends to be highly permeable to K^+ and less so to Na^+ and Ca^{++}; therefore, a net diffusion of K^+ flows out of the cell, leaving behind negatively charged proteins. As a result, the interior of the cell becomes electronegative, and two opposing forces are established: a chemical force due to a concentration gradient and a counteracting electrostatic force established by the negatively charged ions within the cell.

At equilibrium, the chemical and electrostatic forces are equal, and there is no net flow of ions across the

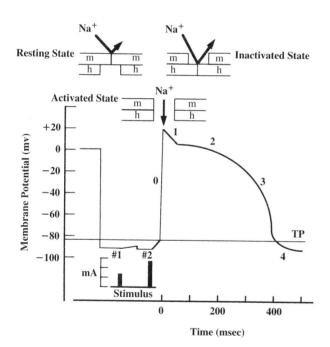
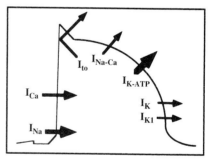

I_{Na}	= Fast Inward Sodium Current
I_{Ca}	= "L" Type Calcium Current
I_{to}	= Transient Outward Current
$I_{Na\text{-}Ca}$	= Sodium-Calcium Exchange Current
$I_{K\text{-}ATP}$	= ATP Sensitive Potassium Current
I_{K1}	= Inward Rectifying Potassium Current
I_K	= Delayed Rectifying Potassium Current

FIGURE 16.1

Transmembrane action potential of a Purkinje fiber as recorded with an intracellular microelectrode. When the electrode tip penetrates the fiber, a resting membrane potential of −90 mV is recorded. The application of a subthreshold stimulus (#1) produces a depolarizing current that fails to result in excitation of the myocardial cell. The application of a threshold stimulus (#2) reaches the threshold potential (TP) and results in an inward current and an action potential. Major transmembrane currents carried by specific ions entering the cell through selective ion channels are depicted to the right. Antiarrhythmic agents alter the electrophysiologic properties of the cardiac cells by modulating one or more of the transmembrane currents, especially the fast inward sodium current and the transmembrane currents carried by the potassium ion (I_K and $I_{K\text{-}ATP}$). I_{NA} = fast inward sodium current; I_{CA} = "L"-type calcium current; I_{to} = transient outward current; $I_{Na\text{-}Ca}$ = sodium-calcium exchange current; $I_{K\text{-}ATP}$ = adenosine triphosphate-sensitive potassium current; I_K = inward rectifying potassium current; I_K = delayed rectifying potassium current.

sarcolemmal membrane. The membrane potential at which this occurs may be calculated using the Nernst equation:

$$E_x = -61 \log([x]_i/[x]_o)$$

In this equation, x is the ion in question, $[x]_i$ is the concentration inside the cell, and $[x]_o$ is the concentration outside the cell. For potassium, using a $[K]_i$ of 140 mM and a $[K]_o$ of 4 mM, the E_K is equal to –94 mV, which is almost identical to the normal resting membrane potential of −90 mV. The contribution of other ionic species to the resting membrane potential is smaller because of the low transmembrane permeability at hyperpolarized resting membrane potentials.

An examination of the relationship of $[K^+]_o$ and $[K^+]_i$ in the Nernst equation shows that an increase in the $[K^+]_o$ will result in a decrease in the membrane resting potential (less negative). Changes in the extracellular concentration of another ion ($Na^+, Ca^{++}, Mg^{++}, Cl^-$) may also modify the resting potential.

To produce membrane depolarization, a current stimulus of sufficient intensity to exceed the outward K^+ current must be applied to the cell. If the depolarizing stimulus raises the membrane potential above a threshold value, sodium channels within the sarcolemmal membrane change their conformation and open their ion-selective pore, allowing Na^+ to enter the cell driven by the electrochemical gradient. The open sodium channels raise the membrane potential toward the equilibrium potential of sodium (+65 mV) and set into motion the intricate and precisely coordinated series of ion channel openings and closings leading to the characteristic action potential.

The action potential has been divided into five phases, rapid depolarization (phase 0), early repolarization (phase 1), plateau (phase 2), rapid repolarization (phase 3) and finally the resting phase in myocytes or slow diastolic depolarization (phase 4). The last is a property in cells with the potential for automaticity (defined later). A brief outline of each of these phases in the normal myocyte is given next.

Ionic Basis for the Membrane Action Potential
Phase 0: Rapid Depolarization

Phase 0 of the action potential encompasses the rapid depolarization of the myocyte induced principally by the opening of voltage gated sodium channels. The sodium channels open rapidly in response to membrane depolarization and close within 1 to 2 milliseconds in a time-dependent fashion. The conformation of the channels changes, and they enter an inactivated state in which they cannot be recruited to participate in generating a subsequent action potential for a defined inter-

val. The interval during which the myocyte cannot be stimulated is the *absolute refractory period*. After the myocyte returns to a hyperpolarized resting potential, the channels cycle through the inactivated state back to the rested or closed conformation and again are available to open in response to a stimulus of sufficient intensity. The rate of recovery of the Na^+ channels from voltage-dependent inactivation is one determinant of the cell's ability to generate a subsequent action potential. The refractory period defines the maximal rate at which the cardiac cells will respond to applied stimuli and propagate impulses to neighboring cells. The density of available sodium channels in the cell membrane also determines the rate at which an impulse is conducted from one cell to another. The maximal upstroke velocity of phase 0 (V_{max}) is a major determinant of the speed of impulse conduction within the myocardium and therefore is important in initiation and maintenance of arrhythmia. Genetic mutations in the sodium channel resulting in a sustained inward leak current have been identified and underlie one form of the long QT syndrome (LQTS 3).

Phase 1

At the peak of the action potential upstroke, a short rapid period of repolarization occurs and the membrane potential returns toward 0 mV. This produces a spike and dome configuration of the action potential and is a result of the inactivation of the I_{Na} and activation of a short-lived outward current called the transient outward current (I_{to}). I_{to} is composed of two distinct channels carried by either potassium or chloride. The distribution of I_{to} is heterogeneous throughout the myocardium and varies from species to species. I_{to} is present in both the atrium and the ventricular myocardium. Within the ventricle, I_{to} is present in the epicardium and absent in the endocardium. Consequently, the epicardium repolarizes more rapidly than the endocardium; this is the basis for the QRS complex and the T-wave on the surface electrocardiogram having an identical axis as opposed to an opposite axis. Abnormalities in the function of I_{to} have been implicated in Brugada syndrome, a potentially lethal genetic disease resulting in ventricular tachycardia and fibrillation.

Phase 2: Action Potential Plateau

Phase 2 is characterized by a net balance between inward (depolarizing) and outward (repolarizing) ion currents maintaining the myocyte in a depolarized state. During this phase, Ca^{++} enters the cell, causing Ca^{++} release from intracellular stores and linking electrical depolarization with mechanical contraction. Interestingly, the current flow during the plateau phase is small, and therefore, perturbations in any of the currents participating in this phase (either through genetic mutations or pharmacologically) may result in profound alterations in the action potential. Ca^{++} enters the cell through voltage-dependent channels highly selective for Ca^{++} that open when the membrane is depolarized above −40 mV. The channel (L-type calcium channel) possesses slow inactivation kinetics resulting in a long-lasting current.

Outward repolarizing K$^+$ currents oppose the effect of the inward I$_{Ca}$$^{++}$ on the plateau phase. This current is carried predominantly through delayed rectifier potassium channels (I$_K$). These channels are voltage sensitive, with slow inactivation kinetics. Three distinct subpopulations of I$_K$ with differing activation and inactivation kinetics have been described. A rapidly activating subset (I$_{Kr}$), a slowly inactivating subset (I$_{Ks}$), and an ultra–rapidly activating subset to date are identified only in atrial tissue (I$_{Kur}$).

Phase 3: Late Phase of Repolarization

Termination of phase 2 of the action potential plateau occurs when time-dependent, voltage-dependent, and intracellular Ca^{++}–dependent inactivation of I$_{Ca}$$^{++}$ results in the unopposed repolarizing effects of the outward K$^+$ currents. The combination of these effects results in rapid repolarization with a return to the hyperpolarized resting membrane potential. Pharmacological interventions that inhibit I$_K$ prolong the membrane action potential by de-

laying repolarization. Mutations in the genes encoding the various subtypes of I$_K$ inhibit proper channel function and result in the LQTS.

Phase 4

In normal atrial and ventricular myocytes, phase 4 is electrically stable, with the resting membrane potential held at approximately −90 mV and maintained by the outward potassium leak current and ion exchangers previously described. It is during phase 4 that the Na$^+$ channels necessary for atrial and ventricular myocyte depolarization recover completely from inactivation. In myocytes capable of automaticity, the membrane potential slowly depolarizes during this period to initiate an action potential (discussed later).

Automaticity

Automaticity can be defined as the ability of a cell to alter its resting membrane potential toward the excitation threshold without the influence of an external stimulus. The characteristic feature of cells with automaticity is a slow decrease in the membrane potential during diastole (phase 4) such that the membrane potential reaches threshold (Figure 16.2). During phase 4 in these pacemaker cells, the background potassium leak current decreases and an inward depolarizing current (I$_f$) is

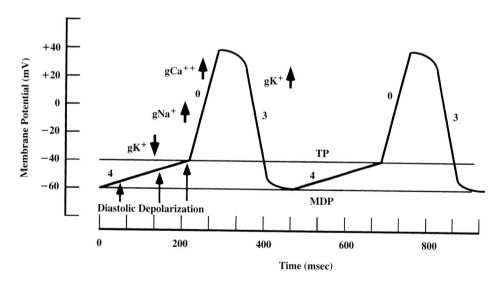

FIGURE 16.2

Transmembrane action potential of a sinoatrial node cell. In contrast to other cardiac cells, there is no phase 2 or plateau. The *threshold potential* (*TP*) is −40 mV. The maximum diastolic potential (MDP) is achieved as a result of a gradual decline in the potassium conductance (gK$^+$). Spontaneous phase 4 or diastolic depolarization permits the cell to achieve the TP, thereby initiating an action potential (g = transmembrane ion conductance). Stimulation of pacemaker cells within the sinoatrial node decreases the time required to achieve the TP, whereas vagal stimulation and the release of acetylcholine decrease the slope of diastolic depolarization. Thus, the positive and negative chronotropic actions of sympathetic and parasympathetic nerve stimulation can be attributed to the effects of the respective neurotransmitters on ion conductance in pacemaker cells of the sinuatrial node. gNa$^+$ = Na$^+$ conductance.

activated. In combination, this results in slow depolarization of the myocyte. If the membrane potential depolarizes above the threshold for the opening of I_{Ca}^{++}, an action potential is generated.

Myocytes within the sinoatrial node possess the most rapid intrinsic rate of automaticity; therefore, the sinoatrial node serves as the normal pacemaker of the heart. Specialized cells within the atria, atrioventricular (A-V) node, and His-Purkinje system are capable of spontaneous depolarization, albeit at a slower rate. *The more rapid rate of depolarization of the sinoatrial nodal cells normally suppresses all of the other cells with the potential for automaticity.* The other cells will become pacemakers when their own intrinsic rate of depolarization becomes greater than that of the sinoatrial node or when the pacemaker cells within the sinoatrial node are depressed. When impulses fail to conduct across the A-V node to excite the ventricular myocardium (heart

block), spontaneous depolarization within the His-Purkinje system may become the dominant pacemaker maintaining cardiac rhythm and cardiac output.

The rate of pacemaker discharge within these specialized myocytes is influenced by the activity of both divisions of the autonomic nervous system. Increased sympathetic nerve activity to the heart, the release of catecholamines from the adrenal medulla, or the exogenous administration of adrenomimetic amines will cause an increase in the rate of pacemaker activity through stimulation of β-adrenoceptors on the pacemaker cells (Figure 16.3).

The parasympathetic nervous system, through the vagus nerve, inhibits the spontaneous rate of depolarization of pacemaker cells. The release of acetylcholine from cholinergic vagal fibers increases potassium conductance (gK^+) in pacemaker cells, and this enhanced outward movement of K^+ results in a more negative po-

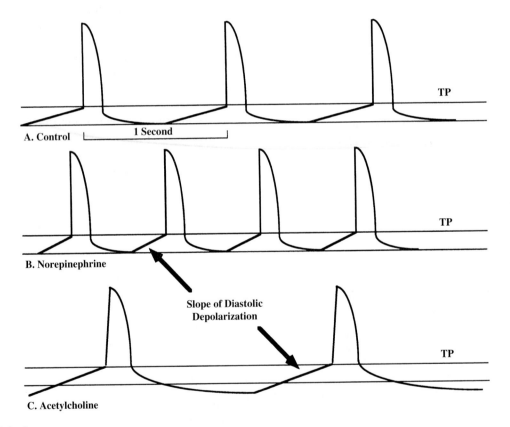

FIGURE 16.3

Effects of norepinephrine and acetylcholine on *spontaneous diastolic depolarization (automaticity)* in a pacemaker cell for the sinoatrial node. The pacemaker cell discharges spontaneously when the threshold potential (TP) is attained. The rate of spontaneous discharge is determined by the initial slope of the membrane potential and the time required to reach the threshold potential. A. Control recording showing the spontaneous diastolic depolarization. B. The effect of norepinephrine is to increase the slope of diastolic depolarization. The frequency of spontaneous discharge is increased. This effect is mediated through the activation of β-adrenoceptors in sinoatrial nodal cells. C. Acetylcholine stimulates muscarinic receptors in sinoatrial nodal cells. There is a decrease in the slope of diastolic depolarization as well as hyperpolarization of the cell. The time to reach the threshold potential is prolonged, with the net effect being a decrease in the rate of spontaneous depolarization.

tential, or hyperpolarization, of the sinoatrial cells. Thus, during vagal stimulation, the threshold potential of the sinoatrial node pacemaker cells is achieved more slowly and the heart rate is slowed.

Cardiac Conduction

The cardiac impulse begins in the sinoatrial node in the high lateral right atrium near the junction of the superior vena cava and the right atrium. Excitation leaves the sinoatrial node and spreads throughout the atrium. The myocytes (both atrial and ventricular) are long thin structures linked electrically via low-resistance pores known as gap junctions. The gap junctions are heterogeneously dispersed throughout the sarcolemmal membrane, although they are mainly concentrated on the ends of the myocytes. This distribution leads to polarity of the myocyte, with end-to-end conduction occurring at a more rapid rate than side-to-side (*anisotropic*) conduction. The difference in conduction velocity is up to a factor of three and may be important in supporting certain types of arrhythmias.

After the excitatory wave has spread throughout the atrium, it enters the atrioventricular (A-V) node. Importantly, the atrium and ventricle are electrically isolated from one another by a fibrous ring encircling the atrioventricular groove with the only connection occurring through the A-V node. If additional connections exist between the atrium and ventricle (accessory pathway), the potential for arrhythmia is present (atrioventricular reciprocating tachycardia), such as occurs with the Wolff-Parkinson-White syndrome. Conduction velocity slows significantly as the electrical signal enters the AV-node, where cellular depolarization depends on I_{Ca}^{++} rather than I_{Na}. The delay in ventricular excitation allows the atria to contract and enhances the filling of the ventricle. After passing through the A-V node, the electrical signal is carried via the right and left bundle branches to the body of the right and left ventricles.

The principal determinant of conduction velocity within the myocardium is the maximum rate of depolarization (V_{max}) of phase 0 of the action potential in individual myocytes. The number of sodium channels that are recruited to open by a depolarizing stimulus determines the V_{max} in atrial and ventricular muscle. Changes in the configuration of the sodium channel in the sarcolemmal membrane at resting membrane potentials, which are more positive (depolarized) than −75mV, cause the channels to enter an inactivated state in which they cannot participate in an action potential. As a result, there is a reduction in the peak sodium current leading to a reduction in upstroke velocity, action potential amplitude, excitability, and conduction velocity. This has important ramifications for the genesis of arrhythmias. *One common clinical cause of depolarization of myocardial tissue is ischemia resulting from coronary artery disease.*

Refractory Period

Depolarized cardiac cells are transiently unresponsive to any activation stimuli. During this interval, most Na$^+$ and some Ca^{++} channels are inactivated, and the cardiac myocytes are said to be refractory. The refractory period is subdivided into three phases, absolute, effective, and relative. *The absolute refractory period* is the time from the onset of the action potential until a stimulus is able to evoke a local nonconducted response. During this period, the cell is completely refractory to any stimulus regardless of its intensity. The *effective refractory period (ERP)* begins with the onset of the action potential, incorporates the absolute refractory period, and ends when an excitatory stimulus is able to generate a conducted signal. The ERP is determined as the shortest interval between two stimuli of equal intensity that results in the generation of a propagated response. The *relative refractory period* begins with the completion of the ERP and continues through the time in which a signal may be conducted slowly, prior to obtaining normal propagation of the signal. Since the cell is not fully repolarized during the relative refractory period, a stronger than normal stimulus is needed to produce depolarization and conduction of a propagated impulse.

Pharmacological agents that impair the function of channels normally active during phase III repolarization exert their effects by prolonging the refractory period of the tissue, thereby prolonging the interval before the myocardial cells are capable of responding to a subsequent stimulus that will propagate in a normal manner. As the myocytes repolarize, they enter a relative refractory period during which they again can undergo depolarization. Normal conduction velocity resumes when cells are stimulated, having fully recovered at the end of the relative refractory period. *Thus, the membrane potential at which excitation of the cell occurs determines conduction velocity. Conducted impulses generated during the relative refractory period will propagate slowly and may contribute to the genesis of cardiac arrhythmias.*

Mechanisms of Arrhythmias

Disturbances in the orderly formation and conduction of the cardiac impulse may result in heart rates that are either too fast (tachycardia) or too slow (bradycardia). In general, bradyarrhythmias result from the failure of impulse generation within the sinoatrial node or failure of the excitatory wavefront to conduct from the atrium to the ventricle through the atrioventricular node. *In general, bradyarrhythmias are not amenable to long-term pharmacological therapy and may require permanent cardiac pacing.* Tachyarrhythmias, conversely, frequently may be palliated with long-term medical therapy. The mechanisms supporting tachycardias may be classified broadly into three groups: (1) abnormal automaticity, (2) triggered activity, or (3) reentry.

Enhanced Automaticity

Automaticity, as outlined earlier, describes a cell's ability to raise spontaneously (depolarize) the resting membrane potential above the threshold value to initiate an action potential. Enhanced automaticity resulting in tachycardia may result from an increase in the slope of phase 4 depolarization or a decrease (less negative) in the resting membrane potential. Activation of β-adrenoceptors, hypokalemia, and stretching of cardiac cells all increase the slope of phase 4 depolarization and may serve as the trigger for enhanced automaticity. It is also possible for tissue that normally does not have pacemaking capabilities to develop inappropriate spontaneous diastolic depolarization and serve as an ectopic focus for impulse generation.

Triggered Activity

Triggered activity occurs when after-depolarizations induced by a preceding action potential raise the resting membrane potential above the threshold value, leading to an additional action potential. After-depolarizations may be categorized as early, occurring during phase III of the action potential before achieving full repolarization, or delayed, occurring after full repolarization of the membrane. After-depolarizations may stimulate an isolated extrapropagated impulse or lead to sustained repetitive activity. The crucial difference between triggered activity and abnormal automaticity is that triggered activity depends on a preceding action potential and cannot be self-induced. After-depolarizations or triggered activity are often associated with excessive increases in intracellular [Ca^{++}]. The potential for development of triggered activity is accentuated in the presence of an increase in extracellular [Ca^{++}] that would increase the amount of ionized calcium entering the cell during depolarization. Furthermore, conditions or pharmacological interventions favoring prolongation of the plateau (phase 3) of the action potential and prolongation of the QT interval of the electrocardiogram would increase intracellular [Ca^{++}] and the potential for proarrhythmia.

Early after-depolarizations are purported to be the mechanism giving rise to *torsades de pointes*. Conditions or drugs known to prolong the action potential, especially by interventions that decrease the outward potassium currents, facilitate development of torsades de pointes tachyarrhythmias. Early after-depolarizations may develop in association with hypokalemia, hypoxia, acidosis, and a wide range of pharmacological agents that interfere with outward currents or enhance inward currents. Antiarrhythmic agents, in particular sotalol,

quinidine, and dofetilide, may give rise to after-depolarizations and torsades de pointes tachyarrhythmia in persons with underlying cardiac abnormalities or alterations in plasma electrolytes. Conditions leading to bradycardia also may facilitate development of torsades de pointes tachyarrhythmia.

Early after-depolarizations and the associated ventricular arrhythmia can be prevented or suppressed by the appropriate adjustment of plasma potassium and/or magnesium concentrations. Lidocaine or procainamide may be effective for termination of the arrhythmia.

Delayed after-depolarizations (Figure 16.4) may occur in the presence of a rapid heart rate, digitalis glycosides, hypokalemia, hypercalcemia and catecholamines. Each of these influences ultimately leads to an increase in intracellular ionized calcium that is known to activate an inward ionic current. The inward ionic current activates a nonselective channel that normally is involved with the transport of sodium but that under pathophysiological conditions may permit the movement of sodium or potassium ions. Upon reaching threshold, the calcium-induced oscillatory potentials lead to the production of a sustained ventricular arrhythmia. Delayed after-depolarizations, in contrast to early after-depolarizations, are more likely to produce triggered tachyarrhythmias during periods of short pacing cycle lengths (rapid heart rates). Exercise-induced ventricular tachycardia in persons without overt cardiac disease exemplifies such a situation. The electrophysiological abnormality is catecholamine dependent and calcium sensitive. The arrhythmia may respond to L-type calcium channel antagonists or inhibitors of the cardiac β-adrenoceptor. Each of these approaches would serve to reduce the tissue calcium concentration.

Reentry

Reentry is an abnormality of impulse conduction wherein an excitatory wavefront circulates around an inexcitable region. Figures 16.5 and 16.6 show a normally propagated and a reentrant event in injured ventricular myocardium, respectively. As illustrated in Figure 16.5, the wave of excitation passes through homogeneous tissue involving the Purkinje system (P$_1$ and P$_2$) and enters normal ventricular myocardium. As indicated in the figure, the wave of excitation conducts around an inexcitable barrier, collides within the tissue, and extinguishes within the ventricular myocardium. *A normally propagating impulse will enter ventricular myocardium nearly simultaneously at multiple regions where Purkinje fibers terminate in the walls of both ventricles.* The sequence of activation of the ventricular myocardium is rapid (~0.04 second). The net result is orderly activation of all ventricular myocardial fibers, giving rise to normal-appearing action potentials in the respective regions and a normal electrocardiogram.

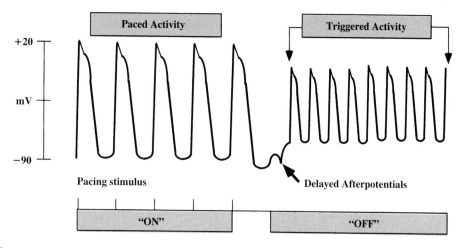

FIGURE 16.4

An example of *triggered activity* developing in Purkinje tissue. The appearance of a *delayed after-depolarization (DAD)* after the fifth paced impulse is followed by a burst of triggered activity that maintains the rapid rate of impulse formation despite the cessation of electrical pacing. Triggered activity from DADs occurs in Purkinje fibers or ventricular muscle when the tissues are exposed to toxic concentrations of digitalis, catecholamines, or other interventions that increase intracellular calcium concentrations. Whereas DADs occur after the cell has achieved its maximum diastolic potential, the phenomenon of *early afterdepolarization (EADs)* occurs before complete repolarization has taken place. EADs can occur after exposure to drugs that prolong the action-potential duration and may account for the *proarrhythmic action* (discussed in the text) of several antiarrhythmic drugs.

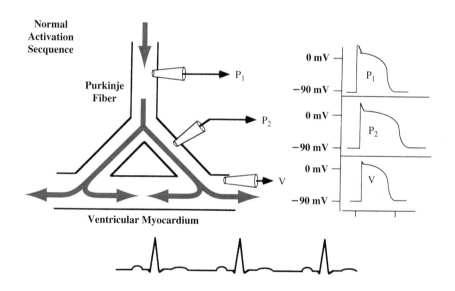

FIGURE 16.5

Schematic representation of normal activation and impulse transmission through the His-Purkinje system with final entry into ventricular myocardium. Intracellular recording electrodes are placed in the proximal Purkinje network (P_1), in the Purkinje branch on the right of the diagram (P_2), and in ventricular myocardium (V). The inset to the right illustrates the membrane action-potential recordings from the respective microelectrodes. The action-potential duration, and thus the effective refractory period, is longest in the more distal portion of the Purkinje branch immediately before insertion into the ventricular myocardium. Under normal conditions, the impulses within the terminal Purkinje network conduct with relatively equal velocities so as to activate the ventricular myocardium in a uniform manner. The longer duration of the effective refractory period in the terminal Purkinje fiber prevents the impulse, traversing within ventricular myocardium, from reentering the Purkinje network in the retrograde direction. The many wave fronts of excitation invading the ventricular myocardium from multiple insertions of the Purkinje network will collide in the ventricular myocardium and terminate. The net result is a homogeneous and nearly simultaneous activation of the entire ventricular myocardium within 400 msec. The electrocardiographic tracing below illustrates a normal sinus rhythm in which there is a repetitive and coordinated activation of the entire heart. One conducted sinoatrial impulse entering the ventricle from the atrioventricular node distributes over the His-Purkinje system to elicit one QRS complex indicating depolarization of the ventricular myocardium.

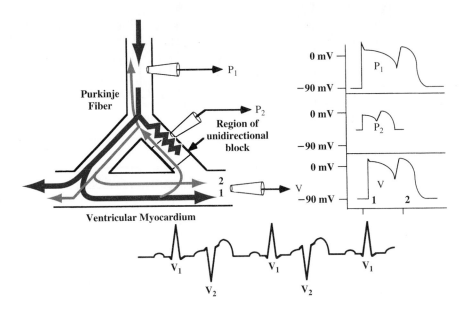

FIGURE 16.6

Conduction disorders due to *reentry* as might occur in the ischemic or postinfarcted myocardium. See Fig. 16.5 for a description of the format. As in the previous figure, *antegrade conduction* occurs in a normal manner over the proximal Purkinje system (P_1) and in the distal Purkinje network on the left of the diagram. However, the Purkinje network on the right (P_2) has been subjected to injury. The intracellular recordings from the respective electrodes indicate that the resting membrane potential from P_2 is decreased due to the presence of injury at this site. Therefore, the impulse conducts slowly and decrementally, and finally is blocked in the area of injury (*unidirectional block*). The ventricular myocardium, however, has been depolarized from normally conducting Purkinje fibers at remote insertion sites. The excitatory impulses traversing within the ventricular myocardium will reenter the distal portion of the Purkinje network (right side of diagram) and conduct slowly in the retrograde direction through the area of unidirectional block. The appropriate conditions are established by the conduction velocities and refractory periods in the respective tissues. The retrograde impulse can reenter the proximal Purkinje system and initiate reexcitation of the proximal and distal Purkinje network as well as the ventricular myocardium if each of these sites has recovered its excitability from the previous depolarization. The reentry impulse may give rise to a *premature coupled ventricular complex* in which the normally conducted impulse (V_1) is followed with precise timing by a *reentry ventricular complex* (V_2). The reentry impulses could occur more frequently so that the cardiac rhythm becomes dominated by the activity in the reentry pathway, thus leading to a rapid, repetitive series of ventricular complexes (*ventricular tachycardia*) in which the ventricular rate becomes rapid (>100 beats min) and may degenerate into ventricular fibrillation. The object of antiarrhythmic drug therapy is to reduce the frequency of hemodynamically disturbing premature ventricular impulses and to prevent the establishment of a sustained and rapidly conducting reentrant rhythm capable of becoming lethal.

In the undamaged myocardium, cardiac impulses travel rapidly antegrade through the Purkinje fibers to deliver the excitatory electrical impulse to the ventricular myocardium. During the normal activation sequence, retrograde conduction from ventricular myocardium to the conducting fibers is prevented by the longer duration of the membrane action potential and thus the refractory period in the Purkinje fibers.

In the presence of myocardial ischemia, propagation of cardiac impulses may be interfered with and a functional unidirectional block may occur. Impulses may fail to conduct longer in the anterograde direction to excite the more distal ventricular myocardium. Thus,

the terminal segments of the Purkinje fibers within the affected region may be activated by impulses passing from the ventricular myocardium to conduct in a retrograde direction (impulse 1, Fig. 16.6), albeit at a slower rate of conduction. In some situations, the retrograde impulse will enter an area of normal myocardium sufficiently repolarized that it is no longer refractory, and a propagated action potential will result. The generation of an action potential may produce an increased rate of ventricular activation and may become self-sustaining. The latter phenomenon is known as a *reentrant,* or *circus, rhythm.* If propagation is too rapid through the region of myocardial damage, the retrograde impulse will attempt to reenter the normal region while the tissue is refractory. This will give rise to bidirectional block, terminating the reentrant wave front. Therefore, for *reentry* to occur, there must be a region of *unidirectional block* and *slow conduction*. The delay in conduction permits the tissue ahead of the advancing wave front to regain its excitability, sustaining the reentry circuit. As shown in Figure 16.6, the reentrant wave front gives rise to a second depolarizing impulse (2) in the ventricular myocardium and in each of the branches of the Purkinje network (P_1 and P_2). The net result of the reentrant wave is depicted in the electrocardiogram (ECG), in which coupled ventricular premature complexes (V_2) follow each normal (V_1) complex.

It is estimated that 80 to 90% of clinical arrhythmias have a reentry mechanism. One explanation of how an antiarrhythmic agent may abolish reentry is by converting unidirectional block to bidirectional block. A second mechanism to explain the action of antiarrhythmic drugs is that they can prevent reentry by increasing the ERP of the cardiac fibers within or surrounding the region of the reentrant circuit.

CLASSIFICATION OF ANTIARRHYTHMIC DRUGS

Antiarrhythmic drugs have historically been segregated by the Vaughn Williams classification system into four main groups, based on their predominant mechanism of action. This is a good starting point for organizing one's thinking about the various antiarrhythmic drugs, but it is a great oversimplification and does not address several drugs that have electrophysiological effects characteristic of more than one group. Thus, although the grouping of antiarrhythmic agents into four classes is convenient, such a classification falls short of explaining the underlying mechanisms by which many drugs ultimately exert their therapeutic antiarrhythmic effect. Also, certain agents do not fall neatly into the four classes; these are discussed at the end of the chapter.

Class I Drugs

Class I antiarrhythmic drugs are characterized by their ability to block the voltage-gated sodium channel. The class I agents may block the channel when it is in either the open or the inactivated state. Inhibition of the sodium channel results in a decrease in the rate of rise of phase 0 of the cardiac membrane action potential and a slowing of the conduction velocity. Additionally, class I drugs, through inhibition of the sodium channel, require that a more hyperpolarized membrane potential (more negative) be achieved before the membrane becomes excitable and can propagate an excitatory

stimulus. As a result, the ERP of fast-response fibers is prolonged. Although many class I antiarrhythmic drugs possess local anesthetic actions and can depress myocardial contractile force, these effects are usually observed only at higher plasma concentrations.

The antiarrhythmic drugs in class I suppress both normal Purkinje fiber and His bundle automaticity in addition to abnormal automaticity resulting from myocardial damage. Suppression of abnormal automaticity permits the sinoatrial node again to assume the role of the dominant pacemaker.

The antiarrhythmic agents that belong to class I are divided into three subgroups (Table 16.1) with slightly different properties. Class IA drugs slow the rate of rise of phase 0 (V_{max}) of the action potential and prolong the ventricular ERP. Members of this class impair the function of the membrane sodium channel, thereby decreasing the number of channels available for membrane depolarization. Class IA drugs do not alter the resting membrane potential. Because they decrease V_{max}, class IA drugs slow conduction velocity. Members of this class directly decrease the slope of phase 4 depolarization in pacemaker cells, especially those that arise outside of the sinoatrial node.

Members of class IB have a minimal effect on the rate of depolarization and are characterized by their ability to decrease the duration of action potential and ERP of Purkinje fibers. Members of this class have a minimal effect on conduction velocity in ventricular myocardium and are without apparent effect on refractoriness.

The drugs in class IC produce a marked depression in the rate of rise of the membrane action potential and have minimal effects on the duration of membrane action potential and ERP of ventricular myocardial cells.

Class II Drugs

Class II antiarrhythmic drugs competitively inhibit β-adrenoceptors and inhibit catecholamine-induced stimulation of cardiac β-receptors. In addition, some members of the group (e.g., propranolol and acebutolol) cause electrophysiological alterations in Purkinje fibers that resemble those produced by class I antiarrhythmic drugs. The latter actions have been called membrane-stabilizing effects.

Class III Drugs

Class III antiarrhythmic drugs prolong the membrane action potential by delaying repolarization without altering phase 0 of depolarization or the resting membrane potential. Class III drugs have a significant risk of proarrhythmia because of the prolongation of action potential and the induction of torsades de pointes.

TABLE 16.1 Classification of Antiarrhythmic Drugs

Antiarrhythmic Class	Representative Drug	Principal Pharmacological Effects
IA	Quinidine Procainamide Disopyramide Moricizine[a]	Decrease V_{max} of phase 0, increase refractory period, moderately decrease conduction velocity, decrease fast inward sodium current, inhibit potassium repolarization current.
IB	Lidocaine Phenytoin Tocainide Moricizine[a] Mexiletine	Minimally change V_{max} of phase 0, decrease cardiac action potential duration, decrease inward sodium current in ventricular muscle, increase outward potassium current.
IC	Flecainide Propafenone	Markedly decrease V_{max} of phase 0, profoundly decrease ventricular conduction velocity, markedly inhibit inward sodium current. High potential for proarrhythmia.
II	Propranolol Metoprolol Nadolol Acebutolol Atenolol Pindolol Timolol Sotalol Esmolol[b]	β-Adrenoceptor antagonist, cardiac membrane stabilization, indirect effect on sinoatrial node to decrease rate of spontaneous diastolic depolarization. Indirect effect on A-V node to decrease conduction velocity and prolong ERP.
III	Amiodarone Bretylium Sotalol	Prolong ventricular action potential, prolong refractoriness, inhibit potassium repolarization currents. Prolong QTc interval. Potential for proarrhythmia (torsades de pointes tachyarrhythmia).
IV	Ibutilide Dofetilide Verapamil Diltiazem Bepridil[c]	Inhibit the slow inward calcium current, minimal effect (decrease) on ventricular action potential, major effects on the atrioventricular node to slow conduction velocity and increase the ERP.

[a]Mixed class IA/IB drug.
[b]Ultra–short-acting β-adrenoceptor blocking agent.
[c]May also show class III activity.

Class IV Drugs

Class IV drugs block the slow inward Ca⁺⁺ current (L-type calcium channel) in cardiac tissue. The most pronounced electrophysiological effects are exerted on cardiac cells that depend on the Ca^{++} channel for initiating the action potential, such as those found in the sinoatrial and A-V nodes. The administration of class IV drugs slows conduction velocity and increases refractoriness in the A-V node, thereby reducing the ability of the A-V node to conduct rapid impulses to the ventricle. This action may terminate supraventricular tachycardias and can slow conduction during atrial flutter or fibrillation.

CLASS IA

Quinidine

Quinidine is an alkaloid obtained from various species of *Cinchona* or its hybrids, from *Remijia pedunculata*, or from quinine. Quinidine is the dextrorotatory isomer of quinine.

Quinidine (*Quinidex*) was one of the first clinically used antiarrhythmic agents. Because of the high incidence of ventricular proarrhythmia associated with its use and numerous other equally efficacious agents, quinidine is now used sparingly. Quinidine shares all of the pharmacological properties of quinine, including antimalarial, antipyretic, oxytocic, and skeletal muscle relaxant actions.

Electrophysiological Actions

Quinidine's effect on the electrical properties of a particular cardiac tissue depends on the extent of parasympathetic innervation, the level of parasympathetic tone, and the dose. The anticholinergic actions of quinidine predominate at lower plasma concentrations. Later, when steady-state therapeutic plasma concentrations have been achieved, the drug's direct electrophysiological actions predominate. The direct and indirect electrophysiological actions are summarized in Table 16.2.

TABLE 16.2 Cardiac Electrophysiological Effects of Class I Antiarrhythmic Drugs

Drug	Class	Atria	S-A Node	A-V Node	His-Purkinje	Ventric Muscle	APD	ERP
Quinidine	IA	D	—	D	D	D	Increased	Increased
Procainamide	IA	D	—	D	D	D		Increased
Disopyramide	IA	D	—	D/I[a]	—	D	Increased	Increased/ decreased[a]
Moricizine	IA	—	—	D	D			
Lidocaine	IB	D	—	D	D	D	Decreased (His-Purkinje)	No effect
Phenytoin	IB	—/D	—	I			Decreased	Decreased
Tocainide	IB				D		Decreased	Decreased
Mexiletine	IB				D		Decreased	Decreased
Encainide	IC		D	D	D	D		
Flecainide	IC	D	—	I	D	D		
Propafenone	IC	D	D	D	D	D		Increased

[a]Dependent upon degree of anticholinergic action.
K, decrease in conduction velocity; I, increase in conduction velocity; —, no known conduction effects; APD, action potential duration; ERP, effective refractory period (ventricular).

Sinoatrial Node and Atrial Tissue

The indirect effect of quinidine on the sinoatrial node is a result of the drug's potential to exert an anticholinergic action resulting in a slight increase in heart rate. Higher concentrations of quinidine have a direct effect of depressing the rate of spontaneous diastolic depolarization.

Quinidine administration results in a dose-dependent depression of membrane responsiveness in atrial muscle fibers. The maximum rate of phase 0 depolarization and the amplitude of phase 0 are depressed equally at all membrane potentials. Quinidine also decreases atrial muscle excitability in such a way that a larger current stimulus is needed for initiation of an active response. These actions of quinidine often are referred to as its local anesthetic properties.

A-V Node

Both the direct and indirect actions of quinidine are important in determining its ultimate effect on A-V conduction. The indirect (anticholinergic) properties of quinidine prevent both vagally mediated prolongation of the A-V node refractory period and depression of conduction velocity; these effects lead to enhancement of A-V transmission. Quinidine's direct electrophysiological actions on the A-V node are to decrease conduction velocity and increase the ERP.

His-Purkinje System and Ventricular Muscle

Quinidine can depress the automaticity of ventricular pacemakers by depressing the slope of phase 4 depolarization. Depression of pacemakers in the His-Purkinje system is more pronounced than depression of sinoatrial node pacemaker cells.

Quinidine also prolongs repolarization in Purkinje fibers and ventricular muscle, increasing the duration of the action potential. As in atrial muscle, quinidine administration results in postrepolarization refractoriness, that is, an extension of refractoriness beyond the recovery of the resting membrane potential. The indirect (anticholinergic) properties of quinidine are not a factor in its actions on ventricular muscle and the His-Purkinje system.

Serum K^+ concentrations have a major influence on the activity of quinidine on cardiac tissue. Low extracellular K^+ concentrations antagonize the depressant effects of quinidine on membrane responsiveness, whereas high extracellular K^+ concentrations increase quinidine's ability to depress membrane responsiveness. This dependency may explain why hypokalemic patients are often unresponsive to the antiarrhythmic effects of quinidine and are prone to develop cardiac rhythm disorders.

Electrocardiographic Changes

At normal therapeutic plasma concentrations, quinidine prolongs the PR, the QRS, and the QT intervals. QRS and QT prolongations are more pronounced with quinidine than with most other antiarrhythmic agents. The magnitude of these changes is related directly to the plasma quinidine concentration.

Hemodynamic Effects

Although myocardial depression is not a problem in patients with normal cardiac function, in patients with compromised myocardial function, quinidine may depress cardiac contractility sufficiently to result in a decrease in cardiac output, a significant rise in left ventricular end-diastolic pressure, and overt heart failure. Quinidine can relax vascular smooth muscle directly as well as indirectly by inhibition of α_1-adrenoceptors. The depressant effects of quinidine on the cardiovascular system are most likely to occur after IV administration, and therefore, quinidine should not be employed routinely in the emergency treatment of arrhythmias. Because of its potential to cause marked depression of myocardial contractility and to decrease peripheral vascular resistance, parenteral administration of quinidine is seldom indicated.

Pharmacokinetics

The pharmacokinetic characteristics of quinidine:

Oral bioavailability	Almost complete absorption
Onset of action	1–3 hours
Peak response	1–2 hours
Duration of action	6–8 hours
Plasma half-life	6 hours
Primary route of metabolism	Hepatic; active metabolite
Primary route of excretion	10–50% renal (unchanged)
Therapeutic serum concentration	2–4 μg /mL

Clinical Uses

Primary indications for the use of quinidine include (1) abolition of premature complexes that have an atrial, A-V junctional, or ventricular origin; (2) restoration of normal sinus rhythm in atrial flutter and atrial fibrillation after controlling the ventricular rate with digitalis; (3) maintenance of normal sinus rhythm after electrical conversion of atrial arrhythmias; (4) prophylaxis against arrhythmias associated with electrical countershock; (5) termination of ventricular tachycardia; and (6) suppression of repetitive tachycardia associated with Wolff-Parkinson-White (WPW) syndrome.

Although quinidine often is successful in producing normal sinus rhythm, its administration in the presence of a rapid atrial rate (flutter and possibly atrial fibrillation) can lead to a further and dangerous increase in the ventricular rate secondary to inhibition of basal vagal tone upon the A-V node. For this reason, *digitalis should be used before quinidine when one is attempting to convert atrial flutter or atrial fibrillation to normal sinus rhythm.*

Adverse Effects

The most common adverse effects associated with quinidine administration are diarrhea (35%), upper gastrointestinal distress (25%), and light-headedness (15%). Other relatively common adverse effects include fatigue, palpitations, headache (each occurring with an incidence of 7%), anginalike pain, and rash. These adverse effects are generally dose related and reversible with cessation of therapy. In some patients, quinidine administration may bring on thrombocytopenia due to the formation of a plasma protein–quinidine complex that evokes a circulating antibody directed against the blood platelet. Although platelet counts return to normal on cessation of therapy, administration of quinidine or quinine at a later date can cause the reappearance of thrombocytopenia.

The cardiac toxicity of quinidine includes A-V and intraventricular block, ventricular tachyarrhythmias, and depression of myocardial contractility. Ventricular arrhythmia induced by quinidine leading to a loss of consciousness has been referred to as quinidine syncope. This devastating side effect is more common in women than in men and may occur at therapeutic or subtherapeutic plasma concentrations.

Large doses of quinidine can produce a syndrome known as *cinchonism*, which is characterized by ringing in the ears, headache, nausea, visual disturbances or blurred vision, disturbed auditory acuity, and vertigo. Larger doses can produce confusion, delirium, hallucinations, or psychoses. Quinidine can decrease blood glucose concentrations, possibly by inducing insulin secretion.

Contraindications

One of the few absolute contraindications for quinidine is complete A-V block with an A-V pacemaker or idioventricular pacemaker; this may be suppressed by quinidine, leading to cardiac arrest.

Persons with congenital QT prolongation may develop torsades de pointes tachyarrhythmia and should not be exposed to quinidine.

Owing to the negative inotropic action of quinidine, it is contraindicated in congestive heart failure and hypotension.

Digitalis intoxication and hyperkalemia can accentuate the depression of conduction caused by quinidine.

Myasthenia gravis can be aggravated severely by quinidine's actions at the neuromuscular junction.

The use of quinidine and quinine should be avoided in patients who previously showed evidence of quinidine-induced thrombocytopenia.

Drug Interactions

Quinidine can increase the plasma concentrations of digoxin, which may in turn lead to signs and symptoms of digitalis toxicity. Gastrointestinal, central nervous system (CNS), or cardiac toxicity associated with elevated digoxin concentrations may occur. Quinidine and digoxin can be administered concurrently; however, a downward adjustment in the digoxin dose may be required.

Drugs that have been associated with elevations in quinidine concentrations include acetazolamide, the antacids magnesium hydroxide and calcium carbonate, and the H_2-receptor antagonist cimetidine. Cimetidine inhibits the hepatic metabolism of quinidine. Phenytoin, rifampin, and barbiturates increase the hepatic metabolism of quinidine and reduce its plasma concentrations.

Procainamide

Procainamide (*Pronestyl, Procan SR*) is a derivative of the local anesthetic agent procaine. Procainamide has a longer half-life, does not cause CNS toxicity at therapeutic plasma concentrations, and is effective orally. *Procainamide is a particularly useful antiarrhythmic drug, effective in the treatment of supraventricular, ventricular, and digitalis-induced arrhythmias.*

Electrophysiological Actions

Table 16.2 describes the direct, indirect, and net actions of procainamide on cardiac electrophysiology.

Hemodynamic Effects

The hemodynamic alterations produced by procainamide are similar to those of quinidine but are not as intense. Alterations in circulatory dynamics vary according to the cardiovascular state of the individual. The hypotensive effects of procainamide are less pronounced after intramuscular administration and seldom occur after oral administration.

Pharmacokinetics

The pharmacokinetic characteristics of procainamide:

Oral bioavailability	75–95%
Onset of action	5–10 minutes
Peak response	60–90 minutes
Duration of action	4–10 hours
Plasma half-life	2.5–4.5 hours
Primary route of metabolism	Hepatic; active metabolite
Primary route of excretion	50–60% renal (unchanged)
Therapeutic serum concentration	4–10 μg /mL

Clinical Uses

Procainamide is an effective antiarrhythmic agent when given in sufficient doses at relatively short (3–4 hours) dosage intervals. *Procainamide is useful in the treatment of premature atrial contractions, paroxysmal atrial tachycardia, and atrial fibrillation of recent onset.* Procainamide is only moderately effective in converting atrial flutter or chronic atrial fibrillation to sinus rhythm, although it has value in preventing recurrences of these arrhythmias once they have been terminated by direct current (DC) cardioversion.

Procainamide can decrease the occurrence of all types of active ventricular dysrhythmias in patients with acute myocardial infarction who are free from A-V dissociation, serious ventricular failure, and cardiogenic shock. About 90% of patients with ventricular premature contractions and 80% of patients with ventricular tachycardia respond to procainamide administration.

Although the spectrum of action and electrophysiological effects of quinidine and procainamide are similar, the relatively short duration of action of procainamide has tended to restrict its use to patients who are intolerant of or unresponsive to quinidine.

Adverse Effects

Acute cardiovascular reactions to procainamide administration include hypotension, A-V block, intraventricular block, ventricular tachyarrhythmias, and complete heart block. The drug dosage must be reduced or even stopped if severe depression of conduction (severe prolongation of the QRS interval) or repolarization (severe prolongation of the QT interval) occurs.

Long-term drug use leads to increased antinuclear antibody titers in more than 80% of patients; more than 30% of patients receiving long-term procainamide therapy develop a clinical lupus erythematosus–like syndrome. The symptoms may disappear within a few days of cessation of procainamide therapy, although the tests for antinuclear factor and lupus erythematosus cells may remain positive for several months.

Procainamide, unlike procaine, has little potential to produce CNS toxicity. Rarely, patients may be confused or have hallucinations.

Contraindications

Contraindications to procainamide are similar to those for quinidine. Because of its effects on A-V nodal and His-Purkinje conduction, procainamide should be administered with caution to patients with second-degree A-V block and bundle branch block. Procainamide should not be administered to patients who have shown procaine or procainamide hypersensitivity and should be used with caution in patients with bronchial asthma. Prolonged administration should be accompanied by hematological studies, since agranulocytosis may occur.

Drug Interactions

The inherent anticholinergic properties of procainamide may interfere with the therapeutic effect of cholinergic agents. Patients receiving cimetidine and procainamide may exhibit signs of procainamide toxicity, as cimetidine inhibits the metabolism of procainamide. Simultaneous use of alcohol will increase the hepatic clearance of procainamide. Procainamide may enhance or prolong the neuromuscular blocking activity of the aminoglycosides with the potential of producing respiratory depression. The simultaneous administration of quinidine or amiodarone may increase the plasma concentration of procainamide.

Disopyramide

Disopyramide (*Norpace*) can suppress atrial and ventricular arrhythmias and is longer acting than other drugs in its class.

Electrophysiological Actions

The effects of disopyramide on the myocardium and specialized conduction tissue (Table 16.2) are a composite of its direct actions on cardiac tissue and its indirect actions mediated by competitive blockade of muscarinic cholinergic receptors.

Sinoatrial Node

The direct depressant actions of disopyramide on the sinoatrial node are antagonized by its anticholinergic properties, so that at therapeutic plasma concentrations, either no change or a slight increase in sinus heart rate is observed. Both the anticholinergic and direct depressant actions of disopyramide on sinus automaticity appear to be greater than those of quinidine.

Atrium

Disopyramide reduces membrane responsiveness in atrial muscle and the amplitude of the action potential. Excitability of atrial muscle is decreased. These changes decrease atrial muscle conduction velocity. Action potential duration in atrial muscle fibers is prolonged by disopyramide administration. This occurrence increases ERP. Postrepolarization refractoriness does not occur with disopyramide, and it appears to differ from quinidine and procainamide in this respect.

Abnormal atrial automaticity may be abolished at disopyramide plasma concentrations that fail to alter either conduction velocity or refractoriness. Disopyramide increases atrial refractoriness in patients pretreated with atropine, suggesting that the primary action of disopyramide is a direct one and not a consequence of its anticholinergic effect.

A-V Node

Disopyramide depresses conduction velocity and increases the ERP of the A-V node through a direct action. Its anticholinergic actions, however, produce an increase in conduction velocity and a decrease in the ERP. The net effect of disopyramide on A-V nodal

transmission therefore will be determined by the sum of its direct depression and indirect facilitation of transmission.

His-Purkinje System and Ventricular Muscle

Disopyramide administration reduces membrane responsiveness in Purkinje fibers and ventricular muscle and reduces the action potential amplitude. Even greater depression may occur in damaged or injured myocardial cells. Action potentials are prolonged after disopyramide administration, and this results in an increase in the ERPs of His-Purkinje and ventricular muscle tissue. Unlike procainamide and quinidine, disopyramide does not produce postrepolarization refractoriness.

The effect of disopyramide on conduction velocity depends on extracellular K^+ concentrations. Hypokalemic patients may respond poorly to the antiarrhythmic action of disopyramide, whereas hyperkalemia may accentuate the drug's depressant actions.

Electrocardiographic Changes

The electrocardiographic changes observed after disopyramide administration are identical to those seen with quinidine and procainamide.

Hemodynamic Effects

Disopyramide directly depresses myocardial contractility. The negative inotropic effect may be detrimental in patients with compromised cardiac function. Some patients develop overt congestive heart failure. At usual therapeutic doses, depression of myocardial function is not a problem in most patients with normal ventricular function.

Despite the decrease in cardiac output produced by disopyramide, blood pressure is well maintained by a reflex increase in vascular resistance. Catecholamine administration can reverse the myocardial depression.

Pharmacokinetics

The salient pharmacokinetic features of disopyramide:

Oral bioavailability	87–95%
Onset of action	30 minutes–3.5 hours
Peak response	30 minutes–3 hours
Duration of action	1.5–8.5 hours
Plasma half-life	4–10 hours
Primary route of metabolism	Hepatic, active metabolite
Primary route of excretion	80% renal (50% unchanged); 15% biliary
Therapeutic serum concentration	1–5 μg/mL

Clinical Uses

The indications for use of disopyramide are similar to those for quinidine, except that it is not approved for use in the prophylaxis of atrial flutter or atrial fibrillation after DC conversion. The indications are as follows: unifocal premature (ectopic) ventricular contractions, premature (ectopic) ventricular contractions of multifocal origin, paired premature ventricular contractions (couplets), and episodes of ventricular tachycardia. Persistent ventricular tachycardia is usually treated with DC conversion.

Adverse Effects

The major toxic reactions to disopyramide administration include hypotension, congestive heart failure, and conduction disturbances. These effects are the result of disopyramide's ability to depress myocardial contractility and myocardial conduction. Although disopyramide initially may produce ventricular tachyarrhythmias or ventricular fibrillation in some patients, the incidence of disopyramide-induced syncope in long-term therapy is not known. Most other toxic reactions (e.g., dry mouth, blurred vision, constipation) can be attributed to the anticholinergic properties of the drug.

CNS stimulation and hallucinations are rare. The incidence of severe adverse effects in long-term therapy may be lower than those observed with quinidine or procainamide.

Contraindications

Disopyramide should not be administered in cardiogenic shock, preexisting second- or third-degree A-V block, or known hypersensitivity to the drug. Neither should it be given to patients who are poorly compensated or those with uncompensated heart failure or severe hypotension. Because of its ability to slow cardiac conduction, disopyramide is not indicated for the treatment of digitalis-induced ventricular arrhythmias. Patients with congenital prolongation of the QT interval should not receive quinidine, procainamide, or disopyramide because further prolongation of the QT interval may increase the incidence of ventricular fibrillation.

Because of its anticholinergic properties, disopyramide should not be used in patients with glaucoma. Urinary retention and benign prostatic hypertrophy are also relative contraindications to disopyramide therapy. Patients with myasthenia gravis may have a myasthenic crisis after disopyramide administration as a result of the drug's local anesthetic action at the neuromuscular junction. The elderly patient may exhibit increased sensitivity to the anticholinergic actions of disopyramide.

Caution is advised when disopyramide is used in conjunction with other cardiac depressant drugs, such as verapamil, which may adversely affect atrioventricular conduction.

Drug Interactions

In the presence of phenytoin, the metabolism of disopyramide is increased (reducing its effective concentration) and the accumulation of its metabolites is also increased, thereby increasing the probability of anticholinergic adverse effects. Rifampin also stimulates the hepatic metabolism of disopyramide, reducing its plasma concentration.

Unlike quinidine, disopyramide does not increase the plasma concentration of digoxin in patients receiving a maintenance dose of the cardiac glycoside. Hypoglycemia has been reported with the use of disopyramide, particularly in conjunction with moderate or excessive alcohol intake.

Moricizine

Moricizine (*Ethmozine*) is an antiarrhythmic used to treat documented life-threatening arrhythmias.

Electrophysiological Actions

Moricizine exerts electrophysiological effects that are common to both class IA and IB agents. However, it does not belong in any of the existing drug classes.

Sinoatrial Node
No significant effect of moricizine is noted on the sinus cycle length or on automaticity within the sinoatrial node.

Atria
Moricizine does not affect the atrial refractory period or conduction velocity within atrial muscle.

A-V Node
Moricizine depresses conduction and prolongs refractoriness in the atrioventricular node and in the infranodal region. These changes are manifest in a prolongation of the PR interval on the electrocardiogram.

His-Purkinje System and Ventricular Muscle
The primary electrophysiological effects of moricizine relate to its inhibition of the fast inward sodium channel. Moricizine reduces the maximal upstroke of phase 0 and shortens the cardiac transmembrane action potential. The sodium channel blocking effect of moricizine is more significant at faster stimulation rates; an action referred to as use dependence. This phenomenon may explain the efficacy of moricizine in suppressing rapid ectopic activity. An interesting effect of moricizine is its depressant effect on automaticity in ischemic

Purkinje tissue in contrast to its inability to alter the slope of phase 4 depolarization of spontaneous automatic Purkinje fibers.

Electrocardiographic Changes

The electrocardiographic effects of moricizine include alterations in conduction velocity without an effect on the refractoriness of heart tissue. Moricizine enhances sinus node automaticity and prolongs sinoatrial and His-Purkinje intervals and the QRS. Moricizine prolongs ventricular conduction, thereby widening the QRS complex on the electrocardiogram. It has no significant effects on the QT interval.

The administration of moricizine is not associated with clinically significant hemodynamic effects.

Pharmacokinetics

The characteristics of moricizine:

Oral bioavailability	Not known
Onset of action	Within 2 hours
Peak response	6 hours
Duration of action	10–24 hours
Plasma half-life	1.5–3.5 hours
Primary route of metabolism	Hepatic
Primary route of excretion	56% biliary /fecal; 39% renal
Therapeutic serum concentration	Not established

Clinical Uses

Moricizine is indicated for the treatment of documented ventricular arrhythmias, particularly sustained ventricular tachycardia. Moricizine was evaluated in the CAST II clinical trial for the prevention of postinfarction ventricular premature complexes. It was ineffective and found to be proarrhythmic. Patients in the moricizine arm of the trial exhibited a greater incidence of sudden cardiac death than did controls.

Adverse Effects

The principal adverse gastrointestinal effect of moricizine is nausea (7%). Abdominal discomfort has also been reported. Dizziness (11%) is the most frequently reported CNS-related adverse effect. Such reactions increase in frequency with prolonged drug administration.

As with other antiarrhythmic drugs, moricizine has proarrhythmic activity, which may manifest as new ventricular ectopic beats or a worsening of preexisting ventricular arrhythmias. These effects are most common in patients with depressed left ventricular function and a history of congestive heart failure. Cardiovascular ef-

fects requiring drug withdrawal include conduction defects, sinus pauses, junctional rhythm, and A-V block.

Contraindications

Patients with preexisting second- or third-degree A-V block, cardiogenic shock, or drug hypersensitivity should not be treated with moricizine.

Drug Interactions

Clinically significant interactions with moricizine do not appear to exist.

CLASS IB

Lidocaine

Lidocaine (*Xylocaine*) was introduced as a local anesthetic and is still used extensively for that purpose (see Chapter 27). *Lidocaine is an effective sodium channel blocker, binding to channels in the inactivated state.* Lidocaine, like other IB agents, acts preferentially in diseased (ischemic) tissue, causing conduction block and interrupting reentrant tachycardias.

Electrophysiological Actions
Sinoatrial Node

When administered in normal therapeutic doses (1–5 mg/kg), lidocaine has no effect on the sinus rate.

Atrium

The electrophysiological properties of lidocaine in atrial muscle resemble those produced by quinidine. Membrane responsiveness, action potential amplitude, and atrial muscle excitability are all decreased. These changes result in a decrease in conduction velocity. However, the depression of conduction velocity is less marked than that caused by quinidine or procainamide. Action potential duration of atrial muscle fibers is not altered by lidocaine at either normal or subnormal extracellular K^+ levels. The ERP of atrial myocardium either remains the same or increases slightly after lidocaine administration.

A-V Node

Lidocaine minimally affects both the conduction velocity and the ERP of the A-V node. Lidocaine does not possess anticholinergic properties and will not improve A-V transmission when atrial flutter or atrial fibrillation is present.

His-Purkinje System and Ventricular Muscle

Lidocaine reduces action potential amplitude and membrane responsiveness. Significant shortening of the action potential duration and ERP occurs at lower concentrations of lidocaine in Purkinje fibers than in ventricular muscle. Lidocaine in very low concentrations slows phase 4 depolarization in Purkinje fibers and decreases their spontaneous rate of discharge. In higher concentrations, automaticity may be suppressed and phase 4 depolarization eliminated.

It is difficult to suggest a mechanism for lidocaine's antiarrhythmic action on the basis of its effects on normal ventricular myocardial tissue and His-Purkinje tissue.

Electrocardiographic Changes

Lidocaine does not usually change the PR, QRS, or QT interval, although the QT may be shortened in some patients. The paucity of electrocardiographic changes reflects lidocaine's lack of effect on healthy myocardium and conducting tissue.

Hemodynamic Effects

Lidocaine does not depress myocardial function, even in the face of congestive heart failure, at usual doses.

Pharmacokinetics

The pharmacokinetic characteristics of lidocaine:

Oral bioavailability	30–40%
Onset of action	5–15 minutes intramuscularly (IM); immediate intravenously (IV)
Peak response	Unknown
Duration of action	60–90 minutes IM; 10–20 minutes IV
Plasma half-life	1–2 hours
Primary route of metabolism	90% hepatic
Primary route of excretion	10% renal (unchanged), remainder as metabolites
Therapeutic serum concentration	1.5–5.0 μg/mL

Clinical Uses

Lidocaine is useful in the control of ventricular arrhythmias, particularly in patients with acute myocardial infarction. Lidocaine is the drug of choice for treatment of the electrical manifestations of digitalis intoxication.

Adverse Effects

The most common toxic reactions seen after lidocaine administration affect the CNS. Drowsiness is common, but unless excessive may not be particularly undesirable in patients with acute myocardial infarction. Some patients have paresthesias, disorientation, and muscle twitching that may forewarn of more serious deleterious effects, including psychosis, respiratory depression, and seizures.

Lidocaine may produce clinically significant hypotension, but this is exceedingly uncommon if the drug is given in moderate dosage. Depression of an already damaged myocardium may result from large doses.

Contraindications

Contraindications include hypersensitivity to local anesthetics of the amide type (a very rare occurrence), severe hepatic dysfunction, a history of grand mal seizures due to lidocaine, and age 70 or older. Lidocaine is contraindicated in the presence of second- or third-degree heart block, since it may increase the degree of block and can abolish the idioventricular pacemaker responsible for maintaining the cardiac rhythm.

Drug Interactions

The concurrent administration of lidocaine with cimetidine but not ranitidine may cause an increase (15%) in the plasma concentration of lidocaine. This effect is a manifestation of cimetidine reducing the clearance and volume of distribution of lidocaine. The myocardial depressant effect of lidocaine is enhanced by phenytoin administration.

Phenytoin

Phenytoin (*Dilantin*) was originally introduced for the control of convulsive disorders (see Chapter 32) but has now also been shown to be effective in the treatment of cardiac arrhythmias. Phenytoin appears to be particularly effective in treating ventricular arrhythmias in children.

Electrophysiological Actions
Sinoatrial Node

Most clinically used concentrations of phenytoin do not significantly alter sinus rate in humans. However, the hypotension that may follow IV administration of phenytoin can result in an increase in sympathetic tone and therefore an increased sinus heart rate.

Atrium

Phenytoin, like lidocaine, usually does not alter the action potential duration or ERP of atrial tissue except at very high concentrations. Atrial conduction velocity is either unchanged or slightly depressed.

A-V Node

Phenytoin lacks the anticholinergic properties of quinidine, disopyramide, and procainamide. However, the direct actions of phenytoin on the A-V node facilitate transmission.

His-Purkinje System

The electrophysiological effects of phenytoin on the His-Purkinje system resemble those of lidocaine; that is, action potential duration and ERPs are shortened. Phenytoin decreases the rate of phase 4 depolarization in Purkinje tissue and reduces the rate of discharge of ventricular pacemakers.

Electrocardiographic Changes

Because phenytoin improves A-V conduction and shortens the action potential duration of ventricular myocardium, it may decrease the PR and QT intervals of the surface electrocardiogram.

Hemodynamic Effects

The effects of phenytoin on the cardiovascular system vary with the dose, the mode and rate of administration, and any cardiovascular pathology. Rapid administration can produce transient hypotension that is the combined result of peripheral vasodilation and depression of myocardial contractility. These effects are due to direct actions of phenytoin on the vascular bed and ventricular myocardium. If large doses are given slowly, dose-related decreases in left ventricular force, rate of force development, and cardiac output can be observed, along with an increase in left ventricular end-diastolic pressure.

Pharmacokinetics

The pharmacokinetic characteristics of phenytoin:

Oral bioavailability	Slow and variable
Onset of action	1–2 hours
Peak response	1.5–6 hours
Duration of action	Variable
Plasma half-life	22 hours
Primary route of metabolism	Hepatic
Primary route of excretion	5% renal (unchanged); remainder as metabolites
Therapeutic serum concentration	10–18 μg/mL

Clinical Uses

Phenytoin, like lidocaine, is more effective in the treatment of ventricular than supraventricular arrhythmias. It is particularly effective in treating ventricular arrhythmias associated with digitalis toxicity, acute myocardial infarction, open-heart surgery, anesthesia, cardiac catheterization, cardioversion, and angiographic studies.

Phenytoin finds its most effective use in the treatment of supraventricular and ventricular arrhythmias associated with digitalis intoxication. The ability of phenytoin to improve digitalis-induced depression of A-V conduction is a special feature that contrasts with the actions of other antiarrhythmic agents.

Adverse Effects

The rapid IV administration of phenytoin can present a hazard. Respiratory arrest, arrhythmias, and hypotension have been reported. Other adverse reactions and potential drug interactions are discussed in Chapter 32.

Contraindications

Phenytoin either should not be used or should be used cautiously in patients with hypotension, severe bradycardia, high-grade A-V block, severe heart failure, or hypersensitivity to the drug.

Because of the increase in A-V transmission observed with phenytoin administration, it should not be given to patients with atrial flutter or atrial fibrillation. Phenytoin will probably not restore normal sinus rhythm and may dangerously accelerate the ventricular rate.

Drug Interactions

Plasma phenytoin concentrations are increased in the presence of chloramphenicol, disulfiram, and isoniazid, since the latter drugs inhibit the hepatic metabolism of phenytoin. A reduction in phenytoin dose can alleviate the consequences of these drug–drug interactions.

Tocainide

Tocainide (*Tonocard*) is an orally effective antiarrhythmic agent with close structural similarities to lidocaine.

Electrophysiological Actions

In healthy volunteers, tocainide produced a slight depression in His-Purkinje conduction as well as a slightly delayed enhancement of A-V node conduction during atrial pacing. No significant alterations in heart rate, right ventricular ERP or the excitation thresholds of atrial or ventricular muscle were observed in these subjects.

Hemodynamic Effects

The acute hemodynamic effects are slight and transient and are observed most often during or immediately after drug infusion.

Pharmacokinetics

The pharmacokinetic characteristics of tocainide:

Oral bioavailability	Approximately 100%
Onset of action	Not known
Peak response	0.5–2 hours
Duration of action	8 hours
Plasma half-life	15 hours

Primary route of metabolism	Hepatic
Primary route of excretion	Renal (40% unchanged)
Therapeutic serum	3–11 µg /mL concentration

Clinical Uses

Tocainide is indicated for the treatment of symptomatic ventricular arrhythmias refractory to more conventional therapy. Serious noncardiac adverse effects limit its use to patients with life-threatening arrhythmias.

Adverse Effects

Light-headedness, dizziness, or nausea occurs in approximately 15% of patients, paresthesias and numbness in 9%, and tremor in 8%. These adverse effects are generally mild in intensity, transient, and dose related. Overall, however, approximately 20% of patients prescribed tocainide discontinue therapy because of such effects. Serious immune-based side effects, such as pulmonary fibrosis, have been reported, and blood dyscrasias, such as agranulocytosis and thrombocytopenia, may occur in up to 0.2% of patients.

Contraindications

Patients who are hypersensitive to tocainide or to local anesthetics of the amide type should not be exposed to tocainide. The presence of second- or third-degree heart block in the absence of an artificial pacemaker also contraindicates the use of tocainide.

Drug Interactions

When used with other class IB antiarrhythmic drugs, tocainide toxicity may be increased without significant gain in antiarrhythmic efficacy.

Mexiletine

Mexiletine (*Mexitil*) is an antiarrhythmic agent with pharmacological and antiarrhythmic properties similar to those of lidocaine and tocainide. Like tocainide, mexiletine is available for oral administration.

Electrophysiological Actions

As with other members of class IB, mexiletine slows the maximal rate of depolarization of the cardiac membrane action potential and exerts a negligible effect on repolarization. Mexiletine demonstrates a rate-dependent blocking action on the sodium channel, with rapid onset and recovery kinetics suggesting that it may be more useful for the control of rapid as opposed to slow ventricular tachyarrhythmias.

Hemodynamic Effects

Although its cardiovascular toxicity is minimal, mexiletine should be used with caution in patients who are hypotensive or who exhibit severe left ventricular dysfunction.

Pharmacokinetics

The pharmacokinetic characteristics of mexiletine:

Oral bioavailability	90%
Onset of action	0.5–2 hours
Peak response	2–3 hours
Duration of action	8–12 hours
Plasma half-life	10–12 hours
Primary route of metabolism	Hepatic
Primary route of excretion	Primarily biliary; 10% renal
Therapeutic serum concentration	0.5–2 µg /mL

Clinical Uses

Mexiletine is useful as an antiarrhythmic agent in the management of patients with either acute or chronic ventricular arrhythmias. While it is not at present an indication for use, there is interest in using mexiletine to treat the congenital long QT syndrome when an abnormality in the SCN5A gene (LQTS 3) has been found.

Adverse Effects

A very narrow therapeutic window limits mexiletine use. The first signs of toxicity manifest as fine tremor of the hands, followed by dizziness and blurred vision. Hypotension, sinus bradycardia, and widening of the QRS complex have been noted as the most common unwanted cardiovascular effects of IV mexiletine. The side effects of oral maintenance therapy include reversible upper gastrointestinal distress, tremor, light-headedness, and coordination difficulties. These effects generally are not serious and can be reduced by downward dose adjustment or administering the drug with meals. Cardiovascular adverse effects, which are less common, include palpitations, chest pain, and angina or anginalike pain.

Contraindications

Mexiletine is contraindicated in the presence of cardiogenic shock or preexisting second- or third-degree heart block in the absence of a cardiac pacemaker. Caution must be exercised in administration of the drug to patients with sinus node dysfunction or disturbances of intraventricular conduction.

Drug Interactions

An upward adjustment in dose may be required when mexiletine is administered with phenytoin or rifampin, since these drugs stimulate the hepatic metabolism of mexiletine, reducing its plasma concentration.

CLASS IC

Flecainide

Flecainide (*Tambocor*) is a fluorinated aromatic hydrocarbon examined initially for its local anesthetic action and subsequently found to have antiarrhythmic effects. Flecainide inhibits the sodium channel, leading to conduction slowing in all parts of the heart, but most notably in the His-Purkinje system and ventricular myocardium. It has relatively minor effects on repolarization. Flecainide also inhibits abnormal automaticity.

Electrophysiological Actions
Sinoatrial Node

Flecainide decreases the sinus cycle length but results in a clinically insignificant decrease in heart rate.

Atrium

Flecainide decreases the maximal rate of depolarization in atrial tissue and shifts the membrane responsiveness curve to the right.

A-V Node

The atrioventricular conduction time, measured as the A–H interval, is prolonged by flecainide as is the His-Purkinje or H–V interval.

His-Purkinje System and Ventricular Muscle

Flecainide slows conduction in the His-Purkinje system and ventricular muscle to a greater degree than in the atrium. Flecainide may also cause block in accessory A-V connections, which is the principal mechanism for its effectiveness in treating A-V reentrant tachycardia.

Electrocardiographic Changes

Flecainide increases the PR, QRS, and to a lesser extent, QTc intervals. The rate of ventricular repolarization is not affected, and the QT interval prolongation is caused by the increase in the QRS duration.

Hemodynamic Effects

Flecainide produces modest negative inotropic effects that may become significant in the subset of patients with compromised left ventricular function.

Pharmacokinetics

The pharmacokinetic characteristics of flecainide:

Oral bioavailability	85–90%
Onset of action	1–2 hours
Peak response	1.5–6 hours
Duration of action	1–2 days
Plasma half-life	12–30 hours
Primary route of metabolism	Hepatic
Primary route of excretion	10–50% renal; 5% fecal
Therapeutic serum concentration	0.2–1.0 μg /mL

Clinical Uses

Flecainide is effective in treating most types of atrial arrhythmias. It is also used for life-threatening ventricular arrhythmias. However, flecainide should be used with extreme caution in any patient with structural heart disease. Flecainide crosses the placenta, with fetal levels reaching approximately 70% of maternal levels. In many centers, it is the second-line drug after digoxin for therapy of fetal arrhythmias. Because of the high incidence of proarrhythmia, initiation of therapy or significant increases in dosing should be performed only on inpatients.

Adverse Effects

Most adverse effects occur within a few days of initial drug administration. The most frequently reported effects are dizziness, light-headedness, faintness, unsteadiness, visual disturbances, blurred vision (e.g., spots before the eyes, difficulty in focusing), nausea, headache, and dyspnea.

Worsening of heart failure and prolongation of the PR and QRS intervals are likely to occur with flecainide, and an increased risk of proarrhythmia has been reported.

Contraindications

Flecainide is contraindicated in patients with preexisting second- or third-degree heart block or with bundle branch block unless a pacemaker is present to maintain ventricular rhythm. It should not be used in patients with cardiogenic shock.

Drug Interactions

In patients whose condition has been stabilized by flecainide, the addition of cimetidine may reduce the rate of flecainide's hepatic metabolism, increasing the potential for toxicity. Flecainide may increase digoxin concentrations on concurrent administration.

Propafenone

Propafenone (*Rythmol*) exhibits predominantly class IC properties with conduction slowing due to sodium channel blockade. Additionally, propafenone is a weak β-receptor and L-type calcium channel blocker.

Electrophysiological Actions

As with all members of its class, propafenone has its major effect on the fast inward sodium current. The IC agents depress V_{max} over a wide range of heart rates and shift the resting membrane potential in the direction of hyperpolarization. The IC agents bind slowly to the sodium channel and dissociate slowly. Therefore, they exhibit rate-dependent block. Inhibition of the sodium channel throughout the cardiac cycle will result in a decrease in the rate of ectopy and trigger ventricular tachycardia.

Sinoatrial Node

Propafenone causes sinus node slowing that could lead to sinoatrial block. It may lengthen the sinus node recovery time with minimal effects on sinus cycle length.

Atrium

The action potential duration and ERP of atrial muscle are both prolonged by propafenone. The electrophysiological effects persist beyond removal of the drug from the tissue. In patients with atrial flutter, fibrillation, or tachycardia, propafenone can slow the atrial rate, resulting in a change from 2:1 or 4:1 A-V block to 1:1 A-V conduction with a subsequent increase in the ventricular rate.

A-V Node

The IV administration of propafenone slows conduction through the A-V node.

His-Purkinje System and Ventricular Muscle

Propafenone slows conduction and inhibits automatic foci.

Electrocardiographic Changes

Propafenone causes dose-dependent increases in the PR and QRS intervals.

Hemodynamic Effects

The IV administration of propafenone is accompanied by an increase in right atrial, pulmonary arterial, and pulmonary artery wedge pressures in addition to an increase in vascular resistance and a decrease in the cardiac index. A significant decrease in ejection fraction may be observed in patients with preexisting left ventricular dysfunction. In the absence of cardiac abnormalities, propafenone has no significant effects on cardiac function.

Pharmacokinetics

The pharmacokinetic characteristics of propafenone:

Oral bioavailability	Nearly complete
Onset of action	1 hour
Peak response	2–3 hours
Duration of action	8–12 hours
Plasma half-life	2–10 hours
Primary route of metabolism	Hepatic
Primary route of excretion	18.5–38% renal (unchanged)
Therapeutic serum concentration	<1 μ/mL

Clinical Uses

Approved indications for propafenone include treatment of supraventricular arrhythmias and life-threatening ventricular arrhythmias in the absence of structural heart disease. Propafenone has been shown to increase mortality in patients with structural heart disease, and so extreme caution must be used in this subset of patients. As with flecainide, the patient should be hospitalized for initiation of therapy.

Adverse Effects and Drug Interactions

Concurrent administration of propafenone with digoxin, warfarin, propranolol, or metoprolol increases the serum concentrations of the latter four drugs. Cimetidine slightly increases the propafenone serum concentrations. Additive pharmacological effects can occur when lidocaine, procainamide, and quinidine are combined with propafenone.

As with other members of class IC, propafenone may interact in an unfavorable way with other agents that depress A-V nodal function, intraventricular conduction, or myocardial contractility.

Overall, 21 to 32% of patients have adverse effects. The most common are dizziness or light-headedness, metallic taste, nausea, and vomiting; the most serious are proarrhythmic events.

Contraindications

Propafenone is contraindicated in the presence of severe or uncontrolled congestive heart failure; cardiogenic shock; sinoatrial, A-V, and intraventricular disorders of conduction; and sinus node dysfunction, such as sick sinus syndrome. Other contraindications include severe bradycardia, hypotension, obstructive pulmonary disease, and hepatic and renal failure. Because of its weak β-blocking action, propafenone may cause possible dose-related bronchospasm. This problem is greatest in patients who are slow metabolizers.

CLASS II

Table 16.3 summarizes the cardiac electrophysiological effects of class II, III, and IV agents, and Table 16.4 summarizes the actions of the β-receptor blocking agents

TABLE 16.3   Cardiac Electrophysiological Effects of Class II–IV Antiarrhythmic Drugs

Drug	Class	SA Node[a]	Atria	A-V Node	His-Purkinje	Ventricular Muscle	APD Atria/Ventricle	ERP Atria/Ventricle
							Conduction Velocity	
Propranolol	II	D	D	D	–	–	–	–
Acebutolol	II	D	D	D	–	–	–	–
Esmolol	II	D	D	D	–	–	–	–
Sotalol	II/III	D	–	D	–	–	Increase[b]	Increase
Bretylium	III	I/D	–	I/D	–	–	Increase	Decrease Increase
Dofetilide	III	–	–	–	–	–	Increase[b]	Increase
Ibutilide	III	D±	–	D±	–	–	Increase[b]	Increase
Amiodarone	III	D	D	D	–	–	Increase[b]	Increase
Verapamil	IV	D	–	D	–	–	Decrease	–
Diltiazem	IV	D	–	D	–	–	Decrease	–

a*Spontaneous phase 4 depolarization.*
b *Increase in the QTc interval.*
SA, sinoatrial; D, decrease in conduction velocity; I, increase in conduction velocity; –, no significant effect with clinically relevant doses; ±, minimal effect.

that make up the class II drugs. Bear in mind the complete spectrum of cardiovascular effects of these agents when prescribing their use. For example, while patients with a normally functioning cardiovascular system may tolerate adrenergic blockade of the heart, patients with compensated heart failure, who depend on adrenergic tone to maintain an adequate cardiac output, may undergo acute congestive heart failure if prescribed any of the class II drugs. Table 16.5 summarizes the clinical use of the β-adrenoceptor blocking drugs in the treatment of cardiac arrhythmias.

Propranolol

Propranolol (*Inderal*) is the prototype β-blocker (see Chapter 11). It decreases the effects of sympathetic stimulation by competitive binding to β-adrenoceptors.

Electrophysiological Actions

Propranolol has two separate and distinct effects. The first is a consequence of the drug's β-blocking properties and the subsequent removal of adrenergic influences on the heart. The second is associated with its direct myocardial effects (membrane stabilization). The latter action, especially at high clinically employed doses, may account for its effectiveness against arrhythmias in which enhanced β-receptor stimulation does not play a significant role in the genesis of the rhythm disturbance.

Sinoatrial Node

Propranolol slows the spontaneous firing rate of nodal cells by decreasing the slope of phase 4 depolarization.

Atrium

Propranolol has local anesthetic properties and exerts actions similar to those of quinidine on the atrial membrane action potential. Membrane responsiveness and action potential amplitude are reduced, and excitability is decreased; conduction velocity is reduced. Because these concentrations are similar to those that produce β-blockade, it is impossible to determine whether the drug acts by specific receptor blockade or via a membrane-stabilizing effect.

A-V Node

The depressant effects of propranolol on the A-V node are more pronounced than are the direct depressant effects of quinidine. This is due to propranolol's dual actions of β-blockade and direct myocardial depression. Propranolol administration results in a decrease in A-V conduction velocity and an increase in the A-V nodal refractory period. Propranolol does not display the anticholinergic actions of quinidine and other antiarrhythmic agents.

His-Purkinje System and Ventricular Muscle

Propranolol decreases Purkinje fiber membrane responsiveness and reduces action potential amplitude. His-Purkinje tissue excitability also is reduced. These changes result in a decrease in His-Purkinje conduction velocity. However, these electrophysiological alterations are observed at propranolol concentrations in excess of those normally used in therapy. The most striking electrophysiological property of propranolol at usual therapeutic concentrations is a depression of catecholamine-stimulated automaticity.

TABLE 16.4 General Clinical Uses of Individual Antiarrhythmic Drugs

Drugs	Therapeutic Uses
Acebutolol	Ventricular arrhythmias, ventricular ectopy
Adenosine	Supraventricular tachycardia
	Wolff-Parkinson-White syndrome
Amiodarone	Hemodynamically unstable ventricular tachycardia
	Ventricular fibrillation
Bretylium	Ventricular arrhythmias after cardiac surgery
	Ventricular fibrillation
Diltiazem	Paroxysmal supraventricular tachycardia
	Atrial fibrillation
Disopyramide	Premature ventricular contractions
	Atrial arrhythmias, episodic ventricular tachycardia
Dofetilide	Atrial fibrillation and flutter
Esmolol	Atrial fibrillation and flutter, automatic tachycardias
Flecainide	Ventricular tachycardia
Ibutilide	Atrial fibrillation and flutter
Lidocaine	Post–myocardial infarct arrhythmias
	Ventricular tachycardia
Magnesium sulfate	Sustained ventricular arrhythmias
	Torsades de pointes of magnesium depletion or glycoside toxicity
Mexiletine	Premature ventricular contractions
	Ventricular tachycardia
Moricizine	Ventricular tachycardia
Phenytoin	Digitalis-induced cardiac arrhythmias
Procainamide	Atrial tachycardia, ventricular tachycardia
	Premature ventricular contractions
Propafenone	Atrial fibrillation, ventricular tachycardia
	Premature ventricular contractions
Propranolol	Supraventricular arrhythmias
	Postoperative ventricular arrhythmias
	Wolff-Parkinson-White syndrome
Quinidine	Atrial arrhythmias, ventricular tachycardia
Sotalol	Ventricular arrhythmias, ventricular fibrillation
Tocainide	Premature ventricular contractions
	Ventricular tachycardia
Verapamil	Paroxysmal supraventricular tachycardia
	Atrial fibrillation

Electrocardiographic Changes

Propranolol prolongs the PR interval but does not change the QRS interval. It may shorten the QT interval.

Hemodynamic Effects

The blockade of cardiac β-adrenoceptors prevents or reduces the usual positive inotropic and chronotropic actions of catecholamine administration on cardiac sympathetic nerve stimulation. Blockade of β-receptors prolongs systolic ejection periods at rest and during exercise. Both alterations tend to increase myocardial oxygen consumption. However, these alterations are offset by factors that tend to reduce oxygen consumption, such as decreased heart rate and decreased force of contraction. The decrease in oxygen demand produced by a decrease in heart rate and a decrease in force of contraction is usually greater than the increase in oxygen demand that results from increased heart size and increased ejection time. The net result is that oxygen demand is decreased.

Pharmacokinetics

The pharmacokinetic characteristics of propranolol:

Oral bioavailability	30–40%
Onset of action	1–2 hours
Peak response	1.0–1.5 hours
Duration of action	6–24 hours
Plasma half-life	3–5 hours
Primary route of metabolism	Hepatic
Primary route of excretion	Renal
Therapeutic serum concentration	0.02–1 µg /mL

Clinical Uses

Propranolol is indicated in the management of a variety of cardiac rhythm abnormalities that are totally or partially due to enhanced adrenergic stimulation. In selected cases of sinus tachycardia caused by anxiety, pheochromocytoma, or thyrotoxicosis, β-blockade will reduce the spontaneous heart rate.

Propranolol alone or in conjunction with digitalis can help control the ventricular rate in patients with atrial flutter or atrial fibrillation. Patients with supraventricular extrasystoles and intermittent paroxysms of atrial fibrillation may benefit from β-receptor blockade with propranolol.

The arrhythmias associated with halothane or cyclopropane anesthesia have been attributed to the interaction of the anesthetic with catecholamines, and they have been suppressed by IV administration of 1 to 3 mg propranolol. An increase in circulating catecholamines also has been observed in patients with acute myocardial infarction and has been correlated with the development of arrhythmias.

Clinically, tachyarrhythmias associated with digitalis excess (including supraventricular and ventricular extrasystoles) and ventricular tachycardia have been suppressed by propranolol. Although propranolol is highly effective in the treatment of digitalis-induced arrhythmias, phenytoin and lidocaine are preferred.

Long-term treatment with β-adrenoceptor blocking agents is clearly associated with an increased rate of

TABLE 16.5 Efficacy of β-Adrenoceptor Blocking Agents in the Control of Cardiac Rhythm Disorders

Rhythm Disorder	Efficacy of β-Adrenoceptor Blocking Agent
Supraventricular arrhythmias	
Sinus tachycardia	First treat the underlying cause, e.g., hyperpyrexia, hypovolemia. β-Adrenoceptor blockade is most effective in decreasing the heart rate by inhibiting SA response to enhanced adrenergic stimulation. Do not use as the initial drug in tachycardia associated with pheochromocytoma.
Atrial fibrillation	Sinus rhythm is unlikely to be restored. However, the effect of β-adrenoceptor blockade on the A-V node will decrease the ventricular response to the atrial tachyarrhythmia. Effect is enhanced by the simultaneous use of digoxin or verapamil.
Atrial flutter/tachycardia	β-Adrenoceptor blockers will reduce the ventricular rate by inhibition of transmission through the A-V node as a result of inhibition of adrenergic influences. May be useful for the prevention of recurrent episodes of tachyarrhythmia.
Ventricular arrhythmias	
Premature ventricular complexes	Effective in mitral valve prolapse, hypertrophic cardiomyopathy, digitalis-related ectopic activity, and ventricular complexes associated with exercise or induced by ischemia.
Ventricular tachycardia	Most effective against arrhythmias associated with digitalis toxicity and exercise, particularly if the latter is related to ischemia.
Ventricular fibrillation	Postmyocardial infarct patients show increased survival if treated with a β-adrenoceptor antagonist. The beneficial effect may be related to the decrease in heart rate and the antiischemic benefits of β-adrenoceptor blockade.

SA, sinoatrial.

survival in patients with ischemic heart disease who have recovered from an acute myocardial infarction. Propranolol is the drug of choice for treating patients with the congenital long QT syndrome.

Adverse Effects

The toxicity associated with propranolol is for the most part related to its primary pharmacological action, inhibition of the cardiac β-adrenoceptors. This topic is discussed in detail in Chapter 11. In addition, propranolol exerts direct cardiac depressant effects that become manifest when the drug is administered rapidly by the IV route. Glucagon immediately reverses all cardiac depressant effects of propranolol, and its use is associated with a minimum of side effects. The inotropic agents amrinone (*Inocor*) and milrinone (*Primacor*) provide alternative means of augmenting cardiac contractile function in the presence of β-adrenoceptor blockade (see Chapter 15). Propranolol may also stimulate bronchospasm in patients with asthma.

Since propranolol crosses the placenta and enters the fetal circulation, fetal cardiac responses to the stresses of labor and delivery will be blocked. Additionally, propranolol crosses the blood-brain barrier and is associated with mood changes and depression. School difficulties are commonly associated with its use in children. Propranolol may also cause hypoglycemia in infants.

Contraindications

Propranolol is contraindicated for patients with depressed myocardial function and may be contraindicated in the presence of digitalis toxicity because of the possibility of producing complete A-V block and ventricular asystole. Patients receiving anesthetic agents that tend to depress myocardial contractility (ether, halothane) should not receive propranolol. Propranolol should be used with extreme caution in patients with asthma.

Up-regulation of β-receptors follows long-term therapy, making abrupt withdrawal of β-blockers dangerous for patients with ischemic heart disease.

Acebutolol

Acebutolol (*Sectral*) is a cardioselective β₁-adrenoceptor blocking agent that also has some minor membrane stabilizing effects on the action potential.

Electrophysiological Actions

Acebutolol's effects on the atria, sinoatrial and AV nodes, His-Purkinje system, and ventricular muscle are similar to those of propranolol.

Hemodynamic Effects

Acebutolol reduces blood pressure in patients with essential hypertension primarily through its negative inotropic and chronotropic effects.

Pharmacokinetics

The pharmacokinetic characteristics of acebutolol:

Oral bioavailability	70%
Onset of action	1–3 hours

Peak response	3–8 hours
Duration of action	12–24 hours
Plasma half-life	3–4 hours
Primary route of metabolism	Hepatic
Primary route of excretion	Renal (30–40%); biliary/fecal (50–60%)
Therapeutic serum concentration	Not established

Clinical Uses

Acebutolol is effective in the management of the patient with essential hypertension, angina pectoris, and ventricular arrhythmias. Antiarrhythmic effects are observed with the patient both at rest and taking exercise.

Adverse Effects

Adverse effects include bradycardia, gastrointestinal upset, dizziness, and headache.

Contraindications

Acebutolol should not be administered in cardiogenic shock, uncontrolled heart failure, or severe bradycardia or to patients with known hypersensitivity to the drug.

Esmolol

Esmolol (*Brevibloc*) is a short-acting intravenously administered β_1-selective adrenoceptor blocking agent. It does not possess membrane-stabilizing activity or sympathomimetic activity.

Electrophysiological Actions

Esmolol's electrophysiological actions are similar to those of propranolol.

Hemodynamic Effects

Esmolol decreases arterial pressure, heart rate, ventricular contractility, and pulmonary vascular resistance.

Pharmacokinetics

The pharmacokinetic characteristics of esmolol:

Oral bioavailability	100%
Onset of action	15–30 minutes
Peak response	2–5 minutes
Duration of action	20–30 minutes
Plasma half-life	3.7 hours
Primary route of metabolism	Hepatic
Primary route of excretion	Renal
Therapeutic serum concentration	0.4–1.2 μg /mL

Clinical Uses

Esmolol is used in the treatment of supraventricular tachyarrhythmias for rapid control of ventricular rate and reduction of myocardial oxygen consumption. Discontinuation of administration is followed by a rapid reversal of its pharmacological effects because of esmolol's rapid hydrolysis by plasma esterases.

Adverse Effects and Contraindications

The most frequently reported adverse effects are hypotension, nausea, dizziness, headache, and dyspnea. As with many β-blocking drugs, esmolol is contraindicated in patients with overt heart failure and those in cardiogenic shock.

CLASS III

Bretylium

Bretylium (*Bretylol*) was introduced for the treatment of essential hypertension but subsequently was shown to suppress the ventricular fibrillation often associated with acute myocardial infarction.

Electrophysiological Actions

The net effects of bretylium on the electrical and mechanical properties of the heart are a composite of the direct actions of the drug on cardiac tissues and indirect actions mediated through the drug's effects on the sympathetic nervous system.

Sinoatrial Node

Bretylium administration produces an initial brief increase in sinus node automaticity that is probably the result of a drug-induced release of catecholamines from sympathetic nerve terminals. No change or a slight decrease in sinus heart rate is observed after the initial phase of catecholamine release.

Atria

At therapeutic concentrations, the only significant effect of bretylium is to prolong the action potential. This results in prolongation of the ERP of the atrial muscle.

A-V Node

Moderate doses increase conduction velocity and decrease the A-V nodal refractory period; this effect may result from the initial drug-induced catecholamine release. The net effect of bretylium on A-V transmission during chronic therapy is unknown.

His-Purkinje System and Ventricular Muscle

The most prominent electrophysiological action of bretylium is to raise the intensity of electrical current necessary to induce ventricular fibrillation. This action, which is more prominent with bretylium than with any other available antiarrhythmic agent, can be observed in both normal and ischemic hearts.

Hemodynamic Effects

A unique property of bretylium as an antiarrhythmic agent is its positive inotropic action. This effect, related to its actions on the sympathetic nervous system, includes an initial release of neuronal stores of norepinephrine followed shortly by a prolonged period of inhibition of direct or reflex-associated neuronal norepinephrine release. The onset of bretylium-induced hypotension is delayed 1 to 2 hours because the initial catecholamine release maintains arterial pressure before this time.

Pharmacokinetics

The pharmacokinetic characteristics of bretylium:

Oral bioavailability	Not applicable
Onset of action	5–10 mm
Peak response	6–9 hours (TM)
Duration of action	6–24 hours
Plasma half-life	6.9–8.1 hours
Primary route of metabolism	None
Primary route of excretion	Renal (unchanged)
Therapeutic serum concentration	0.5–2.5 µg /mL

Clinical Uses

Bretylium is not to be considered a first-line antiarrhythmic agent. However, because of its ability to prolong the refractory period of Purkinje fibers and to elevate the electrical threshold to ventricular fibrillation, *bretylium has been found useful in the treatment of life-threatening ventricular arrhythmias,* especially when conventional therapeutic agents, such as lidocaine or procainamide, prove to be ineffective. In addition, bretylium is known to facilitate the reversal of ventricular fibrillation by precordial electrical shock. Its use should be limited to no longer than 5 days.

Adverse Effects

The most important side effect associated with the use of bretylium is hypotension, a result of peripheral vasodilation caused by adrenergic neuronal blockade (a guanethidinelike action). Nausea, vomiting, and diarrhea have been reported with IV administration and can be minimized by slow infusion. Longer-term problems include swelling and tenderness of the parotid gland, particularly at mealtime.

Contraindications

The associated initial release of catecholamines may result in an excessive pressor response and stimulation of cardiac force and pacemaker activity. The resulting increase in myocardial oxygen consumption in a patient with ischemic heart disease may lead to ischemic pain (angina pectoris). Patients in a state of circulatory shock probably should not be administered bretylium because of its delayed sympatholytic action.

Amiodarone

Amiodarone (*Cordarone*) is an iodine-containing benzofuran derivative identified as a class III agent because it predominantly prolongs action potentials. Amiodarone also blocks sodium and calcium channels and is a noncompetitive β-receptor blocker. Amiodarone is effective for the treatment of most arrhythmias. Toxicity associated with amiodarone has led the U. S. Food and Drug Administration (FDA) to recommend that it be reserved for use in patients with life-threatening arrhythmias.

Electrophysiological Actions

The most notable electrophysiological effect of amiodarone after long-term administration is prolongation of repolarization and refractoriness in all cardiac tissues, an action that is characteristic of class III antiarrhythmic agents.

Sinoatrial Node

Amiodarone decreases the slope of phase 4 depolarization. The rate of spontaneous discharge of the sinoatrial node is increased by amiodarone as well as by its metabolite, desethylamiodarone. The depressant action of amiodarone on sinoatrial pacemaker function is, in addition to β-receptor blockade, related to an inhibition of the slow inward current carried by the calcium ion.

Amiodarone prolongs the action potential in atrial muscle and increases the absolute and effective refractory periods.

Amiodarone, like its major metabolite desethylamiodarone, increases A-V nodal conduction time and refractory period.

His-Purkinje System and Ventricular Muscle

The dominant effect on ventricular myocardium that has been chronically exposed to either amiodarone or desethylamiodarone is a prolongation in the action potential with an associated increase in the refractory period and a modest decrease in V_{max} as a function of stimulus frequency. Amiodarone inhibits the delayed outward potassium current, a finding consistent with the observation of a prolonged action potential. Both amiodarone and its metabolite significantly decrease the action potential duration and shorten the ERP in Purkinje fibers, at the same time prolonging action potential in ventricular muscle.

Electrocardiographic Changes

Amiodarone's predominant electrocardiographic changes include prolongation of the PR and QT intervals, development of U waves, and changes in T-wave contour.

Hemodynamic Effects

Amiodarone relaxes vascular smooth muscle; one of its most prominent effects is on the coronary circulation, reducing coronary vascular resistance and improving regional myocardial blood flow. In addition, its effects on the peripheral vascular bed lead to a decrease in left ventricular stroke work and myocardial oxygen consumption. Therefore, amiodarone improves the relationship between myocardial oxygen demand and oxygen supply. IV administration may be associated with profound hypotension requiring volume expansion therapy.

Pharmacokinetics

The pharmacokinetic characteristics of amiodarone are extremely complex:

Oral bioavailability	35–65%
Onset of action	2–3 days, up to 2–3 months
Peak response	3–7 hours after IV administration
Duration of action	Variable, weeks to months
Plasma half-life	2–10 days; 26–107 days with chronic administration
Primary route of metabolism	Hepatic, active metabolites
Primary route of excretion	Biliary
Therapeutic serum concentration	0.5–2 μg /mL

Clinical Uses

Amiodarone is regarded as one of the most efficacious antiarrhythmic agents because of its usefulness in the management of a variety of cardiac rhythm disorders with minimal tendency for induction of torsades de pointes tachyarrhythmia. Its use, however, is limited by the multiple and severe noncardiac side effects that it produces.

Amiodarone is available as an IV formulation as well as an oral preparation. IV amiodarone is indicated for initiating treatment and for prophylaxis of frequently recurring ventricular fibrillation and hemodynamically unstable ventricular tachycardia in patients refractory to other therapy. IV administration also can be used to treat patients with ventricular tachycardia or ventricular fibrillation for whom oral amiodarone is indicated, but who are unable to take oral medication.

Amiodarone may elicit life-threatening side effects in addition to presenting substantial management difficulties associated with its use. The oral formulation of amiodarone is indicated only for the treatment of life-threatening recurrent ventricular arrhythmias (e.g., recurrent ventricular fibrillation and/or recurrent hemodynamically unstable ventricular tachycardia) that have not responded to other potentially effective antiarrhythmic drugs or when alternative interventions could not be tolerated. Despite its efficacy as an antiarrhythmic agent, there is no evidence from clinical trials that the use of amiodarone favorably affects survival.

Initiation of treatment with amiodarone should be done in the hospital setting and only by physicians familiar with the management of patients with life-threatening arrhythmias; this is because of the life-threatening nature of the arrhythmias and the possibility of interactions with previous therapy and of exacerbation of the arrhythmia.

Amiodarone is effective in maintaining sinus rhythm in most patients with paroxysmal atrial fibrillation and in many patients with persistent atrial fibrillation. It is also effective in preventing recurrences of A-V nodal reentry and atrial tachyarrhythmias and in the prevention of reentrant rhythms and atrial fibrillation in patients with Wolff-Parkinson-White syndrome. Also, it is the most efficacious therapy for postoperative junctional ectopic tachycardia.

Adverse Effects

Amiodarone's most significant adverse effects include hepatitis, exacerbation of arrhythmias, worsening of congestive heart failure, thyroid dysfunction, and pulmonary fibrosis. Pulmonary fibrosis is frequently fatal and may not be reversed with discontinuation of the drug. Interestingly, despite significant prolongation of the QT interval, the risk of torsades de pointes is relatively low.

Patients with underlying sinus node dysfunction tend to have significant worsening of nodal function, frequently requiring pacemaker implantation. Corneal microdeposits develop in most adults receiving amiodarone. As many as 10% of patients complain of halos or blurred vision. The corneal microdeposits are reversible with stoppage of the drug.

Photosensitization occurs in 10% of patients. With continued treatment, the skin assumes a blue-gray coloration. The risk is increased in patients of fair complexion. The discoloration of the skin regresses slowly, if at all, after discontinuation of amiodarone.

Amiodarone inhibits the peripheral and possibly intrapituitary conversion of thyroxine (T_4) to triiodothyronine (T_3) by inhibiting 5'-deiodination. The serum concentration of T_4 is increased by a decrease in its clearance, and thyroid synthesis is increased by a reduced suppression of the pituitary thyrotropin T_3. The concentration of T_3 in the serum decreases, and reverse T_3 appears in increased amounts. Despite these changes, most patients appear to be maintained in an euthyroid state. Manifestations of both hypothyroidism and hyperthyroidism have been reported.

Tremors of the hands and sleep disturbances in the form of vivid dreams, nightmares, and insomnia have been reported in association with the use of amiodarone. Ataxia, staggering, and impaired walking have been noted. Peripheral sensory and motor neuropathy or severe proximal muscle weakness develops infrequently. Both neuropathic and myopathic changes are observed on biopsy. Neurological symptoms resolve or improve within several weeks of dosage reduction.

Contraindications

Amiodarone is contraindicated in patients with sick sinus syndrome and may cause severe bradycardia and second- and third-degree atrioventricular block. Amiodarone crosses the placenta and will affect the fetus, as evidenced by bradycardia and thyroid abnormalities. The drug is secreted in breast milk.

Drug Interactions

Amiodarone increases the hypoprothrombinemic response to warfarin (an oral anticoagulant) by reducing its metabolism. Patients receiving digoxin may undergo an increase in serum digoxin concentrations when amiodarone is added to the treatment regimen. Amiodarone interferes with hepatic and renal elimination of flecainide, phenytoin, and quinidine.

Sotalol

In addition to class III actions, sotalol (*Betapace*) possesses β-adrenoceptor blocking properties. The β-blocking effects are most evident at low doses, with action potential prolongation predominating at higher doses. The D-isomer of sotalol, which is devoid of β-blocking action, may increase mortality in post-infarcted patients.

Electrophysiological Actions
Sinoatrial Node and Atrium

Pacemaker activity in the sinoatrial node is decreased because of β-adrenoceptor blockade and a removal of sympathoadrenal influences on spontaneous diastolic depolarization. Sotalol increases the refractory period of atrial muscle.

A-V Node
Sotalol decreases conduction velocity and prolongs the ERP in the A-V node, an action held in common with other β$_1$-adrenoceptor blocking agents.

His-Purkinje System and Ventricular Muscle
The actions of sotalol on the delayed rectifier potassium current prolong the ERP in His-Purkinje tissue. As with other members of class III, the electrophysiological action of sotalol is characterized by prolongation of repolarization and an increase in the ERP of ventricular muscle.

Electrocardiographic Changes

Administration of sotalol is associated with dose- and concentration-dependent slowing of the heart rate and prolongation of the PR interval. The QRS duration is not affected with plasma concentrations within the therapeutic range. The corrected QT interval is prolonged as a result of the increase in the ERP of ventricular myocardium.

Hemodynamic Effects

The hemodynamic effects of sotalol are related to its β-adrenoceptor antagonist activity. Accordingly, decreases in resting heart rate and in exercise-induced tachycardia are seen in patients receiving sotalol. A modest reduction in systolic pressure and in cardiac output may occur. The reduction in cardiac output is a consequence of lowering the heart rate, since stroke volume is unaffected by sotalol treatment. In patients with normal ventricular function, cardiac output is maintained despite the decrease in heart rate because of the simultaneous increase in the stroke volume.

Pharmacokinetics

The pharmacokinetic characteristics of sotalol:

Oral bioavailability	50%o
Onset of action	0.5 hours
Peak response	1–2 hours
Duration of action	12–24 hours
Plasma half-life	4 hours
Primary route of metabolism	Hepatic (80%)
Primary route of excretion	Renal (20% unchanged); 40% metabolite
Therapeutic serum concentration	1–4 μg/mL

Clinical Uses

Sotalol possesses a broad spectrum of antiarrhythmic effects in ventricular and supraventricular arrhythmias. It has value in the management of patients with paroxys-

mal supraventricular arrhythmias, in terminating the reentrant arrhythmia in which the atrioventricular node serves as the reentrant pathway, and possibly in terminating supraventricular tachyarrhythmias associated with an accessory pathway.

Adverse Effects

Side effects of sotalol include those attributed to both β-adrenoceptor blockade and proarrhythmic effects. This arrhythmia is a serious threat, as it may lead to ventricular fibrillation. Adverse effects attributable to its β-blocker activity include fatigue, dyspnea, chest pain, headache, nausea, and vomiting.

Contraindications

The contraindications that apply to other β-adrenoceptor blocking agents also apply to sotalol. In addition, hypokalemia and drugs known to prolong the QT interval may be contraindicated, as they enhance the possibility of proarrhythmic events.

Drug Interactions

Drugs with inherent QT interval–prolonging activity (i.e., thiazide diuretics and terfenadine) may enhance the class III effects of sotalol.

Dofetilide

Dofetilide (*Tikosyn*) is a "pure" class III drug. It prolongs the cardiac action potential and the refractory period by selectively inhibiting the rapid component of the delayed rectifier potassium current (IKr).

Electrophysiological Actions

Dofetilide's mechanism of action involves blockade of the cardiac ion channel that carries the rapid component of the delayed rectifier potassium current, IKr. Dofetilide inhibits IKr with no significant effects on other repolarizing potassium currents (e.g., IKs, IK1) over a wide range of concentrations. At plasma concentrations within the therapeutic range, dofetilide has no effect on sodium channels or on either α_1- or β-adrenoceptors.

Dofetilide blocks IKr in all myocardial tissues. It blocks open channels, and its binding and release from the channels is voltage dependent. The effects of dofetilide are exaggerated when the extracellular potassium concentration is reduced, which is important, as many patients may be receiving diuretics concurrently. Conversely, hyperkalemia decreases the effects of dofetilide, which may limit its efficacy when local hyperkalemia occurs, such as during myocardial ischemia. Dofetilide demonstrates reverse use dependence, that is, less influence on the action potential at faster heart

rates. This is likely due to a greater influence of other repolarizing currents such as the slowly activating component of the delayed rectifier current (IKs).

Sinoatrial Node

Dofetilide induces a minor slowing of the spontaneous discharge rate of the sinoatrial node via a reduction in the slope of the pacemaker potential and hyperpolarization of the maximum diastolic potential.

Atrium

Dofetilide prolongs the plateau phase of the action potential, thereby lengthening the refractory period of the myocardium. The effects on atrial tissue appear to be more profound than those observed in the ventricle. The reason for this is unclear. There is no effect on the voltage-gated sodium channel and as such no effect on the conduction velocity.

A-V Node

There is no effect on conduction through the A-V node.

His-Purkinje System and Ventricular Muscle

Dofetilide increases the ERP of ventricular myocytes and Purkinje fibers. The ERP-prolonging effect on the ventricular tissue is somewhat less than that in atrial tissue.

Electrocardiographic Changes

There are no changes in the PR or QRS intervals, which reflects a lack of effect on the conduction velocity. The QT interval is prolonged as a result of an increase in both the effective and functional refractory periods in the His-Purkinje system and the ventricles. The increase in the QT interval is directly related to the dofetilide dose and plasma concentration.

Hemodynamic Effects

Dofetilide does not significantly alter the mean arterial blood pressure, cardiac output, cardiac index, stroke volume index, or systemic vascular resistance. There is a slight increase in the delta pressure/delta time (dP/dt) of ventricular myocytes.

Pharmacokinetics

The pharmacokinetic characteristics of dofetilide are summarized below. Although the absorption of dofetilide is delayed by ingestion of food, the total bioavailability is not affected. Dosing requires adjustment in patients with renal insufficiency.

Oral bioavailability	>90%
Onset of action	0.5 hour

Peak response	23 hours
Duration of action	8–10 hours
Plasma half-life	7–10 hours
Primary route of metabolism	Hepatic (CYP3A4)
Primary route of excretion	Renal (80% unchanged; 20% metabolites)
Therapeutic serum concentration	Not established

Clinical Uses

Dofetilide is approved for the treatment of atrial fibrillation and atrial flutter. Because of the lack of significant hemodynamic effects, dofetilide may be useful in patients with CHF who are in need of therapy for supraventricular tachyarrhythmias. Dofetilide is not indicated for use in the setting of ventricular arrhythmias.

Adverse Effects

The incidence of noncardiac adverse events is not different from that of placebo in controlled clinical trials. The principal cardiac adverse effect is the risk of torsades de pointes due to QT prolongation. The risk is approximately 3%, and most cases are observed in the first 3 days of therapy. As such, initiation of therapy should be performed with the patient in hospital.

Contraindications

Contraindications include baseline prolongation of the QT interval, use of other QT-prolonging drugs; history of torsades de pointes; a creatinine clearance of less than 20 mL/minute; simultaneous use of verapamil, cimetidine, or ketoconazole; uncorrected hypokalemia or hypomagnesemia; and pregnancy or breast-feeding.

Drug Interactions

Verapamil increases serum dofetilide levels, as do drugs that inhibit cationic renal secretion, such as ketoconazole and cimetidine, raise serum levels.

Ibutilide Fumarate

Ibutilide (*Corvert*) is a structural analog of sotalol and produces cardiac electrophysiological effects similar to those of the antiarrhythmic agents in class III.

Electrophysiological Actions

Ibutilide prolongs action potential in isolated adult cardiac myocytes and increases both atrial and ventricular refractoriness *in vivo.* An additional action is blockade of outward potassium currents. Thus, ibutilide acts by blocking the rapid component of the delayed rectifier current (IKr) as well as by activation of a slow inward current carried predominantly by sodium.

Sinoatrial Node
Although there is evidence that ibutilide causes a modest slowing of the sinus rate, there is no significant change in heart rate.

Atrium
Ibutilide causes an increase in the atrial refractory period, an effect seen at rapid heart rates.

A-V Node
Ibutilide slows conduction through the A-V node; however, there is no change in the PR interval on ECG.

His-Purkinje System and Ventricular Muscle
Ibutilide increases the ERP of ventricular myocytes and Purkinje fibers but has no clinically significant effect on QRS duration.

Electrocardiographic Changes

There are no changes in the PR or QRS intervals, which reflects a lack of effect on the conduction velocity. Although there is no relationship between the plasma concentration of ibutilide and its antiarrhythmic effect, there is a dose-related prolongation of the QT interval. The maximum effect on the QT interval is a function of both the dose of ibutilide and the rate of infusion.

Hemodynamic Effects

Ibutilide has no significant effects on cardiac output, mean pulmonary arterial pressure, or pulmonary capillary wedge pressure in patients with or without compromised ventricular function.

Pharmacokinetics

The pharmacokinetic characteristics of ibutilide are summarized next. The pharmacokinetics are highly variable between patients. Because of extensive first-pass metabolism, ibutilide is not suitable for oral administration.

Oral bioavailability	>90%
Onset of action	Minutes
Peak response	Minutes
Plasma half-life	3–4 hours (range 2–12 hours)
Primary route of metabolism	Hepatic
Primary route of excretion	Renal
Therapeutic serum concentration	Not applicable

Clinical Uses

Ibutilide is approved for the chemical cardioversion of recent-onset atrial fibrillation and atrial flutter. Ibutilide appears to be more effective in terminating atrial flutter than atrial fibrillation. It can also lower the defibrillation threshold for atrial fibrillation resistant to chemical cardioversion.

Adverse Effects

The major adverse effect associated with the use of ibutilide is the risk of torsades de pointes due to QT prolongation. Other reported adverse cardiovascular events (all <2%) include hypotension and hypertension, bradycardia and tachycardia, and varying degrees of A-V block. The incidence of noncardiac adverse events with the exception of nausea does not differ from that of placebo.

Contraindications

Contraindications to the use of ibutilide include baseline prolongation of the QT interval, use of other QT-prolonging drugs, history of torsades de pointes, hypersensitivity to ibutilide, uncorrected hypokalemia or hypomagnesemia, and pregnancy or breast-feeding.

Drug Interactions

Ibutilide has significant drug interactions.

CLASS IV

Verapamil

Verapamil (*Isoptin, Covera*), in addition to its use as an antiarrhythmic agent, has been employed extensively in the management of variant (Prinzmetal's) angina and effort-induced angina pectoris (see Chapters 17 and 19). It selectively inhibits the voltage-gated calcium channel that is vital for action potential genesis in slow-response myocytes, such as those found in the sinoatrial and A-V nodes.

Electrophysiological Actions
Sinoatrial Node

Spontaneous phase 4 depolarization, a characteristic of normal sinoatrial nodal cells, relies on progressive inhibition of an outward potassium current and an increase in a slow inward current that is carried by Na^+ and Ca^{++} ions. Verapamil decreases the rate of rise and slope of the slow diastolic depolarization, the maximal diastolic potential, and the membrane potential at the peak of depolarization in the sinoatrial node.

Atrium

Verapamil fails to exert any significant electrophysiological effects on atrial muscle.

A-V Node

Verapamil impairs conduction through the A-V node and prolongs the A-V nodal refractory period at plasma concentrations that show no effect on the His-Purkinje system.

His-Purkinje System and Ventricular Muscle

The most important electrocardiographic change produced by verapamil is prolongation of the PR interval, a response consistent with the known effects of the drug on A-V nodal transmission. Verapamil has no effect on intraatrial and intraventricular conduction. The predominant electrophysiological effect is on A-V conduction proximal to the His bundle.

Hemodynamic Effects

Usual IV doses of verapamil are not associated with marked alterations in arterial blood pressure, peripheral vascular resistance, heart rate, left ventricular end-diastolic pressure, or contractility.

Pharmacokinetics

The pharmacokinetic characteristics of verapamil:

Oral bioavailability	20–35%
Onset of action	1–2 hours
Peak response	1–2 hours
Duration of action	8–10 hours
Plasma half-life	2.8–7.4 hours
Primary route of metabolism	Hepatic; active metabolite
Primary route of excretion	Renal (30% unchanged)
Therapeutic serum concentration	0.125–0.4 μg /mL

Clinical Uses

Verapamil is useful for slowing the ventricular response to atrial tachyarrhythmias, such as atrial flutter and fibrillation. Verapamil is also effective in arrhythmias supported by enhanced automaticity, such as ectopic atrial tachycardia and idiopathic left ventricular tachycardia.

Adverse Effects

Orally administered verapamil is well tolerated by most patients. Most complaints are of constipation and gastric discomfort. Other complaints include vertigo, headache, nervousness, and pruritus.

Contraindications

Verapamil must be used with extreme caution or not at all in patients who are receiving β-adrenoceptor blocking agents. Normally, the negative chronotropic effect of verapamil will in part be overcome by an increase in reflex sympathetic tone. The latter is be prevented by simultaneous administration of a β-adrenoceptor blocking agent, which exaggerates the depressant effects of verapamil on heart rate, A-V node conduction, and myocardial contractility. The use of verapamil in children less than 1 year of age is controversial.

Diltiazem

The antiarrhythmic actions and uses of diltiazem (*Cardizem;* see Chapter 19) are similar to those of verapamil. *Diltiazem is effective in controlling the ventricular rate in patients with atrial flutter or atrial fibrillation.* The pharmacology of diltiazem is discussed in detail in Chapter 19.

MISCELLANEOUS ANTIARRHYTHMIC AGENTS

Digitalis Glycosides and Vagomimetic Drugs

Digitalis glycosides, especially digoxin (*Lanoxin*), because of their positive inotropic effects, are widely used for treating patients with congestive heart failure. They also continue to be used for the management of patients with supraventricular arrhythmias. Since the digitalis glycosides are discussed elsewhere (see Chapter 15), a full discussion of their mechanism of action is not provided here.

Digitalis glycosides enhance the inotropic state by increasing the intracellular calcium concentration. Intracellular calcium overload is also the mechanism for proarrhythmia associated with digitalis intoxication. The direct effect of digitalis on the electrophysiology of the myocytes is to increase the slope of phase 4 depolarization, an effect that enhances automaticity.

The principal antiarrhythmic effect is achieved via prominent vagotonic actions. The vagotonic influence leads to inhibition of Ca^{++} currents in the A-V node and activation of acetylcholine-sensitive potassium channels in the atrium (these channels are not present in the ventricle). This results in a slowing of conduction through the A-V node, a hyperpolarization of the resting membrane potential, and a shortening of the refractory period in atrial tissue. The principal antiarrhythmic actions are associated with the effects on the A-V node. Digitalis can therefore be used on reentrant arrhythmias that use the A-V node as one limb of the circuit and for limiting A-V conduction during rapid atrial arrhythmias, such as in atrial fibrillation.

Digitalis glycosides have theoretical advantages over other medications that limit conduction through the A-V-node, such as β-blockers and Ca^{++} channel blockers, by providing a positive rather than negative inotropic effect on the ventricles. The effects on the A-V node are limited, however, in states of heightened sympathetic tone, such as during advanced heart failure.

Adenosine

Adenosine (*Adenocard*) is an endogenous nucleoside that is a product of the metabolism of adenosine triphosphate. It is used for the rapid termination of supraventricular arrhythmias following rapid bolus dosing.

Electrophysiological Actions

Adenosine receptors are found on myocytes in the atria and sinoatrial and A-V nodes. Stimulation of these receptors acts via a G-protein signaling cascade to open an acetylcholine-sensitive outward potassium current. This leads to hyperpolarization of the resting membrane potential, a decrease in the slope of phase 4 spontaneous depolarization, and shortening of the action potential duration.

The effects on the A-V node may result in a conduction block and the termination of tachycardias that use the A-V node as a limb of a reentrant circuit. Adenosine does not affect the action potential of ventricular myocytes because the adenosine-stimulated potassium channel is absent in ventricular myocardium.

Electrocardiographic Changes

The most profound effect of adenosine is the induction of an A-V block within 10 to 20 seconds of administration. Mild sinus slowing may be observed initially followed by sinus tachycardia. There is no effect on the QRS duration or QT interval. Rarely, an adenosine bolus injection is accompanied by atrial fibrillation or ventricular tachyarrhythmias.

Hemodynamic Effects

The administration of a bolus dose of adenosine is associated with a biphasic pressor response. There is an initial brief increase in blood pressure followed by vasodilation and secondary tachycardia.

Pharmacokinetics

The pharmacokinetic characteristics of adenosine:

Oral bioavailability	Not measured
Onset of action	10 seconds (IV)
Peak response	Not measured
Duration of action	10–20 seconds
Plasma half-life	<10 seconds
Primary route of metabolism	Red blood cells
Primary route of excretion	Renal; inactive metabolites
Therapeutic serum concentration	Not applicable

Clinical Uses

Adenosine is approved for the acute management and termination of supraventricular tachyarrhythmias, in-

cluding A-V nodal reentrant tachycardia and A-V recip-rocating tachycardia. Adenosine may be helpful in the diagnosis of atrial flutter.

Adverse Effects

Adverse reactions to the administration of adenosine are fairly common; however, the short half-life of the drug limits the duration of such events. The most common adverse effects are flushing, chest pain, and dyspnea. Adenosine may induce profound bronchospasm in patients with known reactive airway disease. The mechanism for bronchospasm is unclear, and the effect may last for up to 30 minutes despite the short half-life of the drug.

Contraindications

Patients with second- or third-degree A-V block should not receive adenosine. As indicated previously, the use of adenosine in asthmatic patients may exacerbate the asthmatic symptoms.

Drug Interactions

Metabolism of adenosine is slowed by dipyridamole, indicating that in patients stabilized on dipyridamole the therapeutically effective dose of adenosine may have to be increased. Methylxanthines antagonize the effects of adenosine via blockade of the adenosine receptors.

Magnesium Sulfate

Magnesium sulfate may be effective in terminating refractory ventricular tachyarrhythmias, particularly polymorphic ventricular tachycardia. Digitalis-induced arrhythmias are more likely in the presence of magnesium deficiency. Magnesium sulfate can be administered orally, intramuscularly, or, preferably, intravenously,

when a rapid response is intended. The loss of deep tendon reflexes is a sign of overdose.

Drug–Device Interactions

The first implantable cardioverter–defibrillator (ICD) was placed in 1982. Since that time, their use has expanded exponentially. Several large clinical trials have demonstrated the superiority of ICDs compared with pharmacological therapy for the secondary prevention of arrhythmic death and possibly as primary therapy for patients at risk for ventricular arrhythmias.

Combination therapy employing both antiarrhythmic drugs and ICDs is becoming more common. While the antiarrhythmic drugs have multiple positive effects on the overall therapy, they may alter the frequency of ICD discharge and the ability of the device to detect ventricular tachycardia. A serious concern is the potential for a given drug to increase the defibrillation threshold, thereby rendering the device ineffective.

In general, drugs that block the sodium channel and shorten the action potential tend to increase the defibrillation threshold. Drugs that prolong repolarization also tend to decrease this threshold. These changes have obvious important ramifications for patients with ICDs.

Effects of antiarrhythmic drugs on defibrillation thresholds:

No change	Increase	Decrease
Quinidine	Amiodarone	Sotalol
Procainamide	Flecainide	Dofetilide
Disopyramide	Lidocaine	
Digitalis	Propafenone	
β-blockers	Mexiletine	

Study QUESTIONS

1. A 45-year-old woman has had recurrent episodes of atrial fibrillation. She is receiving phenytoin and quinidine to control the atrial fibrillation. She is also taking a low dose of diazepam for insomnia and estrogen replacement therapy. You learn today that she has been receiving ciprofloxacin for a urinary track infection. The reason for her appointment today is that she has been having ringing in the ears, headache, nausea, and blurred vision. She tells you that she is also having trouble hearing the television. You suspect drug toxicity. The most likely agent is
    (A) Ciprofloxacin
    (B) Estrogen
    (C) Phenytoin
    (D) Diazepam
    (E) Quinidine

2. You are asked to treat a 55-year-old patient for continuing ventricular arrhythmias. The patient is receiving timolol drops for glaucoma, daily insulin injections for diabetes mellitus, and an ACE inhibitor for hypertension. You decide to use phenytoin instead of procainamide because of what pharmacological effect of procainamide?
    (A) The local anesthetic effect of procainamide would potentiate diabetes.
    (B) The anticholinergic effect of procainamide would aggravate glaucoma.

(C) The hypertensive effects of procainamide would aggravate the hypertension.

(D) The local anesthetic effect of procainamide would aggravate the hypertension.

(E) The cholinergic effects of procainamide would aggravate the diabetes.

3. Exercise-induced ventricular tachycardia in persons without overt cardiac disease is an example of delayed after-depolarizations and is characterized by an increase in intracellular ionized calcium. This type of arrhythmia is known to often respond well to which of the following combinations?

(A) β-Blocker and ACE inhibitor

(B) Calcium channel antagonist and ACE inhibitor

(C) α-Blocker and ACE inhibitor

(D) β-Blocker and calcium channel antagonist

(E) α-Blocker and calcium channel antagonist

4. Antiarrhythmic drugs are classified in four main groups based on their predominant mechanism of action. Antiarrhythmic agents in which class suppress abnormal automaticity and permit the sinoatrial node to again assume the role of the dominant pacemaker?

(A) Class I

(B) Class II

(C) Class III

(D) Class IV

5. Although most antiarrhythmic drugs (and indeed most drugs) are chemically synthesized, some compounds that occur endogenously in humans are useful. Indicate which of the following agents occurs endogenously and is a useful antiarrhythmic agent.

(A) Phenytoin

(B) Digoxin

(C) Adenosine

(D) Quinine

(E) Lidocaine

ANSWERS

1. **E.** Quinidine. These are the classic signs of cinchonism and are adverse effects of quinidine and quinine, constituents of the cinchona tree. Some of these effects could be seen as toxic effects of phenytoin. However, auditory acuity is associated with cinchonism and not with phenytoin toxicity. Nausea but not the other effects could be associated with ciprofloxacin. Excessive drowsiness would be expected if diazepam were involved. These effects would not be expected with the estrogen replacement therapy.

2. **B.** Anticholinergic agents, such as procainamide and disopyramide, are relatively contraindicated in patients with glaucoma. Procainamide is hypotensive rather than hypertensive. The local anesthetic activity of procainamide would have no adverse interaction with the diabetes mellitus.

3. **B.** Each of these approaches would reduce the tissue calcium concentration and prevent arrhythmias. Agents with α-blocking capacity would have no effect on calcium. Agents with ACE inhibitory activity would likewise have no effect on calcium.

4. **A.** Class I agents suppress both normal Purkinje fiber and His bundle automaticity in addition to abnormal automaticity resulting from myocardial damage. Class II drugs block β-adrenoceptors; class III drugs prolong the membrane action potential by delaying repolarization; and class IV drugs block the slow inward movement of calcium ions.

5. **C.** Adenosine is a product of the metabolism of adenosine triphosphate. Phenytoin and lidocaine are totally synthetic, while digoxin occurs naturally in plants and quinine occurs in the cinchona tree.

SUPPLEMENTAL READING

Carmeliet E and Mubagwa K. Antiarrhythmic drugs and cardiac ion channels: mechanisms of action. Prog Biophys Molec Biol 1998;70:1–72.

Cavero I et al. Drugs that prolong QT interval as an unwanted effect: Assessing their likelihood of inducing hazardous cardiac dysrhythmias. Expert Opinion Pharmacotherapy 2000;1:947–973.

Hohnloser SH. Proarrhythmia with class III antiarrhythmic drugs: Types, risks, and management. Am J Cardiol 1997;80(8A):82G–89G.

Huikuri HV, Castellanos A, and Myerburg RJ. Sudden death due to cardiac arrhythmias. N Engl J Med 2001;345:1473–1482.

Link MS et al. Antiarrhythmic drug therapy for ventricular arrhythmias: Current perspectives. J Cardiovasc Electrophys 1996;7:653–670.

Nattel S and Singh BN. Evolution, mechanisms, and classification of antiarrhythmic drugs: Focus on class III actions. Am J Cardiol 1999;84(9A):11R–19R.

Reiffel JA. Drug choices in the treatment of atrial fibrillation. Am J Cardiol 2000;85(10A):12D–19D.

Roden DM and George AL Jr. The cardiac ion channels: Relevance to management of arrhythmias. Annu Rev Med 1996;47:135–148.

Singh BN and Sarma JS. What niche will newer class III antiarrhythmic drugs occupy? Curr Cardiol Rep 2001;3(4):314–323.

CASE Study   Long QT Syndrome

A previously healthy 14-year-old athletic girl complained to her physician of a 6-day history of cough, with 2 days of fever, headache, and mild dyspnea. Several of her schoolmates had similar symptoms and were treated with antibiotics. Her physical examination revealed soft crackles at the bases of her lungs bilaterally. A chest radiograph demonstrated mild interstitial haziness at the bases. A diagnosis of community-acquired pneumonia was made, and she was given a prescription for 10 days of erythromycin. On the second day of therapy while at home, she suddenly lost consciousness while preparing breakfast and developed convulsive seizures on the floor. The emergency medical team was called and found her unresponsive. No pulse was detectable and the initial heart rhythm is shown below. Cardiopulmonary resuscitation was initiated and then DC cardioversion was performed with a return to sinus rhythm. Lidocaine was administered and she was transported to the local hospital. Her presenting ECG is shown below. What is her diagnosis?

ANSWER: Long QT syndrome. LQTS is caused by an abnormality in the function of specific ion channels responsible for myocardial repolarization. This may result from congenital mutations in the DNA encoding the ion channels (inherited form) or may be acquired from pharmacological therapy or other illness (increased intracerebral pressure, for example). In this patient's case, an abnormally long heart rate corrected QT interval was present on her ECG, diagnostic of a cardiac repolarization abnormality. After stopping the erythromycin, she was found to have an underlying long QT interval that was exacerbated by the erythromycin. A detailed family history confirmed the diagnosis when it was revealed that her mother had fainted on several occasions, and her first cousin (maternal) drowned while swimming in a lake 3 summers previously. Her physicians began β-blocker therapy and recommended placing an implantable cardioverter–defibrillator. Several medications prolong cardiac repolarization. The alteration in repolarization normally results from blockade of the rapid component of the delayed rectifier potassium current. In susceptible patients, this may lead to a profound prolongation of the QT interval and place them at risk

for developing polymorphic ventricular tachycardia (torsades de pointe), which may degenerate into ventricular fibrillation and death. In this patient's case, a thorough investigation of all her relatives should be performed to search for family members with abnormal ECGs. In addition to the β-blocker and ICD therapy that was instituted, the patient was given a list of drugs to avoid because of their known QT-prolonging effects. A resource for patients with LQTS including a comprehensive list of QT interval prolonging drugs can be found on the internet at www.SADS.org.

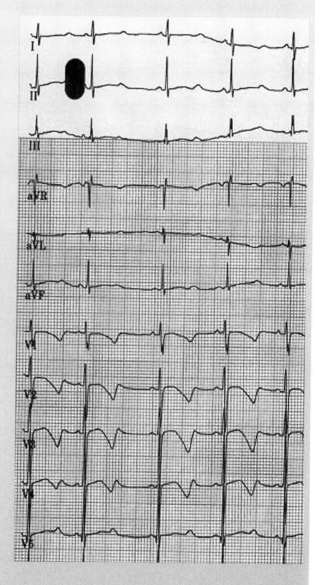

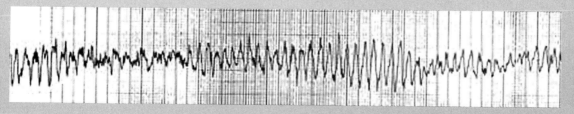

17 Antianginal Drugs

Garrett J. Gross

DRUG LIST

Angina pectoris is a clinical manifestation that results from coronary atherosclerotic heart disease. An acute anginal attack (secondary angina) is thought to occur because of an imbalance between myocardial oxygen supply and demand owing to the inability of coronary blood flow to increase in proportion to increases in myocardial oxygen requirements. This is generally the result of severe coronary artery atherosclerosis. Angina pectoris (variant, primary angina) may also occur as a result of vasospasm of large epicardial coronary vessels or one of their major branches. In addition, angina in certain patients may result from a combination of coronary vasoconstriction, platelet aggregation, plaque rupture, and an increase in myocardial oxygen demand (crescendo or unstable angina).

Antianginal drugs may relieve attacks of acute myocardial ischemia by increasing myocardial oxygen supply or by decreasing myocardial oxygen demand or both. Three groups of pharmacological agents have been shown to be effective in reducing the frequency, severity, or both of primary or secondary angina. These agents include the nitrates, β-adrenoceptor antagonists, and calcium entry blockers. To understand the beneficial actions of these agents, it is important to be familiar with the major factors regulating the balance between myocardial oxygen supply and demand. These factors are summarized in Table 17.1.

THE THERAPEUTIC OBJECTIVES IN THE USE OF ANTIANGINAL DRUGS

The major therapeutic objectives in the treatment of angina are aimed at terminating or preventing an acute attack and increasing the patient's exercise capacity. These objectives can be achieved by reducing overall myocardial oxygen demand or by increasing oxygen supply to ischemic areas. A decrease in myocardial oxygen demand can be attained through use of the organic nitrates, calcium entry blockers, and β-adrenoceptor blocking agents. Increases in myocardial oxygen supply are more difficult to achieve, especially when coronary blood vessels are partially or totally obstructed. However, redistribution of blood flow to the subendocardium of

TABLE 17.1	Major Determinants of Myocardial Oxygen Supply and Demand

Oxygen Supply	Oxygen Demand
Coronary blood flow	Wall tension
Aortic diastolic pressure	Ventricular volume
Endocardial–epicardial flow	Radius or heart size
Coronary collateral blood flow	Systolic pressure (afterload)
Large coronary artery diameter	Diastolic pressure (preload)
	Heart rate
	Contractility

ischemic areas has been documented in experimental animals following nifedipine (*Adalat, Procardia*), diltiazem (*Cardizem*),verapamil (*Calan*), amlodipine (*Norvasc*), nitroglycerin (*Nitrostat, Tridil, Nitro-Dur*), or propranolol (*Inderal*) administration. Increases in collateral flow to ischemic areas also have been observed in experimental animals and humans after treatment with certain calcium entry blockers and organic nitrates.

When coronary vasospasm occurs, the balance between oxygen supply and demand can be restored by relieving the spasm, thereby restoring normal coronary blood flow. Acute vasospasm has been successfully aborted through the use of nitroglycerin. In contrast, calcium entry blockers and long-acting nitrates have proved effective in the chronic therapy of coronary vasospasm.

SPECIFIC ANTIANGINAL DRUGS

Organic Nitrates

Organic nitrates have been used in the therapy of angina pectoris routinely for more than 140 years, and their use is increasingly favored in a variety of other cardiac conditions, such as decompensated congestive heart failure and acute myocardial infarction. The prototype of these agents is nitroglycerin. Other common organic nitrates are isosorbide mononitrate (*Ismo*), isosorbide dinitrate (*Isordil, Sorbitrate*) and pentaerythritol tetranitrate (*Peritrate*). With the exception of nitroglycerin, which is a liquid having a high vapor pressure, these compounds are solid at room temperature. All organic nitrates are very lipid soluble.

Mechanism of Vasodilator Action

The mechanism of action of nitroglycerin and other organic nitrates is thought to involve an interaction with nitrate receptors that are present in vascular smooth muscle. Intact vascular endothelium is not necessary for

the vasodilator action of the nitrates to be produced. The nitrate receptor possesses sulfhydryl groups, which reduce nitrate to inorganic nitrite and nitric oxide (NO). The formation of nitrosothiols, and possibly free NO, has been proposed to stimulate intracellular soluble guanylate cyclase, which leads to an increase in intracellular cyclic guanosine monophosphate (GMP) formation (Fig. 17.1). The increase in GMP results in vascular smooth muscle relaxation, possibly through inhibition of calcium entry via L-type calcium channels, decreased calcium release from the sarcoplasmic reticulum, or via an increase in calcium extrusion via a sarcolemmal Ca^{++}-adenosine triphosphatase (ATPase).

Absorption, Metabolism, and Excretion

Nitroglycerin is a lipid-soluble substance that is rapidly absorbed across the sublingual or buccal mucosa. Its onset of action occurs within 2 to 5 minutes, with maximal effects observed at 3 to 10 minutes. Little residual activity remains 20 to 30 minutes after sublingual administration. The plasma half-life of nitroglycerin, given

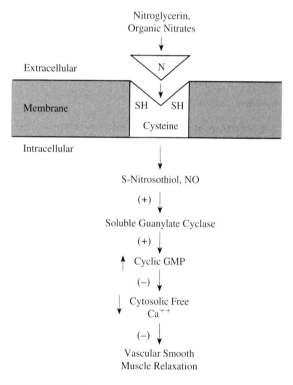

FIGURE 17.1

Proposed mechanism by which nitroglycerin and the organic nitrates produce relaxation in vascular smooth muscle. Nitrates induce endothelial cells to release NO or a nitrosothiol (endothelium-derived releasing factor, or EDRF). EDRF activates the enzyme guanylate cyclase, which causes the generation of cyclic guanosine monophosphate (GMP), producing a decrease in cytosolic free calcium. The end result is vascular smooth muscle relaxation. SH, sulfhydryl.

sublingually or by spray, is estimated to be 1 to 3 minutes. Isosorbide dinitrate and pentaerythritol tetranitrate also can be administered sublingually or buccally. These compounds have a slower onset and slightly longer duration of action than sublingually or buccally administered nitroglycerin.

Nitroglycerin and other organic nitrate esters undergo first-pass metabolism and are rapidly metabolized in the liver by the enzyme glutathione organic nitrate reductase. Although the metabolites of nitroglycerin are virtually inactive as vasodilators, two metabolites of isosorbide dinitrate, isosorbide 2-mononitrate and isosorbide 5-mononitrate, do retain some vasodilator and antianginal activity. Isosorbide mononitrate can be administered orally and does not undergo any first-pass metabolism. The latter esters and their metabolites are water soluble and are readily excreted by the kidney.

Pharmacological Actions

There is little doubt concerning the effectiveness of nitroglycerin in the treatment of angina pectoris. However, the exact mechanism by which the drug acts to reduce myocardial ischemia is still controversial (Fig. 17.2). Although nitroglycerin dilates both peripheral capacitance and resistance vessels, the effect on the venous capacitance system predominates. Dilation of the capacitance vessels leads to pooling of blood in the veins and to diminished venous return to the heart (decreased preload). This reduces ventricular diastolic volume and pressure and shifts blood from the central to the peripheral compartments of the cardiovascular system. These effects of nitroglycerin and other organic nitrates are similar to those of mild phlebotomy, which has been shown clinically to relieve acute anginal attacks by decreasing circulating blood volume.

According to Laplace's law, a reduction in ventricular pressure and heart size results in a decrease in the myocardial wall tension that is required to develop a given intraventricular pressure and therefore decreases oxygen requirement. Since blood flow to the subendocardium occurs primarily in diastole, the reduction in left ventricular end diastolic pressure induced by nitroglycerin reduces extravascular compression around the subendocardial vessels and favors redistribution of

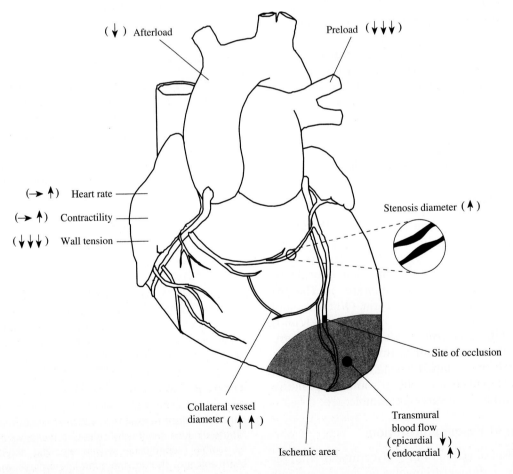

FIGURE 17.2
Major actions of the nitrates on the ischemic heart and peripheral circulation. ↓, decrease; ↑, increase; →, unchanged; ↑↓, variable effect.

coronary blood flow to this area. This effect of nitroglycerin on the distribution of coronary flow is important because the subendocardium is particularly vulnerable to ischemia during acute anginal attacks.

At higher concentrations, nitroglycerin also relaxes arteriolar smooth muscle, which leads to a decrease in both peripheral vascular resistance and aortic impedance to left ventricular ejection (decreased afterload). The decreased resistance to ventricular ejection may also reduce myocardial wall tension and oxygen requirements.

Thus, nitroglycerin relieves the symptoms of angina by restoring the balance between myocardial oxygen supply and demand. Oxygen demand is lowered as a consequence of the reduction in cardiac preload and afterload, and this results in a decrease in myocardial wall tension. Oxygen supply to the subendocardium of ischemic areas is increased because extravascular compression around the subendocardial vessels is reduced. In addition, nitroglycerin may increase blood flow to ischemic areas by its direct vasodilator effect on eccentric epicardial coronary artery stenoses and collateral blood vessels and by its action to inhibit platelet aggregation. Other organic nitrates are thought to exert the same beneficial actions as nitroglycerin.

Nitrate-induced Late Preconditioning

Recent findings suggest a potential new action of nitrates in the treatment of patients with ischemic heart disease. Administration of intravenous (IV) or transdermal nitroglycerin to conscious rabbits exerts a protective effect against myocardial infarction that persists for 72 hours; this effect has been termed late preconditioning. The magnitude of this effect was also found to persist in animals that displayed tolerance to the vascular effects of nitroglycerin. Although this effect of nitroglycerin has not been demonstrated unequivocally in patients receiving long-term nitrate therapy, these results are provocative and may support new uses of nitrates in patients or benefits that have until now remained unrecognized.

Clinical Uses

Sublingual or buccal nitroglycerin is used either to terminate an acute attack of angina or for short-term prevention of angina. Nitroglycerin is also the mainstay of therapy for relieving acute coronary vasospasm because of its rapid onset of action. When taken at the onset of chest pain, the effects of nitroglycerin appear within 2 to 5 minutes; however, the true duration of action is difficult to establish in patients with secondary angina, since the onset of pain causes patients to reduce their physical activity, and this alone can ameliorate the symptoms. Isosorbide dinitrate and pentaerythritol tetranitrate also can be taken sublingually, shortly before antici-

pated physical or emotional stress, to prevent anginal attacks.

Nitroglycerin ointment applied to the skin acts within 15 minutes and may produce its effects for 2 to 6 hours. Sustained-release transdermal nitroglycerin has been shown to deliver an antianginal effect for 2 to 4 hours following small doses and up to 24 hours after larger doses.

Orally administered long-acting nitrates, including nitroglycerin and various nitrate esters, nitroglycerin ointment, and transdermal nitroglycerin, were developed with the goal of providing a nitrate preparation that would have prolonged pharmacological activity for prophylactic therapy of angina pectoris. Considerable controversy surrounds the therapeutic use of the orally active agents because of their extensive first-pass metabolism, and many clinicians consider them to be ineffective. More recently, however, numerous clinical investigations have demonstrated the efficacy of transdermal nitroglycerin, although tolerance can be a problem with prolonged transdermal exposure to nitroglycerin. The drugs and dosage forms of organic nitrates available for therapeutic use, their usual dose, onset of action, and duration of action are summarized in Table 17.2.

Tolerance and Dependence

Repeated and frequent exposure to organic nitrates is accompanied by the development of tissue tolerance to the drug's vasodilating effects. When nitroglycerin formulations (e.g., transdermal patches, sustained-release oral dosing, or ointments) that produce sustained plasma and tissue levels are used, tolerance may occur within 24 hours. The mechanism underlying the phenomenon of nitrate tolerance is not as yet completely understood but may be related to a nitrate-induced oxidation of sulfhydryl groups via the formation of free radicals, a decrease in the sensitivity of vascular smooth muscle soluble guanylate cyclase, or activation of the renin–angiotensin system.

To help avoid nitrate tolerance, clinicians should employ the smallest effective dose and administer the compound infrequently. A daily nitrate-free period is also recommended, particularly with use of the transdermal patches or ointment. A better understanding of the pharmacokinetic profile achieved with these sustained-release formulations should result in more effective dosing regimens.

Since depletion of tissue stores of sulfhydryl groups has been proposed to play an important role in nitrate tolerance, some investigators have administered sulfhydryl-containing compounds in an attempt to reverse or prevent the development of tolerance. The most commonly used agent is *N*-acetylcysteine (NAC), which is hydrolyzed in vivo to cysteine. Although some

TABLE 17.2 Dosage Forms and Pharmacokinetics of Nitrates Most Commonly Used in Angina Pectoris

Drug and Dosage Form	Usual Dose (mg)	Onset of Action (min)	Duration of Action (hr)
Nitroglycerin			
Sublingual	0.3–0.6	2–5	0.16–0.50
Transmucosal (buccal)	1–3	2–5	3–6
Oral	3–20	20–45	2–8
Ointment (2%)	1–5 (0.5–2 inches)	15–60	3–8
Transdermal	5–30 (per 24 hr)	30–60	12–24
Intravenous	5–300 mEq/min	Immediate	Transient
Isosorbide dinitrate			
Sublingual	2.5–10	3–20	1–2
Oral, chewable	5–60	30–60	2–10
Oral, sustained release	40	30–60	6–10
Isosorbide mononitrate			
Oral	20	15–30	6–12
Erythrityl tetranitrate			
Sublingual	5–10	5–15	2–3
Oral, chewable	10–30	30	2–6
Pentaerythritol tetranitrate			
Oral	10–20	30	2–6
Oral, sustained release	30–80	30–60	4–12

investigators have shown a positive effect with NAC, the antinitrate tolerance effect of this compound has not been universally confirmed. Thus, further well-controlled clinical studies are necessary to establish the effectiveness of sulfhydryl-containing compounds at preventing or reversing nitrate tolerance.

Industrial exposure to organic nitrates induces both tolerance and physical dependence. The state of dependence becomes manifest when exposure to nitrates is withdrawn suddenly. For example, munitions workers who have become dependent on nitroglycerin have been reported to undergo angina, myocardial infarction, or even sudden death following removal from contact with nitroglycerin. Some of these patients showed symptoms of ischemic heart disease, even though their coronary arteriography was judged to be normal. Since it is possible that coronary vasospasm plays a role in the pathogenesis of angina that occurs in nitrate-dependent individuals, these patients should be cautioned to watch for increased chest pain when they withdraw from medication or discontinue their exposure.

Adverse Effects

Vascular headache, postural hypotension, and reflex tachycardia are common side effects of organic nitrate therapy. Fortunately, tolerance to nitrate-induced headache develops after a few days of therapy. Postural hypotension and tachycardia can be minimized by proper dosage adjustment and by instructing the patient to sit

down when taking rapidly acting preparations. An effective dose of nitrate usually produces a fall in upright systolic blood pressure of 10 mm Hg and a reflex rise in heart rate of 10 beats per minute. Larger changes than these should be avoided, because a reduction in myocardial perfusion and an increase in cardiac oxygen requirements may actually exacerbate the angina.

Since nitrite ions oxidize the iron atoms of hemoglobin and convert it to methemoglobin, there may be a loss in oxygen delivery to tissues. While methemoglobinemia does not follow therapeutic doses of organic nitrates, it can be observed after overdosage or accidental poisoning.

Cautions

Chest pain that is not relieved by two or three tablets within 30 minutes may be due to an acute myocardial infarction. In addition, nitrate administration may result in an increase in intracranial pressure, and therefore, these drugs should be used cautiously in patients with cerebral bleeding and head trauma.

β-Adrenoceptor Blocking Agents

β-Adrenoceptor blockade is a rational approach to the treatment of angina pectoris, since an increase in sympathetic nervous system activity is a common feature in acute anginal attacks. Based on their ability to reduce oxygen demand, all β-blockers tested so far have also been shown to be effective in the treatment of secondary angina. Administration of these compounds results in a decrease in frequency of anginal attacks, a reduction in nitroglycerin consumption, an increased exercise tolerance on the treadmill, and a decreased magnitude of ST segment depression on the electrocardiogram during exercise. Propranolol is the prototype of this class of compounds

β-Blockers approved for clinical use in secondary angina in the United States include propranolol and nadolol (*Corgard*), compounds that block both β_1- and β_2-adrenoceptors equally, while atenolol (*Tenormin*) and metoprolol (*Lopressor*) are cardioselective β_1-receptor antagonists.

Mechanism of Action

The myocardial response to exercise includes an increase in heart rate and myocardial contractility. These effects are mediated in part by the sympathetic nervous system. Propranolol and other β-adrenoceptor blockers antagonize the actions of catecholamines on the heart and thereby attenuate the myocardial response to stress or exercise (Fig. 17.3). The resting heart rate is reduced by propranolol, but not to the same extent as is the decrease in exercise-induced tachycardia. Overall, propranolol reduces myocardial oxygen consumption for a given degree of physical activity.

Arterial blood pressure (afterload) is also reduced by propranolol. Although the mechanisms responsible for this antihypertensive effect are not completely understood, they are thought to involve (1) a reduction in cardiac output, (2) a decrease in plasma renin activity, (3) an action in the central nervous system, and (4) a resetting of the baroreceptors . Thus, propranolol may exert a part of its beneficial effects in secondary angina by decreasing three of the major determinants of myocardial oxygen demand, that is, heart rate, contractility, and systolic wall tension.

Propranolol and other β-blockers also have been shown to produce an increase in oxygen supply to the subendocardium of ischemic areas. The mechanism responsible for this effect is most likely related to the

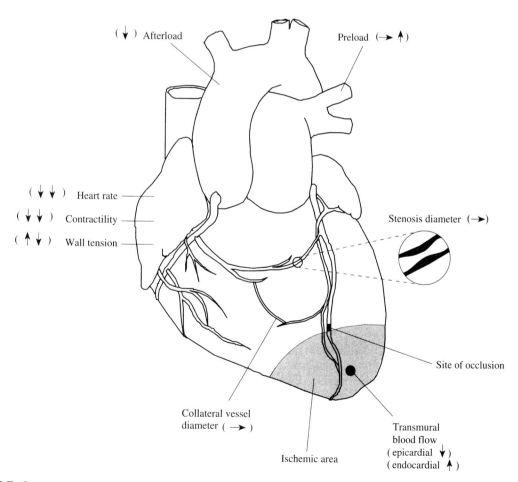

FIGURE 17.3

A schematic drawing indicating the major actions of the β-blockers on the ischemic heart and peripheral circulation. ↓, decrease; ↑, increase; →, unchanged; ↑↓, variable effect.

TABLE 17.3   Doses and Pharmacokinetics of β-Receptor Antagonists Used in the Treatment of Angina Pectoris

Compound	Usual Daily Dose (mg)	Oral Bioavailability (%)	Plasma $t_{1/2}$ (hr)	First-pass Metabolism (%)
Propranolol	40–80	25–30	3–6	90
Nadolol	40	30–40	12–24	0
Metoprolol	50–100	40–45	3–4	50
Atenolol	50	50–55	5–10	0

ability of β-blockers to reduce resting heart rate and increase diastolic perfusion time. Because subendocardial blood flow and flow distal to severe coronary artery stenosis occur primarily during diastole, this increase in diastolic perfusion time, due to the bradycardiac effect of propranolol and other β-blockers, would be expected to increase subendocardial blood flow to ischemic regions. β-Blockers have no significant effect on coronary collateral blood flow. Finally, there is evidence that β-blockers can inhibit platelet aggregation.

Absorption, Metabolism, and Excretion

Propranolol is well absorbed from the gastrointestinal tract, but it is avidly extracted by the liver as the drug passes to the systemic circulation (first-pass effect). This effect explains the large variation in plasma levels of propranolol seen after oral drug administration.

Because of these interindividual variations in the kinetics of propranolol, the therapeutic dose of this drug is best determined by titration. End points of titration include relief of anginal symptoms, increases in exercise tolerance, and plasma concentration of propranolol between 15 and 100 ng/mL. For additional details on the pharmacokinetics of propranolol and other β-receptor antagonists approved for clinical use in the treatment of angina pectoris, see Table 17.3 and Chapter 11.

Clinical Uses

By attenuating the cardiac response to exercise, propranolol and other β-blockers increase the amount of exercise that can be performed before angina develops. Although propranolol does not change the point of imbalance between oxygen supply and demand at which angina occurs, it does slow the rate at which the imbalance point is reached.

Propranolol is particularly indicated in the management of patients whose angina attacks are frequent and unpredictable despite the use of organic nitrates. Propranolol may be combined with the use of nitroglycerin, the latter drug being used to control acute attacks of angina. The combined use of propranolol and organic nitrates theoretically should enhance the therapeutic effects of each and minimize their adverse effects (Table 17.4).

Propranolol and nadolol also have been used successfully in combination with certain calcium entry blockers, particularly nifedipine, for the treatment of secondary angina. Caution should be used, however, when combining a β-blocker and a calcium channel blocker, such as verapamil or diltiazem, since the negative inotropic and chronotropic effects of this combination may lead to severe bradycardia, arteriovenous nodal block, or decompensated congestive heart failure.

TABLE 17.4   Effects of Nitrates, β-Receptor Antagonists, and Calcium Entry Blockers on Determinants of Cardiac Oxygen Supply and Demand

Determinant	Nitrates	β-Receptor Blockers	Calcium Entry Blockers
Wall tension	↓	±	↓
Ventricular volume	↓	↑	±
Ventricular pressure	↓	↓	↓
Heart size	↓	↑	±
Heart rate	↑ (reflex)	↓	±
Contractility	↑ (reflex)	↓	±
Endocardial-epicardial blood flow ratio	↑	↑	↑
Collateral blood flow	↑	→	↑

Table 17.3 and Chapter 11 provide additional details concerning the most commonly used β-blockers (i.e., propranolol, nadolol, atenolol, and metoprolol) in the treatment of angina pectoris.

Adverse Effects

Abrupt interruption of propranolol therapy in individuals with angina pectoris has been associated with reappearance of angina, acute myocardial infarction, or death due to a sudden increase in sympathetic nervous system tone to the heart. The mechanisms underlying these reactions are unknown, but they may be the result of an increase in the number of β-receptors that occur following chronic β-adrenoceptor blockade (up-regulation of receptors). When it is advisable to discontinue propranolol administration, such as before coronary bypass surgery, the dosage should be tapered over 2 to 3 days.

Calcium Entry or Calcium Channel Blockers

The calcium entry blockers or calcium channel blockers are a group of orally active drugs that have been approved for use in the treatment of vasospastic and ef-

fort-induced angina. These compounds block L-type voltage-dependent calcium channels in vascular smooth muscle and the heart, block platelet aggregation, and are particularly effective in the prophylaxis of coronary vasospasm or variant angina. In addition, these compounds are used in the chronic treatment of secondary angina. Two members of this group, verapamil (*Calan*) and diltiazem (*Cardiazem*), also have been approved for use in the therapy of certain supraventricular tachyarrhythmias (see Chapter 16). Other potential clinical uses of these compounds include systemic and pulmonary hypertension and Raynaud's syndrome

A detailed discussion of the pharmacology of this important class of drugs can be found in Chapter 19. Their major hemodynamic effects on the primary determinants of myocardial oxygen supply and demand are summarized in Figure 17.4. A comparison of the effects of all three classes of antianginal drugs on these important parameters is summarized in Table 17.4.

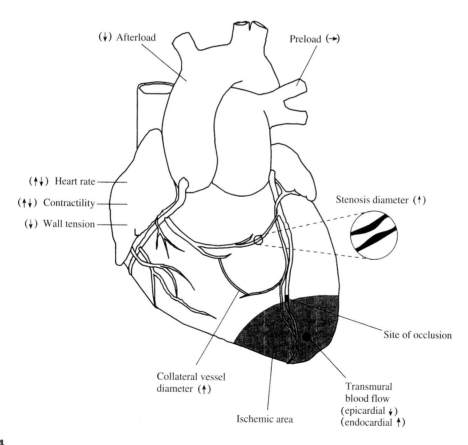

FIGURE 17.4

Major actions of the calcium antagonists on the ischemic heart and coronary circulation. ↓, decrease; ↑, increase; →, unchanged; ↑↓, variable effect.

Study QUESTIONS

1. A patient comes to your office with effort-induced angina and resting tachycardia. You choose the following drug to treat the patient because it slows heart rate by blocking L-type calcium channels in the SA node:
   (A) Verapamil
   (B) Propranolol
   (C) Nitroglycerin
   (D) Isosorbide dinitrate
   (E) Metoprolol

2. Which of the following hemodynamic effects of nitroglycerin are primarily responsible for the beneficial results observed in patients with secondary angina?
   (A) Reduction in the force of myocardial contraction
   (B) Reduction in systemic vascular resistance (afterload)
   (C) Increased heart rate
   (D) Reduction in venous capacitance (preload)
   (E) Increased blood flow to the subepicardium

3. A woman is prescribed a combination of drugs consisting of a nitroglycerin patch and a β-blocker, such as propranolol, to treat her attacks of secondary angina. Which effect of propranolol would counteract an adverse effect of nitroglycerin?
   (A) A decrease in preload
   (B) A decrease in afterload
   (C) A decrease in heart rate
   (D) An increase in myocardial contractile force
   (E) A reduction in coronary vasospasm

4. A patient who has been taking propranolol for a long period for secondary angina comes to your office complaining of increased frequency of chest pains on exertion. You decide to stop the propranolol and give him diltiazem because you suspect he has a mixture of secondary and primary angina. Why would diltiazem be more likely to relieve the angina if your new diagnosis is accurate?
   (A) Diltiazem produces a decrease in heart rate.
   (B) Diltiazem dilates coronary blood vessels in spasm.
   (C) Diltiazem produces AV blockade.
   (D) Diltiazem reduces myocardial contractility.
   (E) Diltiazem reduces afterload.

5. Metoprolol would produce which beneficial effect in a patient with secondary angina?
   (A) A decrease in preload
   (B) An increase in collateral blood flow
   (C) An increase in afterload
   (D) An increase in diastolic filling time

(E) An increase in blood flow through a concentric stenosis

ANSWERS

1. **A.** Verapamil is an L-type calcium channel blocker. Nitroglycerin and isosorbide are both organic nitrates and have no direct effect on L-type calcium channels at the SA node, while propranolol and metoprolol are β-adrenoceptor blockers and will slow heart rate by blocking the actions of norepinephrine and epinephrine on β-receptors at the SA node.

2. **D.** Nitroglycerin can reduce preload, which in turn reduces wall tension and increases subendocardial blood flow. Nitroglycerin also reduces afterload, but this is a small effect compared to the reduction in preload. Its effects on heart rate and contractility are minimal, and if anything reflex tachycardia and increase in contractility would be detrimental effects of too much nitroglycerin.

3. **C.** Nitroglycerin can increase heart rate via an increase in sympathetic tone to the heart due to an excessive decrease in blood pressure; propranolol would block the β-receptors responsible for the tachycardia. Propranolol does not decrease preload, and its effect to decrease afterload would exacerbate the decrease in afterload produced by nitroglycerin. Propranolol does not increase myocardial contractile force and could actually increase the incidence of vasospasm by unmasking α-adrenoceptors in the coronary blood vessels.

4. **B.** Both diltiazem and propranolol would produce the effects listed in A, C, D, and E. Only diltiazem would dilate vessels in spasm. Propranolol would tend to produce vasoconstriction, not vasodilation.

5. **D.** An increase in time spent in diastole would increase subendocardial blood flow. Metoprolol does not decrease preload or increase afterload; in fact the opposite is likely to occur. Metoprolol does not affect collateral blood flow or flow through a concentric stenosis.

SUPPLEMENTAL READING

Fung HL and Bauer JA. Mechanisms of nitrate tolerance. Cardiovasc Drug Ther 1994;8:489.

Knight CJ et al. Different effects of calcium antagonists, nitrates and beta blockers on platelet function: Possible importance for the treatment of unstable angina. Circulation 1997;95:125–132.

Kurz S et al. Evidence for a causal role of the renin-angiotensin system in nitrate tolerance. Circulation 1999;99:3181–3187.

Munzel T et al. Effects of a nitrate-free interval on tolerance, vasoconstrictor sensitivity and vascular superoxide production. J Am Coll Cardiol 2000;36;628–634.

Parker JD and Parker JO. Drug therapy: Nitrate therapy for stable angina pectoris. N Engl J Med 1998;338:520–531.

Torfgard KE and Ahlner J. Mechanisms of action of nitrates. Cardiovasc Drug Ther 1994;8:701–717.

CASE Study Treatment of Coronary Vasospasm

A 60-year-old man comes into the office complaining of chest pains that primarily occur in the early morning and do not appear to be associated with stress or exercise. Following coronary angiography and a positive ergonovine test you determine that this patient has angina pectoris as a result of coronary artery spasm. How would you (1) treat the patient to alleviate the acute attacks when they occur and (2) treat chronically to prevent their reoccurrence?

ANSWER: Treat the patient with sublingual nitroglycerin for the acute attacks because of its rapid onset of action and its powerful vasodilating effect on the large epicardial conductance coronary arteries, which are normally the primary site of the spasm. For the chronic treatment there are two possibilities, an oral calcium channel blocker, such as amlodipine or verapamil, or a long-acting nitrate preparation, such as the transdermal form of nitroglycerin given once a day at bedtime to prevent the early morning episodes. β-Adrenoceptor blockers are not used for patients with coronary vasospasm, as they may worsen the condition.

18

The Renin–Angiotensin–Aldosterone System and Other Vasoactive Substances

Lisa A. Cassis

 DRUG LIST

GENERIC NAME	PAGE	GENERIC NAME	PAGE
Benzapril	212	Losartan	213
Candesartan	213	Moexipril	212
Captopril	210	Quinapril	212
Enalapril	212	Perindopril	212
Eprosartan	213	Ramipril	212
Fosinopril	212	Spironolactone	214
Irbesartan	213	Telmisartan	213
Lisinopril	212	Valsartan	213

THE RENIN–ANGIOTENSIN SYSTEM

The renin–angiotensin system is important for the regulation of vascular smooth muscle tone, fluid and electrolyte balance, and the growth of cardiac and vascular smooth muscle. A normally functioning renin–angiotensin system contributes to the routine control of arterial blood pressure. A variety of basic and clinical investigations have resulted in a broader understanding of the role of the renin–angiotensin system in the cardiovascular pathophysiology of hypertension, congestive heart failure, and more recently, atherosclerosis. Whether or not abnormal activity of the renin–angiotensin system contributes to the primary etiology of these diseases, *pharmacological inhibition of the renin–angiotensin system has proved to be a valuable therapeutic strategy in the treatment of hypertension and congestive heart failure.*

The classical renin–angiotensin system comprises a series of biochemical steps (Fig. 18.1) leading to the production of a family of structurally related peptides (e.g., angiotensin II, angiotensin III, and other smaller peptides with bioactivity). Sites for pharmacological intervention in this system include the enzymatic steps catalyzed by renin, angiotensin-converting enzyme (ACE), and angiotensin receptors that mediate a particular physiological response.

Renin

Renin is an enzyme that is synthesized and stored in the renal juxtaglomerular apparatus and that catalyzes the formation of a decapeptide, *angiotensin I,* from a plasma protein substrate. Renin has a narrow substrate specificity that is limited to a single peptide bond in angiotensinogen, a precursor of angiotensin I. Renin is considered to control the rate-limiting step in the ultimate production of angiotensin II. Control of renin secretion by the juxtaglomerular apparatus is important in determining the plasma renin concentration.

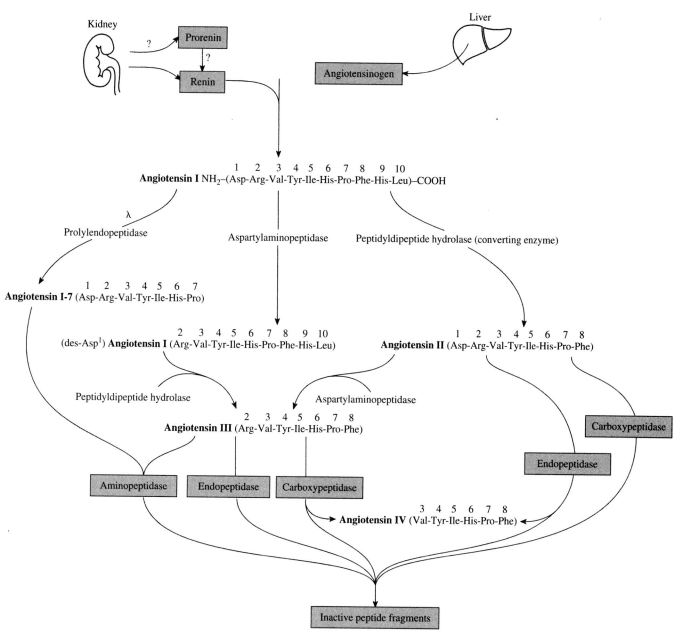

FIGURE 18.1
Synthesis and structures of the angiotensins.

Three generally accepted mechanisms are involved in the regulation of renin secretion (Fig. 18.2). The first depends on renal afferent arterioles that act as stretch receptors or baroreceptors. Increased intravascular pressure and increased volume in the afferent arteriole inhibits the release of renin. The second mechanism is the result of changes in the amount of filtered sodium that reaches the macula densa of the distal tubule. Plasma renin activity correlates inversely with dietary sodium intake. The third renin secretory control mechanism is neurogenic and involves the dense sympathetic innervation of the juxtaglomerular cells in the afferent arteriole; renin release is increased following activation of α_1-adrenoceptors by the neurotransmitter norepinephrine.

Angiotensin II, the primary end product of the renin–angiotensin system, acts on the juxtaglomerular cells to inhibit the release of renin; this process is therefore a negative feedback mechanism. The half-life of renin in the circulation is 10 to 30 minutes, with inactivation occurring primarily in the liver. Small amounts of renin are eliminated by the kidneys. Pure human renin

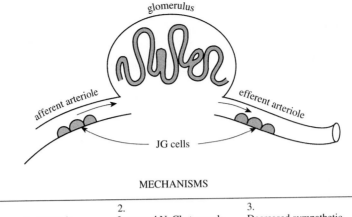

MECHANISMS

1.	2.	3.
Increased pressure in afferent arteriole leads to decreased renin release by JG cells.	Increased NaCl at macula densa in distal tubule leads to decreased renin release by JG cells.	Decreased sympathetic nerve activity in afferent arteriole leads to decreased renin release.

FIGURE 18.2
Mechanisms of regulation of renin secretion from the kidney. JG, juxtaglomerular.

has been used to develop specific inhibitors of the enzyme. Low-molecular-weight orally effective renin inhibitors are under development.

Angiotensinogen

Human plasma contains a glycoprotein called *angiotensinogen*, which serves as the only known substrate for renin. Angiotensinogen must undergo proteolysis before active portions of the protein are sufficiently unmasked to exert biological effects. Angiotensinogen is synthesized in many organs, including the liver, brain, kidney, and fat. Its gene transcription and plasma concentrations increase following treatment with adrenocorticotropic hormone (ACTH), glucocorticoids, thyroid hormone, and estrogens, as well as during pregnancy and inflammation and after nephrectomy. Angiotensinogen also has been found in large quantities in cerebrospinal and amniotic fluid. Mutations in the angiotensinogen gene have been reported to be linked to human hypertension.

Angiotensin-Converting Enzyme: A Peptidyl Dipeptide Hydrolase

Metabolism of angiotensinogen by renin produces the decapeptide *angiotensin I*. This relatively inactive peptide is acted on by a dipeptidase-converting enzyme to produce the very active octapeptide *angiotensin II*. In addition to converting enzyme, angiotensin I can be acted on by prolyl endopeptidase, an enzyme that removes the first amino acid to form angiotensin 1-7, a peptide primarily active in the brain. ACE has been

identified in vascular endothelial cells, epithelial cells of the proximal tubule and small intestine, male germinal cells, and the central nervous system. The lung vascular endothelium contains the highest concentration of ACE, and therefore, the lung serves as the major organ for the production of circulating angiotensin II. Although ACE was originally thought to be specific for the conversion of angiotensin I to II, it is now known to be a rather nonspecific peptidyl dipeptide hydrolase that can cleave dipeptides from the carboxy terminus of a number of endogenous peptides (e.g., substance P, bradykinin). Peptides with penultimate prolyl residues are not cleaved by converting enzyme; this accounts for the biological stability of angiotensin II. Inhibition of converting enzyme results in an elevated pool of angiotensin I. A mutation deletion in the ACE gene has been linked to a higher risk factor for hypertension, left ventricular hypertrophy, and myocardial infarction.

The Angiotensins

The amino acid composition of the peptides and enzymes involved in the synthesis and metabolism of the angiotensins is shown in Figure 18.1. Angiotensin I is believed to have little direct biological activity and must be converted to angiotensin II or angiotensin 1-7 before characteristic responses of the renin–angiotensin system are manifested. Angiotensin I and II are metabolized at their animo terminus by *aspartyl aminopeptidase*, an enzyme in plasma and numerous tissues. Angiotensin II is rapidly metabolized by aspartyl aminopeptidases, endopeptidases, and carboxypeptidases, while angiotensin III is hydrolyzed by aminopeptidases, endopeptidases, and carboxypeptidases (Fig. 18.1). The biological activity of angiotensin III ranges from one-fourth to equipotent with angiotensin II, depending on the response being monitored. The smallest biologically active peptide in this system is angiotensin IV, which exerts unique actions in the central nervous system and periphery that are distinct from those of angiotensin II.

ANGIOTENSIN RECEPTORS

In 1988, a series of reports described the ability of imidazole acetic acid derivatives to act as antagonists at the angiotensin receptor. During the course of characterization of these compounds, it became apparent that certain tissues contained different subtypes of angiotensin receptors. Angiotensin receptors have been classified into two subtypes, AT1 and AT2. Each receptor subtype has been cloned and sequenced, with only 32% homology in the protein sequences for the two receptors. The AT1 receptor uses G proteins as signal transducers and is coupled through traditional second-messenger systems that involve phospholipase C and calcium mobilization, inhibition of adenylyl cyclase, stimulation of mitogen-activated protein kinases and the JAK/STAT pathway, and activation of Jun-kinase. In contrast, the signaling cascades of the AT2 receptor involve the activation of phosphorylases, which inhibit phosphorylation steps of certain types of cell growth.

The distribution of the AT1 and AT2 receptor subtypes is species and tissue specific. *The major biological functions of angiotensin II (cardiovascular regulation) are mediated through the AT1 receptor.* In contrast, despite the increased presence of AT2 receptors in fetal tissues, a lack of AT2 receptors appears to be compatible with life. Current evidence suggests that in general, stimulation of the AT2 receptor appears to oppose those physiological actions of angiotensin II that are mediated through the AT1 receptor.

Angiotensin IV, the smallest bioactive peptide product of the renin–angiotensin system, interacts with a unique receptor termed the *angiotensin IV receptor;* this receptor exhibits minimal affinity for angiotensin II or angiotensin III.

PHARMACOLOGICAL ACTIONS

While the following discussion addresses the pharmacology of angiotensin II that is mediated through the AT1 receptor, most of these responses also follow administration of angiotensin III. Generally, angiotensin III is less potent than angiotensin II. Angiotensin 1-7 is considered to be biologically active and has been demonstrated to exert effects that are similar to, opposite of, or totally distinct from those of angiotensin II.

Vascular Smooth Muscle Contraction

The intravenous injection of angiotensin II results in a sharp rise in systolic and diastolic pressures. The response is consistently reproducible when small doses of angiotensin II are injected; however, larger amounts of the peptide produce *tachyphylaxis* (loss of response on repeated administration). The mechanism underlying tachyphylaxis to angiotensin II is unknown, but it may involve receptor internalization and/or desensitization. Subcutaneous and intramuscular injections are much less potent and have a longer duration of action than do comparable doses given intravenously. Infusions that cause an immediate pressor response tend to result in tachyphylaxis over several hours. On a molar basis, angiotensin II is about 40 times as potent as norepinephrine. The pressor response to angiotensin II is caused by its direct receptor-mediated effect on vascular smooth muscle. The peptide stimulates the formation of the second messenger inositol 1,4,5-triphosphate, which results in a release of intracellular Ca^{++} and ultimately smooth muscle contraction.

Heart Rate and Contractility

The administration of angiotensin II to an animal with intact baroreceptor reflexes results in reflex bradycardia in response to the marked vasoconstriction. When baroreceptor reflexes are depressed (barbiturate anesthesia) or if vagal tone is inhibited (atropine or vagotomy), angiotensin directly induces cardiac acceleration.

Angiotensin II stimulates the influx of Ca^{++} into cardiac muscle cells and can exert a direct inotropic effect at cardiac muscle. In addition, angiotensin II can stimulate the sympathoadrenal system and thereby increase myocardial contractility. In contrast to its effects on vascular smooth muscle, the ability of angiotensin to increase the contractile force of the heart is far less potent. Therefore, in spite of the positive chronotropic and inotropic effects produced by angiotensin II, cardiac output is rarely increased. In fact, angiotensin II may decrease cardiac output through reflex bradycardia induced by the rise in peripheral resistance that it causes. In contrast, centrally administered angiotensin II increases both blood pressure and cardiac output.

Vascular Permeability

Angiotensin II can cause a net fluid accumulation in tissues and has been shown to increase the permeability of the endothelium in large arteries and to widen the interendothelial spaces in the aorta and in coronary, mesenteric, and peripheral arteries. This response to angiotensin II probably reflects the effect of elevated pressure on the endothelial permeability barrier. The peptide also stimulates the release of the vasodilator prostacyclin from arterial endothelial cells.

Growth

Angiotensin II alters the growth of vascular smooth muscle, cardiac myocytes, and cardiac fibroblasts through mechanisms related to increased cell proliferation (hyperplasia) and protein deposition (hypertrophy). These actions of angiotensin II on cell growth involve interactions with other growth factors and are relevant to the pathophysiology of both hypertension and congestive heart failure.

Central Nervous System

Administration of angiotensin II into the vertebral circulation increases peripheral blood pressure. This hypertensive action, mediated by the central nervous system, is primarily the result of an increase in central efferent sympathetic activity going to the periphery. The area postrema of the caudal medulla appears to be the structure responsible for the central cardiovascular actions of angiotensin II.

Angiotensin II produces changes in body hydration and thirst by a direct action in the central nervous system. The administration of angiotensin II into the septal, anterior hypothalamic, and medial preoptic areas stimulates drinking behavior in several species. Part of the volume response also may be caused by the antinatriuretic and antidiuretic effects of angiotensin II.

Angiotensin II, administered into the central nervous system, increases the release of luteinizing hormone, adrenocortical hormone, thyroid-releasing hormone, β-endorphin, vasopressin, and oxytocin from the anterior pituitary. In contrast, centrally administered angiotensin II inhibits the release of anterior pituitary growth hormone and prolactin.

Sympathetic Nervous System

Angiotensin II, acting at presynaptic receptors on noradrenergic nerve terminals, potentiates the release of norepinephrine during low-frequency sympathetic nerve stimulation. Aside from its action on the nerve terminals of postganglionic sympathetic neurons, angiotensin II can directly stimulate sympathetic neurons in the central nervous system, in peripheral autonomic ganglia, and at the adrenal medulla.

Adrenal Cortex and Aldosterone Secretion

Angiotensin II stimulates aldosterone synthesis and secretion from the glomerulosa cells of the adrenal cortex. The aldosterone secretion induced by angiotensin II in humans is not accompanied by an increase in glucocorticoid plasma levels. Chronic administration of angiotensin II will maintain elevated aldosterone secretion for several days to weeks unless hypokalemia ensues.

ANTAGONISTS OF THE RENIN–ANGIOTENSIN SYSTEM

A summary of the agents that inhibit the renin–angiotensin system and their sites of action is provided in Figure 18.3.

Renin Inhibitors

The acid protease inhibitor *pepstatin* and some analogues of angiotensinogen can competitively inhibit the formation of angiotensin I by human renin. Highly specific renin inhibitors may prove beneficial as antihypertensive agents or in the treatment of congestive heart failure. Despite extensive efforts to develop renin inhibitors, most compounds capable of inhibiting renin are large peptidelike molecules that lack adequate physical chemical properties to permit oral absorption.

Angiotensin-Converting Enzyme Inhibitors

Many of the orally active ACE inhibitors are prodrugs. These include perindopril, quinapril, benazepril, ramipril, enalapril, trandolapril, and fosinopril.

Captopril

Captopril (*Capoten*) is an orally effective ACE inhibitor with a sulfhydryl moiety that is used in binding to the active site of the enzyme. Captopril blocks the blood pressure responses caused by the administration of angiotensin I and decreases plasma and tissue levels of angiotensin II.

Pharmacological Actions

Treatment with captopril reduces blood pressure in patients with renovascular disease and in patients with essential hypertension. The decrease in arterial pressure is related to a reduction in total peripheral resistance. Most studies demonstrate a good correlation between the hypotensive effect of inhibitors and the degree of blockade of the renin–angiotensin system. Many of the pharmacological effects of captopril are attributable to the inhibition of angiotensin II synthesis. However, ACE is a relatively nonselective enzyme that also catabolizes a family of kinins to inactive products (Fig. 18.4). Bradykinin, one of the major kinins, acts as a vasodilator through mechanisms related to the production of nitric oxide and prostacyclin by the vascular endothelium. Thus, administration of the ACE inhibitor captopril not only inhibits angiotensin II production but also prevents the breakdown of bradykinin. Increases in bradykinin concentrations after administration of ACE inhibitors contribute to the therapeutic efficacy of these compounds in the treatment of hypertension and congestive heart failure. However, alterations in bradykinin

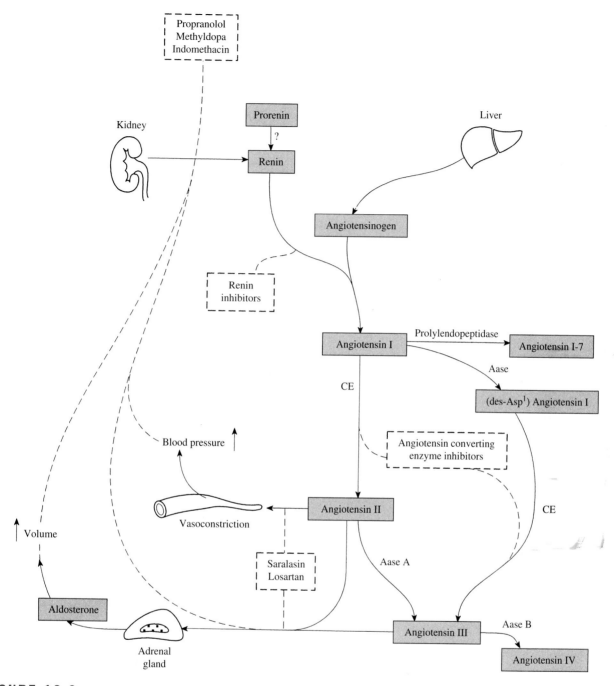

FIGURE 18.3
Agents that inhibit the renin–angiotensin–aldosterone system and points at which they act. CE, converting enzyme; Aase, aspartyl aminopeptidase.

concentrations are also thought to contribute to cough and angioedema sometimes seen after ACE inhibition.

The hypotensive response to captopril is accompanied by a fall in plasma aldosterone and angiotensin II levels and an increase in plasma renin activity. Serum potassium levels are not affected unless potassium supplements or potassium-sparing diuretics are used concomitantly; this can result in severe hyperkalemia.

There is no baroreflex-associated increase in heart rate, cardiac output, or myocardial contractility in response to the decrease in pressure, presumably because captopril decreases the sensitivity of the baroreceptor reflex.

Captopril enhances cardiac output in patients with congestive heart failure by inducing a reduction in ventricular afterload and preload. Converting enzyme inhibitors have been shown to decrease the mass and wall

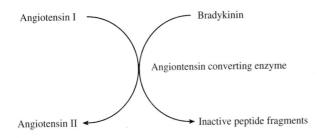

FIGURE 18.4
Interrelationship between the renin–angiotensin system and bradykinin.

thickness of the left ventricle in both normal and hypertrophied myocardium. ACE inhibitors lack metabolic side effects and do not alter serum lipids.

Pharmacokinetics

The onset of action following oral administration of captopril is about 15 minutes, with peak blood levels achieved in 30 to 60 minutes. Its apparent biological half-life is approximately 2 hours, with its antihypertensive effects observed for 6 to 10 hours. The kidneys appear to play a major role in the inactivation of captopril.

Clinical Uses

Captopril, as well as other ACE inhibitors, is indicated in the treatment of hypertension, congestive heart failure, left ventricular dysfunction after a myocardial infarction, and diabetic nephropathy. In the treatment of essential hypertension, captopril is considered first-choice therapy, either alone or in combination with a thiazide diuretic. Decreases in blood pressure are primarily attributed to decreased total peripheral resistance or afterload. An advantage of combining captopril therapy with a conventional thiazide diuretic is that the thiazide-induced hypokalemia is minimized in the presence of ACE inhibition, since there is a marked decrease in angiotensin II–induced aldosterone release.

If the patient is asymptomatic, captopril can be used as monotherapy in the treatment of congestive heart failure. The use of ACE inhibitors in the treatment of congestive heart failure is supported by results from large-scale clinical trials demonstrating a general reduction in the relative risk of death. In symptomatic patients captopril should be used in conjunction with a diuretic because of the weak natriuretic properties of ACE inhibitors. In combination, captopril will reduce afterload and preload and prevent diuretic-induced activation of the renin–angiotensin system. Finally, ACE inhibitors may slow the progression of congestive heart failure by limiting left ventricular hypertrophy.

In the treatment of diabetic nephropathy associated with type I insulin-dependent diabetes mellitus, captopril decreases the rate of progression of renal insufficiency and retards the worsening of renal function.

Adverse Actions

Approximately 10% of the patients treated with captopril report a dose-related maculopapular rash that often disappears when the dosage of captopril is reduced. Other common adverse effects are fever, a persistent dry cough (incidence as high as 39%), initial dose hypotension, and a loss of taste that may result in anorexia. These effects are reversed when drug therapy is discontinued. More serious toxicities include a 1% incidence of proteinuria and glomerulonephritis; less common are leukopenia and agranulocytosis. Since food reduces the bioavailability of captopril by 30 to 40%, administration of the drug an hour before meals is recommended. All converting enzyme inhibitors are contraindicated in patients with bilateral renal artery disease or with unilateral renal artery disease and one kidney. Use under these circumstances may result in renal failure or paradoxical malignant hypertension.

Prodrug Angiotensin-converting Enzyme Inhibitors

Most orally effective inhibitors of peptidyl dipeptide hydrolase are prodrug ester compounds that must be hydrolyzed in plasma to the active moiety before becoming effective. These drugs include benazepril (*Lotensin*), enalapril (*Vasotec*), fosinopril (*Monopril*), moexipril (Univasc), quinapril (*Accupril*), perindopril (*Aceon*), and ramipril (*Altace*). The ester group promotes absorption of the compound from the gastrointestinal tract. In contrast to captopril, the recommended dosing interval for these prodrug compounds is once to twice daily. These compounds are otherwise generally similar to captopril in their mechanism of action and indicated uses.

All prodrug ACE inhibitors are indicated for use as first-choice agents in the treatment of hypertension and congestive heart failure. In addition, results from clinical trials demonstrate that ramipril, a prodrug ACE inhibitor, can reduce the rate of death, myocardial infarction, and stroke in a broad range of high-risk patients who did not have heart failure. These results suggest that ACE inhibitors may be useful in the management of ischemia and atherosclerosis.

While essentially all ACE inhibitors have a similar mechanism of action and therefore exhibit similar efficacy in the treatment of hypertension and congestive heart failure, these drugs differ slightly in their pharmacokinetic profiles. Enalapril, lisinopril, and quinapril are excreted primarily by the kidney, with minimal liver metabolism, while the other prodrug compounds are metabolized by the liver and renally excreted. Thus, in patients with renal insufficiency, the half-life of renally excreted ACE inhibitors is prolonged. In addition, patients with impaired liver function may have a compromised ability to convert prodrug to the active drug moiety, so the efficacy of the compounds may be reduced. In addition, compounds dependent on liver metabolism for elimination may exhibit an increase in plasma half-life. An additional property that distinguishes among these prodrugs is their individual abilities to bind tightly to tissue ACE, as opposed to the circulating form of the enzyme. Of the prodrug inhibitors, quinapril and perindopril bind most tightly.

All ACE inhibitors are contraindicated during pregnancy. Their administration to pregnant women during the second and third trimesters of pregnancy has been associated with fetal and neonatal injury, including fetal death. A summary of the ACE inhibitors and their properties is provided in Table 18.1.

Angiotensin Receptor Antagonists

Angiotensin II can bind with high affinity to two distinct receptors, termed the angiotensin type 1 (AT1) and the angiotensin type 2 (AT2) receptor. These receptors belong to a superfamily of G protein–coupled receptors that contain seven transmembrane regions. The amino acid sequence of these receptors is highly conserved across species. The AT1 and AT2 receptors share only 34% homology, have distinct signal transduction pathways, and are not necessarily found on the same cell type or tissue. As previously discussed, most of the physiological effects of angiotensin II are mediated through effects at the AT1 receptor.

TABLE 18.1 Properties of Angiotensin-Converting Enzyme Inhibitors

Inhibitor (trade name)	Contains Sulfhydryl Groups	Form	
		Prodrug	Nonprodrug
Captopril (Capoten)	X		X
Quinapril (Accupril)		X	
Ramipril (Altace)		X	
Fosinopril (Monopril)	X		X
Benzapril (Lotensin)		X	
Enalapril maleate (Vasotec)		X	
Lisinopril (Prinivil, Zestril)			X

Mechanism of Action and Pharmacological Actions

Losartan (*Cozaar*) was the first imidazole AT1 receptor antagonist developed and is a selective competitive antagonist to angiotensin II. Other AT1 receptor antagonists approved for the treatment of hypertension include valsartan (*Diovan*), irbesartan (*Avapro*), candesartan cilexetil (*Atacand*), telmisartan (*Micardis*), and eprosartan (*Teveten*). These antagonists share some pharmacological characteristics, including a high affinity for the AT1 receptor, little to no affinity for the AT2 receptor, high protein binding, and the ability to produce an almost insurmountable blockade of the AT1 receptor. Although all of the AT1 receptor antagonists are competitive blocking drugs, they only slowly dissociate from the receptor, and their effects cannot be easily overcome.

The administration of an AT1 receptor antagonist results in a decrease in total peripheral resistance (afterload) and cardiac venous return (preload). All of the physiological effects of angiotensin II, including stimulation of the release of aldosterone, are antagonized in the presence of an AT1 receptor antagonist. Reductions in blood pressure occur independently of the status of the renin–angiotensin system, making these drugs effective antihypertensives even in patients with normal to low activity of the renin–angiotensin system. Following the chronic administration of an AT1 receptor antagonist, plasma renin activity increases as a result of removal of the angiotensin II negative feedback.

Pharmacokinetic Profiles of AT1 Receptor Antagonists

While all AT1 receptor antagonists share the same mechanism of action, they differ in their pharmacokinetic profiles. Losartan is well absorbed following oral administration and undergoes significant first-pass liver metabolism to an active metabolite, EXP3174. This metabolite is a long-acting (6–8 hours) noncompetitive antagonist at the AT1 receptor that contributes to the pharmacological effects of losartan. Production of the long-acting metabolite accounts for the sustained antihypertensive properties of losartan following chronic therapy, which would otherwise eventually be overwhelmed by removal of the negative feedback system (inhibition of renin release) for angiotensin II production. Following oral administration, 6% of losartan is excreted unchanged in the urine.

Valsartan has a higher affinity for the AT1 receptor than losartan, does not have an active metabolite, and has a slightly longer duration of action than losartan. Irbesartan exhibits high bioavailability and high affinity for the AT1 receptor, does not have an active metabolite, and has a considerably longer duration of action than losartan. Candesartan cilexetil has an active metabolite with a long duration of action, is a prodrug, and exhibits an AT1 receptor affinity 80 times that of losartan. Telmisartan is the longest-acting AT1 receptor antagonist and has no active metabolites. In contrast, eprosartan has the shortest half-life of the AT1 receptor antagonists and has been suggested to exhibit selective blockade of some effects of angiotensin II more than others.

Clinical Uses of AT1 Receptor Antagonists

Angiotensin type 1 receptor antagonists are effective as monotherapy in the treatment of hypertension. While all of the AT1 receptor antagonists are effective in the treatment of hypertension, several comparative studies have suggested that longer-acting AT1 receptor antagonists, such as irbesartan, candesartan, and telmisartan, may be more effective than the shorter-acting antagonists at providing 24-hour control of blood pressure. In large-scale clinical trials, AT1 receptor antagonists did not exhibit a clear advantage over ACE inhibitors in reducing morbidity and mortality from congestive heart failure. Therefore, the use of AT1 receptor antagonists in the treatment of congestive heart failure is generally restricted to patients who do not tolerate ACE inhibitors.

Adverse Effects of AT1 Receptor Antagonists

All AT1 receptor antagonists have adverse effects that are not significantly different from those of a placebo, although first-dose hypotension may occur. Unlike ACE inhibitors, AT1 receptor antagonists do not produce a cough, suggesting that this side effect may be related to the buildup of bradykinin levels that occurs as a result of converting enzyme inhibition rather than to a reduction in angiotensin II levels. An additional difference between AT1 receptor antagonists and ACE inhibitors is that angiotensin II is capable of interacting at the AT2 receptor in patients treated with an AT1 receptor antagonist (but not following inhibition of ACE). The clinical significance of this difference is not understood.

Finally, additional enzymes have been identified that are capable of forming angiotensin II from angiotensin I, suggesting that inhibition of ACE may not be sufficient for the total elimination of angiotensin II. In contrast, AT1 receptor antagonists are capable of blocking the effects of angiotensin II regardless of its enzymatic route of formation. All AT1 receptor antagonists, like the ACE inhibitors, are contraindicated during pregnancy.

ALDOSTERONE

Aldosterone, produced by the adrenal cortex, acts at epithelial cells in the distal tubule of the nephron to increase the reabsorption of sodium and is therefore considered an important hormone in the regulation of electrolyte balance. Aldosterone exerts its effects at the nephron through mineralocorticoid receptors, which translocate to the nucleus upon aldosterone binding and exert genomic effects leading to increased sodium reabsorption. In addition to the epithelial effects of aldosterone at mineralocorticoid receptors, nonepithelial cells, including cardiac muscle and vascular smooth muscle cells and cells in the brain, can respond to aldosterone and result in left ventricular hypertrophy, cardiac and vascular fibrosis, and stimulation of sympathetic nervous system activity.

Spironolactone (*Aldactone*), an antagonist of the aldosterone mineralocorticoid receptor, is used to treat primary aldosteronism, essential hypertension, and congestive heart failure (see Chapter 21). In the treatment of hypertension resulting from adrenal adenoma (primary aldosteronism) and in patients with essential hypertension, spironolactone lowers blood pressure primarily through blockade of epithelial mineralocorticoid receptors in the kidney, reductions in sodium and water reabsorption, and diuresis. The use of spironolactone in the treatment of essential hypertension is typically restricted to patients who do not respond appropriately to other agents and is often used in combination drug therapy. In large-scale clinical trials in patients with severe heart failure, administration of spironolactone markedly reduced morbidity and mortality without reducing blood pressure. Spironolactone is used to treat patients with moderate to severe heart failure who exhibit symptoms and ventricular dysfunction despite treatment with an ACE inhibitor or a diuretic.

Adverse effects of spironolactone therapy include hyperkalemia, gastrointestinal problems, gynecomastia (breast enlargement in males), and impotence. Gynecomastia and impotence arising from spironolactone treatment are results of significant blockade of the androgen and mineralocorticoid receptors. Novel selective mineralocorticoid receptor antagonists, such as eplerenone, are in clinical trials.

OTHER VASOACTIVE SUBSTANCES

Bradykinin

The kallikrein–kinin system is an enzymatic pathway giving rise to two predominant vasoactive peptides, kallidin and bradykinin. Kallikrein, the enzyme responsible for the formation of these peptides, exists in plasma and tissues. However, circulating levels of the end products, kallidin and bradykinin, are quite low because the kallikrein enzymes are present largely in inactive forms. In addition, the short half-life of these peptides (15 seconds) also contributes to low plasma levels. In general, the kinins produce relaxation of vascular smooth muscle and vasodilation. Bradykinin causes vascular smooth muscle relaxation by stimulating the endothelium to release prostacyclin and nitric oxide. Blood flow to the brain, heart, viscera, skeletal muscle, and glands is increased. In nonvascular smooth muscle, bradykinin will produce a contractile response.

Other actions of kinins include activation of clotting factors simultaneously with the production of bradykinin. In the kidney, bradykinin production results in an increase in renal papillary blood flow, with a secondary inhibition of sodium reabsorption in the distal tubule. In the peripheral nervous system, bradykinin is important for the initiation of pain signals. It is also associated with the edema, erythema, and fever of inflammation.

Bradykinin exerts its physiological effects via two receptors, the B1 and B2 receptors, with most of its physiological effects being mediated by the B2 receptor. The precise function of the B1 receptor is unclear; however, some of the chronic inflammatory responses to bradykinin may be mediated through actions at this receptor.

Bradykinin antagonists of the B2 receptor are currently in development and may find utility in the treatment of pain associated with burns and such chronic inflammatory disorders as arthritis, asthma, and chronic pain.

Endothelin

Endothelins are a family of vasoactive peptides secreted by endothelial cells. The three major endothelin peptides are all composed of 21 amino acids. *Endothelins are the most potent vasoconstrictors known.* Contraction of vascular smooth muscle in response to endothelin is associated with an increase in intracellular calcium. Increases in endothelin levels have been reported in patients with vasospastic, hypoxic, and ischemic diseases. The two identified isoforms of endothelin receptors have differing affinity for the three endothelin peptides. Selective and nonselective endothelin receptor antagonists are in development for potential use in the treatment of hypertension and other disorders associated with increased vascular resistance.

Natriuretic Peptides

Natriuretic peptides are naturally occurring substances in the body that oppose the activity of the renin–angiotensin system. The natriuretic peptide family consists of atrial natriuretic peptide (ANP), brain natriuretic peptide (BNP), and C-type natriuretic peptide (CNP). All three natriuretic peptides are synthesized from cleavage of a larger precursor polypeptide. In the ventricles and brain, the synthesis of BNP predominates; ANP is synthesized by cardiac myocytes predominately in the atria; and CNP is synthesized in the brain, blood vessels, and kidney.

All three peptides exhibit similar biological activities; however, they differ in the potency of individual responses. The target organs of the natriuretic peptides include the kidneys, blood vessels, brain, and adrenal cortex. These peptides exhibit potent diuretic, natriuretic, and vasodilator effects. Natriuretic peptides promote endothelial permeability and the movement of water from the intravascular to the extravascular space. In the kidney, natriuretic peptides increase the glomerular filtration rate through vasodilation of the afferent arteriole and constriction of the efferent arteriole, inhibition of the reabsorption of sodium in the proximal and distal tubule, and inhibition of renin synthesis. In the brain, natriuretic peptides are involved in the regulation of central control of cardiovascular functions. These biological effects of natriuretic peptides come together to reduce venous return and total peripheral resistance, thereby improving cardiac performance and reducing blood pressure.

The release of ANP from the heart is regulated acutely by stretch of atrial myocytes and has been used as a marker for cardiovascular diseases, including congestive heart failure and hypertension. In addition, recent results demonstrate an increase in the circulating concentration of ANP following stroke and linkage of the ANP gene to patients who have strokes. Two types of atrial natriuretic receptors have been identified in target tissues, including guanylate cyclase–linked receptors (subdivided into types A and B) and a receptor thought to serve as a clearance mechanism for the removal of circulating ANP. Analogues that act as ANP agonists are being developed for use in hypertension and congestive heart failure.

In addition, a new class of drugs, termed vasopeptidase inhibitors, inhibit the enzymatic activity of ACE and neutral endopeptidase, the enzyme responsible for the breakdown of natriuretic peptides. The end result is a reduction in the synthesis of angiotensin II and an increase in the circulating level of natriuretic peptides such as ANP. Omapatrilat, a vasopeptidase inhibitor, is under study for the treatment of hypertension and congestive heart failure.

Nitric Oxide

Nitric oxide is a small, unstable free radical that acts as a biological messenger in many physiological responses. Because it can diffuse freely in all directions from its site of origin, regulation of the activity of nitric oxide is primarily through control of its synthesis. Formation of nitric oxide occurs through oxidation of the amino acid L-arginine, a reaction catalyzed by the enzyme nitric oxide synthase (NOS), to produce nitric oxide and L-citrulline. The forms of NOS differ in their cellular location and expression (constitutive expression versus inducible expression). Activation of synthesis of the inducible form of NOS results in continued synthesis of nitric oxide for several hours. Inhibitors of NOS are analogues of arginine, including L-Nw nitroarginine (L- NNA) and L-Nw methylarginine (L-NMA), both of which decrease nitric oxide synthesis.

Physiological sites proposed for nitric oxide action include the immune system, where nitric oxide acts as a cytostatic agent, is tumoricidal, and can inhibit viral replication. In the cardiovascular system, nitric oxide is the biological mediator of vasodilator responses to agents such as acetylcholine and bradykinin, which act as receptors on endothelial cells to activate NOS and stimulate nitric oxide production. Diffusible nitric oxide then activates guanylate cyclase in vascular smooth muscle cells, leading to the production of cyclic guanosine monophosphate (GMP) and vasodilation. In the brain, stimulation of N-methyl-D-aspartate receptors on neurons leads to activation of the brain form of NOS and stimulates production of nitric oxide. The function of brain nitric oxide is thought to involve actions as a retrograde neurotransmitter whereby nitric oxide diffuses back to the presynaptic neuron to activate guanylate cyclase and increase cyclic GMP levels. Through these retrograde actions nitric oxide is thought to play a role in the neural circuitry involved in memory.

Even though nitric oxide is the physiological mediator of a variety of responses, excess nitric oxide is toxic to many cells as a result of its role in the production of peroxynitrite and resultant lipid oxidation. Inhibitors of the NOS enzyme are in clinical trials for the treatment of hypotension associated with septic shock. Administration of low concentrations of nitric oxide through respiratory ventilators has been implemented to treat persistent pulmonary hypertension of the newborn.

Study QUESTIONS

1. An accurate statement regarding the actions of both ACE inhibitors and AT1 receptor antagonists is that
   (A) Both classes of drugs increase bradykinin.
   (B) Angiotensin II can act at the AT2 receptor with both classes of drugs.
   (C) Both classes of drugs reduce total peripheral resistance.
   (D) Both classes of drugs decrease circulating angiotensin II levels.
   (E) Both classes of drugs are first-choice treatments for congestive heart failure.

2. Angiotensin II can
   (A) Increase the synthesis and release of aldosterone
   (B) Reduce the activity of the sympathetic nervous system
   (C) Be a potent positive inotropic at the heart
   (D) Relax vascular smooth muscle
   (E) Reduce the growth of cardiovascular cell types

3. The most potent vasoconstrictor known is
   (A) Bradykinin
   (B) Angiotensin II
   (C) Angiotensin IV
   (D) Natriuretic peptide
   (E) Endothelin

4. The mechanism of action of captopril is
   (A) Angiotensin receptor antagonist
   (B) ACE inhibitor
   (C) Aldosterone receptor antagonist
   (D) Bradykinin antagonist

5. L-Argenine serves as a precursor for
   (A) Bradykinin
   (B) L-Citrulline
   (C) Nitrous oxide
   (D) Atrial natriuretic peptide

ANSWERS

1. **C.** ACE inhibitors increase circulating bradykinin levels, while AT1 receptor antagonists have no effect on circulating bradykinin. The ability of converting enzyme inhibitors to increase bradykinin levels is thought to contribute to the benefits of this class of drugs in the treatment of hypertension and heart failure. With an ACE inhibitor, the actions of angiotensin II at both the AT1 and the AT2 receptor is decreased; however, with an AT1 receptor antagonist, angiotensin II can act at the AT2 receptor. Only ACE inhibitors decrease circulating angiotensin II levels; the level of angiotensin II may actually increase with an AT1 receptor antagonist because of removal of the endocrine feedback loop. ACE inhibitors have proven benefits in the treatment of congestive heart failure, while AT1 receptor antagonists are reserved for therapy of patients who have significant adverse effects from converting enzyme inhibition.

2. **A.** Angiotensin II has diverse physiological effects, including stimulating the synthesis and release of aldosterone from the adrenal cortex. This effect of angiotensin II results in fluid and water retention. The other answers are incorrect in that angiotensin II

stimulates the sympathetic nervous system, is a weak inotropic, contracts vascular smooth muscle, and increases the growth status of cardiovascular cell types.

3. **E.** Bradykinin and natriuretic peptide are vasodilators. Both angiotensin II and angiotensin IV are vasoconstrictors but not nearly as potent as any endothelin peptide.

4. **B.** Compounds that act as ACE inhibitors are particularly useful for the treatment of hypertension and congestive heart failure.

5. **C.** Nitric oxide is an important compound that acts as a biological messenger in many physiological responses. L-Citrulline is a product of the oxidation of L-argenine in the formation of nitric oxide. Bradykinin is formed from a precursor kininogen.

Atrial natriuretic peptide is synthesized by cleavage of a larger precursor polypeptide.

SUPPLEMENTAL READING

Bhoola K et al. Bioregulation of kinins: Kallikreins, kininogens, and kininases. Pharmacol Rev 1992;44:1–80.

Brown NJ and Vaughan DE. Angiotensin-converting enzyme inhibitors. Circulation 1998;97:1411–1420.

Burnier M. Angiotensin II type 1 receptor blockers. Circulation 2001;103:904–912.

Corti R et al. Vasopeptidase inhibitors: A new therapeutic concept in cardiovascular disease? Circulation 2001;104:1856–1892.

Saavedra JM and Timmermans PBMWM. Angiotensin Receptors. New York: Plenum, 1994.

CASE Study   Congestive Heart Failure with Complications

A. D. has refused to go for a yearly physical examination for more than 15 years despite a family history of cardiovascular disease. Over the past 6 months, A. D. has had to cut down and then eliminate his weekly soccer games because of extreme shortness of breath. Exasperated over his inability to exercise, A. D. goes to a primary care physician and is diagnosed with moderate to severe hypertension with a markedly enlarged heart. Unfortunately, A. D. has significant liver impairment from a previous bout of hepatitis. Based on knowledge of the renin–angiotensin system and the specifics concerning drugs targeted against this system, provide a rationale for use of two drugs to treat the cardiovascular disease in this patient.

ANSWER: This patient has congestive heart failure from long-standing hypertension. In addition, the patient has compromised liver function, limiting the choice of drug. Drugs that inhibit the renin–angiotensin system, specifically ACE inhibitors, are indicated in the treatment of both hypertension and congestive heart failure. Therefore, an ACE inhibitor is a rational pharmacological approach in this patient. However, the compromised liver function requires caution with any drug that requires liver metabolism for formation of the active drug moiety (i.e., prodrugs), or for drugs that are primarily eliminated by liver metabolism. With the exception of captopril and lisinopril, all of the available ACE inhibitors are prodrugs and require liver metabolism for elimination. Therefore, either captopril or lisinopril would be an appropriate ACE inhibitor in the treatment of this patient. AT1 receptor antagonists are indicated for the treatment of hypertension and when converting enzyme inhibitors are contraindicated in the therapy of congestive heart failure. Of this class of compounds, eprosartan, valsartan, and telmisartan do not require liver metabolism to produce an active compound.

19 Calcium Channel Blockers

Vijay C. Swamy and David J. Triggle

 DRUG LIST

GENERIC NAME	PAGE	GENERIC NAME	PAGE
Amlodipine	218	Nifedipine	218
Diltiazem	218	Nimodipine	218
Felodipin	218	Nisoldapine	218
Isradipine	220	Verapamil	218
Nicardipine	218		

The agents commonly called the *calcium channel blockers* comprise an increasing number of agents, including the prototypical verapamil (*Calan, Isoptin*), nifedipine (*Adalat, Procardia*), and diltiazem (*Cardizem*). These agents are a chemically and pharmacologically heterogeneous group of synthetic drugs, but they possess the common property of selectively antagonizing Ca^{++} movements that underlie the process of excitation–contraction coupling in the cardiovascular system. *The primary use of these agents is in the treatment of angina, selected cardiac arrhythmias, and hypertension.*

Although the Ca^{++} channel blockers are potent vasodilating drugs, they lack the fluid-accumulating properties of other vasodilators and the persistent activation of the sympathetic and renin–angiotensin–aldosterone axes. Furthermore, the broad potential range of activities, both within and without the cardiovascular system, suggests that they may be clinically useful in disorders from vertigo to failure of gastrointestinal smooth muscle to relax .

A number of second-generation analogues are known, particularly in the nifedipine (1,4-dihydropyridine) series, including nimodipine (*Nimotop*), nicardip-ine (*Cardene*), felodipine (*Plendil*), nisoldipine (*Sular*), and amlodipine (*Norvasc*). These agents differ from nifedipine principally in their potency, pharmacokinetic characteristics, and selectivity of action. Nimodipine has selectivity for the cerebral vasculature; amlodipine exhibits very slow kinetics of onset and offset of blockade; and felodipine and nisoldipine are vascular-selective 1,4-dihydropyridines.

CALCIUM ANTAGONISM

The concept of calcium antagonism as a specific mechanism of drug action was pioneered by Albrecht Fleckenstein and his colleagues, who observed that verapamil and subsequently other drugs of this class mimicked in reversible fashion the effects of Ca^{++} withdrawal on cardiac excitability. These drugs inhibited the Ca^{++} component of the ionic currents carried in the cardiac action potential. Because of this activity, these drugs are also referred to as *slow channel blockers, calcium channel antagonists, and calcium entry blockers.*

The actions of these drugs must be viewed from the perspective of cellular Ca^{++} regulation (Fig. 19.1). Ca^{++} is fundamentally important as a messenger, linking cellular excitation and cellular response. This role is made possible by the high inwardly directed Ca^{++} concentration and electrochemical gradients, by the existence of specific high-affinity Ca^{++} binding proteins (e.g., calmodulin) that serve as intracellular Ca^{++} receptors, and by the existence of Ca^{++}-specific influx, efflux, and sequestration processes. Calcium, in excess, serves as a mediator of cell destruction and death during myocardial and neuronal ischemia, neuronal degeneration, and cellular toxicity. The control of excess Ca^{++} mobilization is thus an important contributor to cell and tissue protection.

The available Ca^{++} channel blockers exert their effects primarily at voltage-gated Ca^{++} channels of the plasma membrane. There are at least several types of channels—L, T, N, P/Q and R—distinguished by their electrophysiological and pharmacological characteristics. The blockers act at the L-type channel at three distinct receptor sites (Fig. 19.2). These different receptor interactions underlie, in part, the qualitative and quantitative differences exhibited by the three principal classes of channel blockers.

Cellular stimuli that involve Ca^{++} mobilization by processes other than that at the L-type voltage-gated channels will be either completely or relatively insensitive to the channel blockers. This differential sensitivity contributes to the variable sensitivity of vascular and

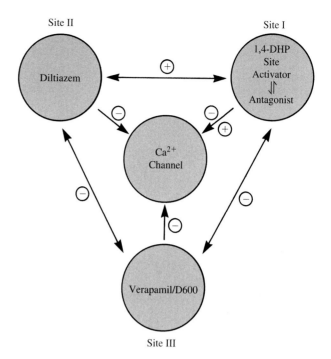

FIGURE 19.2

The principal receptors or drug binding sites at the calcium channel. These sites are linked to the opening and closing of the channel and to each other by activating (+) or inhibiting (−) allosteric mechanisms. The 1,4-DHP site is a receptor site for a number of 1,4-dihydropyridine compounds; D600 is the designation for a close chemical relative of verapamil.

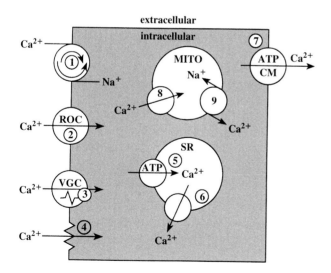

FIGURE 19.1

Cellular calcium regulation. Depicted are several sites that control calcium entry, efflux, and sequestration. *1.* Na$^+$, Ca^{++} exchange. *2.* Receptor-operated channels. *3.* Voltage-gated channels. *4.* Leak pathways. *5, 6.* Entry and efflux in sarcoplasmic reticulum. *7.* Plasma membrane pump. *8, 9.* Entry and efflux in mitochondria. ATP, adenosine triphosphate; CM, cell membrane.

nonvascular smooth muscle to the actions of these drugs, for example, the regional vascular selectivity and the general lack of activity of these agents in respiratory or gastrointestinal smooth muscle disorders.

The Selectivity of Action of Calcium Channel Blockers

Although the available Ca^{++} channel blockers exert their effects through an interaction at one type of channel, they do so at different sites. Figure 19.2 shows that the channel blockers act at three discrete receptor sites to mediate channel blockade indirectly rather than by a direct or physical channel block. The existence of the different receptor sites is one basis for the different pharmacological profiles exhibited by these agents.

The activity of the Ca^{++} channel blockers increases with increasing frequency of stimulation or intensity and duration of membrane depolarization. *This use-dependent activity is consistent with a preferred interaction of the antagonists with the open or inactivated states of the Ca^{++} channel rather than with the resting state.* This activity is not shared equally by all Ca^{++} blockers and so may provide a further basis for the therapeutic differences between them. For example, verapamil and diltiazem are approximately equipotent in cardiac and vascular smooth muscle, whereas nifedipine and all other agents of the 1,4-dihydropyridine class are significantly more active in vascular smooth muscle. Furthermore, different members of the 1,4-dihydropyridine class have different degrees of vascular selectivity. These differences are broadly consistent with the observation that verapamil and diltiazem act preferentially through the open channel state, and nifedipine and its analogues act through the inactivated state.

The clinically available calcium channel antagonists have also proved to be invaluable as molecular probes with which to identify, isolate, and characterize calcium channels of the voltage-gated family. In particular, the 1,4-dihydropyridines with their high affinity, agonist–antagonist properties, and selectivity have become defined as molecular markers for the L-type channel.

Synthetic drugs of comparable selectivity and affinity to the 1,4-dihydropyridines do not yet exist for the other channel types, T, N, P/Q, and R; these remain characterized by complex polypeptide toxins of the aga- and conotoxin classes. Neuronal pharmacology, including that of the central nervous system (CNS), is dominated by the N, P/Q, and R channels. This underscores the normally weak effect of L-channel antagonists on CNS function. Drugs that act at the N, P, and R channels with comparable selectivity and affinity to the 1,4-dihydropyridines may be expected to offer major potential for a variety of CNS disorders, including neuronal damage and death from ischemic insults.

The Ca^{++} channel blockers also differ in the extent of their additional pharmacological properties. Verapamil and to a lesser extent diltiazem possess a number of receptor-blocking properties, together with Na^+ and K^+ channel–blocking activities, that may contribute to their pharmacological profile. Nifedipine and other 1,4-dihydropyridines are more selective for the voltage-gated Ca^{++} channel, but they may also affect other pharmacological properties because their nonpolar properties may lead to cellular accumulation. Together with their channel-blocking properties, these properties may contribute to the recently described antiatherogenic actions seen in experimental and clinical states.

PHARMACOLOGICAL EFFECTS ON THE CARDIOVASCULAR SYSTEM

The effects of the prototypical calcium channel blockers are seen most prominently in the cardiovascular system (Table 19.1), although calcium channels are widely distributed among excitable cells. The following calcium channel–blocking drugs are clinically the most widely used compounds in this very extensive class of pharmacological agents: amlodipine, diltiazem, isradipine, nifedipine, nicardipine, nimodipine, and verapamil.

Vascular Effects

Vascular tone and contraction are determined largely by the availability of calcium from extracellular sources (influx via calcium channels) or intracellular stores. *Drug-induced inhibition of calcium influx via voltage-gated channels results in widespread dilation and a decrease in contractile responses to stimulatory agents.* In general, arteries and arterioles are more sensitive to the relaxant actions of these drugs than are the veins, and some arterial beds (e.g., coronary and cerebral vessels) show greater sensitivity than others. Peripheral vasodilation and the consequent fall in blood pressure are commonly accompanied by reflex tachycardia when nifedipine and its analogues are used; this is in contrast to verapamil and diltiazem, whose effects on peripheral vessels are accompanied by cardiodepressant effects.

Cardiac Effects

Calcium currents in cardiac tissues serve the functions of inotropy, pacemaker activity (sinoatrial (SA) node), and conduction at the atrioventricular (A-V) node. In principle, the blockade of calcium currents should result in decreased function at these sites. In clinical use, how-

TABLE 19.1 Cardiovascular Effects of Calcium Channel Blockers*

	Nifedipine	Diltiazem	Verapamil
Blood pressure	−	−	−
Vasodilation	+++	++	++
Heart rate	++	−	±
Contractility	0/+	0	0/−
Coronary vascular resistance	−	−	−
Blood flow	+++	+++	++

Key: + = increase; − = decrease; 0 = no significant effect.
*Changes are those seen commonly following oral doses used in therapy of hypertension or angina.
The magnitude of response is indicated by number of symbols.

ever, dose-dependent depression is seen only with verapamil and diltiazem and not with nifedipine, reflecting mainly differences in the kinetics of their interaction at calcium channels (see section on calcium antagonism). *Characteristic cardiac effects include a variable slowing of the heart rate, strong depression of conduction at the A-V node, and inhibition of contractility, especially in the presence of preexisting heart failure.*

THERAPEUTIC APPLICATIONS

The calcium channel–blocking drugs have been investigated for an unusually wide number of clinical applications. Verapamil-induced improvement of diastolic function has proved to be beneficial in the treatment of hypertrophic cardiomyopathy. Vasodilatory properties of these drugs are used in the treatment of peripheral vasoconstrictive disorders (Raynaud's disease) and in relieving vasospasm following subarachnoid hemorrhage. There is ongoing interest in investigating protective effects on renal function and in the ability to reduce deleterious vascular changes in diabetes mellitus. Similarly, the potential benefit afforded by their selective vasodilatory action (especially the second-generation agents) in the management of heart failure is an area of interest. These drugs are of some benefit in a variety of noncardiovascular conditions characterized by hyperactivity of smooth muscle (e.g., achalasia). However, their main applications are as follows.

Hypertension

The calcium channel–blocking drugs are effective antihypertensive agents and enjoy widespread use as single medication or in combination. *Their effectiveness is related to a decrease in peripheral resistance accompanied by increases in cardiac index.* The magnitude of their effects is determined partly by pretreatment blood pressure levels; maximum blood pressure lowering generally is seen 3 to 4 weeks after the start of treatment. These drugs possess some distinct advantages relative to other vasodilators, including the following:

1. Their relaxant effect on large arteries results in greater compliance, which is beneficial in older persons.
2. Tolerance associated with renal retention of fluid does not occur; an initial natriuretic effect is often observed, especially with the nifedipine group of blockers.
3. They do not have significant effects on the release of renin or cause long-term changes in lipid or glucose metabolism.
4. Postural hypotension, first-dose effect, and rebound phenomenon are not commonly seen.

Their antihypertensive efficacy is comparable to that of β-adrenergic blockers and angiotensin-converting enzyme (ACE) inhibitors. The choice of a calcium channel blocker, especially for combination therapy, is largely influenced by the effect of the drug on cardiac pacemakers and contractility and coexisting diseases, such as angina, asthma, and peripheral vascular disease.

Ischemic Heart Disease

The effectiveness and use of calcium channel blockers in the management of angina are well established (see Chapter 17); their benefit in postinfarction stages is less certain. Efficacy in angina is largely derived from their hemodynamic effects, which influence the supply and demand components of the ischemic balance (1) by increasing blood flow directly or by increasing collateral blood flow and (2) by decreasing afterload and reducing oxygen demand. *All three agents are useful in the management of stable exertional angina,* with their vasodilatory and cardiac effects making beneficial contributions. Given the differences in their relative effects (Table 19.1), the response of the patient can vary with the agent used and the preexisting cardiac status.

All agents are also effective in the control of variant (Prinzmetal's) angina, in which spasm of the coronary arteries is the main factor. Their usefulness in the more complex unstable (preinfarction) angina is less definite, depending on the hemodynamic status and the susceptibility of the patient to infarction.

Cardiac Arrhythmias

The prominent depressant action of verapamil and diltiazem at the SA and A-V nodes finds use in specific arrhythmias. *They are of proven efficacy in acute control and long-term management of paroxysmal supraventricular tachycardia* (see Chapter 16). Their ability to inhibit conduction at the A-V node is employed in protecting ventricles from atrial tachyarrhythmias, often in combination with digitalis or propranolol.

PHARMACOKINETICS

A comparison of the pharmacokinetic properties of these agents is listed in Table 19.2. All three drugs are well absorbed following oral administration. Verapamil and diltiazem undergo greater first-pass metabolism relative to nifedipine, resulting in lower bioavailability of the former two drugs. Hepatic metabolism of nifedipine is complete, yielding inactive metabolites; this is unlike verapamil and diltiazem, whose metabolites have pharmacological activity. Verapamil is metabolized stereoselectively in favor of the more active (−) enantiomer, thus requiring higher plasma concentrations after oral administration.

TABLE 19.2 Pharmacokinetics of Calcium Channel Blockers

	Verapamil	Nifedipine	Diltiazem
Absorption, oral (%)	>90	>90	>90
Bioavailability (%)	20	60–80	~40
Onset of action: oral (min)	90–120	<20	<30
Peak effect	5 hr	1–2 hr	3–5 hr
Protein binding (%)	90	90	90
Plasma half-life	4–8 hr	5 hr*	5 hr
Metabolism	80% 1st-pass active metabolites	Inactive metabolites	60% of 1st dose: 10% steady state
Excretion			
Renal (%)	70	90	30
Fecal (%)	15	10	70

*Six to 11 hours after oral tablets: above value for capsules.

TOXICITY

The common side effects seen in chronic therapy (Table 19.3) are mostly related to vasodilation—headaches, dizziness, facial flushing, hypotension, and so forth. High doses of verapamil in elderly patients are known to cause constipation. Serious side effects, especially following the intravenous use of verapamil, include marked negative inotropic effects and depression of preexisting sick sinus syndrome, A-V nodal disease, and enhancement of the action of other cardiodepressant drugs. Their use is generally contraindicated in obstructive conditions (e.g., aortic stenosis). No consistent or significant changes in lipid and glucose levels have been reported with chronic therapy. Non–sustained release formulations of nifedipine are contraindicated in hypertension because of sympathetic rebound that may aggravate existing left ventricular dysfunction.

TABLE 19.3 Adverse Effects of Calcium Channel Blockers

	Verapamil	Diltiazem	Nifedipine
Tachycardia	0	0	+
Decreased heart rate*	+	+	0
Depressed A-V nodal conduction*	+++	++	0
Negative inotropy	++	+	0
Vasodilation (flushing, edema, hypotension, headaches)	+	+/0	+++
Constipation, nausea	++	+	+/0

Key: + = increase; 0 = no change.
*Marked effect in presence of sick sinus syndrome and A-V nodal disease.

Study QUESTIONS

1. Which of the following statements most accurately characterize the cellular action of the calcium channel blockers?
(A) Their interaction with membrane phospholipids results in a nonselective decrease of ion transport.
(B) They inhibit the Na^+–Ca^{++} exchanger in cardiac and smooth muscle.
(C) They interact at three distinct sites at the L-type voltage-gated calcium channels.
(D) Their interaction with the sodium pump results in an inhibition of calcium transport.

2. Which of the following calcium channel blockers would be most likely to suppress atrial tachyarrhythmias involving the A-V node?
(A) Nifedipine
(B) Verapamil
(C) Nicardipine
(D) Amlodipine

3. All of the following statements are applicable with regard to the systemic effects caused by nifedipine EXCEPT:
(A) It typically causes peripheral vasodilation.
(B) It often elicits reflex tachycardia.
(C) It causes coronary vasodilatation and an increase in coronary blood flow.
(D) Its benefit in the management of angina is related to the reduction in preload that it induces.

4. All of the following statements regarding the pharmacokinetics of calcium channel blockers are correct EXCEPT
(A) They are characterized by significant amount (~ 90%) of protein binding.
(B) They undergo significant first-pass metabolism.
(C) Their half-life is not altered by hepatic cirrhosis.
(D) They can be administered orally.

5. All of the following adverse effects are likely to occur with long-term use of calcium channel blockers EXCEPT
(A) Skeletal muscle weakness
(B) Flushing
(C) Dizziness
(D) Headache

ANSWERS

1. **C.** The available blockers act primarily at voltage-gated calcium channels of the L type. The three prototypes, verapamil, nifedipine, and diltiazem, act at three discrete sites at this channel.
2. **B.** The other three drugs (dihydropyridines) are characterized by relatively selective vasodilator effects with little if any cardiac effects at doses employed clinically for hypertension or angina.
3. **D.** The vasodilatory effects of nifedipine are largely restricted to arteries (and consequently the afterload). It does not alter venous tone (and thus preload) significantly.
4. **C.** Since they are metabolized in the liver, hepatic cirrhosis can be expected to alter their half-life.
5. **A.** Skeletal muscles depend on the mobilization of intracellular stores of calcium for their contractile responses rather than transmembrane flux of calcium through the calcium channels. Therefore, skeletal muscle weakness is not likely to occur.

SUPPLEMENTAL READING
Abernathy DR and Schwartz JB. Calcium-antagonist drugs. N Engl J Med 1999;34:1447–1457.
Epstein M (Ed.). Calcium Antagonists in Clinical Medicine (3rd Ed.). Philadelphia: Hanley & Belfus, 2002.
Kizer JR and Kimmel SE. Epidemiologic review of the calcium channel blocker drugs: An up-to-date perspective on the proposed hazards. Arch Intern Med 2001;161:1145–1158.
Taira N. Differences in cardiovascular profile among calcium antagonists. Am J Cardiol 1987;59:24B–29B.
Triggle DJ. Mechanisms of action of calcium channel antagonists. In Epstein EM (Ed.). Calcium Antagonists in Clinical Medicine (3rd Ed.). Philadelphia: Hanley & Belfus, 2002.
Tulenko TN et al. The smooth muscle membrane during atherogenesis: A potential target in atheroprotection. Am Heart J 2001;141(2Suppl): S1–S11.

CASE **Study**   **Nifedipine-Induced Vasodilatation**

A 65-year-old recently retired man is being evaluated for elevated blood pressure. He occasionally has angina precipitated by physical exertion and rapidly controlled by sublingual use of nitroglycerin. His blood pressure is 160/100 mm Hg. He is advised to take nifedipine 80 mg/day, which he does, in divided doses of 20 mg (capsules). He develops flushing, dizziness, and nervousness shortly (<30 minutes) after taking the drug, and these symptoms persist for approximately 1 hour. The number of anginal episodes have increased during this period. QUESTION: How do the properties of nifedipine relate to the above development?

ANSWER: Nifedipine, unless formulated for slow, sustained release, is characterized by relatively rapid onset of vasodilatory effects. This man's side effects reflect the rapid and intense fall in blood pressure and consequent reflex increases in sympathetic tone. The increase in anginal episodes also is a result of drug-induced periodic increases in heart rate.

20 Antihypertensive Drugs

David P. Westfall

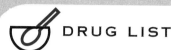

DRUG LIST

GENERIC NAME	PAGE	GENERIC NAME	PAGE
Clonidine	236	Minoxidil	229
Diazoxide	229	Phentolamine	231
Guanabenz	236	Phenoxybenzamine	231
Guanethidine	233	Prazosin	231
Guanfacine	236	Propranolol	233
Hydralazine	228	Reserpine	234
α-Methyldopa	235	Sodium nitroprusside	230
Metyrosine	235		

Hypertension is one of the most serious concerns of modern medical practice. It is estimated that in the United States, as many as 60 million people are hypertensive or are being treated with antihypertensive drugs. Among the growing population of elderly Americans, some 15 million have high blood pressure. The level of blood pressure in itself is not a chief concern, since individuals with high blood pressure may be asymptomatic for many years. What is of prime significance is that *hypertension has been shown convincingly to be the single most important contributing factor to cardiovascular disease,* the leading cause of morbidity and untimely death in the United States.

The actual level of pressure that can be considered hypertensive is difficult to define; it depends on a number of factors, including the patient's age, sex, race, and lifestyle. As a working definition, many cardiovascular treatment centers consider that a diastolic pressure of 90 mm Hg or higher or a systolic pressure of 140 mm Hg or higher represents hypertension. In this chapter, reference is made to the stages of hypertension according to the recommendations of the Sixth Joint National Committee on the Detection, Evaluation, and Treatment of High Blood Pressure. Hypertension is considered to be *stage I, or mild,* if diastolic pressure is 90 to 99 mm Hg and/or systolic pressure is 140 to 159 mm Hg. *Stage II,* or *moderate,* hypertension is diastolic pressure of 100 to 109 mm Hg and/or systolic pressure of 160 to 179 mm Hg. *Stage III,* or *severe,* hypertension exists when diastolic pressure is 110 mm Hg or greater and/or systolic pressure is 180 mm Hg or greater.

These values should not be considered as absolutes but rather as indicators for facilitating discussion, particularly in relation to the indications for use of specific drugs. Since in general terms *hypertension* can be defined as the level of blood pressure at which there is risk, the ultimate judgment concerning the severity of hypertension in any given individual must also include a consideration of factors other than diastolic or systolic pressure.

The aim of therapy is straightforward: *reduction of blood pressure to within the normal range.* When hypertension is secondary to a known organic disease, such as renovascular disease or pheochromocytoma, therapy is directed toward correction of the underlying malady. Unfortunately, about 90% of cases of hypertension are of unknown etiology. The therapy of *primary,* or *essential hypertension,* as these cases are generally called, is often empirical.

There are three general approaches to the pharmacological treatment of primary hypertension. The first involves the use of diuretics to reduce blood volume. The second employs drugs that interfere with the renin–angiotensin system, and the third is aimed at a drug-induced reduction in peripheral vascular resistance, cardiac output, or both. A reduction in peripheral vascular resistance can be achieved directly by relaxing vascular smooth muscle with drugs known as vasodilators or indirectly by modifying the activity of the sympathetic nervous system.

The directly acting vasodilators, with the exception of calcium channel antagonists and sympathetic nervous system depressants, receive the bulk of attention in this chapter. Other chapters offer additional information on diuretics (see Chapter 21), the renin–angiotensin system (see Chapter 18), adrenergic receptor antagonists (see Chapter 11), and the calcium channel antagonists (Chapter 19).

DIURETICS

The exact mechanisms by which diuretics lower blood pressure are not entirely understood. Initially, diuretics produce a mild degree of Na^+ depletion, which leads to a decrease in extracellular fluid volume and cardiac output. The effectiveness of diuretic therapy in mild hypertension may also involve either interference with or blunting of cardiovascular reflexes. Regardless of the details, there is general agreement that the blood pressure–lowering effects of diuretics do ultimately depend on the production of diuresis. *High salt intake or low rates or glomerular filtration will eliminate the antihypertensive effects of the drugs.*

The value of diuretics lies in their ability to reverse the Na^+ retention commonly associated with many antihypertensive drugs that probably induce Na^+ retention and fluid volume expansion as a compensatory response to blood pressure reduction.

When diuretic therapy is indicated for the treatment of primary hypertension, the thiazide-type compounds (e.g., chlorothiazide, hydrochlorothiazide) are generally the drugs of choice. *They can be used alone or in combination with other antihypertensive agents.* Approximately 30% of patients with mild hypertension may be treated effectively with thiazide therapy alone.

Thiazide diuretics are not the drugs of choice in patients with renal insufficiency. In this situation, the loop diuretics furosemide and bumetanide are recommended; they have greater intrinsic natriuretic potency than do the thiazides and do not depress renal blood flow.

In situations of known renin–angiotensin–aldosterone involvement, such as in hypertension secondary to renal disease (i.e., renovascular hypertension), diuretics probably should not be used because they further elevate plasma renin.

The K^+-sparing action of spironolactone, triamterene, and amiloride serves as the basis for their occasional use in the therapy of primary hypertension. The drugs can be employed in conjunction with other types of diuretics to help alleviate the K^+ loss caused by them. Under these conditions, K^+ balance is improved while natriuresis is maintained.

Additional information concerning details of diuretic pharmacology is found in Chapter 21.

VASODILATORS

The drugs discussed in this section produce a direct relaxation of vascular smooth muscle and thereby their actions result in vasodilation. This effect is called *direct* because it does not depend on the innervation of vascular smooth muscle and is not mediated by receptors, such as adrenoceptors, cholinoreceptors, or receptors for histamine, that are acted on by classical transmitters and mediators.

The vasodilators decrease total peripheral resistance and thus correct the hemodynamic abnormality that is responsible for the elevated blood pressure in primary hypertension. In addition, because they act directly on vascular smooth muscle, the vasodilators are *effective in lowering blood pressure, regardless of the etiology of the hypertension.* Unlike many other antihypertensive agents, the vasodilators do not inhibit the activity of the sympathetic nervous system; therefore, orthostatic hypotension and impotence are not problems. Additionally, most vasodilators relax arterial smooth muscle to a greater extent than venous smooth muscle, thereby further minimizing postural hypotension.

Although vasodilators would appear to be ideal drugs for the treatment of hypertension, their effectiveness, particularly when they are used chronically, is severely limited by neuroendocrine and autonomic reflexes that tend to counteract the fall in blood pressure. How these reflexes compromise the fall in blood pressure produced by the vasodilators is shown in Fig. 20.1. The diagram does not show all of the possible interrelationships but rather is meant to draw attention to the most prominent reflex changes. These reflexes include an augmentation of sympathetic nervous activity that leads

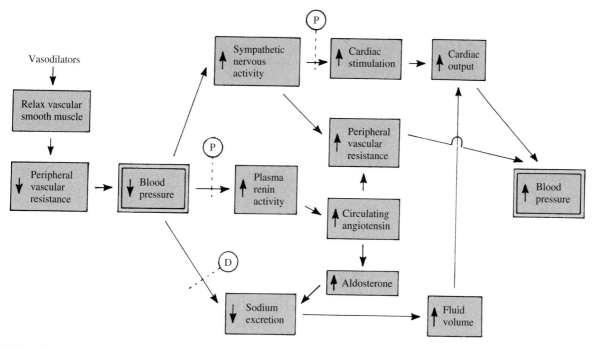

FIGURE 20.1

Neuroendocrine pathways that are activated when vasodilators decrease blood pressure. These pathways lead ultimately to an increase in blood pressure and thus compromise the effectiveness of the vasodilators. The effectiveness can be preserved by coadminstration of propranolol (P) and a diuretic (D).

to an increase in heart rate and cardiac output. Large increases in cardiac output occurring as a result of vasodilator therapy will substantially counter the drug-induced reduction of blood pressure. Increased reflex sympathetic input to the heart also augments myocardial oxygen demand; this is especially serious in patients with coronary insufficiency and little cardiac reserve.

Plasma renin activity is elevated after treatment with vasodilators. The hyperreninemia appears to be due in part to enhanced sympathetic nervous activity. Elevated renin levels lead to an increase in the concentration of circulating angiotensin, a potent vasoconstrictor (see Chapter 18) and thus an increase in peripheral vascular resistance.

Thus, it seems that the lack of sympathetic nervous system inhibition produced by the vasodilators, which is advantageous in some ways, can also be a disadvantage in that reflex increases in sympathetic nerve activity will lead to hemodynamic changes that reduce the effectiveness of the drugs. *Therefore, the vasodilators are generally inadequate as the sole therapy for hypertension.* However, many of the factors that limit the usefulness of the vasodilators can be obviated when they are administered in combination with a β-*adrenoceptor antagonist,* such as propranolol, and a *diuretic.* Propranolol reduces the cardiac stimulation that occurs in response to increases in sympathetic nervous activity, and the

large increase in cardiac output caused by the vasodilators will be reduced. Propranolol also reduces plasma renin levels, and that is an additional benefit. The reduction in Na^+ excretion and the increase in plasma volume that occurs with vasodilator therapy can be reduced by concomitant treatment with a diuretic. These relationships are shown in Fig. 20.1.

Mechanism of Action

Available evidence suggests that a single unifying mechanism does not exist but rather that various vasodilators may act at different places in the series of processes that couple excitation of vascular smooth muscle cells with contraction. For example, the vasodilators known as calcium channel antagonists block or limit the entry of calcium through voltage-dependent channels in the membrane of vascular smooth muscle cells. In this way, the calcium channel blockers limit the amount of free intracellular calcium available to interact with smooth muscle contractile proteins (see Chapter 14).

Other vasodilators, such as diazoxide and minoxidil, cause dilation of blood vessels by activating potassium channels in vascular smooth muscle. An increase in potassium conductance results in hyperpolarization of the cell membrane, which will cause relaxation of vascular smooth muscle.

Another group of drugs, the so-called nitrovasodilators, of which nitroprusside is an example, activate soluble guanylate cyclase in vascular smooth muscle, which brings about an increase in the intracellular levels of cyclic guanosine monophosphate (cGMP). Increases in cGMP are associated with vascular smooth muscle relaxation. The action of the nitrovasodilators appears to be quite similar to that of the endogenous vasodilator released by a variety of stimuli from endothelial cells of blood vessels. This substance, originally named endothelial-derived relaxing factor, or EDRF, is nitric oxide or a closely related nitrosothiol compound. *The knowledge that the nitrovasodilators generate nitric oxide in vivo suggests that this substance may be the final common mediator of a number of vascular smooth muscle relaxants.*

This chapter describes four vasodilators in detail. Two of these agents, *hydralazine* and *minoxidil*, are effective orally and are used for the chronic treatment of primary hypertension. The other two drugs, *diazoxide* and *sodium nitroprusside*, are effective only when administered intravenously. They are generally used in the treatment of hypertensive emergencies or during surgery.

Hydralazine

The vasodilation produced by hydralazine (*Apresoline*) depends in part on the presence of an intact blood vessel endothelium. This implies that hydralazine causes the release of nitric oxide, which acts on the vascular smooth muscle to cause relaxation. In addition, hydralazine may produce vasodilation by activating K^+ channels.

Absorption, Metabolism, and Excretion

Hydralazine is well absorbed (65–90%) after oral administration. Its peak antihypertensive effect occurs in about 1 hour, and its duration of action is about 6 hours.

The major pathways for its metabolism include ring hydroxylation, with subsequent glucuronide conjugation and *N*-acetylation. Hydralazine exhibits a first-pass effect in that a large part of an orally administered dose is metabolized before the drug reaches the systemic circulation. The first-pass metabolism occurs in the intestinal mucosa (mostly *N*-acetylation) and the liver. The primary excretory route is through renal elimination, and about 80% of an oral dose appears in the urine within 48 hours. About 10% is excreted unchanged in the feces.

Approximately 85% of the hydralazine in plasma is bound to plasma proteins. Although this does not appear to be a major therapeutic concern, the potential for interactions with other drugs that also bind to plasma proteins does exist. The plasma half-life of hydralazine in patients with normal renal function is 1.5 to 3 hours.

Interestingly, the half-life of the antihypertensive effect is somewhat longer than the plasma half-life. This may occur because hydralazine is specifically accumulated in artery walls, where it may continue to exert a vasodilator action even though plasma concentrations are low.

The plasma half-life of hydralazine may be increased fourfold or fivefold in patients with renal failure. If renal failure is present, therefore, both the antihypertensive and toxic effects of hydralazine may be enhanced. Since *N*-acetylation of hydralazine is an important metabolic pathway and depends on the activity of the enzyme *N*-acetyltransferase, genetically determined differences in the activity of this enzyme in certain individuals (known as slow acetylators) will result in higher plasma levels of hydralazine; therefore, the drug's therapeutic or toxic effects may be increased.

Pharmacological Actions

Hydralazine produces widespread but apparently not uniform vasodilation; that is, vascular resistance is decreased more in cerebral, coronary, renal, and splanchnic beds than in skeletal muscle and skin. Renal blood flow and ultimately glomerular filtration rate may be slightly increased after acute treatment with hydralazine. However, after several days of therapy, the renal blood flow is usually no different from that before drug use.

In therapeutic doses, hydralazine produces little effect on nonvascular smooth muscle or on the heart. Its pharmacological actions are largely confined to vascular smooth muscle and occur predominantly on the arterial side of the circulation; venous capacitance is much less affected. Because cardiovascular reflexes and venous capacitance are not affected by hydralazine, postural hypotension is not a clinical concern. Hydralazine treatment does, however, result in an increase in cardiac output. This action is brought about by the combined effects of a reflex increase in sympathetic stimulation of the heart, an increase in plasma renin, and salt and water retention. These effects limit the hypotensive usefulness of hydralazine to such an extent that *it is rarely used alone.*

Clinical Uses

Hydralazine is generally reserved for moderately hypertensive ambulatory patients whose blood pressure is not well controlled either by diuretics or by drugs that interfere with the sympathetic nervous system. It is almost always administered in combination with a diuretic (to prevent Na^+ retention) and a β-blocker, such as propranolol (to attenuate the effects of reflex cardiac stimulation and hyperreninemia). *The triple combination of a diuretic, β-blocker, and hydralazine constitutes a unique hemodynamic approach to the treatment of hypertension,* since three of the chief determinants of blood pressure are affected: cardiac output (β-blocker), plasma volume (diuretic), and peripheral vascular resistance (hydralazine).

Although hydralazine is available for intravenous administration and has been used in the past for hypertensive emergencies, it is not generally employed for this purpose. The onset of action after intravenous injection is relatively slow, and its actions are somewhat unpredictable in comparison with those of several other vasodilators.

Adverse Effects

Most side effects associated with hydralazine administration are due to vasodilation and the reflex hemodynamic changes that occur in response to vasodilation. These side effects include headache, flushing, nasal congestion, tachycardia, and palpitations. More serious manifestations include myocardial ischemia and heart failure. These untoward effects of hydralazine are greatly attenuated when the drug is administered in conjunction with a β-blocker.

When administered chronically in high doses, hydralazine may produce a rheumatoidlike state that when fully developed, resembles disseminated lupus erythematosus.

Minoxidil

Minoxidil (*Loniten*) is an orally effective vasodilator. It is more potent and longer acting than hydralazine and does not accumulate significantly in patients with renal insufficiency. It depends on in vivo metabolism by hepatic enzymes to produce an active metabolite, minoxidil sulfate. Minoxidil sulfate activates potassium channels, resulting in hyperpolarization of vascular smooth muscle and relaxation of the blood vessel.

Absorption, Metabolism, and Excretion

Peak concentrations of minoxidil in the blood occur 1 hour after oral administration, although the therapeutic effect may take 2 or more hours to manifest. This is probably related to the time it takes to convert minoxidil to minoxidil sulfate. The antihypertensive action after an oral dose of minoxidil lasts 12 to 24 hours. The long duration of action allows the drug to be administered only once or twice a day, a regimen that may be beneficial for compliance. Interestingly, the therapeutic half-life is considerably longer than the plasma half-life. This may be, as has been suggested for hydralazine, a result either of accumulation of the drug and its active metabolite in arterial walls or a longer plasma half-life of the sulfated metabolite, or both.

The ultimate disposition of minoxidil depends primarily on hepatic metabolism and only slightly on renal excretion of unchanged drug. Because of this, pharmacological activity is not cumulative in patients with renal failure.

Pharmacological Actions

The hemodynamic effects of minoxidil are generally similar to those of hydralazine, with the noteworthy exception that a greater decrease in peripheral vascular resistance and consequently a larger reduction in blood pressure can be achieved with minoxidil. Minoxidil produces no important changes in either renal blood flow or glomerular filtration rate. It has little or no effect on venous capacitance and does not inhibit the reflex activation of the sympathetic nervous system. Orthostasis and other side effects of sympathetic blockade are therefore not a problem. As with hydralazine, there is a significant increase in cardiac output that is secondary to reflex increases in sympathetic activity, hyperreninemia, and salt and water retention. These effects can substantially reduce the effectiveness of minoxidil when it is used alone. The addition of a β-blocker and a diuretic to the therapeutic regimen will preserve minoxidil's antihypertensive action while attenuating some of the undesirable side effects.

Clinical Uses

The major indications for the use of minoxidil are (1) severe hypertension that may be life threatening and (2) hypertension that is resistant to milder forms of therapy. Compromises in renal function do not prolong either the plasma or the therapeutic half-life of minoxidil, and therefore, it seems to be particularly important for hypertensive patients with chronic renal failure.

Adverse Effects

Signs of toxicity common to vasodilator therapy in general also occur with minoxidil; they are attributable to vasodilation and reflex increases in sympathetic nerve activity. These include headache, nasal congestion, tachycardia, and palpitations. These effects do not have great clinical importance, since minoxidil is almost always administered in combination with a β-blocker, which antagonizes the indirect cardiac effects. A more troublesome side effect, particularly in women, is the growth of body hair, possibly due to a direct stimulation of the growth and maturation of cells that form hair shafts. Apparently, minoxidil activates a specific gene that regulates hair shaft protein. In any case, this particular side effect has been capitalized upon, and minoxidil is now marketed as *Rogaine* for the treatment of male pattern baldness.

Diazoxide

Diazoxide (*Hyperstat*) is chemically similar to the thiazide diuretics. It is devoid of diuretic activity and causes Na^+ and water retention. Diazoxide is a very potent vasodilator and is available only for intravenous use in the treatment of hypertensive emergencies. The mechanism by which diazoxide relaxes vascular smooth muscle is related to its ability to activate potassium channels and produce a hyperpolarization of the cell membrane.

Absorption, Metabolism, and Excretion

Diazoxide lowers blood pressure within 3 to 5 minutes after rapid intravenous injection, and its duration of action may be 4 to 12 hours. Interestingly, if diazoxide is either injected slowly or infused its hypotensive action is quite modest. This is believed to be due to a rapid and extensive binding of the drug to plasma proteins. Both the liver and kidney contribute to its metabolism and excretion. The plasma half-life is therefore prolonged in patients with chronic renal failure.

Pharmacological Actions

The hemodynamic effects of diazoxide are similar to those of hydralazine and minoxidil. It produces direct relaxation of arteriolar smooth muscle with little effect on capacitance beds. Since it does not impair cardiovascular reflexes, orthostasis is not a problem. Its administration is, however, associated with a reflex increase in cardiac output that partially counters its antihypertensive effects. Propranolol and other β-blockers potentiate the vasodilating properties of the drug. Diazoxide has no direct action on the heart. Although renal blood flow and glomerular filtration may fall transiently, they generally return to predrug levels within an hour.

Clinical Uses

Diazoxide is administered intravenously for the treatment of *hypertensive emergencies,* particularly malignant hypertension, hypertensive encephalopathy, and eclampsia. It is effective in 75 to 85% of the patients to whom it is administered and rarely reduces blood pressure below the normotensive range.

In patients with coronary insufficiency, a β-blocker can be given in conjunction with diazoxide to decrease the cardiac work associated with reflex increases in sympathetic stimulation of the heart. However, β-blockers potentiate the hypotensive effect of diazoxide, and therefore, the dose of the vasodilator should be lowered. The dose of diazoxide should also be lowered if the patient has recently been treated with guanethidine or another drug that depresses the action of the sympathetic nervous system. Such drugs permit a greater hypotensive effect because they reduce the increase in cardiac output that normally partially counteracts the fall in pressure.

Diazoxide appears to have a direct antinatriuretic action. This direct action, coupled with the neuroendocrine reflexes that are activated by a decrease in peripheral vascular resistance, leads to severe retention of Na$^+$ and water. Since tolerance to diazoxide can develop rapidly, it is frequently administered in conjunction with a diuretic.

Adverse Effects

Since diazoxide is not often used for long-term treatment, toxicities associated with chronic use are rare. The chief concern is the side effects associated with the increased workload on the heart, which may precipitate myocardial ischemia and Na$^+$ and water retention. These undesirable effects can be controlled by concurrent therapy with a β-blocker and a diuretic.

Diazoxide may cause hyperglycemia, especially in diabetics, so if the drug is used for several days, blood glucose levels should be measured.

When used in the treatment of toxemia, diazoxide may stop labor, because it relaxes uterine smooth muscle.

Sodium Nitroprusside

Sodium nitroprusside (*Nipride*) is a potent directly acting vasodilator capable of reducing blood pressure in all patients, regardless of the cause of hypertension. It is used only by the intravenous route for the treatment of *hypertensive emergencies.* The pharmacological activity is caused by the nitroso moiety. The actions of the drug are similar to those of the nitrites and nitrates that are used as antianginal agents (see Chapter 17). The action of the nitrovasodilators depends on the intracellular production of cGMP.

Absorption, Metabolism, and Excretion

The onset of the hypotensive action of sodium nitroprusside is rapid, within 30 seconds after intravenous administration. If a single dose is given, the action lasts for only a couple of minutes. Therefore, sodium nitroprusside must be administered by continuous intravenous infusion. After the infusion is stopped, blood pressure returns to predrug levels within 2 to 3 minutes.

Nitroprusside is metabolically degraded by the liver, yielding thiocyanate. Because thiocyanate is excreted by the kidney, toxicities due to this compound are most likely in patients with impaired renal function.

Pharmacological Actions

In contrast to hydralazine, minoxidil, and diazoxide, sodium nitroprusside relaxes venules as well as arterioles. Thus, it decreases both peripheral vascular resistance and venous return to the heart. This action limits the increase in cardiac output that normally follows vasodilator therapy. Sodium nitroprusside does not inhibit sympathetic reflexes, so heart rate may increase following its administration even though cardiac output is not increased. Renal blood flow remains largely unaffected by sodium nitroprusside, because the decrease in renal vascular resistance is proportional to the decrease in mean arterial pressure. As with all vasodilators, plasma renin activity increases.

Clinical Uses

Sodium nitroprusside is used in the management of hypertensive crisis. Although it is effective in every form of hypertension because of its relatively favorable effect on cardiac performance, sodium nitroprusside has special importance in the treatment of severe hypertension with acute myocardial infarction or left ventricular failure. Because the drug reduces preload (by venodilation) and afterload (by arteriolar dilation), it improves ventricular performance and in fact is sometimes used in patients with refractory heart failure, even in the absence of hypertension.

Adverse Effects

The most commonly encountered side effects of sodium nitroprusside administration are nausea, vomiting, and headache, which quickly dissipate when the infusion is terminated. When sodium nitroprusside treatment extends for several days, there is some danger of toxicity owing to the accumulation of its thiocyanate metabolite. Thiocyanate intoxication includes signs of delirium and psychosis; hypothyroidism also may occur. If nitroprusside is administered for several days, thiocyanate levels should be monitored.

Close supervision is required when nitroprusside is used because of the drug's potency and short duration of action.

DRUGS THAT IMPAIR SYMPATHETIC NERVOUS SYSTEM FUNCTIONING

The drugs discussed in this section reduce blood pressure by depressing the activity of the sympathetic nervous system. This is accomplished in four ways: (1) by reducing the number of impulses traveling in the sympathetic nerves, (2) by inhibiting neurotransmitter release, (3) by depleting the stores of norepinephrine, and (4) by antagonizing the actions of norepinephrine on effector cells. The sites of action of these drugs are diverse and may best be appreciated by considering the sympathetic arc concerned with blood pressure regulation (Fig. 20.2).

While there may be some involvement of the adrenergic nervous system in primary hypertension, there is no clear evidence that a malfunction of this system is causally involved in primary hypertension. Therefore, *even though drugs may depress the sympathetic system and thus lower blood pressure, it should not be assumed that this therapeutic approach corrects the cause of the elevated pressure.* Only in a few specific cases, such as pheochromocytoma, can hypertension be directly related to abnormalities in the functioning of the sympathetic system.

ADRENOCEPTOR ANTAGONISTS

The adrenoceptor-blocking agents are described in detail in Chapter 11, although their use in the treatment of hypertension is briefly described here. Drugs of this group are subdivided into α-adrenoceptor antagonists (α-blockers) and β-adrenoceptor antagonists (β- blockers).

α-Blocking Drugs

Phenoxybenzamine and phentolamine have been available for a number of years and are sometimes referred to as classical α-blockers. The frequency of their use for the treatment of primary hypertension has greatly diminished in recent years because of the development of drugs such as prazosin that are relatively selective for α_1-receptors. α_1-Receptor–selective antagonists will not potentiate the release of norepinephrine from sympathetic nerves. Thus, the stimulation of the heart and renin release, actions that limit the usefulness of classical α-blockers, are less with α_1-selective antagonists.

Unlike the vasodilators, which have a more prominent effect on arterial beds than on venous beds, the α-blockers prevent vasoconstriction in both vascular beds. Because of the venous dilation, postural hypotension is a feature of α-blockade, although less so with prazosin than with the classical α-blockers.

Prazosin and its derivatives that are selective for α_1-adrenoceptors are quite useful for the management of primary hypertension. The α_1-receptor–selective antagonists can be used alone in mild hypertension. When hypertension is moderate or severe, prazosin is generally administered in combination with a thiazide and a β-blocker. The antihypertensive actions of prazosin are considerably potentiated by coadministration of thiazides or other types of antihypertensive drugs.

Prazosin may be particularly useful when patients cannot tolerate other types of antihypertensive agents or when blood pressure is not well controlled by other drugs. Since prazosin does not significantly influence blood uric acid or glucose levels, it can be used in hypertensive patients whose condition is complicated by gout or diabetes mellitus. Prazosin treatment is associated with favorable effects on plasma lipids. Thus, it may be of particular importance in managing patients with hyperlipidemia.

Further information about the pharmacokinetics, adverse reactions, and preparations of α-blockers is given in Chapter 11.

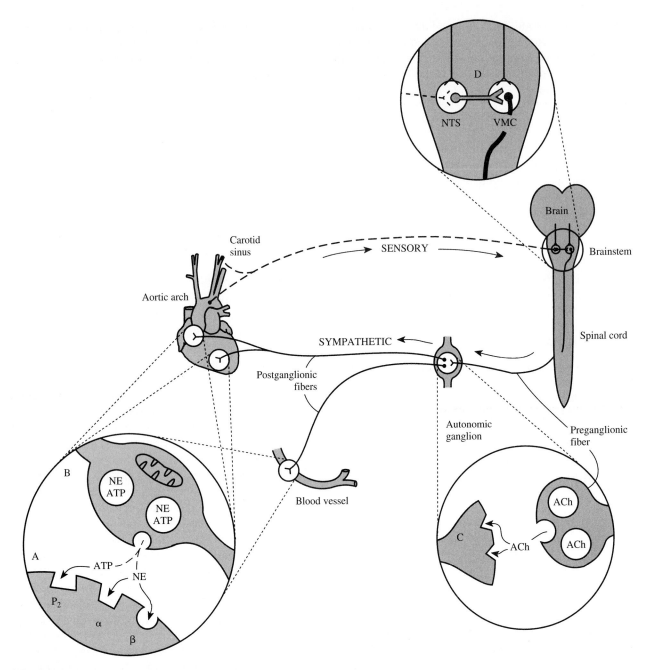

FIGURE 20.2

Sympathetic arc involved in blood pressure regulation and sites where drugs may act to influence the system. *A.* Receptors on effector cell. *B.* Adrenergic varicosity. *C.* Nicotinic receptors (postganglionic fibers). *D.* Brainstem nuclei. NTS, nucleus of the tractus solitarii; VMC, vasomotor center; ACh, acetylcholine; NE, norepinephrine; α, α-adrenoceptors; β, β-adrenoceptors; P_2, P_2-purinoceptors; ATP, adenosine triphosphate.

β-*Blocking Drugs*

β-Blockers competitively antagonize the responses to catecholamines that are mediated by β-receptors (see Chapter 11). These drugs have a number of clinical uses, including treatment of cardiac arrhythmias (see Chapter 10) and angina pectoris (see Chapter 17), for which their therapeutic benefit is directly related to the blockade of β-receptors in the myocardium.

β-Blockers are also used in the treatment of hypertension, although this seems to be somewhat paradoxical in that blockade of vascular smooth muscle β-receptors might be expected to unmask or leave unopposed responses to catecholamines that occur through vascular α-receptors. Unopposed α-mediated responses would be expected to increase, rather than decrease, blood pressure. Nevertheless, β-*blockers have proved to be quite effective antihypertensive agents,* and they have an important place in the treatment of primary hypertension.

The mechanism by which β-blockers produce a sustained reduction in blood pressure in patients with primary hypertension is not completely understood, but it may include such actions as reduction in renin release, antagonism of central nervous system (CNS) β-receptors, or antagonism of presynaptic facilitatory β-receptors on sympathetic nerves.

Decreases in heart rate and cardiac output are the most obvious results of administration of β-blockers. Initially, blood pressure is not much affected, since peripheral vascular resistance will be reflexly elevated as a result of the drug-induced decrease in cardiac output. The reduction of blood pressure that occurs in chronic treatment correlates best with changes in peripheral vascular resistance rather than with a drug-induced variation in heart rate or cardiac output.

The reduction in plasma volume produced by β-blockers contrasts with the increased volume seen with other types of antihypertensives. Tolerance to the antihypertensive actions of β-blockers therefore is less of a problem than with the vasodilating drugs. An additional difference from the vasodilators is that *plasma renin activity is reduced, rather than increased, by propranolol (Inderal).* Orthostatic hypotension does not occur with β-blockers.

The β-blockers are quite popular antihypertensive drugs. They are well tolerated, and serious side effects are seldom observed. When used alone over several weeks, β-blockers produce a significant reduction in blood pressure in approximately 30% of patients with mild to moderate hypertension. Thus, β-*blockers can be employed as a first step in the management of high blood pressure. However, they are often used in conjunction with a diuretic when therapy with a single agent is not satisfactory.* The combination of a β-blocker, thiazide diuretic, and vasodilator provides significant control of moderate to severe hypertension in approximately 80% of patients.

From a hemodynamic viewpoint, there are several obvious advantages to using a β-blocker in combination with a vasodilator. Reflex-mediated cardiac stimulation is a common feature of vasodilator treatment and can severely limit its antihypertensive effectiveness. A β-blocker will reduce the cardiac stimulation and thus preserve the effectiveness of the vasodilator. Conversely, the vasodilator will prevent the increase in peripheral vascular resistance that occurs on initiation of treatment with a β-blocker. Furthermore, vasodilator treatment initiates reflexes that lead to an increase in plasma renin

activity. Thus, β-blockers, such as propranolol, that reduce plasma renin activity are of obvious value.

Although the β-blockers are well-tolerated drugs and patient compliance is good, there may be problems with their administration, particularly in patients with decompensated hearts and cardiac conductance disturbances. These potential problems and the adverse effect of β-blockers are described in detail in Chapter 11.

ADRENERGIC NEURON-BLOCKING DRUGS

The adrenergic neuron-blocking drugs are antihypertensive because *they prevent the release of transmitters from peripheral postganglionic sympathetic nerves.* The contraction of vascular smooth muscle due to sympathetic nerve stimulation is thereby reduced, and blood pressure decreases. Guanethidine is the prototypical member of this class.

Guanethidine

Guanethidine (*Ismelin*) is a powerful antihypertensive agent that is quite effective in the treatment of moderate to severe hypertension. It is most frequently used in the treatment of severe hypertension that is resistant to other agents.

Guanethidine exerts its effects at peripheral sympathetic nerve endings following its active transport into the nerve varicosities by the neuronal amine transport system. This is the same uptake system that transports norepinephrine into the varicosity (see Chapter 9). The accumulation of guanethidine in adrenergic neurons, through an as yet unexplained mechanism, disrupts the process by which action potentials trigger the release of stored norepinephrine and other cotransmitters from nerve terminals. It is this action of guanethidine that is primarily responsible for its antihypertensive properties. Parasympathetic function is not altered, a fact that distinguishes guanethidine from the ganglionic blocking agents (see Chapter 14).

Guanethidine is suitable for oral use, and this is its usual route of administration. However, absorption from the gastrointestinal tract is variable. The half-life of guanethidine is 5 days, with about one-seventh of the total administered dose eliminated per day. The slow elimination contributes to the cumulative and prolonged effects of the drug.

Guanethidine reduces blood pressure by its ability to diminish vascular tone; both the arterial and venous sides of the circulatory system are involved. The resulting venous pooling contributes to orthostatic hypotension, a prominent feature of guanethidine treatment. The reduction in blood pressure is more prominent when the patient is standing than recumbent.

A reduction in cardiac output attributable to a decreased venous return and the inability of sympathetic nerve impulses to release enough transmitters to stimulate the heart occur during the early stages of guanethidine therapy.

With the possible exception of minoxidil, guanethidine is the most potent orally effective antihypertensive drug. Because guanethidine produces a number of side effects that are due primarily to the imbalance between sympathetic and parasympathetic function it produces, it is generally reserved for the treatment of severe hypertension.

A common and troublesome side effect is postural hypotension. Sexual impotence does occur, and male patients may have difficulty ejaculating. Symptoms of unopposed parasympathetic activity include such gastrointestinal disturbances as diarrhea and increased gastric secretion.

Guanethidine may aggravate congestive heart failure or actually precipitate failure in patients with marginal cardiac reserve, owing to its ability to produce vascular volume expansion, edema, and a reduced effectiveness of sympathetic cardiac stimulation.

Guanethidine is contraindicated in patients with pheochromocytoma because the drug may release catecholamines from the tumor. The concomitant use of monoamine oxidase (*MAO*) inhibitors and guanethidine is also to be avoided, since this combined drug treatment eliminates two of the principal mechanisms for terminating the actions of the catecholamines and certain other adrenomimetic drugs, that is, biotransformation and neuronal uptake. Dangerously high concentrations of catecholamines at receptor sites are possible.

The tricyclic antidepressants (e.g., desipramine and amitriptyline) and some phenothiazines block the sympathetic neuronal amine uptake system; they thereby would also block the uptake of guanethidine and thus reduce its hypotensive effectiveness. Conversely, guanethidine competitively inhibits the uptake of drugs that are substrates for neuronal uptake, such as the indirectly acting adrenomimetics, or sympathomimetics (see Chapter 10).

DRUGS THAT INTERFERE WITH NOREPINEPHRINE STORAGE

Reserpine (*Serpasil*) is the prototypical drug interfering with norepinephrine storage. Reserpine lowers blood pressure by reducing norepinephrine concentrations in the noradrenergic nerves in such a way that less norepinephrine is released during neuron activation. Reserpine does not interfere with the release process per se as does guanethidine.

Under normal circumstances, when an action potential invades the sympathetic nerve terminal, a portion of the released norepinephrine is recycled. This event requires two successive steps: (1) transfer of norepinephrine across the neuronal membrane into the cytosol by an energy-dependent carrier-mediated active process, and (2) transfer of the recaptured amine from the cytosol into the noradrenergic storage vesicles, where it is stored until needed. *Reserpine inhibits only the second uptake process.* As a consequence of this inhibition of vesicular uptake, norepinephrine cannot be stored intraneuronally, and much of the cytosolic amine is metabolized by MAO.

In addition to impairing norepinephrine storage and thereby enhancing its catabolism, reserpine impairs the vesicular uptake of dopamine, the immediate precursor of norepinephrine. Since dopamine must be taken up into the adrenergic vesicles to undergo hydroxylation and form norepinephrine, reserpine administration impairs norepinephrine synthesis. *The combined effects of the blockade of dopamine and norepinephrine vesicular uptake lead to transmitter depletion.*

Reserpine also interferes with the neuronal storage of a variety of central transmitter amines such that significant depletion of norepinephrine, dopamine, and 5-hydroxytryptamine (serotonin) occurs. This central transmitter depletion is responsible for the sedation and other CNS side effects associated with reserpine therapy. The depletion of brain amines also may contribute to the antihypertensive effects of reserpine.

The chief use of reserpine is in the treatment of mild to moderate hypertension. As with other sympathetic depressant drugs, tolerance to the antihypertensive effects of reserpine can occur, owing to a compensatory increase in blood volume that frequently accompanies decreased peripheral vascular resistance. Reserpine, therefore, should be used in conjunction with a diuretic.

Because of its sedative properties, reserpine offers special benefit to hypertensive patients who exhibit symptoms of agitated psychotic states and who may be unable to tolerate therapy with phenothiazine derivatives.

The most troublesome untoward effects of treatment with reserpine involve the CNS. Sedation and depression are the most common, although nightmares and thoughts of suicide also occur. Reserpine treatment, therefore, is contraindicated in patients with a history of severe depression. The occasional report of reserpine-induced extrapyramidal symptoms, which are similar to those seen in patients with Parkinson's disease, is believed to be a result of dopamine depletion from neurons in the CNS.

Peripheral nervous system side effects are the result of a reserpine-induced reduction of sympathetic function and unopposed parasympathetic activity; symptoms include nasal congestion, postural hypotension, diarrhea, bradycardia, increased gastric secretion, and occasionally impotence. Because of the increased gastric secretion, reserpine is contraindicated for patients with peptic ulcer. In patients with little cardiac reserve, reserpine must be administered with caution because of its ability to interfere with sympathetic stimulation of the heart.

DRUGS THAT INTERFERE WITH NOREPINEPHRINE SYNTHESIS

Metyrosine (*Demser*) is an example of this class of drugs. Chemically, metyrosine is α-methyl tyrosine. The drug blocks the action of tyrosine hydroxylase, the rate-limiting enzyme in the synthesis of catecholamines. Unlike α-methyldopa, metyrosine is not itself incorporated into the catecholamine synthetic pathway. The ultimate action of the drug is to decrease the production of catecholamines.

Metyrosine is well absorbed from the gastrointestinal tract and is excreted in the urine largely as unchanged drug.

Metyrosine is not employed for the treatment of essential hypertension but rather is used for the management of pheochromocytoma. It is useful for preoperative treatment and for long-term therapy when surgery is not feasible.

Sedation is the most common adverse effect of metyrosine. Other CNS disturbances, such as anxiety, confusion, and disorientation, have also been reported. Symptoms of sympathetic nervous system depression in general, such as nasal congestion and dryness of mouth, can also occur.

GANGLIONIC BLOCKING AGENTS

The basis for the antihypertensive activity of the ganglionic blockers lies in their ability to block transmission through autonomic ganglia (Fig. 20.2C). This action, which results in a decrease in the number of impulses passing down the *postganglionic* sympathetic (and parasympathetic) nerves, decreases vascular tone, cardiac output, and blood pressure. *These drugs prevent the interaction of acetylcholine (the transmitter of the preganglionic autonomic nerves) with the nicotinic receptors on postsynaptic neuronal membranes of both the sympathetic and parasympathetic nervous systems.*

The ganglionic blocking agents are extremely potent antihypertensive agents and can reduce blood pressure regardless of the extent of hypertension. Unfortunately, blockade of transmission in both the sympathetic and parasympathetic systems produces numerous untoward responses, including marked postural hypotension, blurred vision, and dryness of mouth, constipation, paralytic ileus, urinary retention, and impotence. Owing to the frequency and severity of these side effects and to the development of other powerful antihypertensive agents, the ganglionic blocking agents are rarely used.

The orally effective ganglionic blocking agents in fact are not recommended for the treatment of primary hypertension. However, certain intravenous preparations, such as the short-acting agent trimethaphan camsylate (*Arfonad*), are used occasionally for hypertensive emergencies and in surgical procedures in which hypotension is desirable to reduce the possibility of hemorrhage.

A more complete description of trimethaphan and other ganglionic blocking agents can be found in Chapter 14.

CENTRALLY ACTING HYPOTENSIVE DRUGS

Two important antihypertensive agents, α-methyldopa and clonidine, act predominantly in the *brain* (Fig. 20.2D). Although the details of their actions may differ in some respects, *their antihypertensive activity is ultimately due to their ability to decrease the sympathetic outflow from the brain to the cardiovascular system.*

α-Methyldopa

The spectrum of activity of α-methyldopa (*Aldomet*) lies between those of the more potent agents, such as guanethidine, and the milder antihypertensives, such as reserpine. α-Methyldopa is a structural analogue of dihydroxyphenylalanine (dopa) and differs from dopa only by the presence of a methyl group on the α-carbon of the side chain.

Mechanism of Action

A number of theories have been put forward to account for the hypotensive action of α-methyldopa. Current evidence suggests that for α-methyldopa to be an antihypertensive agent, it must be converted to α-methylnorepinephrine; however, *its site of action appears to be in the brain rather than in the periphery.* Systemically administered α-methyldopa rapidly enters the brain, where it accumulates in noradrenergic nerves, is converted to α-methylnorepinephrine, and is released. *Released α-methylnorepinephrine activates CNS α-adrenoceptors whose function is to decrease sympathetic outflow.* Why α-methylnorepinephrine decreases sympathetic outflow more effectively than does the naturally occurring transmitter is not entirely clear.

Absorption, Metabolism, and Excretion

Approximately 50% of an orally administered dose of α-methyldopa is absorbed from the gastrointestinal tract. Both peak plasma drug levels and maximal blood pressure–lowering effects are observed 2 to 6 hours after oral administration. A considerable amount of unchanged α-methyldopa and several conjugated and decarboxylated metabolites can be found in the urine.

Pharmacological Actions

The primary hemodynamic alteration responsible for the hypotensive effects of α-methyldopa remains in dispute. When the patient is supine, the reduction in blood pressure produced by α-methyldopa correlates best with a decrease in peripheral vascular resistance, cardiac output being only slightly reduced. When the patient is upright, the fall in blood pressure corresponds more closely with a reduced cardiac output.

An important aspect of α-methyldopa's hemodynamic effects is that renal blood flow and glomerular filtration rate are not reduced. As occurs with most sympathetic depressant drugs and vasodilators, long-term therapy with α-methyldopa leads to fluid retention, edema formation, and plasma volume expansion. While data conflict somewhat, it is generally thought that α-methyldopa suppresses plasma renin activity.

Clinical Uses

α-Methyldopa is not generally believed to be suitable for monotherapy of primary hypertension. Because plasma volume increases as the duration of α-methyldopa therapy is extended, the drug should be used in conjunction with a diuretic; this will produce a significantly greater fall in blood pressure than would occur with either drug used alone. Because α-methyldopa lowers blood pressure without compromising either renal blood flow or the glomerular filtration rate, *it is particularly valuable in hypertension complicated by renal disease.* However, if end-stage renal failure accompanies severe hypertension, α-methyldopa may not be effective.

The presence of α-methyldopa and its metabolites in the urine reduces the diagnostic value of urinary catecholamine measurements as an indicator of pheochromocytoma, since these substances interfere with the fluorescence assay for catecholamines.

Adverse Effects

The most commonly encountered side effects of α-methyldopa are sedation and drowsiness. These CNS effects are probably the result of reductions in brain catecholamine levels. Other side effects, also typical of sympathetic depression, are dry mouth, nasal congestion, orthostatic hypertension, and impotence.

Autoimmune reactions associated with α-methyldopa treatment include thrombocytopenia and leukopenia. Since a few cases of an α-methyldopa–induced hepatitis have occurred, the drug is contraindicated in patients with active hepatic disease. Flulike symptoms also are known to occur.

Clonidine and Related Drugs

Clonidine (*Catapres*) is effective orally and is used primarily for the treatment of moderate hypertension. It is structurally related to the α-adrenoceptor antagonists phentolamine and tolazoline. *Clonidine, however, is not an α-blocker, but is actually an α-agonist.* Its antihypertensive effectiveness appeared paradoxical until it was recognized that clonidine activated central α_2-receptors, thus reducing sympathetic outflow to the periphery.

Guanabenz (*Wytensin*) and guanfacine (*Tenex*) are two drugs with considerable structural similarity to clonidine. These agents also are central α_2-agonists and exhibit an antihypertensive profile similar to that of clonidine.

Mechanism of Action

The antihypertensive activity of clonidine can be ascribed solely to a decrease in the sympathetic activity transmitted from the brain to the peripheral vasculature. After clonidine administration, direct measurements of sympathetic nerve activity show that electrical discharge is reduced in a number of sympathetic nerves, including the cardiac, splanchnic, and cervical nerves.

It is generally agreed that clonidine acts in the same general area in the brain as does α-methyldopa, that is, somewhere in the medulla oblongata. The principal difference between clonidine and α-methyldopa is that clonidine acts *directly* on α_2-receptors, whereas α-methyldopa first must be converted by synthetic enzymes to α-methylnorepinephrine.

Absorption, Metabolism, and Excretion

Clonidine is well absorbed after oral administration. Peak plasma levels occur between 2 and 4 hours after drug administration and correlate well with pharmacological activity. The plasma half-life in patients with normal renal function is 12 hours. Urinary excretion of clonidine and its metabolites accounts for almost 90% of the administered dose, and fecal excretion accounts for the rest. Approximately 50% of an administered dose is excreted unchanged; the remainder is oxidatively metabolized in the liver.

Pharmacological Actions

An acute intravenous injection of clonidine may produce a transient pressor response that apparently is due to stimulation of peripheral vascular α-receptors. The pressor response does not occur after oral administration, because the drug's centrally mediated depressor action overrides it.

The decrease in blood pressure produced by clonidine correlates better with a decreased cardiac output than with a reduction in peripheral vascular resistance. The reduction in cardiac output is the result of both a decreased heart rate and reduced stroke work; the latter effect is probably caused by a diminished venous return.

Renal blood flow and glomerular filtration are not decreased, although renal resistance is diminished. Like α-methyldopa, it is a useful agent for hypertension complicated by renal disease. Plasma renin activity is reduced by clonidine, presumably as a result of a centrally mediated decrease in sympathetic stimulation of the juxtaglomerular cells of the kidney.

Clinical Uses

The primary indication for clonidine use is in mild and moderate hypertension that has not responded adequately to treatment with a diuretic or a β-blocker. Since clonidine causes sodium and water retention and plasma volume expansion, it generally is administered in combination with a diuretic. A vasodilator can be added to the clonidine–diuretic regimen in the treatment of resistant forms of hypertension. Such drug combinations can be quite effective, since the reflex increases in heart rate and cardiac output that result from vasodilator administration are reduced or negated by clonidine-induced decreases in heart rate and cardiac output.

For severely hypertensive patients, clonidine has been used in combination with a diuretic, a vasodilator, and a β-blocker. Some care must be taken, however, because the coadministration of clonidine and a β-blocker may cause excessive sedation. Clonidine is especially useful in patients with renal failure, since its duration of action is not appreciably altered by renal disease and it does not compromise renal blood flow.

Adverse Effects

It is estimated that about 7% of patients receiving clonidine discontinue the drug because of side effects. Although the symptoms are generally mild and tend to subside if therapy is continued for several weeks, as many as 50% of the patients complain of drowsiness and dryness of mouth. Other untoward effects include constipation, nausea or gastric upset, and impotence. These effects are characteristic of interference with the functioning of the sympathetic nervous system.

A potentially dangerous effect is *rebound hypertension,* which follows abrupt withdrawal of clonidine therapy. This posttreatment hypertension appears to be the result of excessive sympathetic activity. The genesis of the syndrome is not well understood. A contributing factor may be development of supersensitivity in either the sympathetic nerves or the effector organs of the cardiovascular system due to the clonidine-caused chronic reduction in sympathetic activity. Thus, when the drug is abruptly withdrawn, an exaggerated response to "normal" levels of activity may occur. If treatment with clonidine is terminated gradually, rebound hypertension is unlikely. Patients should be warned of the danger of abruptly discontinuing clonidine treatment.

Study QUESTIONS

1. A 55-year-old patient has been referred to you. She complains about a skin rash and a cough. In the course of history taking, she tells you that she takes high blood pressure medication but she doesn't remember the name. You suspect a drug toxicity. Which of the following antihypertensive agents is the patient most likely taking?
   (A) Captopril
   (B) Nifedipine
   (C) Prazosin
   (D) Propanolol
   (E) Clonidine
2. Which of the following compounds depends least upon the release of EDRF (nitric oxide) from endothelial cells to cause vasodilation?
   (A) Bradykinin
   (B) Histamine
   (C) Minoxidil
   (D) Hydralazine
   (E) Acetylcholine

3. Which of the following antihypertensive drugs is contraindicated in a hypertensive patient with a pheochromocytoma?
   (A) Metyrosine
   (B) Labetalol
   (C) Prazosin
   (D) Phenoxybenzamine
   (E) Guanethidine
4. Which of the following antihypertensive agents would decrease renin release?
   (A) Prazosin
   (B) Clonidine
   (C) Captopril
   (D) Nitroprusside
   (E) Diazoxide

ANSWERS

1. **A.** Although many drugs can evoke a reaction such as a rash, a rash and a dry cough are well-recognized side effects of angiotensin converting enzyme

(ACE) inhibitors, such as captopril. Up to 20% of these patients may develop a cough with ACE inhibitors. The cause is not known for certain, but it may be related to the accumulation in the lungs of bradykinin or other inflammatory mediators. Inhibiting ACE leads to an increase in bradykinin, which is normally broken down by this enzyme. The rash was originally attributed to a sulfhydryl group in captopril but is known to occur with other non–sulfhydryl-containing ACE-inhibitors.

2. **C.** The vasodilation caused by bradykinin, histamine, hydralazine, and acetylcholine depends in part upon nitric oxide release from the endothelium. Minoxidil activates K^+ channels, which results in vascular smooth muscle hyperpolarization and thereby relaxation.

3. **E.** Guanethidine does not normally cause release of catecholamines from the adrenal medulla. However, it may provoke the release of catecholamines from pheochromocytoma. This action plus its ability to antagonize neuronal uptake of catecholamines could trigger a hypertensive crisis. The other drugs are good choices to lower blood pressure in a patient with pheochromocytoma: metyrosine, by decreasing synthesis; labetalol, by blocking both the α- and β-effects of the catecholamines; prazosin and especially phenoxybenzamine, by introducing a fairly long α-blockade.

4. **B.** Clonidine is an antihypertensive because it decreases sympathetic outflow from the CNS to the periphery and therefore reduces the sympathetically induced stimulation of renin release. The sympathetic effect on renin release is mediated by β-receptors, so prazosin, an α-blocker would not decrease release. Captopril is an ACE inhibitor and is likely to enhance renin release, although it would prevent the effects of renin by reducing the formation of angiotensin II. Nitroprusside and diazoxide are directly acting vasodilators and will promote renin release reflexively.

SUPPLEMENTAL READING

Dosh SA. The treatment of adults with essential hypertension. J Fam Pract 2002:51;74–80.

Friedman AL. Approach to the treatment of hypertension in children. Heart Dis 2002; 4;47–50.

Hansson L. "Why don't you do as I tell you?" Compliance and antihypertensive regimens. Int J Clin Pract 2002;56:191–196.

Kaplan NM. Kaplan's Clinical Hypertension (8th Ed.). Philadelphia: Lippincott Williams & Wilkins, 2002.

Drugs for hypertension. Med Lett Drugs Ther 1995;37:45–50.

Edvmsson L and Uddman R. (eds.). *Vascular Innervation and Receptor Mechanisms.* San Diego: Academic, 1993.

Sixth Report of the Joint National Committee on Prevention, Detection, Evaluation, and Treatment of High Blood Pressure. Arch Intern Med 1997;157:2413–2446.

C A S E **Study**   Hypertensive Emergency

A 50-year-old woman is seen in the emergency department complaining of a severe headache, shortness of breath, and ankle edema. Her vision is blurry and her blood pressure is 200/140 mm Hg. A blood test reveals azotemia and proteinuria. A chest radiograph reveals an enlarged cardiac silhouette. Is this a hypertensive emergency, and if so what pharmacological treatment might be considered?

ANSWER: This patient appears to be have malignant hypertension and signs of congestive heart failure. The azotemia and proteinuria are signs of renal disease and often portend deteriorating renal function. The enlarged heart and ankle edema are signs of heart failure, as is the shortness of breath. The blood pressure is very high, and this should be treated as an emergency. With blood pressure this high and the ominous clinical signs, this patient needs to be hospitalized and receive drug therapy to lower the blood pressure. The physician in a case such as this would likely choose intravenous therapy to get control of the blood pressure quickly. Although there are a number of choices, sodium nitroprusside should be at the top of the list. Diazoxide is also a good choice. Nitroprusside has a rapid onset of action, within seconds of starting an infusion. It may benefit this patient to improve cardiac output by reducing afterload and preload. Other antihypertensives that could be considered in this situation are labetalol, a combined α- and β-blocker, and nicardipine, a calcium channel antagonist. An advantage of these agents is that they can be administered intravenously, and once the patient is stabilized, one can switch to an oral formulation.

21

Diuretic Drugs

Peter A. Friedman and William O. Berndt

DRUG LIST

By selectively regulating solute or fluid reabsorption, the kidneys play the major role in maintaining the volume and composition of extracellular fluid. Many diseases, including congestive heart failure, hepatic cirrhosis, and Cushing's syndrome (glucocorticoid excess), are associated with or cause significant alterations in extracellular fluid balance. *Diuretics inhibit renal sodium transport and thereby interfere with the normal regulatory activity of the kidney.* In some instances, administration of a diuretic drug is the primary treatment indicated, while in others it is one of several drugs that are used as part of a treatment regimen. In either case, an ideal diuretic would be one that caused the excretion of "extra" urine with an electrolyte composition similar to that of normal plasma. No such diuretic exists. Thus, although diuretic therapy provides welcome relief from pulmonary congestion, ascites, edema, and hypertension, it also invites complications of organ hypoperfusion that may be accompanied by marked distortions of plasma composition.

This chapter includes an overview of the features of fluid balance and renal function that are essential to understanding diuretic action, a discussion of the uses of diuretics for treating abnormalities of fluid balance, and a detailed description of the various classes of diuretics. The practitioner who is armed with the knowledge of the mechanism of action of diuretic drugs and with appropriate recognition and respect for their potential side effects can use these compounds with a high degree of efficacy and safety.

BODY WATER AND ELECTROLYTE METABOLISM

Body fluids are partitioned between the intracellular fluids (ICF), which constitute two-thirds of total body water, and extracellular fluids (ECF), which constitute one-third of total body water. The ECF consists of plasma and interstitial fluid plus lymph. The ionic composition differs substantially between ECF and ICF (Table 21.1). Sodium is the primary cation in ECF, whereas potassium is the principal intracellular cation.

The concentrations and distribution of electrolytes are not fixed, because cell membranes are permeant to ions and to water. Movement of ions and water in and out of cells is determined by the balance of thermodynamic forces, which are normally close to equilibrium. Selective changes of ion concentrations cause movement of water in or out of cells to compensate for these alterations. The kidneys are a major site where changes in salt or water are sensed. The loss of fluids due to illness or disease may alter intracellular and extracellular electrolyte concentrations, with attendant changes in fluid movement in or out of cells. Changes of extracellular or intracellular ion concentrations, particularly for potassium, sodium, and calcium, can have profound effects on neuronal excitability and contractility of the heart and other muscles.

Glomerular Filtration

Urine formation begins with the ultrafiltration of blood at the glomerulus. None of the available diuretics exerts its effects by altering the rate of glomerular filtration. Some agents, discussed later, reduce the glomerular filtration rate (GFR). However, this generally is an undesired or adverse reaction. Furthermore, at reduced GFRs, the delivery of sodium to the loop of Henle and the distal convoluted tubule, where the most efficacious classes of diuretics act, may be sufficiently compromised to reduce the action of the drugs. *Understanding the*

process of filtration is important to understanding the pharmacokinetics of diuretic action because most of these agents exert their inhibitory effect by blocking the entry of sodium from the urine into the cell. Therefore, these diuretics have to be present at sufficient concentrations within the tubular fluid to exert their inhibitory action on sodium transport. Most diuretics are variably bound to albumin and therefore are only partially filtered. They gain access to the tubular fluid by secretion into the proximal tubule (discussed later). In conditions of hemorrhage or liver disease resulting in hypoalbuminemia, the concentration of albumin is reduced and the fraction of bound diuretic is altered. Although this may suggest that more of the diuretic is unbound (or free) and filtered at the glomerulus, this does not occur. The decrease in Starling forces, which govern the rate of fluid filtration across the glomerular and other capillaries, now results in greater entry of fluid into the interstitial space.

Most estimates of diuretic binding to albumin assume that the protein itself is not altered as part of the disease process. In renal failure, however, the number of binding sites on the protein may change, which in turn affects the pharmacokinetics and dynamics of the response to an administered diuretic. Another setting associated with diminished effective diuretic concentrations occurs in *nephrotic syndrome*. In this disease, protein escaping from the glomerulus into the tubules binds the diuretic within the lumen. The bound drug is unavailable to exert its inhibitory effect on sodium transport.

Tubular Reabsorption and Secretion

Two additional processes that participate in urine formation are reabsorption and secretion. Reabsorption defines movement of solute or water from the tubule lumen to the blood, whereas secretion denotes transport from the blood to the tubule lumen. For many solutes, such as organic acids, transport proceeds in both directions. Net transport is determined by the dominant flux. As described later, the tubular secretion of some diuretics is critical for their action. The nephron sites where ions and organic solutes are transported are spatially separated. Figure 21.1 illustrates the various nephron segments, the primary sites of solute transport, and the magnitude of sodium reabsorption. In some instances, as with sodium, several transport mechanisms mediate its reabsorption. Importantly, each mechanism is spatially separated within different nephron segments. This is important in understanding diuretic action, which is specific to particular sodium transport mechanisms. Furthermore, some common side effects caused by diuretics, such as potassium wasting, develop as a direct consequence of the mechanism and the particular location of diuretic action at sites upstream from

TABLE 21.1	Approximate Electrolyte Content of Body Fluids	
Ions	Extracellular Fluid (mEq/L)	Intracellular Fluid (mEq/L)
Cations		
Sodium	140.0	10
Potassium	4.5	125
Magnesium	1.7	40
Anions		
Bicarbonate	25.0	10
Chloride	100.0	25
Phosphate	3.0	150
Protein	15.0	40

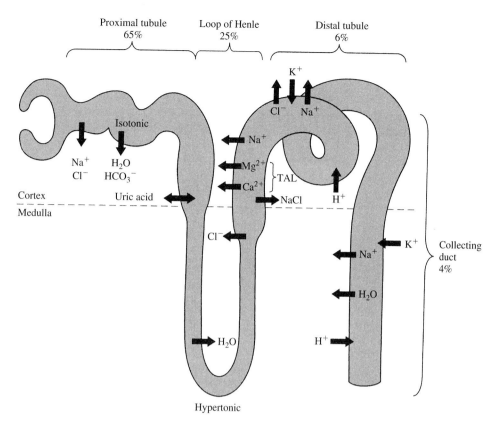

FIGURE 21.1

A nephron, showing the major sites and percentage (in braces) of sodium absorption along with other features of solute transport. The filtered load = GFR (180 L/day) ×plasma Na$^+$ (140 mEq/L) or 25,200 mEq/day. About 1% of this amount is excreted in voided urine. Sites where tubular fluid is isosmotic, hypertonic, or hypotonic relative to plasma are shown. PCT, proximal convoluted tubule; LH, loop of Henle; DCT, distal convoluted tubule; CCD, cortical collecting duct; TAL, thick ascending loop.

the distal nephron. The emphasis of the following sections is on the tubular transport properties that affect or are influenced by diuretics.

Proximal Tubule

The majority (two-thirds) of filtered Na$^+$ is reabsorbed by proximal tubules. A number of transport mechanisms, including Na$^+$–H$^+$ exchange, Na$^+$–phosphate cotransport, Na$^+$–glucose, Na$^+$–lactate, and Na$^+$–amino acid cotransport, participate in Na$^+$ reabsorption. *Na$^+$–H$^+$ exchange is the primary mechanism of Na$^+$ transport in the proximal tubules* (Fig. 21.2). Na$^+$ and HCO$_3^-$ enter the proximal tubule after being filtered at the glomerulus. Na$^+$ diffusion from the lumen into the cell is coupled to the extrusion of a hydrogen ion into the lumen. In the lumen, the H$^+$ combines with HCO$_3^-$ to form carbonic acid (H$_2$CO$_3$), which in the presence of the zinc metalloenzyme *carbonic anhydrase* is rapidly converted to H$_2$O and CO$_2$. The CO$_2$ generated in this reaction readily diffuses into proximal tubule cells, and the process reverses. That is, the CO$_2$ that was generated

combines with intracellular water and in the presence of cytoplasmic carbonic anhydrase forms carbonic acid. The carbonic acid in turn is dehydrated to HCO$_3^-$ and H$^+$. The HCO$_3^-$ is transported across the basolateral membranes into the blood, while the H$^+$ becomes available for another cycle of Na$^+$–H$^+$ exchange. The net result of this process is the reabsorption of Na$^+$ and HCO$_3^-$. *Carbonic anhydrase plays a pivotal role both in the cytoplasm and in the lumen in mediating Na$^+$–H$^+$ exchange and thus in some 40% of total proximal Na$^+$ and H$_2$O absorption.* If this enzyme is inhibited, Na$^+$ absorption is slowed because of the accumulation of H$_2$CO$_3$ in the lumen and the lack of H$^+$ within the cell that can be exchanged for Na$^+$. Similarly, HCO$_3^-$ reabsorption is reduced with a concomitant increase of HCO$_3^-$ excretion.

Several additional noteworthy features of proximal Na$^+$ transport are relevant to diuretic action. First, since several transport proteins mediate proximal Na$^+$ reabsorption, no single diuretic would be expected to inhibit all these processes. Consequently, inhibition of any one mechanism leaves the others unaffected and able to

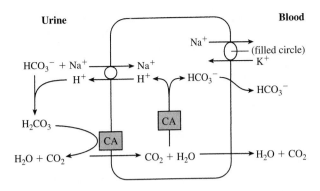

FIGURE 21.2

Carbonic anhydrase-mediated Na$^+$/H$^+$ exchange in proximal convoluted tubule. Na$^+$/H$^+$ exchange across apical cell membranes is shown by the open circle. Carbonic anhydrase (CA) is present in a membrane-bound form in the apical membrane and a soluble form within the cytoplasm. The Na$^+$/K$^+$-ATPase is shown by the filled circle at the basolateral membrane.

continue to absorb the remaining Na$^+$. Second, Na$^+$ that escapes proximal tubular transport is delivered to more distal nephron segments, where compensatory reabsorption reduces the impact of diminished upstream Na$^+$ recovery. *Hence, although most Na$^+$ is reabsorbed by proximal tubules, diuretics inhibiting its transport in this nephron segment have only a modest effect in reducing overall Na$^+$ reabsorption.*

Most of the K$^+$ that is filtered at the glomerulus is reabsorbed by proximal tubules. K$^+$ appearing in the voided urine was secreted by distal and terminal nephron segments (discussed later).

Another significant feature of the proximal tubule is that it is the site of organic acid transport. This is important in understanding both the pharmacokinetics of many of the diuretics, most of which are weak organic acids, and also certain of the side effects induced by these drugs. For instance, uric acid, which is the end product of purine metabolism in humans, is both reabsorbed and secreted by the organic acid transport pathway (see Chapter 37).

An important functional characteristic of the proximal tubule is that fluid reabsorption is isosmotic; that is, proximal reabsorbed tubular fluid has the same osmotic concentration as plasma. Solute and water are transported in the same proportions as in the plasma because of the high water permeability of the proximal tubule. Thus, the total solute concentration of the fluid in the proximal convoluted tubule does not change as the fluid moves toward the descending loop of Henle. The corollary of this high water permeability is that *unabsorbable or poorly permeable solutes in the luminal fluid retard fluid absorption by proximal tubules.* This is an important consideration for understanding the actions of osmotic diuretics.

Loop of Henle
Descending Thin Limb

The descending thin limb of Henle's loop begins at the end of the proximal straight tubule and continues past the hairpin bend in Henle's loop to the start of the thick ascending limb. *Descending thin limbs are virtually devoid of Na$^+$–K$^+$-ATPase and therefore do not participate in active sodium reabsorption.* Moreover, the descending thin limb is highly impermeable to sodium and urea. Although the descending thin limb is not a site of diuretic action per se, its permeability contributes importantly to the action of osmotic agents because of its high water permeability. The presence of unabsorbable solute in the lumen retards water absorption and thereby contributes to the osmotic diuresis. Furthermore, drugs and other compounds in the tubular fluid are concentrated as a result of the removal of water as the descending thin limb of long-looped nephrons passes through the hypertonic renal medulla. The elevation of drug concentrations for agents working at downstream segments may aid in raising the drug concentrations to the levels necessary for diuretic action. These elevated concentrations would not be achieved in the systemic circulation. The selective increase in the concentration of these drugs within the tubular fluid may account for the relatively selective action of these compounds on the kidney, even though the same sodium transport proteins are present in other tissues.

Thick Ascending Limb

The thick ascending limb is a major site of salt absorption and a principal locus of action of an important group of diuretics. Approximately 25% of the filtered sodium is reabsorbed by the thick ascending limb of Henle's loop. Sodium transport in this nephron segment is mediated by Na$^+$–K$^+$–2Cl$^-$ cotransport (Fig. 21.3). This transporter is present only on the apical, or urine, side of the tubule cells. Although K$^+$ is taken up by the transporter, little net K$^+$ reabsorption occurs in the thick ascending limb because much of the absorbed K$^+$

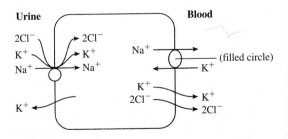

FIGURE 21.3

Na$^+$-K$^+$-2Cl$^-$ cotransport in thick ascending limbs. This transport protein is shown by the open circle on the apical cell membrane. Although K$^+$ enters the cell on the cotransporter, little net K$^+$ reabsorption occurs because much of the K$^+$ is recycled back to the urine from the cell.

is recycled across the apical cell membrane back into the urine. The recirculation of K^+ is important to the generation of the electropositive voltage within the lumen, which serves as a driving force for passive transport of Na^+, Ca^{++}, and Mg^{++} through the tight junctions joining adjacent cells. Hence, *although K^+ is transported by the Na^+–K^+–2Cl cotransporter, the primary solute absorbed into the blood is NaCl.*

Sodium reabsorption in thick ascending limbs depends on the amount, or load, of salt delivered from upstream segments. *The amount of sodium reabsorbed by the thick ascending limb increases as more is delivered.* In situations such as severe volume contraction, when abnormally large amounts of sodium are reabsorbed by proximal tubules, little sodium reaches the thick ascending limb. In this setting the diuretic action of agents that block Na^+–K^+–$2Cl^-$ cotransport is impaired. This is attributable to the reduction of sodium in the tubular fluid of the thick ascending limb.

The reabsorption of NaCl by the thick ascending limb is not accompanied by water because of the low hydraulic permeability of this nephron segment. Consequently, *the tubular fluid becomes dilute as it passes through the thick ascending limbs.* This process contributes to normal urinary dilution. Moreover, when Na^+ transport in thick ascending limbs is inhibited, urinary dilution will diminish.

The thick ascending limb is also an important site for the reabsorption of Ca^{++} and Mg^{++}. These cations are mostly passively reabsorbed through the paracellular pathway between adjacent cells. The driving force for their transport is the transepithelial voltage, which is established by the rate of Na^+ reabsorption. Thus, changes in voltage cause proportionate changes in the rate and magnitude of Ca^{++} and Mg^{++} reabsorption.

Distal Convoluted Tubule

Sodium reabsorption continues in the distal convoluted tubule, which accounts for some 6 to 8% of the transport of sodium. The entry of Na^+ across the apical cell membrane is mediated by Na^+–Cl^- cotransport (Fig. 21.4). This protein is a distinct gene product that differs from the Na^+–K^+–$2Cl^-$ cotransporter in thick ascending limbs.

The permeability properties of the distal convoluted tubule are regulated by antidiuretic hormone (ADH, or *vasopressin*). In hypotonic conditions, ADH secretion by the posterior pituitary is suppressed and the distal convoluted tubule is impermeant to water. Conversely, in hypertonic or volume-contracted states, ADH is released by the posterior pituitary and increases the permeability and water reabsorption by the distal convoluted tubule.

The distal convoluted tubule, along with the collecting duct, is an important site of K^+ transport. The direc-

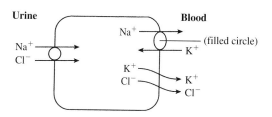

FIGURE 21.4

Na^+-Cl^- cotransport in distal convoluted tubules. This transport protein, shown by the open circle on the apical cell membrane, does not require K^+ for its function. It is a different gene product than the Na^+-K^+-$2Cl^-$ cotransporter. Na^+-Cl^- cotransport is limited largely, if not entirely, to the distal convoluted tubules.

tion (reabsorptive or secretory) and magnitude of K^+ transport is governed by the metabolic state of the individual, the amount and rate of Na^+ and fluid flow through the distal convoluted tubule, and the action of aldosterone. As noted earlier, the main source of urinary K^+ is tubular secretion by distal convoluted tubules and collecting ducts. K^+ secretion also increases during alkalosis and with elevated dietary K^+ intake. *Increases in the rate or amount of Na^+ absorption or of the rate of fluid flow through the distal convoluted tubule stimulate K^+ secretion into the tubular fluid.* These observations are especially important because they account for the elevated K^+ losses that attend the use of diuretics acting in more proximate segments, such as thick ascending limbs and distal convoluted tubules.

In distal convoluted tubules, calcium is transported by an active transport mechanism through rather than between cells. Moreover, in distal convoluted tubules there is a reciprocal relation between the direction and magnitude of calcium on Na^+ transport. As Na^+ absorption increases, calcium decreases, and conversely, reductions of Na^+ absorption are accompanied by elevated calcium reabsorption. This interaction has important implications for diuretics acting in the distal convoluted tubule.

Collecting Ducts

The collecting ducts, which consist of cortical and medullary segments, reabsorb the final 5 to 7% of the filtered Na^+. The epithelium forming the collecting ducts consists of two distinct cell types: *principal cells* and *intercalated cells*. The relative preponderance of the two cell types varies along the length of the collecting duct and between nephron segments. Principal cells are responsible for the reabsorption of Na^+ and the secretion of K^+ (Fig. 21.5). Na^+ enters the principal cell from the tubular fluid through a unique and highly selective epithelial Na^+ channel, ENaC. Intercalated cells reabsorb HCO_3^- and K^+ and secrete H^+. Normally, H^+ is secreted into the urine and HCO_3^- is reabsorbed, while

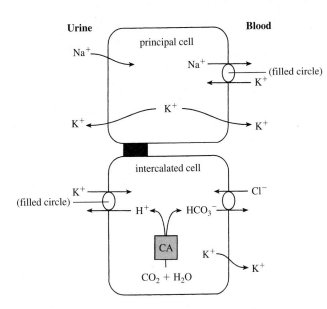

FIGURE 21.5

Principal and intercalated cells of the collecting ducts. Principal (top) cells reabsorb Na^+ and the secreted K^+. Na^+ entry across apical cell membranes is mediated by a Na^+ channel. Na^+ exit across basolateral cell membranes is effected by the Na^+/K^+-ATPase, shown by the filled circle in the principal cell. The rates of Na^+ reabsorption and K^+ secretion are regulated by aldosterone. Intercalated (bottom) cells reabsorb K^+ and HCO_3^- and secretes H^+. K^+ entry and H^+ secretion are mediated by an H^+/K^+ ATPase, which is shown by the filled circle in the apical cell membrane of the intercalated cell.

little net K^+ transport occurs under K^+-replete conditions.

Aldosterone stimulates the rates of Na^+ reabsorption and K^+ secretion. This is relevant to the action of spironolactone, a diuretic that is a competitive inhibitor of aldosterone (discussed later). It is also pertinent because administration of diuretics can cause secondary hyperaldosteronism, which may exaggerate the potassium wasting that is a consequence of the increased delivery of Na^+ and enhanced flow through distal convoluted tubules and collecting ducts.

ADH can significantly modify the total urine volume along with its solute concentration. In the absence of ADH, the collecting ducts are essentially impermeable to water. Little fluid is reabsorbed, and the final urine is dilute with respect to plasma. In other words, the clearance of solute-free water (C_{H_2O}) is greater than the osmolar clearance (C_{osm}). ADH increases water permeability, allowing reabsorption of fluid from the tubules into the interstitium. The driving force for water transport is the osmotic gradient between the medullary interstitium and the tubular fluid. NaCl and urea are the two major solutes accounting for the hypertonicity. The NaCl in the interstitium results from the reabsorption of

Na^+ by thick ascending limbs. Thus, in the absence of ADH, Na^+ reabsorption contributes to medullary interstitial hypertonicity, water abstraction from the collecting ducts, and the formation of concentrated urine. Diuretics blocking Na^+ reabsorption by thick ascending limbs will therefore attenuate the formation of dilute urine (C_{H_2O}) in hypotonic states when ADH is absent or low. Conversely, in hypertonic conditions, when ADH levels are high and diuretics are blocking Na^+ reabsorption by the thick ascending limbs, the generation of concentrated urine is reduced, and C_{osm} is greater than C_{H_2O}.

DIURETIC DRUGS

Many drugs can enhance urine flow. For example, by increasing cardiac output in the patient with congestive heart failure, digitalis administration will mobilize edema fluid and diuresis. The term *diuretic*, however, is generally restricted to agents that act directly on the kidney. *From a therapeutic point of view, diuretics are considered to be substances that aid in removing excess extracellular fluid and electrolytes.* In the main, they accomplish this by decreasing salt and water reabsorption in the tubules.

Carbonic Anhydrase Inhibitors

In the late 1930s, it was reported that sulfanilamide and other *N*-unsubstituted sulfonamides could induce diuresis characterized by excretion of an alkaline urine that is high in sodium bicarbonate. It was soon realized that these compounds inhibited *carbonic anhydrase,* an enzyme highly concentrated in renal tissue, and that this enzyme was important for the tubular reabsorption of bicarbonate. The common structural motif of carbonic anhydrase inhibitors is an unsubstituted sulfonamide moiety. These findings led to the synthesis of a series of compounds capable of inhibiting carbonic anhydrase, the most useful of which was acetazolamide (*Diamox*), which is considered the prototype of this class of diuretics. Although the clinical use of carbonic anhydrase inhibitors has greatly diminished since the 1960s, when their use was increasingly supplanted by the more potent thiazide diuretics (discussed later), they have been vitally important in helping to delineate the physiological role of carbonic anhydrase in electrolyte conservation and acid-base balance. Acetazolamide (*Diamox*), dichlorphenamide (*Daranide*), and methazolamide (*Neptazane*) are the carbonic anhydrase inhibitors available in the United States.

Inhibition of proximal tubule brush border carbonic anhydrase decreases bicarbonate reabsorption, and this accounts for their diuretic effect. In addition, carbonic anhydrase inhibitors affect both distal tubule and collecting duct H^+ secretion by inhibiting intracellular carbonic anhydrase.

Renal excretion of Na^+, K^+, and HCO_3^- is increased by carbonic anhydrase inhibition. Diuresis following carbonic anhydrase inhibition consists primarily of Na^+ and HCO_3^-, with only a small increase of Cl^- excretion. This so-called bicarbonate diuresis is unique to carbonic anhydrase inhibitors. The fractional excretion of Na^+ is generally limited to 5%, as a consequence of downstream compensatory Na^+ reabsorption. Although distal nephron sites recapture much of the Na^+, they possess only a limited ability to absorb HCO_3^-. Fractional K^+ excretion, however, can be as much as 70%. *Potassium loss is particularly marked following carbonic anhydrase inhibition,* both because of the presence of poorly reabsorbable HCO_3^- accompanying Na^+ and because of the inhibition of the Na^+–H^+ exchange mechanism. Elevated urinary HCO_3^- excretion leads to the formation of alkaline urine and to metabolic acidosis as a result of both HCO_3^- loss and impaired H^+ secretion.

The main therapeutic use of carbonic anhydrase inhibitors is not for the production of diuresis but in the treatment of glaucoma. This is true especially of the topically applied compound dorzolamide (*Trusopt*). Because the formation of aqueous humor in the eye depends on carbonic anhydrase, acetazolamide has proved to be a useful adjunct to the usual therapy for lowering intraocular pressure. Although acetazolamide has been used in the treatment of epilepsy, particularly absence epilepsy, it is not known whether the beneficial results are due to carbonic anhydrase inhibition or to the resulting acidosis. Oral carbonic anhydrase inhibitors are also useful in preventing or treating acute mountain sickness. Adverse reactions are minor; they include loss of appetite, drowsiness, confusion, and tingling in the extremities. Animal studies have shown some teratogenic potential, so the use of carbonic anhydrase inhibitors is not recommended during the first trimester of pregnancy.

Thiazide Diuretics

Thiazide diuretics consist of two distinct groups: those containing a benzothiadiazine ring, such as hydrochlorothiazide and chlorothiazide, referred to as thiazide diuretics, and those that lack this heterocyclic structure but contain an unsubstituted sulfonamide group. The latter are called thiazidelike diuretics; they include metolazone, xipamide, and indapamide. The major thiazide and thiazidelike drugs available in the United States are bendroflumethiazide, benzthiazide, chlorothiazide, hydrochlorothiazide, hydroflumethiazide, methyclothiazide, polythiazide, and trichlormethiazide; and chlorthalidone, indapamide, metolazone, and quinethazone, respectively.

Despite the structural distinctions, the drugs share the functional attribute of increasing sodium and chloride excretion by inhibiting Na^+–Cl^- cotransport in distal convoluted tubules.

Although chlorothiazide and its subsequently developed congeners (Table 21.2) retain the sulfamyl group SO_2NH_2, which is necessary for carbonic anhydrase inhibition, their primary effect does not rely on carbonic anhydrase inhibition.

The thiazidelike compounds, including chlorthalidone (*Hygroton*), quinethazone (*Hydromox*), and metolazone (*Zaroxolyn*) have similar mechanisms of action, but they differ substantially from one another in their duration of action, the degree of carbonic anhydrase inhibition, and the dose required for maximum natriuretic activity.

Mechanism of Action

Thiazide diuretics act in the distal convoluted tubule, where they block Na^+–Cl^- cotransport (Fig. 21.4). The Na^+–Cl^- cotransport takes place on the luminal surface of distal convoluted tubules. Thus, to exert their diuretic action, the thiazides must reach the luminal fluid. Since the thiazide diuretics are largely bound to plasma proteins and therefore are not readily filtered across the glomeruli, access to the luminal fluid is accomplished by the proximal tubule organic acid secretory system. The drugs then travel along the nephron, presumably being concentrated as fluid is abstracted, until they reach their site of inhibitory action in the distal convoluted tubule.

Especially at higher doses, administration of some of the thiazides results in some degree of carbonic anhydrase inhibition. However, *at usual doses, only chlorothiazide shows any appreciable carbonic anhydrase inhibitory activity.*

Renal Response

When administered at maximal doses, chlorothiazide markedly increases excretion of Na^+, K^+, Cl^-, and HCO_3^-. Maximal diuresis may approach values as high

TABLE 21.2 Some Commonly Prescribed Thiazide and Thiazidelike Diuretics

Generic Name	Trade Names
Bendroflumethiazide	Naturetin
Benzthiazide	Aquatag, Exna
Chlorothiazide	Diuril
Hydrochlorothiazide	Esidrix, HydroDIURIL
Hydroflumethiazide	Saluron, Diucardin
Methyclothiazide	Enduron, Aquatensen
Polythiazide	Renese
Trichlormethiazide	Naqua, Metahydrin
Chlorthalidone	Hygroton
Indapamide	Lozol
Metolazone	Zaroxolyn, Diulo
Quinethazone	Hydromox

as 10% of the filtered load, although fractional Na^+ excretions of 5% are more common. At usual clinical doses, however, the thiazide diuretics generally increase excretion of Na^+ and Cl^-, with an accompanying loss of K^+. Thus, unlike that of the carbonic anhydrase inhibitors, the diuresis produced by thiazide and thiazidelike diuretics is of NaCl and not $NaHCO_3$. The urinary K^+ wasting induced by the thiazides is primarily a consequence of the increased Na^+ delivered to the distal tubule as discussed earlier.

Two renal responses are unique to the thiazide and thiazidelike diuretics. With these compounds, Na^+ excretion is increased, while Ca^{++} excretion is decreased, primarily and directly because of increased distal Ca^{++} reabsorption, secondarily and indirectly because of a compensatory elevation of proximal solute absorption, making this class of diuretics useful in treating hypercalciuria. This effect, which may not be evident upon initial administration of the drug, is particularly beneficial in individuals who are prone to calcium stone formation.

A second unusual action of this class of diuretics is their utility in treating nephrogenic diabetes insipidus. Patients who have an adequate supply of ADH but whose kidneys fail to respond to ADH excrete large volumes of very dilute urine, not unlike those who have an ADH deficiency. The thiazides reduce glomerular filtration modestly and decrease positive free water formation (C_{H_2O}), that is, production of dilute urine. These actions combine to cause patients with nephrogenic diabetes insipidus to excrete a somewhat reduced urine volume with increased osmolality.

Absorption and Elimination

Orally administered thiazides are rapidly absorbed from the gastrointestinal tract and begin to produce diuresis in about 1 hour. Approximately 50% of an oral dose is excreted in the urine within 6 hours. These compounds are organic acids and are actively secreted into the proximal tubular fluid by the organic acid secretory mechanism. There also appears to be an extrarenal pathway for their elimination involving the hepatic–biliary acid secretory system that is particularly important for thiazide elimination when renal function is impaired.

The thiazides have a variable effect on elimination of uric acid, which also is secreted by the renal acid secretory mechanism. Administration of thiazide diuretics, especially at low doses, may elevate serum uric acid levels and cause goutlike symptoms. Following large doses, thiazides may compete with uric acid for active reabsorption and thereby may promote uric acid elimination rather than impair it (see Chapter 37).

Clinical Uses

Thiazides, especially hydrochlorothiazide (*Dyazide, Esidrix, HydroDIURIL, Oretic*), are useful adjunctive

therapy in controlling the edema associated with congestive heart failure, cirrhosis, premenstrual tension, and hormone therapy. They are widely used in the treatment of hypertension whether or not it is accompanied by edema (see Chapter 20). They can be used in patients with renal disease; however, their diuretic activity is proportional to the residual tubular functional capacity of the kidney. The thiazides do not prevent toxemia in pregnancy, nor are they useful in the treatment of it.

Adverse Effects

Thiazides should be used cautiously in the presence of severe renal and hepatic disease, since azotemia and coma may result. *The most important toxic effect associated with this class of diuretics is hypokalemia,* which may result in muscular and central nervous system symptoms, as well as cardiac sensitization (see Hypokalemia). Periodic examination of serum electrolytes for possible imbalances is strongly recommended. Appropriate dietary and therapeutic measures for controlling hypokalemia are described later in this chapter. The thiazides also possess some diabetogenic potential, and although pancreatitis during thiazide therapy has been reported in a few cases, the major mechanism contributing to the potential for glucose intolerance is not known.

Hypokalemia and Potassium-sparing Diuretics
Hypokalemia

The chronic use of some diuretics may require the oral administration of potassium supplements or potassium-sparing diuretics that reduce urinary K^+ excretion. This is true especially for patients with congestive heart failure and cirrhosis, who are particularly sensitive to K^+ loss. The presence or absence of clinical symptoms of hypokalemia is quite closely related to serum K^+ concentrations, and even small changes in extracellular K^+ can have marked effects. Most patients begin to show symptoms when serum K^+ levels fall below 2.5 mEq/L (from a normal value of approximately 5 mEq/L).

Neurological symptoms include drowsiness, irritability, confusion, loss of sensation, dizziness, and coma. Other important symptoms of hypokalemia are muscular weakness, cardiac arrhythmias, tetany, respiratory arrest, and increased sensitivity of the myocardium to digitalislike drugs.

Treatment

Hypokalemia can be treated by supplying additional K^+ through the diet, drug treatment, or both. Replacement should be gradual, with frequent evaluation of both serum K^+ concentrations and cardiac activity (electrocardiographic monitoring). K^+ supplements can be administered in several forms. KCl is generally preferred over other forms such as bicarbonate, citrate, or gluconate, since most patients exhibit concurrent metabolic alkalosis. KCl corrects both the hypokalemia and the alkalosis. When hypokalemia is not attended by metabolic alkalosis, other forms of K^+ supplementation may be preferred. Since KCl solutions have a rather bitter and unpleasant taste, this salt was formerly given as an enteric-coated tablet. However, the rapid release of KCl from the tablet after it entered the small intestine was responsible for a severe local ulceration, hemorrhage, and stenosis, especially when there was a delay in gut transit time; therefore, the enteric-coated tablets have been withdrawn.

Sugar-coated products have been marketed that contain KCl in a wax matrix (*Slow-K* and *Kaon-Cl*) and are purportedly slow- and controlled-release preparations. Available evidence indicates that these slow-release forms of KCl are occasionally capable of causing local tissue damage and therefore probably should be used with caution for K^+ supplementation. Solutions of potassium gluconate, like the tablets, also have been associated with intestinal ulceration. Microencapsulated KCl preparations (*Micro-K, K-Dur*) that are neither enteric coated nor contained within a wax matrix appear to be superior to the wax matrix formulation.

Consumption of potassium-rich foods is the easiest and most generally advised means of counteracting a K^+ deficit. Table 21.3 lists foods that are suitable for K^+ supplementation.

In general, a normal diet plus about 40 mEq per day of K^+ is adequate to prevent hypokalemia. If K^+-rich foods prove inadequate in replacing large quantities of the electrolyte or if the increased caloric intake that is part of the dietary supplementation is not desirable, oral *liquid* therapy is the formulation of choice. A listing of these solutions is given in Table 21.4. Although patients may find many of these products unpalatable, their further dilution with water or fruit juice can be

TABLE 21.3 **Foods Rich in Potassium (approximately 0.5 g portion)**

Prune juice (1 cup)
Orange juice (1 cup)
Grapefruit juice (1 cup)
Prunes (7)
Banana (1)
Dates (7)
Figs (4)
Raisins (0.5 cup)
Apricots (6)
Sweet potato (1)
White potato (1)

TABLE 21.4 **Potassium Supplementation**

Product	Manufacturer	Dosage Form
Kaochlor	Adria	Liquid
Kay Ciel elixir	Berlex	Liquid
Potassium Triplex	Lilly	Liquid
KCL 10%	Purepac	Liquid
KCL 20%	Stanlabs	Liquid
K-Lor	Abbott	Powder[a]
K-Lyte	Mead Johnson	Tablets[a]

[a]This product, although supplied as a solid dose, is dissolved in water before ingestion.

helpful. Finally, the addition of a K^+-sparing diuretic to the therapeutic regimen may prove useful.

The three principal potassium-sparing diuretic agents produce similar effects on urinary electrolyte composition. Through actions in the distal convoluted tubule and collecting duct, they cause mild natriuresis and a decrease in K^+ and H^+ excretion. Despite their similarities, these agents actually constitute two groups with respect to their mechanisms of action.

Aldosterone Antagonists: Spironolactone

The mechanism by which Na^+ is reabsorbed in coupled exchange with H^+ and K^+ in the collecting duct has been discussed previously; that is, Na^+-driven K^+ secretion is partially under mineralocorticoid control. Aldosterone and other compounds with mineralocorticoid activity bind to a specific mineralocorticoid receptor in the cytoplasm of late distal tubule cells and of principal cells of the collecting ducts. This hormone–receptor complex is transported to the cell nucleus, where it induces synthesis of multiple proteins that are collectively called aldosterone-induced proteins. The precise mechanisms by which these proteins enhance Na^+ transport are incompletely understood. However, the net effect is to increase Na^+ entry across apical cell membranes and to increase basolateral membrane Na^+–K^+–ATPase activity and synthesis.

Mechanism of Action

Spironolactone (*Aldactone*) is structurally related to aldosterone and acts as a competitive inhibitor to prevent the binding of aldosterone to its specific cellular binding protein. Spironolactone thus blocks the hormone-induced stimulation of protein synthesis necessary for Na^+ reabsorption and K^+ secretion. *Spironolactone, in the presence of circulating aldosterone, promotes a modest increase in Na^+ excretion associated with a decrease in K^+ elimination.* The observations that spironolactone is ineffective in adrenalectomized patients and that the actions of spironolactone can be reversed by raising circulating aldosterone blood levels (surmountable antagonism) support the conclusion that spironolactone acts by competitive inhibition of the binding of aldosterone with receptor sites in the target tissue. *Spironolactone acts only when mineralocorticoids are present.*

Pharmacokinetic Properties

Spironolactone is poorly absorbed after oral administration and has a delayed onset of action; it may take several days until a peak effect is produced. It has a somewhat slower onset of action than triamterene and amiloride (discussed later), but its natriuretic effect is modestly more pronounced, especially during long-term therapy. Spironolactone is rapidly and extensively metabolized, largely to the active metabolite *canrenone.* Canrenone and potassium canrenoate, its K^+ salt, are available for clinical use in some countries outside the United States. Canrenone has a half-life of approximately 10 to 35 hours. The metabolites of spironolactone are excreted in both the urine and feces. New selective aldosterone receptor antagonists (SARA), such as eplerenone, have been developed but have not yet been introduced into clinical practice. Eplerenone and canrenone exhibit fewer steroidlike side effects (gynecomastia, hirsutism).

Clinical Uses

Spironolactone has been used clinically in the following conditions:

1. *Primary hyperaldosteronism.* Used as an aid in preparing patients with adrenal cortical tumors for surgery.
2. *Hypokalemia.* Used in patients with low serum K^+ resulting from diuretic therapy with other agents. Its use should be restricted to patients who are unable to supplement their dietary K^+ intake or adequately restrict their salt intake or who cannot tolerate orally available KCl preparations.
3. *Hypertension and congestive heart failure.* Although spironolactone may be useful in combination with thiazides, the latter remain the drugs of first choice. Fixed-dose combinations of spironolactone and a particular thiazide (e.g., *Aldactazide*) generally offer no therapeutic advantage over either component given separately and tend to restrict the ability of the clinician to determine the optimal dosage of each drug for a particular patient.
4. *Cirrhosis and nephrotic syndrome.* Spironolactone is a mild diuretic and may be useful in treating the edema that occurs in these two clinical conditions, that is, when excessive K^+ loss is to be avoided.

Adverse Effects

Serum electrolyte balance should be monitored periodically, since potentially fatal *hyperkalemia* may occur, especially in patients with impaired renal function or excessive K^+ intake (including the K^+ salts of coadministered drugs, e.g., potassium penicillin). Spironolactone can induce hyponatremia and in cirrhotic patients, metabolic acidosis. A variety of gastrointestinal disturbances may accompany spironolactone administration. These include diarrhea, gastritis, gastric bleeding, and peptic ulcers. Spironolactone is contraindicated in patients with peptic ulcers. Spironolactone may also cause elevated blood urea nitrogen, drowsiness, lethargy, ataxia, confusion, and headache. Gynecomastia and menstrual irregularity in males and females, respectively, can occur. Painful *gynecomastia* (directly related to dosage level and duration of therapy), which is generally reversible, may necessitate termination of therapy. Animal studies demonstrating tumorigenic potential support the clinical judgment that spironolactone alone or in combination should not be used for most patients who require diuretic therapy and its unnecessary use should be avoided.

Nonsteroidal Potassium-sparing Drugs: Triamterene and Amiloride

Triamterene (*Dyrenium*) or amiloride (*Midamor*) administration results in changes in urinary electrolyte patterns that are qualitatively similar to those produced by spironolactone. The mechanism by which these agents bring about the alterations in electrolyte loss, however, is quite different. *Triamterene and amiloride produce their effects whether or not aldosterone or any other mineralocorticoid is present.* The action of these two drugs is clearly unrelated to endogenous mineralocorticoid activity, and *these drugs are effective in adrenalectomized patients.*

Mechanism of Action

Both agents appear to affect Na^+ reabsorption in the cortical collecting duct. A site in the connecting tubule also may be involved. Although amiloride has been more extensively studied than triamterene, *both diuretics specifically block the apical membrane epithelial Na^+ channel (ENaC)* (Fig. 21-5). The reduced rate of Na^+ reabsorption diminishes the gradient that facilitates K^+ secretion. K^+ secretion by the collecting duct principal cells is a passive phenomenon that depends on and is secondary to the active reabsorption of Na^+.

In addition to their effects on distal Na^+ and K^+ transport, *all of the K^+-sparing diuretics inhibit urinary H^+ secretion by the late distal tubule and cortical collecting duct.* The mechanism of this inhibitory action is not totally clear.

Pharmacokinetic Properties

Both triamterene and amiloride are effective after oral administration. Diuresis ensues within 2 to 4 hours after administration, although a maximum therapeutic effect may not be seen for several days. Both drugs cause a modest (2–3%) increase in Na^+ and HCO_3^- excretion, a reduction in K^+ and H^+ loss, and a variable effect on Cl^- elimination. Approximately 80% of an administered dose of triamterene is excreted in the urine as metabolites; amiloride is excreted unchanged.

Clinical Uses

Triamterene can be used in the treatment of congestive heart failure, cirrhosis, and the edema caused by secondary hyperaldosteronism. It is frequently used in combination with other diuretics except spironolactone. Amiloride, but not triamterene, possesses antihypertensive effects that can add to those of the thiazides.

These K^+-sparing diuretics have low efficacy when used alone, since only a small amount of total Na^+ reabsorption occurs at more distal sites of the nephron. These compounds are *used primarily in combination* with other diuretics, such as the thiazides and loop diuretics, to prevent or correct hypokalemia. The availability of fixed-dose mixtures of thiazides with nonsteroidal K^+-sparing compounds has proved a rational form of drug therapy. Both triamterene and amiloride are available alone or in combination with hydrochlorothiazide.

Adverse Effects

Because the actions of triamterene and amiloride are independent of plasma aldosterone levels, their prolonged administration is likely to result in hyperkalemia. Both amiloride and triamterene are contraindicated in patients with hyperkalemia. Triamterene should not be given to patients with impaired renal function. Potassium intake must be reduced, especially in outpatients. A folic acid deficiency has been reported to occur occasionally following the use of triamterene.

High-Ceiling, or Loop, Diuretics

The compounds known as *high-ceiling* or *loop diuretics* are the most efficacious agents available for inducing marked water and electrolyte excretion. They can increase diuresis even in patients who are already responding maximally to other diuretics. The drugs in this group available for use in the United States include furosemide (*Lasix*), bumetanide (*Bumex*), torsemide (*Demadex*), and ethacrynic acid (*Edecrin*). Although these agents differ somewhat, they share a common primary site of action, which underlies their effectiveness.

Mechanism of Action

The site of action of loop diuretics is the thick ascending limb of the loop of Henle, and diuresis is brought about by inhibition of the Na^+–K^+–$2Cl^-$ transporter. This seg-

ment of the nephron is critical for determining the final magnitude of natriuresis. As much as 20% of the filtered Na^+ may be reabsorbed by the loop of Henle. The importance of the loop is further emphasized by the realization that drugs that primarily inhibit proximal Na^+ and fluid reabsorption have their natriuretic response reduced by the ability of the ascending limb to augment its rate of Na^+ reabsorption in the presence of an increased tubular Na^+ load. Thus, *any agent that greatly impairs active reabsorption in the thick ascending limb may induce a very large Na^+ and water loss.* Furthermore, the relatively limited capacity of the distal tubule and collecting duct for Na^+ reabsorption makes it impossible to recapture much of the suddenly increased tubular Na^+ reaching them.

Since the thick ascending limb is responsible for initiating events that lead to the hyperosmolar medullary interstitium (and therefore providing the driving force for water reabsorption from the collecting ducts under the influence of ADH), it is this nephron segment that underlies urinary concentration. Thus, drugs that interfere with this concentrating function will have marked effects on urinary output.

Diuretic Response

During the peak effect of the loop diuretics, urine flow is greatly augmented, as is the excretion of Na^+ and Cl^-, corresponding to as much as 20 to 30% of their filtered load. K^+ loss also occurs as an indirect effect of the large Na^+ load reaching the distal tubules and is 2 to 5 times above normal levels of K^+ excretion. With low or moderately effective doses, these drugs do not appreciably affect HCO_3^- or H^+ excretion.

Furosemide (*Lasix*), torsemide (*Demadex*), and bumetanide (*Bumex*) possess some carbonic anhydrase inhibiting activity (about one-tenth that of chlorothiazide). This property may account for the increased bicarbonate and phosphate excretion seen after large doses of these diuretics. The elevated HCO_3^- loss probably indicates some proximal tubular effects for furosemide and bumetanide.

Pharmacokinetic Properties

All of the loop diuretics are available for both oral and parenteral administration. Their onset of action is rapid, usually within 30 minutes after oral and 5 minutes after intravenous administration. They produce peak diuresis in about 2 hours, with a total duration of diuretic action of approximately 6 to 8 hours. Loop diuretics are extensively bound to plasma proteins and are eliminated in the urine by both glomerular filtration and tubular secretion. Approximately a third of an administered dose is excreted by the liver into the bile, from where it may be eliminated in the feces. Only small amounts of these compounds appear to be metabolized by the liver.

The loop diuretics must be present in the tubular fluid before they can become effective. Because of their extensive binding to plasma proteins, filtration across the glomerular capillaries is restricted. Like the thiazides, however, the loop diuretics are weak organic acids that are substrates for the organic acid secretory system in the proximal tubule. A consequence of this active secretion is that the presence of other organic acids or certain forms of renal disease may impair the therapeutic usefulness of the loop diuretics.

Clinical Uses

Because diuresis may be extensive, loop diuretics should be administered initially in small doses; multiple doses, if needed, should be given in early morning and early afternoon. During the remainder of the day, when the drug is not acting, the body can begin to compensate for any derangements in fluid and electrolyte balance that may have occurred as a result of drug therapy. These drugs should be restricted to patients who require greater diuretic potential than can be achieved by other diuretic drugs. In addition to being used in the usual edematous states associated with congestive heart failure, cirrhosis, or renal disease, the loop diuretics can be used in emergencies, such as acute pulmonary edema, when rapid onset of action is essential. They are not recommended for use during pregnancy.

Adverse Effects

Frequent serum electrolyte analysis is essential during therapy with the high-ceiling diuretics. Overdose may result in a rapid reduction of blood volume, dizziness, headache, orthostatic hypotension, hyponatremia, and hypokalemia. Nausea, vomiting, diarrhea, and loss of appetite are especially common with ethacrynic acid.

Ototoxicity has been reported during therapy with all loop diuretics. This effect seems to be dose related and is most common in patients with renal insufficiency. Deafness is usually reversed when these drugs are discontinued, but irreversible hearing loss has been reported after administration of ethacrynic acid, and this has led to a marked decrease in its use.

Furosemide, torsemide, and bumetanide are sulfonamide derivatives, hence chemically related to the thiazides. They share the thiazides' adverse effects of serum uric acid elevation and diabetogenic potential. Ethacrynic acid (*Edecrin*) is chemically unrelated to other diuretics and does not appear to have diabetogenic potential.

Osmotic Diuretics

Osmotic diuretics owe their effects to the physical retention of fluid within the nephron rather than to direct action on cellular sodium transport. These compounds are not electrolytes, and they are freely filtered at the glomerulus and not reabsorbed to a significant extent. Ideally, these drugs should be water-soluble compounds, well absorbed after oral administration, freely filtered at the glomerulus, poorly reabsorbed by the tubule, and devoid of pharmacological effects. The prototype is mannitol (*Osmitrol*), an unmetabolizable polysaccharide derivative of sucrose. Other clinically available osmotic diuretics include glycerin (*Glycerol, Osmoglyn,* and the topical agent *Ophthalgan*), isosorbide (*Ismotic*), and urea (*Ureaphil, Urevert*). Since these osmotic agents act in part to retard tubule fluid reabsorption, *the amount of diuresis produced is proportional to the quantity of osmotic diuretic administered.* Therefore, unless large quantities of a particular osmotic diuretic are given, the increase in urinary volume will not be marked.

Ideally, the distribution of osmotic diuretics should be largely confined to the vascular system, although this can lead to excessive expansion of the vascular compartment. Such an overexpansion could precipitate pulmonary edema or increase cardiac work or both. This is largely the result of rapid transfer of fluid from the interstitial to the vascular compartment. Practically speaking, however, few osmotic diuretics are available for therapeutic use. *These agents, therefore, should be given cautiously to patients with compromised cardiac function.*

Mechanism of Action

The renal response to osmotic diuretics is probably due to the interplay of several factors. The primary effect involves an *increased fluid loss* caused by the osmotically active diuretic molecules; this results in reduced Na^+ and water reabsorption from the proximal tubule.

An additional contributing factor to the diuresis induced by osmotic diuretics is the *increase in renal medullary blood flow* that follows their administration. This medullary hyperemia reduces the cortex–medullary osmolar gradient by carrying away interstitial Na^+ and urea. This partial reduction of the osmolar gradient impairs normal reabsorption of tubular water, which occurs from the descending limb of Henle and the collecting duct.

Finally, there is an additional *increase in electrolyte excretion* due to impairment of ascending limb and distal tubule Na^+ reabsorption; this occurs as a result of lowered tubular Na^+ concentration and the increased tubular fluid flow rate.

Individual Agents
Mannitol

Mannitol (*Osmitrol*) is a six-carbon sugar that does not undergo appreciable metabolic degradation. It is not absorbed from the gastrointestinal tract and therefore must be given intravenously. Humans do not reabsorb it in the proximal tubules.

Mannitol is particularly useful in clinical conditions characterized by hypotension and decreased glomerular filtration. These symptoms are usually the result of some physical trauma or surgical procedure. Mannitol is useful in maintaining kidney function in these conditions, since even at reduced rates of filtration, a sufficient amount of the sugar may enter the tubular fluid to exert an osmotic effect and thus continue urine formation. However, if circulatory failure is profound and glomerular filtration is severely compromised or absent, not enough mannitol may reach the tubules to be effective. The ability to maintain urine flow when renal shutdown might otherwise be expected aids in preventing kidney tubular damage. In addition, mannitol has been used to reduce cerebral edema during neurosurgery, to reduce intraocular pressure before surgery for glaucoma, and to promote the elimination of ingested toxic substances.

The major characteristics of the renal response to mannitol diuresis include a fall in urine osmolality and a decrease in the osmolality of the interstitial fluid of the renal medulla. *The quantity of urine formation and Na^+ excretion is generally proportional to the amount of mannitol excreted.* Although there is a significant inhibition of proximal water reabsorption, the effects of mannitol on proximal Na^+ reabsorption are not marked.

The major adverse reactions associated with mannitol administration are headache, nausea, vomiting, chest pain, and hyponatremia. Too rapid an administration of large amounts may cause an excessive shift of fluid from the intracellular to the extracellular compartment and result in congestive heart failure.

Glycerin

The primary use of anhydrous glycerin (*Ophthalgan*) is as an osmotic agent that is applied topically to reduce corneal edema. Orally administered glycerin (*Glycerol, Osmoglyn*) is used to reduce intraocular pressure and vitreous volume before ocular surgery.

Urea

The use of urea (*Ureaphil, Urevert*) has declined in recent years owing both to its disagreeable taste and to the increasing use of mannitol for the same purposes. When used to reduce cerebrospinal fluid pressure, urea is generally given by intravenous drip. Because of its potential to expand the extracellular fluid volume, urea is contraindicated in patients with severe impairment of renal, hepatic, or cardiac function or active intracranial bleeding.

Isosorbide

Isosorbide (*Ismotic*) is an orally effective, osmotically active drug that is most commonly used for the emergency treatment of acute angle-closure glaucoma. It should not be confused with isosorbide dinitrate, an antianginal drug.

USES OF DIURETICS

The ability of certain drugs to increase both fluid and electrolyte loss has led to their use in the clinical management of fluid and electrolyte disorders, for example, edema. *Regardless of the cause of the syndrome associated with edema, the common factor is almost invariably an increased retention of Na^+.* The aim of diuretic therapy is to enhance Na^+ excretion, thereby promoting negative Na^+ balance. This net Na^+ (and fluid) loss leads to contraction of the overexpanded extracellular fluid compartment.

Congestive Heart Failure

Diuretics may have considerable value in reducing the edema associated with congestive heart failure; however, each patient must be evaluated individually, since diuresis is not considered mandatory in all patients. Digitalis and salt restriction may be sufficient to decrease the associated symptoms of pulmonary congestion and peripheral edema. *In patients who require a diuretic as adjunctive therapy, the usual choice should be a thiazide or thiazide-type diuretic rather than one of the loop diuretics (e.g., bumetanide or furosemide).* This is true especially in mild congestive heart failure. The more efficacious compounds probably should be reserved for those who fail to respond to one of the thiazides. A K^+-sparing diuretic also can be given with the thiazide to maintain serum K^+ levels, which might otherwise be depleted. Hypokalemia predisposes patients to digitalis intoxication.

Hypertension

The use of diuretic drugs, either alone or in combination with other agents, in the management of mild to moderate hypertension is frequent. Diuresis and restriction of salt intake are often sufficient for all hypertensive patients except those with severe, malignant, or complicated hypertension. The mechanisms by which the diuretics lower arterial pressure are not precisely known, although it is thought that the initial response is due to a reduction of plasma volume with a consequently diminished cardiac output. However, after a few weeks, the initial degree of extracellular volume reduction is not maintained, probably owing to a gradual increase in aldosterone production (i.e., increased Na^+ retention and K^+ loss). Nonetheless, the antihypertensive effect is sustained.

Although the arterial pressure in hypertensive patients is related to intravascular volume, the changes in plasma volume are primarily caused by alterations in total body Na^+. *Strict dietary Na^+ restriction can lower arterial pressure in hypertensive patients, whereas a large Na^+ intake will reverse the hypotensive effects of thiazide diuretics.* It appears quite plausible that all of the hypotensive effects of the diuretics can be attributed to some aspect of Na^+ depletion, that is, either directly on extracellular fluid volume or perhaps indirectly through the effects of Na^+ loss on autonomic nervous function (e.g., diminished norepinephrine storage capacity in sympathetic nerves) or vascular smooth muscle reactivity.

Diuretics are frequently used in combination with other antihypertensive agents. The appropriateness of this combination becomes even more apparent when it is realized that nondiuretic antihypertensives (e.g., hydralazine or diazoxide) produce some increase in plasma volume that if not corrected, would lead to an eventual decrease in their activity (see Chapter 20).

Hepatic Ascites

Cirrhosis and other liver diseases may result in the formation of excessive amounts of fluid in the abdomen (*ascites*). The primary causes of ascites are usually elevation of pressure in the portal vein and a decreased amount of hepatic plasma protein production. Both factors tend to reduce the ability of the vascular compartment to retain fluid. The resultant ascites may contribute to decreased appetite and respiratory difficulties, among other symptoms. When these symptoms are present, careful reduction in the fluid volume through the use of diuretics is desirable.

Since patients with cirrhosis vary widely in their response to diuretics, conservative initial diuretic therapy is called for. *The mainstay of treatment, however, remains restriction of dietary Na^+.* A common finding in patients with cirrhosis is decreased glomerular filtration, despite the increase in total blood volume caused by the extensive pooling of blood in the splanchnic vessels. Diminished renal perfusion leads to increased aldosterone secretion, which in turn increases Na^+ retention and K^+ loss. Thus, in addition to diuretics, most patients require K^+ supplementation. *The thiazides remain the drugs of first choice.* The use of a high-ceiling drug, such as furosemide, leads more frequently to such complications as hypokalemia, hyponatremia, and azotemia. K^+-sparing diuretics may be useful adjunctive (but not sole) agents if extensive hypokalemia is present.

Pulmonary Edema

The usual cause of pulmonary edema is acute left ventricular failure. The sequelae of events after left heart failure roughly follow the pattern of reduced stroke volume, leading to increased end-systolic and diastolic volume, which elevates left ventricular end-diastolic pressure. Pressure then increases in the left atrium, pulmonary vein, and finally in the pulmonary capillaries. Elevated pressure in the pulmonary capillaries results in the passing of more fluid into the pulmonary interstitial space, and this compromises gas exchange, diminishes total lung gas volume, and increases airway resistance. *With acute pulmonary edema of cardiac origin, the traditional treatment has included administration of the efficacious, rapidly acting loop diuretics.* These agents, given parenterally, can reduce total blood volume rapidly and thus may help to prevent recurrence of pulmonary congestion. The value of immediate and vigorous use of the loop diuretics has been questioned. The problems of excessive fluid and K^+ loss indicate a conservative approach to diuresis even in this medical emergency.

Increased Intracranial Pressure

A rise in intracranial pressure results in the appearance of a number of symptoms, including headache, vomiting, edema of the optic discs, changes in vital signs, and possibly death. Dehydrating measures, including the use of diuretics, can help lower the pressure, particularly if the elevated intracranial pressure is of a nontraumatic origin. *The parenteral administration of a hypertonic solution of one of the osmotic diuretics, urea or mannitol, can relieve the pressure through its osmotic effects.* The oral administration of glycerol also has been used in neurosurgical procedures when increases in intracranial pressure are anticipated.

Renal Edema
Nephrotic Syndrome

Nephrotic syndrome is characterized by proteinuria and edema due to some form of glomerulonephritis. The resulting fall in plasma protein concentration decreases vascular volume, which leads to diminished renal blood flow. This in turn causes secondary aldosteronism characterized by Na^+ and water retention and K^+ depletion. Rigid control of dietary Na^+ is essential. *Therapy of the nephrotic syndrome using a thiazide (possibly with a K^+-sparing diuretic) to control the secondary aldosteronism, is a useful initial approach to treatment.* Since nephrotic edema is frequently more difficult to control than cardiac edema, it may be necessary to switch to a loop diuretic (and spironolactone) to obtain adequate diuresis.

Chronic Renal Failure

The loop diuretics are usually required in treating chronic renal failure, since drugs with lesser intrinsic activity are not sufficiently effective when tubular function has been compromised greatly. Larger than normal amounts of furosemide are frequently employed, and thus it is especially important to monitor the patient for excessive volume depletion. Intermittent therapy may be the best approach.

Acute Renal Failure

The principal rationale for the use of diuretics in acute renal failure is to prevent complete renal shutdown. Whether renal failure is caused by some underlying disease or by drug-induced renal toxicity, the continued production of even a small amount of urine is probably important in reducing further kidney tubular damage. *Most commonly employed are the osmotic diuretics, with intravenous mannitol generally being the agent of choice.* Osmotic diuresis is possible only if glomerular damage, tubular damage, or both have not progressed too far.

Premenstrual Edema and Edema of Pregnancy

Many women retain fluid during pregnancy and during the last days of the menstrual cycle. Breast fullness and subcutaneous swelling or puffiness are the most commonly observed symptoms; they are largely the result of elevated circulating hormone levels in the blood. Estrogens possess some mineralocorticoid activity, and thus, when present in relatively high concentrations, may produce some expansion of the extracellular fluid compartment. Excessive premenstrual edema frequently responds well to thiazide therapy. *Recent experience has diminished enthusiasm for use of any diuretics in pregnant women.* Since the edema of pregnancy is frequently well tolerated, concerns of compromised uteroplacental perfusion, possible ineffectiveness of diuretics in preeclampsia, and the risk of adverse effects of diuretics on the baby (e.g., thiazides can both cross the placental barrier and appear in breast milk, producing electrolyte disturbances and thrombocytopenia in newborns) have led to diminished routine use of these agents in pregnancy.

Resistance to Diuretic Administration

Since the effectiveness of many diuretics ultimately depends on establishing a negative Na^+ balance to mobilize edema fluid, *restriction of dietary Na^+ intake is generally an essential part of diuretic therapy.* Therefore, one cause of therapeutic failure or apparent patient refractoriness to diuretics could be the patient's continued ingestion of large quantities of NaC1.

Some of the older diuretic drugs were self-limiting; that is, prolonged administration resulted in a gradual diminution of their effectiveness. This problem was corrected through the use of intermittent diuretic therapy. Such a program of several days of diuresis followed by several days of drug withdrawal delayed refractoriness to the drug by preventing excessive disturbances in body electrolyte composition.

Many diuretics (e.g., thiazides and loop diuretics) must reach the tubular lumen before they begin to be effective. Because these compounds are organic acids and are bound to plasma proteins, they reach the luminal fluid by secretion. Any disease condition or drug that impairs *secretion* will affect the access of the diuretics to the luminal fluid and hence to their ultimate site of action (e.g., distal tubule or ascending loop). For example, renal dysfunction may lead to a buildup of *endogenous* organic acids that decrease drug secretion and thereby alter the patient's expected response to the diuretic. Patients with azotemia frequently require large doses of organic acid diuretics to achieve a satisfactory response. The concomitant administration of other drugs that are substrates for the organic acid secretory system (e.g., probenecid or penicillin) may result in an apparent resistance to diuretic action. It should now be obvious that *in addition to disease and electrolyte imbalances, the pharmacodynamic handling of the diuretics themselves may be a factor in diuretic resistance.*

Although most individuals respond well to the usual doses of loop diuretics, a small number of patients are refractory to these drugs. These patients may be vulnerable to ototoxicity or other adverse effects if larger amounts of the diuretic are employed. Compensatory proximal tubular sodium absorption may contribute to or be responsible for the resistance to loop diuretics. Combinations of diuretics may be used as an alternative approach to treating diuretic resistance once it has been verified that satisfactory Na^+ restriction is being followed and that the drug is being adequately absorbed. Administration of a carbonic anhydrase inhibitor may be sufficient to enhance Na^+ delivery to thick ascending limbs, where its reabsorption can be blocked by loop diuretics. Alternatively, thiazide diuretics may be combined with the loop diuretic to limit absorption by distal convoluted tubules. The thiazidelike diuretic metolazone, which has some proximal tubule effects unrelated to carbonic anhydrase, appears to be the most effective of the thiazide and thiazidelike drugs in this regard.

Excessive Diuresis

Excessively vigorous diuresis may lead to intravascular dehydration before removal of edema fluid from the rest of the extracellular compartment. This is especially dangerous if the patient has significant liver or kidney disease. *Once the initial correction of fluid and electrolyte derangement has been achieved, the effect sought is maintenance of homeostasis, not dehydration.* Drug dosage, frequency of administration, and Na^+ intake should be adjusted to achieve homeostasis.

If diuresis has been too vigorous, as may occur after injudicious use of loop diuretics, or if extensive fluid and electrolyte loss has occurred following severe diarrhea or vomiting, replacement therapy may be required. A number of available solutions resemble extracellular fluid and are useful for the repair of water and electrolyte deficits (Table 21-5).

Since the 1950s, diuretic therapy has changed dramatically. Earlier, the major diuretics were acid-forming salts, xanthines, organomercurial compounds, and carbonic anhydrase inhibitors. Either because of toxicity or lack of efficacy, these agents are rarely if ever used.

TABLE 21.5 Solutions Resembling Extracellular Fluid

Solution	Manufacturer
Normosol-R	Abbott
Plasma-Lyte	Baxter
Inosol D-CM	Abbott
Polysal	Cutter
Lactated Ringer's	(Several)

Most of these solutions contain electrolytes in the following mEq range: sodium (130–150), potassium (4–12), chloride (98–109), bicarbonate (50–55), calcium (3–5), and magnesium (0–3).

Study QUESTIONS

1. When a patient is treated with a thiazide diuretic for hypertension, all of the following are likely EXCEPT:
   (A) The fall of blood pressure that occurs in the first 2 weeks of therapy results from a decrease of extracellular volume.
   (B) The sustained fall in blood pressure that occurs after several weeks of therapy is due to a decrease of intravascular resistance.
   (C) After the blood pressure is reduced, hypokalemia remains a complication.
   (D) Hyperuricemia may occur.
   (E) Hypoglycemia may occur.

2. Furosemide increases the excretion of all of the following EXCEPT:
   (A) Na^+
   (B) K^+
   (C) Ca^{++} and Mg^{++}
   (D) Uric acid

3. Which of the following drugs is an appropriate initial antihypertensive therapy in an otherwise healthy adult with mild hypertension?
   (A) Bumetanide
   (B) Triamterene
   (C) Hydrochlorothiazide
   (D) Aldactone

4. When furosemide is administered to a patient with pulmonary edema, there is often symptomatic relief within 5 minutes of starting treatment. This relief is primarily due to:
   (A) A rapid diuretic effect
   (B) An increase in venous capacitance
   (C) A direct effect on myocardial contractility
   (D) Psychological effects

5. All of the following statements are true regarding patients with renal insufficiency who exhibit a reduced diuretic response EXCEPT:

(A) When the GFR drops below 30 mL/minute, thiazide diuretics are virtually useless.
(B) The combination of a thiazide plus a potassium-sparing diuretic may yield an adequate diuretic response.
(C) An 80-mg dose of IV furosemide followed an hour later by a 500-mg dose of IV chlorothiazide will probably yield the highest possible response.
(D) Metolazone is contraindicated.

ANSWERS

1. **E.** There is no evidence that the thiazides have any effect on blood sugar. Initial reductions of blood pressure are due to decreased extracellular volume and cardiac output. The beneficial effect of the sustained reduction of blood pressure is due to reduced vascular resistance. Extracellular volume remains modestly reduced and cardiac output returns to pretreatment levels. Hypokalemia does not ameliorate over time and is associated with an increased risk of ventricular fibrillation and malignant arrhythmias. The magnitude of hypokalemia produced by thiazide and thiazidelike diuretics is dose dependent. However, the degree to which individual patients are affected varies, though chronic administration of even small doses causes some K^+ depletion. Hyperuricemia is thought to have two causes. One is competition of the thiazide class of diuretics, which are weak organic acids, with uric acid for secretion by proximal tubules. This leads to diminished uric acid excretion. Serum concentrations of uric acid are further elevated by the reduced extracellular volume. Diuretic-induced hyperuricemia may cause acute gouty attacks.

2. **D.** Increased Na^+ excretion is a direct consequence of diuretic treatment. In thick ascending limbs, the site of furosemide action, calcium and magnesium transport is largely determined by the magnitude of

sodium absorption. Decreases of Na^+ absorption are accompanied by diminished Ca^{++} and Mg^{++} absorption. K^+ wasting is due to increased K^+ secretion by late distal tubules and collecting ducts. Uric acid excretion decreases as a consequence of competition for the proximal tubule organic acid secretory mechanism.

3. **C.** Although still highly controversial, the initial use of a thiazide diuretic for monotherapy has been recommended by the Joint National Committee on Detection, Evaluation and treatment of High Blood Pressure. Triamterene and Aldactone are rarely used alone and exhibit no antihypertensive activity. A recent study found that the loop diuretics bumetanide and furosemide effectively reduced blood pressure. Serum lipid levels were less affected than with thiazide diuretics or chlorthalidone. However, thiazide diuretics are a more conservative and approved approach for the initial treatment of hypertension that avoid the more dramatic fluid and electrolyte shifts that occur with loop diuretics.

4. **B.** Intravenous furosemide causes a significant decrease in pulmonary capillary wedge pressure and right atrial pressure, concomitantly decreasing stroke volume and increasing vascular resistance. This effect in many cases occurs before diuresis begins.

5. **D.** Metolazone would be expected to be very effective, particularly in combination with a loop diuretic.

SUPPLEMENTAL READING

Bleich M and Greger R. Mechanism of action of diuretics. Kidney Int 1997;51:S11–S15.

Brater DC. The use of diuretics in congestive heart failure. Semin Nephrol 1994;14:479–482.

Brater DC. Pharmacology of diuretics. Am J Med Sci 2000;319: 38–50.

Capasso G et al. Clinical complications of diuretic therapy. Kidney Int 1997;51: S16–S20.

Ellison DH. Diuretic drugs and the treatment of edema: From clinic to bench and back again. Am J Kidney Dis 1994;23:623–643.

Morrison RT. Edema and principles of diuretic use. Med Clin N Am 1997;81:689–704.

Puschett JB. Diuretics and the therapy of hypertension. Am J Med Sci 2000;319:1–9.

Reyes AJ and Taylor SH. Diuretics in cardiovascular therapy: The new clinicopharmacological bases that matter. Cardiovasc Drugs Ther 1999;13:371–398.

Rose BD. Diuretics. Kidney Int 1991;39:336–352.

Rose BD. Resistance of diuretics. Clin Invest 1994;72:722–724.

Suki WN. Use of diuretics in chronic renal failure. Kidney Int 1997;51:S33–S35.

Valtin H and Schafer JA. Renal Function (3rd ed.). Boston: Little, Brown, 1995.

CASE Study Furosemide Resistance

A 26-year-old woman with nephrotic syndrome comes to your office because of worsening edema. Her medications include clonidine 0.1 mg orally twice daily and furosemide 200 mg orally twice daily. On physical examination, her blood pressure is 120/85 mm Hg, and she has generalized massive edema (anasarca). The rest of the examination is unremarkable.

Labatory Studies

Serum creatinine	1.9 mg/dL
Serum albumin	2.0 g/dL
24-hour urine protein excretion	13.0 g
24-hour urine sodium excretion	74.0 mEq

Which of the following factors may contribute to resistance to furosemide in this patient?

(A) Reduced bioavailability

(B) Reduced active tubular secretion of furosemide by the proximal tubule organic acid secretory mechanism

(C) Sequestration of furosemide by intraluminal albumin thereby reducing its inhibition of the Na-K-2Cl cotransporter

(D) Increased reabsorption of sodium downstream to the thick ascending limb of Henle's loop

(E) All of the above

E. Intestinal absorption of furosemide is reduced in patients with anasarca due to edema of the intestinal mucosa. All loop diuretics are highly protein bound; therefore the GFR of these agents is negligible. Availability at the luminal site depends on the activity of the organic acid secretory pump in the proximal tubule. In this patient, secretion of loop diuretics is limited because of reduced renal blood flow and accumulation of organic acids in renal insufficiency, which can compete with furosemide for proximal tubule secretion. In animals, albumin in the tubular fluid binds furosemide, preventing its access to the Na-K-2Cl cotransporter. After prolonged use of furosemide, hypertrophy of the distal tubule epithelial cells occurs, indicating compensatory increased reabsorptive capacity.

22

Anticoagulant, Antiplatelet, and Fibrinolytic (Thrombolytic) Drugs

Jeffrey S. Fedan

 DRUG LIST

GENERIC NAME	PAGE	GENERIC NAME	PAGE
Abciximab	263	Eptifibatide	263
Antihemophilic factor	265	Factor VIIa	265
Ardeparin	260	Factor IX concentrate	265
Alteplase	264	Heparin (unfractionated)	259
Aminocaproic acid	265	Heparin (low molecular weight)	260
Anistreplase	265	Lipirudin	262
Anti-inhibitor coagulant complex	265	Phytonadione	261
Antithrombin III	262	Protamine	260
Aprotinin	265	Reteplase	265
Argatroban	262	Streptokinase	264
Aspirin	262	Tenecteplase	265
Bivalirudin	262	Ticlopidine	263
Clopidogrel	263	Tinzaparin	260
Dalteparin	260	Tirofiban	263
Danaparoid	260	Tranexamic acid	265
Desmopressin	265	Urokinase	264
Dipyridamole	263	Warfarin	260
Enoxaparin	260		

Little intravascular coagulation of blood occurs in normal physiological conditions. Hemostasis involves the interplay of three procoagulant phases (*vascular, platelet,* and *coagulation*) that promote blood clotting to prevent blood loss (Fig. 22.1). The fibrinolytic system prevents propagation of clotting beyond the site of vascular injury and is involved in clot dissolution, or *lysis* (Fig. 22.2).

HEMOSTATIC MECHANISMS

Endothelial cells maintain a nonthrombogenic lining in blood vessels. This results from several phenomena, including (1) the maintenance of a transmural negative electrical charge, which is important in preventing adhesion of circulating platelets; (2) the release of plasminogen activators, which activate the fibrinolytic pathway; (3) the activation of protein C, which degrades

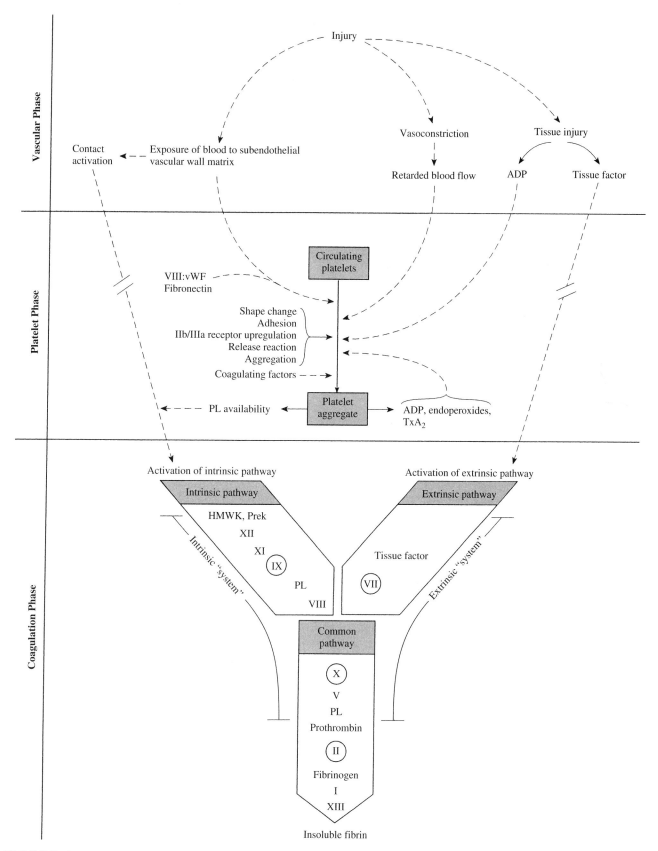

FIGURE 22.1

Hemostatic mechanisms showing the relationships among the vascular, platelet, and coagulation phases. Action is denoted by broken arrows, transformation by solid arrows. Circled factors are those that require vitamin K for activity. Proteins C and S, which degrade factors Va and VIIIa and require vitamin K for activity, are not shown. This figure is a highly simplified summary; see supplemental reading for further details. PL, platelet phospholipid; HMWK, high molecular weight kininogen; PreK, prekallikrein; ADP, adenosine diphosphate; vWF, Von Willebrand factor; TxA_2, thromboxane A_2. (Modified with permission from Wintrobe MM et al. Clinical Hematology (7th ed.). Philadelphia: Lea & Febiger, 1974:390, 422.)

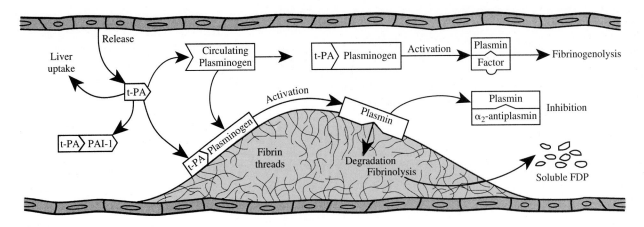

FIGURE 22.2

The fibrinolytic system in blood vessels showing the physiological mechanisms of activation of plasminogen on fibrin to cause fibrinolysis and the pathophysiological mechanism in the blood to cause fibrinogenolysis. The release of t-PA from vascular endothelium and the inhibitory effect of α_2-antiplasmin on plasmin activity are depicted. PAI-1, plasminogen activator inhibitor-1; FDP, fibrin degradation products; factor, coagulation factor. (Modified with permission from Wiman B and Hamsten A. The fibrinolytic enzyme system and its role in the etiology of thromboembolic disease. Semin Thromb Hemost 1990;16:207.)

coagulation factors, a process involving thrombin and its endothelial cofactor (thrombomodulin); (4) the production of heparinlike proteoglycans, which inhibit coagulation; and (5) the release of prostacyclin (PGI_2), a potent inhibitor of platelet aggregation.

In normal individuals, injury severe enough to cause hemorrhage initiates coagulation. Vasoconstriction, combined with increased tissue pressure caused by extravasated blood, results in a reduction, or stasis, of blood flow. Stasis favors the restriction of thrombus formation to the site of injury. The extravasation of blood exposes platelets and the plasma clotting factors to subendothelial collagen and endothelial basement membranes, which result in activation of the clotting sequence. Several substances that participate in coagulation are released or become exposed to blood at the site of injury. These include adenosine diphosphate (ADP), a potent stimulus to platelet aggregation, and *tissue factor*, a membrane glycoprotein cofactor of factor VII.

Platelet aggregation is the most important defense mechanism against leakage of blood from the circulation. Ordinarily, unstimulated platelets do not adhere to the endothelial cell surface. Following disruption of the endothelial lining and exposure of blood to the subendothelial vessel wall, platelets come into contact with and adhere within seconds to factor VIII:vWF polymers and fibronectin. The platelets change shape and then undergo a complex secretory process termed the *release reaction.* This results in the release of ADP from platelet granules and activation of platelet phospholipase A_2. This enzyme, cyclooxygenase, and thrombox-

ane synthetase sequentially convert arachidonic acid into cyclic endoperoxides and thromboxane A_2 (TxA$_2$). In contrast to endothelial cells, platelets lack PGI_2 synthetase. Upon platelet activation with mediators of aggregation (ADP, serotonin, TxA$_2$, epinephrine, thrombin, collagen, platelet activating factor), the integrin platelet receptor for plasma fibrinogen, glycoprotein IIb/IIIa (GPIIb/IIIa), is expressed. The arginine–glycine–aspartic acid (RDG) tripeptide in the α-chain of fibrinogen mediates binding of fibrinogen to the GPIIb/IIIa complex. Fibrinogen, forming a bridge between platelets, and the binding of fibrinogen and Von Willebrand's factor to activated platelets via GPIIb/IIIa are key events in platelet–platelet interactions and play a major role in thrombus formation. Aggregation of circulating platelets to those already adherent amplifies the release reaction.

Other substances liberated from platelets during the release reaction include serotonin (which may promote vasospasm in coronary vessels), platelet factor 4 (a basic glycoprotein that can neutralize the anticoagulant action of circulating heparin), platelet-derived growth factor (a mitogen that initiates smooth muscle cell proliferation and may be involved in atherogenesis), and factors that are also found in the plasma (factor V, factor VIII:vWF, and fibrinogen). During aggregation, the rearrangement of the platelet membrane makes available a phospholipid surface (*platelet factor 3*) that along with Ca^{++} is required for the activation of several clotting factors. *The platelet aggregate becomes a hemostatic plug and is the structural foundation for the assembly of the fibrin network.*

COAGULATION SYSTEMS

Two interrelated processes, the *intrinsic* and *extrinsic* coagulation systems (Fig. 22.1), converge on a common pathway that leads to the activation of factor X, the formation of thrombin (factor IIa), and the conversion by thrombin of the soluble plasma protein fibrinogen into insoluble fibrin. The extrinsic pathway appears to be important for initiating fibrin formation, while the intrinsic pathway is involved in fibrin growth and maintenance; both systems constitute the coagulation cascade. This series of linked and overlapping reactions involves conversion of proenzymes (designated by roman numerals) into serine proteases (designated by roman numeral followed by the suffix -a), and cofactors that speed the protease reactions (factors Va and VIIa).

Exposure of blood to tissue factors activates the extrinsic system, beginning with the proteolytic conversion of factor VII into factor VIIa. Degradation of factors V and VIII:C by protein C at locations distant from the site of vascular injury aids in the localization of clot formation. The coagulation cascade is capable of tremendous amplification as the protease reactions progress. Many of the activated coagulation factors feed back positively in the extrinsic, intrinsic, and common pathways and accelerate the reactions. Either deficiency in a single clotting factor or therapy with the drugs described in this chapter will result in abnormal hemostasis.

ANTICOAGULANT DRUGS

Anticoagulant drugs inhibit the development and enlargement of clots by actions on the coagulation phase. They do not lyse clots or affect the fibrinolytic pathways.

Heparin

Two types of heparin are used clinically. The first and older of the two, standard (unfractionated) heparin, is an animal extract. The second and newer type, called low-molecular-weight heparin (LMWH), is derived from unfractionated heparin. The two classes are similar but not identical in their actions and pharmacokinetic characteristics.

Standard (Unfractionated) Heparin

Heparin (*heparin sodium*) is a mixture of highly electronegative acidic mucopolysaccharides that contain numerous *N*- and *O*-sulfate linkages. It is produced by and can be released from mast cells and is abundant in liver, lungs, and intestines.

Mechanism of Action

The anticoagulation action of heparin depends on the presence of a specific *serine protease inhibitor* (serpin) of thrombin, antithrombin III, in normal blood.

Heparin binds to antithrombin III and induces a conformational change that accelerates the interaction of antithrombin III with the coagulation factors. Heparin also catalyzes the inhibition of thrombin by heparin cofactor II, a circulating inhibitor. Smaller amounts of heparin are needed to prevent the formation of free thrombin than are needed to inhibit the protease activity of clot-bound thrombin. Inhibition of free thrombin is the basis of low-dose prophylactic therapy.

Absorption, Metabolism, and Excretion

Heparin is prescribed on a unit (IU) rather than milligram basis. The dose must be determined on an individual basis. Heparin is not absorbed after oral administration and therefore must be given parenterally. *Intravenous administration results in an almost immediate anticoagulant effect.* There is an approximate 2-hour delay in onset of drug action after subcutaneous administration. Intramuscular injection of heparin is to be avoided because of unpredictable absorption rates, local bleeding, and irritation. Heparin is not bound to plasma proteins or secreted into breast milk, and it does not cross the placenta.

Heparin's action is terminated by uptake and metabolism by the reticuloendothelial system and liver and by renal excretion of the unchanged drug and its depolymerized and desulfated metabolite. The relative proportion of administered drug that is excreted as unchanged heparin increases as the dose increases. Renal insufficiency reduces the rate of heparin clearance from the blood.

Pharmacological Actions

The physiological function of heparin is not completely understood. It is found only in trace amounts in normal circulating blood. It exerts an antilipemic effect by releasing lipoprotein lipase from endothelial cells; heparinlike proteoglycans produced by endothelial cells have anticoagulant activity. Heparin decreases platelet and inflammatory cell adhesiveness to endothelial cells, reduces the release of platelet-derived growth factor, inhibits tumor cell metastasis, and exerts an antiproliferative effect on several types of smooth muscle.

Therapy with heparin occurs in an inpatient setting. *Heparin inhibits both in vitro and in vivo clotting of blood.* Whole blood clotting time and activated partial thromboplastin time (aPTT) are prolonged in proportion to blood heparin concentrations.

Adverse Effects

The major adverse reaction resulting from heparin therapy is hemorrhage. Bleeding can occur in the urinary or gastrointestinal tract and in the adrenal gland. Subdural hematoma, acute hemorrhagic pancreatitis, hemarthrosis, and wound ecchymosis also occur. The incidence of life-threatening hemorrhage is low but variable. Heparin-induced thrombocytopenia of immediate and delayed onset may occur in 3 to 30% of patients. The immediate type is transient and may not involve platelet destruction, while the delayed reaction involves the production of heparin-dependent antiplatelet antibodies and the clearance of platelets from the blood. Heparin-associated thrombocytopenia may be associated with irreversible aggregation of platelets (white clot syndrome). Additional untoward effects of heparin treatment include hypersensitivity reactions (e.g., rash, urticaria, pruritus), fever, alopecia, hypoaldosteronism, osteoporosis, and osteoalgia.

Contraindications, Cautions, and Drug Interactions

Absolute contraindications include serious or active bleeding; intracranial bleeding; recent brain, spinal cord, or eye surgery; severe liver or kidney disease; dissecting aortic aneurysm; and malignant hypertension. Relative contraindications include active gastrointestinal hemorrhage, recent stroke or major surgery, severe hypertension, bacterial endocarditis, threatened abortion, and severe renal or hepatic failure.

Drugs that inhibit platelet function (e.g., aspirin) or produce thrombocytopenia increase the risk of bleeding when heparin is administered. *Oral anticoagulants and heparin produce synergistic effects.* Many basic drugs precipitate in the presence of the highly acidic heparin (e.g., antihistamines, quinidine, quinine, phenothiazines, tetracycline, gentamicin, neomycin).

Heparin Antagonist

The specific heparin antagonist protamine can be employed to neutralize heparin in cases of serious hemorrhage. Protamines are basic low-molecular-weight, positively charged proteins that have a high affinity for the negatively charged heparin molecules. The binding of protamine to heparin is immediate and results in the formation of an inert complex. Protamine has weak anticoagulant activity.

Low-Molecular-Weight Heparin

Low-molecular-weight fragments produced by chemical depolymerization and extraction of standard heparin consist of heterogeneous polysaccharide chains of molecular weight 2,000 to 9,000. The LMWH molecules contain the pentasaccharide sequence necessary for binding to antithrombin III but not the 18-saccharide sequence needed for binding to thrombin. Compared to standard heparin, LMWH has a 2- to 4-fold greater antifactor Xa activity than antithrombin activity.

LMWH has greater bioavailability than standard heparin, a longer-lasting effect, and dose-independent clearance pharmacokinetics. The predictable relationship between anticoagulant response and dose allows

anticoagulant control without laboratory tests. LMWH is more effective than standard heparin in preventing and treating venous thromboembolism. The incidence of thrombocytopenia after administration of LMWH is lower than with standard heparin. Adverse drug reactions like those caused by standard heparin have been seen during therapy with LMWH, and overdose is treated with protamine.

LMWH is available for subcutaneous administration as enoxaparin (*Lovenox*), dalteparin (*Fragmin*), ardeparin (*Normiflo*), and tinzaparin (*Innohep*). Danaparoid (*Orgaran*), a heparinoid composed of heparin sulfate, dermatan sulfate, and chondroitin sulfate, has greater factor Xa specificity than LMWH. Bleeding due to danaparoid is not reversed by protamine.

Orally Effective Anticoagulants

The orally effective anticoagulant drugs are fat-soluble derivatives of 4-hydroxycoumarin or indan-1,3-dione, and they resemble vitamin K. *Warfarin is the oral anticoagulant of choice.* The indandione anticoagulants have greater toxicity than the coumarin drugs.

Mechanism of Action

Unlike heparin, *the oral anticoagulants induce hypocoagulability only in vivo.* They are vitamin K antagonists. Vitamin K is required to catalyze the conversion of the precursors of vitamin K–dependent clotting factors II, VII, IX, and X. This involves the posttranslational γ-carboxylation of glutamic acid residues at the N-terminal end of the proteins. The γ-carboxylation step is linked to a cycle of enzyme reactions involving the active hydroquinone form of vitamin K (K_1H_2). The regeneration of K_1H_1 by an epoxide reductase is blocked by the oral anticoagulants. *These drugs thus cause hypocoagulability by inducing the formation of structurally incomplete clotting factors.*

Commercial warfarin is a racemic mixture of S- and R-enantiomers; S-warfarin is more potent than R-warfarin.

Absorption, Metabolism, and Excretion

Warfarin is rapidly and almost completely absorbed after oral administration and is bound extensively (>95%) to plasma proteins. Since it is the unbound drug that produces the anticoagulant effect, displacement of albumin-bound warfarin by other agents may result in bleeding. Although these drugs do not cross the blood-brain barrier, they can cross the placenta and may cause teratogenicity and hemorrhage in the fetus.

Warfarin is inactivated by hepatic P450 isozymes; hydroxylated metabolites are excreted into the bile and then into the intestine. Hepatic disease may potentiate the anticoagulant response.

Pharmacological Actions

Warfarin is used both on an inpatient and outpatient basis when long-term anticoagulant therapy is indicated. The onset of anticoagulation is delayed, the latency being determined in part by the time required for absorption and in part by the half-lives of the vitamin K–dependent hemostatic proteins. *The anticoagulant effect will not be evident in coagulation tests such as prothrombin time until the normal factors already present in the blood are catabolized;* this takes 5 hours for factor VII and 2 to 3 days for prothrombin (factor II). The anticoagulant effect may be preceded by a transient period of hypercoagulability due to a rapid decrease in protein C levels. More rapid anticoagulation is provided, when necessary, by administering heparin.

Warfarin is administered in conventional doses or minidoses to reduce bleeding. The dose range is adjusted to provide the desired end point.

Adverse Effects

The principal adverse reaction to warfarin is hemorrhage. Prolonged therapy with the coumarin-type anticoagulants is relatively free of untoward effects. Bleeding may be observable (e.g., skin, mucous membranes) or occult (e.g., gastrointestinal, renal, cerebral, hepatic, uterine, or pulmonary). Rarer untoward effects include diarrhea, small intestine necrosis, urticaria, alopecia, skin necrosis, purple toes, and dermatitis.

Contraindications, Cautions, and Drug Interactions

Oral anticoagulants are ordinarily contraindicated in the presence of active or past gastrointestinal ulceration; thrombocytopenia; hepatic or renal disease; malignant hypertension; recent brain, eye, or spinal cord surgery; bacterial endocarditis; chronic alcoholism; and pregnancy. These agents also should not be prescribed for individuals with physically hazardous occupations.

Minor hemorrhage caused by oral anticoagulant overdosage can be treated by discontinuing drug administration. Oral or parenteral vitamin K_1 (phytonadione) administration will return prothrombin time to normal by 24 hours. This period is required for de novo synthesis of biologically active coagulation factors. *Serious hemorrhage may be stopped by administration of fresh frozen plasma or plasma concentrates containing vitamin K–dependent factors.*

Dietary intake of vitamin K and prior or concomitant therapy with a large number of pharmacologically unrelated drugs can potentiate or inhibit the actions of oral anticoagulants. Laxatives and mineral oil may reduce the absorption of warfarin. The patient's prothrombin time and international normalized ratio (INR) should be monitored when a drug is added or removed from therapy. Selected drug interactions involving oral anticoagulants are summarized in Table 22.1.

TABLE 22.1 Drug Interactions Involving Oral Anticoagulants

Drugs That Increase Oral Anticoagulant Effects

Acetaminophen	Chloral hydrate	Fenoprofen	Lovastatin	Propranolol
Alcohol (acute intoxication)	Chlorpropamide	Fluconazole	Mefenamic acid	Quinidine, quinine
	Chymotrypsin	Fluoroquinolones	Metronidazole	Ranitidine
Allopurinol	Cimetidine	Fluoxetine	Micolazole	Sulfamethoxazole-trimethoprim
Amiodarone	Clarithromycin	Fluvastatin	Nabumetone	
Anabolic and androgenic steroids	Clofibrate	Gemcitabine	Nalidixic acid	Sulfinpyrazone
	Cotrimoxazole	Gemfibrozil	Naproxen	Sulindac
Aspirin	Dextran	Glucagon	Omeprazole	Tamoxifen
Azapropazone	Diazoxide	Heparin	Oral hypoglycemics	Ticlopidine
Bromelains	Diflunisal	Ibuprofen	Pentoxifylline	Tolmetin
Cephalosporins	Disulfiram	Indomethacin	Phenylbutazone	Tolterodine
Carboplatin/Etoposide	Ethacrynic acid	Inhalation anesthetics	Phenytoin	Tricyclic antidepressants
Celecoxib	Felbamate	Isoniazid	Piroxicam	Troglitazone
Chenodiol	Fenofibrate	Levamisole/Fluorouracil	Propafenone	Vitamin E

Drugs That Decrease Oral Coagulant Effects

Alcohol (chronic abuse)	Barbiturates	Dextrothyroxine	Nafcillin	Sucralfate
Aminoglutethimide	Carbamazepine	Ginseng	Oral contraceptives	Trazodone
Antacids	Chlordiazepoxide	Griseofulvin	Penicillins (large doses)	Vitamin K (large doses)
Antihistamines	Cholestyramine	Haloperidol	Primidone	
Azathioprine	Corticosteroids	Meprobamate	Rifampin	

Oral anticoagulants also may potentiate hypoglycemia caused by oral hypoglycemic agents, and may enhance phenytoin toxicity.

Direct Thrombin Inhibitor Anticoagulants

Two drugs that are direct inhibitors of thrombin but that do not involve antithrombin III or vitamin K in their mechanism of action have been approved to provide intravenous anticoagulation in patients with heparin-induced thrombocytopenia. Lepirudin (*Refludan*) and bivalirudin (*Angiomax*), which are analogues of the leech peptide anticoagulant hirudin, bind in a 1:1 complex with thrombin to inhibit its protease activity. Argatroban (*Acova, Novastan*), a synthetic analogue of arginine, interacts reversibly with and inhibits thrombin's catalytic site. Both drugs have a short half-life. Lipuridin is cleared following metabolism and urinary excretion of changed and unchanged drug; hepatic metabolism of argatroban is a therapeutic advantage in patients with renal insufficiency. No antagonists for these drugs are available.

CLINICAL INDICATIONS FOR ANTICOAGULANT THERAPY

Anticoagulant therapy provides prophylactic treatment of venous and arterial thromboembolic disorders. *Anticoagulant drugs are ineffective against already formed thrombi,* although they may prevent their further propagation. Generally accepted major indications for anticoagulant therapy with heparin and warfarin include the following:

Deep Vein Thrombosis

Venous stasis resulting from prolonged bed rest, cardiac failure, or pelvic, abdominal, or hip surgery may precipitate thrombus formation in the deep veins of the leg or calf and may lead to fatal pulmonary embolism. Heparin may also be used prophylactically following surgery.

Arterial Embolism

Since arterial emboli formation involves platelet aggregation and leukocyte and erythrocyte infiltration into the fibrin network, the treatment and prophylaxis of arterial thrombi are more difficult. Arterial embolism is treated more successfully with heparin than with the oral anticoagulants. Anticoagulants are useful for prevention of systemic emboli resulting from valvular disease (rheumatic heart disease) and from valve replacement.

Atrial Fibrillation

Restoration of sinus rhythm in atrial fibrillation may dislodge thrombi that have developed as a result of stasis in the enlarged left atrium. The risk of stroke and systemic arterial embolism is decreased by anticoagulation in such patients.

Unstable Angina and Myocardial Infarction

In patients with unstable angina and severe ischemia requiring hospital admission, therapeutic doses of heparin along with antiplatelet therapy (discussed later) are thought to provide additive protection of the patient against myocardial reinfarction. *Thrombolytic drugs are more effective than anticoagulants in treating coronary thromboembolism and in establishing reperfusion of occluded arteries after an infarction.* Anticoagulants in combination with antiplatelet drugs reduce the incidence of thrombus formation and reocclusion after coronary arterial bypass surgery and percutaneous coronary angioplasty.

Disseminated Intravascular Coagulation

Disseminated intravascular coagulation is characterized by widespread systemic activation of the coagulation system, consumption of coagulation factors, occlusion of small vessels by a coat of fibrin, and a hypocoagulation state with bleeding. In conjunction with management of the underlying factor or factors leading to the disorder and coagulation factor and platelet replacement, bleeding may be managed with intravenous (IV) heparin, LMWH, and antithrombin III (*Thrombate*).

ANTIPLATELET DRUGS

The formation of platelet aggregates and thrombi in arterial blood may precipitate coronary vasospasm and occlusion, myocardial infarction, and stroke and contribute to atherosclerotic plaque development. *Drugs that inhibit platelet function are administered for the relatively specific prophylaxis of arterial thrombosis and for the prophylaxis and therapeutic management of myocardial infarction and stroke.* After an infarction or stroke, antiplatelet therapy must be initiated within 2 hours to obtain significant benefit. The antiplatelet drugs are administered as adjuncts to thrombolytic therapy, along with heparin, to maintain perfusion and to limit the size of the myocardial infarction. Recently, antiplatelet drugs have found new importance in preventing thrombosis in percutaneous coronary intervention procedures (angioplasty and stent). Administration of an antiplatelet drug increases the risk of bleeding.

Aspirin inhibits platelet aggregation and prolongs bleeding time. It is useful for preventing coronary thrombosis in patients with unstable angina, as an adjunct to thrombolytic therapy, and in reducing recurrence of thrombotic stroke. It acetylates and irreversibly inhibits cyclooxygenase (primarily cyclooxygenase-1) both in platelets, preventing the formation of TxA_2, and in endothelial cells, inhibiting the synthesis of PGI_2 (see

Chapter 26). While endothelial cells can synthesize cyclooxygenase, platelets cannot. *The goal of therapy with aspirin is to selectively inhibit the synthesis of platelet TxA_2 and thereby inhibit platelet aggregation.* This is accomplished with a low dose of aspirin (160 to 325 mg per day), which spares the endothelial synthesis of PGI_2. If ibuprofen is taken concurrently, it will bind reversibly to cyclooxygenase and prevent the access of aspirin to its acetylation site and thus antagonize the ability of aspirin to inhibit platelets. Dipyridamole (*Persantine*), a coronary vasodilator, is a phosphodiesterase inhibitor that increases platelet cyclic adenosine monophosphate (cAMP) concentrations. It also may potentiate the effect of PGI_2, which stimulates platelet adenylate cyclase. However, dipyridamole itself has little effect on platelets in vivo. Dipyridamole in combination with warfarin is beneficial in patients with artificial heart valves; it is also useful in combination with aspirin (*Aggrenox*) for the secondary prevention of stroke.

Ticlopidine (*Ticlid*) and clopidogrel (*Plavix*) are structurally related drugs that irreversibly inhibit platelet activation by blocking specific purinergic receptors for ADP on the platelet membrane. This action inhibits ADP-induced expression of platelet membrane GPIIb/IIIa and fibrinogen binding to activated platelets. Ticlopidine and clopidogrel are useful antithrombotic drugs. Oral ticlopidine is indicated for prevention of thrombotic stroke in patients who cannot tolerate aspirin and for patients who have had thrombotic stroke. Inhibition of ADP-induced platelet aggregation occurs within 4 days, and the full effect requires approximately 10 days. Ticlopidine is taken with food, is well absorbed, binds extensively to plasma proteins, and is metabolized by the liver. Gastrointestinal disturbances, neutropenia, and agranulocytosis have been observed. Clopidogrel produces fewer side effects than ticlopidine.

Pharmacological agents, such as abciximab (*ReoPro*), eptifibatide (*Integrillin*), and tirofiban (*Aggrastat*), that interrupt the interaction of fibrinogen and Von Willebrand's factor with the platelet GPIIb/IIIa complex are capable of inhibiting aggregation of platelets activated by a wide variety of stimuli. These drugs are given intravenously. The chimeric monoclonal antibody abciximab binds to the GPIIb/IIIa complex, preventing interactions of fibrinogen and Von Willebrand's factor with the integrin receptor. Abciximab is used in conjunction with angioplasty and stent procedures and is an adjunct to fibrinolytic therapy (discussed later). Patients who have murine protein hypersensitivity or who have received abciximab previously may produce an immune response after second administration. Eptifibatide, a cyclic peptide, and tirofiban, a small nonpeptide molecule, both bind reversibly to the GPIIb/IIIa complex and competitively prevent the interaction of the clotting factors with this receptor.

FIBRINOLYTIC SYSTEM

The fibrinolytic system (Fig. 22.2) is involved in restricting clot propagation in the blood and in the removal of fibrin as wounds heal. Treatment of patients with fibrinolytic (thrombolytic) drugs that activate the fibrinolytic system is not a substitute for the anticoagulant drugs. *The purpose of thrombolytic therapy is rapid lysis of already formed clots.*

Fibrinolysis is initiated by the activation of the proenzyme *plasminogen* (present in clots and in plasma) into plasmin, a protease enzyme not normally present in blood. Plasmin catalyzes the degradation of fibrin. The conversion of plasminogen to plasmin is initiated normally by the plasminogen activators, tissue-type plasminogen activator (t-PA) and single-chain urokinase-type plasminogen activator (scu-PA). t-PA and scu-PA are serine protease enzymes synthesized by the endothelium and released into the circulation. The endothelium also releases plasminogen activator inhibitor-1 (PAI-1), which complexes with and inactivates t-PA in the plasma.

t-PA and scu-PA bind with high affinity to fibrin on the clot surface. Circulating plasminogen binds to the plasminogen activator–fibrin complex to form a ternary complex consisting of fibrin, activator, and plasminogen. Therefore, the specificity of t-PA and scu-PA binding to fibrin normally localizes plasmin protease activity to thrombi.

Circulating plasmin is rapidly neutralized by α_2-antiplasmin, a physiological serine protease inhibitor that forms an inert complex with plasmin. In contrast, fibrin-bound plasmin is resistant to inactivation by α_2-antiplasmin. Under normal circumstances plasma t-PA is inactive because it is inhibited by PAI-1, while t-PA that is bound to fibrin is unaffected by PAI-1. In addition, plasma t-PA has a very rapid turnover in blood (half-life 5 to 8 minutes). For these reasons, fibrinolysis is normally restricted to the thrombus.

Activation of the fibrinolytic system with thrombolytic drugs can disturb the balance of these regulatory mechanisms and elevate circulating plasmin activity. Plasmin has low substrate specificity and degrades fibrinogen (fibrinogenolysis), plasminogen, and coagulation factors. The systemic unphysiological activation of the fibrinolytic system with thrombolytic drugs causes consumption of the coagulation factors, a lytic state, and bleeding.

Thrombolytic (Fibrinolytic) Drugs

Thrombolytic drugs cause lysis of formed clots in both arteries and veins and reestablish tissue perfusion.

Mechanism of Action

Thrombolytic drugs are plasminogen activators. The ideal thrombolytic agent is one that can be administered intravenously to produce clot-selective fibrinolysis without activating plasminogen to plasmin in plasma. Older (first generation) thrombolytic agents are not clot selective, and appreciable systemic fibrinogenolysis accompanies successful clot lysis. Newer (second generation) thrombolytic agents bind to fibrin and activate fibrinolysis more than fibrinogenolysis. Third-generation agents have improved fibrin specificity and pharmacokinetic properties.

Pharmacological Actions and Clinical Uses

Thrombolytic drugs are indicated for the management of severe pulmonary embolism, deep vein thrombosis, and arterial thromboembolism and are especially important therapy after myocardial infarction and acute ischemic stroke. Thrombolysis must be accomplished quickly after myocardial or cerebral infarction, since clots become more difficult to lyse as they age. Recanalization after approximately 6 hours provides diminishing benefit to the infarcted area. The incidence of rethrombosis and reinfarction is greater when thrombolytic drugs with shorter plasma half-lives are used. Concurrent administration with heparin followed by warfarin, as well as antiplatelet drugs, is advocated to reduce reocclusion. Adjunctive anticoagulant and antiplatelet drugs may contribute to bleeding during thrombolytic therapy.

Adverse Effects

The principal adverse effect associated with thrombolytic therapy is bleeding due to fibrinogenolysis or fibrinolysis at the site of vascular injury. Hypofibrinogenemia may occur and should be monitored with laboratory tests. At effective thrombolytic doses, the second- and third-generation agents cause less extensive fibrinogenolysis, but bleeding occurs with a similar incidence for all agents. Life-threatening intracranial bleeding may necessitate stoppage of therapy, administration of whole blood, platelets or fresh frozen plasma, protamine (if heparin is present), and an antifibrinolytic drug (discussed later).

Contraindications

The contraindications to the use of thrombolytic drugs are similar to those for the anticoagulant drugs. Absolute contraindications include active bleeding, cardiopulmonary resuscitation (trauma to thorax is possible), intracranial trauma, vascular disease, and cancer. Relative contraindications include uncontrolled hypertension, earlier central nervous system surgery, and any known bleeding risk.

First-Generation Thrombolytic Drugs

Streptokinase (*Streptase, Kabikinase*), a nonenzymatic protein from Lancefield group C β-hemolytic strepto-

cocci, is an *indirectly acting* activator of plasminogen. It forms a 1:1 complex with plasminogen, which results in a conformational change and exposure of an active site that can convert additional plasminogen into plasmin. The systemic administration of streptokinase can produce significant lysis of acute deep vein and pulmonary emboli and acute arterial thrombi. Intravenous or intracoronary artery (IC) streptokinase is effective in establishing recanalization after myocardial infarction and in increasing short-term survival. The greatest benefit of streptokinase appears to be achieved by early intravenous drug administration. Complications associated with the administration of streptokinase include hemorrhage, pyrexia, and allergic or anaphylactic reactions. Patients may be refractory to streptokinase during therapy because of preexisting or streptokinase-induced antibodies. Streptokinase has two half-lives. The faster one (11 to 13 minutes) is due to drug distribution and inhibition by circulating antibodies, and the slower one (23 to 29 minutes) is due to loss of enzyme activity.

Urokinase (*Abbokinase*) is a two-polypeptide chain serine protease that does not bind avidly to fibrin and that directly activates both circulating and fibrin-bound plasminogen. The plasma half-life of urokinase is approximately 10 to 20 minutes. Urokinase is derived from human cells and thus is not antigenic. Urokinase produces a significant resolution of recent pulmonary emboli.

Second- and Third-generation Thrombolytic Drugs

The principal physiological activator of plasminogen in the blood, tissue-type plasminogen activator (t-PA, alteplase) (*Activase*), has a high binding affinity for fibrin and produces, after IV administration, a fibrin-selective activation of plasminogen. This selectivity is not absolute; circulating plasminogen also may be activated by large doses or lengthy treatment. After intravenous administration, alteplase is more efficacious than streptokinase in establishing coronary reperfusion. At equieffective thrombolytic doses, alteplase causes less fibrinogenolysis than streptokinase, but bleeding occurs with a similar incidence. The rate of rethrombosis after t-PA is greater than after streptokinase, possibly because alteplase is rapidly cleared from the blood (half-life is 5 to 10 minutes), and several administrations may be warranted. Reocclusion may be lessened by administration of heparin and antiplatelet drugs. Alteplase is a product of recombinant DNA technology and consists predominantly of the single-chain form (recombinant human tissue-type plasminogen activator, rt-PA). Upon exposure to fibrin, rt-PA is converted to the two-chain dimer.

Two genetically engineered variants of human t-PA have better pharmacological properties than alteplase. Reteplase (*Retavase*) contains only the peptide domains required for fibrin binding and protease activity. These changes increase potency and speed the onset of action. Reteplase may penetrate further into the fibrin clot than alteplase. The half-life of the drug remains short, however. Tenecteplase (TNK-tPA) (*TNKase*) has a longer half-life than alteplase, binds more avidly to fibrin, and in contrast to many other thrombolytic agents, may be administered as an IV bolus.

Anistreplase (*Eminase*) consists of streptokinase in a noncovalent 1:1 complex with plasminogen. Anistreplase is catalytically inert because of acylation of the catalytic site of plasminogen. However, the affinity of plasminogen binding to fibrin is maintained. It has a long catalytic half-life (90 minutes), and the time required for nonenzymatic deacylation lengthens its thrombolytic effect after IV injection. Anistreplase is more effective than streptokinase in establishing coronary reperfusion, but it causes considerable fibrinogenolysis and is antigenic.

Antifibrinolytic Drugs

Hyperplasminemia resulting from thrombolytic therapy exposes fibrinogen and other coagulation factors, plasminogen, and α_2-antiplasmin to nonspecific proteolysis by plasmin, a process normally regulated by α_2-antiplasmin. Consumption of these factors and extensive fibrin dissolution leads to hemorrhage. The binding of plasminogen to fibrin involves interactions with lysine-binding sites in plasminogen. These interactions are blocked by antifibrinolytic drugs such as aminocaproic acid (*Amicar*) and tranexamic acid (*Cyklokapron*); plasminogen activation primarily and plasmin proteolytic activity are inhibited.

In addition to being an *antidote to fibrinogenolysis* during thrombolytic therapy, antifibrinolytic drugs are used orally and intravenously to control bleeding following surgery. They also are useful adjuncts to coagulation factor replacement during dental surgery in hemophiliac patients. Antifibrinolytic drugs are contraindicated if intravascular coagulation is present. These drugs *may* cause nausea.

Agents for Controlling Blood Loss

Cardiopulmonary bypass, with extracorporeal circulation during cardiac artery bypass graft or heart valve replacement surgery, causes transient hemostatic defects in blood cells and perioperative bleeding. The protease inhibitor aprotinin (*Trasylol*) inhibits kallikrein (coagulation phase) and plasmin (fibrinolysis) and protects platelets from mechanical injury. The overall effect after infusion is a decrease in bleeding.

Several biological agents are used intravenously to maintain coagulability in the face of factor deficiencies in hemophilia or Von Willebrand's disease patients. Manufacture of these substances involves extraction from human blood or recombinant technology. They include antihemophilic factor (factor VIII) (*Alphanate, Bioclate,* others) for hemophilia A patients, factor IX concentrate (*Bebulin, AlphaNine, Mononine,* others) for hemophilia B patients, and factor VIIa (*NovoSeven*) for hemophilia and Von Willebrand patients. An increase in factor VIII levels by desmopressin (*DDAVP, Concentraid,* others), an analog of vasopressin, is useful for managing bleeding in hemophilia A and mild Von Willebrand's disease patients. Anti-inhibitor coagulant complex (*Autoplex, FEIBA*) provides activated vitamin K–dependent clotting factors to return coagulability to the blood in hemophilia patients and other patients with acquired inhibitors to clotting factors.

Study Questions

1. Which of the following statements describe why warfarin is not used to prevent blood coagulation in blood collection devices used at blood donating centers?
   (A) Warfarin does not bind to plastic tubing or glass.
   (B) The anticoagulant effect of warfarin occurs only in vivo.
   (C) Warfarin is a prodrug, which must be activated in the liver into the active compound.
   (D) The gastric enzymes needed to convert R-warfarin into S-warfarin are unstable near plastic.
   (E) Warfarin is chemically unstable and is degraded unless made fresh and used immediately.

2. All of the following statements about warfarin are true EXCEPT which one?
   (A) An adverse drug reaction may occur if warfarin is displaced from plasma protein binding sites.
   (B) Warfarin crosses the placenta.
   (C) Drugs that are metabolized by the liver can alter the anticoagulant effect of warfarin.
   (D) Warfarin is eliminated from the body unchanged in the urine.
   (E) Warfarin is a vitamin K antagonist.

3. Which of the following is an adverse effect associated with pharmacotherapy using heparin?
   (A) An increase in the number of circulating platelets
   (B) Thrombocytopenia
   (C) Purple toe syndrome
   (D) Teratogenicity to the fetus
   (E) An increase in the circulating level of antithrombin III

4. Which of the following is a drug that blocks the ADP receptor on the antiplatelet membrane?
   (A) Aspirin
   (B) Abciximab
   (C) Dipyridamole
   (D) Clopidogrel
   (E) Eptifibatide

5. The thrombolytic drug reteplase is improved over older drugs like streptokinase in what respect?
   (A) Reteplase may be taken orally.
   (B) Reteplase is antigenic.
   (C) Reteplase binds to fibrin.
   (D) Bleeding does not occur with reteplase.
   (E) Reteplase produces less thrombocytopenia.

ANSWERS

1. **B.** Warfarin does not produce an anticoagulant effect in vitro. It inhibits coagulation of blood only in vivo, because the effect depends upon warfarin's effect in the liver on the production of clotting factors. Warfarin does not require conversion into an active drug. It inhibits the post-ribosomal carboxylation of glutamic acid residues in the vitamin K-dependent clotting factors. Therefore, heparin rather than warfarin is used when blood is collected from donors and stored.

2. **D.** Warfarin is metabolized in the liver by P450 enzyme system and is appreciably metabolized before it is eliminated. Adverse drug reactions are seen in patients taking warfarin if a second drug displaces warfarin from its protein binding sites in the blood or induces or inhibits the hepatic P450 system. Warfarin can cross the placenta and exert anticoagulant and other effects in the fetus at normal doses given to the mother.

3. **B.** Thrombocytopenia is a frequent side effect association with heparin. This reduction in the level of circulating platelets increases bleeding. Purple toes are encountered during warfarin therapy. Heparin may be administered to pregnant mothers without risk to the fetus. Heparin requires antithrombin III for its anticoagulant action, but does not increase the level of this protein in the blood.

4. **C.** Aspirin inhibits platelet cyclooxygenase. Abciximab, a monoclonal antibody, binds to and inhibits the platelet glycoprotein IIb/IIIa receptor. Dipyridamole inhibits platelet cyclic AMP phosphodiesterase and raises cyclic AMP levels. Eptifibatide binds to the glycoprotein IIb/IIIa complex.

5. **C.** Reteplase binds to fibrin to cause a selective activation of fibrin-bound plasminogen. All fibrinolytic drugs are administered IV. Streptokinase is antigenic, whereas reteplase is not. Thrombocytopenia is not normally caused by thrombolytic drugs.

SUPPLEMENTAL READING

Bennett JS. Novel platelet inhibitors. Annu Rev Med 2001;52:161–184.

Collen D. The plasminogen (fibrinolytic) system. Thromb Haemost 1999;82:259–270.

Diener HC. Stroke prevention: Antiplatelet and antithrombolytic therapy. Haemostasis 2000;30:14–26.

Ferguson JJ and Zaqqa M. Platelet glycoprotein IIb/IIIa receptor antagonists: Current concepts and future directions. Drugs 1999;58:965–982.

Goldhaber SZ. A contemporary approach to thrombolytic therapy for pulmonary embolism. Vasc Med 2000;5:115–123.

Hirsh J et al. Oral anticoagulants: Mechanism of action, clinical effectiveness, and optimal therapeutic range. Chest 2001;19:8S–21S.

Hirsh J et al. Heparin and low-molecular-weight heparin: Mechanisms of action, pharmacokinetics, dosing, monitoring, efficacy, and safety. Chest 2001;119:64S–94S.

Lever R and Page CP. Novel drug development opportunities for heparin. Nature Rev Drug Disc 2002;1:140–148.

Levine GN, Ali MN, and Schafer AI. Antithrombotic therapy in patients with acute coronary syndromes. Arch Intern Med 2001;61:937–948.

Mannucci PM and Poller L. Venous thrombosis and anticoagulant therapy. Br J Haematol 2001;14:258–270.

Mousa SA. Antiplatelet therapies: Recent advances in the development of platelet glycoprotein IIb/IIIa antagonists. Curr Interv Cardiol Rep 1999;1:243–252.

Shord SS and Lindley CM. Coagulation products and their uses. Am J Health Syst Pharm 2000;57:1403–1417.

Sinnaeve P and Van de Werf F. Thrombolytic therapy: State of the art. Thromb Res 2001;103:S71–79.

Verstraete M. Third-generation thrombolytic drugs. Am J Med 2000;109:52–58.

Vorchheimer DA. Current state of thrombolytic therapy. Curr Cardiol Rep 1999;1:212–220.

Weitz JI. Low-molecular-weight heparins. N Engl J Med 1997;337:688–698.

CASE Study Treatment of Thrombosis

A 23-year old pregnant woman who has been administered IV heparin for treatment of deep vein thrombosis has developed heparin-induced thrombocytopenia. Altering therapy by removing heparin and adding warfarin is not a viable option, because warfarin can cross the placenta and exert an anticoagulant effect in the fetus. Suggest a treatment approach.

ANSWER: Treatment of thrombosis can be initiated during pregnancy with infusion of argatroban, a direct inhibitor of thrombin. This drug does not cross the placenta and has not been reported to produce effects in the fetus. Argatroban is discontinued at the time of delivery, and thrombosis is then managed postpartum for 2 months with warfarin.

23

Hypocholesterolemic Drugs and Coronary Heart Disease

Richard J. Cenedella

 DRUG LIST

GENERIC NAME	PAGE	GENERIC NAME	PAGE
Atorvastatin	271	Gemfibrozil	274
Cerivastatin	272	Lovastatin	269
Cholestyramine	272	Niacin	272
Clofibrate	274	Pravastatin	269
Colestipol	272	Probucol	274
Fenofibrate	274	Simvastatin	269
Fluvastatin	272		

PREVENTION OF CORONARY HEART DISEASE AS THE GOAL

Atherosclerosis is the primary cause of coronary heart disease. Markedly lowering blood cholesterol can halt and even reverse to some extent the progression of atherosclerosis. For these reasons, prevention should be the goal, with the focus on decreasing elevated blood cholesterol. About 20% of Americans between 20 and 75 years of age have blood total cholesterol levels above 240 mg/dL, a level requiring management, and up to 40% of some middle aged groups have this elevation.

Although hypercholesterolemias are linked to specific genetic mutations, most have a multifactorial basis that can respond to lifestyle changes. Even though the physician is justified in immediately prescribing a cholesterol-lowering drug to patients with very high blood cholesterol and additional risk factors, strong advice should also be given on the need and benefits of adding life style changes. These changes include reduction of body weight; decreased dietary total fat, choles-

terol, saturated fatty acids, and trans fatty acids; and increased exercise and stress management. In fact, a recent study employing intensive lifestyle changes in patients with coronary heart disease achieved a 37% lowering of LDL (low-density lipoprotein) cholesterol, a 91% decline in anginal episodes, and a decline in coronary artery stenosis within a year—all without drugs. A prescription for lifestyle changes should accompany the one for a hypocholesterolemic drug.

WHEN TO TREAT HYPERCHOLESTEROLEMIAS?

Principal risk factors for heart disease are elevated levels of LDL cholesterol, a family history of heart disease, and hypertension. Other risks include being male, smoking, low levels of high density lipoprotein (HDL) cholesterol, diabetes mellitus, hyperhomocystinemia, high levels of lipoprotein a (Lpa), and high blood levels of C-reactive protein. (Table 23.1). C-Reactive protein is a marker for cellular inflammation.

TABLE 23.1 Treatment Guidelines for Patients with Hypercholesterolemia

Treatment guidelines	LDL cholesterol[a]	
	Initiation level (mg/dL)	Minimal goal (mg/dL)
Dietary treatment		
Without CHD or two other risk factors[b]	≥160	<160[c]
Without CHD and with two or more other risk factors[b]	≥130	<130[d]
With CHD	>100	<100
Drug treatment		
Without CHD or two other risk factors[b]	≥190	<160
Without CHD and with two or more other risk factors[b]	≥160	<130
With CHD	>130	<100

LDL, low-density lipoproteins; CHD, coronary heart disease.
[a]Classification: <130 mg/dL is the desirable LDL cholesterol level; 130-159 mg/dl is borderline-high-risk; >160 mg/dl is high-risk.
[b]Patients have a lower initiation level and goal if they are at high risk because they already have definite CHD or because they have any two of the following factors: male sex, family history of premature CHD, cigarette smoking, hypertension, low high-density lipoprotein (HDL) cholesterol (<35 mg/dL), hyperhomocysteinemia (>16 µM), high plasma levels of Lpa (>30 mg/dL), diabetes mellitus, definite cerebrovascular or peripheral vascular disease, or severe obesity.
[c]Roughly equivalent to total cholesterol level <240 mg/dL.
[d]Roughly equivalent to total cholesterol level <200 mg/dL.
Adapted with permission from *Arch Intern Med* **148:**36, 1988, with permission.
Report of the National Cholesterol Education Program Expert Panel on detection, evaluation, and treatment of high blood cholesterol in adults.

Homocysteine blood levels (>15 µmol/L) promote atherosclerosis, perhaps by stimulating proliferation of arterial wall smooth muscle cells. Supplementing the diet with folic acid can reduce high levels. Lpa is a modified LDL particle that is both atherogenic and prothrombic.

Although development and clinical expression of coronary heart disease (CHD) are determined by the interaction of numerous risk factors, lowering blood cholesterol is the major approach to prevention and suppression of heart disease, the number one cause of death in Western society. The risk of CHD is directly proportional to blood cholesterol levels (Fig. 23.1), and a lowering of cholesterol, specifically LDL cholesterol, deceases the incidence of heart attacks.

The results of several large clinical trials using the statin drugs (discussed later) show that the tested drugs decreased the risk of both primary and secondary cardiovascular events. The incidence of myocardial infarction and death from cardiovascular disease was reduced in patients with hypercholesterolemia who never had a

heart attack (primary prevention) and in those with heart disease (secondary prevention). Furthermore, the statins decreased the risk of a first heart attack in subjects with even average LDL cholesterol levels. In addition to decreased clinical expression of heart disease, aggressive lowering of blood cholesterol with the statin drugs can partially reverse atherosclerosis in the sense of reducing the degree of stenosis (closure) of coronary arteries. Guidelines for initiation and goals of treatment of hypercholesterolemias are outlined in Table 23.1.

MANAGEMENT OF HYPERLIPIDEMIAS WITH DRUGS

Drug Treatment of Polygenic and Familial Hypercholesterolemia

Statins

Mechanism of Action
The statin family of six closely related hypocholesterolemic drugs are all potent competitive inhibitors of the enzyme 3-hydroxy-3-methylglutaryl coenzyme A reductase (HMG CoA reductase), the rate-limiting enzyme in cholesterol biosynthesis. The liver is their target organ, and decreased hepatic cholesterol synthesis ultimately leads to increased removal of LDL particles from the circulation. As a consequence, all other hypocholesterolemic drugs have been relegated to secondary status.

Clinical trials with lovastatin (*Mevacor*), simvastatin (*Zocor*) and pravastatin (*Pravachol*) provided much of the evidence supporting the observation that lowering

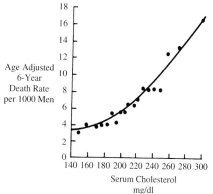

Key points
(1) The risk increases steadily and particularly above 200 mg/dl.
(2) The magnitude of the increased risk is large—fourfold at the top 10% as compared to the bottom 10%.

FIGURE 23.1
Relationship of serum cholesterol to deaths from coronary heart disease in 36,662 men aged 35–37 years during an average followup period of 6 years. Each point represents the median value for 5% of the population. (From Report of the Expert Panel on Detection, Evaluation and Treatment of High Blood Cholesterol in Adults. NIH Publication 88-2925, 1988).

of blood cholesterol lowers the risk of CHD. Reductions in CHD risk appear to be due to multiple consequences of inhibiting the cholesterol synthesis pathway. Drug-induced inhibition of hepatic cholesterol synthesis leads to lowering of liver cholesterol concentrations and feedback up-regulation at the gene level of both HMG CoA reductase and the LDL receptor (mechanisms IV and VII in Fig. 23.2). As long as the statin is present at adequate concentration in the liver, the extra HMG CoA reductase activity is not expressed. However, the increased hepatic LDL receptor protein results in increased rates of removal of LDL particles from the circulation by the liver, lowering of

blood LDL-cholesterol levels, slowing of atherosclerosis, and decreased risk of heart attack. An overview of lipoprotein metabolism and the sites where drugs can influence plasma lipoprotein levels is provided in Figure 23.2.

The reduced risk of CHD achieved with the statins may also be due to drug actions independent of lowering blood cholesterol. Many important molecules besides cholesterol are generated by intermediates in the complex cholesterol synthesis pathway. These include the isoprenes geranylgeranyl and farnesyl, which are covalently attached to some proteins (isoprenylation) and target them to membranes where they function. The re-

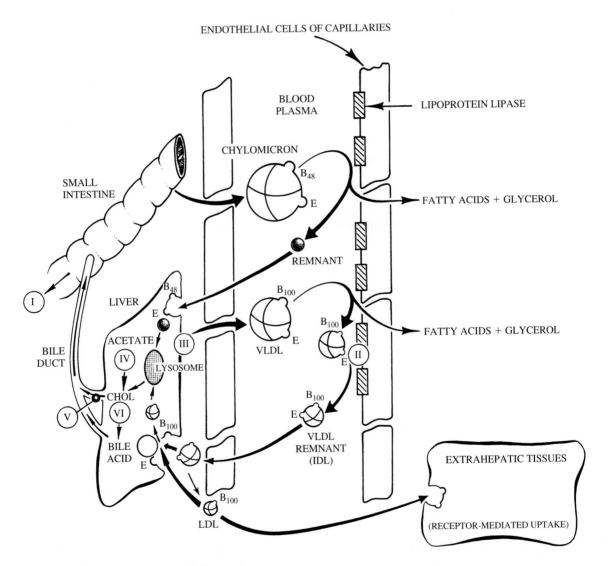

FIGURE 23.2
Partial summary of lipoprotein metabolism in humans. I to VII are sites of action of hypolipidemic drugs. I, stimulation of bile acid and/or cholesterol fecal excretion; II, stimulation of lipoprotein lipase activity; III, inhibition of VLDL production and secretion; IV, inhibition of cholesterol biosynthesis; V, stimulation of cholesterol secretion into bile fluid; VI, stimulation of cholesterol conversion to bile acids; VII, increased plasma clearance of LDL due either to increased LDL receptor activity or altered lipoprotein composition. CHOL, cholesterol; IDL, intermediate-density lipoprotein.

ported capacities of statins to inhibit proliferation of arterial wall smooth muscle cells and to improve endothelial cell functions may be due to inhibited protein isoprenylation in these cells secondary to HMG CoA reductase inhibition.

Clinical Uses

With the possible exception of atorvastatin, the statins are used to lower LDL cholesterol in familial or polygenic (multifactorial) hypercholesterolemia (type IIa) and in combination with triglyceride-lowering drugs to treat combined hyperlipidemia (type IIb) when both LDL and VLDL (very low density lipoproteins) are elevated (Table 23.2). However, the statins probably should not be given with the fibrates (triglyceride-lowering drugs, discussed later), since this combination may greatly increase statin toxicity. Atorvastatin, the most potent of the available statins (Fig. 23.3), has also been shown to lower blood triglycerides significantly.

This effect may be due to decreasing hepatic cholesterol and cholesterol ester levels to such an extent that hepatic formation of VLDL is impaired. The statins also have been claimed to reduce blood cholesterol levels modestly in some patients with homozygous familial hypercholesterolemia, a condition often fatal in childhood or in early adulthood.

The statins may lower the risk of CHD by decreasing inflammation, an important component of atherogenesis. Lovastatin decreased elevated plasma levels of C-reactive protein, a marker for cellular inflammation, and acute coronary events in patients with relatively low plasma cholesterol levels. Recent studies also suggest that use of statins may decrease the risk of stroke, dementia, and Alzheimer's disease and may improve bone

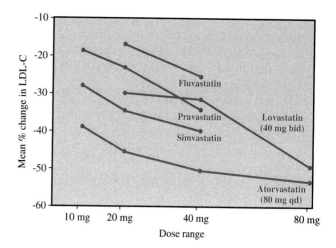

FIGURE 23.3

Comparison of the potency of statins. Percent reduction by various statins in plasma LDL-cholesterol after 8 weeks of treatment of male and female patients with plasma LDL-cholesterol above 160 mg/dL. (Adapted from Jones et al. Comparative Dose Efficacy Study of Atorvastatin vs. Simvastatin. American Journal of Cardiology 81, 582–587, 1998. With permission from Excerpta Medica Inc.)

density in postmenopausal women. These broad actions may be related to the hypocholesterolemic, antiproliferative, antiinflammatory, or antioxidant properties of the statins or some combination of these properties.

Adverse Effects

The statins generally appear to be well tolerated, with muscle pain and liver dysfunction seen in 1 to 2% of patients. However, the consequences of 20 to 30 years of continuous use are unknown. This fact has been

TABLE 23.2   Classification of Hyperlipoproteinemias

Disorders	Type[a]	Lipoprotein(s) Elevated	Main Lipid(s) Elevated	Mechanism	Increased Risk
Polygenic or familial hypercholesterolemia	IIa	LDL	Chol	Deficient LDL receptor activity. Abnormal Apo B_{100}. High-fat diet, excess calories, inactivity.	CHD, stroke
Familial combined hyperlipidemia	IIb	LDL, VLDL	Chol, TG	Increased VLDL production, increased conversion of VLDL to LDL.	CHD, stroke
Familial dyslipo-proteinemia	III	IDL (β-VLDL)	Chol, TG	Decreased plasma clearance of VLDL and chylomicron remnants due to abnormal Apo E (E_2 for normal E_3).	CHD, stroke
Familial hypertri-glyceridemia	IV	VLDL	TG	Overproduction of VLDL; low LPL activity.	Pancreatitis, CHD if HDL is low

[a]Types I and V are not shown. Type I is a rare elevation of chylomicrons treatable only by diet (removing long chained fatty acids). Type V involves elevation of both chylomicrons and VLDL and can be viewed as an extreme type IV.
Chol, cholesterol; TG, triglyceride; CHD, coronary heart disease; LDL, low density lipoproteins; LPL, lipoprotein lipase; VLDL, very low density lipoprotein; HDL, high-density lipoprotein; IDL, intermediate-density lipoprotein.

dramatically reinforced by the recent recognition of a potentially fatal consequence of statin use. A relatively common side effect of the statins (perhaps 1% of patients) is myositis, that is, inflammation of skeletal muscle accompanied by pain, weakness, and high levels of serum creatine kinase. Rhabdomyolysis, i.e., disintegration of muscle with urinary excretion of myoglobin and kidney damage, was considered to be a rare and extreme toxic outcome. However, cerivastatin (*Baycol*) has now been withdrawn from the market by its manufacturer (Bayer) because of 31 deaths linked to fatal rhabdomyolysis. The risk of muscle damage is said to increase with simultaneous use of the triglyceride-lowering fibrates. Pravastatin may be less toxic than other statins because it does not readily penetrate extrahepatic cells and may be more confined to the liver after oral dosage.

Drug Interactions

Most of the statins (lovastatin, simvastatin, atorvastatin, and cerivastatin) are metabolized by the cytochromal P450 3A4 system of intestines and liver to more water-soluble metabolites that are excreted in both the bile and urine. Drugs that inhibit P450 3A4, such as itraconazole, cyclosporine, and erythromycin, can vastly (10-fold) increase plasma statin levels and thus increase the risk of toxicity. Unexpectedly, grapefruit juice can inhibit intestinal metabolism of the statins and can result in an 8- to 10-fold increase in simvastatin serum levels. Since fluvastatin is metabolized by cytochrome P450 2C9, which is also responsible for metabolism of warfarin, warfarin toxicity may be increased if these drugs are simultaneously given. Grapefruit juice should obviously not be consumed within several hours of statin administration. Drugs that induce the P450 3A4 system, such as barbiturates, can accelerate statin metabolism and suppress statin blood levels.

Other Hypocholesterolemic Drugs

Resins

Mechanism of Action

Prior to the introduction of the statins in the mid to late 1980s, the bile acid–sequestering drugs cholestyramine (*Questran*) and colestipol (*Colestid*) were primary drugs for lowering plasma cholesterol. Today they are second-line drugs that can safely be given with a statin to enhance cholesterol lowering or as an alternative for patients intolerant to a statin or concerned with statin's potential for toxicity. Alone, the resins can achieve 20 to 25% reductions in LDL cholesterol, but when used with a statin, such as lovastatin, reductions of 50% and more can be seen.

These drugs are basically anion exchange resins that remain in the gut, bind intestinal bile acids, and greatly increase their fecal excretion (mechanism I in Fig. 23.2).

The lowered concentration of bile acids returning to the liver by the enterohepatic circulation results in derepression of 7-α-hydroxylase, the rate-limiting enzyme for conversion of cholesterol to bile acids. This results in increased use of cholesterol to replace the excreted bile acids and lowering of hepatic cholesterol (mechanism VI in Fig. 23.2). Thus, similar to the statins, the ultimate actions of the bile acid–sequestering resins are up-regulation of transcription of the LDL receptor gene, increased hepatic receptor activity, and lowering of plasma LDL cholesterol (mechanism VII in Fig. 23.2).

Clinical Uses

The bile acid sequestering resins lower elevated LDL cholesterol and therefore are useful in the treatment of type IIa hyperlipoproteinemia. However, because the resins can raise plasma VLDL in some patients, they are not recommended for treatment of combined hyperlipidemias (type IIb) when both LDL cholesterol and VLDL triglycerides are high or in other conditions of elevated triglycerides.

Adverse Effects

The resins are interesting drugs because they have profound metabolic effects without truly entering the body. Perhaps for this reason they are relatively safe, with constipation being the chief complaint. Because the resins are given as the chloride salt and the chloride is exchanged for the negatively charged bile salt, bile acid resins can lead to hyperchloremic acidosis in vulnerable patients (children and patients with kidney failure).

Drug Interactions

The principal precaution with use of the bile acid resins is the possibility of impaired absorption of other drugs given orally at the same time. Cholestyramine and colestipol can bind many other drugs, such as digitoxin, phenobarbital, chlorothiazide, and warfarin, and delay or prevent their absorption. For this reason, other drugs should always be taken at least 1 hour before or 4 to 6 hours after the resin. The resins can also decease absorption of fat-soluble vitamins.

Nicotinic Acid (Niacin)

Nicotinic acid has three special features as a hypolipidemic drug: it has multiple beneficial effects on serum lipoproteins, it is the least expensive, and it is the least well tolerated.

Mechanism of Action

Nicotinic acid decreases formation and secretion of VLDL by the liver (mechanism III in Fig. 23.2). This action appears secondary to its ability to inhibit fatty acid mobilization from adipose tissue. Circulating free fatty acids provide the main source of fatty acids for hepatic triglyceride synthesis, and lowering triglyceride synthesis lowers VLDL formation and secretion by the liver. Since plasma VLDL is the source of LDL, lowering VLDL can ultimately lower LDL. In addition, nicotinic acid shifts LDL particles to larger (more buoyant) sizes. The larger LDL particles are thought to be less atherogenic. Nicotinic acid can also significantly increase plasma HDL levels; the mechanism is unknown.

Clinical Uses

Used alone, nicotinic acid can decrease plasma LDL cholesterol levels by 15 to 30%. It can also be used in combination therapy with the statins or the bile acid–sequestering resins to augment reduction of very high LDL levels. Because nicotinic acid can lower plasma triglycerides by 40% or more, it is useful in treating familial hypertriglyceridemia type IV (Table 23.3), and in combination with the statins it is useful in treating combined hyperlipidemia type IIb. As described later with the fibrates, patients with high plasma triglycerides plus low HDL are at increased risk for CHD. Nicotinic acid is useful for treating these patients, since it can both lower triglycerides and raise HDL.

Adverse Effects

Compliance with nicotinic acid therapy can be poor because the drug can produce an intense cutaneous flush. This can be reduced by beginning the drug in stepped doses of 250 mg twice daily and increasing the dose monthly by 500 to 1000 mg per day to a maximum of 3000 mg per day. Taking nicotinic acid on a full stomach (end of meal) and taking aspirin before dosage can reduce the severity of flushing. Time-release forms of nicotinic acid may also decrease cutaneous flushing. Nicotinic acid can cause gastrointestinal (GI) distress,

liver dysfunction (especially at high doses), decreased glucose tolerance, hyperglycemia, and hyperuricemia. Thus, it is contraindicated in patients with hepatic dysfunction, peptic ulcer, hyperuricemia, or diabetes mellitus. A paradox associated with nicotinic acid is that it is the most widely available hypolipidemic drug (it is sold over the counter), yet its use requires the closest management by the physician.

When to Treat Hypertriglyceridemias

The guidelines for use of drugs to treat familial hypertriglyceridemia type IV are less well defined than those for hypercholesterolemia. One should account for plasma HDL in deciding to treat hypertriglyceridemias with the intent of decreasing the risk for CHD. Moderate hypertriglyceridemia (200–500 mg/dL) without low HDL may not be an independent risk factor for CHD. However, the results of a recent clinical trial indicate that hypertriglyceridemia is an independent risk factor for ischemic stroke. Results of the Helsinki Heart Study showed that the reduced risk of CHD with use of gemfibrozil (discussed later) was correlated with elevation of HDL plus reduction of VLDL triglyceride rather than reduction of LDL cholesterol. Gemfibrozil has little effect on plasma LDL.

Low HDL cholesterol (<35 mg/dL) is an independent risk factor for CHD. HDL appears to antagonize atherogenesis by at least two mechanisms. HDL can mobilize cholesterol from extrahepatic cells (such as arterial wall foam cells) and transport it to the liver for disposal (reverse cholesterol transport); HDL also has antioxidant properties. HDL contains the potent antioxidant enzyme paraoxonase, which may protect LDL lipids from oxidation. Thus, hypertriglyceridemia with

TABLE 23.3 Summary of Major Hypolipidemic Drugs

Drug	Reduced CHD Risk	Lipoprotein Affected	Hyperlipoproteinemia Treated		Principal Adverse Effects
			Singly	In Combination	
Statins	Yes	Reduces LDL	II$_a$	II$_b$ with niacin	Myositis, liver dysfunction, rhabdomyolysis with cerivastatin
Bile acid–sequestering resins	Yes	Reduces LDL	II$_a$	Severe II$_a$ with statin or niacin	GI distress, hyperchloremic acidosis
Nicotinic acid (niacin)	Yes	Reduces LDL Reduces VLDL Raises HDL	II$_a$, II$_b$ IV	II$_b$ with fibrates; severe IV with fibrates	Cutaneous flush, GI distress, liver dysfunction, hyperglycemia, hyperuricemia
Fibrates	Yes	Reduces VLDL Reduces IDL Raises HDL	III, IV	II$_b$ with niacin; severe IV with niacin	GI distress, myositis, gallstone risk, erectile dysfunction

concurrent low HDL cholesterol should be treated to reduce the risk of CHD. Treatment of hypertriglyceridemia independent of HDL levels may also be worthwhile to decrease the risk of ischemic cerebrovascular disease. Very high plasma triglycerides (>1000 mg/dL) are clearly a risk factor for pancreatitis and must be treated for this reason.

As with drugs that lower LDL cholesterol, dietary plus other lifestyle changes should accompany drug therapy of hypertriglyceridemia. Reduction of body weight to ideal is probably the single most important dietary goal. Because patients with familial hypertriglyceridemia may have increased liver capacity to synthesize fat from carbohydrate, attention should be given to restricting excessive carbohydrate and alcohol.

Fibrates

Mechanism of Action

The three structurally related fibrates available in the United States are gemfibrozil (*Lopid*), fenofibrate (*Tricor*) and clofibrate (*Atromid-S*). They share common uses and toxicities. The fibrates typically lower VLDL triglyceride by 40% or more and elevate plasma HDL cholesterol by 10 to 15%. The reduction of plasma triglycerides in humans appears due to increased lipoprotein lipase (LPL) activity. The fibrates activate a nuclear receptor (transcription factor) termed peroxisomal proliferation activated receptor (PPAR) that is a member of the steroid hormone receptor superfamily. PPAR increases transcription of the LPL gene and decreases transcription of the apolipoprotein CIII gene (apo CIII). Since LPL is responsible for catabolism of VLDL triglyceride and apo CIII is an inhibitor of LPL activity, the combined consequences of these changes are increased LPL activity and enhanced removal of triglyceride from the circulation (mechanism II in Fig. 23.2).

The elevation of HDL levels by fibrates may be due to two drug actions: induced synthesis of apo-A1, the principal apoprotein of HDL, and increased assembly of new HDL particles in the circulation. Surface components of VLDL contribute to formation of HDL, as the VLDL particles are reduced in size through the action of LPL. The increased rate of catabolism of VLDL caused by the fibrates would provide more components for assembly of HDL particles.

Clinical Uses

The fibrates are mainly used to treat two hyperlipidemias, familial hypertriglyceridemia (type IV) and dysbetalipoproteinemia (type III). They are also useful in the treatment of hypertriglyceridemia associated with type II diabetes (secondary hyperlipidemia). The fibrates are the drugs of choice in treating hypertriglyceridemias, particularly those associated with low levels of HDL cholesterol. The fibrates additionally appear to shift LDL particles to larger, hence less atherogenic, species.

Type III or dysbetalipoproteinemia is a rare condition in which cholesterol-enriched VLDL remnants, called β-VLDL, accumulate in the plasma. They are atherogenic particles. Dysbetalipoproteinemia is a genetic condition associated with expression of an unusual form of apolipoprotein E (apo E2 versus the normal E3) that leads to reduced plasma clearance of these lipoproteins by the liver. Through stimulation of LPL and perhaps other lipases, the fibrates accelerate clearance of these β-lipoproteins. Both plasma cholesterol and triglyceride levels are elevated in dysbetalipoproteinemia and in combined hyperlipidemia, type IIb. However, the drug treatments are different for the two conditions. Type IIb hyperlipoproteinemia requires use of agents that lower both LDL and VLDL particles; for example, a statin plus niacin, niacin alone, or niacin in combination with a fibrate. Care should be taken in distinguishing between types IIb and III as the cause of the elevated cholesterol plus triglyceride. This can be achieved by examining the profile of the elevated plasma lipoproteins separated by electrophoresis. A broad β-band is seen in type III but distinct β- and pre-β-bands are seen in type IIb.

Adverse Effects

The fibrates are generally well tolerated, with GI distress being the most likely complaint. Other adverse effects include myositis and erectile dysfunction, particularly with clofibrate. There is ongoing concern about the fibrates increasing the risk of gallstones, although the extent of risk is unclear. Because clofibrate was associated with increased mortality in early clinical trials, it should be considered as a second-line drug.

Drug Interactions

The fibrates potentiate the actions of the coumarin anticoagulants, such as warfarin, so care should be taken to reduce the dose of simultaneously administered anticoagulants, and plasma prothrombin should be frequently measured until the level stabilizes. As mentioned earlier, great care should be given to combining a statin with a fibrate, since this combination may increase the risk of myositis and perhaps rhabdomyolysis. Table 23.4 summarizes major interactions of drugs that lower cholesterol.

Other Approaches to Prevention of Coronary Heart Disease with Drugs

Probucol

Probucol (*Lorelco*) is a hypocholesterolemic drug with few side effects that modestly (15–30%) decreases elevated plasma LDL cholesterol levels. The marginal

TABLE 23.4 **Summary of Major Drug Interactions**

Drug	Interactions and Special Precautions
Statins	Inhibition of cytochromal P450 3A4 can greatly increase serum statin levels. Grapefruit juice inhibits intestinal P450 3A4 and raises serum statins. Fluvastatin may increase warfarin toxicity because both compete with P450 2C9 for metabolism. Cerivastatin can cause fatal rhabdomyolysis; risk with other statins unclear.
Bile acid resins	Interferes with absorption of many drugs (give other drugs 1 hr before or 6 hr after the resin). May interfere with absorption of fat-soluble vitamins.
Nicotinic acid (niacin)	Cutaneous flush can limit compliance. Giving niacin after meals and use of aspirin may decrease flushing. Gradually increase niacin dose to maximum.
Fibrates	Potentates coumarin anticoagulants. Therefore, reduce dose of anticoagulant and monitor plasma prothrombin. Use clofibrate as second-line drug because it increased death rate in an early study. Avoid use with statins, since the combination may increases risk of myositis and rhabdomyolysis.

LDL-lowering action plus reports that it can lower HDL cholesterol resulted in its discontinuation as a hypocholesterolemic drug. However, it still may reduce the risk of CHD because it is a powerful antioxidant.

The oxidation hypothesis of atherosclerosis states that oxidation of lipids in LDL is required for LDL uptake by macrophages and smooth muscle cells in the intima of arteries, leading to their transformation to foam cells, an early event in atherogenesis. A recent clinical trial reported that use of probucol decreased the rate of restenosis of coronary arteries by 50% in patients who underwent angioplasty. Fluvastatin also has potent antioxidant properties that may contribute to its antiatherosclerotic effects. These findings suggest that reducing high plasma lipids may not be the only approach to retarding the progression of atherosclerosis and decreasing the risk of coronary heart disease.

Study QUESTIONS

Use the following information to answer questions 1 through 4:

A 54-year white man (5′, 11″; 189 lb) has a plasma total triglyceride of 105 mg/dL and total cholesterol of 431 mg/dL. Plasma HDL is 53 mg/dL. Electrophoresis of his plasma lipoproteins shows an intense β-band; all others are normal. He is taking itraconazole for a persistent fungal infection. He had two older brothers who both died of myocardial infarction at 57 and 63 years of age.

1. What hyperlipoproteinemia does this patient most likely have?
   (A) Type IIa
   (B) Type IIb
   (C) Type III
   (D) Type IV

2. What is the most likely biochemical basis of this patient's hyperlipidemia?
   (A) Abnormal apolipoprotein E content of serum β-lipoproteins.
   (B) Increased transcription of the HMG CoA reductase gene in liver.
   (C) Overproduction of VLDL particle by the liver.
   (D) Reduced hepatic LDL-receptor activity.
   (E) Reduced lipoprotein lipase activity.

3. What drugs would be contradicted in this patient if his use of itraconazole was not discontinued?
   (A) Cholestyramine
   (B) Gemfibrozil
   (C) Niacin
   (D) Probucol
   (E) Simvastatin

4. If the patient was treated with cerivastatin, what adverse effects would be of greatest potential concern?
   (A) Constipation
   (B) Hepatic dysfunction
   (C) Hyperglycemia
   (D) Intense cutaneous flush
   (E) Rhabdomyolysis

Use the following information to answer questions 5 through 8:

A 42-year-old white woman (5′, 4″; 207 lb) has a plasma total triglyceride of 1042 mg/dL and total cholesterol of 368 mg/dL. Plasma HDL cholesterol is 72 mg/dL. Electrophoresis of the plasma lipoproteins shows a intense pre-β-band; all others are normal or absent. Blood glucose is normal. She is not taking any medications.

5. What hyperlipoproteinemia does this patient most likely have?
   - (A) Type IIa
   - (B) Type IIb
   - (C) Type III
   - (D) Type IV
6. What is the greatest health risk to this patient based upon the provided information?
   - (A) Coronary heart disease
   - (B) Decreased digestion of dietary fat
   - (C) Hepatic disease
   - (D) Pancreatitis
   - (E) Stroke
7. Which of the following individual drugs or drug combinations can safely be used to produce maximum lowering of her elevated plasma lipids?
   - (A) Atorvastatin
   - (B) Atorvastatin + gemfibrozil
   - (C) Cholestyramine + niacin
   - (D) Cholestyramine + gemfibrozil
   - (E) Niacin + gemfibrozil
8. If the patient is given fenofibrate to treat her condition, what enzyme or receptor activity will most increased?
   - (A) Cholesterol 7-α-hydroxylase
   - (B) Cytochrome P450 2C9
   - (C) HMG CoA reductase
   - (D) Lipoprotein lipase
   - (E) Low-density lipoprotein receptor

ANSWERS

1. **A.** Type IIa or familial hypercholesterolemia. Because triglycerides are normal, the contribution of VLDL cholesterol to the total cholesterol is slight (about 105/5, or 21 mg) and taking into account HDL cholesterol, it is clear LDL accounts for the increase in cholesterol. This is confirmed by an intense β-lipoprotein band on electrophoresis. High LDL cholesterol without elevation of other lipids defines type IIa. The condition is probably genetic because of the premature death of his brothers due to heart attacks.
2. **D.** Reduced hepatic LDL-receptor activity. Familial hypercholesterolemia is most often due to deficient LDL-receptor activity. A less likely possibility, although not considered in this question, is reduced LDL clearance from the circulation due to defective apolipoprotein B_{100}.
3. **E.** Simvastatin. Itraconazole inhibits cytochrome P450 3A4. This cytochrome is responsible for metabolism of simvastatin. Therefore, itraconazole can increase serum level of simvastatin and increase its toxicity.
4. **E.** Rhabdomyolysis. Cerivastatin increases the risk of death from rhabdomyolysis.
5. **D.** Type IV. The patient's very high triglycerides are due to elevated VLDL, because electrophoresis

showed only an intense pre-β-band. The high cholesterol is due to VLDL being composed of about 20% cholesterol and not to elevated LDL. VLDL cholesterol is about 208 mg/dL (1042/5) and 72 mg/dL for HDL. LDL cholesterol (about 88 mg/dL) must account for the remainder.

6. **D.** Pancreatitis. Extremely high plasma triglycerides, as in this patient, present a serious risk of acute pancreatitis.
7. **E.** Niacin + gemfibrozil. Niacin and gemfibrozil each can reduce plasma triglycerides. In combination a greater reduction should be observed. Although atorvastatin is reported to lower triglycerides, it is mainly a hypocholesterolemic drug. A statin should not be combined with a fibrate. Cholestyramine is a hypocholesterolemic drug that may aggravate hypertriglyceridemia, and therefore, it should not be used in this patient.
8. **D.** Lipoprotein lipase. Fenofibrate is a hypotriglyceridemic drug that lowers plasma triglycerides by increasing the activity of lipoprotein lipase, the enzyme responsible for disassembly of triglycerides in serum lipoproteins (VLDL, IDL and chylomicrons).

SUPPLEMENTAL READING

Choice of lipid-regulating drugs. Med Lett 2001;43 (Issue 1105):43–48.

Collins R, Peto R, and Armitage J. The MCR/BHF: Heart Protection Study: preliminary results. Int J Clin Pract 2002;56:53–56.

Contemporary management of lipid disorders: The evolving importance of statin therapy. Clin Courier 1998;28 (No. 35):1–7.

Downs JR et al. Primary prevention of acute coronary events with lovastatin in men and women with average cholesterol levels. Results of AFCAPS/TEX-CAPS. JAMA 1998;279:1615–1622.

Knopp RH. Drug treatment of lipid disorders. N Engl J Med 1999;341:498–511.

Ornish D et al. Intensive lifestyle changes for reversal of coronary heart disease. JAMA 1998;280:2001–2007.

Ross R. Atherosclerosis: An inflammatory disease. N Engl J Med 1999;340:115–126.

Sacks FM et al. The effect of pravastatin on coronary events after myocardial infarction in patients with average cholesterol levels. N Engl J Med 1996;335:1001–1009.

Shepherd J et al. Prevention of coronary heart disease with pravastatin in men with hypercholesterolemia. N Engl J Med 1995;333:1301–1307.

Tanne D et al. Blood lipids and first-ever ischemic stroke/transient ischemic attack in the Benzafibrate Infarction Prevention (BIP) Registry: High triglycerides constitute an independent risk factor. Circulation 2001;104:2892–2897.

CASE Study   A Plan for Therapy

Mrs. Jones, a sedentary 52-year-old black woman, complains of chest pain upon exertion. The patient is divorced with two daughters, 28 and 31 years old. She provides full-time care for three grandchildren aged 1 to 4. Her mother is living, 78 years old, but her father died of a myocardial infarction at age 53. She has one older brother, 59 years old, who is said to be in good health. The patient neither smokes nor takes alcohol. She consumes a typical American diet of about 40% calories from fat and participates in no regular exercise. She is taking no medication. She says that "taking care of the kids is a handful." Provide a diagnosis and possible treatment plan.

Physical findings
Height: 62 inches
Weight: 173 pounds
Blood pressure:
    144/98 mmHg

Fasting blood chemistry
Total cholesterol: 246 mg/dL
LDL cholesterol: 177 mg/dL
HDL cholesterol: 53 mg/dL
Triglyceride: 131 mg/dL
Glucose: 108 mg/dL

ANSWER: The patient has heterozygous familial hypercholesterolemia (type IIa) that is aggravated by lifestyle factors (obesity, high fat diet, stress, no exercise). Her LDL cholesterol is markedly elevated; other lipids are normal; she has angina; and she has a family history of heart disease. Her hypertension would probably improve with a decrease in body weight.

TREATMENT PLAN: Based upon the criteria for initiating drug therapy of hypercholesterolemia, the physician decides to begin treatment with 40 mg per day of pravastatin. The patient is also referred to a dietitian for advice on diet and weight control.

OUTCOMES: Two months later the patient is reexamined. Her body weight is 164 pounds and blood LDL cholesterol is 114 mg/dL. Her blood pressure is 136/92. She is encouraged to continue to lose weight and take the cholesterol-lowering drug. She complains of the drug cost.

FOLLOW-UP: When the patient is examined 3 months later, her body weight and blood pressure continue to improve (157 pounds, 128/87 mm Hg) but her LDL cholesterol has increased to 167 mg/dL. She says she has stopped taking the drug because she can't afford it. The physician explains that there is a much less expensive cholesterol drug called niacin, but it can produce a bad itch if not taken in the proper way. The physician begins the patient on 250 mg/day of time-release niacin and advises her to take the medicine after her major meal and to take aspirin if she has skin problems. The physician sees her regularly over the next several months, gradually increasing the niacin dose to 2 g/day. She seems to tolerate the drug well (liver enzymes are unchanged, glucose and other blood chemistries are normal). Her blood LDL cholesterol stabilizes at about 130 mg/dL. The physician encourages her to continue losing weight and to exercise regularly to augment the reduction in her blood cholesterol.

IV

DRUGS AFFECTING THE CENTRAL NERVOUS SYSTEM

24

Introduction to Central Nervous System Pharmacology

Charles R. Craig

REVIEW OF BASIC NEUROSCIENCE

The functional unit of the central nervous system (CNS) is the neuron, and most neuropharmacological agents have the neuron as their primary site of action. CNS neurons are capable of transmitting information to and receiving information from other neurons and peripheral end organs, such as muscle cells, glandular cells, and specialized receptors, for example, those involved with proprioception, temperature sensing, and so on.

The depolarization associated with an action potential results in the calcium-facilitated release of a specific chemical substance at the synapse between two neurons (see Chapter 2). This chemical substance or *neurotransmitter* is released, diffuses across the synaptic cleft, and interacts with the membrane of the second neuron to initiate a local change in the ionic composition and a local altered potential difference in the second neuron. This potential difference change is known as a *postsynaptic potential,* and the direction of the potential change may be either *depolarizing* or *hyperpolarizing*. A depolarizing postsynaptic potential is called an *excitatory postsynaptic potential* (EPSP). If the magnitude of depolarization produced by EPSPs in the second neuron is great enough, an action potential produced in the second neuron will be transmitted in an all-or-none fashion through the neuron and its processes. If, on the other hand, a hyperpolarizing potential (known as an *inhibitory postsynaptic potential,* or IPSP) is produced, it will inhibit the formation of depolarizing action potentials.

Most cells normally receive a large excitatory input with a more or less constant generation of action potentials. The net result of generated IPSPs will be to decrease the number of nerve impulses per unit of time. By these mechanisms, neurotransmitters producing ei-

ther an EPSP (*excitatory neurotransmitter*) or an IPSP (*inhibitory transmitter*) directly influence the number of action potentials generated by the neurons with which they interact.

Morphologically, many synapses in the CNS appear to be quite similar to those for the peripheral autonomic nervous system. Electron microscopic studies have verified the similarities and have shown the presence of several types of storage vesicles in the areas of synapses. Neurons may synthesize, store, and release one or more transmitters. Many more synapses exist in the CNS than in the periphery, and many more neurotransmitters appear to be involved.

The several ways in which pharmacological agents can either increase or decrease neurotransmission are illustrated in Fig. 24.1. The agent can increase the amount of transmitter at the synapse and thereby produce an exaggerated effect. This can be accomplished by (1) increasing the rate of transmitter synthesis, (2) increasing the rate of transmitter release, or (3) prolonging the time the transmitter is in the synapse. This last mechanism can be accomplished either by inhibiting enzymatic breakdown or by inhibiting the reuptake of a previously released transmitter.

In contrast, an agent can produce a diminished response by (1) decreasing synthesis of transmitter, (2) increasing transmitter metabolism, (3) promoting an increased neuronal uptake, or (4) blocking access of the transmitter to its receptor. The first three processes tend to diminish the amount of transmitter in the synaptic cleft. Some agents (including several useful drugs) possess most of these capabilities at norepinephrine, dopamine, serotonin, histamine, and acetylcholine (ACh) synapses. Several important drugs interfere with

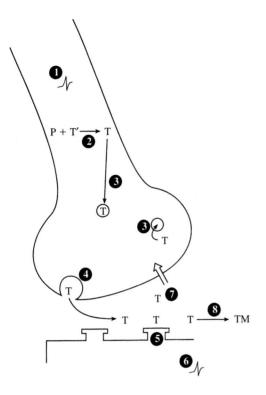

FIGURE 24.1
Sites where drugs may act to alter neurotransmission. The steps are depicted for a typical neurotransmitter (T). Some neurotransmitters do not follow this scheme. Site 1 is an action potential; site 2, synthesis of T from T'; site 3, storage of T in vesicles; site 4, release of T in response to the action potential; site 5, binding of T to receptor; site 6, intracellular response to action of T at site 5; site 7, reuptake of T across neuronal membrane; site 8, metabolism of T to an inactive metabolite, TM.

other CNS transmitter systems, particularly some of the amino acid transmitters, in some of the above-mentioned ways to produce their effects.

In the mammalian CNS powerful inhibitory systems function continually to slow the number of action potentials generated. The effects of stimulating an excitatory pathway can appear to be exaggerated if normal inhibitory influences to that region are diminished. Correspondingly, an inhibitory pathway will appear exaggerated if part of the excitatory influence to that system has been removed.

CENTRAL NERVOUS SYSTEM NEUROTRANSMITTERS

A large number of CNS neurotransmitters have been either tentatively or positively identified. While a detailed discussion of the various central neurotransmitters and the criteria for their identification is beyond the scope of this text, a summary of the most important mammalian central neurotransmitters follows.

Acetylcholine

The discovery that ACh was a transmitter in the peripheral nervous system formed the basis for the theory of neurotransmission. ACh is also a neurotransmitter in the mammalian brain; however, only a few cholinergic tracts have been clearly delineated. ACh is an excitatory neurotransmitter in the mammalian CNS. There is good evidence that ACh (among other neurotransmitters) is decreased in certain cognitive disorders, such as Alzheimer's disease.

Dopamine

Quantitatively, dopamine is the most important of the biogenic amine neurotransmitters in the CNS. The three major distinct dopaminergic systems in the mammalian brain are categorized according to the lengths of the neurons. There is a system comprising ultrashort neurons within amacrine cells of the retina and periglomerular cells in the olfactory bulb. Of the several intermediate-length dopaminergic neuronal systems, the best studied are neurons in the tuberobasal ventral hypothalamus that innervate the median eminence and the intermediate lobe of the pituitary. These neurons are important in the regulation of various hypothalamohypophysial functions, including prolactin release from the anterior pituitary. The best-categorized of the dopamine neuronal systems are the long projections from nuclei in the substantia nigra and ventral tegmental areas to the limbic cortex; other limbic structures, including the amygdaloid complex and piriform cortex; and the neostriatum (primarily the caudate and putamen). In Parkinson's disease, the primary biochemical feature is a marked reduction in the concentration of dopamine in this long projection system (see Chapter 31).

Several classes of drugs, notably the antipsychotics, discussed in Chapter 34, interfere with dopaminergic transmission. In general, dopamine appears to be an inhibitory neurotransmitter. Five dopamine receptors have been identified; the most important and best studied are the D_1- and D_2-receptor groups. The D_1-receptor, which increases cyclic adenosine monophosphate (cAMP) by activation of adenylyl cyclase, is located primarily in the region of the putamen, nucleus accumbens, and in the olfactory tubercle. The D_2-receptor decreases cAMP, blocks certain calcium channels, and opens certain potassium channels.

Norepinephrine

Most central noradrenergic neurons are located in the nucleus locus ceruleus of the pons and in neurons of the reticular formation. Fibers from these nuclei innervate a large number of cortical, subcortical, and spinomedullary fields. Many functions have been ascribed to the central noradrenergic neurons, including a role in affective disorders (see Chapter 33), in learning and memory, and in sleep–wake cycle regulation. The mammalian CNS contains both α- and β-adrenoceptors.

Epinephrine

Epinephrine is found only in very low concentrations in the mammalian CNS, and it is unlikely to play a major role as a neurotransmitter.

Serotonin

Serotonin (5-hydroxytryptamine, or 5HT) is present in the brain as well as in the periphery. In humans, about 90% of the total serotonin in the body is in enterochromaffin cells in the gastrointestinal tract; the remaining 10% occurs primarily in the platelets and brain. The physiological significance of the vast amounts of serotonin constantly synthesized and metabolized in the periphery still remains an enigma. Brain serotonin has been implicated as a potential neurotransmitter in the mediation of a wide variety of phenomena (see Actions).

Synthesis and Fate

Dietary tryptophan is the source of the formation of serotonin. Enzymes and cofactors necessary for serotonin synthesis are present in both the enterochromaffin cells of the gastrointestinal tract and neurons in the brain. Tryptophan is initially hydroxylated to form 5-hydroxytryptophan. Decarboxylation of the latter compound results in the formation of serotonin (Fig. 24.2).

The enzymes responsible for the metabolism of serotonin are present in all of the cells containing this amine and in the liver. Serotonin is initially oxidatively deaminated to form 5-hydroxyindoleacetaldehyde; this compound is subsequently rapidly oxidized to the major metabolite 5-hydroxyindoleacetic acid, which is excreted in the urine. Much of the serotonin released in the brain at synapses is taken back into the initial neuron by an active reuptake mechanism to be released again.

Actions and Site of Actions

Most of the serotonin in the brain is in the brainstem, specifically in the raphe nuclei; considerable amounts also are present in areas of the hypothalamus, the limbic system, and the pituitary gland. Current evidence indicates that serotonin is involved in the regulation of several aspects of behavior, including sleep, pain perception, depression, sexual activity, and aggressiveness. Some of the most important antidepressant agents are believed to prevent the reuptake of serotonin (see Chapter 33). Serotonin also may be involved in temperature regulation and in the hypothalamic control of the release of pituitary hormones.

In addition to its presumed role as a neurotransmitter within the brain, serotonin is synthesized in the pineal gland, where it is a precursor for the synthesis of melatonin, a hormone that influences endocrine activity, presumably by an action within the hypothalamus.

The mammalian brain appears to have an abundance of sites with which serotonin interacts. Fourteen

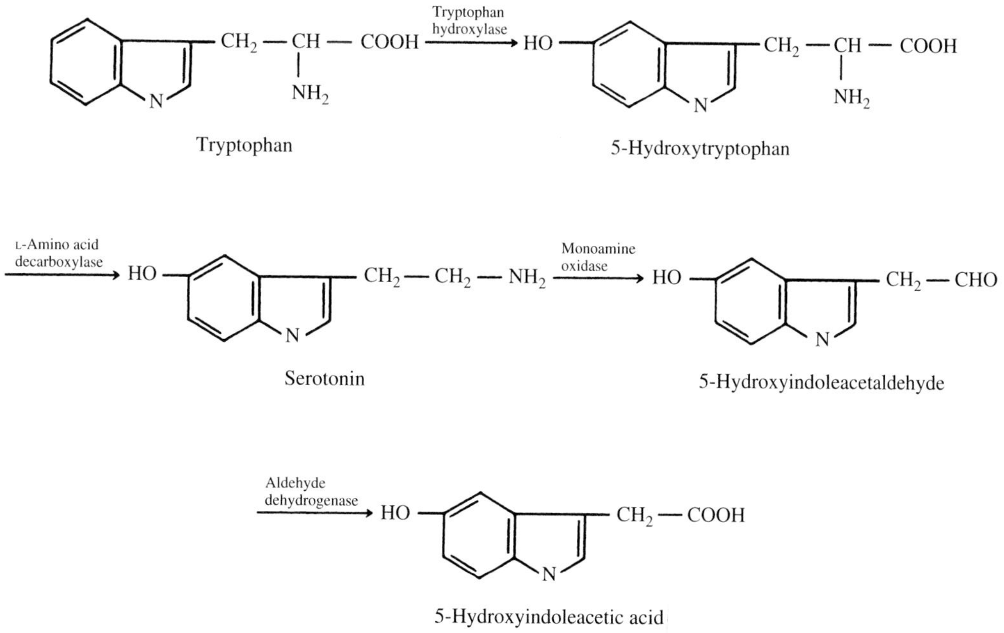

FIGURE 24.2
Steps involved in the synthesis and metabolic degradation of serotonin.

distinct mammalian receptor subtypes for serotonin have been established, not all of which have been identified in the brain. They are characterized as $5\text{-}HT_1$, $5\text{-}HT_2$, . . . $5\text{-}HT_7$ subsets. There are at least five subtypes of the $5\text{-}HT_1$ subset and three receptor subtypes for the $5\text{-}HT_2$ subset. The interested reader may explore the various subsets and subtypes in the work by Hoyer et al. listed at the end of this chapter.

Amino Acid Neurotransmitters

A large number of amino acids serve as neurotransmitters in the mammalian CNS.

γ-Aminobutyric Acid

γ-Aminobutyric acid (GABA) is the major inhibitory neurotransmitter in the mammalian CNS. GABA is primarily synthesized (Fig. 24.3) from glutamate by the enzyme L-glutamic acid-l-decarboxylase (GAD); it is subsequently transaminated with α-ketoglutarate by $GABA_A$-oxoglutarate transaminase (GABA-T) to yield glutamate and succinic semialdehyde.

Two types of GABA receptors have been identified in mammals, a $GABA_A$- and a $GABA_B$-receptor. The $GABA_A$-receptor (or recognition site), when coupled with GABA, induces a shift in membrane permeability, primarily to chloride ions, causing hyperpolarization of the neuron. This GABA receptor appears to be part of a macromolecule that contains, in addition to the $GABA_A$-receptor, benzodiazepine and barbiturate binding sites and the chloride ionophore (chloride channel). See Figure 24.4.

A number of drugs are thought to exert their CNS effect by altering $GABA_A$-receptor activity. The 1,4-benzodiazepines, β-carbolines, barbiturates, alcohols, and general anesthetics appear to facilitate GABA transmission by interacting at this macromolecular complex. Vigabatrin, a newly approved anticonvulsant, elevates brain GABA by inhibiting the breakdown enzyme GABA-T. Several CNS convulsants, including bicuculline, picrotoxinin, and pentylenetetrazol, are antagonists at the GABA receptor. Since GABA agonists

have been shown to be anticonvulsants and GABA antagonists are convulsants, there is much interest in the role of GABA in epilepsy (see Chapter 32). The $GABA_B$-receptor, in contrast, is not modulated by benzodiazepines, is not linked to chloride movement, and is not nearly as well characterized as is the $GABA_A$-receptor. The $GABA_B$-receptor is coupled to K^+ channels and is activated by the antispastic agent baclofen.

Glycine

Glycine is another inhibitory CNS neurotransmitter. Whereas GABA is located primarily in the brain, glycine is found predominantly in the ventral horn of the spinal cord. Relatively few drugs are known to interact with glycine; the best-known example is the convulsant agent strychnine, which appears to be a relatively specific antagonist of glycine.

Glutamic Acid and Aspartic Acid

These two excitatory amino acids (EAAs) are widely distributed throughout the mammalian CNS. Their administration leads to rapid depolarization of neurons and an increase in firing rate. There are two distinct classes of EAA receptors: ionotropic receptors and metabotropic receptors. The ionotropic receptors directly gate ion channels, while the metabotropic receptors are coupled to intracellular G proteins. Receptors are named according to their sensitivity to the action of selective agonists (Table 24.1). The best-characterized receptor is known as the NMDA (N-methyl-D-aspartate) receptor, which directly gates a Mg^{++} cation channel that is also permeable to Ca^{++} and Na^+. Compounds that block the NMDA receptor complex may attenuate the neuronal damage following anoxia, such as occurs during a stroke; much of the neuronal damage associated with strokes may be related to the release of glutamic acid, aspartic acid, or both. Similarly, neuronal damage may occur as a result of seizures, and this also may be related to excessive EAA release. Antagonists of the NMDA receptor complex are being studied for possible uses in strokes and other types of hypoxia.

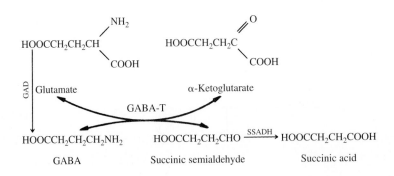

FIGURE 24.3
Steps in the synthesis and metabolism of GABA.

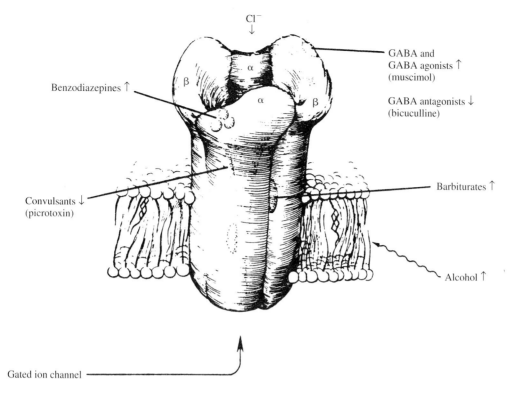

FIGURE 24.4

The $GABA_A$ receptor complex. This model is not meant to indicate the subunit assembly or location and stoichiometry of the various recognition sites associated with the subunits. Arrows indicate the enhancement ($\uparrow$) or inhibition ($\downarrow$) of GABAergic function by various agents. (Reprinted with permission from Schwartz RD. The $GABA_A$ receptor-gated ion channel: Biochemical and pharmacological studies of structure and function. Biochem Pharmacol 37:3370, 1988. Copyright 1988, Pergamon Press PLC.)

Histamine

Histamine occurs in the brain, particularly in certain hypothalamic neurons, and evidence is strong that histamine is a neurotransmitter. Distribution of histamine, its synthetic enzyme (histidine decarboxylase), and methyl histamine (the major brain metabolite) is not uniform. Possible roles for histamine in the regulation of food and water intake, thermoregulation, hormone release, and sleep have been suggested. Additional information on histamine can be found in Chapter 38.

Other Possible Amino Acid Neurotransmitters

Several additional amino acids are considered to be neurotransmitter candidates. Among these are taurine, α- and β-alanine, 2-phenylethylamine, and imidazole-4-acetic acid. No available drugs are known to act via these amino acids.

Peptides as Neurotransmitters

A large number of endogenous peptides are produced by neurons that appear to possess the essential charac-

teristics of neurotransmitters (e.g., their release is Ca^{++}dependent, they are localized in specific neurons, and their release induces changes in postsynaptic neuronal systems).

The names of the agents can be terribly misleading to the beginning student. Many of the peptides have

TABLE 24.1 Receptors for Excitatory Amino Acids

Receptor Designation	Function
Ionotropic NMDA	Produces excitation by increasing Ca^{++} conductance; generates slow component of EPSP
AMPA	Generates fast component of EPSP
Kainate	Specific distribution, similar pharmacologically to AMPA
Metabotropic 1S,3R-ACPD	Linked to IP_3 formation

NMDA, N-methyl-D-aspartate; AMPA, α-amino-3-hydroxy-5-methyl-isoxazole-4-proprionic acid; 1S,3R-ACPD, L-amino-cyclopentane-1S,3R-dicarboxylic acid; IP_3, inosine triphosphate

been around for many years and were named according to their known effects when they were discovered. Examples are gastrin and cholecystokinin (CCK), compounds that were historically known as gut hormones. It is important, therefore, to realize that the names of the neuroactive peptides may bear no resemblance to their function in the brain. Many of the neuroactive peptides exist as families of chemically related compounds or occur within larger precursor molecules (or propeptides). However, several forms may be "active," and several slightly different structures may confer subtle changes in selectivity. Many neuroactive peptides appear to coexist and be released along with one or more of the "traditional" neurotransmitters, such as ACh, dopamine, or serotonin.

More than two dozen peptides are being studied as probable central neurotransmitters, and likely many more compounds remain to be discovered. Therefore, this chapter makes no attempt to cover them all. A few of the most important peptide transmitters are discussed briefly, with still others listed in Table 24.2. For additional information, see the supplemental reading list at the end of this chapter.

Substance P

The first neuropeptide to be isolated and characterized is known as substance P. Although this 11–amino acid peptide (undecapeptide) has been known for more than 60 years, its exact physiological role is still not clear. Substance P occurs in high concentrations in neurons projecting into the *substantia gelatinosa* layer of the spinal cord from dorsal root ganglia, among many other areas of the brain. Substance P can directly depolarize motor neurons in a manner analogous to that of other excitatory neurotransmitters. It is probable that substance P is released from small unmyelinated nerve fibers in response to painful stimulation. Levels of sub-

TABLE 24.2 **Known or Suspected Peptide Neurotransmitters**

Family (compound)	Number of Amino Acids	Special Characteristics
Vasopressin (antidiuretic hormone)	9	Inhibitory to neurons; may facilitate learning and memory
Oxytocin	9	Inhibitory; very similar to vasopressin
Tachykin peptides		
Substance P	11	Levels of substance P are reduced in Huntington's chorea; pain transmission
Neurokinin A	10	
Neurokinin B	13	
Neurotensin	30	Lowers body temperature; coexists in neurons with dopamine and norepinephrine
Glucagon-related peptides		
Vasoactive intestinal peptide	28	May be involved in pain pathways; concentrated in neocortex; produces vasodilation high levels in hypothalamus and median eminence
Growth hormone releasing hormone	24	
Opioid peptides		
Proopiomelanocortin peptides		
β-Endorphin	30	Most potent of endogenous opioid compounds
Enkephalin pentapeptides		
Met^5-enkephalin	5	Distributed widely throughout CNS
Leu^5-enkephalin	5	
Prodynorphin peptides		
Dynorphin A	8	Extended forms of Leu^5-enkephalin
Dynorphin B	8	
Somatostatin	28	Inhibits basal growth hormone release, causes decreased spontaneous motor activity and sleep disturbances, deficit in cerebrospinal fluid of patients with Alzheimer's disease
Cholecystokinin	8	Coexists with dopamine in nucleus accumbens and with GABA intracortical neurons; may have a role in regulating appetite
Angiotensin II	8	In periphery: induces secretion of aldosterone and modifies blood pressure; centrally: induces drinking behavior
Calcitonin gene-related peptide	37	Causes vasodilation
Corticotropin-releasing factor	41	Regulates corticotropin secretion; produces "anxiogenic" response
Neuropeptide Y	36	One of the most abundant neuropeptides; produces increased feeding, hypothermia; may act at multiple receptors

stance P in the substantia nigra are markedly reduced in the neurological disease Huntington's chorea.

Vasopressin and Oxytocin

Historically vasopressin and oxytocin, two nonapeptides, were the first peptide "neurohormones" to be considered; they are stored in the neurohypophysis and released into the bloodstream upon an appropriate stimulus. In the periphery, oxytocin stimulates the contraction of epididymal and uterine smooth muscle (see Chapter 62) and vasopressin (antidiuretic hormone) facilitates the reabsorption of water from the kidney tubules. In addition to these well-accepted roles as neurohormones, there is convincing evidence that these compounds function as neurotransmitters; they both possess potent inhibitory actions on neurohypophyseal neurons. The significance of their neurotransmitter function is not yet clear.

Endogenous Opioid Peptides

A seminal discovery during the 1960s and 1970s was the presence of endogenous substances in mammalian brain that appeared to possess the pharmacological qualities of morphine and other opioid analgesics. It had been known for quite awhile that most "drug receptors" were in fact receptors for endogenous transmitters. It was surprising, therefore, when tissue from mouse brain was shown to avidly bind opioids, such as morphine and heroin, in a stereoselective manner. As Avram Goldstein, one of the pharmacologists involved in discovering the endogenous opioids, noted, "It seemed unlikely, *a priori,* that such highly stereospecific receptors should have been developed by nature to interact with alkaloids from the opium poppy."[1] A series of peptides, occurring naturally in brain and possessing pharmacological properties similar to those of morphine, have been described. At least three separate families of peptides have opioid properties (Table 24.2), and the different classes of peptides reside in separate distinct neurons. It is likely that the endogenous opioid peptides coexist in neurons with other nonopioid neurotransmitters. The initial hope that these endogenous agents or synthetic derivatives of them would be found to retain the analgesic activity of the opioids but be devoid of respiratory depression and/or addictive properties has now somewhat abated.

BLOOD-BRAIN BARRIER

Not all substances in the bloodstream can readily gain entry into the brain. This apparent barrier to drugs and other chemicals is relative rather than absolute, and in fact there are several barriers to substances entering the brain from the systemic circulation. The term *blood-brain barrier* is usually applied to the lack of passage of certain drugs or other exogenously administered chemicals into the brain.

One important property that determines entry to the brain from the systemic circulation is molecular weight. Compounds with molecular weights of about 60,000 and above tend to remain within the circulatory system. Furthermore, the portion of an administered drug that is bound to plasma proteins is unavailable for distribution to the brain (as well as to other tissues and organs), in part because of the high molecular weight of the plasma protein–drug complex.

There are two physicochemical factors particularly important in allowing a drug to enter the CNS. First, for compounds that are mainly un-ionized at plasma pH (pK$_a$ 7.4 or higher), the drug's *solubility in lipids is an important determinant.* A lipid-soluble agent can more easily penetrate lipid membranes, such as those found in the CNS. The proportion of drug that is un-ionized is another important determinant. These two properties cannot be completely separated, since un-ionized drugs are generally more lipid soluble than ionized ones.

Location of the Blood-Brain Barrier

The capillaries of the brain are the most likely location of the blood-brain barrier. Brain capillaries differ in several important respects from capillaries in other body locations (Fig. 24.5). For example, the endothelial cells of brain capillaries are so closely joined to each other that passage of substances cannot readily occur through the intercellular clefts between adjacent cells; furthermore, brain capillaries do not contain fenestrae (pores). Fenestrae are prominent in many capillaries, especially those in renal glomeruli and in the chorioid plexus. The ability of a drug to leave a capillary by diffusion appears to be directly related to the number of capillary pores. Compared with capillaries at other sites, brain capillaries also appear to possess very few pinocytotic vesicles, which are believed to play a role in the transport of large molecules through capillary walls.

Brain capillaries contain many more mitochondria than do other capillaries, and it is probable that the mitochondria supply energy for active transport of water-soluble nutrient substances into the brain. A large number of lipid-insoluble endogenous substances are known to be transported into the brain. These

[1]Goldstein A. Opioid peptides (endorphins) in pituitary and brain. Science 1976; 193:1081–1086.

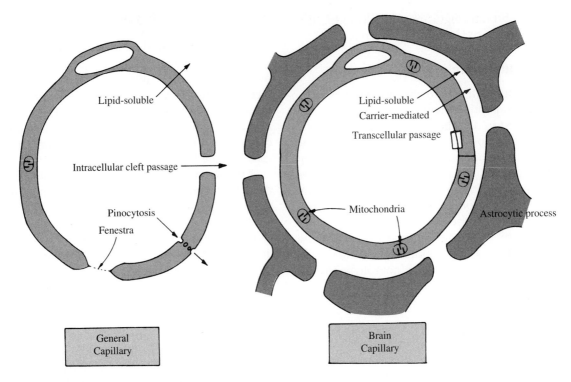

FIGURE 24.5

Major differences between a general (nonneural) and brain capillary. In the brain capillary, the intercellular clefts are sealed shut by tight junctions. There are also reduced pinocytosis and no fenestrae. Exchange of compounds between the circulation and the brain must take place in the cells of the capillary wall, the major barriers of which are the inner and outer plasma membranes of the capillary endothelial cells. (Reprinted with permission from Oldendorf WA. Permeability of the blood-brain barrier. In Tower DB [ed.]. The Nervous System. Vol. 1 New York: Raven, 1975.)

substances include glucose, amino acids, simple carboxylic acids, and purines.

Significance of the Blood-Brain Barrier

It is likely that the blood-brain barrier serves primarily to preserve the internal environment of the brain and prevent sudden increases in concentration of a variety of water-soluble ionized substances, including many circulating neurotransmitters, such as norepinephrine, epinephrine, ACh, serotonin, and dopamine. The concentration in the brain of these bioactive substances appears to be carefully regulated. On the other hand, the biochemical precursors of these transmitters can pass relatively easily, although usually by active transport, from the blood to the brain, and this ensures an adequate supply of locally synthesized transmitters. By and large, the precursors are inactive biologically or have only minimal biological activity. The amino acid transmitters GABA, glycine, glutamic acid, and aspartic acid are actively taken up by the brain capillaries, but ordinarily the transport system for these amino acids is close to saturation. Therefore, a sudden increase in blood concentration of these substances would have little effect on brain levels. Peptide transmitters will not readily penetrate the brain from the circulation, and they are synthesized in the brain.

The blood-brain barrier is not found in all parts of the brain. Certain small areas, including the *area postrema* beneath the floor of the fourth ventricle, an area in the *preoptic recess,* and portions of the floor of the third ventricle surrounding the stalk of the pituitary, appear to be devoid of this barrier.

The ability of the blood-brain barrier to exclude entry of a number of drugs into the brain has several therapeutic implications. Many drugs, most notably certain antibiotics, are relatively excluded from the brain. In the treatment of infectious diseases of the CNS, the physician must, in addition to establishing the organism's drug sensitivity, either select an agent that can get to the site of the infection or use a route (intrathecal) that bypasses the barrier. In the human fetus and newborn, the barrier is not as well developed as it is in later life. This fact also must be taken into consideration when one is prescribing drugs during pregnancy and for neonates (see Chapter 6).

Study QUESTIONS

1. The neurotransmitter serotonin is derived from which precursor amino acid?
   (A) Dopamine
   (B) Tyrosine
   (C) Tryptophan
   (D) Dopa
   (E) Glutamine

2. The major inhibitory neurotransmitter in the mammalian CNS is
   (A) Acetylcholine
   (B) Norepinephrine
   (C) Glycine
   (D) γ-Aminobutyric acid
   (E) Glutamic acid

3. The location of the blood-brain barrier is considered to be
   (A) At the level of the brain capillaries
   (B) At the level of glia
   (C) At the level of neurons
   (D) At the level of dendrites

4. Identify the major excitatory neurotransmitter system in the mammalian CNS.
   (A) γ-Aminobutyric acid
   (B) Histamine
   (C) Substance P
   (D) Glutamate/aspartate
   (E) Serotonin

5. Agents that potentiate the actions of GABA in the brain will likely have which of the following effects?
   (A) Elevate blood pressure
   (B) Provide sedation
   (C) Cause seizures
   (D) Relieve pain

6. What is the number of neurotransmitters in the mammalian CNS?
   (A) 3
   (B) 6
   (C) 15
   (D) more than 20

ANSWERS

1. **C.** Dopamine is a precursor for norepinephrine and a neurotransmitter. Tyrosine is a precursor of dopamine and norepinephrine. Dopa (dihydroxyphenylalanine) is a precursor of dopamine and subsequently also of norepinephrine. Glutamine can be converted to the neurotransmitter glutamic acid.

2. **D.** Acetylcholine and norepinephrine are important neurotransmitters in the peripheral autonomic nervous system but are not nearly as prominent in the CNS. Glycine is a major inhibitory neurotransmitter in the spinal cord but not the rest of the CNS. Glutamic acid is a major excitatory neurotransmitter in the mammalian CNS.

3. **A.** The site of the blood-brain barrier was hotly debated for many years until electron micrographs clearly showed that endothelial cells lining brain capillaries are so closely joined to each other that passages of substances cannot readily occur through the intercellular clefts located between adjacent cells and that this constitutes a barrier to the passage of many substances from the blood to the parenchyma of the brain.

4. **D.** GABA is the major inhibitory neurotransmitter in the mammalian CNS. Histamine is a CNS neurotransmitter, but has limited distribution. This is also true for serotonin. Substance P is an excitatory neurotransmitter in the spinal cord.

5. **B.** Since GABA is an inhibitory neurotransmitter, agents that potentiate its action are likely to be CNS depressants with sedative activity. GABA has no significant effect on blood pressure and will decrease the incidence of seizures. It has no direct ability to relieve pain.

6. **D.** The exact number of agents identified as neurotransmitters in the mammalian CNS is not established, but it is certainly more than 20. More and more compounds are being established as neurotransmitters as scientists who concentrate on this area.

SUPPLEMENTAL READING

Carlsson A et al. Interactions between monoamines, glutamate, and GABA in schizophrenia: new evidence. Annu Rev Pharmacol Toxicol 2001; 41:237–260.

Cowan WM, Harter DH, and Kandel ER. The emergence of modern neuroscience: Some implications for neurology and psychiatry. Annu Rev Neurosci 2000; 23:343–391.

Cherubini E and Conti F. Generating diversity at GABAergic synapses. Trends Neurosci 2002;24:155–162.

Dunzendorfer S and Wiedermann CJ. Neuropeptides and the immune system: focus on dendritic cells. Crit Rev Immunol 2001;21:523–557.

Dautzenberg FM and Hauger RL. The CRF peptide family and their receptors: yet more partners discovered. Trends Pharmacol Sci 2002;23:71–78.

Hoyer D et al. International Union of Pharmacology Classification of receptors for 5-hydroxytryptamine (serotonin) Pharmacol Rev 1994;46:157–203.

Law A, Gauthier S, and Quirion R. Say NO to
Alzheimer's disease: The putative links between ni-
tric oxide and dementia of the Alzheimer's type.
Brain Res Brain Res Rev 2001;35:73–996.

Leurs R, Watanabe T, and Timmerman H. Histamine
receptors are finally "coming out." Trends
Pharmacol Sci 2001;22:337–339.

Strange PG. Antipsychotic drugs: Importance of
dopamine receptors for mechanisms of therapeutic
actions and side effects. Pharmacol Rev
2001;53:119–133.

Yehuda S, Rabinovitz, S, Carasso RL, and Mostofsky
DI. Fatty acids and brain peptides. Peptides
1998;19:407–419.

CASE Study   Drugs and the Newborn

A mother calls to tell you that her week-old baby is having convulsions. She says the baby exhibited signs of a serious ear infection soon after birth. A physician prescribed penicillin G that apparently was well tolerated. The signs and symptoms of the ear infection appeared to be greatly reduced, but the baby began to have convulsions about an hour after receiving the last injection of penicillin. What would you advise the mother to do?

ANSWER: Penicillin G is a potent antagonist of the inhibitory neurotransmitter γ- GABA. Since penicillin G normally does not penetrate the blood-brain barrier to any extent, this is not usually a problem. However, the blood-brain barrier is not fully developed at birth, and substances that normally are excluded from entering the CNS may enter the immature brain of the newborn. Seizures are a manifestation of several GABA antagonists, including penicillin G. Since the mother indicates that the seizures have almost ceased, you instruct her not to administer any more penicillin and to bring her child to your office as soon as she can.

25 | General Anesthesia: Intravenous and Inhalational Agents

David J. Smith and Michael B. Howie

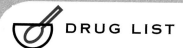

DRUG LIST

Anesthesia usually involves a loss of memory and awareness, along with insensitivity to painful stimuli, during a surgical procedure. Many drugs aid anesthesiologists in the management and comfort of their patients during the perioperative period. These compounds vary in their chemical and physical characteristics and in their usual routes of administration. There are inhalational agents, including volatile liquids and gases, and intravenously administered drugs.

While many of the individual compounds produce anesthesia, each one's unique pharmacokinetic and pharmacological characteristics will determine the way the practitioner uses the agent. This chapter focuses on these characteristics so that their influence on the anes-thesiologist's choice of anesthetic technique will be understood.

Contemporary anesthetic management requires (1) rapid loss of consciousness, which eliminates awareness, memory of pain, anxiety, and stress throughout the surgical period; (2) a level of analgesia sufficient to abolish the reflex reactions to pain, such as muscular movement and cardiovascular stimulation; (3) minimal and reversible influence on vital physiological functions, such as those performed by the cardiovascular and respiratory systems; (4) relaxation of skeletal muscle to facilitate endotracheal intubation, provide the surgeon ready access to the operative field, and reduce the dose of anesthetic required to produce immobility; (5) lack of operating room safety hazards, such as flammability and explosiveness; and (6) prompt patient recovery to psychomotor competence, facilitating the clinician's assessment of the patient and the patient's ability to become physiologically self-supporting.

While none of the anesthetic drugs discussed in this chapter possesses all of the features required for ideal anesthetic management (a summary of these features is presented in Table 25.1), the patient's needs are usually met with the use of anesthetic drugs and/or adjunctive agents, such as neuromuscular blocking drugs, opioids, and vasoactive substances. *Balanced anesthesia* is a term used to describe the multidrug approach to managing the patient's anesthetic needs. Balanced anesthesia takes advantage of each drug's beneficial effects while minimizing each agent's adverse qualities.

PHARMACOKINETIC CHARACTERISTICS INFLUENCING THE CLINICAL APPLICATION OF INTRAVENOUS AND INHALATIONAL ANESTHETICS

Intravenous anesthetics are generally employed to induce anesthesia, to provide supplemental anesthesia, or to permit anesthesia for short operative procedures. The inhalational anesthetics are most often used for longer-term maintenance of the anesthetic state. Although intravenous (IV) agents produce anesthesia rapidly, most are metabolized slowly, so recovery may be prolonged when an IV anesthetic is used as the primary drug during a long surgical procedure. In contrast, while the anesthetic partial pressure of an inhalational agent is

TABLE 25.1 General Anesthetics

Agent	Induction rate (minutes)	Anesthesia	Eliminate reflex reaction to pain	Muscle paralysis	Blood pressure[a]	Ventilation[a]	Note
Intravenous							
Thiopental (sodium pentothal)	<1	Yes	No	No	Decrease	Depressed	
Etomidate (Amidate)	<1	Yes	No	No	Minimal change	Minimal change	↓ adrenocortical response to stress
Midazolam (Versed)	<1	Yes	No	No	Minimal change	Minimal change	Water-soluble benzodiazepine
Propofol (Diprivan)	<1	Yes	No	No	Decrease	Decrease	↓ opioid requirement; antiemetic; rapid recovery via extrahepatic metabolism
Ketamine (Ketalar)	<1	Dissociative	Yes	No	Slight decrease	Minimal change	emergence delirium; IM or IV
Sufentanil (Sufenta)	<1	Incomplete amnesia?	Yes	No	Minimal change	Decrease	Anesthesia supplemented because of concern for partial awareness
Inhalational Gases							
N$_2$O	3–5	Incomplete	Yes	No	No Change	No Change	Laughing gas
Cyclopropane	3–5	Yes	Some	Some	Increase	Decrease	Flammable; explosive
Inhalational Volatile Liquids							
Sevoflurane (Ultane)	3–5	Yes	Some	Some	Decrease	Decrease	Pleasant smell; (?) nephrotoxic byproduct; combative behavior, disorientation
Desflurane (Suprane)	3–5	Yes	Some	Some	Decrease	Decrease	Bad odor; airway irritation, ↑ sympathetic outflow
Halothane (Fluothane)	10–30	Yes	Some	Minimal	Decrease	Decrease	Rare liver dysfunction
Enflurane (Ethrane)	10–30	Yes	Some	Some	Decrease	Decrease	Myoclonic
Isoflurane (Forane)	10–30	Yes	Some	Some	Decrease	Decrease	Popular inhalational agent, largely owing to cardiovascular safety
Methoxyflurane (Penthrane)	>60	Yes	Some	Minimal	Decrease	Decrease	Excessive fluoride production
Ether	>60	Yes	Yes	Yes	Increase	Increase	Flammable and explosive

[a]Effects are those commonly observed in healthy patients. Poor-risk patients with significant systemic disease should be monitored for reactions of greater clinical significance.

achieved slowly, the patient recovers at a clinically acceptable rate.

Distribution of Intravenous Drugs

Intravenously administered anesthetic drugs are especially well suited to accomplish the first requirement of anesthetic management, rapid induction of unconsciousness. These compounds generally induce anesthesia within one or two circulation times after their administration because they rapidly achieve initial high concentration in the central nervous system (CNS). These drugs enter the brain because they are quite lipid soluble and consequently diffuse rapidly through all biological membranes, including the blood-brain barrier. In addition, since the brain tissue receives a large proportion of the cardiac output, a large proportion of an intravenously administered anesthetic will be distributed to the CNS. Tissues with lower blood flow per unit mass will receive and therefore remove proportionally less anesthetic during the initial phase of drug distribution. This concept is illustrated for thiopental in Fig. 25.1. All IV anesthetic drugs in use show this early pattern of distribution. The use of IV anesthetics permits the patient to pass rapidly through the initial stages of anesthesia, and sleep is induced quickly.

The initial unequal tissue–drug distribution cannot persist, however, because physicochemical forces tend to require an eventual establishment of concentration equilibria with other less well perfused organs. Therefore, as the drug continues to be removed from the blood by the less richly perfused tissues or eliminated by metabolism and excretion or both, plasma levels will fall, and the concentration of anesthetic in the brain will decline precipitously.

Tissues with an intermediate blood flow per unit of mass, such as skeletal muscle and skin, are among the first to participate in drug redistribution. In fact, it is the patient's skeletal muscle tissue groups that will contain the largest proportion of the initial dose of anesthetic when the patient awakens (Fig. 25.2). Most of the IV drugs used to induce anesthesia are slowly metabolized and excreted and depend on redistribution to terminate their pharmacological effects. The rate of initial redistribution following the administration of a single IV bolus of drug is defined by the half-life ($t_{1/2\alpha}$), and is generally about 8 minutes for most anesthetics. It can be said, therefore, that redistribution of IV anesthetics to skeletal muscle accounts for the return to consciousness after a single sleep dose of these agents. Patients generally awaken 15 to 30 minutes after a single IV injection of most of the commonly used IV anesthetics.

Poorly perfused tissues (adipose tissue, connective tissue, and bone) require hours to come into equilibrium with plasma drug concentrations (Fig. 25.1). Since the accumulation of anesthetic in body fat is relatively small soon after its IV administration, it is common clinical practice to calculate drug dosage on the basis of lean body mass rather than on total body weight. Thus, an obese patient may receive the same dose of IV anesthetic as a patient of normal body weight.

Since the distribution of blood flow is the dominant factor controlling both tissue drug levels and the accumulation of IV anesthetics, changes in cardiac output can be expected to influence the pharmacological effects of the IV anesthetics. Because blood flow to the brain is preserved, a greater proportion of the total dose of anesthetic will be delivered to the brain during times of diminished cardiac output, such as in congestive heart failure or hemorrhage. At such times, smaller

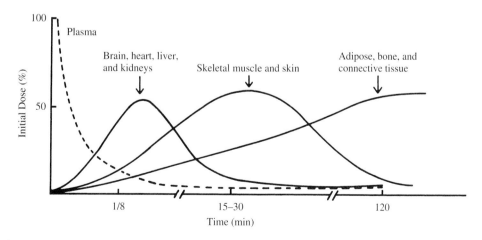

FIGURE 25.1

The distribution of thiopental in body tissues and organs following intravenous injection. Note the redistribution of the drug, with time, to tissues with lower rates of blood flow. (Reprinted with permission from Price HL et al. The uptake of thiopental by body tissues and its relation to the duration of narcosis. Clin Pharmacol Ther 1:16, 1960.)

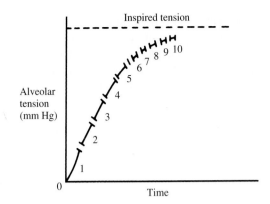

FIGURE 25.2
Alveolar tension of a hypothetical anesthetic gas of low solubility after 10 breathing cycles. Alveolar tension approaches inspired tension.

doses of anesthetic must be administered to avoid excessive CNS depression. The use of significantly lower doses of IV anesthetic drug also should be a consideration in elderly patients, since they have low cardiac output, low lean body mass, and frequently a reduced capacity for drug clearance.

The effect of increased cardiac output on the administered dose of anesthetic is opposite that discussed for reduced cardiac output. Intensely anxious patients and those who have such diseases as thyrotoxicosis usually require larger doses of anesthetic to induce anesthesia.

Metabolism and Excretion of Intravenous Drugs

Clearance of IV anesthetics from the body eventually requires metabolism and excretion. Since *drugs with long elimination half-lives ($t_{1/2\beta}$) will have slow rates of clearance,* their use by repeated IV bolus or continuous infusion to maintain anesthesia has been restricted. Long-term application with limited concern for the pharmacokinetics of the agents may lead to delayed awakening, as large quantities of these drugs may accumulate in reservoir tissues, such as skeletal muscle and fat. Thus, after lengthy anesthetic administration, drug plasma levels will remain high as the compound diffuses from these tissue reservoirs. On the other hand, if the duration of an infusion remains short, awakening may be nearly the same with drugs exhibiting short and long elimination half-lives. With a shorter infusion, the quantities of drug accumulated in reservoir tissues are not sufficient to maintain high plasma and brain levels. Thus, length of infusion is a context in which the duration of drug action is considered. The term *context sensitive half-time* has been coined to express the effect of duration of infusion (the context) on plasma levels of infused drugs.

Administration of Intravenous Anesthetics by Controlled Infusion

The recent advent of computer-assisted IV drug administration has made more practical the maintenance of anesthesia with anesthetics with relatively short half-lives (e.g., propofol and short-acting phenylpiperidine opioids). The technique called *total intravenous anesthesia* (TIVA) is done with short-acting drugs so that rapid recovery occurs even after long infusions. The loading and maintenance doses of each agent can be programmed by taking their individual pharmacokinetic profiles into consideration. Thus, dosage is automatically adjusted for factors that may alter drug distribution, parameters controlling drug clearance, and the duration of the procedure, to maintain a plasma level that is just adequate for the appropriate depth of anesthesia. Many practitioners, however, still prefer to titrate the infusion of intravenous drugs to effect without the use of computer programming.

The shorter-acting drugs seem to have increasing applications in outpatient surgery, which now accounts for nearly 60% of all elective procedures, and for minor inpatient procedures (e.g., wound repair, bronchoscopy, angiography). Patients generally receive lower doses of drugs so that operative procedures are tolerable, avoiding the substantial depression of cardiorespiratory systems that may occur with the higher doses required for hypnosis. Sedative doses of benzodiazepines and propofol are among the most common; they are frequently administered in combination with short-acting opioids. The term for such a technique is *conscious sedation.* Other techniques may also be employed. For example, when an opioid is combined with a neuroleptic drug, such as the butyrophenone droperidol (*Inapsine*), the technique is called *neuroleptanalgesia.* An inhalational drug, such as nitrous oxide (N_2O), may be added during intervals of the operative procedure when complete anesthesia is desired (i.e., neuroleptanesthesia).

INTRAVENOUS ANESTHETIC AGENTS

Important pharmacological characteristics for anesthetic management using IV anesthetics are shown in Table 25.1. The principal use of these drugs is to induce anesthesia. In typical anesthetic management, the last event that the patient remembers is the insertion of the needle. Patients are often unaware that other anesthetics, most frequently in the form of inhalational drugs, are necessary to maintain the anesthesia.

Ultra–Short-Acting Barbiturates

Among the barbiturates (see Chapter 30), three compounds, thiopental sodium (*Pentothal Sodium*), thiamylal sodium (*Surital*), and methohexital sodium (*Brevital*

Sodium), are useful as induction agents, as supplemental drugs only during short periods when surgery requires increased depth of anesthesia, or as maintenance hypnotics for short surgical procedures. These drugs are termed *ultra–short-acting* agents, since their rapid entry into the CNS is followed by relatively rapid redistribution of the drug to indifferent tissues, such as skeletal muscle. Because of their slow rate of metabolism, these agents, when used in large repeated doses or by continuous infusion, cause persistent hypnosis or subtle mental cloudiness.

Pharmacological Actions

All three IV barbiturates rapidly produce unconsciousness. Since unconsciousness is attended by amnesia without either analgesia or skeletal muscle relaxation, anesthetized patients may react to painful stimuli but are unaware and do not remember the procedure. For example, patients undergoing short surgical procedures with thiopental alone may respond to surgical maneuvers with facial grimaces or arm and leg movements and with potentially dangerous changes in blood pressure and heart rhythm. Consequently, induction of anesthesia may be nearly the only indication for thiopental. However, if thiopental is to be used to maintain anesthesia for short operative procedures, analgesia should be provided with other drugs.

Thiopental remains the most popular IV induction agent. Its rapid and pleasant induction of anesthesia and its relatively low cost are among the reasons for its high acceptance rate by both the patient and the practitioner. Also, it does not induce obstructive secretions in the airway, produces little or no emesis, and does not sensitize the myocardium to endogenous catecholamines that may be released in response to the stress of surgery. It can, however, cause cardiovascular depression.

Although the pharmacological actions of the IV barbiturates are similar, methohexital in particular may provide some advantages in selected situations. Its duration of action is only half as long, and it exerts fewer cumulative effects than does thiopental. The occasional requirement of intraoperative communication between the patient and surgeon is easily satisfied with methohexital because of its short duration of action. For example, it can be used for basal sedation in the few moments that a very painful stimulus is applied, and then, as consciousness is quickly regained, the surgeon can assess the results by talking to the patient.

Adverse Effects

Cardiovascular depression may occur after the administration of barbiturates by IV bolus. The hemodynamic changes are transient in the healthy patient with good cardiovascular reserve, but they may be prolonged and/or not well tolerated in elderly patients or those with poorly compensated myocardial function. For example, thiopental decreases myocardial contractility and dilates capacitance vessels, thereby reducing venous return to the heart. The healthy normovolemic patient may compensate for these changes by an increase in heart rate to maintain stroke volume and blood pressure. The patient with myocardial disease or hypovolemia may not be capable of appropriate compensation. Serious ischemic impairment of the myocardium may occur in patients with coronary artery disease.

Respiratory depression also may occur after the administration of barbiturates by IV bolus. Respiration may be further compromised by barbiturate-induced laryngospasm, as it is with most anesthetics.

There is some tendency of the ultra–short-acting barbiturates to precipitate at biological pH once they are injected, especially if the injection solution is not given slowly enough to allow the drug to be diluted by the venous blood. If inadvertent intraarterial injection occurs and drug precipitates are formed, arterial thrombosis, vasospasm, local ischemia, and possibly tissue sloughing may occur. Methohexital precipitation is less common, since it is a more potent barbiturate and can be provided in a more dilute solution. Barbiturate solutions must not be coadministered with acidic solutions, such as those containing meperidine, morphine, or ephedrine.

Most of the adverse reactions associated with the use of the intravenous barbiturates are predictable and therefore can be controlled or avoided. Some reactions, such as hypersensitivity, are entirely unpredictable. Particularly patients with asthma, urticaria, or angioedema may acquire allergic hypersensitivity to the barbiturates. Acute intermittent porphyria is an absolute contraindication to the use of barbiturates.

Benzodiazepines

Midazolam (*Versed*), diazepam (*Valium*), and lorazepam (*Ativan*) are benzodiazepine derivatives that are useful in anesthesia. Midazolam is the most popular of these agents for the induction of anesthesia. Its popularity is related to its aqueous solubility and to its short duration of action, which permits a prompt return of psychomotor competence. Unlike midazolam, lorazepam and diazepam are not water soluble and must be formulated in propylene glycol; the latter is irritating to the vasculature on parenteral administration.

Benzodiazepines are useful as orally administered premedications. They are also used intravenously in doses that produce conscious sedation rather than hypnosis. Sedated patients tolerate unpleasant procedures (e.g., wound repair, bronchoscopy, angiography) while maintaining cardiorespiratory function and the ability to respond to tactile stimulation or verbal commands.

Midazolam has a shorter half-life ($t_{1/2\beta} = 1.3$–2.2 hours) than either diazepam ($t_{1/2\beta} = 30$ hours) or lorazepam and is not converted in the liver to active metabolites, as is diazepam. Thus, use of midazolam results in a more rapid return to psychomotor competence. Doses may need to be lowered by at least 30% in older patients and in those premedicated with opioids or other sedative drugs.

Pharmacological Actions

The benzodiazepines, when given by slow IV infusion to induce anesthesia, have minimal influences on the cardiovascular and respiratory systems. Thus, they may be logical substitutes for barbiturates in poor-risk patients who cannot tolerate cardiovascular depression. In other respects, they appear pharmacologically similar to the barbiturates. IV administration causes unconsciousness without analgesia; skeletal muscle relaxation is inadequate for intubation or short surgical procedures. Consequently, when these characteristics of anesthetic management are desired, benzodiazepines must be coadministered with appropriate analgesic drugs and neuromuscular blocking agents.

The popularity of the benzodiazepines as an anesthetic supplement in cardiac surgery is related to their amnesic potential. They can ensure unawareness during the initial period, when the anesthetics are being diluted in the fluid of the bypass circuit. Lorazepam is often chosen for this purpose because it is longer acting and more potent than either midazolam or diazepam. Benzodiazepine administration may cause amnesia even when used in doses that do not produce unconsciousness. Antegrade amnesia may occur with the doses that are used to relieve preoperative anxiety.

Benzodiazepine Antagonist

Flumazenil (*Romazicon*) is a benzodiazepine antagonist that specifically reverses the respiratory depression and hypnosis produced by the benzodiazepine receptor agonists. Its block of the amnesic effect of the agonists is less reliable. Flumazenil is particularly useful when an overdose of benzodiazepines has occurred. It is also employed when a benzodiazepine has been used to produce conscious sedation and rapid recovery of psychomotor competency is desirable. To avoid resedation, flumazenil may require administration by intravenous infusion.

Etomidate

The pharmacological properties of etomidate (*Amidate*) are similar to those of the barbiturates, although its use may provide a greater margin of safety because of its limited effects on the cardiovascular and respiratory systems. Since it has a relatively short elimination half-life ($t_{1/2\beta} = 2.9$ hours), in addition to its use as an induc-

tion agent, etomidate has been used as a supplement to maintain anesthesia in some critically ill patients. Etomidate is rapidly hydrolyzed in the liver.

Pharmacological Actions

A primary advantage of etomidate is its ability to preserve cardiovascular and respiratory stability; both cardiac output and diastolic pressure are well maintained. Use of etomidate may offer some advantage to the patient with compromised myocardial oxygen or blood supply or both, since it produces mild coronary vasodilation. Thus, coronary vascular resistance decreases with no change in perfusion pressure. Preservation of diastolic perfusion pressure may be particularly important when myocardial blood supply cannot be increased by autoregulation.

Adverse Effects

Etomidate may cause pain on injection and may produce myoclonic muscle movements in approximately 40% of patients during its use as an induction anesthetic. In addition, etomidate can suppress the adrenocortical response to stress, an effect that may last up to 10 hours.

Propofol

Propofol (*Diprivan*) is rapidly acting, has a short recovery time, and possesses antiemetic properties. A rapid onset of anesthesia (50 seconds) is achieved, and if no other drug is administered, recovery will take place in 4 to 8 minutes. The recovery is attributed to redistribution of the drug and rapid metabolism to glucuronide and sulfate conjugates by the liver and extrahepatic tissues, such as intestine and kidney.

Rapid recovery and its antiemetic properties make propofol anesthesia very popular as an induction agent for outpatient anesthesia. Propofol can also be used to supplement inhalational anesthesia in longer procedures. Both continuous infusion of propofol for conscious sedation and with opioids for the maintenance of anesthesia for cardiac surgery are acceptable techniques.

Pharmacological Actions

Propofol is primarily a hypnotic drug with substantial cardiorespiratory depressant actions and with no ability to produce neuromuscular blockade. While propofol lacks analgesic properties, its use permits lower doses of opioids. Likewise, less propofol is required for adequate hypnosis when it is administered with opioids. Thus, it is said that propofol and opioids interact synergistically.

Adverse Effects

The dose of propofol should be reduced in older patients; however, it does have a relatively linear dose-response characteristic, and patients generally can be safely titrated. The pain on injection, especially when small veins are used, can be considerably reduced if lidocaine 20 mg is administered first.

Anesthesia induction with propofol causes a significant reduction in blood pressure that is proportional to the severity of cardiovascular disease or the volume status of the patient, or both. However, even in healthy patients a significant reduction in systolic and mean arterial blood pressure occurs. The reduction in pressure appears to be associated with vasodilation and myocardial depression. Although propofol decreases systemic vascular resistance, reflex tachycardia is not observed. This is in contrast to the actions of thiopental. The heart rate stabilization produced by propofol relative to other agents is likely the result of either resetting or inhibiting the baroreflex, thus reducing the tachycardic response to hypotension.

Since propofol does not depress the hemodynamic response to laryngoscopy and intubation, its use may permit wide swings in blood pressure at the time of induction of anesthesia. Propofol should be used with utmost caution in patients with cardiac disease.

Ketamine

Ketamine is a cyclohexanone derivative whose pharmacological actions are quite different from those of the other IV anesthetics. The state of unconsciousness it produces is trancelike (i.e., eyes may remain open until deep anesthesia is obtained) and cataleptic; it has frequently been characterized as dissociative (i.e., the patient may appear awake and reactive but does not respond to sensory stimuli). The term *dissociative anesthesia* is used to describe these qualities of profound analgesia, amnesia, and superficial level of sleep.

Pharmacological Actions

Slow IV administration of ketamine does not cause gradual loss of airway reflexes, apnea, or general muscular relaxation. The onset of the ketamine-induced "anesthetic state" is accompanied by a gradual, mild increase in muscle tone (which greatly resembles catatonia), continued maintenance of pharyngeal and laryngeal reflexes, and opening of the eyes (usually accompanied by nystagmus). Although reflexes may be maintained, the airway still must be protected, since ketamine sensitizes laryngeal and pharyngeal muscles to mucous or foreign substances, and laryngospasm may occur.

Ketamine also can be contrasted to other intravenous drugs in its ability to cause cardiovascular stimulation rather than depression. The observed increases in heart rate and blood pressure appear to be mediated through stimulation of the sympathetic nervous system. In a healthy, normovolemic, unpremedicated patient, the initial induction dose of ketamine maintains or stimulates cardiovascular function. In contrast, patients with

poor cardiac reserve, compromised autonomic control, or hypovolemia may undergo a precipitous fall in blood pressure after induction of anesthesia with ketamine. If selection of the patient and preoperative preparation are carefully done, however, ketamine may be an excellent drug for the induction of anesthesia in individuals who cannot tolerate compromise of their cardiovascular system.

The analgesia induced by ketamine also is a property that separates it from other IV anesthetic drugs. Analgesia is obtained without a deep level of anesthesia. When subdissociative doses of ketamine are given either IV or intramuscularly (IM), they provide adequate analgesia for postoperative pain relief as well as analgesia for brief operations on the skin, such as debridement of third-degree burns. Because it can be regarded as a nearly complete anesthetic (hypnosis and analgesia), does not require anesthesia equipment, and is relatively protective of hemodynamics, ketamine also can be very useful outside of normal operating room conditions, such as may be found during painful radiographic procedures.

A most important advantage of ketamine over other anesthetic agents is its potential for administration by the IM route. This is particularly useful in anesthetizing children, since anesthesia can be induced relatively quickly in a child who resists an inhalation induction or the insertion of an IV line. Ketamine has a limited but useful role as an IM induction agent and in pediatrics.

Adverse Effects

The most serious disadvantage to the use of ketamine is its propensity to evoke excitatory and hallucinatory phenomena as the patient emerges from anesthesia. Patients in the recovery period may be agitated, scream and cry, hallucinate, or experience vivid dreams. These episodes may be controlled to some extent by maintaining a quiet reassuring atmosphere in which the patient can awaken or if necessary by administering tranquilizing doses of diazepam.

Other reported side effects include vomiting, salivation, lacrimation, shivering, skin rash, and an interaction with thyroid preparations that may lead to hypertension and tachycardia. Ketamine also may raise intracranial pressure and elevate pulmonary vascular resistance, especially in children with trauma or congenital heart disease. Increases in intraocular pressure also may occur, and vigilance is required if ketamine is used in ocular surgery.

Intravenous Anesthetic Techniques Managed with Opioids

Opioid analgesics have always been important for the control of pain in the preoperative and postoperative periods. They are also used to supplement anesthesia when other anesthetic drugs do not adequately control pain reactions. Recently, the more potent and rapidly acting phenylpiperidine opioids have been used as induction agents or as the primary drug for the maintenance of anesthesia (opioid anesthesia), particularly when hemodynamic stability is essential. The high doses required to produce unconsciousness do not depress the myocardium, nor do they cause a significant reduction in blood pressure. Doses must be at least 10 times those used for the control of pain in ambulatory patients; thus, the anesthetic approach is often referred to as high-dose opioid. The opioids most commonly used are the highly potent, short-acting phenylpiperidine compounds (see Chapter 26), such as fentanyl (*Sublimaze*), sufentanil citrate (*Sufenta*), alfentanil (*Alfenta*) and remifentanil (*Ultiva*). Compared to fentanyl and sufentanil, alfentanil has a shorter duration of action because of pharmacokinetic characteristics that favor its sequestration in plasma (i.e., high protein binding and relatively low lipid solubility).

Remifentanil, recently approved for use in the United States and Europe, is the first truly ultra–short-acting opioid. Remifentanil's unique ester linkage allows it to be rapidly degraded to an inactive carboxylic acid metabolite by nonspecific esterases found in tissue and red blood cells. Since it is not a good substrate for plasma pseudocholinesterase, deficiency of the enzyme does not influence its duration of action. Also, hepatic and renal insufficiencies do not influence remifentanil's pharmacokinetics, so it is useful when liver or kidney failure is a factor. Because of its rapid clearance following infusion, remifentanil has gained popularity as an agent for maintenance of anesthesia when an IV technique is practical.

Although opioid anesthesia is particularly useful in patients with compromised myocardial function, the opioids depress respiration by inhibiting the responsiveness of the medullary respiratory center to PCO_2 and alter the rhythm of breathing. Consequently, it is necessary to assist ventilation intraoperatively. Since respiratory depression may extend into the postoperative period as a result of drug accumulation in the tissues, the use of opioids whose clearances are slow, remain most appropriate for patients who are expected to require postoperative ventilatory care.

Less potent opioids have fallen into disfavor because of the prominence of the untoward effects they produce when given in high doses. Meperidine hydrochloride (*Demerol*) causes tachycardia, while morphine produces hypotension and bronchoconstriction as a consequence of its histamine-releasing action.

Opioid-induced muscle rigidity is a frequent complication of this form of anesthesia. It is most common with phenylpiperidine drugs and occurs even after low doses of fentanyl, such as those used in certain diagnostic or minor surgical procedures where a pain-free but communicative patient is required (i.e., neuroleptanalgesia; conscious sedation). Rigidity affects the chest wall and abdomen and thus significantly interferes with breathing. The problem may result from an opioid-induced stimulation of spinal reflexes or interference with basal ganglia integration; the rigidity can be controlled through the use of neuromuscular blocking agents (e.g., pancuronium) and ventilatory support.

One of the most serious drawbacks of opioid anesthesia is the possibility of inadequate anesthetic depth. Signs of inadequate anesthesia include sweating, pupillary dilation, wrinkling of the forehead, and opening of the eyes. Most important, however, awareness or incomplete amnesia may occur. Consequently, additional doses of the opioids are appropriate when signs of light anesthesia manifest. Furthermore, many clinicians supplement the high-dose opioid technique with inhalational anesthetics or hypnotics, such as benzodiazepines (midazolam for shorter cases; the longer-acting drug lorazepam for cases longer than 4 hours) or more recently, propofol. Unfortunately, the use of many of these supplemental drugs may result in some loss of cardiovascular stability.

α_2-Adrenoceptor Agonists

α_2-Adrenoceptor agonists have received attention for their ability to produce sedation and analgesia. Their sedative properties may be related to action on α_2-receptors in the locus ceruleus, and analgesia likely occurs via α_2-receptors in the spinal cord and locus ceruleus. Agents used when sedation is desirable include oral clonidine (*Catapres*) and IV dexmedetomidine (*Precedex*), which has recently been approved in the United States for sedation in intensive care units. A solution of clonidine (*Duraclon*) is also available to provide or as a supplement for epidural analgesia. Hypnosis sufficient for surgical anesthesia is not adequate when the α_2-adrenoceptor agonists are used alone, and cardiovascular side effects, including bradycardia and hypotension, limit the doses that can be used. As adjunctive drugs they significantly reduce the dose requirement for opioids and anesthetics during surgery.

INHALATIONAL ANESTHETICS

The inhalational anesthetics can be divided into two classes based on their physical properties. N_2O and cyclopropane are gases at room temperature and are supplied in gas tanks that are regulated by the anesthesia machine. The others are liquids that are volatile following the application of low heat, which is supplied by a vaporizer attached to the anesthesia machine. The halogenated hydrocarbons are among the most potent volatile anesthetics.

Pharmacokinetic Characteristics

The use of inhalational anesthetics is generally reserved for maintenance of anesthesia. The development of an anesthetic concentration in the brain occurs more slowly with inhalational anesthetics than with IV drugs. Once an anesthetic level has been achieved, however, it is easily adjusted by controlling the rate or concentration of gas delivery from the anesthesia machine. The rate of recovery from a lengthy procedure in which inhalational agents are used is reasonably rapid, since inhalational anesthetics are eliminated by the lungs and do not depend on a slow rate of metabolism for their tissue clearance. Thus, inhalational drugs meet the requirement for a relatively prompt return of the patient's psychomotor competence.

Pharmacokinetic factors that influence the distribution of gases control the establishment of anesthetic concentrations in tissue. Thus, factors influencing gas distribution in tissues are important to the anesthesiologist, who must control anesthetic delivery and adjust for physiological influences and/or pathological conditions that can alter the accumulation of the gas. Unlike most drugs whose equilibration with tissues involves concentration gradients, partial pressure gradients control the equilibration of gases between various tissue compartments.

Development of the Partial Pressure of a Gas in Solution

Henry's law explains the behavior of gases in solutions and can be extended to body tissues. In many ways, inhalation anesthetic agents appear to be inert gases that interact with tissues and liquids physically rather than chemically. Therefore, laws governing the physical association of gases and liquids are of paramount importance to an understanding of the pharmacokinetics of these drugs. Henry's law describes the regulation of a gas concentration in a liquid when the association of these two phases is through physical interaction alone. The law states that at equilibrium, the concentration of gas physically dissolved in a liquid is directly proportional to the partial pressure (or tension) of the agent and its affinity for the molecules of the liquids (or its solubility in the liquid).

For a clear understanding of Henry's law, it is important to consider each of its component parts.

Partial Pressure of Gas Molecules in a Liquid

Inherent in Henry's law is the concept that when a liquid is exposed to a gas, a partial pressure equilibrium will be achieved between the gas and liquid phases. Thus, molecules of the gas that are physically dissolved in the liquid will exert tension that is equal to the partial pressure of the gas above the liquid. It is not necessary that a defined gas space, such as a bubble, exist before pressure can be generated. Individual molecules of gas become surrounded and separated by liquid or tissue molecules. Furthermore, since they are inert and do not combine chemically with the solvent, the gas molecules remain independent and therefore are free to undergo random molecular motion and exert pressure equal to that in the gas phase.

Practically speaking, this concept explains the basis for the establishment of partial pressure equilibrium of anesthetic gas between the lung alveoli and the arterial blood. Gas molecules will move across the alveolar membrane until those in the blood, through random molecular motion, exert pressure equal to their counterparts in the lung. Similar gas tension equilibria also will be established between the blood and other tissues. For example, gas molecules in the blood will diffuse down a tension gradient into the brain until equal random molecular motion (equal pressure) occurs in both tissues.

Affinity of Gas Molecules for Solvent Molecules

A primary force opposing random molecular motion is the affinity of gas molecules for the tissue in question (a second factor in Henry's law that expresses the degree of solubility of that agent in the tissue). If a particular gas has a strong affinity for the molecules of a solvent, its random molecular motion will be impeded by a great number of collisions with the solvent molecules. Therefore, it will require a greater volume of an agent of high affinity (or greater solubility) to enter a tissue to generate the same partial pressure as does an agent of low affinity (or lower solubility).

Concentration of Anesthetic Gas in a Tissue

The anesthesiologist can control brain concentration of gas only by modifying the partial pressure of the agent that is delivered to the alveoli. The gas then diffuses across the alveolus to the blood and ultimately into the CNS. The final concentration of gas in the tissue is a function of the partial pressure and the affinity for the tissue (i.e., Henry's law).

A Concept of Anesthetic Dose Based on Partial Pressure–Minimum Alveolar Concentration

Since the anesthesiologist has control over the partial pressure of anesthetic delivered to the lung, it can be manipulated to control the anesthetic gas concentration in the brain, hence the level of unconsciousness. For this reason, anesthetic dose is usually expressed in terms of the alveolar tension required at equilibrium to produce a defined depth of anesthesia. The dose is determined experimentally as the partial pressure needed to eliminate movement in 50% of patients challenged with a standardized skin incision. The tension required is defined as the minimum alveolar concentration (MAC) and is usually expressed as the percentage of inhaled gases that is represented by anesthetic gas at 1 atm.

Various anesthetic agents require widely different partial pressures to produce the same depth of anesthesia (Table 25.2). Methoxyflurane, for example, with a MAC of 0.16%, is the most potent agent listed in the table. Only 0.16% of the molecules of inspired gas need be methoxyflurane. N_2O is the least potent agent, with a MAC that exceeds 100%. Thus, a level of unconsciousness needed to eliminate movement is seldom achieved with N_2O.

Clinical Application and Interpretation of MAC

MAC is a valuable index for clinical anesthesia, but it is seldom employed without taking other factors into consideration. For example, inhibiting movement in only 50% of patients is not acceptable. Consequently, if an inhalational agent were being used alone—that is, without the administration of other anesthetics or analgesic drugs—the anesthesiologist would employ a multiple of its MAC value to ensure immobility. MAC is frequently multiplied by a factor of 1.3 to achieve nearly 100% clinical efficacy. On the other hand, useful clinical results may be achieved with doses of anesthetics below MAC levels. For example, mild analgesia and amnesia often occur with doses of inhalational agents that are near 0.5 MAC. In this state, it may even be possible to communicate with patients intraoperatively, while their recall is limited.

Anesthetics are infrequently used without the administration of other drugs. Many of these drug combinations can interact to alter MAC requirements. For example, inhalational anesthetics used in combination appear to have an additive effect on the level of unconsciousness. Therefore, when a combination of inhalational agents is used (e.g., N_2O with halothane), MAC values for the individual agents can be reduced appropriately. In this regard, an acceptable anesthetic maintenance tension for N_2O and halothane in the inspired air may be 40% and 0.5%, respectively.

The MAC requirement also is reduced by the coadministration of other CNS depressants, such as barbiturates or opioid analgesics. CNS stimulants, such as amphetamine, may elevate the partial pressure needed for anesthesia.

Factors Affecting the Rate of Development of Anesthetic Concentration in the Lung

Gases diffuse from areas of high partial pressure to areas of low partial pressure; thus, the tension of anesthetic in the alveoli provides the driving force to establish brain tension. In fact, the tension of anesthetic in all body tissue will tend to rise toward the lung tension as equilibrium is approached. Consequently, factors that control or modify the rate of accumulation of anesthetic in the lung (e.g., rate of gas delivery, uptake of gas from the lung into the pulmonary circulation) will simultaneously influence the rate at which tension equilibria in other body compartments is established.

Graphs of the alveolar tension plotted against time are used in this chapter to illustrate the changes in lung partial pressure as anesthetic is inhaled. Only a fraction of total lung gases are exchanged during one breathing cycle. Therefore, the volume of gases already in the lung dilutes the first breath of anesthetic (breathing cycle 1 in Fig. 25.3). In subsequent breathing cycles, the alveolar tension will continue to rise toward the inspired level along an exponentially declining curve. The net change of anesthetic tension becomes smaller with each breathing cycle, and the curve of alveolar tension will approach the inspired level more slowly.

The alveolar tension–time curve always declines in an exponential manner, but the position of the curve can be greatly affected by the rate of delivery of anesthetic gases and the rate of their uptake into the pulmonary circulation. For this reason, it is important to consider factors that modify or regulate delivery and uptake.

Effect of the Alveolar–Arterial Tension Gradient on Alveolar Tension of Anesthetic Gas

Tissues, including the brain, that have a high blood flow per unit mass (Fig. 25.1) equilibrate with the alveolar tension of anesthetic gases first. Tissues with lower blood flow require a longer time and continue to accumulate anesthetic gas during the maintenance phase of

TABLE 25.2	Minimum Alveolar Concentration in Oxygen[a]
Nitrous oxide	>100.00[b]
Desflurane	6.00
Sevoflurane	2.05
Enflurane	1.68
Isoflurane	1.15
Halothane	0.75
Methoxyflurane	0.16

[a]Expressed as the percent of lung gases that are anesthetic gas at 1 atm.
[b]MAC value greater than 100 indicates that hyperbaric conditions are required to produce anesthesia.
Adapted with permission from Eger EI II (ed.). Anesthetic Uptake and Action. Baltimore: Williams & Wilkins, 1974: 5; Eger EI. Isoflurane: A review. Anesthesiology 1981;55:559.

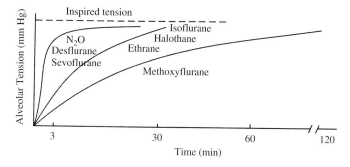

FIGURE 25.3

The rate of rise in alveolar tension of several anesthetic agents.

anesthesia, that is, after patients become unconscious. As body tissues become saturated with anesthetic molecules, blood returning to the lung will have increasingly high anesthetic tension, and the alveolar–arterial tension gradient will be reduced. Since the gradient controls the rate of diffusion across the alveolar capillary membrane, uptake is also reduced and the rate of rise of the alveolar tension of anesthetic is accelerated.

Effect of Solubility of Various Agents

The inhalational anesthetics have distinctly different solubility (affinity) characteristics in blood as well as in other tissues. These solubility differences are usually expressed as coefficients and indicate the number of volumes of a particular agent distributed in one phase, as compared with another, when the partial pressure is at equilibrium (Table 25.3). For example, isoflurane has a blood-to-gas partition coefficient (often referred to as the Ostwald solubility coefficient) of approximately 1.4. Thus, when the partial pressure has reached equilibrium, blood will contain 1.4 times as much isoflurane as an equal volume of alveolar air. The volume of the various anesthetics required to saturate blood is similar to that needed to saturate other body tissues (Table 25.3); that is, the blood–tissue partition coefficient is usually not more than 4 (that of adipose tissue is higher).

The solubility of anesthetic agents is a major factor for the rate of induction of anesthesia, or the time required to establish a level of unconsciousness adequate for surgery. Agents with limited plasma solubility and a low rate of uptake (e.g., N_2O, cyclopropane, sevoflurane, and desflurane) will equilibrate rapidly with tissues. For an agent that is highly soluble in plasma (e.g., methoxyflurane), the rate of rise of alveolar tension to the inspired level and the equilibration of the gas with brain will be delayed by a higher initial uptake into plasma from the alveoli. This phenomenon is often counterintuitive to students. However, with gases, partial pressure is the controlling factor for equilibration between tissues, and even though uptake is high, partial

pressure in the tissues and lung rises slowly, as large quantities of a highly soluble gas must be accumulated to establish the desired tension (Henry's law).

To illustrate the effect of solubility on the rate of induction of anesthesia, we can consider a situation in which individual agents are delivered to patients at their equivalent MAC values. Under these conditions, regardless of the agent being employed, a similar level of anesthesia will be achieved. In contrast, induction rates, illustrated as the time required for the alveolar tension to rise to the inspired level (Fig. 25.3), can be seen to be quite different. A patient receiving a MAC of N_2O, desflurane, or sevoflurane will be unconscious within 3 minutes. However, halothane, enflurane, and isoflurane, which have significant blood and tissue solubilities, will require at least 30 minutes before surgical anesthesia is established. Methoxyflurane, a highly soluble agent, requires several hours and may be clinically impractical if administered in this way.

Effect of Pulmonary Perfusion

The rate of pulmonary perfusion (in healthy individuals, essentially equivalent to the cardiac output) also affects the rate of induction of anesthesia. Since more blood will pass through the pulmonary capillary bed when the cardiac output is high, it follows that a greater total transfer of any anesthetic agent across the alveolus will

TABLE 25.3 **Partition Coefficients of Some Anesthetic Gases at 37° C**

Anesthetic Gas	Blood/Gas	Tissue/Blood
Cyclopropane	0.41	1.16 muscle
		0.76 brain
Desflurane	0.42	2.00 muscle
		1.30 brain
Nitrous oxide	0.47	1.15 muscle
		1.06 brain
Sevoflurane	0.69	3.10 muscle
		1.70 brain
Isoflurane	1.40	4.00 muscle
		2.60 brain
Enflurane	1.80	1.70 muscle
		1.45 brain
Halothane	2.30	3.40 muscle
		3.50 brain (white)
		2.30 brain (gray)
		2.60 liver
Diethyl ether	12.10	1.14 brain
		0.98 muscle
Methoxyflurane	12.00	2.30 brain (white)
		1.70 brain (gray)
		1.30 muscle

Adapted from Eger EI II (ed.). Anesthetic Uptake and Action. Baltimore: Williams & Wilkins, 1974:82.

occur in these conditions. Also, tissues normally receiving a smaller proportion of the total cardiac output receive a greater amount when cardiac output is high and will accumulate a larger proportion of the anesthetic crossing the alveolar membrane. Ultimately, greater uptake will slow the rate of rise of the alveolar tension–time curve, and anesthetic induction with an individual agent may be slower when the cardiac output and perfusion of the lung are high. In low cardiac output states, the reverse is true. The rate of uptake will be lower, and the alveolar tension will rise toward the inspired tension more quickly. To minimize the effect of cardiac output on the rate of induction of anesthesia, agents of lower solubility would be preferred clinically.

Effect of the Rate of Ventilation and Inspired Gas Concentration

Frequently it is desirable to overcome the slow rate of rise of alveolar tension associated with such factors as the high blood solubility of some anesthetics and increased pulmonary blood flow. Since both of these factors retard tension development by increasing the uptake of anesthetic, the most effective way to alleviate the problem is to accelerate the input of gas to the alveoli. A useful technique to increase the input of anesthetic to the lung is to elevate the minute alveolar ventilation. This maneuver, which causes a greater quantity of fresh anesthetic gas to be delivered to the patient per unit of time, is most effective with highly soluble agents (Fig. 25.4).

Increasing the inspired tension of an anesthetic gas above the maintenance tension (i.e., near the MAC value) is also an effective means of quickly establishing effective alveolar tension. This maneuver, frequently referred to as overpressure, parallels the concept of loading dose. As the desired depth of anesthesia or level of alveolar tension is achieved, the delivered tension of anesthetic must be returned to the maintenance (MAC) level to avoid overdosing the patient.

Other Factors Affecting the Alveolar Tension of Anesthetic Agents

Special factors influence the rate of rise of the alveolar tension to the inspired level when anesthetics are delivered in high concentration. These factors particularly significant when N_2O is used, since it is often required in concentrations exceeding 25% in the inspired air.

Concentration Effect

When anesthetics are delivered in high concentration, the alveolar tension will rise rapidly. Thus, if 75% N_2O is being delivered in the inspired air, the 75% tension in blood will be established more quickly than if 40% N_2O were being inhaled and a 40% N_2O tension were desired in blood. This phenomenon is illustrated in

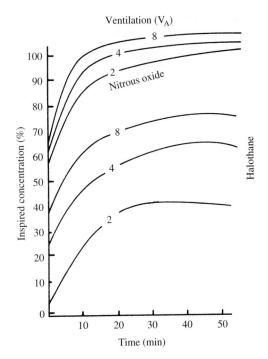

FIGURE 25.4

The alveolar rate of rise toward the inspired concentration (F_A/F_1) is accelerated by an increase in alveolar ventilation from 2 to 4 and from 4 to 8 liters per minute (constant cardiac output). The increase is greatest with the more soluble agent, halothane, and smaller with the least soluble anesthetic, nitrous oxide. (Reprinted with permission from Eger EI II [ed.]. Anesthetic Uptake and Action. Baltimore: Williams & Wilkins, 1974.)

Figure 25.5. An explanation is that when high inspired tensions of anesthetics are used, particularly if they are highly soluble, a large uptake from the alveoli will occur. Consequently, the lung volume may tend to shrink, causing negative pressure. However, the shrinkage is opposed by the pulling in of fresh gases from nonrespiratory conducting airway passages between inspirations, thus effectively increasing the total ventilation. Since greater uptake will occur with 75% N_2O than with 40%, the effect will be greater at higher inspired anesthetic tensions.

Second Gas Effect

The alveolar tension of other anesthetic gases also rises more rapidly (second gas effect) when an anesthetic such as N_2O is present in high concentration. These gases are also subject to the increased inflow (pulling in of fresh gases) as N_2O is taken up into the blood.

Diffusion Hypoxia

Diffusion hypoxia may be encountered at the end of an anesthetic administration with N_2O. The mechanism underlying diffusion hypoxia is essentially the reverse of the concentration effect; that is, when anesthetic administration is stopped, large volumes of N_2O move from the blood into the alveolus, diluting oxygen and expanding lung expiratory volume. To avoid diffusion hypoxia, the anesthesiologist may employ 100% oxygen rather than room air after discontinuing administration of the anesthetic gas mixture.

Halogenated Hydrocarbon Anesthetics

Sevoflurane, desflurane, enflurane, isoflurane, halothane, and methoxyflurane are considered to be quite potent halogenated hydrocarbon anesthetics, since they produce surgical levels of anesthesia at low inspired partial pressures. None of the halogenated hydrocarbons, however, possess all of the pharmacological properties that are considered desirable for an anesthetic agent, so they are often given with other anesthetics and adjunctive drugs to provide effective and safe anesthetic management. The use of these drug combinations is referred to as balanced anesthesia.

Balanced Anesthesia with Inhalational Anesthetic Agents

An anesthetic plan based on the concept of balanced anesthesia may proceed as follows. First, since anesthetic partial pressure for an inhalational agent in the brain is not attained rapidly, patients are usually anesthetized with an IV agent. A bolus of an IV anesthetic provides unconsciousness long enough to establish the anesthetic brain tension of most of the inhalational drugs. Second, a supplemental analgesic (i.e., an opioid or the inhalational gas N_2O) is required because halogenated hydrocarbons exhibit varying and often inadequate degrees of analgesia, so patients may respond to strongly noxious surgical manipulations with movement and reflex cardiovascular changes. Third, since the neuromuscular

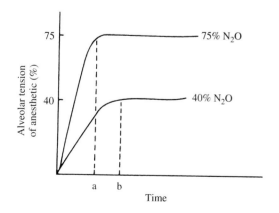

FIGURE 25.5
The effect of two concentrations of N_2O on the alveolar tension of anesthetic with time.

blockade provided by the halogenated hydrocarbons is incomplete, neuromuscular blocking agents, such as succinylcholine or the curariform drugs, must be used to provide paralysis adequate for surgical access. Fourth, the anesthetic plan is also designed to minimize any undesirable cardiovascular and respiratory responses to these drugs. This includes using drug combinations that minimize the dose of the halogenated hydrocarbon. For example, N_2O 25 to 40%, which by itself produces minimal cardiovascular depression, is frequently used with about half of the MAC of a particular halogenated hydrocarbon; this tends to preserve cardiovascular stability. Since MACs are additive, unconsciousness is adequate when a combination of inhalational agents is used.

Halothane

Halothane (*Fluothane*) depresses respiratory function, leading to decreased tidal volume and an increased rate of ventilation. Since the increased rate does not adequately compensate for the decrease in tidal volume, minute ventilation will be reduced; plasma $PaCO_2$ rises, and hypoxic drive is depressed. With surgical anesthesia, spontaneous ventilation is inadequate, and the patient's ventilation must be controlled.

Halothane administration can result in a marked reduction in arterial blood pressure that is due primarily to direct myocardial depression, which reduces cardiac output. The fall in pressure is not opposed by reflex sympathetic activation, however, since halothane also blunts baroreceptor and carotid reflexes. Systemic vascular resistance is unchanged, although blood flow to various tissues is redistributed. Halothane also sensitizes the heart to the arrhythmogenic effect of catecholamines. Thus, maintenance of the patient's blood pressure with epinephrine must be done cautiously.

It is clinically significant that *cerebral* blood flow increases as a result of a direct relaxant action of halothane on cerebral vasculature. Intracranial pressure may rise to a level at which it can become dangerous in patients with intracranial pathology. Although the *coronary* arteries are dilated, coronary blood flow decreases because of the overall reduction in systemic blood pressure. Thus, the balance between myocardial perfusion and oxygen demand (which is reduced with halothane) should be taken into account for patients with cardiac disease.

Similar disturbances in intracranial pressure and coronary blood flow occur with most of the halogenated hydrocarbons. In addition, renal blood flow, filtration, and urine output decrease with the use of halothane. These changes also occur with other inhalational agents that reduce arterial blood pressure.

Halothane and all other halogenated hydrocarbons cause some relaxation of skeletal muscle. The relaxation is not adequate when muscle paralysis is a requirement of the operative procedure, but halothane's action will potentiate the effect of neuromuscular blocking drugs, reducing their dose requirement.

Although recovery from anesthesia does not rely on metabolic factors, halothane and many of the halogenated hydrocarbons undergo some biotransformation. Halothane is oxidized in the liver to trifluoroacetic acid, Br⁻, and Cl⁻. In the absence of oxygen, reductive intermediates of halothane metabolism may form and damage liver tissue. These intermediates have been implicated in a controversial syndrome of halothane hepatitis. This rare syndrome (1:35,000 anesthetics) is histologically indistinguishable from viral hepatitis. The likelihood of liver dysfunction increases with repeated administrations of halothane, and antibodies to hepatocytes are obtained from patients who develop liver dysfunction following halothane. It has been suggested that liver necrosis may be a hypersensitivity reaction, perhaps initiated by the reactive intermediates formed during halothane metabolism. It seems prudent to limit the use of halothane in patients with liver dysfunction that resulted from a previous exposure to the anesthetic.

Methoxyflurane

Methoxyflurane (*Penthrane*) is the most potent inhalational agent available, but its high solubility in tissues limits its use as an induction anesthetic. Its pharmacological properties are similar to those of halothane with some notable exceptions. For example, since methoxyflurane does not depress cardiovascular reflexes, its direct myocardial depressant effect is partially offset by reflex tachycardia, so arterial blood pressure is better maintained. Also, the oxidative metabolism of methoxyflurane results in the production of oxalic acid and fluoride concentrations that approach the threshold of causing renal tubular dysfunction. Concern for nephrotoxicity has greatly restricted the use of methoxyflurane.

Enflurane

Enflurane (*Ethrane*) depresses myocardial contractility and lowers systemic vascular resistance. In contrast to halothane, it does not block sympathetic reflexes, and therefore, its administration results in tachycardia. However, the increased heart rate is not sufficient to oppose enflurane's other cardiovascular actions, so cardiac output and blood pressure fall. In addition, enflurane sensitizes the myocardium to catecholamine-induced arrhythmias, although to a lesser extent than with halothane. Enflurane depresses respiration through mechanisms similar to halothane's and requires that the patient's ventilation be assisted.

Neuromuscular transmission is depressed by enflurane, resulting in some skeletal muscle paralysis. Although muscle relaxation is inadequate for many surgical procedures, the anesthetic enhances the action of neuromuscular blocking agents, thereby lowering the dose of the paralytic agent needed and minimizing side effects.

Deep anesthesia with enflurane is associated with the appearance of seizurelike electroencephalographic (EEG) changes. Occasionally frank tonic–clonic seizures are observed. Consequently, other inhalational agents are usually given to patients with preexisting seizure disorders.

Another concern associated with the use of enflurane is its biotransformation, which leads to increased plasma fluoride. Following lengthy procedures in healthy patients, fluoride may reach levels that result in a mild reduction in renal concentrating ability. Thus, enflurane should be used cautiously in patients with clinically significant renal disease.

Isoflurane

Isoflurane (*Forane*) is a structural isomer of enflurane and produces similar pharmacological properties: some analgesia, some neuromuscular blockade, and depressed respiration. In contrast, however, isoflurane is considered a particularly safe anesthetic in patients with ischemic heart disease, since cardiac output is maintained, the coronary arteries are dilated, and the myocardium does not appear to be sensitized to the effects of catecholamines. Also, blood pressure falls as a result of vasodilation, which preserves tissue blood flow. Isoflurane causes transient and mild tachycardia by direct sympathetic stimulation; this is particularly important in the management of patients with myocardial ischemia.

Unlike enflurane, isoflurane does not produce a seizurelike EEG pattern. Furthermore, the metabolic transformation of isoflurane is only one-tenth that of enflurane, so fluoride production is quite low. Among the halogenated hydrocarbons, isoflurane is one of the most popular, since it preserves cardiovascular stability and causes a low incidence of untoward effects.

Desflurane

Desflurane (*Suprane*) shares most of the pharmacological properties of isoflurane. Desflurane has low tissue and blood solubility compared with other halogenated hydrocarbons, and its anesthetic partial pressure is thus established more rapidly. Recovery is similarly prompt when the patient is switched to room air or oxygen. Desflurane's popularity for outpatient procedures stems from its rapid onset and prompt elimination from the body by exhalation. A disadvantage is that desflurane irritates the respiratory tract; thus, it is not preferred for induction of anesthesia using an inhalational technique. However, desflurane may be used to maintain anesthesia after induction with an alternative IV or inhalational agent, preserving the advantage of rapid recovery.

Desflurane, like other halogenated hydrocarbon anesthetics, causes a decrease in blood pressure. The reduced pressure occurs primarily as a consequence of decreased vascular resistance, and since cardiac output is well maintained, tissue perfusion is preserved.

Desflurane stimulates the sympathetic nervous system and causes abrupt transient tachycardia during induction or as the concentration of the agent is raised to meet the patient's changing needs.

Desflurane causes an increase in the rate of ventilation, a decrease in tidal volume, and a decrease in minute volume as inspired concentrations only slightly exceed 1 MAC. Thus should anesthesiologists require desflurane to be administered near or above MAC levels, patients are likely to have marked reductions in PCO_2.

Sevoflurane

Sevoflurane (*Ultane*) is the most recently introduced inhalation anesthetic. It has low tissue and blood solubility, which allows for rapid induction and emergence and makes it useful for outpatient and ambulatory procedures. It has the advantage of not being pungent, a characteristic that permits a smooth inhalation induction, and is particularly useful in pediatric anesthesia.

Hypotension is produced by sevoflurane as systemic vasodilation occurs and cardiac output decreases. Since it does not directly produce tachycardia, it is a useful alternative to consider in patients with myocardial ischemia. However, a concern for reflex-induced tachycardia remains.

Sevoflurane undergoes hepatic biotransformation (about 3% of the inhaled dose), and it is somewhat degraded by conventional CO_2 absorbents. The degradation product from the absorbent has been reported to be nephrotoxic, although the report is controversial and not substantiated by more recent studies. Sevoflurane's actions on skeletal muscle and on vascular regulation within the CNS are similar to those described for the other halogenated hydrocarbon anesthetics.

Nonhalogenated Inhalational Anesthetics

In contemporary surgical settings, the only useful nonhalogenated inhalational anesthetic is N_2O. Earlier agents, ether and cyclopropane, have fallen out of favor, since they present a serious safety hazard due to their flammability and explosiveness. They remain interesting from a historical point of view, since they were among the first developed.

Nitrous Oxide: An Inhalational Gas

N_2O (commonly called laughing gas) produces its anesthetic effect without decreasing blood pressure or cardiac output. Although it directly depresses the myocardium, cardiac depression is offset by an N_2O–mediated sympathetic stimulation. Likewise, respiration is maintained. Tidal volume falls, but minute ventilation is supported by a centrally mediated increase in respiratory rate. However, since the respiratory depressant effect of N_2O are synergistic with drugs such as the opioids and benzodiazepines, N_2O should not be considered benign.

Deep levels of anesthesia are unattainable, even when using the highest practical concentrations of N_2O (N_2O 60–80% with oxygen 40–20%). Although unconsciousness occurs at these inspired levels, patients exhibit signs of CNS excitation, such as physical struggling and vomiting. If the airway is unprotected, vomiting may lead to aspiration pneumonitis, since the protective reflexes of the airway are depressed.

On the other hand, lower inspired concentrations (25–40%) of N_2O produce CNS depression without excitatory phenomena and are more safely used clinically. CNS properties of low inspired tension of N_2O include periods of waxing and waning consciousness, amnesia, and extraordinarily effective analgesia. N_2O 25% produces the gas's maximum analgesic effect. With this concentration, responses to painful surgical manipulations are blocked as effectively as they would be with a therapeutic dose of morphine. Such low inspired concentrations of N_2O are used in dentistry and occasionally for selected painful surgical procedures (i.e., to relieve the pain of labor). Since the tissue solubility of N_2O is low, the CNS effects are rapid in onset, and recovery is prompt when the patient is returned to room air or oxygen.

The most common use of N_2O is in combination with the more potent volatile anesthetics. It decreases the dosage requirement for the other anesthetics, thus lowering their cardiovascular and respiratory toxicities. For example, an appropriate anesthetic maintenance tension for N_2O and halothane would be N_2O 40% and halothane 0.5%. With this combination in a healthy patient, anesthesia is adequate for major surgery, and the dose-dependent cardiac effects of halothane are reduced.

MECHANISM OF ANESTHETIC ACTION

Among the earliest proposals to explain the mechanism of action of anesthetics is the concept that they interact physically rather than chemically with lipophilic membrane components to cause neuronal failure. However, this concept proposes that all anesthetics interact in a common way (the unitary theory of anesthesia), and it is being challenged by more recent work demonstrating that specific anesthetics exhibit selective and distinct interactions with neuronal processes and that those interactions are not easily explained by a common physical association with membrane components. Proposals for the production of anesthesia are described next.

Anesthesia from Physical Interactions with Lipophilic Membrane Components

The idea that a physical interaction is important stems from experimental observations made in the late nineteenth and early twentieth centuries, when it was recognized that noble gases such as xenon, which do not chemically interact with tissues, produce unconsciousness. Also, anesthesia produced at ambient atmospheric pressure can be attenuated by physically raising the pressure to 100 atm, a phenomenon known as pressure reversal. Finally, a clear correlation exists between anesthetic potency and the physical parameter lipid solubility, suggesting that anesthesia may be produced when anesthetics physically dissolve into the cell membrane's lipid biophase (Meyer Overton rule). Such a correlation is shown in Fig. 25.6, where anesthetic potency is expressed as MAC and lipid solubility is estimated as the oil–gas partition.

Membrane conformational changes are observed on exposure to anesthetics, further supporting the importance of physical interactions that lead to perturbation of membrane macromolecules. For example, exposure of membranes to clinically relevant concentrations of anesthetics causes membranes to expand beyond a critical volume (critical volume hypothesis) associated with normal cellular function. Additionally, membrane structure becomes disorganized, so that the insertion of anesthetic molecules into the lipid membrane causes an increase in the mobility of the fatty acid chains in the phospholipid bilayer (membrane fluidization theory) or prevent the interconversion of membrane lipids from a gel to a liquid form, a process that is assumed necessary for normal neuronal function (lateral phase separation hypothesis).

Anesthesia from Selective Interactions of Anesthetics with Cellular Components

While current observations do not rule out that anesthetics may require a hydrophobic environment near the site of their action, they do suggest that various agents may also have distinct interactions with tissues. For example, enantiomers of newer agents have selective and unique actions, even though they have identical physical properties; for example, stereoisomers of isoflurane are differentially potent but have identical oil–gas partition coefficients.

Contemporary research has shown that at clinically relevant concentrations, various anesthetics interact specifically with different components of the GABA$_A$-receptor–chloride ionophore and enhance chloride conductance, some directly and others by enhancing the action of GABA. Inhalational agents directly activate the chloride channel as well as facilitate the action of GABA, while barbiturates, propofol, benzodiazepines, and etomidate primarily enhance the action of GABA by interacting with specific receptor sites (Fig. 25.7). Also, anesthetics enhance other processes known to inhibit neuronal function, such as the glycine receptor–gated chloride channel. A smaller number of anesthetics, including ketamine, N_2O, and xenon, produce neuronal inhibition by antagonizing excitatory neuronal transmission mediated via the N-methyl-D-aspartic acid (NMDA) receptor. In addition, some inhalational drugs activate K^+ channels and so contribute to hyperpolarization and reduced neuronal excitability; they also inhibit the function of the protein complex involved in neurotransmitter release.

Clearly much must be explained of the complex changes in the CNS that eventually produce unconsciousness. Although physical interactions of anesthetics with hydrophobic membrane components may lead to conformational changes that alter neuronal function, specific interactions at critical receptors and ion channels are also likely to contribute to anesthesia. Thus, structurally and pharmacologically diverse anesthetic drugs produce unconsciousness through qualitatively different mechanisms and through actions occurring at anatomically distinct sites in the nervous system.

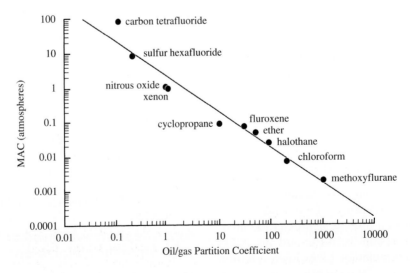

FIGURE 25.6
A comparison of the minimum alveolar concentration (MAC) with the oil–gas partition coefficient of several inhalational anesthetic agents.

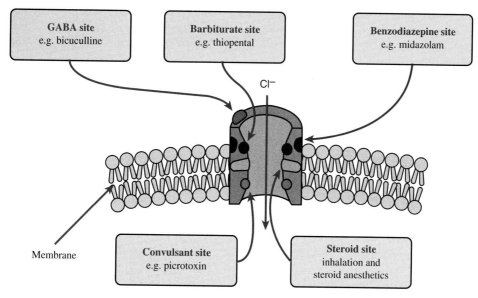

FIGURE 25.7
The GABA_A-receptor–chloride ionophore sites of drug action.

Study QUESTIONS

1. A patient whose anesthesia is being managed only with isoflurane (Forane) delivered at an inspired concentration near the MAC occasionally moves and exhibits facial grimacing, apparently in response to surgical manipulation of the bowel. These responses are
(A) Natural consequences of physical manipulations that induce noxious sensory input to the CNS
(B) An indication that neuromuscular blocking agents should be administered without delay
(C) Not likely to be blocked by coadministering an analgesic drug such as morphine
(D) Signs suggesting that the patient should be given twice the MAC of isoflurane
(E) Not avoidable because the bowel is unusually sensitive to physical manipulation.

2. A hypotensive patient suspected of having internal bleeding is given a dose lower than the usual amount of an intravenous anesthetic. An acceptable level of anesthesia occurs. How is it possible to achieve anesthesia in this patient with a dose of anesthetic that may be inadequate in a normotensive patient with adequate blood volume?
(A) Enzymatic activity of hepatic enzymes is compromised when blood pressure is low.
(B) More anesthetic appears in the brain and redistribution of the intravenous drug to tissues with reduced blood flow is compromised when hemorrhagic shock occurs.
(C) The diffusion of lipid-soluble drugs through the blood-brain barrier is enhanced.
(D) Tissues with a characteristically high blood flow per unit mass receive less blood and less anesthetic when blood volume is low.
(E) Anesthetics bind more readily to tissue receptors when hypotension and poor oxygenation occur.

3. With which hypothetical anesthetic would you expect anesthetic partial pressure to be achieved relatively quickly?
(A) An agent that is highly soluble in blood and other body tissues
(B) An agent with a low MAC (in range less than 1% in the inspired air)
(C) An agent with a high Ostwald solubility coefficient
(D) An agent whose rate of rise of partial pressure in the lung is influenced minimally by uptake into the blood.
(E) An agent supplied as a gas rather than one supplied as a volatile liquid

4. Remifentanil (Ultiva) has recently gained popularity as a high-dose opioid anesthesia because
(A) It induces anesthesia in patients faster than any other drug

(B) Phenylpiperidine-type opioids releases histamine from mast cells

(C) It is metabolized by nonspecific esterases in red blood cells and other tissues

(D) It has a long duration of action following intravenous infusion

(E) It does not produce chest wall rigidity

5. Patients with coronary artery disease are particularly challenging for anesthesia, since alterations in vascular responsiveness and myocardial function may put them at risk. In this respect, which statement correctly describes the cardiovascular action of an agent or agents that should be taken into account when planning anesthesia for such patients?

(A) All halogenated hydrocarbon inhalational anesthetics sensitize the myocardium to catecholamine-induced cardiac arrhythmias.

(B) Halogenated hydrocarbon inhalational agents reduce cardiac output equally well.

(C) Sevoflurane (Ultane) directly stimulates sympathetic function.

(D) Reflex sympathetic stimulation is a major component of halothane's (Fluothane) cardiovascular profile.

(E) Several halogenated hydrocarbons produce vascular relaxation to reduce blood pressure.

6. The mechanism of anesthesia remains an active area of research. Which statement best describes significant developments in this area of scientific investigation?

(A) Anesthetics are physically attracted to the aqueous phase of neuronal membranes.

(B) Anesthesia is associated with interactions of the agents with a single unique site on the $GABA_A$ receptor.

(C) Anesthesia ultimately occurs as Cl^- moves out of neuronal cells, an action that makes the cells less excitable.

(D) Although some exceptions occur, a correlation between anesthetic potency and their oil–water partition coefficient suggested a unitary hypothesis for the production of anesthesia.

(E) Enantiomers of inhalational agents provide support for the Meyer Overton rule.

ANSWERS

1. **A.** Unless supplemented with strong analgesic drugs such as opioids, most general anesthetics allow reflex reactions to painful stimuli, which may include movement and autonomic reflex changes. Even though these reflex changes occur, if adequately anesthetized, patients will not experience the noxious stimulus. To give this patient a neuromuscular blocking agent without initially evaluating the adequacy of anesthesia would be a mistake. A lawsuit is almost certain, should the patient be inadequately anesthetized and complain postoperatively of being aware but paralyzed. If it is determined that the patient is receiving adequate anesthesia (i.e., evaluate the delivery of gas, and check other reflexes such as corneal), the use of a neuromuscular blocking drug may be acceptable if movement is interfering with the procedure. Morphine may be a reasonable supplement to anesthetic management to inhibit reflex reactions to noxious stimuli. Raising the inspired concentration of isoflurane may further blunt reflex reactions to noxious stimuli. However, it may not be a wise choice, since multiples of MAC may cause greater instability of physiological functions (i.e. cardiovascular function). Use a balanced anesthetic approach with adjunctive agents. The gut is quite responsive to noxious insult, but the reflex responses are still inhibited with proper analgesics, so muscular movement is avoidable.

2. **B.** Perfusion of the brain is preserved when hemorrhage occurs. Thus, a greater proportion of the initial dose of anesthetic should appear in the brain, and a dose smaller than what is needed for a normovolemic patient is all that is required. Also, since flow to tissues associated with redistribution of the drug and termination of anesthesia is compromised, anesthesia should be deep and extended. Titrate this patient to a safe level of effect. While poor perfusion of the liver may reduce the exposure of drugs to metabolic enzymes, most intravenous anesthetics rely very little on hepatic clearance to terminate the anesthetic effect when a single bolus is administered. Furthermore, the question implies a direct influence of blood pressure on the efficiency of hepatic enzymes, and there is no evidence to support such a contention. Option C is not true. The opposite of option D is true. No evidence exists that binding of anesthetics is altered by these conditions.

3. **D.** Anesthetics with low blood and tissue solubility require minimal uptake from the lung, as alveolar partial pressure equilibrates with tissue. Remember, alveolar partial pressure is the driving force to establish tension gradients throughout the body. Thus, when uptake is low and alveolar tension rises quickly, blood and brain (which receives a high blood flow) equilibrate with gaseous agents quickly, and anesthesia is induced relatively rapidly. A gas that is highly soluble in tissues requires a greater accumulation from the lung before partial pressure equilibria are attained, since with greater uptake the rate of rise of the alveolar tension to the inspired level is slower. Although a relationship exists between MAC and blood solubility with respect to anesthetic concentration in the tissues, the association suggested by choice B is opposite the expectation. Consider the implications of the Meyer Overton rule. An agent with a high Ostwald solubil-

ity coefficient is one of the more soluble agents in tissue, so the explanation of option A applies. Option E has no apparent bearing on the rate of rise of the alveolar partial pressure in brain, alveolus, or any other tissue.

4. **C.** Remifentanil has become popular as a component drug in the technique of total intravenous anesthesia as a consequence of this feature. It is distribution of blood to the brain, not specific pharmacological properties, that primarily controls the rate of induction of anesthesia with IV agents. Phenylpiperidines as a class of opioids are less likely to produce histamine release. Moreover, histamine release may complicate anesthetic management (e.g. bronchoconstriction and hypotension), so if it were an action of remifentanil it would be a negative feature. Remifentanil's duration of action is short because it is rapidly metabolized. Chest wall rigidity is associated with high doses of phenylpiperidine opioids in particular, and no evidence suggests that remifentanil would be any less likely to cause such an effect.

5. **E.** Reduced peripheral vascular resistance occurs with most halogenated hydrocarbons, and reflex tachycardia may be a concern. Halothane may be the clearest exception, since there appears to be a balance between relaxation and constrictor influences in various vascular beds with this agent so that total peripheral resistance changes very little. Halothane is the agent of concern when sensitization of the myocardium to catecholamine-induced arrhythmias may be important, such as during incidences of hypercapnia. Sevoflurane does not directly influence sympathetic function. However, reflex tachycardia can occur. Reflex sympathetic stimulation is blocked by halothane. In fact, this may be an advantage of the drug in physiologically risky patients when swings in blood pressure are likely to be frequent.

6. **D.** Although few contend that a unitary hypothesis will explain anesthesia, the Meyer Overton rule was among the first explanations provided by the scientific community. The correlation remains significant, as it suggests that sites of action for various anesthetics may reside near (or the agent must pass though) hydrophobic tissue components. Also, physical disruption of membrane function may yet be found to play a role for at least some agents. Option A is the reverse of the true interaction. Several sites on the GABA receptor complex may be involved. Cl⁻ moves inward to cause cells to become less excitable. Enantiomers, which have nearly identical physical properties but different potencies, challenge the Meyer Overton rule.

SUPPLEMENTAL READING
Eger EI. Uptake and distribution. In Miller RD (ed.). Anesthesia (5th ed.). Philadelphia: Churchill Livingstone, 2000.

Evers AS and Crowder CM. General Anesthetics. In JG Hardman and LE Limbird (eds.). Goodman and Gilman's the Pharmacological Basis of Therapeutics (10th ed.). New York: McGraw Hill, 2001.

Koblin DD. Mechanism of Action. In Miller RD (ed.). Anesthesia (5th ed.). Philadelphia: Churchill Livingstone, 2000.

Reves JG, Glass PSA, and Lubarsky DA. Non-barbiturate Intravenous Anesthetics. In Miller RD (ed.). Anesthesia (5th ed.). Philadelphia: Churchill Livingstone, 2000.

CASE Study   Bradycardia and β-Blockers

A 77-year-old man is admitted to the hospital for a coronary artery bypass. He has been treated with a β-blocker (Tenormin 100 mg per day), which he took every morning. He is induced with propofol 1 mg/kg, fentanyl 5 μg/kg and vecuronium 8 mg for muscle relaxation. After 3 minutes a decreasing heart rate becomes a worry for the anesthesiologist. The heart rate continues to fall until it reaches 38 BPM. At this point the patient's blood pressure is 80/60 and the anesthesiologist gives atropine 0.4 mg and ephedrine 10 mg. This treatment results in a stable patient. What effects were most likely produced by the anesthesia procedure? Could this have been avoided?

ANSWER: This feature of bradycardia is typical of patients who take β-blockers, which should be continued so they result ultimately in better anesthetic management. The drugs given could have been modified (i.e., etomidate instead of propofol, which does not raise or may cause a slower heart rate). The potent opioids in the fentanyl family all cause vagal transmitted bradycardia. The muscle relaxant vecuronium (norcuron) has no effect on heart rate and could have been replaced by pancuronium, which has a vagolytic effect and will counter bradycardia in the usual induction bolus doses.

26 | Opioid and Nonopioid Analgesics

Sandra P. Welch and Billy R. Martin

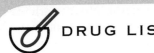

DRUG LIST

THE NATURE OF PAIN

Pain has been described by the International Association for the Study of Pain as an "unpleasant sensory and emotional experience associated with actual or potential tissue damage, or described in terms of such damage." Although pain is a reaction of the body to harmful stimuli and is therefore a protective early warning system, the sensation of pain in postoperative patients, cancer patients, and other chronic pain patients has little positive effect. The stress response to pain can alter the healing process by evoking massive sympathetic discharge that in turn alters blood flow, tissue perfusion, and immune function. In addition, in certain painful conditions the patient has reduced respiratory function. Hence, the term *pain,* derived from the Latin *poena* for punishment, reflects the deleterious effects that can be inflicted upon the body. Since millions of Americans suffer from some form of pain each year, resulting in the expenditure of billions of dollars for various treatment modalities, pain and its underlying causes are a major public health problem.

The nature of pain is highly subjective. Pain has both sensory (somatic) and psychological (affective) components. One person may feel pain in response to noxious stimuli, while another person may disregard the stimuli. The affective (psychological) aspects of pain play a critical role in pain perception. A patient under external stress or other significant psychological problems often cannot handle the additional stress of pain. Anxiety exacerbates the perception of pain. Pain in turn exacerbates anxiety, decreases the comfort of the patient, and results in disturbances in sleeping, eating, and locomotion, creating a cycle of related medical problems. The drugs described in this chapter are used to interrupt such a cycle. *The nonopioid analgesics act to decrease the generation of the mediators of pain at the site of tissue damage, although several of the drugs also have some effects within the central nervous system (CNS). The opioid analgesics are unique in that they not only block the incoming nociceptive signals to the brain but also act at higher brain centers, controlling the affective components of the pain.* The drugs described in this chapter do not constitute the entirety of the armamentarium of therapies for pain relief. Many patients respond best to a combination of therapies. Therapeutic modalities in addition to the drugs described in this chapter include antidepressants, adrenergic agonists (e.g., clonidine), transcutaneous electrical nerve stimulation, physical therapy, massage therapy, acupuncture, meditation, and behavior modification. The treatment regimen is generally based upon the type of pain.

Cells in the substantia gelatinosa (lamina II contains highest levels of opioid binding) of the dorsal horn of the spinal cord respond to incoming nociceptive stimuli and regulate, or gate, the transmission of nociceptive impulses to other pathways within the CNS via the spinothalamic tract. Opioids also can elicit analgesic effects by stimulating the release of norepinephrine from a descending noradrenergic pathway, which extends from the locus ceruleus to the dorsal horn of the spinal cord.

In general, pain can be described as either acute or chronic. *Acute pain,* which does not outlast the initiating painful stimulus, has three generally encountered origins. The most common type of acute pain is of superficial origin from wounds, chemical irritants, and thermal stimuli, such as burns. Acute pain of deep somatic origin usually arises from injection of chemical irritants or from ischemia, such as with myocardial infarction. Acute pain of visceral origin is most often associated with inflammation. *Chronic pain,* by contrast, outlasts the initiating stimulus, which in many cases is of unknown origin. Chronic pain is often associated with diseases such as cancer and arthritis. Treatment of chronic pain presents a challenge to the physician in that the underlying cause is often not readily apparent. Neuropathic pain, a type of chronic pain, responds poorly to opioids. Some causes of neuropathic pain include diabetic neuropathies, shingles (herpes zoster), ischemia following stroke, and phantom limb pain. Neuropathic pain responds well in many cases to therapies other than the use of opioids and nonsteroidal antiinflammatory drugs (NSAIDs).

Pain thus has several etiologies, and transmission of nociceptive inputs from diverse nociceptors occurs via different fiber bundles. Aδ-fibers are the site for rapid transmission of sharp, painful stimuli. Such fibers are myelinated and enter the dorsal horn, from which point the ascending systems of the spinothalamic tract are activated. C-fibers, which also enter the dorsal horn and synapse on spinothalamic tract neurons, are responsible for the slower transmission (fibers are not myelinated) of nociceptive impulses, resulting in a dull, aching sensation. The Aδ-fibers and C-fibers are activated by mechanoreceptors. Aδ-fibers and C-fibers are also activated by other types of nociceptors, such as those responding to heat and chemicals. Current studies on the plasticity of pain-modulating systems that contribute to the chronic long-lasting nature of pain have been reviewed in detail by Julius and Basbaum (2001) and include alterations in numerous intracellular signaling systems beyond the scope of this chapter. However, what is becoming apparent is that novel analgesics may be designed in the future to target the modulation of intracellular targets in pain processing and neuronal plasticity.

The loss of quality of life for a patient with either acute or chronic pain has led to extensive development of various drugs to treat pain. Such drugs eliminate pain by either decreasing the underlying cause of the pain (as do the nonopioid analgesics described later) or decreasing the transmission of nociceptive impulses and pain perception (as do the opioids). Both nonopioid and opioid drugs are described in detail in this chapter.

NONOPIOID ANALGESICS

In general, pain is first treated with the nonopioid analgesics. These drugs are useful for treatment of pain, fever, and inflammation and for reduction of platelet aggregation. Although the NSAIDs are less effective than the opioids in providing pain relief, they do not produce tolerance and physical dependence, as do the opioids. *The mechanism of action of traditional NSAIDs involves blockade of the production of prostaglandins by inhibition of the enzyme cyclooxygenase (COX) at the site of injury in the periphery, thus decreasing the formation of mediators of pain in the peripheral nervous system.* COX was originally thought to be a single enzyme that was responsible for the conversion of arachidonic acid to a variety of prostanoids. The prostanoids produced by COX activity include those that are involved in inflammatory responses in tissue leading to detrimental effects and those that are critical to the maintenance of the gastric mucosal lining and certain renal functions. Thus, inhibition of COX by the NSAIDs may be accompanied by ulceration of the stomach lining and renal damage. In 1991 it was discovered that the COX system consisted of two enzymes, COX-1 and COX-2. COX-1 appears to remain constitutively active and is the site of action of the NSAIDs used prior to the early 1990s. However, COX-2 is not constitutively active and is induced by traumatic tissue injury, although some evidence of low levels of COX-2 constitutive activity exists for certain regions, such as the brain. The discovery of COX-2 led to the hypothesis that the major therapeutic benefit of the COX inhibitors was due to the block of inducible COX-2, while the major problematic side effects of the NSAIDs were due to COX-1 inhibition. Although this hypothesis has undergone several iterations, it does appear that the COX-2 inhibitors can at the very least be described as gut sparing. The original NSAIDs appear to be nonselective for COX-1 and COX-2. Development of novel COX-2 inhibitors has led to the discovery of a class of NSAIDs largely devoid of the gastrointestinal (GI) and renal problems associated with the older NSAIDs. Although the COX-2 drugs are no more efficacious than the older nonselective COX inhibitors, the decrease in side effect profile has provided a new mechanism of long-term antiinflammatory treatment.

Aspirin is one of the most important NSAIDs because it decreases pain at predominantly peripheral sites with little cortical interaction and thus has few CNS effects. The prototypical COX-2 inhibitors are celecoxib (*Celebrex*) and its chemical cousin, rofecoxib (*Vioxx*). In addition to a role in inflammatory processes,

COX-2 seems to play a role in colon cancer and Alzheimer's disease, providing potential additional uses for COX-2-selective drugs.

Salicylates
Chemistry

Aspirin is a weak organic acid and is one of the oldest known drugs for the relief of fever and pain. Aspirin remains the standard to which most NSAIDs are compared for efficacy.

Pharmacokinetics

Aspirin itself is an acid with a pKa of 3.5 and is relatively insoluble in water, while its sodium or calcium salts have enhanced solubility. Aspirin and related salicylates are rapidly absorbed upon oral administration, with most absorption occurring in the small intestine. The pH of the stomach, a secondary site of drug absorption, along with the gastric emptying time of the stomach, determines the rate of absorption of the drug. Thus, food, which alters gastric emptying time and possibly the pH of the stomach, will alter absorption of the drug. Buffering of the drug decreases irritation in the stomach, increases drug solubility, and therefore may increase the rapidity of absorption. Enteric-coated aspirin tablets have a variable rate of dissolution depending on the preparation but are somewhat useful for prevention of stomach ulceration and gastric distress. Absorption of aspirin from rectal suppositories is slower and more variable than from oral administration. The peak plasma concentration of aspirin occurs 1 to 2 hours following oral administration. Aspirin is immediately hydrolyzed by various esterases in the stomach and in the liver to acetate and salicylic acid. Salicylic acid is glucuronidated, conjugated to glycine to form salicyluric acid (the major metabolic pathway), oxidized to gentisic acid (a minor metabolic pathway), or remains free as salicylic acid, which is secreted in the proximal tubule of the kidney. Diflunisal (*Dolobid*) differs from other salicylates in that it is not metabolized to salicylic acid but is rapidly glucuronidated. The conjugated metabolites of salicylates are inactive.

Salicylic acid is highly plasma protein bound, an effect that alters the pharmacokinetics of other drugs taken in combination with aspirin. Salicylates passively diffuse to all tissues, including breast milk, fetal tissues, and the CNS. They tend to accumulate, since increases in dose decrease renal clearance and prolong the half-life of the drug. Clearance at high doses (>2–4 g/day) is via zero order kinetics, and the half-life can approach 15 hours. At lower doses (600–1000 mg/day), clearance depends on the concentration of glucuronide or glycine available for conjugation and is a first-order process (half-life of approximately 3–6 hours). However, renal clearance is highly dependent on the pH of the urine; *the higher the pH of the urine, the greater the clearance of the drug.* Alkalinization of the urine is used to increase clearance of the salicylates in the case of toxicity or overdose.

Mechanism of Action and Pharmacological Effects

Aspirin and related salicylates produce their pharmacological effects predominantly by inhibiting the synthesis of prostaglandins and to a lesser extent synthesis of the thromboxanes (implicated in platelet aggregation). The prostanoids are mediators of inflammatory responses in many cell types. Aspirin is unique among NSAIDs in that it irreversibly acetylates COX-1 and COX-2, which are required for the synthesis of prostanoids from arachidonic acid. COX-2 is induced during inflammation and is therefore considered to mediate most inflammatory responses. Aspirin acetylation of COX-1 permanently inactivates the enzyme, while acetylated COX-2 is capable of producing 15-HETE. *New enzyme must be synthesized to overcome the effects of aspirin,* which in the case of platelets can take as long as 11 days. The metabolite of aspirin, salicylic acid, is a reversible inhibitor of COX. Other NSAIDs have reversible effects at different sites on COX-1 and on COX-2. In addition, aspirin interferes with kinin-induced modulation of the inflammatory response.

Clinical Uses

Aspirin and related salicylates are the primary treatment for mild to moderate pain, such as that associated with headache, joint and muscle pain, and dysmenorrhea. At higher doses aspirin is an effective analgesic in rheumatoid arthritis (see Chapter 36). The analgesic effects of salicylates are thought to be due to the inhibition of prostaglandin synthesis in the periphery and to a less well documented mechanism at cortical areas.

The salicylates are also potent antipyretic agents, with the exception of diflunisal, which is only weakly active. Aspirin acts at two distinct but related sites. It decreases prostaglandin-induced fever in response to pyrogens and induces a decrease in interleukin-1 modulation of the hypothalamic control of body temperature. Thus, the hypothalamic control of body temperature returns, vasodilation occurs, heat dissipates, and fever decreases. Other uses of aspirin include inhibition of platelet aggregation via inhibition of thromboxanes, which has been shown to decrease the incidence of blood clots, myocardial infarction, and transient ischemic attacks.

Overdose and Other Adverse Effects

The major consequence of aspirin overdose, which often occurs in children, results from actions on respira-

tory centers in the medulla. Salicylate-induced stimulation of respiration leads to hyperventilation. In addition, salicylates uncouple oxidative processes leading to increased carbon dioxide production and metabolic acidosis. The onset of acidosis, if not treated less than 1 hour after ingestion of aspirin, will lead to loss of rhythmicity of respiration and eventually loss of breathing. Treatments include alkalinization of the urine, fluid replacement, gastric lavage with activated charcoal, dialysis, and artificial ventilation.

Some patients exhibit hypersensitivity to aspirin in the form of *salicylism,* which is accompanied by ringing in the ears (tinnitus), vertigo, and bronchospasm (especially in asthmatics). The use of salicylate-containing preparations is not the only source of this drug. Those sensitive to salicylates should be aware of salicylates in a number of foods, such as curry powder, licorice, prunes, raisins, and paprika.

The use of aspirin in children and teenagers with either chickenpox or influenza is contraindicated, since there is evidence linking the use of the salicylates in such diseases to Reye's syndrome, a potentially fatal disease accompanied by liver damage and encephalopathy. The mechanism by which the use of salicylates increases the chances for development of Reye's syndrome is not known.

Other potential adverse effects of the drugs include the use of aspirin by patients who anticipate surgery or dental procedures. Such patients should be closely monitored and the salicylate stopped at least 1 week prior to surgery because of the possibility of increased clotting time and excessive bleeding. Similarly, the use of salicylates in pregnant women may increase bleeding upon delivery and prolong delivery. In addition, adverse fetal effects have been documented, such as low birth weight, fetal intracranial bleeding, and possible teratogenic effects. Due to the ulcerogenic effects of the drugs, patients with a history of ulcers or other GI disturbances should be carefully monitored for increased blood in the feces while taking salicylates.

Drug Interactions

The salicylates displace a number of drugs from plasma protein binding sites, thereby leading to potential adverse effects by these agents. Since aspirin is an over-the-counter medication, patients may fail to inform the doctor of their aspirin consumption. Anticoagulants are potentiated by aspirin by (1) displacement of the anticoagulants from plasma proteins and (2) the intrinsic anticoagulant effect of aspirin. Thus, the dosage of drugs such as coumarin and heparin should be reduced in patients taking aspirin. A similar effect is observed in patients taking oral sulfonylureas (*Orinase, DiaBeta*) for non–insulin-dependent diabetes or phenytoin (*Dilantin*) for seizures. Displacement of the sulfonylureas or phenytoin from plasma binding necessitates a decrease in dosage to prevent an acute hypoglycemic event or sedation, respectively. Aspirin enhances the effects of insulin (leading to hypoglycemia), penicillins and sulfonamides (increasing acute toxicity), and corticosteroids. Aspirin increases the hypotensive effects of the cardiac drug nitroglycerin but decreases the effectiveness of the loop diuretics. In patients taking methotrexate for cancer chemotherapy, aspirin may increase retention of the drug, and severe toxicity may result.

Conversely, certain drugs modify the effectiveness or side effects of aspirin. Phenobarbital, occasionally used for seizures, induces liver enzymes that increase the metabolism and excretion of aspirin, β-adrenoceptor–blocking drugs, such as propranolol, and decrease the antiinflammatory effects of aspirin, whereas reserpine decreases its analgesic effects. Antacids decrease the absorption of aspirin. Alcohol consumption in combination with aspirin increases the latter's ulcerogenic effects.

p-Aminophenol Derivatives

Acetaminophen (*Tylenol*) is the active metabolite of both phenacetin and acetanilide but has fewer toxic effects than either precursor. Phenacetin and acetanilide are no longer used therapeutically because they have been linked to methemoglobinemia.

Pharmacokinetics

Acetaminophen, with a pKa of 9.5, is rapidly absorbed from the GI tract following oral administration. Peak plasma concentrations are observed within 30 minutes to 2 hours. Absorption is nearly complete following oral administration but varies with suppository forms of the drug. Acetaminophen is less plasma protein bound than the salicylates, although the amount bound varies from 20 to 50%. Following the use of normal therapeutic doses of acetaminophen, metabolism and conjugation to sulfate or glucuronides occurs, and clearance of these metabolites occurs in the kidney. A minor toxic metabolite is generated by the metabolism of acetaminophen via the P450 mixed-function oxidase system. This toxic metabolite is normally conjugated to glutathione in the liver and excreted via the kidney as conjugated cysteine and mercapturic acid. However, with the depletion of glutathione in certain disease states, such as liver cirrhosis and necrosis, and following chronic use of high doses of acetaminophen, this toxic reactive metabolite can accumulate and induce liver damage.

Mechanism of Action

Acetaminophen is a weak inhibitor of peripheral COX. Its analgesic effects may arise from inhibition of prostanoid synthesis in the CNS or other centrally mediated effects yet to be elucidated. The antipyretic effects of acetaminophen are similar to those of aspirin in that it acts at the level of the hypothalamus to reduce pyrogen-initiated alterations in body temperature by inhibiting prostaglandin synthesis.

Pharmacological Effects and Clinical Uses

Acetaminophen is similar to salicylates in that it is a useful analgesic for mild to moderate pain, with equal efficacy to aspirin, and like aspirin, it is antipyretic. However, *acetaminophen exerts little if any effects on platelet aggregation and is not antiinflammatory*. Thus, it is not useful for patients with arthritis or other inflammatory diseases. It is also not useful as an antithrombotic agent in the prevention of myocardial infarction or transient ischemic attacks. Acetaminophen does not produce the gastric ulceration that can occur with aspirin and is useful in patients who are salicylate sensitive or who have a history of ulcers or other gastric ulcerations.

Adverse Effects, Contraindications, and Drug Interactions

Toxicity from overdose with acetaminophen differs in time course and mechanism from that observed with the salicylates. The onset of toxicity may not occur for several days, and the predominant damage is to the liver. The initial signs of toxicity occur within 12 to 24 hours and include nausea and vomiting. Signs of hepatotoxicity occur within 72 hours. In addition to hepatotoxic effects, renal necrosis and myocardial damage may occur. Oral *N*-acetylcysteine is used to treat acetaminophen toxicity, although many patients are hypersensitive to such treatment. In addition, gastric lavage with activated charcoal can be used immediately after ingestion of the drug to decrease acetaminophen absorption from the stomach.

Acetaminophen is contraindicated in late-stage alcoholism, since chronic alcohol consumption can induce the P450 system, leading to increased production of the toxic metabolite of acetaminophen, hence to liver necrosis. In addition, barbiturates and phenytoin induce the liver P450 system and may decrease the effectiveness of acetaminophen. Acetaminophen crosses the placenta but is nonetheless used in pregnant women with few side effects for the mother or the fetus. Although the drug has been shown to be present in breast milk, no conclusive evidence links the drug to abnormalities associated with consumption of breast milk by the newborn.

Indoles (indomethacin) and Related Compounds
Chemistry and Mechanism of Action

Indomethacin (*Indocin*) is an acetic acid derivative related functionally to sulindac (*Clinoril*), a prodrug with a long half-life, and etodolac (*Lodine*). They are metabolized in the liver and excreted as metabolites in the bile and via the kidney. They are potent inhibitors of COX and thus extremely effective antiinflammatory agents (see Chapter 36).

Clinical Uses, Adverse Effects, and Contraindications

All of these drugs produce analgesic effects, antipyresis, and antiinflammatory effects. Due to the high incidence of gastric irritation, headache, nausea, and other side effects, including hematological effects and coronary vasoconstriction, *they are not useful as an initial treatment for pain.* GI irritation and ulceration occur to a lesser extent with etodolac. Indomethacin is useful in the treatment of acute gout, osteoarthritis, ankylosing spondylitis, and acceleration of the closure of the ductus arteriosus in premature infants. The tocolytic effects of indomethacin to prevent preterm labor are the result of its effects on prostaglandin synthesis. However, the toxicity of the drug limits such application, since it increases fetal morbidity. Indomethacin is contraindicated in pregnancy, in asthmatics, and in those with gastric ulcers or other ulceration of the GI tract. Indomethacin may increase the symptoms associated with depression or other psychiatric disturbances and those associated with epilepsy and Parkinson's disease. The drug should be used with caution in such patients.

Fenamates

Meclofenamate (*Meclomen*) and mefenamic acid (*Ponstel*) exhibit potency and side effects similar to those of other nonsalicylate NSAIDs. However, both drugs produce serious side effects, have a short duration of action, and are not safe for children. Their use is limited to patients who fail to respond to other treatments. They are analgesic, antipyretic, and antiinflammatory agents indicated for mild to moderate pain, treatment of dysmenorrhea, rheumatoid arthritis, and osteoarthritis. These drugs are metabolized via glucuronidation in the liver and excreted via the kidney. Thus, fenamates require normal liver and kidney function for excretion and are contraindicated in patients with either liver or renal failure. Overdose with fenamates leads to seizures that are sometimes insensitive to traditional treatment with benzodiazepines. In cases of overdose with meclofenamate dialysis may be required to restore fluid and electrolyte balance.

Arylpropionic Acid Derivatives
Chemistry and Mechanism of Action

Ibuprofen (*Advil*), flurbiprofen (*Ansaid*), fenoprofen (*Nalfon*), ketoprofen (*Orudis*), and naproxen (*Naprosyn*) are all 2-substituted propionic acid derivatives. They block the production of prostaglandins via inhibition of COX and therefore are similar to the salicylates in that they produce analgesia, antipyresis, and antiinflammatory effects. However, they are more potent than aspirin, with a decreased incidence of side effects such as gastric irritation. Ketoprofen inhibits lipoxygenase and COX, thus decreasing the production of both leukotrienes and prostaglandins. It also decreases lysosomal release of enzymes in inflammatory diseases. *The principal differences among these drugs lie in the time to onset and duration of action.* Naproxen has a long half-life, whereas fenoprofen and ketoprofen have short half-lives. All of the drugs are extensively metabolized in the liver and require adequate kidney function for clearance of the metabolites. The drugs vary in plasma protein binding, but clearly all are bound to a relatively high degree and can interfere with the binding of other drugs that compete for plasma protein binding (as described for aspirin). The one exception is ketoprofen, which although highly bound to plasma proteins, does not appear to alter the binding of other drugs.

Clinical Uses, Adverse Effects, and Contraindications

The arylpropionic acid derivatives are useful for the treatment of rheumatoid arthritis and osteoarthritis, for reduction of mild to moderate pain and fever, and for pain associated with dysmenorrhea. Side effects of the drugs are similar to but less severe than those described for the salicylates. Those who are sensitive to salicylates also may be sensitive to and have adverse reactions when taking ibuprofen and related drugs. Acute hypersensitivity to ibuprofen has been reported in patients with lupus. The hypersensitivity reaction to sulindac can be fatal. The use of sulindac has also been linked to cases of acute pancreatitis. The use of dimethylsulfoxide (DMSO) topically in combination with sulindac has been reported to induce severe neuropathies. The concurrent use of ibuprofen with aspirin reduces the antiinflammatory effects of both drugs. Ibuprofen is contraindicated in patients with aspirin sensitivity leading to bronchiolar constriction and in patients with angioedema. As with all NSAIDs, renal and liver function should be normal for adequate clearance of the drugs.

Pyrazolone Derivatives

Phenylbutazone (*Butazolidin*) is metabolized to oxyphenbutazone (*Phlogistol*), and both compounds have all of the activities associated with the NSAIDs. Their use is accompanied by serious adverse reactions, such as anemia, nephritis, renal failure or necrosis, and liver damage. Because of their toxicity, they are prescribed only for the treatment of pain associated with gout or phlebitis or as a last resort for other painful inflammatory diseases resistant to newer and less toxic treatments. Interactions with a large number of other drugs (similar to those described for aspirin) occur, since phenylbutazone displaces several drugs from plasma protein binding sites. The drug is contraindicated in children and in the elderly with diminished renal function. The consequences of overdose occur slowly and can include liver damage, renal failure, and shock. There is no antidote for overdose. Supportive measures include ventilation, dialysis, and gastric lavage with activated charcoal, as well as the use of benzodiazepines to control convulsions.

Oxicam Derivatives

Piroxicam (*Feldene*) is the prototypical oxicam derivative, with analgesic, antipyretic, and antiinflammatory properties. Its long half-life (45 hours) favors compliance, since only one dose per day is given. Side effects are similar to those encountered with other NSAIDs: gastric disturbances, tinnitus, and headache. Piroxicam is indicated for inflammatory and rheumatoid conditions.

Acetic Acid Derivatives

Diclofenac (*Voltaren*) is a phenylacetic acid derivative that is a potent inhibitor of COX and that has analgesic, antiinflammatory, and antipyretic effects. Its use is accompanied by side effects similar to those of other NSAIDs. Indications for the drug include rheumatoid arthritis, osteoarthritis, and ophthalmic inflammation (use of an ophthalmic preparation).

Ketorolac (*Toradol*) is an NSAID with very mild antiinflammatory and antipyretic activity. It is a potent analgesic for postoperative pain. Its efficacy is equivalent to that of low doses of morphine in the control of pain. For this reason it is often combined with opioids to reduce opioid dose and related side effects while providing adequate pain relief. It is also used to replace the opioids in some patients with opioid sensitivity. The mechanism of action of ketorolac involves the inhibition of COX and decreased formation of prostaglandins. However, some evidence exists that ketorolac may stimulate the release of endogenous opioids as a part of its analgesic activity.

Tolmetin (*Tolectin*) is an antiinflammatory, analgesic, and antipyretic agent that produces the usual gastric distress and ulceration observed with NSAIDs. However, tolmetin is better tolerated than aspirin and produces less tinnitus and vertigo. Tolmetin is a substitute for indomethacin in indomethacin-sensitive patients and is unique among such drugs in that it can be used to treat juvenile arthritis.

Miscellaneous Agents

Oxaprozin (*Daypro*) has pharmacological properties that are similar to those of other propionic acid derivatives. However, it has a very long half-life (more than 40 hours) and therefore can be effective with once-a-day treatment.

Nabumetone (*Relafen*) has antiinflammatory, antipyretic, and analgesic properties. It is converted by liver enzymes to an active metabolite that is a potent COX inhibitor. Although nabumetone shares many of the adverse effects of other NSAIDs, it appears to produce a lower incidence of GI ulceration.

COX-2 Inhibitors
Chemistry

Celecoxib (*Celebrex*) and rofecoxib (*Vioxx*) are the two available COX-2 inhibitors. Both lack a carboxylic group present in most NSAIDs and therefore are able to orient into the COX-2 enzyme in a selective manner that differs from that of other NSAIDs. They have low aqueous solubility that prevents parenteral administration.

Mechanism of Action

As previously discussed, the COX-2 inhibitors have selectivity for inhibition of the COX-2 enzyme, which has low constitutive activity but is highly inducible at sites of tissue injury. In addition to the peripheral role of COX-2 in inflammation, COX-2 may play an important role in the CNS. COX-2 is expressed constitutively in some excitatory neurons in the brain and spinal cord and is induced in traumatic brain injury such as that induced by ischemia and seizures. It has been hypothesized that COX-2 may also be involved in neurodegenerative diseases, since COX-2 inhibitors have shown some positive effects in Alzheimer's disease. Thus, the mechanism of action of COX-2 inhibitors may involve brain and spinal cord sites as well as local sites of injury.

Pharmacological Effects and Clinical Uses

Celecoxib has been approved for the treatment of osteoarthritis and rheumatoid arthritis, and rofecoxib has been approved for the treatment of osteoarthritis, acute pain and primary dysmenorrhea. Celecoxib and rofecoxib do not appear to differ in efficacy for the treatment of osteoarthritis. However, neither drug has efficacy greater than that of the non-selective NSAIDs. Since the COX-2 enzyme appears to play an important role in colon cancer the COX-2 inhibitors may find future uses in the treatment or prevention of colorectal cancer.

Adverse Effects, Contraindications

The major advantage of the COX-2 inhibitors is their decreased GI effects and formation of gastric ulcerations compared with the COX nonselective agents. However, once an ulcer is present, COX-2 is induced in response, and the COX-2 enzyme is essential for wound healing. Therefore, celecoxib and rofecoxib can delay in wound healing and increase the time for ulcer repair and tissue regeneration. Patients with gastric ulcers should be switched if possible to another antiinflammatory to allow ulcers to heal.

Celecoxib is contraindicated during pregnancy, since COX-2 levels must be maintained for ovulation and onset of labor. COX-2 seems to be involved into the regulation of the renin–angiotensin system, and both celecoxib and rofecoxib use are associated with transient sodium retention.

OPIOID ANALGESICS

Chemistry

The basic structure of morphine (Fig. 26.1) can be altered in rather minor ways that drastically change the effects of the drug. Acetylation of the hydroxyl groups leads to the synthesis of heroin (diacetylmorphine),

which has a much greater ability to pass the blood-brain barrier. In the brain, however, heroin is converted to morphine and monoacetyl morphine. Some researchers attribute heroin's potent analgesic effects and rapid onset of action solely to its conversion to morphine. Others contend that heroin produces analgesic effects distinct from the conversion to morphine and thus should be considered as a therapeutically useful analgesic. Heroin is not approved for medical use in the United States, although it is used therapeutically in other nations.

Morphine is glucuronidated in the liver at the phenolic hydroxyl group (C_3). Protection of that group with a methyl group, as occurs in codeine and other codeine derivatives such as oxycodone, renders the molecule less susceptible to glucuronidation and decreases the first-pass effect in the liver. It is for this reason that codeine and its derivatives retain activity following oral

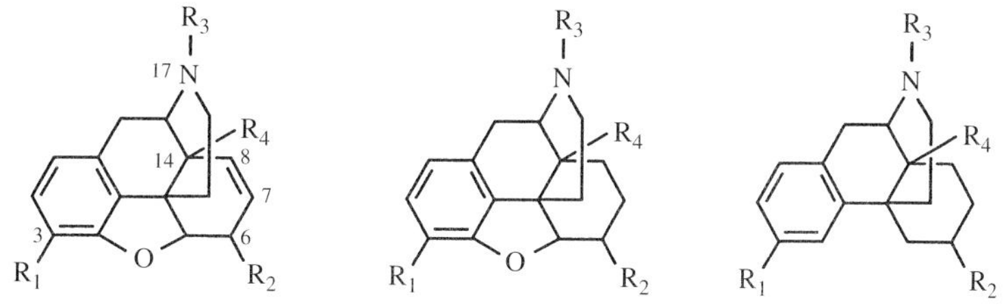

Generic name	Template	R_1	R_2	R_3	R_4
Morphine	A	—OH	—OH	—CH_3	—H
Codeine	A	—OCH_3	—OH	—CH_3	—H
Heroin	A	—$OCOCH_3$	—$OCOCH_3$	—CH_3	—H
Hydrocodone	B	—OCH_3	=O	—CH_3	—H
Oxycodone	B	—OCH_3	=O	—CH_3	—OH
Dihydrocodeine	B	—OCH_3	—OH	—CH_3	—H
Hydromorphone	B	—OH	=O	—CH_3	—H
Oxymorphone	B	—OH	=O	—CH_3	—OH
Levorphanol	C	—OH	—H	—CH_3	—H
Butorphanol	C	—OH	—H	—CH_2◇	—OH
Nalbuphine	B	—OH	—OH	—CH_2◇	—OH
Buprenorphine	B¹	—OH	—OCH_3	—CH_2◁	—OH
Naloxone	B	—OH	=O	—$CH_2CH=CH_2$	—OH
Naltrexone	B	—OH	=O	—CH_2◁	—OH
Nalmefene	B	—OH	=CH_2	—CH_2◁	—OH

FIGURE 26.1
Opioid agonists, mixed agonist–antagonists, and antagonists.

administration to a greater degree than does morphine. However, the glucuronidation of morphine at the hydroxyl moiety on C_6 leads to an active metabolite, morphine-6-glucuronide, which contributes to the activity of morphine and extends its duration of action.

Endogenous Opioids

The *endogenous opioids* are naturally occurring peptides that are the products of four known gene families. The gene responsible for the production of the *endomorphins,* a new class of endogenous opioids, has yet to be identified. The enkephalins, the first opioid peptides identified, were first discovered in the brain and were therefore given the name *enkephalin,* which means from the head. The *dynorphins* were so named because they were thought to be dynamic endorphins, having a wide range of activities in the body, a hypothesis that has proved to be accurate.

The endogenous opioids have been implicated in the modulation of most of the critical functions of the body, including hormonal fluctuations, thermoregulation, mediation of stress and anxiety, production of analgesia, and development of opioid tolerance and dependence. The endogenous opioids maintain homeostasis, amplify signals from the periphery to the brain, and serve as neuromodulators of the body's response to external stimuli. As such, the endogenous opioids are critical to the maintenance of health and a sense of well-being.

Opioid Receptors

Given the diversity of opioid effects, William R. Martin hypothesized that multiple opioid receptors existed. Recently, a number of previously hypothesized opioid receptors have been cloned (μ, δ, and κ). The σ-receptor, once thought to be an opioid receptor, is a nonopioid receptor that mediates some of the dysphoric effects of the opioids. *The cloned opioid receptors are members of the large superfamily of G protein–coupled receptors.* Subtypes of the receptors have been proposed. It has been shown that μ_1-receptors mediate the analgesic and euphoric effects of the opioids and physical dependence on them, whereas μ_2-receptors mediate the bradycardiac and respiratory depressant effects. δ-Receptors, of which at least two subtypes have been identified pharmacologically, mediate spinal analgesic effects and have been implicated in the modulation of tolerance to μ-opioids. Three κ-opioid receptors have been identified and are thought to mediate spinal analgesia, miosis, sedation, and diuresis. The existence of the ϵ-receptor is hypothetical pending cloning of the receptor.

Opioid receptors and their precursor mRNAs are distributed throughout the brain and spinal cord. High levels of opioid binding have been found in the ascending pathways for nociceptive transmission, including the dorsal horn of the spinal cord and in particular the substantia gelatinosa lamina II. Other ascending tracts with high levels of binding include the spinothalamic tracts to the subcortical regions and limbic areas of the brain responsible for the discriminative and sensory aspects of pain and the euphoric effects of the drugs. Limbic areas, including cortical sites and the amygdala, are involved in the anxiolytic effects of the drugs. Binding in the thalamus and hypothalamus is also very high. Binding in the hypothalamus is linked to the modulation of hormone release and to thermoregulation by the opioids and opioid peptides. Some descending pathways possess high levels of opioid receptors believed to be linked to the analgesic effects of the drugs. In addition, the receptor binding in medullary pathways has been linked to inhibitory neurotransmitter release in the dorsal horn.

Opioid binding at medullary sites is consistent with the respiratory depressant effects of the drugs. *Binding in the nucleus accumbens and the resultant release of dopamine by the μ- and δ-opioids is linked to the development of physical dependence.* However, the κ-opioids, which also bind extensively in the nucleus accumbens, are linked to a decrease in dopamine release, possibly explaining their lower abuse liability. The localization of different receptor subtypes within different-size fiber pathways has been established. The μ- and δ-receptors appear associated with the large-diameter fibers, while the κ-receptors appear to be located in the small to medium-size fiber bundles of the dorsal root ganglia. Such differences may explain the modulation of specific types of nociceptive stimuli by the different opioid agonists and opioid peptides.

Pharmacokinetics

Most of the opioids are well absorbed from the GI tract in addition to being absorbed following transcutaneous administration. As described previously, the first-pass effect on drugs like morphine, which have a free hydroxyl group in position 3, is glucuronidation by the liver. In the case of morphine, the conjugation to glucuronide decreases the oral bioavailability of the drug. Following absorption, the drugs distribute rapidly to all tissues, although the distribution is limited by their lipophilicity. Fentanyl (highly lipophilic) distributes to the brain rapidly but also remains in fat, which serves as a slow-releasing pool of the drug. Certain of the drugs, notably methadone and fentanyl, have long half-lives inconsistent with their duration of action. This discrepancy is due to accumulation in various tissue and plasma reservoirs and redistribution from the brain to these reservoirs. Heroin passes readily into the brain. Codeine passes into the brain more readily than morphine, which is slow in crossing the blood-brain barrier. The drugs cross readily into fetal tissues across the placenta and therefore should be used with care during pregnancy and delivery. Moreover, glucuronidation by the fetus is slow, increasing buildup of the drugs and increasing their half-life in the fetus.

The majority of their metabolites are inactive with a few notable exceptions, such as morphine-6-glucuronide, which produces an analgesic effect; normeperidine and norpropoxyphene, which produce excitatory but not analgesic effects; and 6-β-naltexol, which is less active than naltrexone as an antagonist but prolongs the action of naltrexone. Excretion of the metabolites requires adequate renal function, since excretion by routes other than the urine are of minor importance.

Cellular Mechanisms of Action

Opioid receptors are members of the G protein superfamily of receptors. Drug-induced interaction with these receptors is associated with a decrease in activation of the enzyme adenylyl cyclase and a subsequent decrease in cyclic adenosine monophosphate (cAMP) levels in the cell. Binding of opioids to their receptors produces a decrease in calcium entry to cells by decreasing the phosphorylation of the voltage operating calcium channels and allows for increased time for the channels to remain closed. In addition, activation of opioid receptors leads to potassium efflux, and the resultant hyperpolarization limits the entry of calcium to the cell by increasing the negative charge of the membrane to levels at which these calcium channels fail to activate. *The net result of the cellular decrease in calcium is a decrease in the release of dopamine, serotonin, and nociceptive peptides, such as substance P, resulting in blockage of nociceptive transmission.*

Pharmacological Effects
Analgesia

Opioid agonists interact with receptors in the brain and in the spinal cord. The initial binding of opioids in the brain causes the release of the inhibitory neurotransmitter serotonin, which in turn induces inhibition of the dorsal horn neurons. Both the brain and the spinal cord are required for the production of a maximal analgesic effect following systemic administration of opioids, although analgesia can be elicited by spinal administration only. In the spinal cord, morphine inhibits the release of most nociceptive peptides. Morphine also affects descending noradrenergic pathways. Norepinephrine release in response to opioid administration results in an analgesic effect at the spinal level.

Opioids have profound effects upon the cerebrocortical regions that control the somatosensory and discriminative aspects of pain. Thus, the *opioids suppress the perception of pain by eliminating or altering the emotional aspects of pain and inducing euphoria and sleep*

with higher doses. Patients become inattentive to the painful stimuli, less anxious, and more relaxed. Disruption of normal REM sleep occurs with opioid administration. In addition, opioids depress polysynaptic responses but can increase monosynaptic responses and lead to convulsant effects in high doses. In patients with chronic pain, the euphoric effect of opioids, mediated by the μ-receptor, is usually blunted. Some patients feel a dysphoric effect upon the administration of opioids, which is most likely mediated by the σ-receptor.

Medullary Effects

Opioids depress respiration via the μ_2-receptor at the level of the medulla and thereby increase P_{CO_2}. Opioids reduce respiration, an effect that is fatal in the case of overdose, by a dual action. *The opioids decrease both the sensitivity of the medulla to carbon dioxide concentrations and the respiratory rate.* Cardiovascular function and the response to hypoxia are not compromised. By contrast, *tolerance to the respiratory depressant effects of the opioids does not appear to occur,* while tolerance to the emetic effects of the opioids occurs upon repeated administration. The area postrema chemoreceptor trigger zone of the medulla mediates opioid-induced vomiting.

Miosis

Miosis, or the pinpoint pupillary response to the opioids, is diagnostic of the use and abuse of the opioids. No tolerance to such an effect is observed. Miosis is due to disinhibition of the Edinger-Westphal nucleus in the cortex resulting in increased pupillary constrictor tone.

Hypothalamic Effects

The opioids have pronounced effects on the release of hormones from both the pituitary and the hypothalamus. Stimulation of some of the opioid receptors in hypothalamic nuclei decrease the release of dopamine, thus increasing release of prolactin. Opioids bind in the supraoptic nuclei of the hypothalamus and increase the release of antidiuretic hormone (vasopressin).

GI Effects

Morphine and most other opioids produce some degree of constipation by increasing sphincter tone and decreasing gastric motility. Such an effect is uncomfortable for patients required to take opioids chronically. Tolerance to the constipative effects of the opioids does not generally occur. In addition, the decrease in gastric motility increases gastric emptying time and reduces absorption of other drugs. The constriction of sphincters, especially the bile duct, may result in increased pain in certain patients with biliary colic or other GI distress. Constriction of the urinary sphincter can lead to painful urine retention in some patients. The effects of opioids on the GI tract are largely mediated by the parasympathetic release of acetylcholine. All of the opioid receptors have been shown to mediate such GI effects.

Immune Function and Histamine

Opioids induce the release of histamine, which leads to the itching sensation associated with use and abuse of opioids. Bronchiolar constriction is possible. Opioids are also immunosuppressive, having effects on the T-helper and T-suppressor cells.

Antitussive Effects

The opioids block cough by a mechanism that is not yet understood. No stereoselectivity of the opioids for blockade of the cough reflex has been shown. Thus, the isomers of opioids, such as dextrorphan, are as efficacious as the L-isomers as antitussives. *This lack of stereoselectivity prompted the development of the D-isomers of opioids as antitussives since they are devoid of the dependence liability of L-isomers.* Drugs with predominantly antitussive effects are described later in this chapter. Certain of the opioids, such as propoxyphene and meperidine, are relatively devoid of antitussive effects.

Tolerance and Physical Dependence

All of the opioid agonists produce some degree of tolerance and physical dependence. The biochemical mechanisms underlying tolerance and physical dependence are unclear. It is known, however, that intracellular mechanisms of tolerance to opioids include increases in calcium levels in the cells, increased production of cAMP, decreased potassium efflux, alterations in the phosphorylation of intracellular and intranuclear proteins, and the resultant return to normal levels of release of most neurotransmitters and neuromodulators. Tolerance to the analgesic effects of opioids occurs rapidly, especially when large doses of the drugs are used at short intervals. However, tolerance to the respiratory depressant and emetic effects of the opioids occurs more slowly. The miotic and constipative effects of the opioids rarely show tolerance.

Tolerance to one opioid usually renders a patient cross-tolerant to other opioids but not to drugs of other classes. Within the opioid class of drugs, certain drugs with high intrinsic activity (e.g., fentanyl) appear to lack cross-tolerance to opioids of lower intrinsic activity (e.g., morphine), an effect thought to be related to the change in receptor number induced by the chronic opioid administration. Theoretically, a drug with high intrinsic activity would need to occupy fewer receptors to exert an effect and would be less affected by changes in receptor number, which occurs upon chronic administration of drugs with lower intrinsic activity.

The cessation of opioid drug administration leads to an observable abstinence syndrome. In the case of the opioids, signs of withdrawal include chills, fever, sweating, yawning, vomiting, diarrhea, nausea, dizziness, and hypertension. The onset of symptoms occurs 6 to 12 hours after the last drug dose (depending on the kinetics of the drug) and continues for several days, with most of the signs of withdrawal ending by 72 hours after the last dose of the drug. However, signs of withdrawal, including restlessness, anxiety, and drug craving, may be detectable for 6 months to 1 year after cessation of drug use.

In general, the effects observed upon withdrawal from a drug are opposite to those observed when the person is taking the drug, and such is the case with the opioids. The degree of dependence is generally reflected by the severity of withdrawal signs. In addition, drugs with long half-lives, such as methadone, produce a gradual and prolonged withdrawal. The use of methadone replacement for heroin is based upon the pharmacokinetics of methadone. The longer onset and duration of action and the oral bioavailability render the drug useful for the treatment of opioid addiction by decreasing the rapid highs and lows associated with fast-onset, short-duration drugs such as heroin. Drugs with a short duration of action produce a more rapid onset of withdrawal signs.

A derivative of methadone, L-α-acetyl-methadol (LAAM) has been approved for the treatment of opioid addiction. In some addicts whose degree of tolerance is not known, the patient is first given methadone to stabilize the withdrawal signs and is then switched to LAAM. LAAM has an advantage over methadone in that it has a longer duration of action. Dosing is required only three times per week in most addicts to prevent withdrawal.

Babies born to opioid-addicted women also exhibit withdrawal signs, but because of the slower metabolism of opioids in the newborn, the withdrawal signs are more protracted. The babies are often treated with the opium preparation paregoric to reduce withdrawal signs.

Other treatments for opioid addiction are described in detail in Chapter 35.

Morphine
Clinical Uses

Morphine remains the standard by which other analgesic drugs are compared. The predominant effects of morphine are at the μ-opioid receptor, although it interacts with other opioid receptors as well. Morphine is indicated for the treatment of moderate to severe and chronic pain. It is useful preoperatively for sedation, anxiolytic effects, and to reduce the dose of anesthetics. Morphine is the drug of choice for the treatment of myocardial infarction because of its bradycardiac and vasodilatory effects. In addition, morphine is the most commonly used drug for the treatment of dyspnea-associated pulmonary edema. It is thought that morphine reduces the anxiety associated with shortness of breath in these patients along with the cardiac preload and afterload.

The use of morphine via the oral route has drawbacks because of its first-pass effect; however, oral morphine has been recommended for use in cancer patients for its ease of administration. In particular, the long-acting preparations of morphine, such as *MS-Contin* and *Ora-Morph*, are described as the cornerstone of pain treatment in cancer patients, either alone or in combination with nonopioids.

Morphine is the most commonly used analgesic drug administered via the epidural route because it is potent, efficacious, and hydrophilic. The more hydrophilic the drug, the slower the onset and the longer the duration of action following epidural administration. Single-dose or continuous infusion of morphine is used to provide pain relief in thoracic and abdominal surgical patients and in cancer patients at high risk for developing side effects associated with systemic opioids. Since morphine does not produce anesthesia via the epidural route, the patient is able to move about normally; motor function is preserved. The drawback to epidural use of morphine is that certain types of pain are relatively unresponsive, such as that associated with visceral stimuli, as in pancreatitis, and neuropathic pain from nerve deafferentation. In addition, patients can develop respiratory depression and nausea from the rostral flow of the drug to medullary centers, although the effects are much less severe than those observed following the systemic administration of the drug, and can be alleviated by elevation of the head of the patient at a 30-degree angle. Patients may also itch because of histamine release.

Patient-controlled analgesia (PCA) is an alternative method of administration of morphine. The use of an indwelling catheter allows the patient to administer the drug at frequent intervals for pain relief. PCA systems allow patients the freedom to assess the need for their own analgesia and to titrate a dose tailored to their needs. Dependence is rarely observed in patients using PCA for acute pain management.

Adverse Effects and Contraindications

The opioids generally have a high level of safety when used in therapeutic dosages. However, there are several notable exceptions. Morphine and other opioids are contraindicated in patients with hypersensitivity reactions to the opioids. In addition, morphine should not be used in patients with acute bronchial asthma and should not be given as the drug of first choice in patients with pulmonary disease, because it has antitussive effects that prevent the patient from clearing any buildup of mucus in the lungs. Opioids with less antitussive effects, such as meperidine, are better for such situations.

When used via the epidural route, the site for injection must be free of infection. In addition, the use of corticosteroids by the patient should be halted for at least 2 weeks prior to the insertion of the catheter to prevent infection, since morphine increases the immunosuppressive effects of the steroids.

Opioids are contraindicated in head trauma because of the risk of a rise in intracranial pressure from vasodilation and increased cerebrospinal fluid volume. In addition, in such patients the onset of miosis following opioid administration can mask the pupillary responses used diagnostically for determination of concussion.

The clearance of morphine and its active metabolite, morphine-6-glucuronide depends on adequate renal function. The elderly are particularly susceptible to accumulation of the drugs, hence respiratory depression and sedation. Morphine, like all opioids, passes through the placenta rapidly and has been associated with prolongation of labor in pregnant women and respiratory depression in the newborn.

Morphine and other opioids exhibit intense sedative effects and increased respiratory depression when combined with other sedatives, such as alcohol or barbiturates. Increased sedation and toxicity are observed when morphine is administered in combination with the psychotropic drugs, such as chlorpromazine and monoamine oxidase inhibitors, or the anxiolytics, such as diazepam.

Respiratory depression, miosis, hypotension, and coma are signs of morphine overdose. While the IV administration of naloxone reverses the toxic effects of morphine, naloxone has a short duration of action and must be administered repeatedly at 30- to 45minute intervals until morphine is cleared from the body.

Codeine and Other Phenanthrene Derivatives

Like morphine, codeine is a naturally occurring opioid found in the poppy plant. Codeine is indicated for the treatment of mild to moderate pain and for its antitussive effects. It is widely used as an opioid antitussive because at antitussive doses it has few side effects and has excellent oral bioavailability. *Codeine is metabolized in part to morphine, which is believed to account for its analgesic effect.* It is one of the most commonly used opioids in combination with nonopioids for the relief of pain. The administration of 30 mg of codeine in combination with aspirin is equivalent in analgesic effect to the administration of 65 mg of codeine. The combination of the drugs has the advantage of reducing the amount of opioid required for pain relief and abolition of the pain via two distinct mechanisms, inhibition of prostanoid synthesis and opioid inhibition of nociceptive transmission. When given alone, orally administered codeine has about one-tenth to one-fifth the potency of morphine for the relief of pain. In addition, IV codeine has a greater tendency to release histamine and produce vasodilation and hypotension than does morphine. Thus, the use of IV codeine is rare. Codeine is rarely addictive and produces little euphoria.

Adverse effects and drug interactions with codeine are similar to those reported for morphine, although they are less intense. Overdose in children results in the same effects as overdose of morphine, such as respiratory depression, miosis, and coma; these symptoms are treated with naloxone administration.

Hydrocodone (*Hycodan*), oxycodone (*Roxicodone*), dihydrocodeine, hydromorphone (*Dilaudid*), and oxymorphone (*Numorphan*) are derivatives of codeine and morphine. All are indicated for the relief of mild to severe pain or for their antipyretic effects; they are often used in combination with nonopioid analgesics. The drugs vary in potency, but their pharmacological effects do not differ significantly from those of codeine or morphine.

Hydromorphone is eight times as potent as morphine but has less bioavailability following oral administration. Its side effects do not differ from those of morphine but are more intense. Hydromorphone is indicated for use in severe pain and in high doses for relief of pain in opioid-addicted patients.

Oxycodone is nearly 10 times as strong as codeine, with absorption equal to that of orally administered morphine. Neither hydromorphone nor oxycodone is approved for use in children, and hydromorphone is contraindicated in obstetrical analgesia and in asthmatics.

Oxymorphone is 10 times as potent as morphine, with actions similar to those of hydromorphone. Oxymorphone, however, has little antitussive activity, and as such is a useful analgesic in patients with pulmonary disease who need to retain the ability to cough.

Meperidine and Related Phenylpiperidine Derivatives
Clinical Uses and Adverse Effects

Meperidine (*Demerol*) is a phenylpiperidine derivative of morphine that was developed in the late 1930s as a potential anticholinergic agent. It has some anticholinergic side effects that lead to tachycardia, blurred vision, and dry mouth. Meperidine is approximately one-fifth as potent as morphine and is absorbed only half as well when administered orally as parenterally. It has a rapid onset and short duration of action (2 hours), that is, approximately one-fourth that of morphine.

Like morphine, meperidine has an active metabolite, normeperidine, formed by *N*-demethylation of meperidine. Normeperidine is not analgesic but is a proconvulsant and a hallucinogenic agent. For this reason, meperidine use in patients with renal or liver insufficiency is contraindicated because of the decreased clearance of the drug and its metabolite. Convulsant activity has been documented in elderly patients given meperidine and in patients using PCA who have decreased renal function.

Meperidine differs from morphine in that it has far less antitussive effect and little constipative effect. The drug is particularly useful in cancer patients and in pulmonary patients, in whom the cough reflex must remain intact. However, it does have more seizure-inducing activity than morphine. Although meperidine produces spasms of the biliary tract and colon, such spasms are of shorter duration than those produced by morphine.

Meperidine readily passes the placenta into the fetus. However, respiratory depression in the newborn has not been observed, and meperidine clearance in the newborn is rapid in that it does not rely upon conjugation to glucuronides. Meperidine, unlike morphine, has not been associated with prolongation of labor; conversely, it increases uterine contractions.

Symptoms of overdose with meperidine are qualitatively different from those of morphine in that seizures rather than sedation are common. Respiratory depression and miosis are present. While naloxone reverses overdose-associated toxicity, its use in patients who have received large, frequent doses of meperidine may precipitate seizures.

Diphenoxylate (*Lomotil*) is a meperidine derivative used as an antidiarrheal. It exhibits no morphinelike effects at low doses, but it produces mild opioid effects, such as sedation, euphoria, and dependence, at higher doses. Its salts are highly insoluble in water, which reduces recreational use. Preparations often include atropine.

Difenoxin is a metabolite of diphenoxylate with antidiarrheal effects similar to the parent drug. Loperamide (*Imodium*) is a piperidine derivative of diphenoxylate, which acts both at the level of the gut and also in the CNS to reduce GI motility. Its use as an antidiarrheal and its potency are similar to those of diphenoxylate.

Contraindications

Contraindications are similar to those of morphine. In addition, because normeperidine accumulates in renal dysfunction and meperidine accumulates in hepatic dysfunction, meperidine is contraindicated in such patients because of convulsant effects. Similarly, the use of meperidine is contraindicated in patients who have a history of seizures or who are taking medication to prevent seizures. Phenytoin administered for seizures may reduce the effectiveness of meperidine by increasing the metabolism of the drug in the liver. Meperidine is not generally used in patients with cardiac dysfunction, since its anticholinergic effects can increase both heart rate and ectopic beats.

Fentanyl, Sufentanil, and Alfentanil
Clinical Uses and Pharmacological Effects

Fentanyl (*Sublimaze*) and its related phenylpiperidine derivatives are extremely potent drugs. They are used as adjuncts to anesthesia, and fentanyl may be given transdermally as an analgesic and as an oral lozenge for the induction of anesthesia, especially in children who may become anxious if given IV anesthesia.

Fentanyl is 80 to 100 times as potent as morphine. Sufentanil (*Sufenta*) is 500- to 1,000-fold more potent than morphine, while alfentanil (*Alfenta*) is approximately 20 times more potent than morphine. Their onset of action is usually less than 20 minutes after administration. Dosage is determined by the lean body mass of the patient, since the drugs are lipophilic and tend to get trapped in body fat, which acts as a reservoir, prolonging their half-life. In addition, redistribution of the drugs from the brain to fat stores leads to a rapid offset of action. Droperidol, a neuroleptic agent, is generally administered in combination with fentanyl for IV anesthesia.

Fentanyl transdermal patches are available for analgesia in chronic pain and for postsurgical patients. The use of the patch is contraindicated, however, for patients immediately after surgery because of the profound respiratory depression associated with its use. The patches must be removed and replaced every 3 days. The onset of action of transdermal fentanyl is slower than that of oral morphine. Thus, patients may require the use of oral analgesics until therapeutic levels of fentanyl are achieved. Fentanyl lozenges have been used to induce anesthesia in children and to reduce pain associated with diagnostic tests or cancer in adult patients. However, all of the adverse side effects associated with morphine are produced with far greater intensity, but shorter duration, by fentanyl in the patch, the lozenge, or IV administration. Given the abuse liability of fentanyl, controversy exists as to the ethics of marketing a lollipop lozenge form.

Sufentanil is much more potent than fentanyl and is indicated specifically for long neurosurgical procedures. In such patients, sufentanil maintains anesthesia over a long period when myocardial and cerebral oxygen balance are critical.

Fentanyl is commonly used to relieve pain from intubation of premature infants, although the safety of the drug in infants has not been established. Sufentanil has been studied to a limited extent in newborns, and reports indicate that it can be used safely. Tolerance and physical dependence have been demonstrated after prolonged use of fentanyl in the newborn.

Adverse Effects and Contraindications

In addition to all of the adverse effects and contraindications previously described for morphine, the following contraindications apply specifically to these drugs. They are contraindicated in pregnant women because of their potential teratogenic effects. They also can cause respiratory depression in the mother, which reduces oxygenation of fetal blood, and in the newborn; the incidence of sudden infant death syndrome (SIDS) in the newborn is also increased.

Cardiac patients need to be monitored closely when receiving these drugs because of their bradycardiac effects (which can lead to ectopic arrhythmias), and hypotensive effects resulting from prolonged vasodilation. In addition, the drugs stiffen the chest wall musculature, an effect reversed by naloxone.

Levorphanol

Levorphanol (*Levo-Dromoran*) is an L-isomer morphinan derivative of morphine that is five to seven times more potent than morphine. It produces all of the side effects associated with morphine but less nausea. It is indicated for moderate to severe pain as a preoperative anxiolytic. It is often used in combination with thiopental to reduce the latter drug's anesthetic dose and to decrease postoperative recovery time. The D-isomer of levorphanol, dextrorphan, does not possess opioid analgesic activity but is a useful antitussive.

Methadone

Methadone (*Dolophine*) has an analgesic profile and potency similar to that of morphine but a longer duration of action and better oral bioavailability. The kinetic properties of methadone and its derivative, LAAM, have been shown to be useful in the treatment of opioid addiction, as discussed in Chapter 35.

Methadone is a useful analgesic drug for the treatment of moderate to severe pain. Unlike morphine, it is generally not used epidurally because of its long duration of action. It is also rarely or never used in PCA systems or in pregnant women during labor. The side effects and signs of overdose following methadone administration are similar to those observed with morphine. Overdose is treated with naloxone. Clearance of methadone is via the urine and bile as the cyclic N-demethylated drug. The ability to N-demethylate the drug decreases in elderly patients, prolonging the action of methadone. In such patients, dosing intervals should be longer than in younger patients. In addition, the pH of the urine has a major effect on clearance of the drug. Alkalinization of the urine or renal insufficiency decreases excretion of the drug.

Drug interactions and precautions for the use of methadone are similar to those of morphine. In addition, rifampicin and hydantoins markedly increase the metabolism of methadone and can precipitate withdrawal from methadone. Conversely, the tricyclic antidepressants and certain benzodiazepines can inhibit metabolism of methadone, thereby increasing accumulation of the drug, prolonging its half-life, and intensifying its side effects. Continuous dosing with methadone may lead to drug accumulation and to an increased incidence of side effects; methadone is generally not used for PCA. In pregnant heroin-addicted women, substitution of methadone for heroin has been shown to be associated with fewer low-birth-weight newborns and fewer learning and cognition problems later in the life of the child.

Propoxyphene

Propoxyphene (dextropropoxyphene; *Darvon*) is structurally related to methadone but is much less potent as an analgesic. Compared with codeine, propoxyphene is approximately half as potent and is indicated for the treatment of mild pain. *It is not antipyretic or antiinflammatory like aspirin and is less useful than aspirin in most cases of mild pain.* Toxicity from propoxyphene, especially in combination with other sedatives, such as alcohol, has led to a decrease in its use. Death following ingestion of alcohol in combination with propoxyphene can occur rapidly (within 20 minutes to 1 hour). The drug is not indicated for those with histories of suicide or depressive illnesses.

Like meperidine, propoxyphene has an active metabolite, norpropoxyphene, that is not analgesic but has excitatory and local anesthetic effects on the heart similar to those of quinidine. Use of the drug during pregnancy is not safe. Teratogenic effects have been observed in newborns, as have withdrawal signs at birth. As with morphine, propoxyphene requires adequate hepatic and renal clearance to prevent toxicity and drug accumulation. It is thus contraindicated in the elderly patient and those with renal or liver disease.

Propoxyphene interacts with several drugs. The use of sedatives in combination with propoxyphene can be fatal. In addition, the metabolism of the drug is increased in smokers due to induction of liver enzymes. Thus, smokers may require a higher dose of the drug for pain relief. Propoxyphene enhances the effects of both warfarin and carbamazepine and may increase the toxicity associated with both drugs, such as bleeding and sedation, respectively.

The abuse liability of propoxyphene is low because of the extreme irritation it causes at the site of injection. Oral use is the preferred route of administration for this reason.

Opium-Containing Preparations

The use of opium dates to 4,000 B.C. At that time it was used for medicinal and recreational purposes mainly via inhalation. Today few opium-containing preparations are used, since the activity of opium is largely attributed to its morphine content. The preparations in use today are those that have constipative effects useful for the treatment of diarrhea. Preparations include pantopon, an injectable hydrochloride of opium alkaloids, and paregoric, a camphorated tincture of opium. Paregoric can be used to treat infants with opioid withdrawal signs following in utero exposure to opioids.

Heroin

Heroin is the diacetyl derivative of morphine. It is not available in the United States for therapeutic use, although its use as a recreational drug is again on the rise. It is either injected or snorted (taken intranasally). It is most often cut, or diluted, with substances such as quinine, which contribute to the flash, or high. Injection of the drug leads to the eventual collapse of the vessels into which it is injected, leading to the appearance of track marks under the skin. Heroin passes rapidly into the brain and thus has a rapid onset of action. It is then metabolized to morphine. The rapid onset contributes to the abuse liability of the drug. Heroin use in pregnant women can lead to low-birth-weight babies, babies born addicted to heroin, immunosuppression, and an increased incidence of infections in both the mother and newborn; an increased incidence of AIDS also occurs.

Mixed Opioid Agonist–Antagonists or Partial Agonists

The mixed opioid agonist–antagonists are potent analgesics in opioid-naive patients but precipitate withdrawal in patients who are physically dependent on opioids. They are useful for the treatment of mild to moderate pain. They were developed to reduce the addiction potential of the opioids while retaining the analgesic potency of the drugs. Their analgesic effect is generally attributed to an interaction at the κ- and to a lesser extent the μ-opioid receptor.

Interaction at the κ-receptor increases the sedative effects of the drugs. The euphoric effects are due to interaction with the μ-receptor. The dysphoric and psychotomimetic side effects of the drugs are attributed to interaction at the σ-receptor.

The mixed agonist–antagonists and partial agonists differ from morphine in that they (1) produce excitatory and hallucinogenic effects, (2) produce a low degree of physical dependence, (3) induce withdrawal signs that differ from those of morphine, and (4) produce excitatory effects related to the sympathetic discharge of norepinephrine and therefore are positive inotropic agents in the heart.

Pentazocine

Pharmacological Effects

Pentazocine (*Talwin*) is a potent analgesic with antagonistic activity in opioid-addicted patients. It incompletely blocks the effects of morphine in such patients but will precipitate withdrawal. To eliminate abuse of the drug via IV administration, pentazocine is combined with naloxone (*Talwin-NX*). IV administration of Talwin-NX will produce no analgesic or euphoric effects because naloxone blocks the pentazocine moiety. However, the drug will retain its analgesic potency when administered orally, since naloxone is not active orally. Pentazocine produces as much respiratory depression as morphine but does not produce the same degree of constipation or the biliary constriction observed with morphine. Pentazocine may increase GI motility if used in high doses. Unlike morphine, pentazocine increases heart rate and blood pressure by releasing norepinephrine. Pentazocine also may increase uterine contractions in pregnancy.

Pharmacokinetics

Absorption of pentazocine following oral administration is rapid. The onset of action occurs within approximately 15 minutes, and the half-life is 2 to 3 hours. Pentazocine is extensively metabolized in the liver and thus has a high first-pass effect following oral administration; its half-life differs considerably from patient to patient. Oxidation of the methyl groups followed by conjugation to glucuronides in the liver terminates the effects of pentazocine. Excretion occurs through the kidney.

Clinical Uses

Pentazocine is indicated for relief of moderate pain in patients not receiving large doses of opioids. It is also used as premedication for anesthesia and as a supplement to surgical anesthesia.

Adverse Effects

The most common side effect of pentazocine is sedation resulting from an interaction with the κ-receptor. Also observed are sweating, dizziness, psychotomimetic effects, anxiety, nightmares, and headache. Nausea and vomiting are less frequent than with morphine. Respiratory depression and increased heart rate, body temperature, and blood pressure accompany overdose. Naloxone is effective in reducing the respiratory depression but requires the use of higher doses than for morphine overdose.

Contraindications

Most of the contraindications specific to pentazocine stem from its excitatory effects. Other contraindications are similar to those for morphine. Pentazocine is contraindicated in patients with myocardial infarction because it increases heart rate and cardiac load. Similarly, it is contraindicated in epileptic patients because it decreases seizure threshold. In addition, in head trauma patients, it can increase intracranial pressure and brain injury. Pentazocine use in patients with psychoses is contraindicated because of its psychotomimetic side effects.

Drug Interactions

The combination of pentazocine with the antihistamine tripelennamine results in a combination known to drug abusers as T's and blues. This combination produces heroinlike subjective effects, and heroin addicts use it in the absence of heroin. In addition, the use of pentazocine in combination with alcohol or barbiturates greatly enhances its sedative and respiratory depressant effects.

Tolerance and Dependence

Tolerance to the analgesic effects of pentazocine develops. Withdrawal signs are milder than those seen with morphine, and they produce more excitatory effects.

Butorphanol

Butorphanol (*Stadol*) is chemically related to levorphanol but pharmacologically similar in action to pentazocine. As an opioid antagonist it is nearly 30 times as potent as pentazocine and has one-fortieth the potency of naloxone. It is a potent opioid analgesic indicated for the relief of moderate to severe pain. Its potency is 7 times that of morphine and 20 times that of pentazocine as an analgesic. Its onset of action is similar to that of morphine. The side effects and signs of toxicity are similar to those produced by pentazocine. It produces excitatory effects and sedation and precipitates withdrawal in opioid-dependent patients. Although generally administered parenterally because of its low bioavailability following oral administration, it is also unique in that a nasal spray formulation is available. The nasal spray is indicated for the relief of postoperative pain and migraine headache. The low molecular weight of butorphanol, its high lipophilicity, and its lack of vasoconstrictor effects make it particularly suitable for nasal administration.

Nasal administration of butorphanol decreases the onset of action to 15 minutes and decreases the first-pass effect of the drug, which increases bioavailability. Generally the patient sprays a set dose of 1 mg per hour for 2 hours. The duration of action is 4 to 5 hours. The convenience of such administration is a major advantage to patients requiring repeat dosing. The abuse potential following such administration has not been extensively studied, although it is thought to be small. Butorphanol is not a federally controlled ("scheduled") drug, so physicians are not required to obtain the licenses and security safeguards required for other opioid analgesics.

Adverse effects, contraindications, and drug interactions are similar to those for pentazocine and morphine.

Nalbuphine

Nalbuphine (*Nubain*) is a mixed agonist–antagonist that is similar in structure to both the antagonist naloxone and the agonist oxymorphone. It is administered parenterally and is equipotent to morphine and 5 times as potent as pentazocine. Although the pharmacological effects (analgesia, respiratory depression, sedation, and so on) are similar to those produced by pentazocine, nalbuphine produces fewer psychotomimetic effects. It differs from pentazocine in that it has far greater antagonist than agonist effect. Thus, its use is likely to precipitate severe withdrawal in opioid-dependent patients. It is used much as pentazocine is, that is, for moderate to severe pain, postsurgical anesthesia, and obstetrical analgesia. Nalbuphine's abuse potential is less than that of codeine and propoxyphene, although tolerance and dependence have been shown following chronic administration. High doses are perceived by addicts as being like those of the barbiturates. Drug interactions and contraindications are similar to those for pentazocine and morphine.

Buprenorphine

Buprenorphine (*Temgesic*) is a mixed agonist–antagonist and a derivative of the naturally occurring opioid thebaine. Buprenorphine is highly lipophilic and is 25 to 50 times more potent than morphine as an analgesic. The sedation and respiratory depression it causes are more intense and longer lasting than those produced by morphine. Its respiratory depressant effects are not readily reversed by naloxone. It binds to the μ-receptor with high affinity and only slowly dissociates from the receptor, which may explain the lack of naloxone reversal of respiratory depression.

Buprenorphine has more agonist than antagonist effects and is often considered a partial agonist rather than a mixed agonist–antagonist, although it precipitates withdrawal in opioid-dependent patients. Its pharmacological effects are similar to those produced by both morphine and pentazocine. Indications for its use are similar to those of pentazocine, that is, for moderate to severe pain. Sublingual preparations are available, but have a slow onset and erratic absorption.

The abuse potential of buprenorphine is low. While high doses of the drug are perceived by addicts as being

morphinelike, it does reduce the craving for morphine and for the stimulant cocaine. Thus, buprenorphine is a potential new therapy for the treatment of addiction to both classes of drugs.

Drug interactions and contraindications are similar to those described for pentazocine and morphine.

Dezocine

Dezocine (*Dalgan*) is a synthetic aminotetralin derivative with potent agonist–antagonist effects. The onset of activity and potency as an analgesic are comparable to those of morphine. Although the drug requires glucuronidation during metabolism, patients with hepatic insufficiency clear it normally. The main route for clearance is the kidney. Thus, patients with renal dysfunction are prone to buildup of dezocine over time. As an antagonist, dezocine is more potent than pentazocine. As an agonist, dezocine produces analgesia and respiratory depression (which is readily reversed by naloxone), but unlike pentazocine, it has little if any effect on the cardiovascular system.

Dezocine is indicated as an analgesic for moderate to severe pain. In addition, it shows promise in chronic pain states, such as with victims of severe burns. Contraindications and adverse effects of the drug are similar to those described for morphine. No tendency toward abuse has been demonstrated thus far.

Opioid Antagonists

Naloxone and naltrexone are pure opioid antagonists synthesized by relatively minor changes in the morphine structure. Alteration of the substituent on the piperidine nitrogen from a methyl group to a longer side chain changes the drug from an agonist to an antagonist.

Opioid antagonists bind to the opioid receptor with high affinity and have low efficacy. The pure antagonists block the effects of opioids at all opioid receptors. However, as previously discussed, the dose required for naloxone blockade of the μ-receptor versus the κ-opioid receptor is several times as much. All opioid antagonists will precipitate withdrawal in opioid-dependent patients.

Naloxone

Because of its fast onset (minutes), naloxone (*Narcan*) administered IV is used most frequently for the reversal of opioid overdose. However, it fails to block some side effects of the opioids that are mediated by the σ-receptor, such as hallucinations. The rapid offset of naloxone makes it necessary to administer the drug repeatedly until the opioid agonist has cleared the system to prevent relapse into overdose. The half-life of naloxone in plasma is 1 hour. It is rapidly metabolized via glucuronidation in the liver and cleared by the kidney. Naloxone given orally has a large first-pass effect, which reduces its potency significantly. Often an overshoot will follow the administration of naloxone for overdose. The heart rate and blood pressure of the patient may rise significantly. The overshoot is thought to be due to precipitation of acute withdrawal signs by naloxone. Given alone to nonaddicts, naloxone produces no pharmacological effects.

Naloxone is approved for use in neonates to reverse respiratory depression induced by maternal opioid use. In addition, naloxone has been used to improve circulation in patients in shock, an effect related to blockade of endogenous opioids. Other experimental and less well documented uses for naloxone include reversal of coma in alcohol overdose, appetite suppression, and alleviation of dementia from schizophrenia. Side effects of naloxone are minor.

Naltrexone

Naltrexone (*Trexan*) is three to five times as potent as naloxone and has a duration of action of 24 to 72 hours, depending on the dose. It is used orally in the treatment of opioid abstinence. Naltrexone exhibits a large first-pass effect in the liver. However, the major metabolite, 6-β-naltrexol, is also a pure opioid antagonist and contributes to the potency and duration of action of naltrexone. Administration of naltrexone orally blocks the subjective effects of abused opioids and is used to decrease the craving for opioids in highly motivated recovering addicts. However, high doses of the opioids can overcome the naltrexone blockade and lead to seizures or respiratory depression and death. In addition, it has been reported recently that naltrexone can reduce the craving for alcohol in alcoholic patients. Naltrexone also has been used with success in treating apneic episodes in children, an effect hypothesized to be due to blockade of β-endorphin–induced respiratory depression.

Naltrexone can induce hepatotoxicity at doses only five times the therapeutic dose and should be used with care in patients with poor hepatic function or liver damage. Side effects of the use of naltrexone are more frequently observed than following naloxone administration. Such side effects include headache, difficulty sleeping, lethargy, increased blood pressure, nausea, sneezing, delayed ejaculation, blurred vision, and increased appetite.

Nalmefene

Nalmefene (*Revex*) is a long-acting injectable pure opioid antagonist recently introduced in the United States. It binds all opioid receptors and reverses the effects of opioid agonists at those receptors. The onset of action is 2 minutes after IV administration. Hepatic metabolism is slow and occurs via glucuronide conjugation to inactive metabolites. Its half-life of 11 hours is about 5 times that of naloxone. Indications include use in postoperative settings to reverse respiratory depression and in opioid overdose. Due to the long duration of action of nalmefene, however, naloxone may be preferred for treatment of overdose because it produces a shorter duration of withdrawal effects.

Drugs Used Predominantly as Antitussives

Certain opioids are used mainly for their antitussive effects. Such drugs generally are those with substituents on the phenolic hydroxyl group of the morphine structure. The larger the substituent, the greater the antitussive versus analgesic selectively of the drugs.

Dextromethorphan

Dextromethorphan hydrobromide is the D-isomer of levorphanol. It lacks CNS activity but acts at the cough center in the medulla to produce an antitussive effect. It is half as potent as codeine as an antitussive. Anecdotal reports of abuse exist, but studies of abuse potential are lacking. It has few side effects but does potentiate the activity of monoamine oxidase inhibitors, leading to hypotension and infrequently coma. Dextromethorphan is often combined in lozenges with the local anesthetic benzocaine, which blocks pain from throat irritation due to coughing.

Levopropoxyphene

Levopropoxyphene is the L-isomer of the analgesic agonist dextropropoxyphene. Levopropoxyphene is only mildly antitussive and is rarely used. It has no CNS effects. Side effects include dizziness and nausea. It is available as the napsylate derivative (*Novrad*) and is taken orally in the form of a liquid or less frequently as a capsule.

Noscapine

Noscapine is a naturally occurring product of the opium poppy. It is a benzylisoquinoline with no analgesic or other CNS effects. Its antitussive effects are weak, but it is used in combination with other agents in mixtures for cough relief.

Benzonatate

Benzonatate (*Tessalon*) is related to the local anesthetic tetracaine. It anesthetizes the stretch receptors in the lungs, thereby reducing coughing. Adverse reactions include hypersensitivity, sedation, dizziness, and nausea.

Study QUESTIONS

1. Which of the following opioids has an analgesically active metabolite?
   (A) Naloxone
   (B) Meperidine
   (C) Propoxyphene
   (D) Codeine
   (E) Nalmefene
2. Which of the following statements about celecoxib is true?
   (A) It irreversibly acetylates the COX-2 enzyme.
   (B) It inhibits both the inducible and constitutive COX-2 enzyme.
   (C) It produces no GI bleeding.
   (D) It is indicated only for the disease, osteoarthritis.
   (E) It increases healing of GI ulcers.
3. Morphine produces an analgesic effect due to
   (A) A block of potassium efflux from a neuron
   (B) An increase in c–AMP accumulation in a neuron
   (C) A decrease in intracellular calcium in a neuron
   (D) Interaction with a G_s protein in the neuron
   (E) An increase in calcium channel phosphorylation in the neuron
4. κ-Opioid receptor activation is required to observe
   (A) Respiratory depression
   (B) Bradycardia
   (C) Miosis
   (D) Mydriasis
   (E) Hypocapnia
5. Which of the following statements about fentanyl patches is true?
   (A) They produce no respiratory depression.
   (B) They produce anesthesia and analgesia.
   (C) They produce no constipation.
   (D) They can be used during pregnancy.
   (E) They cannot be used in nonambulatory patients.

ANSWERS

1. **D.** The purpose of this question is to identify first opioids that produce analgesia and then those with a metabolite that compounds the analgesic effects of the drug by being an active analgesic. Naloxone and nalmefene are not analgesics but opioid antagonists. Codeine is metabolized to an active analgesic metabolite, morphine. Meperidine and propoxyphene have nonanalgesic, excitatory, and proconvulsant metabolites.
2. **B.** The purpose of this question is to clarify the uses and limitations of use of the COX-2 selective inhibitor celecoxib. Celecoxib, by inhibiting COX-2 reversibly, will block the activity of both injury-inducible COX-2 and the small amount of constitutive COX-2. COX-2 inhibition has been shown to produce some GI bleeding, albeit less than with the nonselective COX inhibitors. If a patient has ulcerations and bleeding, COX-2 inhibitors will prolong healing by blocking the protective effects of COX-2 in the GI tract. Celecoxib is indicated for both osteoarthritis and rheumatoid arthritis.
3. **C.** The purpose of this question is to clarify the cellular mechanism of analgesia produced by morphine. First, morphine blocks the transmission of nociceptive impulses. In that case, the relevant question is how nociceptive impulses are transmitted via the release of pronociceptive neurotransmitters. The question then is to determine which intracellular process favors a block of release of neurotransmitters. The correct answer is C because calcium is required for neurotransmitter release. Blocking potassium efflux and increasing calcium channel phosphorylation produce functional depolarization and neurotransmitter release. Opioids are coupled to G_i (inhibitory proteins) that decrease cAMP.
4. **C.** The purpose of this question is to clarify the functional significance of the activation of opioid receptor types. Respiratory depression and bradycardia are associated with the μ_2-opioid receptor. Mydriasis is associated with the σ-receptor, which is no longer thought of as opioid. Opioids, via respiratory depression, induce hypercapnia, a build-up of carbon dioxide. The clinically relevant sign of opioid overdose and opioid use is miosis, pinpoint pupils, mediated by κ-receptor activation.
5. **E.** Fentanyl patches have the same effect as fentanyl, only in a time-release manner. Thus, the purpose of the question is delineation of opioid effects—respiratory depression and constipation. The respiratory depression is life-threatening when the patch is used in nonambulatory patients, and it is therefore contraindicated for that purpose. Similarly, fentanyl is a teratogenic drug contraindicated for use during pregnancy. The fentanyl patch does not induce anesthesia (loss of consciousness) but does produce analgesia.

SUPPLEMENTAL READING
Darland T et al. Orphanin FQ/nociceptin: A role in pain and analgesia, but so much more. Trends Neurosci 1998;21:215–221.
Devi LA. Heterodimerization of G-protein-coupled receptors: Pharmacology, signaling and trafficking. Trends Pharmacol Sci 2001;22:532–537.

Julius D and Basbaum AI. Molecular mechanisms of nociception. Nature 2001;413:203–210.

Marnett LJ and Kalgutkar M. Cyclooxygenase 2 inhibitors: Discovery, selectivity and the future. Trends Pharmacol Sci 1999;20:465–469.

Moran TD et al. Cellular neurophysiological actions of nociceptin/orphanin FQ. Peptides 2000;21:969–976.

Tseng, L. Evidence for ε-opioid receptor-mediated β-endorphin-induced analgesia. Trends Pharmacol Sci 2001;22:623–630.

Wallace JL. Selective COX-2 inhibitors: Is the water becoming muddy? Trends Pharmacol Sci. 1999;20: 4–6.

Zadina JE et al. Endomorphins: novel endogenous mu-opiate receptor agonists in regions of high mu-receptor density. Ann NY Acad Sci 1999;897: 136–144.

CASE Study   Opioids and Head Trauma

A 45-year-old woman is found outside her car after hitting a tree. The car appears severely damaged. There is no evidence as to how the woman escaped from the car. It is thought that she was able to open her door and then fell from the car. When she is discovered, she is conscious but disoriented and complaining of severe pain of multiple origins. While in route to the emergency department, her pain increases in intensity. Which opioid might be used to ease her pain immediately upon her arrival at the hospital?

ANSWER: No opioid should be used immediately. The use of an opioid at this stage will block the pupillary responses in her eyes due to miosis, which will detract from immediate diagnosis of a concussion. In addition, opioids will induce hypercapnia due to respiratory depression, vasodilation, bradycardia, and hypotension and make a patient in shock less stable. Such effects will be intensified if the woman was drinking prior to the accident. In addition, opioids increase intracranial pressure via hypercapnia and vasodilation, possibly increasing any damage to the brain. In general a patient in severe pain may be given a general anesthetic agent.

27 Local Anesthetics

J. David Haddox

DRUG LIST

GENERIC NAME	PAGE	GENERIC NAME	PAGE
Benzocaine	334	Mepivacaine	335
Bupivacaine	335	Prilocaine	335
Chloroprocaine	334	Procaine	334
Cocaine	334	Ropivacaine	335
Etidocaine	335	Tetracaine	334
Lidocaine	335		

The first clinical uses of a local anesthetic agent occurred in 1884, when cocaine was employed as a topical agent for eye surgery and to produce a nerve block. These events inaugurated a new era, that of regional anesthesia. New applications were developed, including spinal, epidural, and caudal anesthesia. The search for a better local anesthetic led to chemical synthesis of a number of other compounds that have more selective local anesthetic properties and few systemic side effects.

PROPERTIES OF LOCAL ANESTHETICS

An important property of the ideal local anesthetic is low systemic toxicity at an effective concentration. Onset of action should be quick, and duration of action should be sufficient to allow time for the surgical procedure. The local anesthetic should be soluble in water and stable in solution. It should not deteriorate by the heat of sterilization, and it should be effective both when injected into tissue and when applied topically to mucous membranes. Its effects should be completely reversible.

Although the characteristics of an ideal local anesthetic are easily identifiable, synthesis of a compound possessing all these properties has not been accomplished. The compounds discussed in the following sections fall short of the ideal in at least one aspect. However, the judicious choice of a particular agent for a particular need will permit the practitioner to employ local anesthesia effectively and safely.

Chemistry

The basic components in the structure of local anesthetics are the lipophilic aromatic portion (a benzene ring), an intermediate chain, and the hydrophilic amine portion (Fig. 27.1). The intermediate chain has either an ester linkage from the combination of an aromatic acid and an amino alcohol or an amide linkage from the combination of an aromatic amine and an amino acid. The commonly used local anesthetics can be classified as esters or amides based on the structure of this intermediate chain.

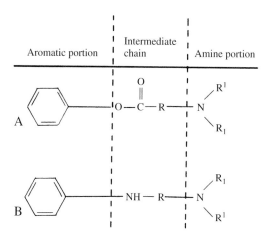

FIGURE 27.1

Model structure of local anesthetics showing aromatic portion, intermediate chain, and amine portion.

Mechanism of Action

The application of a local anesthetic to a nerve that is actively conducting impulses will inhibit the inward migration of Na^+. This elevates the threshold for electrical excitation, reduces the rate of rise of the action potential, slows the propagation of the impulse, and if the drug concentration is sufficiently high, completely blocks conduction. *The local anesthetics interfere with the process fundamental to the generation of the action potential, namely, the large, transient voltage-dependent rise in the permeability of the membrane to Na^+.*

While the physiological basis for the local anesthetic action is known, the precise molecular nature of the process is not completely clear. Almost all local anesthetics can exist as either the uncharged base or as a cation. The uncharged base is important for adequate penetration to the site of action, and the charged form of the molecule is required at the site of action. The cation forms of local anesthetics appear to be required for binding to specific sites in or near the Na^+ channels. The presence of the local anesthetic at these sites interferes with the normal passage of Na^+ through the cell membrane by stopping a conformational change in the subunits of the voltage-gated Na^+ channel.

Studies suggest that the receptor for the local anesthetic is near the inner (axoplasmic) surface of the cell membrane, because quaternary analogues of local anesthetics are quite effective when applied to the inside of the axonal membrane but are inactive when placed on the outside of the membrane. These permanently charged molecules cannot penetrate to the receptor sites.

Nerves that are rapidly depolarizing are inherently particularly susceptible to the effects of local anesthetics. This is termed *frequency-dependent blockade* and is thought to occur because the local anesthetics get to their receptor sites only when the Na^+ channel is open (depolarizing).

Differential Blockade

Peripheral nerve functions are not affected equally by local anesthetics. Loss of sympathetic function usually is followed by loss of temperature sensation; sensation to pinprick, touch, and deep pressure; and last, motor function. This phenomenon is called *differential blockade*. Differential blockade is the result of a number of factors, including the size of the nerve, the presence and amount of myelin, and the location of particular fibers within a nerve bundle. For conduction to be effectively blocked, the local anesthetic must exert its effects over the distance between several nodes of Ranvier. Since the smallest nerves (C fibers) have no myelin, they can be most easily blocked; thus, sympathetic functions often are blocked soon after a local anesthetic is applied to a particular nerve bundle. Small myelinated nerves have correspondingly short distances between nodes of Ranvier and therefore are often blocked next. These nerves subserve temperature and sharp pain sensation. Larger nerves then become blocked, accounting for the loss of function up to and including motor innervation.

Pharmacokinetic Properties
Absorption and Distribution

The rate of absorption of a local anesthetic into the bloodstream is affected by the dose administered, the vascularity at the site of injection, and the specific physicochemical properties of the drug itself. Local anesthetics gain entrance into the bloodstream by absorption from the injection site, direct intravenous injection, or absorption across the mucous membranes after topical application. Direct intravascular injection occurs accidentally when the needle used for infiltration of the local anesthetic lies within a blood vessel, or it occurs intentionally when lidocaine is used for the control of cardiac arrhythmias.

All tissues will be exposed to local anesthetics after absorption, but concentrations will vary among the organs. Although the highest concentrations appear to occur in the more highly perfused organs (i.e., brain, kidney, and lung), factors such as degree of protein binding and lipid solubility also affect drug distribution. The lung can absorb as much as 90% of a local anesthetic during the first pass. Consequently, the lungs can act as a buffer to prevent higher and therefore more toxic concentrations.

Placental transfer of local anesthetics is known to occur rapidly, fetal blood concentrations generally reflecting those found in the mother. However, the quantity of drug crossing to the fetus is also related to the time of exposure, that is, from the time of injection to delivery. Subtle neurobehavioral changes in the neonate are detectable for as long as 8 hours after mepivacaine administration to the mother but are absent following the use of bupivacaine, lidocaine, and chloroprocaine. In general, minimal amounts of chloroprocaine reach the fetus because of its rapid hydrolysis by serum cholinesterase; this feature is its principal advantage in obstetrics.

Metabolism

The metabolic degradation of local anesthetics depends on whether the compound has an ester or an amide linkage. Esters are extensively and rapidly metabolized in plasma by pseudocholinesterase, whereas the amide linkage is resistant to hydrolysis. The rate of local anesthetic hydrolysis is important, since slow biotransformation may lead to drug accumulation and toxicity. In patients with atypical plasma cholinesterase, the use of ester-linked compounds, such as chloroprocaine, procaine and tetracaine, has an increased potential for toxicity. The hydrolysis of all ester-linked local anesthetics leads to the formation of paraaminobenzoic acid (PABA), which is known to be allergenic. Therefore, some people have allergic reactions to the ester class of local anesthetics.

Local anesthetics with an amide linkage (and one ester-lined anesthetic, cocaine) are almost completely metabolized by the liver before excretion. However, the total dose administered and the degree of drug accumulation resulting from the initial and subsequent doses are still a concern.

Clinical Uses

Local anesthetics are extremely useful in a wide range of procedures, varying from intravenous catheter insertion to extensive surgery under regional block. For minor surgery, the patients can remain awake; this is an advantage in emergency surgery, because protective airway reflexes remain intact. Many operative procedures in the oral cavity are facilitated by regional block of specific nerves. If surgery permits, the patient can return home, because he or she is less sedated than would be the case after general anesthesia.

Topical Anesthesia

Local anesthetics are used extensively on the mucous membranes in the nose, mouth, tracheobronchial tree, and urethra. The vasoconstriction produced by some local anesthetics, cocaine especially, adds a very important advantage to their use in the nose by preventing bleeding and inducing tissue shrinkage. Topical anesthesia permits many diagnostic procedures in the awake patient, and when it is combined with infiltration techniques, excellent anesthesia may be obtained for many

surgical procedures in the eye and nose. The practitioner should be cautious when higher volumes are required, since overdosage may cause systemic reactions. Additionally, when the tracheobronchial tree and larynx are anesthetized, normal protective reflexes, which prevent pulmonary aspiration of oral or gastric fluids and contents, are lost.

Infiltration

Infiltration (i.e., the injection of local anesthetics under the skin) of the surgical site provides adequate anesthesia if contiguous structures are not stimulated. Since the onset of local anesthesia is rapid, the surgical procedures can proceed with little delay. Minimally effective concentrations should be used, especially in extensive procedures, to avoid toxicity from overdosage.

Regional Block

Regional block, a form of anesthesia that includes spinal and epidural anesthesia, involves injection near a nerve or nerve plexus proximal to the surgical site. It provides excellent anesthesia for a variety of procedures. Brachial plexus block is commonly used for the upper extremity. Individual blocks of the sciatic, femoral, and obturator nerves can be used for the lower extremity. An amount that is close to the maximally tolerated dose is required to produce blockade of a major extremity.

Spinal Anesthesia

Spinal anesthesia (subarachnoid block) produces extensive and profound anesthesia with a minimum amount of drug. The local anesthetic solution is introduced directly into the spinal fluid, where the nerves are not protected by a perineurium. This produces, in effect, a temporary cord transection such that no impulses are transmitted beyond the level that is anesthetized. The onset is rapid, and with proper drug selection, the anesthesia may last 1 to 4 hours. With careful technique, neurological complications are extremely rare. Procedures as high as upper-abdominal surgery can be performed under spinal anesthesia. Arterial hypotension produced by the local anesthetic is proportional to the degree of interruption of sympathetic tone, and it can produce pooling of blood in the lower extremities, which leads to decreased cardiac filling pressures. Knowing this allows blood pressure to be easily controlled, and hypotension is not usually a deterrent to spinal anesthesia. The sites of action of spinal anesthesia are the spinal nerve roots, spinal ganglia, and (perhaps) the spinal cord.

Lumbar Epidural Anesthesia

Lumbar epidural anesthesia affects the same area of the body as does spinal anesthesia. As the name implies, the drug is deposited outside the dura. In contrast to spinal anesthesia, this method requires a much larger amount of drug. This procedure makes segmental anesthesia possible, whereby the anesthetized area is bordered caudally and cephalad by unaffected dermatomes and myotomes.

The concentration and volume of the local anesthetic solution will affect the extent of the cephalad and caudad spread of the block. The anesthesia can be made continuous by maintaining a small catheter in the epidural space; prolonged effects are obtained by periodically injecting supplemental doses through the catheter or by attaching it to a computer pump. The site of anesthetic action is on the nerves as they leave the intervertebral foramina. However, effective drug concentrations may be found in the spinal fluid, probably gaining entrance through the arachnoid villi. Arterial hypotension occurs by the same mechanism and is managed as in spinal anesthesia.

Epidural anesthesia is especially useful in obstetrics. Excellent analgesia occurs and the patient remains awake. Analgesia by the epidural route can be provided for labor and delivery or for cesarean section. Bupivacaine in lower concentrations has the advantage of providing excellent analgesia while minimally reducing motor strength.

Caudal Anesthesia

In the caudal form of extradural anesthesia, the agent is introduced through the sacral hiatus above the coccyx. It is particularly applicable to perineal and rectal procedures. Anesthetization of higher anatomical levels is not easily obtained, because the required injection volume can be excessive. Although caudal anesthesia has been used extensively in obstetrics, lumbar epidural blockade is now more commonly used because of the lower dose of drug required; in addition, the sacral segments are spared until their anesthesia is required for the delivery.

Intravenous Extremity Block

Excellent and rapid anesthetization of an extremity can be obtained easily. Following insertion of an intravenous catheter in the limb of interest, a rubber bandage is used to force blood out of the limb, and a tourniquet is applied to prevent the blood from reentering; a dilute solution of local anesthetic, most commonly lidocaine, is then injected intravenously. This technique fills the limb's vasculature and carries the anesthetic solution to the nerve by means of the blood supply. Because of the pain produced by a tourniquet after some time, this procedure usually is limited to less than 1 hour. The systemic blood levels of drug achieved after tourniquet release generally remain below toxic levels.

Although it is more easily and therefore more commonly used on the upper extremity, intravenous extremity anesthesia can be used on the leg and thigh.

Sympathetic Block

Blockade of the sympathetic nervous system can be more selectively accomplished than that which occurs during spinal or epidural anesthesia. Cell bodies for preganglionic sympathetic nerves originate in the intermediolateral cell column of the spinal cord, from the first thoracic to the second lumbar segments. The myelinated axons of these cells travel as white communicating rami before joining the sympathetic chain and synapsing in the ganglia. The best location for a sympathetic block is at the sympathetic ganglia, since a block at this level will affect only the sympathetic nerves. For example, local anesthetic blockade of the stellate ganglion (which includes T1) blocks sympathetic innervation to all of the upper extremity and head on the injected side. A block of the sympathetic chain at L2 affects all of the lower extremity. This form of local anesthesia is particularly useful during treatment of a variety of vasospastic diseases of the extremities and for some pain syndromes.

Control of Cardiac Arrhythmias

Procainamide and lidocaine are two of the primary drugs for treating cardiac arrhythmias. Since lidocaine has a short duration of action, it is common to administer it by continuous infusion. Procainamide, because of its amide linkage, has longer action than does its precursor, procaine. Orally active analogues of local anesthetics (e.g., mexiletine) also are used as antiarrhythmics (see Chapter 16).

Use of Vasoconstrictors

The most commonly used vasoconstrictors, the sympathomimetic drugs, are often added to local anesthetics to delay absorption of the anesthetic from its injection site. By slowing absorption, these drugs reduce the anesthetic's systemic toxicity and keep it in contact with nerve fibers longer, thereby increasing the drug's duration of action. Administration of lidocaine 1% with epinephrine results in the same degree of blockade as that produced by lidocaine 2% without the vasoconstrictor.

Many vasoconstrictors are available, but epinephrine is by far the most commonly employed. Because epinephrine can have systemic α- and β-adrenergic effects, precaution is needed when local anesthetics containing this amine are given to a patient with hypertension or an irritable myocardium. Sensitivity to epinephrine may be incorrectly diagnosed as an allergy to local anesthetics. Epinephrine-containing solutions should be used cautiously in persons taking tricyclic antidepressants or monoamine oxidase (MAO) inhibitors, since those drugs may enhance the systemic pressor effects of sympathomimetic amines.

Levonordefrin (*Neo-Cobefrin*) is an active optical isomer of nordefrin that has α_1-adrenergic activity and possesses little or no β-agonist properties. It is used exclusively in some dental anesthetic cartridges as a vasoconstrictor. Its theoretical advantage is that it causes less hypertension and tachycardia than does epinephrine.

Phenylephrine hydrochloride (*Neo-Synephrine*) is a pure α-agonist that is occasionally used for subarachnoid block and is marketed with procaine for use in dentistry. It has little direct cardiac effect.

Adverse Effects

The central nervous and cardiopulmonary systems are most commonly affected by high plasma levels of local anesthetics. Local anesthetics given in initially high doses produce central nervous system (CNS) stimulation characterized by restlessness, disorientation, tremors, and at times clonic convulsions. Continued exposure to high concentrations results in general CNS depression; death occurs from respiratory failure secondary to medullary depression. Treatment requires ventilatory assistance and drugs to control the seizures. The ultra–short-acting barbiturates and the benzodiazepine derivatives, such as diazepam, are effective in controlling these seizures. Respiratory stimulants are not effective. CNS manifestations generally occur before cardiopulmonary collapse.

Cardiac toxicity is generally the result of drug-induced depression of cardiac conduction (e.g., atrioventricular block, intraventricular conduction block) and systemic vasodilation. These effects may progress to severe hypotension and cardiac arrest.

Allergic reactions, such as red and itchy eczematoid dermatitis or vesiculation, are a concern with the ester-type local anesthetics. True allergic manifestations have been reported with procaine. *The amides are essentially free of allergic properties,* but suspected allergic phenomena may be caused by methylparaben, a parahydroxybenzoic acid derivative used as an antibacterial preservative in multiple-dose vials and some dental cartridges. Esters probably should be avoided in favor of an amide when the patient has a history of allergy to a PABA-containing preparation such as certain cosmetics or sunscreens.

ESTERS

Cocaine

Cocaine hydrochloride remains useful primarily because of the vasoconstriction it provides with topical use. Toxicity prohibits its use for other than topical anesthesia.

Cocaine has a rapid onset of action (1 minute) and a duration of up to 2 hours, depending on the dose or concentration. Lower concentrations are used for the eye, while the higher ones are used on the nasal and pha-

ryngeal mucosa. Epinephrine plus cocaine, although still used occasionally, is hazardous because the catecholamine potentiates the cardiovascular toxicity (e.g., arrhythmia, ventricular fibrillation) of cocaine.

Cardiovascular effects are related to both central and peripheral sympathetic stimulation. Initial bradycardia appears to be related to vagal stimulation; this is followed by tachycardia and hypertension. Larger doses are directly depressant to the myocardium, and death results from cardiac failure.

Cocaine is readily absorbed from mucous membranes, so the potential for systemic toxicity is great. The CNS is stimulated, and euphoria and cortical stimulation (e.g., restlessness, excitement) frequently result. Overdosage leads to convulsions followed by CNS depression. The cortical stimulation it produces is responsible for the drug's abuse (see Chapter 35).

Benzocaine

Benzocaine is a PABA derivative used primarily for topical application to skin and mucous membranes. Its low aqueous solubility allows it to stay at the site of application for long periods. Its minimal rate of absorption after topical administration is associated with a low incidence of systemic toxicity. Benzocaine is contraindicated in patients with known sensitivity to ester-linked anesthetics or PABA-containing compounds.

Chloroprocaine

Chloroprocaine hydrochloride (*Nesacaine*) is obtained from addition of a chlorine atom to procaine, which results in a compound of greater potency and less toxicity than procaine itself. This local anesthetic is hydrolyzed very rapidly by cholinesterase and therefore has a short plasma half-life. Because it is broken down rapidly, chloroprocaine is commonly used in obstetrics. It is believed that the small amount that might get to the fetus continues to be rapidly hydrolyzed, so there may be no residual effects on the neonate.

Procaine

Procaine hydrochloride (*Novocain*) is readily hydrolyzed by plasma cholinesterase, although hepatic metabolism also occurs. It is not effective topically but is employed for infiltration, nerve block, and spinal anesthesia. It has a relatively slow onset and short (1 hour) duration of action. All concentrations can be combined with epinephrine. It is available in dental cartridges with phenylephrine as the vasoconstrictor.

Tetracaine

Tetracaine hydrochloride (*Pontocaine*) is an ester of PABA that is an effective topical local anesthetic agent and also is quite commonly used for spinal (subarachnoid) anesthesia. Epinephrine is frequently added to prolong the anesthesia. Tetracaine is considerably more potent and more toxic than procaine and cocaine. It has approximately a 5-minute onset and 2 to 3 hours of action.

AMIDES

Lidocaine hydrochloride (*Xylocaine*) is the most commonly used local anesthetic. It is well tolerated, and in addition to its use in infiltration and regional nerve blocks, it is commonly used for spinal and topical anesthesia and as an antiarrhythmic agent (see Chapter 16). Lidocaine has a more rapidly occurring, more intense, and more prolonged duration of action than does procaine.

Bupivacaine hydrochloride (*Marcaine, Sensorcaine*) has particularly long action, and some nerve blocks last more than 24 hours; this is often an advantage for postoperative analgesia. Its use for epidural anesthesia in obstetrics has attracted interest because it can relieve the pain of labor at concentrations as low as 0.125% while permitting some motor activity of abdominal muscles to aid in expelling the fetus. The lower concentration minimizes the possibility of cardiac toxicity. Fetal drug concentrations remain low, and drug-induced neurobehavioral changes are not observed in the newborn. Bupivacaine also is approved for spinal anesthesia and is approximately four times more potent and more toxic than mepivacaine and lidocaine. It can be used with or without epinephrine.

Levobupivacaine hydrochloride (*Chirocaine*) is the S-enantiomer of bupivacaine. It too has long action. Animal studies show that it has less CNS and cardiac toxicity than does bupivacaine. It also is slightly more motor sparing than is bupivacaine.

Ropivacaine (*Naropin*) is a recently developed long-acting amide-linked local anesthetic. Its duration of action is similar to that of bupivacaine, but it is slightly less potent and requires higher concentrations to achieve the same degree of block. Its primary advantage over bupivacaine is its lesser degree of cardiotoxicity.

Etidocaine hydrochloride (*Duranest*), although chemically similar to lidocaine, has a more prolonged action. It is used for regional blocks, including epidural anesthesia. It exhibits a preference for motor rather than sensory block; therefore, its use in obstetrics is limited, although fetal drug concentrations remain low. It can be used with or without epinephrine.

Mepivacaine hydrochloride (*Carbocaine*) is longer acting than lidocaine and has a more rapid onset of action (3–5 minutes). Topical application is not effective. It has been widely used in obstetrics, but its use has declined recently because of the early transient neurobehavioral effects it produces. Adverse reactions associated with mepivacaine are generally similar to those produced by other local anesthetics. It can be used with epinephrine or levonordefrin (dental use only).

Prilocaine hydrochloride (*Citanest*) is an amide anesthetic whose onset of action is slightly longer than that of lidocaine; its duration of action is comparable. Prilocaine is 40% less toxic acutely than lidocaine, making it especially suitable for regional anesthetic techniques. It is metabolized by the liver to orthotoluidine, which when it accumulates, can cause conversion of hemoglobin (HB^{++}) to methemoglobin (HB^{+++}). Oxygen transport is impaired in the presence of methemoglobinemia. Treatment involves the use of reducing agents, such as methylene blue, given intravenously, to reconvert methemoglobin to hemoglobin.

TOPICAL AGENTS

EMLA cream (lidocaine 2.5% and prilocaine 2.5%) consists of a *e*utectic *m*ixture of *l*ocal *a*nesthetics. It is used to provide topical anesthetic to intact skin. Other topical preparations are effective only on mucosal surfaces. EMLA has been shown to reduce pain on venipuncture and provide substantial anesthesia for skin graft donor sites. No significant local or systemic toxicity has been demonstrated.

TAC (tetracaine, adrenalin [epinephrine], and cocaine) is a combination topical anesthetic frequently used in pediatric emergency departments for repair of minor lacerations. The usual mixture is tetracaine 0.5%, epinephrine 1:2,000, and cocaine 11.8%. Because of potential complications (seizures), lower concentrations of cocaine and epinephrine in a tetracaine 1% solution have been suggested (TAC III).

Study Questions

1. Local anesthetics interfere with the movement of which ion as a fundamental basis for their action?
   (A) Calcium
   (B) Sodium
   (C) Potassium
   (D) Hydrogen
   (E) Oxygen

2. Sympathetic block is one use of local anesthetics. What is the best location to apply the local anesthetic?
   (A) Nerve cell ending
   (B) Neuromuscular junction
   (C) Sympathetic ganglia
   (D) Spinal cord

3. Frequently vasoconstrictors are combined with local anesthetics to delay absorption of the anesthetic from its injection site. What is the most widely employed agent?
   (A) Dopamine
   (B) Phenylephrine
   (C) Levonordefrin
   (D) Epinephrine
   (E) Cocaine

4. What is the most commonly used local anesthetic?
   (A) Bupivacaine
   (B) Procaine
   (C) Lidocaine
   (D) Etidocaine

5. A 25-year old-woman visits your office with red and itchy eczematoid dermatitis. She had a dental procedure earlier in the day, and the dentist administered a local anesthetic. There were no other findings, although she indicated that she had a history of allergic reactions. Which of the following drugs is most likely involved?
   (A) Cocaine
   (B) Procaine
   (C) Lidocaine
   (D) Bupivacaine
   (E) Etidocaine

ANSWERS

1. **B.** Inhibition of inward migration of Na^+ can result in complete block of conduction and therefore abolition of pain transmission. This block of conduction is not a feature of alteration of any of the other ions.

2. **C.** A block at this level will affect only the sympathetic nerves, not parasympathetic activity.

Application to the nerve cell ending would result only in topical anesthesia, and blockade of the neuromuscular junction could produce respiratory failure. Administration to the spinal cord is too general an answer. The injection must be near a nerve or nerve plexus proximal to the surgical site.

3. **D.** Epinephrine is by far the most commonly employed vasoconstrictor. Phenylephrine is occasionally used with procaine for dental procedures. Levonordefrin is also used rarely in dental procedures. Dopamine has no vasoconstrictor activity. Cocaine is itself a local anesthetic with some vasoconstrictor properties. However, cocaine, because of its abuse potential and toxicity, is seldom used. Its only use is topical.

4. **C.** Lidocaine is well tolerated and has a rapid onset and an adequate duration of action for most procedures. Bupivacaine has a particularly long duration of action. This may be advantageous in certain procedures, but not in most. Procaine has a relatively slow onset of action as well as a short duration of action. Etidocaine shows a preference for motor rather than sensory block; this limits its effectiveness in obstetrics.

5. **B.** Allergic reactions occur only to the ester type of local anesthetics. This is because the metabolism of all ester-linked local anesthetics leads to the formation of PABA, which is known to be allergenic to some individuals. Both cocaine and procaine are esters. However, cocaine is not employed in dental procedures. Therefore, the best choice is procaine.

SUPPLEMENTAL READING

Denson DD and Mazoit JX. Physiology, pharmacology and toxicity of local anesthetics: Adult and pediatric considerations. In P Prithvi Raj P (ed.). Clinical Practice of Regional Anesthesia. New York: Churchill Livingstone, 1991.

McLeod GA, Burke D. Levobupivacaine. Anaesthesia. 2001;56:331.

Tucker CT and Mather LE. Properties, absorption, and disposition of local anesthetic agents. In Cousins MJ and Bridenbaugh PO (eds.). Neural Blockade in Clinical Anesthesia and Management of Pain (2nd ed.). Philadelphia: Lippincott, 1988.

Vercauteren MP et al. Levobupivacaine combined with sufentanil and epinephrine for intrathecal labor analgesia: A comparison with racemic bupivacaine. Anesth Analg 2001;93:996–1000.

CASE **Study**   A Fatality Due to Local Anesthesia

A college athlete is scheduled to undergo open repair of two fractured fingers. She is otherwise healthy, takes no medications, and has no family history of difficulties with anesthesia. The anesthetic management is to be brachial plexus anesthesia with bupivacaine. During injection of the anesthetic, the patient abruptly becomes uncommunicative and loses consciousness. The electrocardiograph deteriorates rapidly, and no blood pressure is obtainable. The trachea is intubated, cardiopulmonary resuscitation is started and advanced life support follows. Despite aggressive treatment, the resuscitation is unsuccessful. What is a possible reason for this outcome in light of the type of anesthesia being used ?

ANSWER: Bupivacaine use for local anesthesia of this type is very safe and commonly done. However, SOMETIMES inadvertent vascular injection results in a large amount of anesthetic in the systemic circulation. Because the heart is beating, the excitable tissue in the heart is being depolarized repetitively. Local anesthetics bind to rapidly depolarizing tissues more than tissues at rest (frequency-dependent block). Also, bupivacaine has a long duration of action because of its long residence time at receptors (sodium channel). Thus, this combination of factors contributed to the catastrophic outcome of this case. Had the same case involved lidocaine, the resuscitation would have likely been successful.

28 Agents Affecting Neuromuscular Transmission

Michael D. Miyamoto

DRUG LIST

GENERIC NAME	PAGE	GENERIC NAME	PAGE
4-Aminopyridine	340	Guanidine	340
Atracurium	343	Mivacurium	343
Baclofen	344	Pancuronium	343
Botulinum toxin A	340	Rapacuronium	343
Cyclobenzaprine	345	Rocuronium	343
Dantrolene	344	Succinylcholine	341
3,4-Diaminopyridine	340	d-Tubocurarine	342
Diazepam	344	Vecuronium	343

Neuromuscular transmission involves the events leading from the liberation of acetylcholine (ACh) at the motor nerve terminal to the generation of end plate currents (EPCs) at the postjunctional site. Release of ACh is initiated by membrane depolarization and influx of Ca^{++} at the nerve terminal (Fig. 28.1). This leads to a complex process involving docking and fusion of synaptic vesicles with active sites at the presynaptic membrane. Because ACh is released by exocytosis, functional transmitter release takes place in a quantal fashion. Each quantum corresponds to the contents of one synaptic vesicle (about 10,000 ACh molecules), and about 200 quanta are released with each nerve action potential.

ACh diffusing across the synaptic cleft may bind to ACh receptors (AChRs) to produce an electrical response, interact with acetylcholinesterase (AChE) and be hydrolyzed, or diffuse into the systemic circulation.

AChRs are located primarily at the peaks of the subsynaptic folds, whereas AChE is distributed uniformly in the basal lamina at the subsynaptic membrane (Fig. 28.1).

The AChR consists of five subunits surrounding an ion-conducting channel (Fig. 28.2). Activation of the binding sites on the two α-subunits results in a conformational change. This allows the simultaneous inflow of Na^+ and Ca^{++} and outflow of K^+, with a net inflow of positive charge. The response to a spontaneously secreted quantum of ACh (that is, activation of several thousand AChRs) is seen as a miniature EPC. With nerve stimulation, many quanta are released synchronously to produce a full-sized EPC, which is the summated response of the 200 or so individual miniature EPCs. The EPC is a local graded current that in normal conditions triggers an action potential in the adjacent muscle membrane (Fig. 28.1).

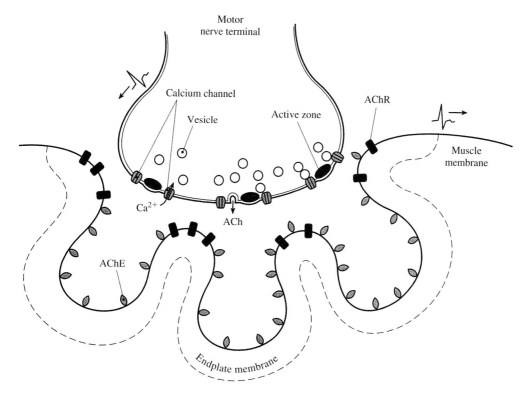

FIGURE 28.1

Neuromuscular transmission. Transmitter release at the motor nerve terminal occurs by exocytosis of synaptic vesicles that contain acetylcholine (ACh). The process is enhanced by an action potential that depolarizes the membrane and allows Ca^{++} entry through channels at the active sites. ACh may be hydrolyzed by acetylcholinesterase (AChE) or bind to receptors (AChRs) located at the peaks of the subsynaptic folds. Simultaneous activation of many AChRs produces an end plate current, which generates an action potential in the adjacent muscle membrane.

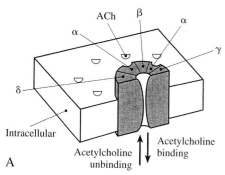

A

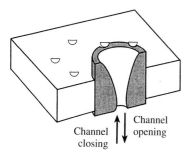

B

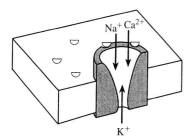

C

FIGURE 28.2

Nicotinic ACh receptor (AChR) at the muscle end plate. **A.** The AChR is a pentameric complex made up of five subunits surrounding a central conducting channel. Embryonic AChR, containing the γ-subunit as shown, is a low-conducting channel. Adult AChR has instead an ε-subunit and is a high-conducting channel. **B.** Cooperative binding of two ACh (ACh) molecules produces a conformational change that results in channel opening. **C.** The open channel allows Na$^+$ and Ca^{++} to enter and K$^+$ to exit simultaneously. The result is a net inflow of positive charge and a membrane depolarization.

Drugs may modify transmission by affecting either the release of transmitter or the interaction of ACh with its receptor. An increase in transmitter release is produced by substances that induce repetitive firing in the motor nerve, prolong the nerve action potential, or promote Ca^{++} influx at the nerve terminal. An increase in the postjunctional response is produced by drugs that inhibit AChE (and thereby increase the synaptic concentration of ACh), whereas a decrease in response is produced by drugs that block the binding sites or ion-conducting channel of the AChR.

Changes in miniature EPC frequency, amplitude, and duration can be used to identify the sites of drug action. *In general, a change in frequency indicates a prejunctional action, while a change in amplitude reflects a postjunctional effect.* Drugs that inhibit AChE give rise to a larger and more prolonged miniature EPC, whereas those that block the AChR binding site produce a decrease in miniature EPC amplitude. Agents that obstruct the open channel of the AChR cause a reduction in miniature EPC amplitude and duration.

ENHANCEMENT OF ACETYLCHOLINE RELEASE

Aminopyridines

The aminopyridines (4-aminopyridine; 3,4-diaminopyridine) accelerate spontaneous exocytosis at central and peripheral synapses. There is also an increase in the number of transmitter quanta released by a nerve action potential. This is probably the result of increased Ca^{++} inflow at the terminals due to a reduction of K^+ conductance and prolongation of the nerve action potential. Muscle strength is increased in patients with the Lambert-Eaton myasthenic syndrome and in others poisoned with botulinum E toxin (discussed later). Improvement in uncontrolled spasms, muscle tone, and pulmonary function is noted in patients with multiple sclerosis or long-standing spinal cord damage. Side effects that limit clinical utility include convulsions, restlessness, insomnia, and elevated blood pressure. Of the two agents, 3,4-diaminopyridine is the more potent and crosses the blood-brain barrier less readily.

Guanidine

Guanidine hydrochloride is the drug of choice in the management of patients with myasthenic syndrome and may be of use in the treatment of botulinum intoxication. Its ability to enhance transmitter release may involve a block of K^+ channels and prolongation of the nerve action potential.

DEPRESSION OF ACETYLCHOLINE RELEASE

Botulinum Toxin

Botulism is most commonly caused by ingestion of a neurotoxin produced by *Clostridium botulinum* in improperly canned food. Poisoning may also occur after wound contamination with the organism. Infant botulism may occur when spores of the organism germinate and manufacture the toxin in the intestinal tract of infants. *Botulinum toxin works by inhibiting ACh release at all cholinergic synapses.*

Botulinum toxins are classified into seven antigenically distinct types, A through G. Each consists of a polypeptide chain of about 150,000 daltons. All but one is nicked by trypsin-type enzymes to yield a light and heavy chain linked by a disulfide bridge. One end of the heavy chain mediates binding to the nerve terminal, and the other initiates internalization of the toxin. The light chain produces the intracellular inhibition of ACh release. This involves a Zn^{++}-dependent endopeptidase action to cleave synaptic target proteins that control vesicle docking and fusion with the prejunctional membrane.

Neuromuscular paralysis occurs 12 to 36 hours after ingestion of the toxin. Early symptoms include diplopia, dysphagia, and dysarthria. Paralysis may descend to include proximal and limb muscles and result in dyspnea and respiratory depression. The toxins do not cross the placental barrier but do enter the central nervous system (CNS). Pupil size may or may not be normal, but mental and sensory functions are not impaired. Recovery from paralysis requires days to weeks.

Reliable antidotes for botulism are not available. In some cases, anticholinesterase drugs may improve muscle strength, albeit temporarily. Guanidine and 4-aminopyridine also have limited usefulness. Management depends primarily on supportive measures, such as administering antitoxin and maintaining respiration.

Botulinum toxin is used clinically in the treatment of blepharospasm, writer's cramp, spasticities of various origins, and rigidity due to extrapyramidal disorders. It is also used to treat gustatory sweating and cosmetically to decrease facial wrinkles. Botulinum toxin A (*Botox, Oculinum*) injected intramuscularly produces functional denervation that lasts about 3 months. Clinical benefit is seen within 1 to 3 days. Adverse effects range from diplopia and irritation with blepharospasm to muscle weakness with dystonias.

Botulinum toxin is the most toxic substance known. One gram of crystalline toxin adequately dispersed can kill a population of a million people, so its use in bioterrorism is a possibility. The toxin can be introduced through inhalation or ingestion but not through dermal exposure. The threat of mass inhalation poisoning is limited by the ability or inability to aerosolize the toxin for widespread dispersion. Contaminating the water or food supply is also a possibility, although the toxin is degraded by standard water treatment and by heating of foods to 85°C (185°F) for 5 minutes. Prior immunization with toxoid vaccine is advisable for personnel at risk, but prophylactic administration of trivalent equine antitoxin is not recommended.

Lambert-Eaton Myasthenic Syndrome

Lambert-Eaton myasthenic syndrome (LEMS) is an autoimmune disease that is often associated with small-cell lung carcinoma. It is characterized by fatigability, hyporeflexia, and autonomic dysfunction. The neuromuscular junction appears normal in morphology, and postjunctional receptor function is unchanged. However, particles at the active zones of nerve terminals that correspond to Ca^{++} channels are reduced in number and disorganized, and patients with LEMS have high titers of antibodies against the prejunctional P/Q-type Ca^{++} channel. Thus, *muscle weakness results from impaired influx of Ca^{++} and diminished release of ACh.* Diagnosis is confirmed by an incremental increase in electromyographic recordings upon repetitive stimulation.

Treatment with guanidine may produce clinical improvement within 3 to 4 days. Side effects include paresthesia, gastrointestinal distress, renal tubular necrosis, and hyperirritability. The most serious effect is bone marrow depression, which is dose-related and potentially fatal. Aminopyridines have been used in clinical studies with some positive results. Corticosteroids and plasmapheresis may also be of some benefit, whereas anticholinesterase agents are only marginally effective.

DEPRESSION OF POSTJUNCTIONAL RESPONSE TO ACETYLCHOLINE

Neurotoxins

α-Bungarotoxin (α-BTX), isolated from snake venom, is a protein that binds selectively and irreversibly to the AChR of muscle. Because binding of the toxin is irreversible, recovery from α-BTX block indicates synthesis and insertion of new AChR into the membrane. Studies using α-BTX show that the AChR is a glycoprotein consisting of five polypeptide subunits (α, β, γ, δ, and ε). The complex is a cylindrical unit about 8 nm in diameter that spans the plasma membrane (Fig. 28.2).

Histrionicotoxin, obtained from a Panamanian frog, is a toxin that attaches to a high-affinity site within the pore of the AChR complex and results in muscular

blockade. Agents that have a similar effect include local anesthetics, barbiturates, and phencyclidine. They reduce the flow of ions and shorten the duration of time the channel is open.

The AChR in muscle is distinct from the AChRs found in the central and autonomic nervous systems (neuronal AChRs). Although both are activated by nicotine, each is blocked by a different antagonist (e.g., α-BTX vs. κ-BTX).

Myasthenia Gravis

The "acquired" form of myasthenia gravis (MG) is an autoimmune disease with an incidence approaching 1 in 10,000. It involves an antibody response against part of the α-subunit of the AChR in muscle. This leads to degradation of AChRs, reduction of synaptic infoldings, and weakness due to diminished postjunctional response. Because anti-AChR antibodies are found in nearly 90% of MG patients, serum testing can serve as a diagnostic tool. MG is often found associated with abnormalities of the thymus, which contains a protein that is immunologically related to muscle AChR.

Standard treatment consists of anti-AChE agents such as pyridostigmine, whose effect is long-lasting and predictable. A short acting anti-AchE, such as edrophonium, can be used to differentiate between a *myasthenic crisis* (insufficient treatment) and a *cholinergic crisis* (overtreatment with anti-AChEs). Thymectomy is a good option for patients under 50 years of age. Immunosuppressive agents, such as corticosteroids and possibly azathioprine or cyclosporine A, are also effective. Plasmapheresis is beneficial, but the effect is transient.

NEUROMUSCULAR BLOCKING AGENTS

Depolarizing Blocker (Succinylcholine)

Succinylcholine chloride (*Anectine*) is the only depolarizing-type blocker that is in widespread clinical use. *It produces neuromuscular block by overstimulation, so that the end plate is unable to respond to further stimulation.* Structurally, succinylcholine is equivalent to two ACh molecules joined back to back. The resulting 10-carbon atom spacing between the two quaternary ammonium heads is important for activation of the two binding sites on the AChR. Because the succinylcholine molecule is "thin," binding to the two sites does not sterically occlude the open channel, and cations are allowed to flow and depolarize the end plate.

Neuromuscular block with succinylcholine occurs by two sequential events. An initial depolarization of the end plate produces muscle action potentials and fasciculation. Maintained depolarization past the threshold for firing produces Na^+ channel inactivation, so that muscle action potentials cannot be generated. This is called *phase I*, or *depolarization block*. In the continued presence of succinylcholine, the membrane becomes repolarized, Na^+ channel inactivation is reversed, and muscle membrane excitability is restored. Nonetheless, the neuromuscular block persists because of desensitization of the AChR. This is known as *phase II*, or *desensitization block*.

Although the mechanism for phase II block is not completely understood, a series of allosteric transitions in the AChR is suspected. One model to describe this has the AChR in equilibrium among four conformations: resting, active, inactive, and desensitized. Agonists stabilize the active and desensitized states, whereas antagonists tend to stabilize the resting and possibly the desensitized state.

Absorption, Metabolism, and Excretion

Succinylcholine is given systemically because the molecule is charged and does not easily cross membranes. It is rapidly hydrolyzed by plasma cholinesterase to succinylmonocholine, which is pharmacologically inactive. Because plasma cholinesterase is synthesized in the liver, neuromuscular block may be prolonged in patients with liver disease. About 10% of succinylcholine is excreted unchanged in the urine. The response to succinylcholine may also be prolonged in individuals with a genetic defect leading to atypical plasma cholinesterase (homozygous incidence of about 1 in 2,500). In this case, the enzyme has a decreased affinity for substrates such as succinylcholine that can be measured by the dibucaine test.

Pharmacological Actions

Succinylcholine acts primarily at the skeletal neuromuscular junction and has little effect at autonomic ganglia or at postganglionic cholinergic (muscarinic) junctions. Actions at these sites attributed to succinylcholine may arise from the effects of choline. Succinylcholine has no direct action on the uterus or other smooth muscle structures. It does not enter the CNS and does not cross the placental barrier. It may, however, release histamine from mast cells. Because succinylcholine works by stimulating rather than blocking end plate receptors, *anti-AChEs will not reverse muscle paralysis and may actually prolong the block.*

Clinical Uses

The principal advantage of succinylcholine is its rapid and ultra-short action. With intravenous (IV) administration, succinylcholine produces flaccid paralysis that occurs in less than 1 minute and lasts about 10 minutes. This makes it suitable for short-term procedures, such as endotracheal intubation, setting of fractures, and pre-

vention of injury during electroconvulsive therapy. Apart from its rapid onset and brief action, succinylcholine has few benefits and many disadvantages.

Adverse Effects and Contraindications

Succinylcholine produces muscle fasciculation, which may result in myoglobinuria and postoperative muscle pain. The amount produced depends on the level of physical fitness. Succinylcholine causes contractions of extraocular muscles, posing the danger of transient elevated intraocular pressure. Succinylcholine may produce hyperkalemia in patients with large masses of traumatized or denervated muscle (e.g., spinal cord injury). Denervated muscle is especially sensitive to depolarizing drugs because of the increased number of AChRs on the sarcolemma (denervation supersensitivity). Succinylcholine also causes prolonged contraction of the diseased muscles of patients with myotonia or amyotrophic lateral sclerosis.

Succinylcholine-induced hyperkalemia may lead to cardiac arrhythmia and arrest when plasma K^+ reaches 7 and 10 mM, respectively. The drug also may precipitate a fulminant attack of malignant hyperthermia in susceptible individuals (not to be confused with neuroleptic malignant hyperpyrexia, which involves dopamine and the CNS). Treatment in either case consists of cooling the body and administering oxygen and dantrolene sodium (discussed later).

Nondepolarizing Blockers: d-Tubocurarine, Atracurium, Mivacurium, Pancuronium, Vecuronium, Rocuronium, and Rapacuronium
Mechanism of Action

With the exception of succinylcholine, all neuromuscular blocking agents are nondepolarizing. These agents prevent excitation of end plate AChRs by acting as reversible competitive antagonists at the binding sites. The prototype for this group is *d*-tubocurarine, an alkaloid used as a South American arrow poison. In general, these compounds have two charged heads (e.g., quaternary ammonium) separated by a "thick" organic moiety (e.g., steroid nucleus). These heads enable attachment of the drug to the two AChR binding sites. However, because of the large intervening moiety, the channel is occluded such that the flow of cations is prevented. Because of the competitive nature of this blockade, *the effect of nondepolarizing blockers can be reversed by anti-AChE agents* and other procedures that increase the synaptic concentration of ACh.

Pharmacological Actions

d-Tubocurarine blocks nicotinic AChRs in muscle end plates and autonomic ganglia but has no effect on mus-

carinic AChRs. It does not affect nerve or muscle excitability or conduction of action potentials. Because it is charged, it penetrates cells poorly and does not enter the CNS. However, if applied directly to brain or spinal cord, it will block nicotinic AChR in those tissues. In humans, *d*-tubocurarine has a moderate onset of action (3-4 minutes) followed by progressive flaccid paralysis. The head and neck muscles are affected initially, then the limb muscles, and finally the muscles of respiration. Recovery from paralysis is in the reverse order.

Clinical Uses

Nondepolarizing blockers are used to relax skeletal muscle for surgical procedures, to prevent dislocations and fractures associated with electroconvulsive therapy, and to control muscle spasms in tetanus. *They do not produce anesthesia or analgesia.*

The degree of blockade can be influenced by body pH and electrolyte balance. Hypokalemia due to diarrhea, renal disease, or use of potassium-depleting diuretics potentiates the effect of nondepolarizing blockers. By contrast, hyperkalemia may oppose the actions of *d*-tubocurarine but enhance the end plate response to succinylcholine. The effectiveness of *d*-tubocurarine is reduced by alkalosis.

Newborn children are extremely sensitive to nondepolarizing muscle relaxants but may require three times as much depolarizing agent as an adult for an equivalent degree of block. Like newborn children, patients with myasthenia gravis are very sensitive to paralysis by *d*-tubocurarine but are resistant to succinylcholine. This altered responsiveness is probably due to the fewer number of *functional* AChRs at the end plate. Since neonates are very sensitive to *d*-tubocurarine, the dosage must be reduced and the degree of block closely monitored.

Adverse Effects and Precautions

d-Tubocurarine may cause bronchospasms and hypotension by release of histamine from mast cells. This may be counteracted by prior treatment with antihistamines. *d*-Tubocurarine produces partial block of sympathetic ganglia and the adrenal medulla, which may also contribute to hypotension.

Inhalation anesthetics, such as isoflurane, enflurane, halothane, and nitrous oxide, potentiate the action of nondepolarizing blockers, either through modification of end plate responsiveness or by alteration of local blood flow. The extent of potentiation depends on the anesthetic and the depth of anesthesia. The dose of muscle relaxant should be reduced when used with these anesthetics.

Certain antibiotics (e.g., aminoglycosides, macrolides, polymyxins, lincomycin) enhance neuromuscular blockade by either decreasing ACh release or blocking the postjunctional response. Procainamide and phenytoin also increase the effects of *d*-tubocurarine-like drugs. The amount of neuromuscular blocker should be decreased accordingly.

Other Nondepolarizing Blockers of Importance

Atracurium besylate (*Tracrium*) is a benzylisoquinolinium compound like *d*-tubocurarine. Its actions are similar to those of *d*-tubocurarine, but its duration of action is shorter (45 minutes) because of spontaneous degradation of the molecule (Hofmann elimination). Because of this, atracurium is useful in patients with low or atypical plasma cholinesterase and in patients with renal or hepatic impairment.

Mivacurium chloride (*Mivacron*) is a newer agent that is chemically related to atracurium. The primary mechanism of inactivation is hydrolysis by plasma cholinesterase. Although it is useful for patients with renal or hepatic disease, some caution is warranted, since these individuals may have reduced plasma cholinesterase as a result of the disease. Mivacurium has an onset of action (1.8 minutes) and duration of effect (20 minutes) only twice that of succinylcholine, and in this respect, it is the most similar to succinylcholine of all of the nondepolarizing agents.

Pancuronium bromide (*Pavulon*) is a synthetic bisquaternary agent containing a steroid nucleus (amino steroid), as denoted by the -curonium suffix. It is five times as potent as *d*-tubocurarine. Unlike *d*-tubocurarine, it does not release histamine or block ganglionic transmission. Like *d*-tubocurarine, it has a moderately long onset (2.9 minutes) and duration of action (110 minutes). Pancuronium and its metabolite are eliminated in the urine.

Vecuronium bromide (*Norcuron*) is chemically identical to pancuronium except for a tertiary amine in place of a quaternary nitrogen. However, some of the drug will exist as the bisquaternary compound, depending on body pH. Vecuronium has a moderate onset of action (2.4 minutes) and a duration of effect of about 50 minutes. Like pancuronium, it does not block ganglia or vagal neuroeffector junctions, does not release histamine, and is eliminated by urinary excretion.

Rocuronium bromide (*Zemuron*) is a recently approved amino steroid neuromuscular blocking agent. It has a rapid onset of action (1 minute), but its duration of action is intermediate (55 minutes), about that of vecuronium. On rare occasions, it may release histamine and cause cardiac irregularities. Rapacuronium bromide (*Raplon*) is the most recent neuromuscular blocking agent approved by the United States Food and Drug Administration (FDA). It is an analogue of vecuronium and is thus categorized as an amino steroid. It has a rapid onset of action (1.5 minutes) and a short to intermediate duration of action (20 minutes). This makes it a suitable alternative to mivacurium or succinylcholine for short procedures. It is eliminated mainly by the liver. Adverse effects are dose dependent; they include tachycardia, hypotension, and bronchospasm. These effects may be related to the ability of the drug to release a small amount of histamine.

PHARMACOLOGY OF ANTISPASTICITY AGENTS

Muscle relaxants have some value for relief of spastic muscle disorders, that is, a state of increased muscle tone that results from an imbalance between central and spinal control of muscle tone. *Spasticity* is the result of a general release from supraspinal control and is characterized by heightened excitability of α- and γ-motor systems and the appearance of primitive spinal cord reflexes. Treatment is difficult, since relief often can be achieved only at the price of increased muscle weakness.

Baclofen

Baclofen (*Lioresal*) is the parachlorophenol analogue of the naturally occurring neurotransmitter γ-aminobutyric acid (GABA).

Mechanism of Action

Baclofen appears to affect the neuromuscular axis by acting directly on sensory afferents, γ-motor neurons, and collateral neurons in the spinal cord to inhibit both monosynaptic and polysynaptic reflexes. The principal effect is to reduce the release of excitatory neurotransmitters by activation of presynaptic $GABA_B$ receptors. This seems to involve a G protein and second-messenger link that either increases K^+ conductance or decreases Ca^{++} conductance.

Absorption, Metabolism, and Excretion

Baclofen is rapidly and effectively absorbed after oral administration. It is lipophilic and able to penetrate the blood-brain barrier. Approximately 35% of the drug is excreted unchanged in the urine and feces.

Clinical Uses

Baclofen is an agent of choice for treating spinal spasticity and spasticity associated with multiple sclerosis. It is not useful for treating spasticity of supraspinal origin. Doses should be increased gradually to a maximum of 100 to 150 mg per day, divided into four doses.

Adverse Effects

Side effects are not a major problem, and they can be minimized by graduated dosage increases. They include lassitude, slight nausea, and mental disturbances (in-

cluding confusion, euphoria, and depression). The drowsiness is less pronounced than that produced by diazepam—an important therapeutic advantage. Hypotension has been noted, particularly following overdose. Elderly patients and patients with multiple sclerosis may require lower doses and may display increased sensitivity to the central side effects. Baclofen may increase the frequency of seizures in epileptics.

Benzodiazepines

Benzodiazepines also possess muscle relaxant activity. Their pharmacology is discussed in Chapter 30. Diazepam (*Valium*) has been used for control of flexor and extensor spasms, spinal spasticity, and multiple sclerosis. The muscle relaxant effect of the benzodiazepines may be mediated by an action on the primary afferents in the spinal cord, resulting in an increased level of presynaptic inhibition of muscle tone. Polysynaptic reflexes are inhibited. The most troublesome side effect is drowsiness, which is dose dependent. Tolerance to both the therapeutic effects and the side effects develops.

Dantrolene Sodium

Dantrolene sodium (*Dantrium*) is used in the treatment of spasticity due to stroke, spinal injury, multiple sclerosis, or cerebral palsy. *It is also the drug of choice in prophylaxis or treatment of malignant hyperthermia.* Susceptibility to malignant hyperthermia is due to a rare genetic defect that allows Ca^{++} release from the sarcoplasmic reticulum to open more easily and close less readily than normal. This leads to a high level of Ca^{++} in the sarcoplasm, which produces muscle rigidity, oxygen consumption, and heat. Dantrolene acts by blocking Ca^{++} release from the sarcoplasmic reticulum and uncoupling excitation from contraction.

Dantrolene is active orally, although its absorption is slow and incomplete. Its biological half-life ($t_{1/2}$) is 8.7 hours in adults. The drug is metabolized by liver microsomal enzymes and is eliminated in the urine and bile. It is given IV when treating an attack of malignant hyperthermia.

The most prominent and often limiting feature of dantrolene administration is dose-dependent muscle weakness. Other side effects are drowsiness, dizziness, malaise, fatigue, and diarrhea. Symptomatic hepatitis is reported in 0.5% of patients receiving it and fatal hepatitis in up to 0.2%. Contraindications include respiratory muscle weakness and liver disease. It is suggested that patients on dantrolene therapy be given regular liver function tests.

Central Skeletal Muscle Relaxants

The central skeletal muscle relaxants are a chemically diverse group of compounds that have limited utility in relieving the signs and symptoms of local muscle spasm. None has been shown to be superior to analgesic–antiinflammatory agents for the relief of acute or chronic muscle spasm, although all are superior to placebo. Most of these drugs have mild sedative properties, and their muscle relaxant activity may be a direct result of sedation. Experimentally, *all centrally active skeletal muscle relaxants preferentially depress spinal polysynaptic reflexes over monosynaptic reflexes.*

Most of the agents have similar actions, and therefore, the same adverse reactions are seen. These consist most commonly of drowsiness, dizziness, and light-headedness. One agent, cyclobenzaprine (*Flexeril*), has a prominent anticholinergic component and frequently causes dryness of the mouth along with sedation and dizziness.

In addition to being employed alone, many of these compounds are available in combination with a nonopioid analgesic, caffeine, or both. Because of their limited utility, they are not be considered individually. Some of the approved agents are listed in Table 28.1.

TABLE 28.1 Some Centrally Acting Skeletal Muscle Relaxants

Generic name	Trade name
Carisoprodol	Rela, Soma
Chlorzoxazone	Paraflex
Cyclobenzaprine	Flexeril
Methocarbamol	Robaxin, Delaxin
Orphenadrine	Norflex

Study QUESTIONS

1. Which of the following agents produces its therapeutic action by causing a nondepolarizing block of end plate receptors at the skeletal neuromuscular junction?
(A) Hexamethonium
(B) Nicotine
(C) Rapacuronium
(D) Scopolamine
(E) Succinylcholine

2. A 50-year-old white man is found to have 90% blockage of his coronary arteries and is prepared for bypass surgery. For preanesthetic medication, he is given atropine to block secretions and a mild sedative to reduce anxiety and induce sedation. He is then given an IV bolus of succinylcholine to facilitate endotracheal intubation. Induction of general anesthesia with enthrane is begun with no major complications. However, shortly thereafter, the patient displays muscle rigidity and a rapid increase in temperature. He is quickly cooled with ice packs, switched to 100% oxygen, and then given an IV bolus of which of the following?
(A) Atropine
(B) Baclofen
(C) Dantrolene
(D) Diazepam
(E) Neostigmine

3. A former respiratory therapist who once called himself the Angel of Death was charged in the deaths of six elderly nursing home patients. Their exhumed bodies all contained a drug that halts breathing, even though the drug was not part of their therapeutic regimen. Toxicological tests identified the drug as a muscle relaxant. Which of the following is the most likely agent used?

(A) Baclofen
(B) Mecamylamine
(C) Pancuronium
(D) Pyridostigmine
(E) Succinylcholine

4. Which of the following adjuvants to anesthesia has the potential to cause hyperkalemia, postoperative muscle pain, muscle fasciculation, and prolonged apnea and paralysis in genetically sensitive patients?
(A) Atracurium
(B) Diazepam
(C) Edrophonium
(D) Rocuronium
(E) Succinylcholine

5. A 45-year-old man in otherwise good health complains of muscle weakness early in the morning but says it is less of a problem as the day goes on. The neurologist performs electromyography and notes no alteration in nerve conduction velocity but does observe facilitation in the compound action potential with repetitive 50-Hz stimulation. This indicates a defect at the prejunctional side of the neuromuscular junction. Which of the following is a possible cause?
(A) Autonomic hyperreflexia
(B) Atypical plasma cholinesterase
(C) Lambert-Eaton myasthenic syndrome
(D) Malignant hyperthermia
(E) Myasthenia gravis

6. Which of the following agents blocks the release of neurotransmitter from all cholinergic nerve endings?
(A) Atracurium
(B) Baclofen

(C) Botulinum toxin
(D) Diazepam
(E) Rocuronium

7. A 45-year-old African-American woman diagnosed with myasthenia gravis was prescribed pyridostigmine with a resulting improvement in muscle strength. Several months later, she felt a loss of strength and increased her dose of pyridostigmine. She now complains of significant muscle weakness. The neurologist administers edrophonium, which produces no significant improvement, and the diagnosis is cholinergic crisis. Treatment should consist of which of the following options?
(A) Replacing pyridostigmine with pancuronium
(B) Replacing pyridostigmine with neostigmine
(C) Giving dantrolene to decrease sarcoplasmic release of calcium
(D) Adding succinylcholine to her regimen
(E) Allowing pyridostigmine to be eliminated

ANSWERS

1. **C.** Rapacuronium is a skeletal muscle relaxant that works by competing with ACh for receptors at the postjunctional membrane. Nicotine and succinylcholine also act at the end plate receptors but cause depolarization. Hexamethonium is a ganglion blocker that has essentially no activity at the end plate receptors, and scopolamine blocks cholinergic muscarinic receptors and thus does not act at the end plate receptors.

2. **C.** The patient has a rare genetic defect that results in susceptibility to malignant hyperthermia. Acute attacks are manifested by heat generation, muscle rigidity, and high oxygen consumption, all of which can lead to lactic acidosis. It has a fatality rate in excess of 70% if left untreated. Attacks can be precipitated by stress or infection but are generally a result of using succinylcholine and certain gaseous anesthetics. These appear to trigger excessive release of Ca^{++} from the sarcoplasmic reticulum due to a defect in the calcium release channels. Dantrolene acts by blocking the release of Ca^{++} and is the standard treatment for this reaction.

3. **C.** Pancuronium is a nondepolarizing neuromuscular blocking agent. The depolarizing neuromuscular blocking agent succinylcholine may also appear to be a viable possibility. However, it can be excluded, since it is rapidly broken down to natural products by plasma cholinesterase and would not have been detected by the toxicological tests. Because of this, succinylcholine and potassium chloride can be used to kill without leaving evidence of a foreign substance. Pyridostigmine is an anticholinesterase that can be used to reverse the effect of nondepolarizing blockers. Mecamylamine is a ganglion blocker that has no effect at the neuromuscular junction, and ba-

clofen is a centrally acting relaxant that would not be effective in causing respiratory paralysis.

4. **E.** Succinylcholine is the only depolarizing neuromuscular blocking in widespread clinical use, particularly as an aid for intubation. Its administration may produce muscle fasciculation and postoperative muscle pain. It can produce hyperkalemia in patients with muscle damage or prolonged paralysis in patients with atypical plasma cholinesterase.

5. **C.** Lambert-Eaton myasthenic syndrome is a rare disorder of autoimmune attack against calcium channels of the presynaptic motor nerve ending. The result is diminished release of ACh manifested as muscle weakness. In these patients, repetitive stimulation promotes facilitation of transmitter release, and this is seen clinically as an improvement in muscle strength with increased physical activity. This is the opposite of myasthenia gravis, the autoimmune attack against postjunctional ACh receptors, in which muscle strength decreases with increased physical activity. Autonomic hyperreflexia is a syndrome found in patients with spinal cord damage in which central inhibition of reflexes is impaired. Atypical plasma cholinesterase does not affect neuromuscular transmission except with regard to breakdown of succinylcholine. Malignant hyperthermia is due to a defect in the contractile apparatus of skeletal muscle and not in neuromuscular transmission.

6. **C.** Botulinum toxin works by preventing exocytosis of ACh from all cholinergic nerve endings. Atracurium and rocuronium are nondepolarizing neuromuscular blockers that act specifically at the postjunctional receptors of the skeletal neuromuscular junction. Baclofen and diazepam are centrally acting muscle relaxants that stimulate presynaptic $GABA_B$ receptors and benzodiazepine sites on postsynaptic $GABA_A$ receptors, respectively.

7. **E.** Cholinergic crisis occurs when patients are overtreated with anticholinesterases, that is,, when acetylcholinesterase at the neuromuscular junction is inhibited and ACh levels increase in the synaptic cleft. An extreme example is seen with organophosphate poisoning, that is, exposure to nerve gases or industrial insecticides such as parathion. This can lead to depolarization and desensitization of the end plate receptors so that they cannot respond to further stimulation by ACh. Unlike the irreversible organophosphates, pyridostigmine has a short to intermediate duration of action, and treatment should be to allow pyridostigmine to be eliminated by normal pathways.

SUPPLEMENTAL READING

Becker R, Alberti O, and Bauer BL. Continuous intrathecal baclofen infusion in severe spasticity after traumatic or hypoxic brain injury. J Neurol 1997;244:160–166.

Booij LHDJ. Neuromuscular transmission and its pharmacological blockade. Part 1: Neuromuscular transmission and general aspects of its blockade. Pharmacy World Sci 1997;19:1–12.

Drachman DB. Immunotherapy in neuromuscular disorders: Current and future strategies. Muscle Nerve 1996;19:1239–1251.

Kaminski HJ and Ruff RL. The myasthenic syndromes. In Schultz SG, Andreoli TE, Brown AM (eds.). Molecular Biology of Membrane Transport Disorders. New York: Plenum, 1996.

Kessler KR and Benecke R. Botulinum toxin: From poison to remedy. Neurotoxicol 1997;18: 761–770.

Leuwer M. Neuromuscular blocking agents and skeletal muscle relaxants. In Dukes MNG, Aronson JK (eds.). Meyler's Side Effects of Drugs. Amsterdam: Elsevier, 2000.

Shapiro RL, Hatheway C, and Swerdlow DL. Botulism in the United States: A clinical and epidemiologic review. Ann Intern Med 1998;129:221–228.

Sparr HJ, Beaufort TM, and Fuchs-Buder T. Newer neuromuscular blocking agents: How do they compare with established agents? Drugs 2001;61:919–942.

Vincent A and Wray D (eds.). Neuromuscular Transmission: Basic and Applied Aspects. New York: Pergamon, 1992.

Vincent A, Palace J, and Hilton-Jones D. Myasthenia gravis. Lancet 2001;357:2122–2128.

Wittbrodt ET. Drugs and myasthenia gravis: An update. Arch Intern Med 1997;157:399–408.

C A S E **Study**   **Generalized Muscle Weakness**

A 30-year-old white woman is referred to a neurologist after complaining of a general loss of strength at the end of the day and drooping eyelids that make reading difficult. Electromyography on the adductor pollicis using train-of-four 50-Hz stimulation reveals a progressive decrease in the compound muscle action potential. After establishing the patient's baseline strength with a tonometer, she is given one-sixth the normal paralytic dose of mivacurium IV, which results in a decrease in measured strength. Subsequent administration of edrophonium results in an improvement in muscle strength to above baseline values. The neurologist prescribes oral pyridostigmine and prednisone, which lead to clinical improvement over the next few weeks. Further laboratory tests disclose that the patient has a thymoma and increased titers of antinuclear antibodies. Following removal of the thymoma, the patient no longer shows signs of muscle weakness and appears to be in remission. What is your diagnosis?

ANSWER: The patient shows classic signs of myasthenia gravis, an autoimmune disease that results from antibody attack against the end plate receptors of skeletal muscle and leads to muscle weakness. The disease may be triggered by disorders of the thymus, which contains a protein antigenically related to skeletal muscle receptors. The train-of-four stimulation is used to differentiate between a prejunctional cause of weakness (such as Lambert-Eaton myasthenic syndrome, which normally shows facilitation in the action potentials) and a postjunctional cause (such as myasthenia gravis). Use of a short-acting nondepolarizing neuromuscular blocker (mivacurium) followed by a short-acting acetylcholinesterase inhibitor (edrophonium) is an almost conclusive test for myasthenia gravis. In many instances, edrophonium alone may be used (the Tensilon test). Pyridostigmine is a long-acting cholinesterase inhibitor that can provide palliative relief, whereas prednisone is used to suppress the autoimmune process. The finding of a thymoma presents the possibility that removal may eliminate the source of the autoimmunity and lead to remission.

29 Central Nervous System Stimulants

David A. Taylor

DRUG LIST

GENERIC NAME	PAGE	GENERIC NAME	PAGE
Amphetamine	350	Pemoline	350
Caffeine	351	Pentylenetetrazol	349
Doxapram	349	Sibutramine	351
Fenfluramine	351	Phentermine	351
Methamphetamine	350	Theobromine	351
Methylphenidate	350	Theophylline	351
Modafenil	351		

Central nervous system (CNS) stimulation is the primary action of a diverse group of pharmacological agents and an adverse effect associated with the administration of an even larger group of drugs. CNS stimulation consists of a range of behaviors including mild elevation in alertness, increased nervousness and anxiety, and convulsions.

In general, any hyperexcitability associated with drug administration (as either a desired or an undesired effect) results from an alteration in the fine balance normally maintained in the CNS between excitatory and inhibitory influences. Thus, the bases for CNS stimulation by this class of drugs reside in adjusting the integration of excitatory and inhibitory influences at the level of the individual neuron. An agent that induces CNS stimulation appears to act by one or more of the following mechanisms: (1) potentiation or enhancement of excitatory neurotransmission, (2) depression or antagonism of inhibitory neurotransmission, and (3) altered presynaptic control of neurotransmitter release.

Although the use of CNS stimulants (also known as *analeptics* or *convulsants*) has declined, certain compounds within this category do possess some clinical utility. Historically, general CNS stimulants were used primarily as respiratory stimulants in the treatment of acute overdosage with CNS depressants (e.g., barbiturates). Several factors have contributed to the almost complete lack of use of CNS stimulants in this clinical situation. First, since the stimulants were not *specific* antagonists of the depressant agents, they frequently were not effective in reversing severe pharmacologically induced CNS depression. Second, the duration of action of the CNS stimulant was generally shorter than that of the depressant. Third, the dose of most CNS stimulants required to reverse severe CNS depression was quite close to the dose that produced convulsions and cardiac arrhythmias. In such cases, the CNS stimulant often exacerbated the clinical picture by producing severe life-threatening complications. Another factor contributing to the decline in CNS stimulant use for drug-induced CNS depression has been the development of generally safer procedures for patient management. Supportive measures (e.g., maintenance of a patent airway, elevation of low blood pressure) often provide greater bene-

TABLE 29.1   Classification of CNS Stimulants

Analeptic Stimulants	Psychomotor Stimulants	Methylxanthines
Doxapram	Amphetamine	Caffeine
Nikethamide	Methamphetamine	Theophylline
Pentylenetetrazol	Methylphenidate	Theobromine
Strychnine	Pemoline	
Picrotoxin	Ephedrine	
Bicuculline	Phentermine	
	Fenfluramine	
	Phenylpropanolamine	

fit to the patient than does the use of analeptic drugs. Tolerance and abuse potential are additional problems associated with the use of such psychomotor stimulants as amphetamine and many of its congeners.

Compounds that possess as their primary action the stimulation of the CNS can be divided into three major categories (Table 29.1) based on either their proposed mechanism of action or their chemical structure. Each class of compounds is discussed in general terms, and individual drugs are mentioned only as appropriate.

ANALEPTIC STIMULANTS

Chemistry and Pharmacokinetics

The analeptic stimulants are a diverse chemical class of agents ranging from plant alkaloids, such as picrotoxin and strychnine, to synthetic compounds, such as pentylenetetrazol and doxapram. The wide range of chemical structures makes this particular class somewhat difficult to categorize with respect to absorption, distribution, and metabolism. However, most analeptic stimulants can be absorbed orally and have short durations of action. The pharmacological effect of most of these compounds is terminated through hepatic metabolism rather than renal excretion of unchanged drug.

Mechanism of Action

Perhaps the most unifying concept concerning the mode of action of these agents comes from studies of the γ-aminobutyric acid (GABA) receptor–chloride ionophore interaction. It has long been recognized that the inhibitory action of many amino acid neurotransmitters (e.g., GABA) involves an increase in chloride conductance. Thus, GABA and other inhibitory amino acids actively promote an increase in chloride influx by activation of the chloride channel in the neuronal membrane. An increase in chloride conductance generally leads to mem-

brane *hyperpolarization* and a reduction in the probability of action potential generation (i.e., inhibition of neuronal activity). With GABA in particular, the interaction appears to occur through specific membrane-associated GABA$_A$-receptors that form an integral part of the chloride channel (see Chapter 24). The chloride channel appears to contain other regulatory sites with high affinity for such agents as the benzodiazepines, picrotoxin, alcohol, neuroactive steroids, and the barbiturates.

Chloride movement across neuronal membranes can be regulated at this ion channel by at least three distinct molecular entities: (1) a GABA-binding site, (2) a benzodiazepine-binding site, and (3) a picrotoxin-binding site. GABA and other agonists open the chloride channel (i.e., increase chloride conductance). Benzodiazepine-induced facilitation of GABA-mediated increases in chloride conduction are antagonized by pentylenetetrazol and possibly by the methylxanthines, while picrotoxin closes the chloride channel. Other agents that appear to promote chloride conductance through this channel include the barbiturates and alcohol.

The existence of the chloride channel as a major site of drug action permits a single molecular event (control of chloride ion movement) to be involved in the mechanism of action of a diverse class of agents.

Strychnine is an analeptic stimulant with a well-defined mechanism of action that is unrelated to interaction with GABA receptors or other sites that modulate the activity of the chloride ionophore. Strychnine appears to be a specific competitive postsynaptic antagonist of glycine. Glycine, like GABA, is a known inhibitory transmitter in the mammalian CNS. Whereas GABA is likely to be more important in the brain, glycine is more important in the spinal cord. Glycine mediates inhibition of spinal cord neurons and is intimately involved in the regulation of spinal cord and brainstem reflexes. *Strychnine directly antagonizes this inhibition, allowing excitatory impulses to be greatly exaggerated.*

Clinical Uses

As indicated, most of the analeptic stimulants were used as pharmacological treatments for overdosage of CNS depressants. Doxapram (*Dopram*) *is sometimes used to counteract postanesthetic respiratory depression and as an aid in chronic obstructive pulmonary disease.* Pentylenetetrazol (*Metrazol*) was used experimentally on rare occasions to "activate" the electroencephalogram. Strychnine is used almost exclusively in animal studies as a tool for studying CNS mechanisms because it is a relatively specific glycine antagonist.

Adverse Effects

Most of the CNS stimulants produce adverse reactions that are extensions of their therapeutic effect. These

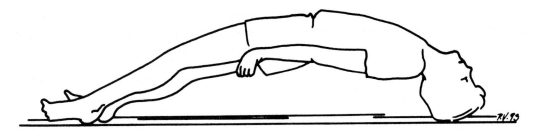

FIGURE 29.1
Patient in opisthotonos.

agents produce convulsions that can be followed by coma and death. Convulsions produced by this class of agents (with the exception of strychnine) are usually tonic–clonic and are uncoordinated. In some cases, the convulsions are preceded by marked stimulation of respiration, tachycardia, and excessive pressor effects.

The uncontrolled excitation that occurs after accidental or intentional strychnine ingestion (in the absence of normal inhibition) results in characteristic convulsions. In humans, in whom extensor muscles are normally dominant, tonic extension of the body and all limbs is observed. This hyperextension is known as *opisthotonos;* at its extreme, it consists of a characteristic posture in which the back is arched and only the back of the head and the heels are touching the surface on which the victim is lying. Figure 29.1 illustrates a patient in opisthotonos. Under the influence of strychnine, all sensory stimuli produce exaggerated responses. The primary therapeutic consideration after strychnine poisoning is to prevent convulsions, which may be fatal. Diazepam and clonazepam (see Chapter 33) appear to be moderately effective in preventing strychnine convulsions, and either of these is the agent of choice. Barbiturates are often used to treat overdoses of all of the analeptic stimulants. Generally, however, antidotal therapy is not required.

PSYCHOMOTOR STIMULANTS

Pharmacokinetics

Many psychomotor stimulants possess activities similar to those of amphetamine and have been discussed previously (see Chapter 10). Of primary importance to our discussion of the psychomotor stimulants are amphetamine (*Adderall, Benzedrine, Dexedrine*), methamphetamine (*Desoxyn*), and methylphenidate (*Concerta, Ritalin, Metadate, Methylin*).

All of these compounds are well absorbed after oral administration, leaving injectable forms with few legitimate applications. Although several catabolic pathways metabolize the amphetamines, a considerable portion of untransformed drug is excreted in the urine. Thus, it is possible to ion-trap this weak organic base by acidifying the urine, thereby reducing its reabsorption in the renal tubules and enhancing its clearance.

Mechanism of Action

There is good evidence that the facilitation of peripheral sympathetic nervous system transmission produced by the amphetamines also occurs in the CNS. The possibility that amphetamines act indirectly (i.e., by releasing monoamines) at monoaminergic synapses in the brain and spinal cord seems likely. However, amphetamine has effects beyond displacement of catecholamines; these include inhibition of neuronal amine uptake, direct stimulation of dopamine and serotonin receptors, antagonism of catecholamine action at certain subtypes of adrenoceptors, and inhibition of monoamine oxidase. Interestingly, none of these actions explains the therapeutic benefit of the amphetamines in hyperkinetic children.

Clinical Uses

The therapeutic indications for the psychomotor stimulants are quite limited. They are beneficial in the treatment of the *hyperkinetic syndrome* (attention deficit–hyperactivity disorder with minimal brain dysfunction). This is generally a childhood disease characterized by hyperactivity, inability to concentrate, and impulsive behavior. Amphetamines and the more extensively used methylphenidate paradoxically are quite effective in calming a large proportion of children with this disorder. Pemoline (*Cylert*) is also used in the treatment of attention deficit disorder with hyperkinetic behavior. The mechanism by which these compounds are effective in this disorder is not known.

Narcolepsy is another medically recognized indication for the use of the psychomotor stimulants. This disorder is characterized by sleep attacks, particularly during the day, sudden loss of muscle tone (*cataplexy*), sleep paralysis, and vivid visual and auditory nightmares that may persist into the waking state. Drugs that influence the central action of adrenomimetic amines remarkably affect narcolepsy. Monoamine oxidase inhibitors (e.g., selegiline) and amphetamines are both quite effective in preventing sleep attacks and improving cataplexy. Modafinil (*Provigil*) is a nonamphetamine compound whose mechanism of action is not known but that has been shown to be successful in the treatment of narcolepsy. However, amphetamine and methylphenidate are still considered among the drugs of choice in this disorder.

Previously, another use of the amphetamines and other centrally acting adrenomimetics has been in the management of obesity and weight reduction. Although the amphetamines have a significant anorexic effect, tolerance to this action develops within a few weeks. In addition, insomnia restricted their use during the latter part of the day. The combined drawbacks of the development of tolerance and potential for drug abuse have convinced much of the medical community that *the use of amphetamines in weight control is inappropriate.*

Fenfluramine (*Pondimin*) and phentermine (*Adipex-P, Fastin*) are anorexigenic drugs that produce *depression* of the CNS and at one time were used (Fen-phen) in the treatment of obesity. Sibutramine (*Meridia*) is also available for the treatment of obesity.

Adverse Effects

The acute effects of psychomotor stimulant overdoses are related to their CNS stimulant properties and may include euphoria, dizziness, tremor, irritability, and insomnia. At higher doses, convulsions and coma may ensue. These drugs are cardiac stimulants and may cause headache, palpitation, cardiac arrhythmias, anginal pain, and either hypotension or hypertension. Dextroamphetamine produces somewhat less cardiac stimulation. Chronic intoxication, in addition to these symptoms, commonly results in weight loss and a psychotic reaction that is often diagnosed as schizophrenia.

These agents produce addiction, including psychological dependence, tolerance, and physical dependence. Psychic dependence also has been seen following high doses of methylphenidate. The abstinence syndrome seen after abrupt discontinuation of amphetamines is neither as dramatic nor as predictable as that observed during withdrawal from the barbiturates or opioids. With the amphetamines, the abstinence syndrome consists primarily of prolonged sleep, fatigue, and extreme hunger (*hyperphagia*). These symptoms may be accompanied by profound and long-lasting depression. Amphetamine abuse is discussed more completely in Chapter 35.

XANTHINES

The compounds known as xanthines, methylxanthines, or xanthine derivatives constitute a particularly interesting class of drugs. Since they possess diverse phar-

macological properties, there is always a question of where most appropriately to discuss them in a pharmacology text. The xanthines are clearly CNS stimulants, although not all have this characteristic equally. While the xanthines have legitimate therapeutic uses, by far the greatest public exposure to them is in xanthine-containing beverages, including coffee, tea, cocoa, and cola drinks. The popularity of xanthine-containing drinks appears to be related to its subtle CNS stimulant effect. It is primarily for this reason that xanthines are listed as CNS stimulants in this text.

Chemistry and Pharmacokinetics

Three xanthines are pharmacologically important: *caffeine, theophylline,* and *theobromine.* All three alkaloids, which occur naturally in certain plants, are widely consumed in the form of beverages (infusions or decoctions) derived from these plants. Coffee primarily contains caffeine (about 100–150 mg per average cup); tea contains caffeine (30–40 mg per cup) and theophylline; and cocoa contains caffeine (15–18 mg per cup) and theobromine. Cola drinks also contain significant amounts of caffeine (about 40 mg/12 oz). *The CNS stimulation associated with these beverages is predominantly due to the caffeine.*

The xanthines are readily absorbed by the oral and rectal routes. Although these agents can be administered by injection (*aminophylline* is a soluble salt of theophylline), *intravascular administration is indicated only in status asthmaticus and apnea in premature infants.* Intramuscular injection generally produces considerable pain at the injection site.

The compounds are extensively metabolized, primarily to uric acid derivatives. There is, however, no indication that methylxanthines aggravate gout.

Mechanism of Action

The mechanism of action of methylxanthine-induced stimulation of the CNS has been the subject of much investigation, and at least two other possible mechanisms of action of the methylxanthines have been suggested. The first derives from the ability of the methylxanthines to act as antagonists of the naturally occurring compound adenosine, a substance that can inhibit both neuronal activity and behavior through direct postsynaptic action on neurons and through indirect action involving presynaptic inhibition of neurotransmitter release. The A1 subtype of the purine receptors mediates these actions of adenosine. Thus, as an equilibrium-competitive antagonist of adenosine, the methylxanthines may produce excitation either by direct blockade of inhibitory effects of adenosine at the neuron or by an antagonism of the presynaptic inhibitory effect of adenosine on the release of an excitatory substance (e.g., acetylcholine).

Another suggested mechanism of action involves the chloride channel. As discussed previously, the chloride channel is intimately associated with neuronal inhibition, and its activity appears to be modulated at many different sites. Caffeine can compete for binding at the benzodiazepine site and would therefore be expected to reduce chloride conductance. Thus, caffeine may act functionally like the analeptic stimulants that limit chloride channel activation.

Clinical Uses
Central Nervous System

Xanthines, primarily as the intramuscularly administered combination of *caffeine* and *sodium benzoate,* have been used in the treatment of CNS depressant overdosage. Black coffee has been used to physiologically antagonize alcohol intoxication, although many physicians believe that this ineffective therapy simply produces a wide-awake drunk.

Many over-the-counter preparations are aimed at relieving fatigue through CNS stimulation. Such compounds are often referred to as wake-up tablets, but these methylxanthine-containing products do little to offset physical fatigue, so they place individuals using them at risk for accidental injuries.

Diuresis

All the xanthines, but especially theophylline, are capable of producing some degree of diuresis in humans. This specific action of the methylxanthines is discussed in greater detail in Chapter 21.

Bronchial Asthma

Theophylline is frequently used as a bronchodilator in the treatment of asthma. The importance of the methylxanthines in the management of bronchial asthma is discussed more fully in Chapter 39. Caffeine as the citrate salt (*Cafcit*) is used for the short-term management of apnea in premature infants (28–33 weeks of gestational age).

Cardiac Uses

Theophylline, given as the soluble ethylenediamine salt aminophylline, offers some help in relieving the paroxysmal dyspnea that is often associated with left heart failure. A major portion of its efficacy may be due to the relief of bronchospasm secondary to pulmonary vascular congestion. Theophylline increases myocardial contractile force and has occasionally been used in the treatment of refractory forms of congestive heart failure. Theophylline also has shown some benefit in the treatment of neonatal apnea syndrome.

Miscellaneous Uses

Xanthines (usually caffeine) are frequently combined with aspirin in the treatment of headaches. In combination with an ergot derivative, methylxanthines have been used to treat migraine. These effects are likely due to their ability to produce vasoconstriction of cerebral blood vessels. Aminophylline is useful in the relief of pain due to acute biliary colic.

Adverse Effects

Toxicity associated with the methylxanthines usually takes the form of nervousness, insomnia, and in severe cases, delirium. Cardiovascular stimulation is seen as tachycardia and extrasystoles. Excessive respiratory stimulation may occur, and diuresis may be prominent.

The intravenous administration of aminophylline (or theophylline) may present some problems if the drug is given too rapidly. In such cases, severe headache, hypotension, and palpitation accompany drug administration. Subsequently the patient may show signs of excessive CNS stimulation, shock, and even death. Children appear to be especially prone to this toxicity.

Abuse of Xanthines

The use of some xanthine-containing beverages is customary in most cultures, and moderate use of such beverages does not appear to cause problems in most people. There is little question, however, that such use is habituating. For example, it has been observed that chronic coffee drinkers who suddenly abstain frequently have headaches and a general feeling of fatigue that may last for several days. Although it has not been established that these symptoms constitute any kind of abstinence syndrome, it remains a possibility. There is no good evidence for the development of tolerance to the CNS stimulant effects of caffeine.

Drug Interactions

An interaction of potential clinical significance involves the xanthines and the coumarin anticoagulants. Xanthines by themselves shorten clotting time by increasing tissue prothrombin and factor V and in this regard may be expected to antagonize the effectiveness of oral anticoagulants. However, the usual therapeutic doses of xanthines cause no significant effect on the patient's response to oral anticoagulants.

Study QUESTIONS

1. Opisthotonos is a convulsive condition that is often associated with the ingestion of strychnine. This condition is associated with all of the following EXCEPT
   (A) Antagonism of the inhibitory amino acid neurotransmitter glycine
   (B) The predominance of glycine as an inhibitory amino acid transmitter in the spinal cord
   (C) Antagonism of the inhibitory amino acid neurotransmitter GABA
   (D) The convulsions lead to tonic extension of the body and all limbs
2. Which of the following classes of agents is useful in the treatment of attention deficit hyperkinetic disorder?
   (A) Analeptic stimulants
   (B) Benzodiazepines
   (C) Xanthines
   (D) Psychomotor stimulants
   (E) Phosphodiesterase inhibitors
3. Which of the following mechanisms of action account for the effects of all analeptic stimulants except strychnine?
   (A) Antagonism of chloride ion influx at the GABA receptor–chloride channel complex
   (B) Increased release of catecholamines from CNS neurons
   (C) Inhibition of cholinesterase leading to increased acetylcholine levels
   (D) Antagonism of CNS adrenoceptors to reduce inhibition produced by catecholamines
   (E) Antagonism of nicotinic receptors that inhibit motor neuron activity
4. The CNS stimulation produced by methylxanthines, such as caffeine, is most likely due to the antagonism of which of the following receptors?
   (A) Glycine receptors
   (B) Adenosine receptors
   (C) Glutamate receptors
   (D) GABA receptors
   (E) Cholinergic muscarinic receptors
5. Cardiac stimulation is an adverse effect associated with the use of the psychomotor stimulants, such as amphetamine. Which of the following mechanisms is most likely responsible for this peripheral effect?
   (A) Inhibition of vagal tone through an action in the CNS
   (B) Indirect sympathomimetic effects in the periphery due to release of norepinephrine
   (C) Inhibition of a GABA-mediated negative chronotropic effect at the heart

(D) Antagonism of muscarinic receptors in the heart
(E) Blockade of ganglionic transmission at sympathetic ganglia in the periphery

ANSWERS

1. **C.** Glycine is the major inhibitory amino acid transmitter in the spinal cord, and strychnine is a relatively selective antagonist of glycine. Strychnine has very little if any action at the GABA receptor–chloride channel complex.
2. **D.** Attention deficit–hyperkinetic disorder and attention deficit disorder are among only a few approved uses of the psychomotor stimulants of the amphetamine type.
3. **A.** Analeptic stimulants, such as pentylenetetrazol and picrotoxin, act by inhibiting chloride influx at the $GABA_A$ receptor–chloride channel complex. This antagonism can occur through interaction with one of several binding sites or allosteric modifiers of receptor–channel function.
4. **B.** Methylxanthines have been proposed to be inhibitors of phosphodiesterase, which would elevate intracellular levels of cAMP. However, the concentration of cAMP that is required for such action is above the threshold of CNS stimulation. Since the methylxanthines are relatively potent antagonists of adenosine and since adenosine has been shown to be a reasonably potent inhibitor of both central and peripheral neurons, the most likely mechanism by which CNS stimulation occurs is through antagonism of adenosine receptors.
5. **B.** Psychomotor stimulants such as amphetamine are also indirectly acting sympathomimetics that increase the release of catecholamines from sympathetic nerve terminals. While amphetamine and other congeners possess additional actions on peripheral sympathetic nerves, this is the most likely explanation for the cardiac stimulation observed following the administration of these agents.

SUPPLEMENTAL READING

Barnard EA. The molecular biology of $GABA_A$ receptors and their structural determinants. In Biggio C, Sanna E, and Costa E (eds.). $GABA_A$ Receptors and Anxiety: From Neurobiology to Treatment. New York: Raven, 1992.
Costa E. From $GABA_A$ receptor diversity emerges a unified vision of GABAergic inhibition. Annu Rev Pharmacol Toxicol 1998;38:321–350.

Daval, J-L, Nehlig A, and Nicolas F. Physiological and pharmacological properties of adenosine: Therapeutic implications. Life Sci 1991;49:1435–1453.

Fredholm BB et al. International Union of Pharmacology. XXV. Nomenclature and classification of adenosine receptors. Pharmacol Rev 2001;53: 527–552.

Linden J. Structure and function of A_1 adenosine receptors. FASEB J 1991;5:2668–2676.

Sieghart W. Structure and pharmacology of γ-aminobutyric acid$_A$ receptor subtypes. Pharmacol Rev 1995;47:181–234.

Smith GB and Olsen RW. Functional domains of GABA$_A$ receptors. Trends Pharmacol Sci 1995;16:162–168.

CASE Study   Daytime Sleepiness

W. M. is a 55-year-old highly successful businessman who often spends long hours at the office or in his automobile traveling to meet new clients and partners. Since his days in college, W. M. has had frequent episodes of daytime somnolence, which he attributed to overwork and fatigue. Over the past several years, the number of daytime episodes has begun to increase, and he recently began to lose mobility in his arms and legs during the periods of somnolence. He also barely avoided a significant automobile accident for which the local sheriff's deputy cited him for failure to maintain control of his vehicle. During questioning by the police, W. M. indicated that he had no memory of any of the events surrounding the incident; he tested negative for any intoxicating substances. As a result of this most recent episode, W. M. has come to you, his family physician, to determine the cause of the excessive daytime sleepiness (EDS) and to find a way to manage this condition. Your examination reveals an individual who is in otherwise excellent health and mentation with no apparent significant pathology. He indicates that he has several periods of EDS during the day and that the frequency of these events is beginning to increase. While he feels well rested upon waking, he is especially concerned about the recent loss of skeletal muscle function and fears that he may be developing some degenerative progressive disease that will leave him disabled and unable to continue working. What types of pathological conditions can lead to excessive somnolence? What is the appropriate therapeutic management of these pathological conditions?

ANSWER: Three disorders are most often associated with EDS. *Sleep apnea* is characterized by pauses in respiration during sleep and usually excessive snoring. Patients with sleep apnea have EDS but often awake without feeling rested. Sleep apnea is managed by treating the nighttime episodes of apnea. *Narcolepsy* is characterized by episodic EDS. Patients with this pathology often exhibit periods of irresistible instantaneous REM sleep and may also progress to cataplexy, or sudden loss of tone in skeletal muscles (usually bilaterally). A final type of disorder that displays periods of EDS is *idiopathic hypersomnia*, in which patients usually have periods of EDS usually associated with non-REM sleep. W. M. most likely has *narcolepsy*, which could be more clearly defined by determining whether he has a specific human leukocyte antigen associated with the disorder (HLA-DR2). Management of narcolepsy is accomplished with psychomotor stimulants of the amphetamine type. *Methylphenidate, modafinil, pemoline,* and *dextroamphetamine* all are effective in managing the EDS periods, while *imipramine* and *clomipramine* can be used to manage any cataplexy.

30 Sedative–hypnotic and Anxiolytic Drugs

John W. Dailey

DRUG LIST

GENERIC NAME	PAGE	GENERIC NAME	PAGE
Alprazolam	357	Lorazepam	357
Buspirone	356	Midazolam	359
Chloral hydrate	361	Oxazepam	357
Chlordiazepoxide	359	Prazepam	357
Clonazepam	359	Propranolol	361
Clorazepate	357	Temazepam	357
Diazepam	359	Triazolam	357
Flurazepam	357	Zephalon	360
Hydroxyzine	361	Zolpidem	360

The primary use of sedative–hypnotic and anxiolytic drugs is to encourage calmness (*anxiolytics* or *sedatives*) or to produce sleep (*sedative–hypnotics*). All people are subject to states of emotional tension and uneasiness. For otherwise healthy individuals, these occasions are usually sufficiently mild and short that pharmacological intervention is unnecessary. However, at times the symptoms of anxiety become quite discomforting and can interfere with a person's ability to function effectively. Anxiety almost invariably accompanies many medical and surgical conditions, and it is often a symptom of psychiatric illness. When the symptoms become intolerable or interfere with the treatment of the underlying disease and if counseling is not sufficient, drug treatment can be considered as a means of helping patients cope with their anxiety.

All central nervous system depressants have some ability to relieve anxiety. However, most of these drugs relieve symptoms of anxiety only at doses that produce noticeable sedation. Drugs used to produce sedation and relieve anxiety are consistently among the most commonly prescribed drugs. Whether they are prescribed too frequently remains a matter of controversy.

Insomnia includes a wide variety of sleep disturbances, such as difficulty in falling asleep, early or frequent awakenings, and remaining unrefreshed after sleep. Use of sedative–hypnotic drugs is one approach to the therapy of insomnia. Other measures include advice to avoid stimulants before retiring, maintenance of a proper diet, initiation of an exercise program, and avoidance of stressful or anxiety-provoking situations.

Most anxiolytic and sedative–hypnotic drugs produce dose-dependent depression of central nervous system function. The ideal anxiolytic drug should calm the patient without causing too much daytime sedation and drowsiness and without producing physical or psychological dependence. Similarly, the ideal hypnotic drug should allow the patient to fall asleep quickly and should maintain sleep of sufficient quality and duration so that the patient awakes refreshed without a drug hangover. Also, both types of drugs should have very low toxicity and should not interact with other medications in such a way as to produce unwanted or dangerous effects.

AZAPIRONES

Buspirone (*BuSpar*) is the first example of a class of anxiolytic agents that can relieve some symptoms of anxiety in doses that do not cause sedation. Buspirone is structurally unrelated to existing psychotropic drugs.

Mechanism of Action

Although buspirone has been shown to interact with a number of neurotransmitter systems in the brain, it appears that its clinically relevant effects are mediated through interactions at the serotonin (5-hydroxytryptamine, 5-HT) 5-HT$_{1A}$ receptor, where it acts as a partial agonist.

Pharmacokinetics

Buspirone is well absorbed from the gastrointestinal tract, and peak blood levels are achieved in 1 to 1.5 hours; the drug is more than 95% bound to plasma proteins. Buspirone is extensively metabolized, with less than 1% of the parent drug excreted into the urine unchanged. At least one of the metabolic products of buspirone is biologically active. The parent drug has an elimination half-life of 4 to 6 hours.

Pharmacological Actions

Buspirone is as effective as the benzodiazepines in the treatment of general anxiety. However, the full anxiolytic effect of buspirone takes several weeks to develop, whereas the anxiolytic effect of the benzodiazepines is maximal after a few days of therapy. In therapeutic doses, buspirone has little or no sedative effect and lacks the muscle relaxant and anticonvulsant properties of the benzodiazepines. In addition, buspirone does not potentiate the central nervous system depression caused by sedative–hypnotic drugs or by alcohol, and it does not prevent the symptoms associated with benzodiazepine withdrawal.

Clinical Uses

Buspirone is effective in general anxiety and in anxiety with depression.

Adverse Effects

Like the benzodiazepines, buspirone appears to be safe even when given in very high doses. The most common side effects are dizziness, light-headedness, and headache. Abuse, dependence, and withdrawal have not been reported, and buspirone administration does not produce any cross-tolerance to the benzodiazepines. Buspirone has been reported to increase blood pressure in patients taking monoamine oxidase inhibitors, and it may increase plasma levels of haloperidol if coadministered with that agent.

BENZODIAZEPINES

The benzodiazepines constitute the most commonly used group of anxiolytics and sedative–hypnotics. Since the first member of this group, *chlordiazepoxide,* was introduced, many congeners have been marketed. Most of these drugs possess anxiolytic, sedative–hypnotic, and anticonvulsant properties. Thus, the clinical indications for specific benzodiazepines are not absolute. and their uses overlaps considerably.

Chemistry

The basic chemical structure of the benzodiazepines consists of a benzene ring coupled to a seven-member heterocyclic structure containing two nitrogens (diazepine) at positions 1 and 4 (Fig. 30.1). Of the 2,000 benzodiazepines that have been synthesized, approximately 15 clinically useful compounds are on the market in the United States (Table 30.1).

Mechanism of Action

The benzodiazepines bind with high affinity to specific macromolecules within the central nervous system. *These benzodiazepine-binding sites (receptors) are closely associated with the receptors for γ-aminobutyric*

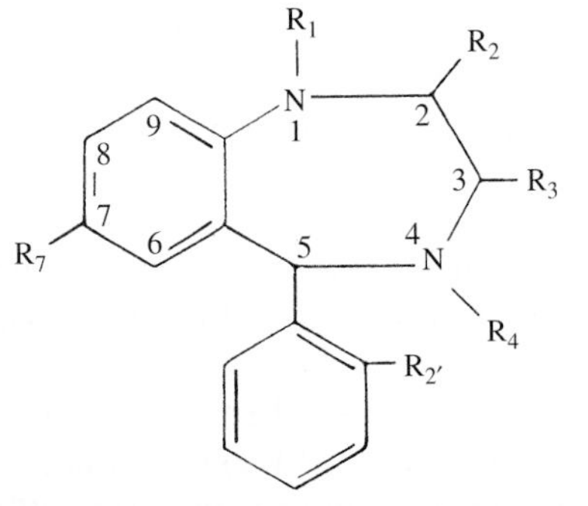

1,4-Benzodiazepine nucleus

FIGURE 30.1
General structure of 1,4 benzodiazepines.

TABLE 30.1 Clinical Uses of the Sedative–Hypnotic and Anxiolytic Drugs

Drugs	Therapeutic Uses
Alprazolam (*Xanax*)	Anxiety
Buspirone (*BuSpar*)	Anxiety
Chloral hydrate (*Noctec, Somnos*)	Insomnia
Chlordiazepoxide (*Librium*)	Anxiety, alcohol withdrawal
Chlorazepate (*Tranxene*)	Anxiety
Diazepam (*Valium*)	Anxiety, muscle relaxation, status epilepticus
Flurazepam (*Dalmane*)	Insomnia
Flumazenil (*Romazicon*)	Reverse benzodiazepine-induced sedation
Hydroxyzine (*Atarax, Vistaril*)	Anxiety
Lorazepam (*Ativan*)	Anxiety
Midazolam (*Versed*)	Anesthesia
Oxazepam (*Serax*)	Anxiety
Prazepam (*Centrax*)	Anxiety
Propranolol (*Inderal*)	Anxiety
Temazepam (*Restoril*)	Insomnia
Triazolam (*Halcion*)	Insomnia
Zolpidem (*Ambien*)	Insomnia
Zaleplon (*Sonata*)	Insomnia

acid (GABA), which is the major inhibitory neurotransmitter in the mammalian brain. Benzodiazepines potentiate GABAergic neurotransmission in essentially all areas of the central nervous system. This enhancement is thought to occur indirectly at the postsynaptic GABA$_A$ receptor complex.

The functional significance of this drug–receptor interaction is that the *receptor complex regulates the entrance of chloride into the postsynaptic cells.* The increase in chloride conductance mediated by GABA is intensified by the benzodiazepines. This facilitation of GABA-induced chloride conductance results in greater hyperpolarization of these cells and therefore leads to diminished synaptic transmission.

Another chemical class of sedative–hypnotic drugs, the *barbiturates,* also binds to receptors associated with the GABA–chloride ionophore, but these drugs appear to prolong rather than intensify GABA's effects. Fig. 24.4 shows the presumed drug receptor–GABA–chloride ionophore relationship.

In addition to the clinically useful benzodiazepines, which act as agonists at the benzodiazepine receptor, at least two other types of ligands also interact with this binding site. These are the benzodiazepine receptor *antagonists* and the *inverse agonists.* For example, flumazenil (*Romazicon*) is a receptor antagonist that selectively blocks the effects of other benzodiazepines at their binding sites; it has clinical application in the treat-

ment of benzodiazepine overdose and in the reversal of benzodiazepine-induced sedation. The inverse agonists are compounds that interact with benzodiazepine receptors and decrease, rather than increase, GABA-mediated changes. They also can antagonize the effects of benzodiazepine agonists and when administered alone, can be anxiogenic and proconvulsant.

Pharmacokinetics

Benzodiazepines are usually given orally and are well absorbed by this route. Since the benzodiazepines are weak bases, they are less ionized in the relatively alkaline environment of the small intestine, and therefore, most of their absorption takes place at this site. For emergency treatment of seizures or when used in anesthesia, the benzodiazepines also can be given parenterally. Diazepam and lorazepam are available for intravenous administration.

The distribution of the benzodiazepines from blood to tissues and back again is a dynamic process with considerable influence on the onset and duration of the therapeutic effects produced by these compounds. Those having greater lipid solubility tend to enter the central nervous system more rapidly and thus tend to produce their effects more quickly. Several of the benzodiazepines have therapeutic effects that are much shorter in duration than would be predicted based on their rates of metabolism and excretion; redistribution away from the central nervous system is of primary importance in terminating their therapeutic effects.

Although tissue redistribution of benzodiazepines may be an important means of terminating the actions of selected members of this class of drugs, many benzodiazepines do undergo extensive biotransformation. Metabolism takes place both by dealkylation (phase 1) and conjugation (phase 2) reactions. In many instances, dealkylation can result in the formation of pharmacologically active compounds. Indeed, *most clinically available benzodiazepines are converted in the liver to one or more active metabolites.* In several cases the active metabolites have a much longer half-life than the parent compound. In one case, acid hydrolysis in the stomach converts an inactive compound (clorazepate) to an active drug (nordazepam). Figure 30.2 shows the biotransformations involved in the metabolism of representative benzodiazepines. The water-soluble metabolites of the benzodiazepines are excreted primarily in the urine.

Since most of the benzodiazepines do undergo biotransformation, it is possible that changes in liver function may alter the duration of the therapeutic effect produced by these drugs. Despite the fact that few clinical studies have demonstrated serious toxicities associated with benzodiazepine administration in individuals with compromised liver function, prudence in the use of

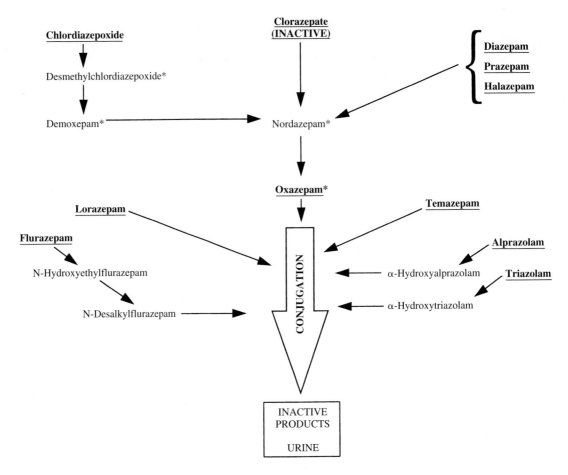

FIGURE 30.2
The metabolism of some benzodiazepines. In some cases, several active metabolites are formed. A result is very long apparent half-lives. In many cases, the ultimate product is oxazepam. *Active metabolic product.

these compounds in the elderly and in individuals with liver disease seems advisable.

One of the great disadvantages associated with many of the sedative and hypnotic drugs (e.g., barbiturates, propanediol carbamates), which have now largely been replaced by the benzodiazepines, is the fact that those drugs are very effective inducers of hepatic drug-metabolizing enzymes. Since the benzodiazepines are only weak inducers of hepatic microsomal enzymes, they cause relatively few clinically significant drug interactions related to metabolism of other drugs.

Pharmacological Actions

Although it is widely claimed that the benzodiazepine drugs have a specific calming or anxiolytic effect, their most prominent and easily quantifiable action is central nervous system depression. In very low therapeutic doses, this depression manifests as relief of anxiety that is often accompanied by a feeling of sluggishness or drowsiness. As the dose is increased, the degree of depression is intensified such that muscle relaxation, hyp-

nosis, and a more intense central nervous system depression occur. This depression is related to the ability of these drugs to facilitate the inhibitory actions of GABA.

A significant advantage of the benzodiazepines over other central nervous system depressants (e.g., the barbiturates) is that they possess a much greater separation between the dose that produces sleep and the dose that produces death. *This increased margin of safety has been one of the major reasons benzodiazepines have largely replaced the barbiturates and other types of sedative–hypnotics in the treatment of anxiety and insomnia.* In addition, benzodiazepine administration is associated with few side effects.

Clinical Uses
Anxiety

Anxiety disorders are among the most common forms of psychiatric illness. Anxiety often accompanies other psychiatric disease and such medical illnesses as angina pectoris, gastrointestinal disorders, and hypertension.

Anxiety that results from fear caused by an acute illness or a stressful event, such as a divorce or the loss of a loved one, is usually self-limiting and can be of relatively short duration. Other disorders that have anxiety as a component are not necessarily associated with a life event, and may persist for considerable periods, even throughout the individual's life.

Both acute and chronic anxiety can be treated with benzodiazepines, although it is anticipated that for most anxiety disorders counseling will also play an important role. Benzodiazepines employed in the treatment of anxiety should be used in the lowest effective dose for the shortest duration so that they will provide maximum benefit to the patient while minimizing the potential for adverse reactions. For most types of anxiety, none of the benzodiazepines is therapeutically superior to any other. Choice of a particular agent is usually made on the basis of pharmacokinetic (Table 30.2) considerations. A benzodiazepine with a long half-life should be considered if the anxiety is intense and sustained. A drug with a short half-life may have advantages when the anxiety is provoked by clearly defined circumstances and is likely to be of short duration.

Insomnia

All of the benzodiazepines will produce sedative–hypnotic effects of sufficient magnitude to induce sleep, provided that the dose is high enough. However, the aim in the treatment of sleep disorders is to induce sleep that is as close as possible to natural sleep so that the patient falls asleep quickly, sleeps through the night, and has sleep of sufficient quality to awake refreshed.

Extensive sleep studies have been conducted with a variety of sedative–hypnotic drugs, and all of these drugs appear to alter the normal distribution of rapid eye movement (REM) and non-REM sleep. Most of the older sedative–hypnotic agents markedly depress REM sleep. In contrast, when the benzodiazepines are used in appropriate doses, they depress REM sleep to a much smaller extent. As with treatment of anxiety, the choice

of a particular benzodiazepine to treat a sleep disturbance is again generally based on pharmacokinetic criteria. While longer-acting compounds may ensure that a patient will sleep through the night, they also may cause cumulative effects resulting in daytime sluggishness or drug hangover. Shorter-acting compounds avoid the hangover problem, but their use may be associated with early awakening and an increase in daytime anxiety.

Epilepsy and Seizures

Nearly all central nervous system depressants have some capacity to suppress seizures by virtue of their depressant activity on the brain and spinal cord. Clonazepam and diazepam are two benzodiazepines that depress epileptiform activity and are used in the treatment of epilepsy and seizure disorders (see Chapter 32).

Sedation, Amnesia, and Anesthesia

Benzodiazepines have the capacity to produce a calming effect and to cause *anterograde amnesia,* in which the patient cannot recall events that took place for some time after the drug was administered. Benzodiazepine-induced sedation and amnesia are deemed useful in the preparation of patients for anesthesia, surgery, and other frightening or unpleasant medical and dental procedures and diagnostic tests. Midazolam is a frequently used anesthetic benzodiazepine (see Chapter 25).

Muscle Relaxation

Benzodiazepines have the capacity to depress polysynaptic reflexes and have been shown to decrease decerebrate rigidity in cats and spasticity in patients with cerebral palsy. What is not clear is whether they can, in humans, relax voluntary muscles in doses that do not cause considerable central nervous system depression. Nevertheless, benzodiazepines, such as diazepam, are often prescribed for patients who have muscle spasms and pain as a result of injury. In these circumstances, the sedative and anxiolytic properties of the drug also may promote relaxation and relieve tension associated with the condition.

Alcohol and Sedative–Hypnotic Withdrawal

Withdrawal from long-term high-dose use of alcohol or sedative–hypnotic drugs can be life threatening if physical dependence is present. Benzodiazepines, such as chlordiazepoxide (*Librium*) and diazepam (*Valium*), are sometimes used to lessen the intensity of the withdrawal symptoms when alcohol or sedative–hypnotic drug use is discontinued. Benzodiazepines are also employed to help relieve the anxiety and other behavioral symptoms that may occur during rehabilitation.

TABLE 30.2	Pharmacokinetic Properties of Selected Benzodiazepines	
Drug	**Time to peak (hr)**	**Elimination half-life (hr)***
Chlordiazepoxide	0.5–2.0	8–20
Diazepam	0.5–1.5	20–60
Flurazepam	0.5–1.0	24–120
Alprazolam	1.0–2.0	12–15
Oxazepam	2.0–4.0	4–12
Triazolam	1.5–2.0	3–5

*Includes parent compounds and active metabolites.

Adverse Effects and Toxicities

Most adverse effects associated with use of the benzodiazepines are related to their ability to produce central nervous system depression. These include drowsiness, excessive sedation, impaired motor coordination, confusion, and memory loss. These effects are most troublesome during the initial week or two of treatment. Subsequently, the patient becomes tolerant and these effects produce less difficulty. Although for most individuals these symptoms are mild, patients should be cautioned against engaging in potentially dangerous tasks such as operating machinery or driving a car during the initial treatment period.

Less common adverse effects include blurred vision, hallucinations, and paradoxical reactions consisting of excitement, stimulation, and hyperactivity. Also, a variety of gastrointestinal complaints occur, and blood dyscrasias have been reported, but these are rare. Benzodiazepine administration during pregnancy, delivery, or lactation has the potential to have adverse effects on the fetus or newborn.

As with other central nervous system depressants, the effects of benzodiazepines are additive with those of ethanol. Patients should be warned that *ethanol-containing beverages may produce a more profound depression when taken simultaneously with a benzodiazepine.*

One of the major reasons for the popularity of the benzodiazepines is their relative safety. Overdoses with the benzodiazepines occur commonly, but fatal toxic occurrences are rare. Fatal intoxications are more likely in children, in individuals with respiratory difficulties, and in individuals who have consumed another central nervous system depressant, such as alcohol. After an overdose, the patient begins a deep sleep that may last for 24 to 48 hours, depending on the dose. However, even with large overdoses, the patient can usually still be aroused.

Tolerance and dependence do occur with the use of benzodiazepines. Discontinuation of drug administration, particularly abrupt withdrawal, can be associated with a variety of symptoms, including rebound insomnia and rebound anxiety. The level of insomnia or anxiety may even exceed that which preceded the treatment. Usually, *a gradual tapering of the dose until it is eventually discontinued lessens the likelihood of a withdrawal reaction,* although in some individuals even this method of drug removal can result in anxiety, apprehension, tension, insomnia, and loss of appetite. More severe symptoms may occur when an individual withdraws from a supratherapeutic dose, particularly if the drug has been taken for months or years. These symptoms can include, in addition to those already mentioned, muscle weakness, tremor, hyperalgesia, nausea, vomiting, weight loss, and possibly convulsions.

Drug Interactions

When used with other sedative–hypnotics or alcohol, the benzodiazepines will produce additive central nervous system depression.

Many benzodiazepines are metabolized by the cytochrome P450 (CYP) enzyme designated CYP3A4. CYP3A4 is inhibited by grapefruit juice and by drugs such as ketoconazole, itraconazole, nefazodone, erythromycin, and ritonavir. Coadministration of these substances along with a benzodiazepine may result in intensification and prolongation of the benzodiazepine effect. Conversely, rifampin, carbamazepine, and phenytoin can induce the CYP3A4 enzyme, and therefore their coadministration can reduce the therapeutic effect of the benzodiazepines.

OTHER BENZODIAZEPINE RECEPTOR AGONISTS

Zolpidem (*Ambien*) and zaleplon (*Sonata*) are structurally unrelated to the benzodiazepines, but both drugs share pharmacological properties with the benzodiazepines. They bind to benzodiazepine receptors and facilitate GABA-mediated inhibition.

In usual sedative doses, zolpidem preserves deep sleep (stages 3 and 4) and has only minor and inconsistent effects on REM sleep. Compared with the benzodiazepines, zolpidem has relatively weak anxiolytic, anticonvulsant, and skeletal muscle relaxant properties at therapeutic doses. Zolpidem has a rapid onset and a relatively short duration of action. It is well absorbed after oral administration, with approximately 70% bioavailability. It undergoes hydroxylation and oxidation to inactive metabolites in the liver. Its elimination half-life is approximately 2.5 hours, which is usually sufficient to provide for a normal 8 hours of sleep without daytime grogginess.

Principal side effects are gastrointestinal and central nervous system symptoms, including drowsiness, dizziness, and diarrhea. Zolpidem may increase the depressant effects of other sedative drugs, such as the antipsychotics, tricyclic antidepressants, and antihistamines.

There is less therapeutic experience with the newer zaleplon than with zolpidem. Zaleplon has a rapid onset and a half-life of approximately 1 hour. It is extensively metabolized by aldehyde dehydrogenase, so that less than 1% of a dose is excreted unchanged. Because of its rapid onset of action and short biological half-life, zaleplon is well suited for treatment of sleep onset insomnia. Its short half-life often does not ensure a full 8 hours of sleep.

SEDATIVES AND ANXIOLYTICS WITH OTHER MAJOR USES

Antihistamines

Several H$_1$ histamine antagonists (e.g., diphenhydramine, promethazine, and hydroxyzine) have been used as sedative–hypnotics, since they produce some degree of sedation. While this sedation is usually considered a side effect of their antihistaminic activity, in some cases the sedation is sufficient to allow the drugs to be used in the treatment of anxiety and sleep disturbances. For these drugs, *the anxiolytic properties are thought to be a direct consequence of their ability to produce sedation.*

Hydroxyzine hydrochloride (*Atarax, Vistaril*) is the antihistamine with the greatest use in the treatment of anxiety. It is often used to reduce the anxiety that is associated with anesthesia and surgery. It also produces sedation, dries mucous membranes (via an anticholinergic mechanism), and has antiemetic activity. A more extensive discussion of the pharmacology of the H$_1$-receptor antagonists is found in Chapter 38.

β-Adrenoceptor Blocking Agents

β-Adrenoceptor antagonists, such as propranolol (*Inderal*), have been widely used in the treatment of cardiovascular diseases (see Chapters 16 and 20). These β-blockers also are useful in some forms of anxiety, particularly those that are characterized by somatic symptoms or by performance anxiety (stage fright). There is general agreement that β-blockers can lessen the severity and perhaps prevent the appearance of many of the autonomic responses associated with anxiety. These symptoms include tremors, sweating, tachycardia, and palpitations.

Antidepressants

Antidepressant drugs, such as the *tricyclic antidepressants* and the *selective serotonin reuptake inhibitors (SSRIs)*, are very important for the treatment of psychotic depression (see Chapter 34). They have been shown to be effective when used in the treatment of several anxiety disorders, including general anxiety, obsessive-compulsive disorder, and several phobias, including agoraphobia. Because the SSRIs are less toxic than the tricyclic antidepressants, their use in the treatment of anxiety is safer and less likely to produce serious side effects.

OLDER SEDATIVE–HYPNOTIC AND ANXIOLYTIC AGENTS

Before the introduction of the benzodiazepines, a number of drugs from different chemical and pharmacological classes were used in the treatment of anxiety and insomnia. However, these drugs are more toxic and produce more serious side effects than do the benzodiazepines. Many also have significant abuse potential. Consequently, most of these compounds are no longer widely used. These drugs include the barbiturates (e.g., pentobarbital, amobarbital), carbamates (e.g., meprobamate), piperidinediones (e.g., glutethimide), and alcohols (e.g., ethchlorvynol).

Chloral hydrate (*Noctec, Somnos*) was developed in the late 1800s and is still used as a sedative–hypnotic agent. It is a hydrated aldehyde with a disagreeable smell and taste that is rapidly reduced in vivo to trichloroethanol, which is considered to be the active metabolite. It produces a high incidence of gastric irritation and allergic responses, occasionally causes cardiac arrhythmias, and is unreliable in patients with liver damage.

NONPRESCRIPTION DRUGS

A wide variety of sedative–hypnotic products that do not require a prescription are available. Most of these over-the-counter products have antihistamines, such as pyrilamine, diphenhydramine, or promethazine, as the active ingredient. In most cases, the dose of the active ingredient is low and the preparations are safe.

Ethanol (ethyl alcohol) has central nervous system depressant properties and is widely used to relieve anxiety and produce sedation. Although some medical practitioners occasionally prescribe an alcoholic beverage for relieving minor anxiety and inducing sleep, individuals frequently self-medicate with ethanol. Many individuals who abuse alcohol may have started using it to relieve symptoms of central nervous system disorders, such as anxiety and depression.

Ethanol produces central nervous system depression over a wide range of doses. Its effects are additive or sometimes more than additive with other central nervous system depressants. Symptoms often associated with acute alcohol intoxication include increase in self-confidence, loss of inhibitions, euphoria, and loss of judgment. With increasing doses motor and intellectual impairment become prominent. Chronic abuse of ethanol leads to severe liver impairment (see Chapter 35).

Study Questions

1. A 21-year-old man is a full-time college student who also works 25 hours per week. Over the past 3 months he has become increasingly anxious. He says he is tired most of the time and has trouble concentrating on his studies. Which of the following drugs would be the most appropriate initial pharmacologic treatment for his anxiety?
(A) Phenobarbital
(B) Alprazolam
(C) Zolpidem
(D) Hydroxyzine
(E) Propranolol

2. A 33-year-old woman has recently undergone a divorce. She reports that although she is exhausted, it usually takes her 2 or more hours to fall asleep at night. Which of the following drugs would help relieve her sleep disturbance while being least disruptive to REM sleep?
(A) Triazolam
(B) Chloral hydrate
(C) Zolpidem
(D) Amobarbital
(E) Hydroxyzine

3. A 54-year-old man is scheduled for an elective colonoscopy that will take approximately 20 minutes. Which of the following drugs would be most likely to produce the desired anesthesia and anterograde amnesia?
(A) Buspirone
(B) Zephalon
(C) Midazolam
(D) Chlordiazepoxide
(E) Hydroxyzine

4. A 33-year-old woman has a 15-year history of alcohol abuse. She comes to the emergency department for treatment of injuries received in a fall. She says she has been drinking heavily and almost continuously for 2 weeks, and she wants to stop. Which of the following drugs would most effectively and safely lessen the intensity of her withdrawal syndrome?
(A) Buspirone
(B) Chlordiazepoxide
(C) Chloral hydrate
(D) Midazolam
(E) Zolpidem

5. A 23-year-old medical student has to make a presentation before his classmates. He is very anxious about this presentation and reports that on one previous occasion the sweating and palpitations that accompany his stage fright were so intense that he was unable to complete his presentation. Pretreatment with which of the following drugs would relieve his symptoms without making him drowsy?
(A) Alprazolam
(B) Zephalon
(C) Chloral hydrate
(D) Propranolol
(E) Diazepam

ANSWERS

1. **B.** The young man's anxiety is probably caused by the stress induced by a full college curriculum along with working 25 hours per week. A benzodiazepine antianxiety agent would help relieve his symptoms.

2. **C.** Zolpidem is effective at relieving sleep-onset insomnia. The other agents listed could also induce sleep, although each would be expected to produce more disruption of sleep rhythm than would zolpidem.

3. **C.** Midazolam, like all benzodiazepines given in sufficient dose, has the capacity to produce anterograde amnesia. It is also available in an injectable form and frequently is used as an anesthetic agent during short procedures.

4. **B.** Chlordiazepoxide, through its metabolites, has a relatively long biological half-life. It will prevent many of the severe symptoms of acute alcohol withdrawal. Buspirone is not a sedative and will not suppress alcohol withdrawal. The other agents have sedative properties and could potentially suppress alcohol withdrawal but each has a much shorter biological half-life than chlordiazepoxide.

5. **D.** As a β-adrenoceptor blocker, propranolol can relieve many of the symptoms of stage fright. For this use it can be taken once a few hours before the performance. Chronic dosing is usually not necessary. The other agents produce sedation.

SUPPLEMENTAL READING

Yuan R, Flockhart DA, and Balian JD. Pharmacokinetic and pharmacodynamic consequences of metabolism-based drug interactions with alprazolam, midazolam and triazolam. J Clin Pharmacol 1999;39,1109–1125.

Dooley M and Plosker GL. Zaleplon: A review of its use in the treatment of insomnia. Drugs 2000;60,413–445.

Doghramji PP. Treatment of insomnia with zaleplon, a novel sleep medication. Int J Clin Pract 2001;55,329–334.

Zohar J and Westenberg HG. Anxiety disorders: A review of tricyclic antidepressants and selective serotonin reuptake inhibitors. Acta Psychiatr Scand Suppl 2000;403,39–49.

CASE Study   Nighttime Anxiety

M. W. is a 22-year-old woman who visits her doctor because she is extremely tired. She reports that although she is exhausted at bedtime, she typically cannot fall asleep for at least an hour or two. She moved to town 2 months ago and has her first full-time job. She likes her job but fears that her supervisors think she is "dumb" because she has made some careless mistakes. After falling to sleep, she sometimes wakes an hour or more before her alarm goes off, usually thinking about her dumb mistakes. Her problems with sleeping began approximately 5 months ago, when she was studying for final examinations in her senior year of college. Aside from a minor dermatological condition, she is in excellent health. What treatment would you recommend for her insomnia and fatigue?

ANSWER: Zolpidem is the best choice. M. W.'s inability to sleep well is probably the result of anxiety caused by several stresses in her life. She is a recent college graduate, has a new job, and has moved to a new town. These events constitute three stressors, which can induce anxiety and sleep loss. The sleep loss and anxiety are usually of relatively short duration. Zolpidem has a quick onset and a half-life of approximately 2.5 hours. If taken at bedtime, it should allow her to fall asleep quickly and sleep though most or all of the night. Its elimination is fast enough that it should not produce residual drowsiness during the day. A week-long trial of zolpidem should help M. W. overcome her sleep disturbance.

31

Drugs Used in Neurodegenerative Disorders

Patricia K. Sonsalla

 DRUG LIST

GENERIC NAME	PAGE	GENERIC NAME	PAGE
Amantadine	370	Pergolide	369
Benztropine	370	Pramipexole	369
Biperiden	370	Procyclidine	370
Bromocriptine	369	Rivastigmine	371
Carbidopa	368	Ropinirole	369
Donepezil	371	Selegiline	369
Entacapone	370	Tacrine	371
Galanthamine	371	Tolcapone	370
Levodopa	367	Trihexyphenidyl	370

Neurodegenerative diseases are a group of disorders characterized by neuronal loss and generally an accumulation of insoluble intracellular or extracellular material in certain brain regions. Most neurodegenerative disorders are of unknown etiology, affect the elderly, are progressive, and damage selected neuronal populations or brain regions. There are some inherited forms of these disorders; however, most are sporadic occurrences (idiopathic) with genetic predisposition, environmental factors, and aging contributing as risk factors.

The neurodegenerative disorders include (1) Alzheimer's disease, the most common cause of dementia, in which the neural injury is primarily in the hippocampus and cortex; (2) Parkinson's disease, a disabling motor impairment disorder due to the loss of nigrostriatal dopamine neurons; (3) Huntington's disease, a motor disease characterized by excessive and abnormal movements resulting from the loss of a specific subset of striatal neurons; (4) amyotrophic lateral sclerosis (ALS), in which progressive weakness and muscle atrophy are due to degeneration of spinal, bulbar, and cortical neurons. This chapter focuses on Parkinson's and Alzheimer's diseases, for which pharmacological intervention can alleviate the clinical symptoms. However, *drugs used in the treatment of neurodegenerative disorders only treat symptoms and do not cure or alter the progression of the disease.*

PARKINSON'S DISEASE

The classic publication in 1817 by James Parkinson defined the triad of distinguishing symptoms that bear his name; this movement disorder is known as Parkinson's

disease or parkinsonism. It generally affects the elderly and is estimated to afflict more than 1% of individuals over the age of 65. A small subset of patients has familial forms of parkinsonism with an autosomal dominant pattern of inheritance. Genetic mutations in three proteins have been identified thus far. These genes encode for α-synuclein, a protein found in abundance in vesicles and synaptic regions, and for parkin and ubiquitin carboxy-terminal hydroxylase, both of which are involved with protein degradation.

Some forms of parkinsonism have been traced to specific entities, such as viral inflammation (e.g., the postencephalitic parkinsonism of the early 1900s), brain trauma, stroke, and poisoning by manganese, carbon monoxide, pesticide, or 1-methyl-4-phenyl,-1,2,3,6-tetrahydropyridine (MPTP). Intoxication with MPTP, a byproduct of the synthesis of an illegal meperidine analogue, produces a condition closely resembling parkinsonism, but there is little evidence that this or a similar toxin exists in the environment. However, the information from research with this toxin has provided important insight into mitochondrial function and has led to the theory that impairment of mitochondrial function (whether of genetic or toxin derivation) may be a relevant risk factor in Parkinson's disease.

Although the causes of some forms of parkinsonism are known, most cases are sporadic and are of unknown origin (idiopathic Parkinson's disease). The causes are likely multifactorial, with genetic predisposition, environmental toxins, and aging contributing to the initiation and progression of the disease. There is a progressive loss of dopamine neurons with age. Relatively smooth functioning of motor control is maintained until neuronal loss is such that it causes an 80% reduction of dopamine in the striatum. At this time, clinical symptoms appear and then worsen with increasing neuronal loss.

Another form of parkinsonism is drug-induced, that is, iatrogenic parkinsonism, which often is a complication of antipsychotic therapy, especially following the use of the butyrophenone and phenothiazine drug classes (see Chapter 34). Unlike idiopathic parkinsonism, striatal content of dopamine is not reduced by administration of these drugs. In contrast, they produce a functional decrease in dopamine activity by blocking the action of dopamine on postsynaptic dopamine receptors.

Clinical Findings

The onset of symptoms of Parkinson's disease is usually gradual. The most prominent features of parkinsonism are tremor, rigidity, and bradykinesia, although the time of onset and the relative severity of each symptom may differ in individual patients. Tremors are often unilateral in onset, present at rest, and cease during voluntary movement. Rigidity, or increased muscle tone, described as jerky resistance that has been likened to the movement of a cogwheel (*cogwheel rigidity*), is also an indication of altered motor control. Bradykinesia, an extreme slowness of movement, is the most disabling feature because it affects all motor systems. Bradykinesia results in a typical stooped posture when the person is standing or walking and a characteristic shuffling gait marked by the absence of normal arm-swinging movements. The absence of facial expression (masklike face) results from loss of facial muscle function. Inability to swallow leads to drooling, while bradykinesia of the muscles in the larynx results in changes in voice quality. Orthostatic hypotension may also be observed and may complicate therapy. Cognitive dysfunction and dementia are also seen in a small percentage of Parkinson's disease patients, especially the elderly.

Pathology

Parkinson's disease is one of the few neurological disorders in which knowledge of the pathology led directly to the rational development of drugs to treat the disease. *The most prominent pathological findings in Parkinson's disease are degeneration of the darkly pigmented dopamine neurons in the substantia nigra, loss of dopamine in the neostriatum, and the presence of intracellular inclusion bodies known as Lewy bodies.* Other neuronal populations are also affected in Parkinson's disease to a much lesser extent, but they may contribute to some of the other pathology seen in parkinsonism (e.g., cognitive decline, depression, and dementia).

In postmortem examination of tissue, the substantia nigra is readily identifiable because of the dark pigmentation in the neurons that is the result of the accumulation of neuromelanin, a substance whose neurochemical composition is not completely known but is thought to derive from oxidized dopamine. Lewy bodies are composed of many cytoskeleton and other proteins, including α-synuclein, ubiquitin, and synaptophysin. It is not clear whether the formation of these inclusions contributes to neuronal degeneration or they are merely a byproduct of degenerating neurons.

Basal Ganglia Anatomy

The basal ganglia can be viewed as modulators of motor function. They are composed of several brain regions, including the neostriatum and the substantia nigra (Fig. 31.1). The neostriatum receives massive excitatory input from the cortex that is mediated by neurons that use glutamate as the neurotransmitter. The dopamine neurons originate in the *substantia nigra pars compacta* and project to the neostriatum, where they synapse on the input glutamatergic terminals and on striatal projection neurons that use the neurotransmitter γ-aminobutyric acid (GABA).

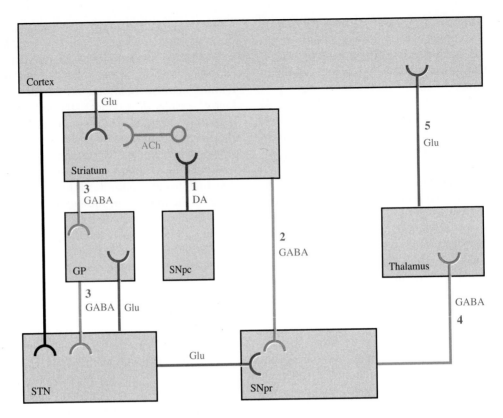

FIGURE 31.1

Basal ganglia and associated circuitry. Several brain regions and numerous neurotransmitters are involved with the function and regulation of neuronal activity within the basal ganglia. In Parkinson's disease, the loss of dopamine neurons projecting from the SNpr to the neostriatum (1) leads to neuronal imbalance in this brain region and alterations in striatal outflow pathways. The direct pathway (2) the striatum to SNpr) becomes less active, whereas the indirect pathway (3) striatum to globus pallidus to STN to SNpr) increases in activity. The consequence is an enhanced activation of SNpr outflow neurons (4), which exert an overall reduction of the thalamic–cortical pathway (5). DA, dopamine; Glu, glutamate, excitatory transmitter; GABA, α-amino butyric acid, inhibitory transmitter; ACh, acetylcholine, excitatory intrastriatal transmitter. GP, globus pallidus; SNpc, substantia nigra pars compacta; SNpr, substantia nigra, pars reticulate; STN, subthalamic nucleus.

Dopamine is a catecholamine (see Chapter 10 and Fig. 31.2) whose actions are mediated by dopamine receptors that are classified as D_1-like (D_1, D_5) or D_2-like (D_2, D_3, D_4). Dopamine actions on D_1 receptors exert an excitatory effect, whereas the actions of dopamine on D_2 receptors inhibit neuronal activity. The loss of striatal dopamine produces an imbalance in information processing in the neostriatum that modifies transmission in other basal ganglia regions. Also important in neural transmission are the striatal interneurons that are found within the confines of the striatum, that use the excitatory neurotransmitter acetylcholine, and that modulate the activity of striatal output neurons.

Possible Mechanisms of Neurodegeneration

The mechanisms responsible for the degeneration of dopamine neurons are not known, but hypotheses include effects such as oxidative stress and excitotoxicity.

The inability of the neurons to eliminate the oxidative load may result in a self-perpetuating cycle of oxidative damage that ultimately leads to neuronal death. One source of oxidative stress may be dopamine metabolism (Fig. 31.2). The excessive excitatory activity in the substantia nigra created by the loss of dopamine actions within the striatum could lead to excitotoxicity that is mediated by glutamate.

Therapy of Parkinsonism

Since there is no cure for parkinsonism, the aim of pharmacological therapy is to provide symptomatic relief. This is obtained through the use of drugs that either increase dopaminergic actions or diminish neuronal outflow from the striatum. These drugs include levodopa, which increases brain dopamine levels; dopamine agonists, which directly stimulate dopamine receptors; monoamine oxidase (MAO) inhibitors, which prevent dopamine metabolism; and anticholinergic agents, which reduce the excitatory activity within the striatum (Fig 31.3).

Levodopa and Carbidopa

Levodopa (*L-DOPA*), the most reliable and effective drug used in the treatment of parkinsonism, can be considered a form of replacement therapy. Levodopa is the biochemical precursor of dopamine (Fig. 31.2). It is used to elevate dopamine levels in the neostriatum of parkinsonian patients. Dopamine itself does not cross the blood-brain barrier and therefore has no CNS effects. However, levodopa, as an amino acid, is transported into the brain by amino acid transport systems, where it

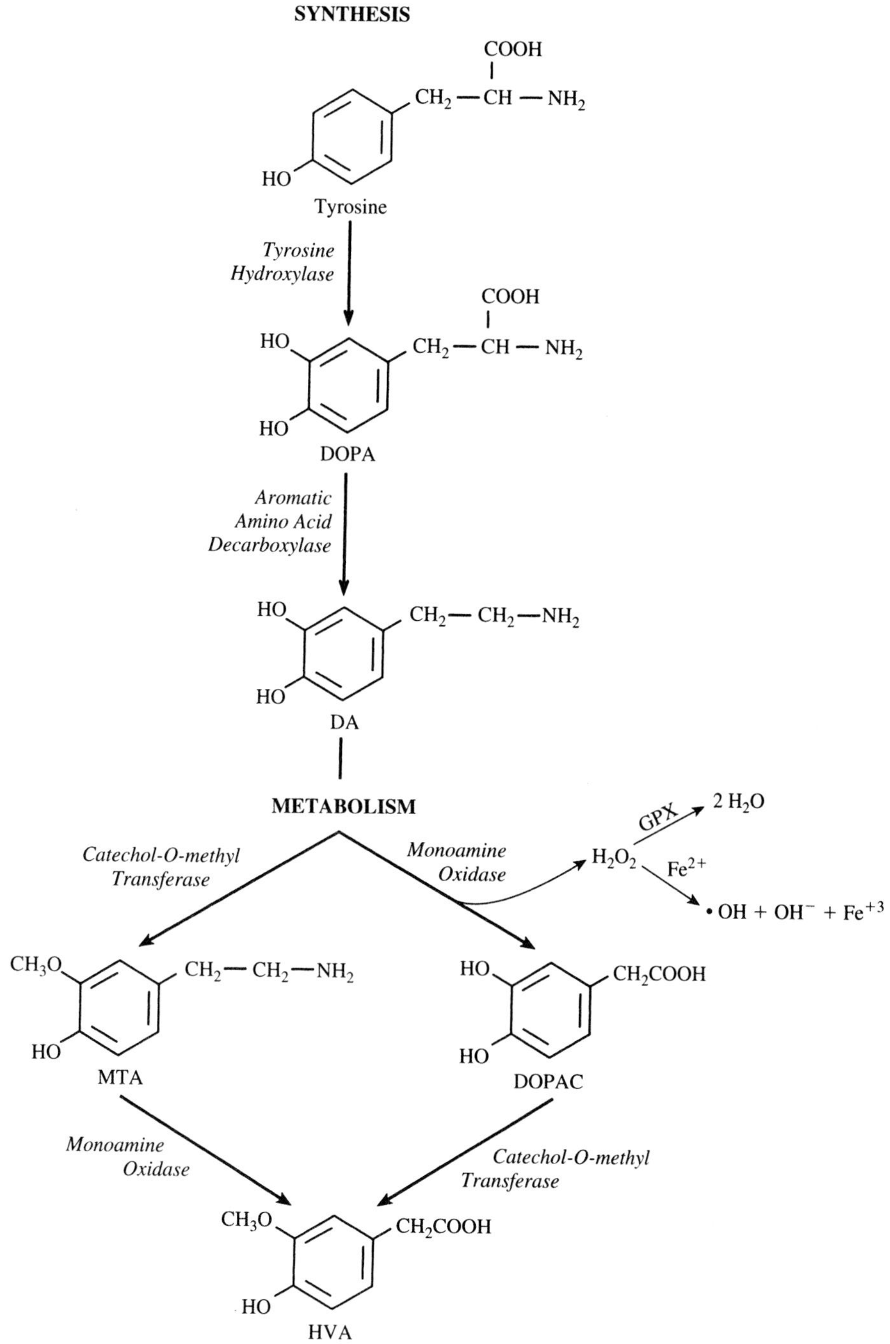

FIGURE 31.2

Pathways in the synthesis and metabolism of dopamine. The metabolism of dopamine produces hydrogen peroxide, which can be converted to water by glutathione peroxidase (GPX) or can in the presence of iron produce reactive hydroxyl radicals. DOPA, dihydroxyphenylalanine; DA, dopamine; MTA, 3-methoxytyramine; DOPAC, dihydroxyphenyl acetic acid; HVA, homovanillic acid; GPX, glutathione peroxidase; H_2O_2, hydrogen peroxide.

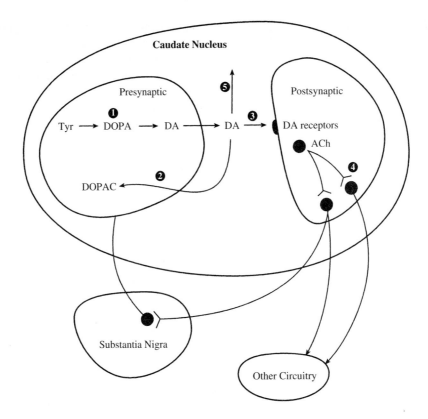

FIGURE 31.3

Pharmacological action of antiparkinsonian drugs. (1) Levodopa, as the immediate precursor of dopamine, increases dopamine production within the basal ganglia. (2) MAO-B inhibitors (selegiline) block a major pathway in dopamine metabolism and thus increase the duration of action of dopamine. (3) Dopamine receptor agonists (pramipexole, pergolide, bromocriptine) directly activate dopamine receptors on postsynaptic neurons. (4) Anticholinergic drugs block the increased excitatory activity of cholinergic interneurons on outflow pathways from the basal ganglia, which is secondary to a loss of inhibitor actions of dopamine on these cholinergic interneurons. (5) COMT inhibitors (with central actions) block an alternate pathway in the metabolism of dopamine.

is converted to dopamine by the enzyme L-aromatic amino acid decarboxylase.

If levodopa is administered alone, it is extensively metabolized by L-aromatic amino acid decarboxylase in the liver, kidney, and gastrointestinal tract. To prevent this peripheral metabolism, levodopa is coadministered with carbidopa (*Sinemet*), a peripheral decarboxylase inhibitor. *The combination of levodopa with carbidopa lowers the necessary dose of levodopa and reduces peripheral side effects associated with its administration.*

Levodopa is widely used for treatment of all types of parkinsonism except those associated with antipsychotic drug therapy. However, as parkinsonism progresses, the duration of benefit from each dose of levodopa may shorten (*wearing-off* effect). Patients can also develop sudden, unpredictable fluctuations between mobility and immobility (*on-off* effect). In a matter of minutes, a patient enjoying normal or nearly normal mobility may suddenly develop a severe degree of parkinsonism. These symptoms are likely due to the

progression of the disease and the loss of striatal dopamine nerve terminals.

Other disturbing behaviors that can be produced by levodopa therapy are the *dyskinesias*. These are excessive and abnormal choreiform movements of the limbs, hands, trunk, and tongue. These dyskinesias eventually occur in 40 to 90% of patients receiving long-term high-dosage levodopa therapy. The mechanism underlying these abnormal movements is unclear, but it may be related to fluctuating plasma levels of levodopa and the presence of hypersensitive dopamine receptors. The dyskinesias can be reduced by lowering the dosage; however, the symptoms of parkinsonism may then reappear. Most patients prefer to tolerate a certain degree of dyskinesia if their mobility can be improved by levodopa therapy.

The most common peripheral side effects are anorexia, nausea, and vomiting (likely due to dopamine's stimulation of the chemoreceptor trigger zone of the area postrema in the medulla oblongata).

Orthostatic hypotension may occur as a result of the peripheral decarboxylation of levodopa and release of dopamine into the circulation. Cardiac arrhythmias occur in some patients and are attributed to the stimulation of cardiac α- and β-adrenoceptors by dopamine.

Centrally mediated adverse effects of levodopa therapy include vivid dreams, delusions, hallucinations, confusion, and sleep disturbances, especially in the elderly. Certain drugs can interfere with the clinical effectiveness or exacerbate the adverse reactions of levodopa therapy. For instance, nonselective MAO inhibitors (phenelzine, tranylcypromine) should not be administered with levodopa, since the combination can precipitate a life-threatening hypertensive crisis and hyperpyrexia. The additive effects of levodopa and adrenomimetic amines demonstrate that extreme care should be exercised in treating the symptoms of asthma or emphysema in patients with Parkinson's disease. Also, levodopa should not be given to patients with narrow-angle glaucoma, since it can produce severe mydriasis that would markedly aggravate the glaucoma. Patients with a history of cardiac arrhythmias or recent cardiac infarction should receive levodopa only when absolutely necessary. Also, proteins ingested with meals may produce sufficient amounts of amino acids to compete effectively with levodopa transport both in the gastrointestinal tract and in the brain. Levodopa therefore should be administered at least 30 minutes before meals.

Dopamine Agonists

Dopamine receptor agonists are considered by many clinicians as the first approach to therapy. They have a long duration of action and are less likely to cause dyskinesias than levodopa. The rationale for the use of dopamine agonists is that they provide a means of directly stimulating dopamine receptors and do not depend on the formation of dopamine from levodopa. As monotherapy, the dopamine agonists are less effective than levodopa but are often used early in the disease to delay initiation of levodopa therapy. When used as an adjunct to levodopa in advanced stages, the dopamine receptor agonists may contribute to clinical improvement and reduce levodopa dosage needs.

The four dopamine agonists used in the United States are bromocriptine (*Parlodel*), pergolide (*Permax*), pramipexole (*Mirapex*), and ropinirole (*Requip*). Bromocriptine, an ergot derivative, is an agonist at the D_2-receptors and a partial D_1-antagonist. Pergolide, also an ergot derivative, is an agonist at both D_1- and D_2-receptor subtypes. The more recently introduced nonergot drugs, ropinirole and pramipexole, are selective agonists at D_2-receptor sites.

All four exert similar therapeutic effects and can produce the same adverse effects seen with levodopa. The differences between the ergot derivatives and the newer agents reside primarily in their adverse effects and tolerability. Postural hypotension, nausea, somnolence, and fatigue are common adverse effects of bromocriptine and pergolide therapy and can limit the use of these drugs.

Because of these adverse effects, the drugs are generally first administered at low doses and then the dose is gradually increased over weeks or months as tolerance to the adverse effects develops. These symptoms are generally less frequent and less severe with pramipexole and ropinirole, which allows for a more rapid achievement of therapeutic response. Also, because pramipexole and ropinirole are better tolerated, they are increasingly used as monotherapy.

Selegiline

Another drug used in the treatment of Parkinson's disease is selegiline (also known as deprenyl, or *Eldepryl*). It is an irreversible inhibitor of MAO-B, an important enzyme in the metabolism of dopamine (Fig. 33.2). Blockade of dopamine metabolism makes more dopamine available for stimulation of its receptors. Selegiline, as monotherapy, may be effective in the newly diagnosed patient with parkinsonism because its pharmacological effect enhances the actions of endogenous dopamine.

Selegiline is also used in conjunction with levodopa–carbidopa in later-stage parkinsonism to reduce levodopa dosage requirements and to minimize or delay the onset of dyskinesias and motor fluctuations that usually accompany long-term treatment with levodopa. It has also been proposed that selegiline may slow the progression of the disease by reducing the formation of toxic free radicals produced during the metabolism of dopamine (Fig.31.2). However, any neuroprotective effect of selegiline in parkinsonian patients remains to be established.

Most of the adverse reactions to selegiline are related to actions of increased levels of dopamine, as discussed earlier. At recommended doses, and unlike the nonselective MAO inhibitors used in the treatment of depression, selegiline has little effect on MAO-A and therefore generally does not cause the hypertension associated with the ingestion of tyramine-enriched foods (see Chapter 20). However, at doses higher than those usually recommended, MAO-A may be inhibited, which increases the risk of a tyramine reaction.

Selegiline should not be coadministered with tricyclic antidepressants or selective serotonin uptake inhibitors because of the possibility of a severe adverse drug reaction (e.g., hyperpyrexia, agitation, delirium, coma).

Anticholinergic Drugs

Before the introduction of levodopa, the *belladonna alkaloids* (e.g., atropine and scopolamine) were the primary agents used in the treatment of parkinsonism. The belladonna alkaloids have been replaced by anticholinergic agents with more selective central nervous system (CNS) effects. Trihexyphenidyl (*Artane*), benztropine mesylate (*Cogentin*), biperiden (*Akineton*), and procyclidine (*Kemadrin*) are useful in most types of parkinsonism.

The efficacy of anticholinergic drugs in parkinsonism is likely due to the ability to block muscarinic receptors in the striatum. In the absence of the inhibitory action of dopamine, the actions of the intrastriatal cholinergic interneurons are unopposed, yielding enhanced stimulation of muscarinic receptors. Blockade of these receptors reduces striatal activity. *The muscarinic antagonists exert only modest antiparkinsonian actions and thus are most commonly used during the early stages of the disease or as an adjunct to levodopa therapy.*

Of the drugs used for treating parkinsonism, the anticholinergics are the only class that can provide benefit in the treatment of the drug-induced parkinsonism seen with antipsychotic therapy. This is because the blockade of dopamine receptors by the antipsychotics leads to increased activity of the striatal neurons. Blockade of the muscarinic receptors reduces this excitatory activity.

The adverse effects of the anticholinergic drugs are due to their antimuscarinic effects in other systems (e.g., cycloplegia, dry mouth, urinary retention, and constipation). Confusion, delirium, and hallucinations may occur at higher doses.

The antihistamine diphenhydramine (*Benadryl*), because it has anticholinergic properties, is used for mild parkinsonism and with the elderly, who may not be able to tolerate the more potent anticholinergics, levodopa, or the dopamine agonists.

Amantadine

Amantadine was originally introduced as an antiviral compound (see Chapter 50), but it is modestly effective in treating symptoms of parkinsonism. It is useful in the early stages of parkinsonism or as an adjunct to levodopa therapy. Its mechanism of action in parkinsonism is not clear, but amantadine may affect dopamine release and reuptake. Additional sites of action may include antagonism at muscarinic and *N*-methyl-D-aspartate (NMDA) receptors. Adverse effects include nausea, dizziness, insomnia, confusion, hallucinations, ankle edema, and livedo reticularis. Amantadine and the anticholinergics may exert additive effects on mental functioning.

Catechol-O-Methyl Transferase Inhibitors

A recently introduced class of drugs for the treatment of parkinsonism is the *catechol-O-methyl transferase (COMT) inhibitors.* COMT metabolizes catechol compounds, including dopamine and levodopa (see Chapter 9), producing the inactive compound 3-*O*-methyl DOPA. The rationale for the use of COMT inhibitors is analogous to that for carbidopa; that is, since COMT is present in the periphery as well as in the CNS, inhibition of peripheral COMT results in an increase in the plasma half-life of levodopa, thereby making more drug available for transfer to the brain. Additionally, compounds that block COMT in the CNS also prolong the brain concentration of levodopa.

The two COMT inhibitors in clinical use are tolcapone (*Tasmar*) and entacapone (*Comtan*). They are used in combination with levodopa–carbidopa. In patients with motor fluctuations, they increase the "on" time. Adverse effects are similar to those observed with levodopa–carbidopa alone. Tolcapone therapy can cause fatal hepatotoxicity and so should be used only in patients who do not respond to other therapies. Patients taking tolcapone require close monitoring of liver enzymes for signs of hepatic changes.

Nonpharmacological Approaches to the Treatment of Parkinsonism

Additional approaches to the treatment of Parkinson's disease include surgical procedures, brain stimulation, and transplantation of dopaminergic cells. In general, surgical procedures are reserved for patients who are refractory to levodopa or who have profound dyskinesias or fluctuations in response to levodopa. Tremor can be abolished by ablation of the ventral intermediate nucleus of the thalamus. Dyskinesias can be effectively controlled by ablation of the posteroventral portion of the globus pallidus. Brain stimulation appears to be a promising technique. High-frequency electrical stimulation of the thalamus, subthalamic nucleus, or globus pallidus can improve various symptoms of parkinsonism and reduce levodopa dosage.

A potentially promising, although very controversial, approach to the treatment of Parkinson's disease is replacement of dopaminergic neurons. The grafting of fetal substantia nigra tissue, which contains the dopamine neurons, into the striatum of parkinsonian patients has been modestly successful. The procedure will remain experimental, however, until the many practical problems and ethical issues associated with the use of fetal tissue are resolved. The discovery of pluripotent stem cells is also being viewed as a possible way of developing dopamine neurons for transplant purposes.

ALZHEIMER'S DISEASE

Alzheimer's disease, the most prevalent form of dementia, afflicts approximately 10% of the population over age 65. The cardinal features of Alzheimer's disease are progressive loss of memory and disordered cognitive function. Alterations in behavior and a decline in language function can also be observed in the early stages of Alzheimer's disease. The impairment in cognitive abilities occurs gradually, with the loss of short-term memory generally preceding loss of long-term distant memory. In the advanced stages, the individual may not recognize spouse or children, and the levels of arousal and alertness are severely impaired. Other signs of Alzheimer's disease include reduced verbal fluency, naming deficits, and impairment of speech exemplified by failure to arrange words in proper order (dysphasia). Ultimately, with progression of the disease, motor function is impaired and the patient may fall into a vegetative state. Death is usually associated with complications of immobility (e.g., pneumonia or pulmonary embolism).

Pathology

The pathological features of Alzheimer's disease include the presence of β-amyloid plaques, τ-enriched neurofibrillary tangles, neuronal loss, and alterations in many neurotransmitter systems. Affected brain regions include the entorhinal cortex; hippocampus; amygdala; association cortices of the frontal, temporal and parietal lobes; and subcortical nuclei that project to these regions. Characteristically, the brains of Alzheimer's disease patients contain two distinct types of insoluble materials that are hallmarks of the brain lesions associated with the disorder: extracellular neuritic plaques containing β-amyloid (Aβ) and intracellular τ-enriched neurofibrillary tangles. As with Lewy bodies in Parkinson's disease, it is unclear whether the tangles and plaques are causal or byproducts of degenerative processes. However, considerable evidence suggests that alterations in Aβ processing may be necessary components of cell destruction.

One theory of the pathogenesis of Alzheimer's disease proposes that increased production or decreased secretion of the Aβ peptides leads to accumulation of these peptides. A second theory proposes that an abnormal τ-protein causes the formation of intracellular neurofibrillary tangles. τ-Proteins are important in the maintenance of cytoskeleton function and axonal transport of proteins. Another theory is that Aβ accumulation is a precipitating factor that is followed by the development of the τ-enriched tangles in the dying neurons.

Therapy of Alzheimer's Disease

The discovery of the loss of the cholinergic neurons and acetylcholine in the brain of Alzheimer's disease patients led to the use of drugs that would enhance the actions of acetylcholine in the brain. Therapeutic agents approved for the treatment of Alzheimer's disease are the *cholinesterase inhibitors*, drugs that block the breakdown of acetylcholine and increase the availability of the neurotransmitter in synapses (see Chapter 12). These drugs are palliative only and do not cure or prevent neurodegeneration.

Available drugs are tacrine (*Cognex*), donepezil (*Aricept*), rivastigmine (*Exelon*), and galanthamine (*Reminyl*). The drugs have a significant but modest effect on the cognitive status of patients, possibly because the drugs do not correct for changes that occur in other neuronal systems.

Adverse effects produced by the drugs include nausea, diarrhea, vomiting, and insomnia. These symptoms are most frequent and severe with tacrine. Hepatotoxicity is associated with tacrine therapy. Because of these significant side effects, tacrine is not widely used.

Future Directions in the Treatment of Alzheimer's Disease

It is becoming clear that Alzheimer's disease is a multifactorial syndrome and that unraveling its causes may be difficult. However, as knowledge of the mechanisms of degeneration are elucidated, this knowledge can be applied to the development of therapies to alleviate the symptoms and hopefully to prevent the disease or inhibit its progression.

Several new directions in therapeutic approaches are being investigated. One is to lower Aβ peptide levels and thus reduce Aβ deposits through the use of molecules that prevent the proteolytic cleavage of amyloid precursor protein or through a novel immunization technique that would use antibodies to remove the Aβ peptides from the cells and brain. Other approaches being examined are targeted at blocking the more downstream effects, such as the use of antiinflammatory agents and antioxidants.

Study QUESTIONS

1. J. S. is a newly diagnosed Parkinson's disease patient who has motor difficulties. Which of the following is the most appropriate treatment for early stage parkinsonism?
   (A) Levodopa–carbidopa
   (B) Pramipexole
   (C) Entacapone
   (D) Clozapine
   (E) Donepezil

2. M. K. is a 60-year-old woman with Parkinson's disease. Her current therapy is levodopa–carbidopa. She complains that she frequently goes from being

fairly mobile to being immobile in only a matter of a few minutes. Her neurologist decides to add tolcapone to her therapy. What blood tests should be performed before and during her treatment with tolcapone?
(A) Red blood cell count
(B) White blood cell count
(C) Serum levels of calcium and phosphorus
(D) Serum levels of creatinine and uric acid
(E) Serum levels of transglutaminase enzymes

3. T. T. is a 75-year-old man whom you have seen off and on for 5 years. His wife accompanies him for his visit. She indicates that he is getting very forgetful and that about 2 weeks ago, he got lost on a trip to the grocery store and she had to go pick him up. You suspect that your patient is in the early stages of Alzheimer's disease. Which of the following would be most appropriate?
(A) Tell T. T. that this is normal for his age and not to worry.
(B) Suggest that he begin adding a daily vitamin to his existing treatment.
(C) Don't tell your patient anything, but arrange for a separate appointment with his wife in which you tell her that T. T. has Alzheimer's disease.
(D) Tell T. T. that this may be an early sign of Alzheimer's disease and offer a prescription to a cholinesterase inhibitor approved for the treatment of Alzheimer's disease.

4. N. C. is a 67-year-old woman with Parkinson's disease. She appears in the emergency department complaining of purplish mottling of the skin on her legs. The most likely drug to be involved is
(A) Levodopa
(B) Levodopa–carbidopa (Sinemet)
(C) Bromocriptine
(D) Amantadine
(E) Tolcapone

5. B. M. is a 45-year-old schizophrenic who finally has his antipsychotic medication adjusted properly and who is doing reasonably well at the moment. He came to your office today exhibiting many signs of parkinsonism, including tremor, rigidity, stooped posture, and shuffling gait. He indicates that even though his schizophrenia is under control, these new symptoms are very unpleasant. What do you do?
(A) Withdraw his antipsychotic medication.
(B) Prescribe levodopa.
(C) Prescribe a muscarinic blocking agent.
(D) Prescribe a dopa agonist.
(E) Prescribe amantadine.

ANSWERS
1. **B.** Pramipexole is a dopamine receptor agonist. This class of drugs is often used in the early stages

of parkinsonism. Ropinirole and pergolide are other drugs in this class that could be used. Some patients also get symptomatic relief from selegiline (MAO inhibitor). Although levodopa–carbidopa would be effective, this therapy is usually delayed until other treatments become ineffective. Entacapone is a COMT inhibitor and is used only in combination with levodopa–carbidopa to inhibit the peripheral metabolism of levodopa. Clozapine is an antipsychotic drug used to treat levodopa-induced psychosis. Donepezil is an anticholinesterase inhibitor that increases acetylcholine actions in the brain. This drug may exacerbate parkinsonism.

2. **E.** The patient is feeling the on-off effects of levodopa therapy, possibly as a result of fluctuating blood and brain levels of levodopa. The rationale for adding tolcapone (a COMT inhibitor) to her therapy is to reduce the peripheral metabolism of levodopa, thus increasing its plasma half-life and its duration of action in the brain. However, tolcapone can produce hepatotoxicity. Therefore, it is important to monitor hepatic function before and during treatment. Increased levels of transglutaminase enzymes (e.g., SGOT [serum glutamic-oxaloacetic transaminase] and SGPT [serum glutamate pyruvate transaminase]) indicate compromised hepatic function. If elevations occur during treatment, tolcapone therapy must be stopped. The patient could then be treated with entacapone, a COMT inhibitor that is not associated with hepatotoxicity. Other approaches to treating the on-off symptoms may also be used. For example, the physician might consider switching the patient to a controlled-release formulation of levodopa–carbidopa, which would provide a more prolonged release of levodopa or adding a dopamine receptor agonist, which has a longer duration of action than levodopa.

3. **D.** The patient should be informed that his symptoms are consistent with early Alzheimer's disease but that he will need testing to rule out other causes of memory impairment. Subsequently he may be offered the opportunity to try one of the agents that is approved for this condition. However, you should indicate that although these agents are not curative, they are beneficial to many patients.

4. **D.** Although not widely used, amantadine may be useful in the early stages of Parkinson's disease or as an adjunct to other agents. Livedo reticularis is a characteristic purple mottling of the skin associated with amantadine.

5. **C.** A is not correct because the signs and symptoms of schizophrenia would soon reappear. The administration of levodopa will not antagonize the signs of Parkinson's disease in this patient because there is no deficit of dopa, only a blockade of dopamine receptors. Likewise the administration of either a

dopa agonist or amantadine will be ineffective. A muscarinic blocking agent will block the increased activity of striatal neurons and antagonize the parkinsonism.

SUPPLEMENTAL READING

Grutzendler J and Morris JC. Cholinesterase inhibitors for Alzheimer's disease. Drugs 2001;61:41–52.

Mark MH. Treatment of Parkinson's disease. Med Lett 2001;14:151–161.

Olanow CW and Tatton WG. Etiology and pathogenesis of Parkinson's disease. Annu Rev Neurosci 1999;22:123–144.

Selkoe DJ. Alzheimer's disease: Genes, proteins and therapy. Physiol Rev 2001;81:741–766.

CASE Study   Early-Stage Parkinsonism

M.S. is a 60-year old architect who designs buildings. His drawings are very detailed and they must be drawn to a specific scale. During the past month he has developed a slight tremor in his right hand that causes some embarrassment but does not interfere with function. He has, however, noticed that his writing and drawing have gotten much smaller, causing problems with his work. His primary care physician has referred him to a neurologist for evaluation. On examination, the neurologist notes some motor rigidity in the right arm. He also observes a slight slowing in the patient's walk and a reduction in the swing of his arms as he walks. What is the diagnosis, and how should the patient be treated?

ANSWER: The patient is in early-stage parkinsonism, most likely idiopathic (Parkinson's disease). Clinically, the disease is very mild and the neurologist might consider not treating him at this point, but because the micrographia interferes with his work, the neurologist decides to prescribe medication. Several drugs can be used to treat early-onset parkinsonism. The most commonly used are the dopamine receptor agonists (pramipexole, ropinirole, pergolide; amantadine is also a possibility, and some people get an acceptable response to selegiline, the MAO inhibitor). Levodopa–carbidopa could also be used; however, most clinicians prefer to delay its use until absolutely needed because of the adverse effects, such as motor fluctuations and dyskinesias, that accompany long-term use of levodopa.

32 Antiepileptic Drugs

Charles R. Craig

DRUG LIST

GENERIC NAME	PAGE	GENERIC NAME	PAGE
Carbamazepine	378	Mephenytoin	378
Clobazam	381	Mephobarbital	381
Clonazepam	380	Metharbital	381
Clorazepate	381	Nitrazepam	381
Diazepam	383	Oxcarbazepine	379
Ethosuximide	381	Phenobarbital	381
Ethotoin	378	Phenytoin	377
Felbamate	382	Primidone	381
Fosphenytoin	383	Tiagabine	381
Gabapentin	382	Topiramate	379
Levetiracetam	382	Valproic acid (Sodium valproate)	379
Lamotrigine	379	Vigabatrin	381
Lorazepam	380	Zonisamide	379

Epilepsy (or epilepsies, since markedly different clinical entities exist) is a common neurological abnormality affecting about 1% of the human population. Epilepsy is a chronic, usually life-long disorder characterized by recurrent seizures or convulsions and usually, episodes of unconsciousness and/or amnesia. Table 32.1 illustrates the major types of epileptic seizures. Patients often exhibit more than one type. In most instances, the cause of the seizure disorder is not known (idiopathic epilepsy), although trauma during birth is suspected of being one cause.

Head trauma, meningitis, childhood fevers, brain tumors, and degenerative diseases of the cerebral circulation are conditions often associated with the appearance of recurrent seizures that may require treatment with anticonvulsant drugs. Seizures also may be a toxic manifestation of the action of central nervous system (CNS) stimulants and certain other drugs. Seizures often occur in hyperthermia (febrile seizures are very common in infants); sometimes in eclampsia, uremia, hypoglycemia, or pyridoxine deficiency; and frequently as a part of the abstinence syn-

TABLE 32.1 Major Seizure Types

Clinical Seizure Type	Key Ictal EEG Manifestations	Major Clinical Manifestations
I. Partial (focal, local) seizures A. Simple partial seizures	Local contralateral discharge	Seizures may be limited to a single limb or muscle group; may show sequential involvement of body parts (epileptic march); consciousness usually preserved; may be somatosensory (hallucinations, tingling, gustatory sensations); may have autonomic symptoms or signs such as epigastric sensations, sweating, papillary dilation
B. Complex partial seizures (psychomotor epilepsy, temporal lobe epilepsy)	Unilateral or bilateral asynchronous focus, most often in temporal region	Impairment of consciousness, may have automatisms, flashback (déjà vu, terror); autonomic activity such as pupil dilation, flushing, piloerection
C. Partial seizures evolving to secondary generalized seizures		May generalize to tonic, clonic, or tonic-clonic
II. Generalized seizures A. Absence seizures (petit mal epilepsy)	3-Hz polyspike and wave	Brief loss of consciousness with or without motor involvement; occurs in childhood with a tendency to disappear following adolescence
B. Myoclonic seizures		Sudden, brief, shocklike contractions of musculature (myoclonic jerks)
C. Clonic seizures	Fast activity (10 Hz or more; slow waves)	Repetitive muscle jerks
D. Tonic seizures	Low-voltage, fast activity	Rigid, violent muscular contraction with limbs fixed
E. Tonic-clonic seizures (grand mal epilepsy)	Fast activity (10 Hz or more) increasing in amplitude during tonic phase; interrupted by slow waves during clonic phase	Loss of consciousness; sudden sharp tonic contractions of muscles, falling to ground, followed by clonic convulsive movements; often postictal depression and incontinence
F. Atonic seizures (astatic)	Polyspikes and wave	Sudden diminution in muscle tone affecting isolated muscle groups or loss of all muscle tone; may have extremely brief loss of consciousness

Modified from the International Classification of Epileptic Seizures. Various methods of seizure classification are used by different authors.

drome of individuals physically dependent on CNS depressants.

The therapeutic goal in epilepsy treatment is complete seizure control without excessive side effects. The prognosis depends in part upon the type of seizure disorder, but overall, only about 40 to 60% of patients become totally seizure free with available drugs. These agents are chemically and pharmacologically diverse, having in common only their ability to inhibit seizure activity without impairing consciousness. The choice of drug or drugs used depends on seizure classification, since a particular drug may be more or less specific for a particular type of seizure; patients having a mixture of seizure types present particular therapeutic difficulties. It is not always clear when to treat with one drug (monotherapy) or more than one drug (polytherapy) in a particular patient. Approximately 25% of patients given a single anticonvulsive agent do not achieve successful seizure control because of an unacceptable level of side effects. Therefore, two or more drugs may be combined in an attempt to provide better seizure control.

Convulsive disorders often begin in childhood, and drug therapy must be continued for decades; therefore,

any adverse reaction is especially significant. A knowledge of interactions between anticonvulsants and other drugs is necessary, since the patient usually must continue anticonvulsant medication regardless of the need for other drugs. Since it may be dangerous to withdraw anticonvulsant medication from a pregnant woman with epilepsy, the teratogenic potential of anticonvulsant drugs also is a consideration in the treatment of women of childbearing age.

The Development of Effective Drug Treatment for Convulsive Disorders

The first effective treatment of seizure disorders was the serendipitous finding in 1857 that potassium bromide could control seizures in some patients. Even though side effects were troublesome, the bromides were widely used for many years. Phenobarbital was introduced as a treatment for epilepsy in 1912 and was immediately shown to be markedly superior to bromides. While other barbiturates were synthesized and used, none were shown to be superior to phenobarbital, and the latter compound is still used. A chemically related nonbarbiturate, phenytoin, was discovered about 20 years later and also remains a valuable drug today. Approaches being used for the identification of new anticonvulsant drugs include the search for agents that block specific cationic channels in neuronal membranes, agents that enhance the activity of the inhibitory neurotransmitter γ-aminobutyric acid (GABA), and agents that are capable of inhibiting the activity of the excitatory neurotransmitters glutamic and aspartic acids.

Mechanism of Action

In epilepsy certain neurons and/or groups of neurons become hyperexcitable and begin firing bursts of action potentials that propagate in a synchronous manner to other brain structures (and in the case of generalized seizures, to practically all areas of the brain). These may be the result of abnormalities in neuronal membrane stability or in the connections among neurons. It is known that the epileptic bursts consist of sodium-dependent action potentials and a calcium-dependent depolarizing potential.

Recent drug development studies have centered on the capacity of known antiepileptic drugs (AEDs) to interact with ion channels, and it is now established that several agents appear to be exerting their effects primarily by inhibiting ion channels. Modulation of neuronal sodium channels decreases cellular excitability and the propagation of nerve impulses. Inhibition of sodium channels appears to be a major component of the mechanism of action of several anticonvulsant drugs.

Much interest is also centered on the role of calcium channels in neuronal activity, since the depolarization associated with burst firing is mediated by the activation of calcium channels. At therapeutically relevant concentrations, the antiabsence drug ethosuximide appears to exert its effect by inhibiting the T-type calcium channels. A portion of valproic acid's activity may also be attributable to this effect.

Disinhibition may play an important role in the generation of epileptic seizures, since a reduction of GABAergic inhibition is necessary to produce the synchronous burst discharges in groups of cells. Compounds that antagonize the activity of GABA (picrotoxinin, penicillin C, bicuculline) are CNS convulsants, while agents that facilitate GABA's inhibition have anticonvulsant activity. Several anticonvulsant drugs act to facilitate the actions of GABA.

Excitatory neurotransmitters also may be involved in the appearance of epilepsy, since the bursting activity typically seen during epileptic discharges may be due in part to the action of glutamate acting on N-methyl-D-aspartate (NMDA) receptor channels to produce depolarization. It is likely that a major part of the anticonvulsant activity of felbamate involves blockade of the NMDA receptor. Table 32.2 summarizes the most likely mechanism of action associated with available anticonvulsant drugs.

CLINICALLY USEFUL DRUGS

Anticonvulsant drugs may be divided into four classes, based on their most likely mechanism of action. Although it may be premature to assign a mechanism of action to some of these compounds, the proposed classes are a convenient way to group the drugs. Furthermore, the classes themselves may have rele-

---

TABLE 32.2   Categorization of Anticonvulsants by Their Proposed Mechanism

Class	Description	Drugs
Type I	Block SRF by enhancing sodium channel inactivation	Phenytoin Carbamazepine Oxcarbazepine Lamotrigine Felbamate[a]
Type II	Multiple actions: enhance GABAergic inhibition, reduce T-calcium currents, and possibly block SRF	Valproic acid Benzodiazepines Phenobarbital Primidone
Type III	Block T-calcium currents only	Ethosuximide Trimethadione
Type IV	Only enhances GABAergic inhibition	Vigabatrin
Noncategorized	Has no known effect on SRF, GABAergic inhibition, or T-calcium currents	Gabapentin[b]

Adapted with permission from designation of classes described by Macdonald RL and Meldrum BS. In Levy RH et al. (eds.). *Antiepileptic Drugs* (4th ed.). New York: Raven, 1995:61-77.
[a]Felbamate probably possesses other actions.
[b]The mechanisms of action of gabapentin are unknown.
SRF, sustained high-frequency repetitive firing.

vance, since compounds in a particular category are often used for the same clinical indication. For a proposed mechanism of action to be considered relevant for a given drug, the effect must occur at concentrations similar to those that are likely to be achieved therapeutically.

Sodium Channel Blocking Agents

Drugs sharing this mechanism include phenytoin (*Dilantin*), carbamazepine (*Tegretol*), oxcarbazepine (*Trileptal*), topiramate (*Topamax*), valproic acid (*Depakene*), zonisamide (*Zonegran*), and lamotrigine (*Lamictal*). All of these agents have the capacity to block sustained high-frequency repetitive firing (SRF) of action potentials. This is accomplished by reducing the amplitude of sodium-dependent action potentials through an enhancement of steady-state inactivation. The sodium channel exists in three main conformations: a resting (R) or activatable state, an open (0) or conducting state, and an inactive (I) or nonactivatable state. The anticonvulsant drugs bind preferentially to the inactive form of the channel. Because it takes time for the bound drug to dissociate from the inactive channel, there is time dependence to the block. Since the fraction of inactive channels is increased by membrane depolarization as well as by repetitive firing, the binding to the I state by antiepileptic drugs can produce voltage-, use-, and time-dependent block of sodium-dependent action potentials. This effect is similar to that of local anesthetic drugs (see Chapter 27) and is shown in Figure 32.1.

These agents are discussed together because their pharmacological properties, clinical indications for the treatment of epilepsy, and presumed mechanisms of action are similar. They differ from each other in several ways, however, and one drug cannot routinely be substituted for another. They differ primarily in their pharmacokinetic properties, their adverse reactions, and their interactions with other drugs. In addition to blocking sodium channels, some possess other therapeutically relevant mechanisms of action as well.

Phenytoin

Phenytoin is a valuable agent for the treatment of generalized tonic–clonic seizures and for the treatment of partial seizures with complex symptoms. The establishment of phenytoin (at that time known as diphenylhydantoin) in 1938 as an effective treatment for epilepsy was more than simply the introduction of another drug for treatment of seizure disorders. Until that time the only drugs that had any beneficial effects in epilepsy were the bromides and barbiturates, both classes of compounds having marked CNS depressant properties. The prevailing view among neurologists of that era was that epilepsy was the result of excessive electrical activ-

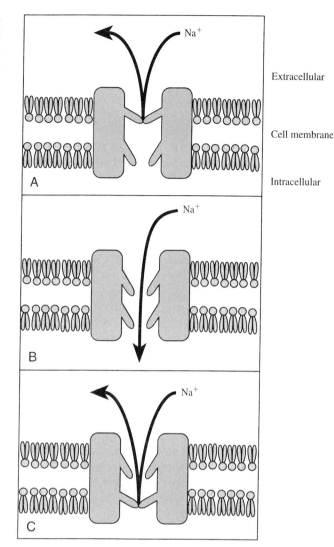

FIGURE 32.1

Mechanism of action of anticonvulsant drugs that act on sodium channels. The sodium channel can normally exist in a closed (**A**), open (**B**), or inactivated (**C**) state. **A.** An activation gate is closed and sodium ions cannot pass through the channel. **B.** The channel activation gate opens rapidly following depolarization and sodium enters freely. Soon after opening, an inactivation gate (**C**) closes, preventing further entry of sodium ions into the cell. Phenytoin and drugs with a similar mechanism of action stabilize and prolong the existence of the inactivated state, and therefore, sodium entry is impeded longer than occurs in the absence of the drug.

ity in the brain and it therefore seemed perfectly reasonable that CNS depressants would be effective in antagonizing the seizures. Consequently, many patients received high doses of barbiturates and spent much of their time sedated. Also, since CNS depression was considered to be the mechanism of action of AEDs, the pharmaceutical firms were evaluating only compounds with profound CNS depressant properties as potential antiepileptic agents. It was, therefore, revolutionary when phenytoin was shown to be as effective as phenobarbital in the treatment of epilepsy without any significant CNS depressant activity. This revolutionized the search for new anticonvulsant drugs as well as immediately improving the day-to-day functioning of epileptic patients.

An understanding of absorption, binding, metabolism, and excretion is more important for phenytoin than it is for most drugs. Following oral administration, phenytoin absorption is slow but usually complete, and it occurs primarily in the duodenum. Phenytoin is highly bound (about 90%) to plasma proteins, primarily plasma albumin. Since several other substances can also bind to albumin, phenytoin administration can displace (and be displaced by) such agents as thyroxine, triiodothyronine, valproic acid, sulfafurazole, and salicylic acid.

Phenytoin is one of very few drugs that displays zero-order (or saturation) kinetics in its metabolism. At low blood levels the rate of phenytoin metabolism is proportional to the drug's blood levels (i.e., first-order kinetics). However, at the higher blood levels usually required to control seizures, the maximum capacity of drug-metabolizing enzymes is often exceeded (i.e., the enzyme is saturated), and further increases in the dose of phenytoin may lead to a disproportionate increase in the drug's blood concentration. Since the plasma levels continue to increase in such a situation, steady-state levels are not attained, and toxicity may ensue. Calculation of half-life ($t_{1/2}$) values for phenytoin often is meaningless, since the apparent half-life varies with the drug blood level.

Acute adverse effects seen after phenytoin administration usually result from overdosage. They are generally characterized by nystagmus, ataxia, vertigo, and diplopia (cerebellovestibular dysfunction). Higher doses lead to altered levels of consciousness and cognitive changes.

A variety of idiosyncratic reactions may be seen shortly after therapy has begun. Skin rashes, usually morbilliform in character, are most common. Exfoliative dermatitis or toxic epidermal necrolysis (Lyellís syndrome) has been observed but is infrequent. Other rashes occasionally have been reported, as have a variety of blood dyscrasias and hepatic necrosis.

The most common side effect in children receiving long-term therapy is gingival hyperplasia, or overgrowth of the gums (occurs in up to 50% of patients). Although the condition is not serious, it is a cosmetic problem and can be very embarrassing to the patient. Hirsutism also is an annoying side effect of phenytoin, particularly in young females. Thickening of subcutaneous tissue, coarsening of facial features, and enlargement of lips and nose (hydantoin facies) are often seen in patients receiving long-term phenytoin therapy.

Peripheral neuropathy and chronic cerebellar degeneration have been reported, but they are rare.

There is evidence that phenytoin is teratogenic in humans, but the mechanism is not clear. However, it is known that phenytoin can produce a folate deficiency, and folate deficiency is associated with teratogenesis.

Only a few well-documented drug combinations with phenytoin may necessitate dosage adjustment. Coadministration of the following drugs can result in elevations of plasma phenytoin levels in most patients: cimetidine, chloramphenicol, disulfiram, sulthiame, and isoniazid (in slow acetylators). Phenytoin often causes a decline in plasma carbamazepine levels if these two drugs are given concomitantly.

Ethotoin and mephenytoin are congeners of phenytoin that are marketed as AEDs in the United States. They are not widely used.

Carbamazepine

Carbamazepine has become a major drug in the treatment of seizure disorders. It has high efficacy, is well tolerated by most patients, and exhibits fewer long-term side effects than other drugs.

Oral absorption of carbamazepine is quite slow and often erratic. Its half-life is reported to vary from 12 to 60 hours in humans. The development of blood level assays has markedly improved the success of therapy with this drug, since serum concentration is only partially dose related. Carbamazepine is metabolized in the liver, and there is evidence that its continued administration leads to hepatic enzyme induction. Carbamazepine-10,11-epoxide is a pharmacologically active metabolite with significant anticonvulsant effects of its own.

Carbamazepine is an effective agent for the treatment of partial seizures and generalized tonic–clonic seizures; its use is contraindicated in absence epilepsy. Carbamazepine is also useful in the treatment of trigeminal neuralgia and is an effective agent for the treatment of bipolar disorders (see Chapter 33).

Like most of the agents that block sodium channels, side effects associated with carbamazepine administration involve the central nervous system (CNS). Drowsiness is the most common side effect, followed by nausea, headache, dizziness, incoordination, vertigo, and diplopia. These effects occur particularly when the drug is first taken, but tolerance often develops over a few weeks. There appears to be little risk of cognitive impairment with carbamazepine.

Carbamazepine causes a variety of rashes and other allergic reactions including fever, hepatosplenomegaly, and lymphadenopathy, but the incidence of serious hypersensitivity reactions is rare. Systemic lupus erythematosus can occur, but discontinuation of the drug leads to eventual disappearance of the symptoms. Idiosyncratic hematological reactions to carbamazepine may occur, but serious blood dyscrasias are rare. Carbamazepine has been shown to exacerbate or precipitate seizures in some patients, particularly those exhibiting generalized atypical absences.

While the number of side effects may be fairly large, most are not serious and can be managed. Severe adverse reactions occur less commonly than with phenytoin and similar drugs. The overall incidence of toxicity seems to be fairly low at usual therapeutic doses.

Most of the drug interactions with carbamazepine are related to its effects on microsomal drug metabolism. Carbamazepine can induce its own metabolism (autoinduction) after prolonged administration, decreasing its clearance rate, half-life, and serum concentrations. The possibility of autoinduction requires the clinician to reevaluate the patient's blood levels after a month of carbamazepine therapy. The autoinduction phenomenon is over in about a month.

Carbamazepine also can induce the enzymes that metabolize other anticonvulsant drugs, including phenytoin, primidone, phenobarbital, valproic acid, clonazepam, and ethosuximide, and metabolism of other drugs the patient may be taking. Similarly, other drugs may induce metabolism of carbamazepine; the end result is the same as for autoinduction, and the dose of carbamazepine must be readjusted. A common drug–drug interaction is between carbamazepine and the macrolide antibiotics erythromycin and troleandomycin. After a few days of antibiotic therapy, symptoms of carbamazepine toxicity develop; this is readily reversible if either the antibiotic or carbamazepine is discontinued.

Cimetidine, propoxyphene, and isoniazid also have been reported to inhibit metabolism of carbamazepine. It is essential to monitor blood levels and adjust the dose if necessary whenever additional drugs are given to patients taking carbamazepine.

Oxcarbazepine

Oxcarbazepine is chemically and pharmacologically closely related to carbamazepine, but it has much less capacity to induce drug-metabolizing enzymes. This property decreases the problems associated with drug interactions when oxcarbazepine is used in combination with other drugs. The clinical uses and adverse effect profile of oxcarbazepine appear to be similar to those of carbamazepine.

Lamotrigine

Lamotrigine has a broad spectrum of action and is effective in generalized and partial epilepsies. Its primary mechanism of action appears to be blockage of voltage-dependent sodium channels, although its effectiveness against absence seizures indicates that additional mechanisms may be active. Lamotrigine is almost completely absorbed from the gastrointestinal tract, and peak plasma levels are achieved in about 2 to 5 hours. The plasma half-life after a single dose is about 24 hours. Unlike most drugs, lamotrigine is metabolized primarily by glucuronidation. Therefore, it appears likely that lamotrigine will not induce or inhibit cytochrome P450 isozymes, in contrast to most AEDs.

Severe skin rashes appear to be the major concern with lamotrigine use. The incidence of rash is greater in children than in adults. Other adverse effects are similar to those of drugs with the same mechanism of action, such as cerebellovestibular changes leading to dizziness, diplopia, ataxia, and blurred vision. Disseminated intravascular coagulation has been reported.

Topiramate

Topiramate is most useful in patients with generalized tonic–clonic seizures and those with partial complex seizures. Topiramate causes a higher incidence of CNS-related side effects (primarily cognitive slowing and confusion) than other AEDs. It does not appear to cause a significant incidence of rashes or other hypersensitivity reactions; however, a significantly higher incidence of kidney stones has been observed in persons receiving topiramate than in a similar untreated population.

Zonisamide

Zonisamide has only recently been approved for use in the United States, although it has been available in Japan for several years. It is effective in partial complex and generalized tonic–clonic seizures and also appears to be beneficial in certain myoclonic seizures. It has a long half-life (about 60 hours) and requires about 2 weeks to achieve steady-state levels. It causes cerebellovestibular side effects similar to those of most other AEDs sharing its mechanism of action. In addition, it appears to cause an increased incidence of kidney stones.

Valproic Acid (Sodium Valproate)

Although it is marketed as both valproic acid (*Depakene*) and as sodium valproate (*Depakote*), it is the valproate ion that is absorbed from the gastrointestinal tract and is the active form.

As with several other AEDs, it is difficult to ascribe a single mechanism of action to valproic acid. This compound has broad anticonvulsant activity, both in experimental studies and in the therapeutic management of human epilepsy. Valproic acid has been shown to block voltage-dependent sodium channels at therapeutically relevant concentrations. In several experimental studies, valproate caused an increase in brain GABA; the mechanism was unclear. There is evidence that valproate may also inhibit T-calcium channels and that this may be important in its mechanism of action in patients with absence epilepsy.

Valproic acid is well absorbed from the gastrointestinal tract and is highly bound (~90%) to plasma protein, and most of the compound is therefore retained within the vascular compartment. Valproate rapidly enters the brain from the circulation; the subsequent decline in brain concentration parallels that in plasma, indicating equilibration between brain and capillary blood. A large number of metabolites have been identified, but it is not known whether they play a role in the anticonvulsant effect of the parent drug. Valproic acid inhibits the metabolism of several drugs, including phenobarbital, primidone, carbamazepine, and phenytoin, leading to an increased blood level of these compounds. At high doses, valproic acid can inhibit its own metabolism. It can also displace phenytoin from binding sites on plasma proteins, with a resultant increase in unbound phenytoin and increased phenytoin toxicity. In this instance, the dosage of phenytoin should be adjusted as required. These examples reinforce the need to determine serum anticonvulsant levels in epileptic patients when polytherapy is employed.

Valproic acid has become a major AED against several seizure types. It is highly effective against absence seizures and myoclonic seizures. In addition, valproic acid can be used either alone or in combination with other drugs for the treatment of generalized tonic–clonic epilepsy and for partial seizures with complex symptoms.

The most serious adverse effect associated with valproic acid is fatal hepatic failure. Fatal hepatotoxicity is most likely to occur in children under age 2 years, especially in those with severe seizures who are given multiple anticonvulsant drug therapy. The hepatotoxicity is not dose related and is considered an idiosyncratic reaction; it can occur in individuals in other age groups, and therefore, valproic acid should not be administered to patients with hepatic disease or significant hepatic dysfunction or to those who are hypersensitive to it. Valproic acid administration has been linked to an increased incidence of neural tube defects in the fetus of mothers who received valproate during the first trimester of pregnancy. Patients taking valproate may develop clotting abnormalities.

Valproic acid causes hair loss in about 5% of patients, but this effect is reversible. Transient gastrointestinal effects are common, and some mild behavioral effects have been reported. Metabolic effects, including hyperglycemia, hyperglycinuria, and hyperammonemia, have been reported. An increase in body weight also has been noted. Valproic acid is not a CNS depressant, but its administration may lead to increased depression if it is used in combination with phenobarbital, primidone, benzodiazepines, or other CNS depressant agents.

Drugs That Primarily Enhance the Action of GABA

A major effort has been directed to the search for agents that can mimic, facilitate, prolong, or enhance the actions of GABA, with the expectation that such compounds will likely be beneficial in the treatment of convulsive disorders. Although there have been some disappointments, in general this appears to be a fruitful approach in the search for better and safer antiepileptic compounds.

Benzodiazepines

Several benzodiazepines are used in the management of epileptic seizures, although only a few are approved for the treatment of seizure disorders in the United States. Since the benzodiazepines share many properties, they will be discussed as a class; individual members will be mentioned for specific indications.

The primary action of the benzodiazepines as anticonvulsants is to enhance inhibition through their interaction with the $GABA_A$ receptor at the benzodiazepine binding site. However, there appears to be an additional action of benzodiazepines: blocking voltage-dependent sodium channels. This effect is not seen at usual doses but is likely a factor in their use in the treatment of status epilepticus (discussed later).

Benzodiazepines are well absorbed, and the oral route is preferred in most situations. In the treatment of status epilepticus, the preferred route is usually intravenous. Benzodiazepines are extensively metabolized by the microsomal drug-metabolizing system; frequently an active compound is broken down to another agent that is also active pharmacologically. This is the reason for the long duration of action of several benzodiazepines.

The benzodiazepines have many clinical indications and are discussed in Chapters 25, 30, 35, and 40. As AEDs, they have their major usefulness in the treatment of absence, myoclonic, and atonic seizures and in the emergency treatment of status epilepticus.

Drowsiness occurs readily and unfortunately is usually a problem at therapeutic doses. The other limiting side effect of the benzodiazepines is the rapid development of tolerance to their anticonvulsant effects.

Although all of the benzodiazepines are similar, certain ones are employed more for the treatment of seizure disorders. Clonazepam was the first benzodiazepine approved in the United States specifically for the treatment of convulsive disorders. Clonazepam is a very long acting compound with potent anticonvulsant activity. Unfortunately, sedation and tolerance tend to limit its usefulness. Drooling and hypersalivation may be troublesome in children and in infants.

Lorazepam is the benzodiazepine of choice for emergency treatment of status epilepticus, serial seizures, and prolonged seizures and for prophylaxis of febrile seizures. The intravenous route is preferable for emergency treatment.

Clorazepate dipotassium is approved in the United States as an adjunct in the treatment of partial complex seizures. It appears to be useful, especially in patients with high seizure frequencies and psychic disturbances.

Other benzodiazepines have been used as AEDs but are not approved for this use in the United States. They include lorazepam (*Ativan*), nitrazepam (*Mogadon*), and clobazam (*Urbanil*). It is unlikely that these drugs offer any advantages over similar agents.

Tiagabine

Tiagabine (*Gabitril*) blocks the reuptake of GABA into neurons and glia, thereby resulting in higher levels of GABA in the synaptic cleft. The ability to increase GABA concentrations is presumed to be involved in the effectiveness of tiagabine in the treatment of seizure disorders. It is primarily used in the treatment of partial complex seizures. Adverse effects of tiagabine administration include dizziness, somnolence, nervousness, nausea, and confusion.

Vigabatrin

Vigabatrin (*Sabril*) is a relatively specific irreversible inhibitor of GABA-transaminase (GABA-T), the major enzyme responsible for the metabolism of GABA in the mammalian CNS. As a result of inhibition of GABA-T, there is an increase in the concentration of GABA in the brain and consequently an increase in inhibitory neurotransmission. Vigabatrin is well absorbed orally and is distributed to all body systems. The major route of elimination for vigabatrin is renal excretion of the parent compound; no metabolites have been identified in humans.

At present, the primary indication for vigabatrin is in the treatment of patients with partial seizures, but it appears to be an effective and generally well tolerated antiepileptic medication for other seizure types as well. It should not be used in patients with absence epilepsy or with myoclonic seizures. Vigabatrin is not approved as an AED in the United States, although it is approved in many other countries.

Phenobarbital and Primidone (Mysoline)

Phenobarbital and primidone are quite similar both chemically and pharmacologically, and much of the anticonvulsant activity of primidone may be ascribed to its metabolic conversion to phenobarbital. As would be expected in such a case, the clinical indications for the two compounds are very similar. There is some indication that primidone may be more effective in the treatment of partial seizures with complex symptoms, but the evidence is not compelling.

The primary mechanism of action of phenobarbital is related to its effect of facilitating GABA inhibition. By binding to an allosteric site on the GABA-benzodiazepine receptor, hence by prolonging the opening of the chloride channels, phenobarbital enhances GABA's inhibitory activity. At somewhat higher concentrations, phenobarbital can block sodium channels, similar to drugs previously discussed, and may block excitatory glutamate responses.

Phenobarbital is effective orally and is distributed widely throughout the body. It is metabolized by microsomal drug-metabolizing enzymes, but up to 50% of the parent drug is excreted unchanged by the kidneys. Primidone is metabolized to phenobarbital and phenylethylmalonamide. The latter metabolite has anticonvulsant activity, but most of the anticonvulsant efficacy of primidone is due to the phenobarbital that is produced.

The major untoward effect of phenobarbital and primidone, when used as anticonvulsants, is sedation. Another side effect of considerable importance, particularly in children, is a possible disturbance in cognitive function. Even when the serum concentration is within the therapeutic range, apparently the ability to concentrate and perform simple tasks is decreased.

At present, phenobarbital and primidone are considered as alternative drugs for the treatment of partial seizures and for generalized tonic–clonic epilepsy. They are judged to be less effective than carbamazepine and phenytoin.

Phenobarbital and primidone are classic agents capable of inducing microsomal drug-metabolizing enzymes (See Chapter 4), and this fact must be considered when using either drug singly or in combination with other agents. Consequently, many interactions can occur between phenobarbital and primidone and a variety of other drugs, and it is necessary, therefore, to monitor drug blood concentrations to ensure that therapeutic levels of all administered agents are being maintained. Phenobarbital and primidone are known to alter blood phenytoin levels. If valproic acid is administered with either phenobarbital or primidone, striking increases in phenobarbital blood levels are frequently observed.

Two other barbiturates, mephobarbital (*Mebaral*) and metharbital (*Gemonil*) continue to be marketed as anticonvulsant drugs, but they are infrequently used.

Agents That Block T-Calcium Channels
Ethosuximide

It is now generally accepted that the specific antiepileptic action of ethosuximide (and the older agent trimethadione, no longer employed) against absence epilepsy is its ability to reduce the low-threshold calcium current (LTCC) or T (transient) current. These currents underlie the 3-Hz spike wave discharges that are characteristic of absence epilepsy. A blockade of

T-calcium current is likely also to be a mechanism used by valproic acid.

The only clinical use for ethosuximide (*Zarontin*) is in the treatment of absence epilepsy. If absence attacks are the only seizure disorder present, ethosuximide alone is effective. If other types of epilepsy are present, ethosuximide can be readily combined with other agents.

For the most part, ethosuximide is a safe drug. Most of the side effects are dose related and consist of nausea, gastrointestinal irritation, drowsiness, and anorexia. A variety of blood dyscrasias have been reported, but serious blood disorders are quite rare.

Agents Whose Mechanism of Action Is Not Known
Felbamate

Felbamate (*Felbatol*) was introduced with the expectation that it would become a major drug in the treatment of epilepsy. Felbamate exhibited few manifestations of serious toxicity in early clinical trials. Soon after its introduction, however, it became apparent that its use was associated with a high incidence of aplastic anemia. Consequently, felbamate is indicated only for patients whose epilepsy is so severe that the risk of aplastic anemia is considered acceptable.

While its mechanism of action has not been clearly established, felbamate shows some activity as an inhibitor of voltage-dependent sodium channels in a manner similar to that of phenytoin and carbamazepine. Felbamate also interacts at the strychnine-insensitive glycine recognition site on the NMDA receptor–ionophore complex. Whether this effect is important to its anticonvulsant activity is not clear.

Gabapentin

Gabapentin (*Neurotonin*) was initially designed to be a rigid analogue of GABA. When it was discovered to have antiepileptic properties, it was assumed that this activity was related to a GABAergic mechanism. However, subsequent studies have failed to show any GABAergic activity of gabapentin. Although it has not yet been possible to ascribe any definite mechanism to its antiepileptic activity, there is recent evidence that it may function as an agonist at $GABA_B$ receptors in the brain.

Gabapentin is recommended as adjunctive therapy in the treatment of partial seizures in adults. When used with other drugs, it appears to be an effective AED; it is usually not effective when employed alone for patients with severe seizures.

Gabapentin is generally well tolerated, with somnolence, dizziness, and ataxia the most commonly reported adverse effects. A low incidence of potentially serious side effects and no significant allergic reactions have been reported.

Levetiracetam

Levetiracetam (*Keppra*) has recently been approved for the treatment of partial-onset seizures. It appears to be safe and effective; its exact therapeutic profile has yet to be determined. It does not appear to share any of the mechanisms of action of agents that have been discussed to this point. It does have a highly specific brain binding site, but the significance of this observation to its mechanism of action has not been elucidated.

ANTICONVULSANT DRUGS AND PREGNANCY

The treatment of epileptic pregnant women poses particularly difficult questions. There is good evidence of an increased risk of congenital malformations in infants born of women taking antiseizure medication during pregnancy, although most such women give birth to normal infants. Because most patients are taking multiple medications and congenital malformations can occur even without medication, it is difficult or impossible to demonstrate a cause and effect relationship for most agents. In some cases the evidence is clearer. Valproic acid has been known to cause spina bifida in a small percentage of cases. Phenytoin has also long been implicated in causing birth defects, and a specific fetal hydantoin syndrome has been suggested. The most common abnormality seen in children of mothers receiving antiepileptic therapy is cleft palate.

Withdrawal of medication from an epileptic pregnant woman is not without its hazards, to the patient and possibly to the fetus. It is not clear whether maternal seizures can directly affect the fetus. If it is feasible, the physician should prescribe only one drug at the lowest effective dosage to minimize teratogenic risks.

The U. S. Food and Drug Administration has developed a use-in-pregnancy rating system that attempts to provide physicians with information that they can use to evaluate the risk to the fetus compared to the benefit to the patient. This classification uses five categories: (A) controlled studies show no risk; (B) no evidence of risk to humans; (C) risk cannot be ruled out; (D) positive evidence of risk; and (X) contraindicated in pregnancy. Using this classification, all approved AEDs are in pregnancy category C except carbamazepine, which is in pregnancy category D. Neither phenytoin nor valproic acid is classified, but both have black box warnings regarding teratogenicity.

A deficiency of folate during gestation has been associated with abnormal fetal growth and development. Since most AEDs cause some degree of folate deficiency, it is considered worthwhile to administer folate daily as a supplement during the period of organogenesis in the first trimester.

Another concern in infants of mothers with epilepsy is a serious hemorrhagic disorder that is associated with a high (25–35%) mortality. This probably results from the finding that many AEDs can act as competitive inhibitors of vitamin K–dependent clotting factors. The competitive inhibition can be overcome by the administration of oral vitamin K supplements to the mother during the last week or 10 days of pregnancy.

TREATMENT OF FEBRILE SEIZURES

Convulsions associated with fever often occur in children 3 months to 5 years of age. Epilepsy later develops in approximately 2 to 3% of children who exhibit one or more such febrile seizures. Most authorities now recommend prophylactic treatment with anticonvulsant drugs only to patients at highest risk for development of epilepsy and for those who have multiple recurrent febrile seizures. Phenobarbital is the usual drug, although diazepam is also effective. Phenytoin and carbamazepine are ineffective, and valproic acid may cause hepatotoxicity in very young patients.

TREATMENT OF STATUS EPILEPTICUS

Status epilepticus is a continuous seizure state that can prove fatal unless the convulsions are terminated. It is a leading cause of death in epileptic patients and must be considered a medical emergency. The choice of drug may not be as important as establishing and correcting the cause of the seizures, maintaining vital functions, and beginning drug treatment as soon as possible. Virtually any general CNS depressant, including general anesthetics, can be used to terminate the seizure state. The pharmacological treatment of choice at present consists of intravenous infusion of either diazepam or lorazepam (the only benzodiazepines available in the United States for parenteral administration) or fosphenytoin.

Fosphenytoin (*Cerebyx*) is a prodrug that is highly soluble in intravenous solutions without solubilizing agents and is supplied in vials for intravenous use. Fosphenytoin is converted to phenytoin following parenteral administration. It is very effective in terminating seizures and will stop most status epilepticus episodes and provide long-term control without any decreased level of consciousness. All of these drugs should be administered slowly to avoid respiratory depression and apnea.

Study QUESTIONS

1. A 10-year-old boy with generalized tonic seizures is seen by his dentist at a routine checkup. The dentist observes that the patient has an overgrowth of gum tissue. The patient was most likely receiving which of the following agents?
(A) ethosuximide
(B) clonazepam
(C) primidone
(D) phenytoin
(E) zonisamide
2. The metabolism of which AED frequently displays zero-order kinetics following moderate to high therapeutic doses?
(A) Carbamazepine
(B) Phenytoin
(C) Valproic acid
(D) Ethosuximide
(E) Zonisamide
3. Many anticonvulsant drugs, as a major part of their mechanism of action, block the sodium channel, but other effective agents do not use this mechanism. Which of the following anticonvulsants has the ability to block T-calcium currents as its primary mechanism of action?

(A) Ethosuximide
(B) Phenytoin
(C) Topiramate
(D) Carbamazepine
(E) Lamotrigine
4. A 14-year-old patient is diagnosed with absence epilepsy. Any of the following drugs could be considered a reasonable choice to prescribe EXCEPT
(A) Ethosuximide
(B) Phenobarbital
(C) Carbamazepine
(D) Valproic acid
5. Which of the following agents has the capacity to inhibit the reuptake of GABA into neurons and glia?
(A) Zonisamide
(B) Vigabatrin
(C) Tiagabine
(D) Ethosuximide
(E) Gabapentin

ANSWERS
1. **D.** This is a rather specific effect of phenytoin. Although the gum tissue can be cut back and in some cases overgrowth prevented with good oral

hygiene, this is a source of embarrassment to the patient and constitutes a deterrent to the use of this agent.

2. **B.** Phenytoin is one of a handful of drugs that demonstrates zero-order (or saturation) kinetics. If a patient is showing signs of toxicity to phenytoin, it is important to measure blood levels, since the likelihood that phenytoin is demonstrating zero-order kinetics is very high.

3. **A.** Ethosuximide has no effect on blocking the sodium channel at therapeutics doses; however, it is very effective in blocking the T-calcium current in the therapeutic dose range. All other choices block the sodium channel at therapeutic doses, and it is acknowledged that this is their sole (or major) mechanism of action.

4. **C.** The only drug listed that would be expected to offer no benefit to a patient with absence seizures is carbamazepine. In fact, there is clinical evidence that it may actually increase the incidence of absence seizure episodes.

5. **C.** Tiagabine is the first agent that has been shown to elevate GABA levels by inhibiting the reuptake of this neurotransmitter at neuronal and glial sites in the brain. Vigabatrin can also elevate GABA levels, but it does so by inhibiting the metabolism of GABA.

SUPPLEMENTAL READING

Adkins JC and Noble S. Tiagabine: A review of its pharmacodynamic and pharmacokinetic properties and therapeutic potential in the management of epilepsy. Drugs 1998;55:437–460.

Bertrand S et al. The anticonvulsant, antihyperalgesic agent gabapentin is an agonist at brain gamma-aminobutyric acid type B receptors negatively coupled to voltage-dependent calcium channels. J Pharmacol Exper Therap 2001;298:15–24.

Ferrendelli JA. Concerns with antiepileptic drug initiation: Safety, tolerability, and efficacy. Epilepsia 2001;42:28–30.

Leppik IE. Issues in the treatment of epilepsy. Epilepsia 2001;42:1–6.

Treiman DM. GABAergic mechanisms in epilepsy. Epilepsia 42:8–12.

CASE Study   Epilepsy and Pregnancy

A 28-year-old woman you have been treating for a seizure disorder tells you that she is 2 months pregnant and thought you should know about it. She has exhibited absence seizures in the past, but currently her episodes are generalized tonic–clonic. She usually has two or three generalized seizures per month. She indicates that she has had only one episode during the past 2 months and wonders if she should stop her medication. She is taking oxcarbazepine, valproic acid, and ethosuximide. Are any of the agents that the patient is taking clearly more teratogenic than others? Is there any significance to the apparent decreased incidence of seizures during pregnancy? How would you propose treating this patient?

ANSWER: Valproic acid has been shown to be implicated in causing birth defects. Ethosuximide has not, but there is little evidence that ethosuximide is effective, since her absence seizures terminated months ago. Oxcarbazepine has not been clearly shown to be teratogenic, but teratogenicity cannot be ruled out, since its close chemical and pharmacological relative carbamazepine has been implicated in causing teratogenicity.

A decrease in seizure frequency is frequently seen during pregnancy. This is not always the case, and the explanations are not established.

Ethosuximide should be discontinued immediately. It is probably appropriate to discontinue the valproic acid over the next week or so. At that time, the dose of oxcarbazepine should be decreased by 50% if there is no increased incidence of seizures following termination of valproic acid. Since the woman has had a relatively long duration of seizure episodes, it is probably not reasonable to discontinue all medication. She should keep a log of her seizure incidence and contact you immediately if the incidence appears to be increasing.

33 Drugs Used in Mood Disorders

Herbert E. Ward and Albert J. Azzaro

 DRUG LIST

GENERIC NAME	PAGE	GENERIC NAME	PAGE
Amitriptyline	389	Mirtazapine	388
Amoxapine	389	Nefazodone	389
Bupropion	388	Nortriptyline	389
Carbamazepine	395	Olanzapine	395
Citalopram	388	Paroxetine	388
Clomipramine	389	Phenelzine	392
Desipramine	389	Protriptyline	389
Doxepin	389	Sertraline	387
Fluoxetine	387	Tranylcypromine	392
Fluvoxamine	386	Trazodone	389
Imipramine	389	Trimipramine	389
Isocarboxazid	392	Valproic acid	395
Lithium	393	Venlafaxine	388
Maprotiline	389		

The most common mood disorders are major depression (unipolar depression) and manic-depressive illness (bipolar disorder). Major depression is a common disorder that continues to result in considerable morbidity and mortality despite major advances in treatment. Approximately 1 in 10 Americans will be depressed during their lifetime. Of the 40,000 suicides occurring in the United States each year, 70% can be accounted for by depression. Antidepressants are now the mainstay of treatment for this potentially lethal disorder, with patients showing some response to treatment 65 to 80% of the time.

Both major depression and manic-depressive disorders are characterized by exaggerated mood associated with physiological, cognitive, and psychomotor disturbances. Major depression generally presents as depressed mood, diminished interest in normal activities, anorexia with significant weight loss, insomnia, fatigue, and inability to concentrate. By contrast, manic episodes associated with manic-depressive illness are characterized by expansive mood, grandiosity, inflated self-esteem, pressured speech, flight of ideas, and poverty of sleep. While each condition is a diagnostic entity unto itself, it can also be secondary to specific medical problems (e.g. hypothyroidism), neurological disease (e.g., Parkinson's disease), and chronic administration of specific medications (e.g., antihypertensives). Attempting to rule out an underlying medical cause for the mood disturbance is essential before additional treatment is initiated.

This chapter covers the basic and clinical pharmacology of each class of agents demonstrating efficacy in the treatment of major depression and manic-depressive illness. The distinguishing features among agents for the treatment of each illness are their side effect profiles and relative toxicity. Physicians should understand both the appropriate agent for the treatment of specific mood disorders and pharmacological factors that allow for the individualization of medication to meet the patient's needs. A list of drugs and their half-lives are shown in Table 33.1.

TABLE 33.1 Half-Lives of Antidepressant Drugs

Drug (trade name)	Half-life (hr)
Heterocyclics	
Amitriptyline (Elavil)	16–26
Nortriptyline (Pamelor)	19–45
Imipramine (Tofranil)	11–25
Desipramine (Norpramin)	20–25
Protriptyline (Vivactil)	67–89
Trimipramine (Surmontil)	8
Doxepin (Sinequan)	11–23
Maprotiline (Ludiomil)	27–58
Amoxapine (Asendin)	8
SSRIs	
Fluoxetine (Prozac)	168–216[a]
Sertraline (Zoloft)	25
Paroxetine (Paxil)	21
Citalopram (Celexa)	35
MAOIs	
Phenelzine (Nardil)	1.5–4.0
Tranylcypromine (Parnate)	1.5–3.5
Isocarboxazid (Marplan)	~4
Miscellaneous agents	
Trazodone (Desyrel)	5–9
Bupropion (Wellbutrin SR)	21[a]
Nefazodone (Serzone)	18[a]
Venlafaxine (Effexor XR)	11[a]
Mirtazapine (Remeron)	30

SSRI, selective serotonin reuptake inhibitor; MAOI, monoamine oxidase inhibitor.
[a]Parent compound and active metabolite.

TREATMENT OF MAJOR DEPRESSION

It is often surprising for the student to learn that mood-elevating agents do not act as stimulants of the central nervous system (CNS). With the exception of varying degrees of sedation, the antidepressants have little effect on behavior early in treatment. During this period patients will, however, have side effects specific to the class and agent being used. Only after 2 to 3 weeks of dosing will a therapeutic benefit on depression emerge. At this point the patient begins to demonstrate elevation in mood and self-esteem. In addition, many of the vegetative signs of the illness (e.g., insomnia, anorexia) abate, and the patient regains an interest in daily activities. Failure to continue the medication, however, will result in an immediate relapse into the depressive state. Therefore, maintenance therapy must be continued for at least 6 months.

The Selective Serotonin Reuptake Inhibitors

In 1987, the FDA approved the drug fluoxetine (*Prozac*) for use in the treatment of major depression. Fluoxetine belongs to a class of agents referred to as *selective serotonin reuptake inhibitors* (SSRIs). The SSRIs now include sertraline (*Zoloft*), fluvoxamine (*Luvox*), paroxetine (*Paxil*), and citalopram (*Celexa*). Fluvoxamine is approved for use only in obsessive-compulsive disorder and is not discussed in this chapter.

With the introduction of the SSRIs, the safety and tolerability of antidepressants improved remarkably. As a class, these medications have little or no affinity for cholinergic, β-adrenergic or histamine receptors and do not interfere with cardiac conduction. They are well tolerated by patients with heart disease and by the elderly, who are especially sensitive to the anticholinergic and orthostatic effects of the tricyclic antidepressant agents (TCAs) and monoamine oxidase inhibitors (MAOIs).

The high degree of selectivity of SSRIs for the nerve terminal serotonin reuptake system has supported the hypothesis that these agents produce their therapeutic action through an ability to modulate serotonin neurotransmission in the brain. Chronic studies in animals have provided evidence for a cascade of altered synaptic events, beginning with inhibition of 5-hydroxytryptamine (5-HT) neuronal reuptake (Fig. 33.1). Increased 5-HT levels activate 5-HT_{1A} autoreceptors and result in a decrease in neuronal firing. Desensitization of this receptor results in enhanced serotonin release. The terminal 5-HT_{1B} autoreceptors normally inhibiting release of serotonin also become desensitized. These events, triggered by a sustained inhibition of the nerve terminal serotonin reuptake system, ultimately cause a potentiation of serotonin neurotransmission at central synaptic

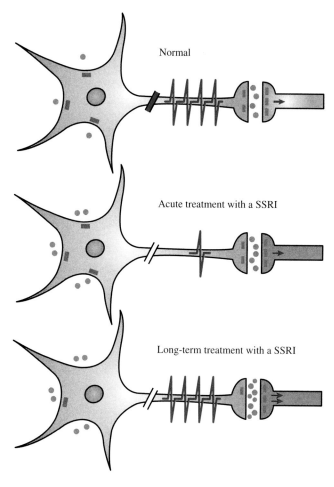

FIGURE 33.1
5-HT neurons depicting the impact of an SSRI on 5-HT neurotransmission. The cell bodies of 5-HT neurons are in the brainstem and give rise to 5-HT projections reaching all brain structures. The rectangles on the cell bodies of 5-HT neurons represent the 5-HT$_{1A}$ autoreceptors, and the ones on the terminals represent the 5-HT$_{1B}$ autoreceptors; their disappearance after long-term treatment is meant to illustrate their desensitization. The rectangles on the postsynaptic neurons represent 5-HT$_{1A}$ receptors in the hippocampus that do not desensitize after long-term treatment. The number of zigzags on the axons and dots represent the firing frequency of the 5-HT neurons and the level of synaptic 5-HT, respectively. (Reprinted with permission from Blier P and Ward H. CNS Spectrum 2002;7:148–153.)

sites. The development of these synaptic events shares the time frame of the delayed appearance of the therapeutic benefit of these agents in depression.

With initiation of therapy with an SSRI, some patients describe anxiety or agitation. This can usually be overcome by reducing the dose and titrating upward more slowly. Insomnia can be a persistent activating side effect that can limit therapy or require the addition of a sedating agent at bedtime. Nausea and loose stools are a frequent side effect and may be lessened by taking the medication with food. As many as one-third of patients taking SSRIs may complain of sexual dysfunction, including decreased libido, delayed ejaculation, and anorgasmia. The SSRIs tend to be weight neutral with the exception of paroxetine (*Paxil*), which is associated with weight gain. No correlation has been made between plasma levels of the SSRIs and efficacy.

Fluoxetine

Fluoxetine (*Prozac*) is given in the morning because of its potential for being activating and causing insomnia. Food does not affect its systemic bioavailability and may actually lessen the nausea reported by some patients. Fluoxetine is highly bound to serum proteins and may interact with other highly protein bound drugs. It is demethylated in the liver to form an active metabolite, norfluoxetine. Inactive metabolites are excreted by the kidney. Doses must be reduced in patients with liver disease.

The slow elimination of fluoxetine and norfluoxetine lead to special clinical concerns when adjusting doses and discontinuing this medication. Steady state is not reached until 4 to 6 weeks, and similarly, complete elimination takes 4 to 6 weeks after discontinuation of the medication. A 4- to 6-week waiting period should be permitted before starting a medication with potential for an interaction with fluoxetine, such as a monoamine oxidase inhibitor (MAOI). Additionally, fluoxetine is a potent inhibitor of cytochrome P450 2D6 and can significantly elevate levels of drugs metabolized by this route. Thus, coadministration of drugs with a narrow therapeutic index, such as TCAs and type 1C antiarrhythmics, including flecainide and propafenone, are a particular concern.

Sertraline

Sertraline (*Zoloft*) has an elimination half-life of 25 hours and can be administered once a day, usually in the morning to avoid insomnia. Sertraline undergoes extensive hepatic metabolism, and doses must be reduced in patients with liver disease. Sertraline may produce more gastrointestinal side effects, such as nausea and diarrhea, than does fluoxetine and is generally thought to be less activating than fluoxetine. It is highly bound to serum proteins (98%) and may alter plasma protein binding of other medications. A 14-day washout period is recommended before starting a MAOI. Sertraline is a weak inhibitor of cytochrome P450 2D6. Intensive therapeutic drug monitoring is indicated when combining sertraline with drugs metabolized by this route that have a narrow therapeutic index, such as the TCAs and the type 1C antiarrhythmics propafenone, encainide, and flecainide.

Paroxetine

Paroxetine (*Paxil*) has an elimination half-life of 21 hours and is also highly bound to plasma proteins, so it requires special attention when administered with drugs such as warfarin. Paroxetine is a potent inhibitor of the cytochrome P450 2D6 isoenzyme and can raise the plasma levels of drugs metabolized via this route. Of particular concern are drugs with a narrow therapeutic index, such as TCAs and the type 1C antiarrhythmics flecainide, propafenone, and encainide. Additionally, paroxetine itself is metabolized by this enzyme and inhibits its own metabolism, leading to nonlinear kinetics. Weight gain is higher with paroxetine than with the other SSRIs, and it tends to be more sedating, presumably because of its potential anticholinergic effects. Additionally, patients have had difficulty with abrupt discontinuation with this agent, reporting a flulike syndrome; this symptom can be avoided by tapering the medication.

Citalopram

Citalopram (*Celexa*) has an elimination half-life of 35 hours and is 80% bound to plasma proteins. Of all of the SSRIs it has the least effect on the cytochrome P450 system and has the most favorable profile regarding drug–drug interactions.

Miscellaneous Antidepressants
Venlafaxine

Venlafaxine (*Effexor*) inhibits the reuptake of both serotonin and norepinephrine at their respective presynaptic sites. This drug does not have significant effects at muscarinic, histamine, or α-adrenergic receptors and therefore is devoid of many of the side effects associated with the TCAs. Venlafaxine and its active metabolite, *O*-desmethyl-venlafaxine, have half lives of 5 and 11 hours respectively, so dosing twice a day is necessary. However, an extended release preparation (*Effexor XR*) now allows for once-daily dosing and better tolerance. Venlafaxine has a side effect profile similar to that of the SSRIs (Table 33.2). Higher doses of venlafaxine result in modest increases in blood pressure in approximately 5% of patients. Venlafaxine has minimal effects on the cytochrome P450 enzyme system.

Bupropion

Bupropion (*Wellbutrin*) is a pharmacologically unique antidepressant, since it is a weak inhibitor of both dopamine and norepinephrine neuronal reuptake. However, its actual antidepressant activity is not well understood. Bupropion is generally well tolerated and does not block muscarinic, histaminergic, or adrenergic receptors. Unlike the SSRIs and venlafaxine, bupropion does not cause sexual side effects. However, it can cause CNS stimulation, including restlessness and insomnia. High doses of bupropion, given as its original formulation, were associated with a risk of seizures in 0.4% of patients. However, this risk is lower with slow-release bupropion (*Wellbutrin SR*). This formulation still requires dosing twice a day, and bupropion is contraindicated in patients with a history of seizures. Bupropion inhibits the cytochrome P450 2D6 isoenzyme and may elevate blood levels of drugs metabolized by this route.

Mirtazapine

Mirtazapine (*Remeron*) enhances both serotonergic and noradrenergic neurotransmission. By blocking presynaptic α2-adrenoceptors, mirtazapine causes release of norepinephrine. Indirectly, through noradrenergic modulation of serotonin systems, mirtazapine also causes increased release of serotonin. It is an antagonist

TABLE 33.2 Common Side Effects of Therapeutic Doses of Antidepressants

Agent	Sedation	Anticholinergic	Orthostasis	Weight Gain	Sexual Dysfunction
SSRIs	+/−	0	0	+/−	+++
TCAs	+++	+++	+++	++	++
Miscellaneous					
Trazodone	+++	0	++	++	+[a]
Bupropion	0	0	0	0	0
Nefazodone	++	0	0	0	0
Venlafaxine	+/-	0	0[b]	0	++
Mirtazapine	++	0	0	++	0
MAOIs	0	+	+++	++	+

TCA, tricyclic antidepressant; SSRI, selective serotonin reuptake inhibitor; MAOI, monoamine oxidase inhibitor.
0, no effect; +, + +, +++ indicate increasing effect.
[a]Priapism.
[b]Venlafaxine can cause a dose-dependent increase in blood pressure.

at the $5-HT_{2A}$, $5HT_{2C}$, $5-HT_3$, and histamine receptors but has minimal affinity for muscarinic or α_1-receptors. Mirtazapine does not inhibit neuronal reuptake of serotonin or norepinephrine. Weight gain and sedation are common side effects (Table 33.2); sedation necessitates dosing at bedtime. Mirtazapine does not have significant effects on cytochrome P450 isoenzymes.

Trazodone

Trazodone (*Desyrel*) was introduced in the early 1980s as a second-generation antidepressant. It blocks the neuronal reuptake of serotonin and is an antagonist at the $5HT_2$-receptor. Also, its major metabolite, *m*-chlorophenylpiperazine (mCPP), is a postsynaptic serotonin receptor agonist. When compared to the TCAs, trazodone is relatively free of antimuscarinic side effects, but it does block the α-adrenoceptor. Common side effects include marked sedation, dizziness, orthostatic hypotension, and nausea (Table 33.2). Priapism is an uncommon but serious side effect requiring surgical intervention in one-third of the cases reported. Because of trazodone's sedating quality, it is often used in low doses to counter the insomnia associated with the newer antidepressants, such as the SSRIs.

Nefazodone

Although nefazodone (*Serzone*) is structurally related to trazodone, it is less sedating. It does not block α_1-adrenoreceptors, and its use is not associated with priapism. Nefazodone inhibits the neuronal reuptake of serotonin and blocks $5HT_{2A}$ receptors. Its short half-life requires dosing twice a day (Table 33.1). Nefazodone is not associated with weight gain or sexual dysfunction. It inhibits the cytochrome P450 3A4 isoenzyme that is responsible for 50% of known oxidative metabolism, and therefore, nefazodone can elevate levels of drugs dependent on this pathway for metabolism.

Tricyclic Antidepressants

In the late 1950s, imipramine was noted to be effective for the symptomatic treatment of depression. A number of chemical congeners of imipramine have been synthesized and tested for antidepressant properties; they are collectively known as TCAs. The TCAs are no longer considered first-line agents in the treatment of depression because of their prominent side effects and the need to monitor drug blood levels to avoid toxicity.

Seven TCA drugs are available in the United States for treatment of major depression. They are generally categorized as tertiary or secondary amines. Tertiary amines include imipramine (*Tofranil*), amitriptyline (*Elavil*), trimipramine (*Surmontil*), and doxepin (*Sinequan*). Desipramine (*Norpramin*), nortriptyline (*Pamelor*), and protriptyline (*Vivactil*) are secondary amines.

Clomipramine (*Anafranil*) also a member of the tricyclic family, possesses similar pharmacology and antidepressant efficacy. This agent, however, has Food and Drug (FDA) approval only for use in the treatment of obsessive-compulsive disorder and is not included in this discussion of antidepressant drugs.

Maprotiline (*Ludiomil*) and amoxapine (*Asendin*) are heterocyclic antidepressant agents that are not members of the tricyclic family. However, their pharmacology is so similar to that of the tricyclic amines that they are included for discussion purposes with this class of agents. Desipramine and nortriptyline are major metabolites of imipramine and amitriptyline, respectively.

Mechanism of Action

The precise molecular mechanism responsible for the antidepressant action of the TCA drugs is unknown, although a number of hypotheses have been generated. Many of these involve alterations in neurotransmission of norepinephrine or serotonin or both.

β-Adrenoceptor down-regulation at central noradrenergic synapses is one popular theory used to explain the antidepressant properties of TCA drugs and other antidepressants. This theory focuses on a cascade of adaptive changes at the noradrenergic synapse that appears to be triggered by inhibition of norepinephrine neuronal reuptake by TCA drugs (Fig. 33.2). Subsensitivity in the β-adrenoceptor–coupled adenylyl cyclase system and associated reductions in β-adrenoceptor density appear to be common features of the antidepressants and of electroconvulsant treatment. Moreover, the time-dependent changes in β-adrenoceptor

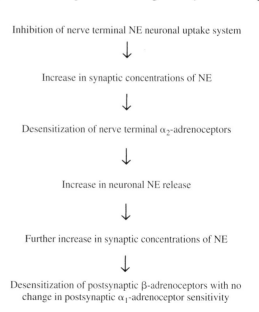

Inhibition of nerve terminal NE neuronal uptake system

↓

Increase in synaptic concentrations of NE

↓

Desensitization of nerve terminal α_2-adrenoceptors

↓

Increase in neuronal NE release

↓

Further increase in synaptic concentrations of NE

↓

Desensitization of postsynaptic β-adrenoceptors with no change in postsynaptic α_1-adrenoceptor sensitivity

FIGURE 33.2
Cascade of adaptive changes occurring at norepinephrine (NE) synapses following chronic TCA drug treatment.

function parallel the time delay associated with clinical efficacy of these drugs (2–3 weeks). These latter findings have added to the attractiveness of this theory. However, at noradrenergic synapses with multiple adrenoceptors (i.e., α_1-, α_2-, and β-adrenoceptors), synaptic transmission through α_1-adrenoceptors will likely be enhanced at the same time that synaptic transmission through α_2- and β-adrenoceptors is reduced (Figure 33.3).

While much emphasis has been placed on alterations in noradrenergic neurotransmission, TCA drugs are not without effect on serotonin (5-HT) neurotransmission. Long-term studies with TCA drugs in animals have demonstrated postsynaptic supersensitivity to serotonin (5-HT$_{1A}$) receptor agonists at serotonin synapses, with an associated enhancement of serotonergic neurotransmission. The sensitization to 5-HT$_{1A}$ agonists is mediated in part by an increase in the density of postsynaptic 5-HT$_{1A}$ receptors. Enhancement of trans-

mission through 5-HT$_{1A}$ receptors appears to be a common phenomenon after chronic administration of all clinically effective antidepressants and electroconvulsive treatment. The occurrence of this 5-HT$_{1A}$ supersensitivity parallels the delayed onset of the therapeutic actions of these agents (2–3 weeks). These observations lend strong support to the hypothesis that enhanced serotonergic neurotransmission is required for the therapeutic benefit from TCA drugs.

It is likely that TCA drugs produce their therapeutic benefits by acting at both serotonin and norepinephrine synapses. The literature also supports the notion of an interdependence of these two monoamine systems in the treatment of depression. The time-dependent changes in the flow of synaptic information through individual receptor subtypes within the norepinephrine and serotonin synapses following chronic TCA administration are summarized in Figure 33.3.

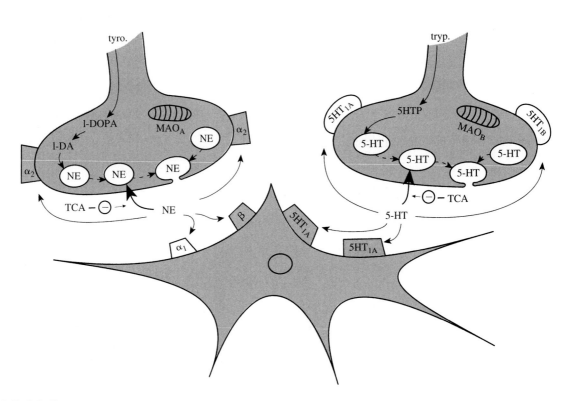

FIGURE 33.3

Flow of information through receptor subtypes at norepinephrine and serotonin synapses following chronic TCA drug administration. A cascade of events leads to altered receptor-mediated physiology of the norepinephrine (NE) and serotonin (5-HT) synapses of the brain following long-term TCA drug administration. The adaptive changes in synaptic physiology are triggered by selective inhibition of the NE and/or 5-HT neuronal reuptake systems. Responses at β- and α_2-adrenoceptors are depressed, whereas responses at 5-HT$_{1A}$ receptors are enhanced. Responses at α_1-adrenoceptors and 5-HT$_{1B}$ receptors remain unchanged. Accordingly, the postsynaptic flow of information at NE and 5-HT synapses will be reduced through β-adrenoceptors but enhanced through 5-HT$_{1A}$ receptors. Although the responsiveness of α_1-adrenoceptors remains unchanged, it is likely that transmission through these postsynaptic sites will be enhanced. In this regard, desensitization of α_2-adrenoceptors will provide greater concentrations of synaptic NE to activate normosensitive postsynaptic α_1-adrenoceptors.

Pharmacokinetics

The TCA drugs are well absorbed from the gastrointestinal tract, are extremely lipid soluble, and bind extensively to plasma proteins. Their half-lives range from 8 to 89 hours (Table 33.1). Several days to weeks are required both to achieve steady-state serum levels and for complete elimination of these agents from the body. Long half-lives make most of these agents amenable to dosing once a day, generally at bedtime.

Drug inactivation generally occurs through oxidative metabolism by hepatic microsomal enzymes. Tertiary amines are converted to secondary amines, which generally possess biological activity and are frequently in serum at levels equal to or greater than that of the parent tertiary amine. A second route of inactivation includes conjugation of hydroxylated metabolites with glucuronic acid.

Adverse Effects

The TCA drugs have lost their place as first-line therapy for depression because of their bothersome side effects (Table 33.2) at therapeutic doses and lethal effects in toxic doses. In addition to their presynaptic effects on the neuronal uptake of norepinephrine and serotonin, they block several postsynaptic receptors. They are potent cholinergic muscarinic receptor antagonists, resulting in symptoms such as dry mouth, constipation, tachycardia, blurred vision and urinary retention. Blockade of histamine receptors (H_1) often results in sedation and weight gain. Antagonism of α_1-adrenoceptors in the vasculature can cause orthostatic hypotension.

TCA drugs have potent membrane-stabilizing properties similar to those of quinidine. Conduction is slowed throughout the heart, and serious ventricular arrhythmias may develop in patients with preexisting conduction abnormalities at therapeutic doses and in all patients at toxic doses. At therapeutic doses, the TCA drugs lower the seizure threshold and at toxic doses can cause life-threatening seizures. Maprotiline has a greater potential for reducing the seizure threshold and should not be used in patients with a seizure disorder. Amoxapine has dopamine receptor antagonist properties (see Chapter 31) and can induce extrapyramidal side effects, gynecomastia, lactation, and neuroleptic malignant syndrome. To increase tolerance to the anticholinergic and orthostatic effects of the TCA drugs, the dose is usually titrated with increasing increments over the first few weeks of therapy.

Drug Interactions

Multiple drug interactions can occur with the TCA drugs. Because of their high degree of binding to plasma proteins, competition for binding sites can exist between TCAs and phenytoin, aspirin, phenothiazines, and other agents that also display avid plasma protein-binding characteristics. Elevation in the serum level of TCAs (with corresponding toxicity) can occur following the administration of one of these second drugs. Elevations in the serum TCA level also can occur following inhibition of hepatic TCA metabolism by antipsychotics, methylphenidate, oral contraceptives, and some SSRIs.

Tricyclic antidepressant drugs can prevent the action of antihypertensive drugs, such as guanethidine and clonidine. This antagonistic action is related to the primary (inhibition of neuronal reuptake) and secondary (adaptive changes) effects of TCA drugs at noradrenergic synapses. A more serious but rare interaction exists between TCA drugs and MAOIs. While both classes of drugs are effective in the treatment of major depression, simultaneous administration of a drug from each class can result in severe CNS toxicity (hyperpyrexia, convulsions, and coma). In TCA-resistant patients, it is advisable to discontinue the TCA drug for 2 to 3 weeks before initiation of a MAOI agent. Finally, TCA drugs potentiate the sedative effects of alcohol, and patients must be cautioned about this interaction.

Therapeutic Drug Monitoring

Safe and effective use of the TCA drugs requires monitoring of serum levels. The importance of this monitoring is based on the relatively narrow range between therapeutic and toxic doses (therapeutic index of 3) of each agent. While annoying side effects (sedation, dry mouth, constipation) begin to occur at subtherapeutic serum concentrations, life-threatening cardiac and CNS effects develop in a dose dependent fashion above serum levels of 500 ng/mL. The metabolism and elimination rates vary 10- to 30-fold among individuals taking TCA drugs. For this reason, it is estimated that only 50% of the patients receiving a standard dose of a TCA drug would achieve an optimal therapeutic serum concentration. Of additional concern, 3 to 5% of patients will be deficient in hepatic enzymes that metabolize the TCA drugs and may develop life-threatening serum levels on standard doses. Therefore, steady-state serum levels of TCA drugs (drawn 10 to 12 hours after the last dose) are monitored to avoid toxicity, monitor compliance, and optimize the therapeutic response.

Monoamine Oxidase Inhibitors

Iproniazid, originally developed for the treatment of tuberculosis, exhibited mood-elevating properties during clinical trials in tuberculosis patients with depression. The distinguishing biochemical feature between iproniazid and other chemically similar antituberculosis compounds was the ability of the former to inhibit MAO. Thus, a series of hydrazine and non–hydrazine-related

MAOI agents was synthesized and tested for antidepressant properties. Three MAOI agents are approved in the United States for use in major depression: isocarboxazid (*Marplan*), phenelzine (*Nardil*), and tranylcypromine (*Parnate*).

The MAOIs are as effective as the heterocyclic antidepressants and the newer agents, such as the SSRIs. However, at least two forms of life-threatening toxicity (hepatotoxicity and dietary tyramine–induced hypertensive crisis) have been associated with their chronic use. For this reason, the MAOIs are not considered first-line agents in the treatment of depression. They are generally reserved for treatment of depressions that resist therapeutic trials of the newer, safer antidepressants. However, a new transdermal formulation of selegiline undergoing clinical trials demonstrates antidepressant efficacy without concerns of liver toxicity or dietary tyramine-induced hypertension.

Mechanism of Action

Monoamine oxidase exists in the human body in two molecular forms, known as type A and type B. Each of these isozymes has selective substrate and inhibitor characteristics. Neurotransmitter amines, such as norepinephrine and serotonin, are preferentially metabolized by MAO-A in the brain. MAO-B is more likely to be involved in the catabolism of human brain dopamine, although dopamine is also a substrate for MAO-A.

Isocarboxazid, phenelzine, and tranylcypromine are irreversible nonselective inhibitors of both MAO-A and MAO-B. However, it appears that inhibition of MAO-A, not MAO-B, is important to the antidepressant action of these agents.

Therapeutic efficacy by selective MAO-A inhibitors (such as clorgyline or moclobemide) in major depressions strongly suggests that MAO inhibition at central serotonin or norepinephrine synapses or both is responsible for the antidepressant properties of these agents. However, since complete MAO-A inhibition is achieved clinically within a few days of treatment, while the antidepressant effects of these drugs are not observed for 2 to 3 weeks, suggests that additional actions must be involved.

In a manner similar to that of the TCAs and SSRIs, MAOIs are known to induce adaptive changes in the CNS synaptic physiology over 2 to 3 weeks. These changes result in both down-regulation of synaptic transmission mediated through noradrenergic α- and β-adrenoceptors and up-regulation or enhancement of synaptic transmission at serotonin synapses ($5HT_{1A}$-receptors). This action on serotonin neurotransmission is the result of desensitized somatodendritic autoreceptors responsible for the regulation of the firing rate of serotonin-containing neurons of the forebrain. Accordingly, these neurons fire at elevated rates, releasing large quantities of serotonin into the synapse. This serotonin is protected from degradation by inhibition of synaptic MAO-A. It is believed that the development of these physiological changes at norepinephrine and serotonin synapses, which parallel the time delay associated with the antidepressant properties of the MAOIs, is the mechanism of action for these agents in the treatment of major depression.

Adverse Effects

The potential for toxicity that is associated with the administration of the MAOIs restricts their use in major depression. Hepatotoxicity is likely to occur with isocarboxazid or phenelzine, since hydrazine compounds can cause damage to hepatic parenchymal cells. This is true particularly for patients identified as slow acetylators (see Chapter 4) of hydrazine compounds. Fortunately, the incidence of hepatotoxicity is low with the available agents.

A greater concern is the potentially lethal cardiovascular effects that can occur in patients who do not comply with their dietary restrictions. Patients who take a MAOI should not eat food rich in tyramine or other biologically active amines. Normally, these amines are rapidly metabolized by MAO-A during gastric absorption by the mucosal cells of the intestinal wall and by MAO-A and MAO-B during passage through the liver parenchyma. If both isozymes of MAO are inhibited, elevated circulating levels of tyramine will be free to interact with the sympathetic noradrenergic nerve terminals innervating cardiac and vascular smooth muscle tissue to produce a pressor effect (see Chapter 10). In these conditions, tyramine can cause an acute elevation in blood pressure, sometimes leading to a hypertensive crisis. Cheeses, wine, and a whole host of other foods rich in tyramine must be avoided. A number of other bothersome side effects, such as tremors, orthostatic hypotension, ejaculatory delay, dry mouth, fatigue, and weight gain, are common at therapeutic doses of MAOIs (Table 33.2).

Drug Interactions

Serious hypertension can occur with concomitant administration of over-the-counter cough and cold medications containing sympathomimetic amines. When switching from a MAOI to another antidepressant, such as a SSRI, a drug-free period of 2 weeks is required to allow for the regeneration of tissue MAO and elimination of the MAOI. When switching from an antidepressant, such as an SSRI, to a MAOI, sufficient time should be allowed for the SSRI to be cleared from the body (at least 5 half-lives) before starting the MAOI. Special note should be taken of fluoxetine's long half-life, requiring at least 5 weeks after discontinuation of fluoxetine at a 20-mg dose and longer at higher doses, before initiation of MAOI therapy. Coadministration of a MAOI and an SSRI or venlafaxine can overstimulate the serotonin receptors in the brainstem and spinal cord (serotonin syndrome), which can be lethal. Serotonin syndrome consists of a constellation of psychiatric, neurological, and cardiovascular symptoms that may include confusion, elevated or dysphoric mood, tremor, myoclonus, incoordination, hyperthermia, and cardiovascular collapse.

TREATMENT OF MANIC-DEPRESSIVE ILLNESS

Lithium

For more than 40 years, Li^+ has been used to treat mania. While it is relatively inert in individuals without a mood disorder, lithium carbonate is effective in 60 to 80% of all acute manic episodes within 5 to 21 days of beginning treatment. Because of its delayed onset of action in the manic patient, Li^+ is often used in conjunction with low doses of high-potency anxiolytics (e.g., lorazepam) and antipsychotics (e.g. haloperidol) to stabilize the behavior of the patient. Over time, increased therapeutic responses to Li^+ allow for a gradual reduction in the amount of anxiolytic or neuroleptic required, so that eventually Li^+ is the sole agent used to maintain control of the mood disturbance.

In addition to its acute actions, Li^+ can reduce the frequency of manic or depressive episodes in the bipolar patient and therefore is considered a mood-stabilizing agent. Accordingly, patients with bipolar disorder are often maintained on low stabilizing doses of Li^+ indefinitely as a prophylaxis to future mood disturbances. Antidepressant medications are required in addition to Li^+ for the treatment of breakthrough depression.

Mechanism of Action

Lithium is a monovalent cation that can replace Na^+ in some biological processes. It can be argued that competition by Li^+ for active Na^+ sites may lead to altered neuronal functions that may account for its antimanic and mood-stabilizing actions. In this regard, the failure of Li^+ to maintain a normal membrane potential because of its lower affinity for the Na^+ pump has been demonstrated. However, this action of Li^+ would not explain its relatively selective effects on the CNS, sparing comparable excitable tissues (e.g. cardiac muscle) in the periphery. Moreover, an action on membrane polarity would be so general that the entire pool of brain neurons would be affected by Li^+. It seems more reasonable that Li^+ produces its psychotropic actions by perturbation of molecular events common to a few CNS synapses that might have been disturbed during the course of the manic-depressive illness.

Recently, attention has focused on the actions of Li^+ on receptor-mediated second-messenger signaling systems of the brain. In this regard, interactions between Li^+ and guanine nucleotide (GTP) binding proteins (G proteins) have been the target of many studies, since G proteins play a pivotal role in the function of many second-messenger signaling systems. Lithium is capable of altering G-protein function. It can diminish the coupling between the receptor recognition site and the G protein. The molecular mechanism involves the competition for Mg^{++} sites on the G protein, which are essential for GTP binding. Guanine nucleotide activates the G protein. Accordingly, in the presence of Li^+, receptor-mediated activation of these G proteins is attenuated. This action of Li^+ has been selectively demonstrated for G proteins associated with β-adrenoceptors and M_1 muscarinic receptors of the CNS (Fig. 33.4).

While it is not possible at present to assign a therapeutic role to this action of Li^+, it is a step toward explaining the stabilizing actions of this drug. Since several neurotransmitter receptors share common G protein–regulated second-messenger signaling systems, Li^+ could simultaneously correct the alterations at individual synapses associated with depression and mania by a single action on the function of specific G proteins.

An additional action of Li^+ is interruption of the phosphatidylinositide cycle through an inhibitory action on inositol phosphate metabolism. By this mechanism, depletion of membrane inositol and the phosphoinositide-derived second-messenger products diacylglycerol and inositol triphosphate ultimately reduces signaling through receptor systems dependent on the formation of these products. It is presently unclear to what extent inhibition of inositol phosphate metabolism contributes to the therapeutic properties of Li^+ in bipolar patients.

Pharmacokinetics and Therapeutic Drug Monitoring

Lithium is readily absorbed from the gastrointestinal tract, reaching a peak plasma level in 2 to 4 hours. Distribution occurs throughout the extracellular fluid with no evidence of protein binding. Passage through the blood-brain barrier is limited, so that cerebrospinal fluid levels are 50% of plasma levels at steady state.

The elimination half-life of Li^+ is estimated at 24 hours, and more than 90% of the dose of Li^+ is excreted into the urine. Renal clearance, however, is only 20%, since Li^+ is actively reabsorbed in the proximal tubule at sites normally used for the conservation of Na^+. Thus, competition between Li^+ and Na^+ for uptake sites can alter the elimination of Li^+ and its concentration in total body water. Na^+ loading enhances Li^+ clearance, while Na^+ depletion promotes Li^+ retention. This important relationship explains the appearance of Li^+ toxicity (discussed later) associated with diet (low Na^+),

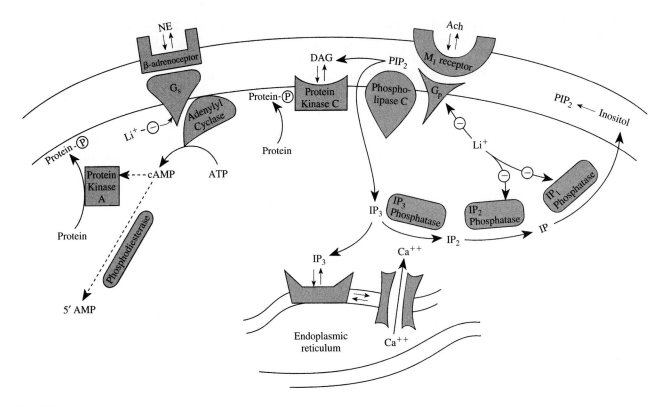

FIGURE 33.4

The actions of Li+ on postsynaptic receptor-mediated second-messenger signaling systems. Lithium can simultaneously alter the flow of synaptic information through several receptor-mediated systems by diminishing coupling between the receptor recognition site and its specific G proteins. This model explains the stabilizing actions of Li+ at both ends of the mood spectrum through a single action at the G-protein level. Attenuating actions of Li+ have been demonstrated through G-protein interactions at the β-adrenoceptor and the acetylcholine M₁ muscarinic receptor systems of the CNS. A second action of Li+ as an inhibitor of inositol diphosphate (IP₂) phosphatase may further attenuate the flow of synaptic information through the M₁ muscarinic receptor by the eventual depletion of membrane phosphatidyl inositol-bis-phosphate (PIP₂). IP₃, inositol triphosphate; DAG, diacylglycerol; ATP, adenosine triphosphate; cAMP, cyclic adenosine monophosphate; 5'-AMP, 5'-adenosine monophosphate; NE, norepinephrine; ACh, acetylcholine.

drugs (diuretics), medical conditions (diarrhea), or physical activities (those that induce sweating) that deplete the body of Na+.

The elimination rate of Li+ from the body is variable. It is quite rapid during the first 10 hours after ingestion, and this period accounts for about 40% of the total Li+ excretion. However, the remaining portion of the Li+ dose is excreted very slowly over 14 days. Because of this biphasic elimination rate, clinically useful serum Li+ concentrations are usually determined 12 hours after the last dose. This period assures a relatively accurate reflection of the Li+ concentration, since it is beyond the most variable portion (rapid elimination phase) of the Li+ elimination profile.

Adverse Effects

The frequency and severity of adverse reactions associated with Li+ therapy are directly related to serum lev-

els. Since Li+ has a low therapeutic index (approximately 3) and a narrow therapeutic window (0.5–1.5 mEq/L), the frequent measurement of serum steady-state concentrations is standard practice in the treatment of bipolar patients.

Adverse reactions occurring at serum trough levels (12 hours after the last dose) below 1.5 mEq/L are generally mild, whereas those seen above 2.5 mEq/L are usually quite severe. Mild toxicity is usually expressed as nausea, vomiting, abdominal pain, diarrhea, polyuria, sedation, and fine tremor. If the serum concentration of Li+ progressively rises above 2 mEq/L, frank neurological toxicity appears, beginning with mental confusion and progressing to hyperreflexia, gross tremor, dysarthria, focal neurological signs, seizures, progressive coma, and even death.

Adverse effects sometimes seen during chronic maintenance of bipolar patients with Li+ include hypothyroidism (approximately 5%) and nephrogenic diabetes insipidus. Both conditions are readily reversible by discontinuation of Li⁺. Routine laboratory monitoring includes TSH (thyroid-stimulating hormone) and serum creatinine measurements to detect hypothyroidism and any change in renal capacity to clear the drug.

Other Mood-Stabilizing Agents

Several anticonvulsant medications have mood-stabilizing properties. Valproic acid and carbamazepine are the best studied to date. In 1995, valproic acid was approved by the FDA for treatment of acute mania and is now considered a first-line agent. Other anticonvulsants under investigation include lamotrigine and topiramate, which are covered in Chapter 32. The atypical antipsychotic agent olanzapine received FDA approval in 2000 for use in acute mania and mixed episodes associated with bipolar disorder; it is covered in Chapter 34.

Study QUESTIONS

1. Which of the following antidepressants is most selective for inhibition of neuronal reuptake of serotonin?
   (A) Mirtazapine (*Remeron*)
   (B) Venlafaxine (*Effexor*)
   (C) Bupropion (*Wellbutrin*)
   (D) Sertraline (*Zoloft*)
   (E) Imipramine (*Tofranil*)
2. In a patient with a seizure disorder, which antidepressant is contraindicated?
   (A) Nefazodone (*Serzone*)
   (B) Fluoxetine (*Prozac*)
   (C) Venlafaxine (*Effexor*)
   (D) Mirtazapine (*Remeron*)
   (E) Bupropion (*Wellbutrin*)
3. Mr. Smith is 28 years old and has no active medical problems. He has been treated with Li⁺ for manic-depressive illness for 1 year, and his mood has been stable. He now reports the gradual onset of fatigue, weight gain, and cold intolerance. Which single laboratory test is most likely to lead to the correct diagnosis?
   (A) TSH (thyroid-stimulating hormone)
   (B) Hepatic function panel
   (C) Glucose tolerance test
   (D) Hematocrit
   (E) Serum prolactin level
4. Which of the following antidepressants requires therapeutic blood monitoring for safe use?
   (A) Paroxetine (*Paxil*)
   (B) Phenelzine (*Nardil*)
   (C) Nortriptyline (*Pamelor*)
   (D) Venlafaxine (*Effexor*)
   (E) Bupropion (*Wellbutrin*)
5. Which of the following statements about antidepressant medications is most appropriate?
   (A) They all have a delay of approximately 48 hours for onset of benefit.
   (B) There are large differences in efficacy among individual agents.

(C) Some benefit is expected in 65 to 80% of patients treated with an antidepressant for major depression.
(D) The major contribution of the newer antidepressants lies in the marked improvement in duration of action.

ANSWERS

1. **D.** Mirtazapine acts at serotonin and adrenergic receptors and does not effect reuptake of neurotransmitters. Venlafaxine is a mixed serotonin–norepinephrine reuptake inhibitor. Bupropion inhibits norepinephrine and dopamine reuptake. Imipramine is a TCA with mixed serotonin and norepinephrine properties. Sertraline belongs to the class of antidepressants know as the SSRIs and selectively blocks neuronal reuptake of serotonin.

2. **E.** Nefazodone, fluoxetine, mirtazapine, and venlafaxine have minimal effects on seizure threshold. Bupropion in its original formulation caused seizures in 4 in 1000 patients. Although this has been reduced with the slow release form of the medication (*Wellbutrin SR*), it remains a contraindication to prescribe this medication to patients with a history of seizures.

3. **A.** Approximately 5% of patients taking lithium over the long term develop hypothyroidism, and thyroid status should be followed as routine care for these patients. Mr. Smith's symptoms are classic for hypothyroidism. Impairment in glucose metabolism, hepatic function, red blood cell production, and prolactin secretion are not typical complications of lithium therapy.

4. **C.** Nortriptyline (*Pamelor*) is a TCA, and as a class these drugs require at least one steady-state blood level to safely and effectively use the medication. Paroxetine, venlafaxine, and bupropion have not had blood levels correlated to response, and their relatively low toxicity does not require therapeutic blood monitoring. Nardil is a MAOI, which can be

lethal in overdose, but blood levels are not used to monitor for efficacy or toxicity.

5. **C.** All agents have a delay of approximately 48 hours. There are no significant differences in efficacy among the individual agents. The major contribution of the newer antidepressants is in their improved safety and tolerability.

SUPPLEMENTAL READING

American Psychiatric Association. Practice guidelines for major depressive disorder (MDD) in adults. Am J Psychiat 2000;157(Suppl 4):1–45.

Blier P and Abbott FV. Putative mechanisms of action of antidepressant drugs in affective and anxiety disorders and pain. J Psychiat Neurosci 2001;26(1):37–43.

Feighner JP. Mechanism of action of antidepressant medications. J Clin Psychiatr 1999;60:4–11.

Goodnick PL and Goldstein BJ. Selective serotonin inhibitors in affective disorders: I. Basic pharmacology. J Psychopharmacol 1998;12:S5–20.

Greden JF. The burden of recurrent depression: causes, consequences, and future prospects. J Clin Psychiatr 2001;62:22:5–9.

Janicak PG, Davis JM, Preskorn SH, and Ayd FJ Jr. Treatment with Antidepressants. In Principles and Practice of Psychopharmacotherapy (3rd ed.). Philadelphia: Lippincott Williams & Wilkins, 2001.

C A S E **Study**   Treatment of Depression

Mary Smith is a 46-year-old secretary who complains to her primary care physician mainly of fatigue. She reports having low energy over the past 2 months and finding it more and more difficult to maintain her home and work responsibilities. Although tired, she is unable to sleep through the night and awakens several times each night. Her appetite has been low and she has lost 10 pounds over this time. Her husband has noticed that she has lost interest in her hobbies and has withdrawn from their friends. He is concerned that she now has to bring office work home because her impaired attention and concentration make it impossible for her to complete her assignments during the workday. On this visit, Ms. Smith is neatly dressed, appropriate in conversation, but worried about why she has become unable to execute her tasks at work and enjoy her family and friends. She becomes tearful when describing this, feels guilty, and describes her mood as down. She expresses concern that she may not get better and has had thoughts of death but no actual plan or intent to end her life. She drinks no alcohol and doesn't use recreational drugs. She has no active medical problems and takes no prescription medications. Ms. Smith has one sister with a history of major depression, successfully treated with sertraline. Her mother was treated for depression with imipramine and phenelzine. Physical examination produces normal findings. Thyroid testing, blood counts, and blood chemistry are normal. Ms. Smith meets the DSM-IV criteria for major depression (depressed mood, loss of interest in pleasurable activities, decreased attention and concentration, fatigue, sleep disturbance, low appetite, weight loss, ideas of death). What pharmacological approach would you recommend?

ANSWER: Because of sertraline's favorable side effect profile and no need for dietary restrictions, it probably should be chosen over the older agents (TCAs and MAOIs). She should be warned about nausea and possibly loose stools, anorgasmia, and insomnia before she begins therapy. It also should be explained that the medication will take at least 2 weeks to begin working and that a complete trial of the medication to assess its efficacy will take 4 to 6 weeks. Since this is her first episode of depression, she should take the medication for 6 to 12 months after her symptoms have remitted before considering discontinuation of drug therapy.

34 | Antipsychotic Drugs

Stephen M. Lasley

DRUG LIST

GENERIC NAME	PAGE	GENERIC NAME	PAGE
Chlorpromazine	399	Pimozide	400
Clozapine	399	Risperidone	399
Dibenzodiazepine	400	Thioridazine	399
Haloperidol	399	Thiothixene	399
Olanzapine	400		

The term *psychosis* refers to a variety of mental disorders characterized by one or more of the following symptoms: diminished and distorted capacity to process information and draw logical conclusions, hallucinations, delusions, incoherence or marked loosening of associations, catatonic or disorganized behavior, and aggression or violence. Antipsychotic drugs lessen these symptoms regardless of the underlying cause or causes. These agents are prescribed for the treatment of mania, some movement disorders, and various types of nonspecific agitated behaviors but are most frequently employed in the therapy of schizophrenia. *Schizophrenia* is the term for a group of disorders marked by chronicity, impaired behavioral function, and disturbances of thinking and affect. The disorder has a prevalence of about 1% in the U. S. population, emerging most commonly during late adolescence or early adulthood.

Antipsychotic drugs have been used clinically for 50 years, and the first agents introduced, such as chlorpromazine, revolutionized the practice of psychiatry. Many newer agents have since been developed, reflecting significant degrees of success in enhancing potency and diminishing undesirable side effects. The terms *antipsychotics* and *neuroleptics* have been applied interchange-

ably to these drugs, but the latter term refers more appropriately to the older agents, whose extrapyramidal side effects (parkinsonism, dyskinesias, akathisia) are more prominent.

THE DISEASE OF SCHIZOPHRENIA

Schizophrenia is a group of heterogeneous, chronic psychotic disorders. Key symptoms include hallucinations, delusions, and abnormal experiences, such as the perception of loss of control of one's thoughts, perhaps to some outside entity. Patients lose empathy with others, become withdrawn, and demonstrate inappropriate or blunted mood. Discrimination of several subtypes of the disease represents only different patterns of symptoms with little value in relating behavior to neuropathology. The disorder has a strong genetic component, as demonstrated by a concordance of 40 to 50% between monozygotic twins, but no objective physiological or biochemical diagnostic tests exist.

Schizophrenic symptoms have been divided into two major categories. *Positive symptoms* are those that can be regarded as an abnormality or exaggeration of normal function (e.g., incoherent speech, agitation). The antipsychotic drugs are generally more effective in controlling these signs. *Negative symptoms* are those that indicate a loss or decrease in function, such as poverty of speech content or blunted affect. Both types of features are observable in most patients. Negative signs are considered to be more chronic and persistent and less responsive to some antipsychotic agents. Although any of these symptoms may undergo partial remission, persistent dysfunction and exacerbations are typical.

Schizophrenic patients appear to have small brains with large ventricular volumes, indicating a relative deficit of neurons. Structural and functional brain imaging studies have strongly suggested that regions of the medial temporal lobe (e.g., hippocampus) have diminished numbers of neurons and also have demonstrated the inability of individuals with schizophrenia to activate the frontal cortex and successfully execute tasks that require frontal cortical function. However, the relationship between behavioral signs, neuropathology, and a postulated functional excess of dopamine (discussed later) is unknown, and no theory of causation is conclusive.

The Dopamine Hypothesis of Schizophrenia

The dopamine hypothesis of schizophrenia is the most fully developed theory of causation for this disorder, and until recently, it has been the foundation for the rationale underlying drug therapy for this disease. The hypothesis is based on multiple lines of evidence suggesting that excessive dopaminergic activity underlies schizophrenia: (1) drugs that increase dopaminergic activity, such as levodopa and amphetamines, either aggravate existing schizophrenia or induce a psychosis indistinguishable from the acute paranoid form of the disorder; (2) traditional antipsychotic drugs strongly block D_2-dopaminergic receptors in the central nervous system (CNS), and clinical efficacy is highly correlated with the potency of individual agents to bind to this receptor; (3) some postmortem studies have reported increases in dopamine receptor density in brains of schizophrenics who were not treated with antipsychotic drugs; and (4) clinical response to antipsychotic drug treatment is correlated with a decrease in homovanillic acid, a primary dopamine metabolite, in cerebrospinal fluid (CSF), plasma, and urine.

However, the dopamine hypothesis does not account for some important observations. If an abnormality of dopamine physiology were solely responsible for the pathogenesis of schizophrenia, antipsychotic drugs would do a much better job in treating patients. As it is, they are only partially effective for most and ineffective for some patients. Moreover, there is evidence that diminished glutamatergic activity also plays a role in

the disease. The primary defect could emanate from nondopaminergic systems that exert a regulatory effect on dopamine neurons, leading to disinhibition of some dopaminergic pathways.

ANTIPSYCHOTIC MECHANISMS OF ACTION

Several lines of evidence demonstrated long ago that antipsychotic drugs blocked the synaptic actions of dopamine and should be classified as dopaminergic antagonists. Three dopaminergic pathways in the brain serve as primary substrates for the pharmacological effects of these agents. The nigrostriatal system consists of neurons with cell bodies in the substantia nigra that project to the caudate and putamen, and it is primarily involved in the coordination of posture and voluntary movement. The mesolimbic–mesocortical system projects from cell bodies in the ventral mesencephalon to the limbic system and neocortex, pathways associated with higher mental and emotional functions. The tuberoinfundibular system connects arcuate and periventricular nuclei of the hypothalamus to the mammotropic cells of the anterior pituitary, thereby physiologically inhibiting prolactin secretion. *The antagonism of dopamine in the mesolimbic–mesocortical system is thought to be the basis of the therapeutic actions of the antipsychotic drugs, while antagonism of the nigrostriatal system is the major factor in the extrapyramidal side effects seen with these agents.* Moreover, antagonism of dopamine's neurohormonal action in the anterior pituitary accounts for the hyperprolactinemia associated with antipsychotic administration. Thus, the same pharmacodynamic action may have distinct psychiatric, neurological, and endocrinological outcomes.

Five subtypes of dopamine receptors have been described; they are the D_1-like and D_2-like receptor groups. All have seven transmembrane domains and are G protein–coupled. The D_1-receptor increases cyclic adenosine monophosphate (cAMP) formation by stimulation of dopamine-sensitive adenylyl cyclase; it is located mainly in the putamen, nucleus accumbens, and olfactory tubercle. The other member of this family is the D_5-receptor, which also increases cAMP but has a 10-fold greater affinity for dopamine and is found primarily in limbic regions. The therapeutic potency of antipsychotic drugs does not correlate with their affinity for binding to the D_1-receptor.

The D_2-dopaminergic receptor decreases cAMP production by inhibiting dopamine-sensitive adenylyl cyclase and opens K^+ channels but can also block Ca^{++} channels. It is located both presynaptically and postsynaptically on neurons in the caudate putamen, nucleus accumbens, and olfactory tubercle. Another member of this family is the D_3-receptor, which also decreases cAMP formation but which has much lower expression, primarily in limbic and ventral striatal areas. The D_4-receptor also inhibits adenylyl cyclase and is found in frontal cortex and amygdala. *The binding affinity of antipsychotic agents to D_2-receptors is very strongly correlated with clinical antipsychotic and extrapyramidal potency.*

The antischizophrenic actions of these drugs may not consist simply of postsynaptic blockade of hyperactive dopamine systems. Such a blockade occurs within hours, while most symptoms improve over weeks. This discrepancy in the latency to therapeutic effect has been hypothesized to be linked to drug-induced changes in dopaminergic activity: after initiation of therapy, dopamine turnover increases, but after continued antipsychotic treatment, tolerance develops and dopamine metabolism returns to normal. This downward adjustment of dopaminergic activity is consistent with the decreased plasma concentrations of the dopamine metabolite homovanillic acid, an observation that correlates temporally with the clinical response to drug treatment.

Antipsychotic drugs also affect other transmitter systems that may contribute both to their antipsychotic actions and to their adverse reactions. Until recently the main focus in drug development was to discover agents that were more potent and selective in blocking D_2-receptors. However, newer atypical antipsychotics, such as clozapine and risperidone, have a weaker affinity for D_2-receptors and bind more strongly to 5-HT$_2$ (5-hydroxytryptamine) serotonergic receptors. Thus, lesser activity at the D_2-receptor relative to other transmitter receptors may diminish untoward side effects such as extrapyramidal toxicity. However, the antipsychotics also have variable antagonist actions at muscarinic, α-adrenergic, and histaminergic receptors in brain and peripheral tissue. The antimuscarinic activities cause blurred vision, dry mouth, and urinary retention and may contribute to excessive sedation. Blocking α-adrenoceptors may lead to sedation, orthostatic hypotension, and light-headedness. The antihistaminergic actions of these drugs probably contribute to drowsiness and sedation also.

PHARMACOLOGY

Phenothiazines are classified on the basis of their chemistry, pharmacological actions, and potency. Chemical classifications include the aliphatic (e.g., chlorpromazine; *Thorazine*), piperidine (e.g., thioridazine; *Mellaril*), and piperazine subfamilies. The piperazine derivatives are generally more potent and pharmacologically selective than the others. The thioxanthenes (e.g., thiothixene; *Navane*) are chemically related to the phenothiazines and have nearly equivalent potency. The

butyrophenone haloperidol (*Haldol*) is structurally distinct from the two preceding groups, offering greater potency and fewer autonomic side effects. The dibenzodiazepine clozapine (*Clozaril*) bears some structural resemblance to the phenothiazine group but causes little extrapyramidal toxicity. The benzisoxazole risperidone (*Risperdal*) is representative of many of the newer agents in having a unique structure relative to the older groups while retaining antipsychotic potency and a better side effect profile.

Pharmacokinetics

Most of the antipsychotics are readily but incompletely absorbed, and many undergo significant first-pass metabolism. The oral bioavailability of chlorpromazine and thioridazine is in the range of 25 to 35%, while that of haloperidol, which is less likely to be metabolized, has an oral bioavailability of about 65%. The antipsychotics are highly lipid soluble and are about 95% bound to proteins. Generally they have a much longer clinical duration of action than could be estimated from their plasma half-lives; this is likely due to their sequestration in fat tissue. Depot preparations are more slowly absorbed and longer acting, and thus can be administered parenterally at intervals up to 3 weeks. The main routes of metabolism are mediated by hepatic oxidative microsomal enzymes and by glucuronidation. Some metabolites, such as 7-hydroxychlorpromazine, retain measurable activity, but this effect is not considered to be clinically important; an exception to this observation is the major metabolite of thioridazine, which is more potent than the parent drug. Since drug blood concentrations of the less potent antipsychotics are lower after several weeks of treatment at the same dose, it is believed that these compounds may weakly induce their own metabolism. Also, the ability to metabolize and eliminate these drugs has been shown to diminish with age. Typical elimination half-lives vary from 12 to 24 hours.

Pharmacological Distinctions

Despite differences in potency, all commonly used antipsychotic drugs have approximately equal efficacy in equivalent doses. However, individual patients may be more responsive to one drug class than another. Prototype or representative members of the antipsychotics are arranged in decreasing order of potency in Table 34.1. While the sedative and autonomic effects of the high-potency drugs are less prominent, these agents are more likely to cause acute extrapyramidal symptoms. Generally, these trends are reversed as potency decreases.

All antipsychotics block D_2-receptors, but the degree of blockade in relation to actions on other receptors varies greatly. For example, chlorpromazine and

TABLE 34.1   Pharmacological Distinctions Among Representative Antipsychotic Drugs

Drug	Chemical Classification	Equivalent Oral Dose (mg)	Side Effects		
			Sedation	Autonomic[a]	Extrapyramidal Reactions[b]
Haloperidol	Butyrophenone	2	+	+	+++
Pimozide[c]	Diphenylbutylpiperidine	2	+	+	+++
Risperidone	Benzisoxazole	4	++	++	++
Thiothixene	Thioxanthene	5	++	++	++
Olanzapine	Thienobenzodiazepine	5	+	++	+
Clozapine	Dibenzodiazepine	75	+++	+++	+/-
Chlorpromazine	Phenothiazine (Aliphatic)	100	+++	+++	++
Thioridazine	Phenothiazine (Piperidine)	100	+++	+++	+

[a]α_1-Antiadrenergic and anticholinergic effects.
[b]Excluding tardive dyskinesia, which appears to be produced to the same degree and frequency by all agents except clozapine.
[c]Pimozide is used principally in the treatment of Tourette's syndrome.

thioridazine block α-adrenoceptors (autonomic side effects) more potently than D_2-receptors and also block 5-HT_2 serotonergic and H_1 histamine receptors (sedative side effects) to a significant extent. However, their affinity for D_1-receptors is weak. Haloperidol and pimozide (*Orap*) act mainly on D_2-receptors (extrapyramidal toxicity) with negligible activity at D_1-receptors. Clozapine, risperidone, and olanzapine (*Zyprex*) show marked clinical differences from the other drugs. Clozapine binds more to D_4, 5-HT_2, α_1-, and H_1-receptors (autonomic and sedative side effects) than to either D_2 (low extrapyramidal activity) or D_1 sites. Risperidone binds primarily to D_2-, 5-HT_2-, and α_1-receptors, retaining high potency with lesser potential for side effects. Current drug development is directed toward a search for atypical antipsychotics like clozapine that have a broad spectrum of effects on other neurotransmitter receptors.

Other Pharmacological Actions

Antipsychotic drugs produce shifts in the pattern of electrographic (EEG) frequencies, usually slowing them and causing hypersynchrony. This slowing is sometimes focal or unilateral, which may pose diagnostic problems, but the frequency and amplitude changes are readily apparent. The hypersynchrony produced by these drugs probably accounts for their activating effect on the EEG in epileptic patients and for the low incidence of seizures in patients with no history of seizure disorders.

Antipsychotics produce striking effects on the reproductive system. Amenorrhea and increased libido have been reported in women, whereas decreased libido and gynecomastia have been observed in men. Some of these actions are undoubtedly the result of a drug-associated blockade of dopamine's tonic normal inhibition of prolactin secretion, but they may also be partially due to an enhanced peripheral conversion of androgens to estrogens.

Orthostatic hypotension and high resting pulse rates can result from the use of the low-potency phenothiazines. Mean arterial pressure, peripheral resistance, and stroke volume are decreased, while pulse rate is increased. Abnormal electrocardiograms (ECGs) have been observed, especially following thioridazine administration. These findings include prolongation of the QT interval and abnormal configurations of the ST segment and T waves, the latter being rounded, flattened, or notched. These effects are readily reversed upon drug withdrawal.

CLINICAL USES

The treatment of schizophrenia is the primary indication for the use of these drugs. The principal goals for the management of a chronic schizophrenic disorder are the minimizing of symptoms and the prevention of exacerbations. Antipsychotic effectiveness is demonstrated by their ability to reduce the rate of relapse in the chronic condition by about two-thirds to three-quarters compared to no treatment. Drug choice is determined mainly by the patient's past responses and the drug's potential for producing adverse effects. The clinical trend is to prescribe the higher-potency atypical agents.

All antipsychotics except clozapine have a similar potential for producing tardive dyskinesia, the most serious adverse effect. Clozapine is reserved for patients who have failed to respond to therapy with at least two other antipsychotics and for those who have disabling tardive dyskinesia. Therapy with clozapine has been reported to salvage up to half of otherwise treatment-refractory patients. Its second-line status follows from its ability to cause seizures and a fatal agranulocytosis in large doses.

Substantial therapeutic margins exist for doses of antipsychotic drugs. Once the disorder is controlled, single daily doses are preferred. Bedtime dosing facilitates compliance and takes advantage of the sedation produced by some agents, and patients have fewer adverse reactions. Use of large doses, or rapidly increasing doses to treat severe conditions, has not proved beneficial because of the incidence of acute dystonic reactions. A parenteral form of haloperidol offers the advantage of greater bioavailability and so can be used for rapid initiation or for long-term maintenance in noncompliant individuals. During maintenance therapy, continual dosing with the smallest possible antipsychotic dose is preferred, as opposed to "as needed" treatment for recurrent episodes. Therapy is typically continued for at least a year after remissions are apparent.

Schizoaffective disorders have depression or mania as a major component in addition to psychosis. Thus, lithium or an antidepressant may have to be added to the regimen. Antipsychotic agents are also used in the initial therapy of mania because the patient's response is more rapid than with lithium. As the condition subsides, the antipsychotic can be withdrawn.

Tourette's syndrome, a heterogeneous behavioral disorder associated with motor and vocal tics of variable form and severity, can be effectively treated with haloperidol. Antipsychotics can also be employed to control disturbed behavior in senile dementia or Alzheimer's disease, since they decrease confusion, agitation, and hyperactivity. Most of these drugs also exhibit a strong antiemetic effect and can sometimes be used clinically for this purpose.

ADVERSE EFFECTS

Antipsychotic drugs are characterized by high therapeutic indices with respect to mortality, but side effects occur routinely at therapeutic doses, mostly as exten-

sions of pharmacological actions (Table 34.2). The characteristic neurological symptoms (discussed next) caused by these agents are particularly troublesome, often limit the tolerated dose, and may interfere with the desired benefits and patient compliance.

Sedation

Sedation is common after use of all antipsychotic drugs and is especially notable with the low-potency phenothiazines; this is a result of their activity at α_1-adrenergic and H_1-histaminergic receptors. However, sedation decreases during long-term treatment, and many patients become tolerant to this effect. Single daily doses given at bedtime minimize this problem.

Extrapyramidal Reactions

Two extrapyramidal conditions, acute dystonia and akathisia, occur early during treatment, while parkinsonism tends to evolve gradually over days to weeks. All three reactions occur most commonly with the high-potency antipsychotics (Table 34.1) and are related to high D_2-receptor occupancy. Acute dystonia, which occurs in about 5% of patients on antipsychotic therapy, consists of uncontrollable movements and distortions of the face, head, and neck. It can be treated with centrally acting antimuscarinic agents, such as benztropine, while antipsychotic therapy is temporarily discontinued. When this reaction subsides, the anticholinergic can be withdrawn.

The incidence of akathisia is about 20%; the syndrome consists of intense motor restlessness and agitation that contribute to a behavioral deterioration. It is frequently unresponsive to anticholinergics and is more effectively treated with benzodiazepines and β-adrenergic antagonists, such as propranolol.

Signs of parkinsonism—akinesia, tremor, rigidity—can develop gradually, but this reaction usually responds favorably to central antimuscarinic agents. As with dystonia, parkinsonism may subside, permitting withdrawal of the antimuscarinic drug.

TABLE 34.2 Significant Adverse Effects of Antipsychotic Drugs

Type	Manifestations	Mechanism
Sedation	Drowsiness, lethargy	α_1-adrenoceptor block, H_1 histamine receptor block
Extrapyramidal reactions	Dystonias, akathisia, parkinsonism	D_2-receptor block
	Tardive dyskinesia	D_2-receptor up-regulation (?)
	Neuroleptic malignant syndrome	Extrapyramidal sensitivity
Autonomic signs	Dry mouth, blurred vision, urinary retention, constipation	Muscarinic cholinoreceptor block
	Orthostatic hypotension, impotence	α_1-Adrenoceptor block
Endocrine signs	Amenorrhea, galactorrhea, infertility, impotence	D_2-receptor block resulting in hyperprolactinemia

Tardive dyskinesia is a late-occurring syndrome of abnormal movements of the face and tongue with widespread choreoathetosis. It is the most serious adverse effect of the antipsychotic drugs. It can be expected to occur in 20 to 40% of chronically treated patients; there is no established treatment, and reversibility may be limited. These reactions are more frequent and severe in the elderly.

Tardive dyskinesia is generally accepted to be a D_2 supersensitivity phenomenon, though research has not unequivocally established this postulate. An appropriate clinical response to these symptoms would be to reduce the dose or discontinue the antipsychotic agent and then eliminate all drugs with central anticholinergic action, such as antidepressants. The rationale is to balance the risks of continuing treatment in a patient with tardive dyskinesia with the benefits of antipsychotic administration. If these steps are not helpful, clozapine therapy can be considered, or diazepam can be employed to enhance GABAergic activity. Prevention of this reaction is important. Generally, antipsychotics should be prescribed in minimally effective doses and their use reserved for time-limited treatment except in the treatment of chronic schizophrenic disorders.

The *neuroleptic malignant syndrome* is a rare medical emergency involving extrapyramidal symptoms that occurs in about 1% of patients receiving antipsychotics. The concern is not the incidence but that about 10% of these cases are fatal. The condition is marked by hyperthermia or fever, diffuse muscular rigidity with severe extrapyramidal effects, autonomic dysfunction such as increased blood pressure and heart rate, and fluctuating levels of consciousness. Neuroleptic malignant syndrome is most common in males, with about 80% of cases occurring in patients under 40 years of age. Treatment should include general supportive measures, such as rehydration and body cooling; antipsychotic therapy should be discontinued. Short-term therapy with dantrolene in combination with antiparkinson agents such as bromocriptine has been employed to control the muscular rigidity and hyperthermia.

Autonomic and Endocrine Effects

Most antipsychotics have both α-adrenergic and cholinergic antagonist activities, and blocking actions at histamine and serotonin receptors also contribute to the autonomic effects of some agents. Postural hypotension and depression of medullary cardiovascular centers resulting from α_1-adrenoceptor blockade is particularly troublesome in elderly or debilitated patients. β_2-Agonists, such as epinephrine, are contraindicated, as they may worsen the hypotension. The anticholinergic effects can be very bothersome but usually subside as tolerance to these effects occurs. Typically, autonomic signs can be controlled by adjustment of dose.

All antipsychotics except clozapine and perhaps olanzapine produce hyperprolactinemia by removing the inhibitory actions of dopamine on prolactin secretion. This results in amenorrhea, galactorrhea, and infertility in women and in loss of libido and impotence in men. Inhibition of the release of follicle-stimulating and luteinizing hormones may also play a role. In addition, weight gain is common, and food intake must be monitored.

Other Adverse Effects

Cholestatic jaundice is observed infrequently, usually during the first few weeks of treatment. This is thought to be a hypersensitivity reaction and is usually mild and self-limited. Cutaneous allergic reactions are occasionally reported. Both types of problems normally disappear upon changing to an antipsychotic from a different chemical class. Photosensitivity usually manifests as an acute hypersensitivity reaction to sun with sunburn or rash, but the condition is generally mild and does not require dosage adjustment.

Opacities of the cornea and lens due to deposition of fine particulate matter are a common complication of chlorpromazine therapy but regress after drug withdrawal. The most serious ocular complication is pigmentary retinopathy associated with high-dose thioridazine administration; it is an irreversible condition leading to decreased visual acuity and possibly blindness.

Agranulocytosis is a potentially catastrophic idiosyncratic reaction that usually appears within the first 3 months of therapy. Although the incidence is extremely low (except for clozapine), mortality is high. Thus, any fever, sore throat, or cellulitis is an indication for discontinuing the antipsychotic and immediately conducting white blood cell and differential counts.

Contraindications for antipsychotic therapy are few; they may include Parkinson's disease, hepatic failure, hypotension, bone marrow depression, or use of CNS depressants. Overdoses of antipsychotics are rarely fatal, except for thioridazine, which is associated with major ventricular arrhythmias, cardiac conduction block, and sudden death. For other agents gastric lavage should be attempted even if several hours have elapsed since the drug was taken, because gastrointestinal motility is decreased and the tablets may still be in the stomach. Moreover, activated charcoal effectively binds most of these drugs and can be followed by a saline cathartic. The hypotension often responds to fluid replacement or pressor agents such as norepinephrine.

DRUG INTERACTIONS

Because of their multiple effects, antipsychotic drugs produce more important pharmacodynamic than pharmacokinetic interactions. The action of other CNS depressants may be enhanced, and concurrent use of tricyclic antidepressants or other agents with anticholinergic activity may cause additive CNS dysfunction and peripheral anticholinergic effects. The hypotensive effects of an antipsychotic may be increased by diuretics, captopril, and other antihypertensive medications. Antipsychotic agents are also susceptible to enhanced metabolism by inducers of microsomal mixed-function oxidases.

Study QUESTIONS

1. Which of the following agents possesses pharmacological actions characterized by high antipsychotic potency, high potential for extrapyramidal toxicity, and a low likelihood of causing sedation?
   (A) Thioridazine
   (B) Haloperidol
   (C) Flumazenil
   (D) Clozapine
   (E) Carbamazepine

2. Tardive dyskinesia after long-term antipsychotic administration is thought to be due to
   (A) A decrease in dopamine synthesis
   (B) Enhanced stimulation of D_2 dopamine autoreceptors
   (C) Loss of cholinergic neurons in striatum
   (D) Up-regulation of striatal dopamine receptors
   (E) Increased tolerance to antipsychotic agents

3. Which neuroleptic agent has the lowest likelihood of producing tardive dyskinesia?
   (A) Imipramine
   (B) Chlorpromazine
   (C) Clozapine
   (D) Fluoxetine
   (E) Thiothixene

4. Which clinical condition poses the greatest concern to a patient on antipsychotic therapy?
   (A) Epilepsy
   (B) Nausea associated with motion sickness
   (C) Manic phase of bipolar disorder
   (D) Hallucinogen-induced psychosis
   (E) Tourette's syndrome

5. Mr. James began haloperidol therapy for schizophrenia and within several weeks developed bradykinesia, rigidity, and tremor. Though his psychoses were well controlled, he was switched to another agent, thioridazine, which proved to be as effective as haloperidol in managing his primary condition and did not result in the undesirable symptoms. The most likely explanation for these observations is that
   (A) Haloperidol acts presynaptically to block dopamine release.
   (B) Haloperidol activates GABAergic neurons in the striatum.

   (C) Haloperidol has a low affinity for D_2-receptors.
   (D) Thioridazine has greater α_1-adrenergic blocking activity than haloperidol.
   (E) Thioridazine has greater muscarinic blocking activity in brain than haloperidol.

6. Which drug may be useful in the management of the neuroleptic malignant syndrome, although it can worsen the symptoms of schizophrenia?
   (A) Risperidone
   (B) Thiothixene
   (C) Haloperidol
   (D) Bromocriptine
   (E) Valproic acid

ANSWERS

1. **B.** The question describes the pharmacological profile of a high-potency classical antipsychotic agent, most likely of the butyrophenone or phenothiazine class. Thioridazine is a low-potency piperidine phenothiazine agent with significant affinity for α_1-adrenergic and muscarinic receptors, having a high potential for sedation as a side effect. Haloperidol is a high-potency butyrophenone with its primary action at the D_2 dopaminergic receptor, so it produces a significant incidence of extrapyramidal toxicity and little sedation. Clozapine is a low-potency atypical antipsychotic that binds primarily to D_4, $5\text{-}HT_2$, and α_1 receptors and possesses very little extrapyramidal toxicity but significant sedative and autonomic side effects. Flumazenil is a benzodiazepine antagonist, and carbamazepine is an anticonvulsant; neither possesses significant antipsychotic properties.

2. **D.** This question concerns the most important extrapyramidal reaction to long-term antipsychotic administration—tardive dyskinesia—and its generally accepted basis. Although some tolerance to the sedative effects of antipsychotics can occur, there is no evidence linking this to tardive dyskinesia. Antipsychotic agents enhance dopamine synthesis acutely by blocking D_2-autoreceptors by which the transmitter normally inhibits dopamine cell firing and synthesis. Long-term treatment with a D_2-receptor antagonist causes depolarization inactivation

of dopamine neurons with diminished transmitter production and release. However, a decrease in dopamine synthesis has not been linked with tardive dyskinesia. On the contrary, lower dopamine tone would more resemble a parkinsonian state, whereas in tardive dyskinesia, antidopaminergic drugs tend to suppress the dyskinetic symptoms, and dopaminergic agonists worsen the condition. Therefore, it is generally accepted that up-regulated dopamine receptors underlie tardive dyskinesia. There is no evidence that the antipsychotics lead to loss of striatal cholinergic neurons.

3. **C.** Tardive dyskinesia is an extrapyramidal reaction that occurs most commonly after long-term administration of high-potency butyrophenone, thioxanthene, or phenothiazine. Thus, thiothixene is not a good choice. Chlorpromazine is a low-potency phenothiazine agent with moderate potential to cause extrapyramidal signs. Clozapine is well known to have the lowest potential for producing tardive dyskinesia during chronic therapy. It has other undesirable side effects, but clinical experience with other newer atypical antipsychotics is not sufficient to establish their potential for causing this disorder. Imipramine and fluoxetine are antidepressants.

4. **A.** The question concerns actions of antipsychotic agents that may have untoward consequences when combined with other coincident or preexisting medical conditions. These drugs have an activating effect on the EEG in epileptic patients and thus may worsen that condition. Generally, the antipsychotics have antiemetic properties but generally are more potent than is necessary to treat motion sickness. The other three conditions listed—C, D, and E—are indications for the use of antipsychotic agents.

5. **E.** The question concerns the emergence of parkinsonian signs relatively early in a patient's therapy for schizophrenia and their elimination by switching treatment to a second agent, thioridazine. Haloperidol has high affinity for D_2-dopaminergic receptors and is well known to have a high potential for causing these kinds of extrapyramidal signs. The drug has no direct action on GABAergic neurons and does not act presynaptically to affect dopamine release. While thioridazine binds to D_2-dopaminergic receptors with an affinity similar to that of haloperidol, it also has much greater antimuscarinic activity. This latter action can compensate for dopamine receptor blockade in the nigrostriatal tract, so that extrapyramidal function is more appropriately maintained. Thioridazine has greater α_1-adrenergic blocking activity than haloperidol, but this is not thought to play a role in elimination of the parkinsonian signs.

6. **D.** The neuroleptic malignant syndrome is an infrequent extrapyramidal reaction with a relatively high rate of lethality. It is marked by muscle rigidity, high fever, and autonomic instability. It may result from too-rapid block of dopaminergic receptors in individuals who are highly sensitive to the extrapyramidal effects of antipsychotic drugs. Management consists of control of fever, use of muscle relaxants, and administration of the dopamine agonist bromocriptine, which is likely to worsen the psychotic symptoms. Choices A to C are antipsychotics and would likely worsen neuroleptic malignant syndrome. Valproic acid has antimanic, antimigraine, and anticonvulsant properties, but it is not used to treat the syndrome in question.

SUPPLEMENTAL READING

Ananth J, Burgoyne KS, Gadasalli R, and Aquino S. How do the atypical antipsychotics work? J Psychiatry Neurosci 2001;26:385–394.

Kane JM. Schizophrenia. N Engl J Med 1996;334:34–41.

Konradi C and Heckers S. Antipsychotic drugs and neuroplasticity: Insights into the treatment and neurobiology of schizophrenia. Biol Psychiatry 2001;50:729–742.

Marder SR. Antipsychotic medications. In Schatzberg, AF and Nemeroff CB (eds.). Textbook of Psychopharmacology. Washington: American Psychiatric, 1998.

Rector NA and Beck AT. A clinical review of cognitive therapy for schizophrenia. Curr Psychiatry Rep 2002;4:83–96.

Tuunainen A, Wahlbeck K, and Gilbody S. Newer atypical antipsychotic medication in comparison to clozapine: A systematic review of randomized trials. Schizophr Res 2002;56:1–10.

CASE Study Refractory Schizophrenia

Ms. Anderson is a 29-year-old single woman who was diagnosed with schizophrenia more than 5 years ago. She started with haloperidol and then after several months switched to thiothixene. While her extrapyramidal signs with these agents were not unacceptable, the frequency of her acute psychotic episodes marked by paranoid delusions was not substantially diminished. Subsequently she was also given a trial of thioridazine with a similar clinical response to those of the earlier agents. What antipsychotic agent would be the most appropriate next choice for this patient? What are the primary concerns with the use of this drug, and what precautions should be taken during therapy with this agent?

ANSWER: Clozapine would be the next best choice in the treatment of this patient. Therapy with this drug has been reported to salvage as many as 50% of otherwise treatment-refractory individuals. Clozapine does not have the status of a first-line agent because of its undesirable side effects. De novo seizures occur in 2 to 5% of treated patients, and agranulocytosis is a problem. The significance of agranulocytosis is not the incidence (1–2%) but the severity: about 10% of these cases are fatal. *As a result, weekly blood counts are mandatory for patients receiving clozapine.* Patients should also be alert for sudden onset of any fever or chills. Other atypical antipsychotics, such as risperidone and olanzapine, are available, but clinical experience with these agents is insufficient to establish their value in treating refractory patients.

35 Contemporary Drug Abuse

Billy R. Martin and William L. Dewey

DRUG LIST

GENERIC NAME	PAGE	GENERIC NAME	PAGE
Alfentanil	408	Marijuana	416
Amobarbital	411	MDA	418
Amphetamine	410	MDMA	418
Buprenorphine	408	Mescaline	417
Butorphanol	408	Methadone	408
Caffeine	410	Methamphetamine	410
Chlordiazepoxide	411	Methylphenidate	410
Cocaine	410	Midazolam	411
Diazepam	411	Morphine	409
Disulfiram	415	Nicotine	411
Ethanol	412	Pentobarbital	411
Fentanyl	408	Phencyclidine	417
Flurazepam	411	Phenmetrazine	410
Heroin	409	Psilocybin	417
Lorazepam	411	Secobarbital	411
LSD	417		

The phrases *substance abuse* and *drug abuse* are often applied to the use of an illegal or *illicit* chemical substance (e.g., LSD, heroin). However, these terms may be applied when a legally obtainable medication is used excessively and for unintended purposes or is diverted to someone else's use. Also, some legal substances (e.g., nicotine, alcohol) are used to the detriment of the individual. Inappropriate use, or abuse, is the excessive *self-administration* of any substance for nonmedical purposes. An additional aspect of drug abuse is the production of hazardous or harmful effects to the individual and/or to society. The etiology of substance abuse is a complicated phenomenon that is sometimes a function of genetics, socioeconomic status, education, peer pressure, thrill seeking, or experimenting behavior and sometimes an inappropriate attempt at *self-medication* to treat a real or perceived disease state. It is also clear that drug abuse is a function of the pharmacology of each drug. Almost all abused substances produce an effect on the brain that is perceived as desirable and will initiate *drug-seeking behavior.*

The professionals in the drug abuse field have such diverse backgrounds that adopting a common terminology for terms such as *addiction* and *dependence* has been difficult. These terms are best defined in the context of the pattern and consequences of drug use. Regardless of the characteristics of the drug-induced *intoxication,* the properties of the drug that are responsible for drug-seeking behavior are often referred to as the *reinforcing properties.* These drugs produce effects that are so desirable that the user is compelled to obtain more of the drug.

Recurrent abuse of a drug may properly be termed an *addiction* when the individual becomes so obsessed with constantly obtaining and using a drug that it becomes a primary goal and disrupts the ability to function in family, social, or career settings. Typically, especially during the initial stages of drug addiction, the primary reinforcing property is the production of *euphoria,* a term indicating anything from happiness or pleasantness to an excitement resembling sexual orgasm. Euphoria is considered to be a *positive reinforcing property,* one that the individual would desire or seek. The evaluation of drugs for their reinforcing properties is an assessment of their *abuse potential.* The craving or desire to obtain additional drug, especially when it is not available, was at one time termed *psychological addiction* or *psychological dependence,* though today these terms are not necessarily descriptive or specific. The term *addiction* should be used to describe recurrent drug abuse, while the term *dependence* (discussed later) refers to another state, a function of drug use, not drug craving per se. *Addiction* has also been used to describe recurrent substance abuse by individuals who realize it is harmful to their health but cannot fulfill their desire to stop, such as with tobacco.

Chronic use of a drug over a long period sometimes produces a state of tolerance that may be classified as pharmacokinetic, pharmacodynamic, or behavioral. The degree of tolerance is generally proportional to the drug dose and the duration of use. In some cases, partial or complete tolerance to the euphoric effect of the drug develops. However, tolerance to many of the other acute effects also generally develops. Termination of drug abuse may create a condition of *drug abstinence,* which coincides with the emergence of a measurable physical syndrome. This *abstinence syndrome* is an indication of *dependence,* is often referred to as drug *withdrawal,* and was once termed *physical dependence* to distinguish it from psychological dependence. It is assumed that adaptation, or tolerance, to repeated administration of drug is responsible for physical dependence. Generally, the severity of the abstinence syndrome or level of dependence is proportional to the degree of tolerance attained. However, the relationship between tolerance and dependence has not been fully resolved; tolerance and dependence can occur separately.

Epidemiological studies indicate that most individuals who abuse any one drug often also abuse, or coabuse, other drugs during the same period. *Polydrug abuse* complicates conclusions drawn from epidemiological and clinical studies. One reason for coabuse of drugs relates to similarities in pharmacological effects. In these cases, once tolerance to the primary drug develops, the individual also has *cross-tolerance* to related classes of drugs. For example, the development of tolerance to one CNS depressant, such as barbiturates, anxiolytic agents, or alcohol, simultaneously produces some degree of tolerance to the other depressants. Users may attempt to ameliorate selected drug effects by coabuse of drugs with opposite pharmacological profiles.

Drugs of abuse are derived from numerous chemical classes, and therefore, it is not surprising that they produce distinctive pharmacological effects. Also, the consequences of acute and chronic use vary considerably among different classes of compounds, as summarized in Table 35.1.

TABLE 35.1 Consequences of Drug Abuse

Substance or Drug Class	Drug	Abuse Potential[a]	Acute Intoxication[b]	Withdrawal Symptoms[c]	Additional Consequences of Use[d]
Sympathomimetic stimulants	Cocaine	++++	Euphoria	+	+++
	Amphetamine	+++			
	Methamphetamine		Increased alertness	Drug craving	Depression
	Phenmetrazine		Increased motor activity	Dysphoria	Toxic psychosis
	Methylphenidate			Sleepiness	Sexual dysfunction
	MDMA			Fatigue	
	MDA			Bradycardia	Cerebrovascular accidents

408 IV DRUGS AFFECTING THE CENTRAL NERVOUS SYSTEM

TABLE 35.1 Consequences of Drug Abuse—cont'd

Substance or Drug Class	Drug	Abuse Potential[a]	Acute Intoxication[b]	Withdrawal Symptoms[c]	Additional Consequences of Use[d]
Tobacco	Nicotine	++	Subtle effects Anxiolytic Mild stimulant Increased alertness	+ Anxiety Restlessness Bradycardia Weight gain	Cardiovascular accidents +++ Cancer Cardiovascular disease Bronchitis
Opioid agonists	Heroin Morphine Methadone LAAM Oxycodone Meperidine Fentanyl Sufentanil Alfentanil Oxymorphone Hydrocodone Hydromorphone Levorphanol	+++	Euphoria Relaxation Anxiolytic Rush Sedation	+++ Opioid craving Irritability Hyperalgesia Cramps Nausea, vomiting Muscle aches Mydriasis Sweating Piloerection Tachycardia Hypertension Fever Is rarely life-threatening	+++ Life expectancy decreased by 50% Increased risk of HIV transmission in IV users
Opioid mixed agonist–antagonists	Pentazocine Nalbuphine Butorphanol Buprenorphine	++	Same as opioid agonists but less intense	Same as opioid agonists but less intense	
Opioids (miscellaneous)	Codeine Propoxyphene	++	Same as opioid agonists but less intense	Same as opioid agonists but less intense	
Alcohol	Ethanol	++	Stimulant at low doses including euphoria and increased talkativeness Depressant at high doses producing ataxia, slurred speech, decreased motor skills	+++ Tremor Nausea Sweating Hypertension Seizure Delirium tremens Life-threatening	+++ Liver disease Fetal alcohol syndrome Life-expectancy decreased by 10 yrs Contributes to highway fatalities
Barbiturates	Secobarbital Pentobarbital Amobarbital	+++	Intoxication similar to alcohol	+++ See alcohol Life-threatening	+++ Death from drug overdose Suicide
Benzodiazepines and other mild tranquilizers	Diazepam Chlordiazepoxide Midazolam Lorazepam Flurazepam Meprobamate Methaqualone	+	Intoxication similar to alcohol	++ Cramps Myoclonic jerks Agitation, anxiety Seizure (rarely)	+
Inhalants	Gasoline Paint thinner Lighter fluid Solvents	++	Intoxication Dizziness Flushing	Some indication of alcohol-like withdrawal	+ Cardiac arrhythmias Liver and kidney damage Provide adolescents easy entry into drug abuse

TABLE 35.1 Consequences of Drug Abuse

Substance or Drug Class	Drug	Abuse Potential[a]	Acute Intoxication[b]	Withdrawal Symptoms[c]	Additional Consequences of Use[d]
Marijuana	Δ-THC	+	Euphoria Heightened sensory perception Hallucinations and motor impairment at high doses	+ Restlessness Irritability Agitation Sleep disturbances Nausea	+ Bronchitis Disruption of short-term memory Impaired motor skills
Hallucinogens	LSD (lysergide) Psilocybin, psilocin DMT, mescaline DOM, STP	+	Distortion of perception, mood, and thought	−	+++ Neurotoxicity Flashbacks Toxic psychosis PCP can be lethal
	PCP (phencyclidine)	+	Severe CNS depression	−	
Anabolic steroids	Testosterone Nandrolone	+/−	No acute behavioral effects	−/+	+ Liver damage Altered sex drive

Severity ratings: −, none; +, low; ++, intermediate; +++, high; ++++, very high.
[a]Abuse potential: abuse liability, reinforcing property, drug-seeking, craving, psychological effect.
[b]Intoxication: acute pharmacological effects.
[c]Withdrawal: withdrawal signs, abstinence syndrome, physiological effect.
[d]Consequence: detrimental personal effect (health), negative societal effects (economic, social).

OPIOIDS

For centuries opium was used for both medicinal and recreational purposes. Derived from the poppy *Papaver somniferum*, it contains numerous opiates, the primary one of which is morphine. The term *opiate* has largely been replaced by *opioid*, which represents all compounds with morphinelike activity and includes morphine, morphine derivatives, and peptides. *Opiate* is used to refer to morphinelike drugs derived from the plant and structurally similar analogues. These drugs are frequently referred to as narcotics, a Greek term for stupor, which is scientifically obsolete. Even in its early history, opium presented a problem when it was smoked or taken orally. The introduction of the hypodermic needle and syringe, however, drastically enhanced the euphoric properties of opioids and thereby altered their abuse liability. In addition, the synthesis of heroin resulted in an opioid that was more potent than morphine and ideally suited for intravenous administration.

Extent and Pattern of Abuse

The abuse of opioids falls into two distinct categories of users, those who initiate use solely for recreational purposes and those who become physically dependent as a result of being treated medically with opioids. As discussed in Chapter 26, the primary use of opioids is for the control of moderate to severe pain. However, few patients receiving opioids for pain management become dependent. Furthermore, dependence is less likely if opioids are used judiciously. Acute pain can be controlled with opioids such as hydromorphone or oxycodone, which have a rapid onset and short duration of action. In contrast, chronic pain is better treated with opioids such as methadone or morphine (e.g., *Duramorph, MS Contin*), which are less likely to produce euphoria because of their slow onset of action. Dependence in patients is most likely to occur in those with pain of unexplained or poorly defined etiology. Avoiding long-term use of opioids in this population reduces the risk of developing dependence. *Development of dependence should not be a consideration in the management of terminal cancer pain.*

The primary illicit opioid is heroin (diacetylmorphine), which was once used almost exclusively by the intravenous route. In recent years, the purity of street heroin has risen to levels that allow it to be smoked or snorted.

Pharmacological Aspects

First-time users frequently experience unpleasant, or dysphoric, effects that may include nausea and vomiting. The frequent user experiences a rush, or warm flushing feeling, in the skin and lower extremities that is often equated with sexual orgasm. This intense euphoria lasts for one to several minutes and is followed by sedation, relaxation, and tranquility lasting up to an hour. This latter period is sometimes called being on the nod. All effects have largely dissipated within 3 to 5 hours, which requires the user to inject at frequent intervals.

Pharmacokinetics plays a very important role in the manner in which opioids are abused. Morphine and many of its derivatives are slowly and erratically absorbed after oral administration, which makes this route suitable for long-term management of pain but not for producing euphoria. In addition, opioids undergo considerable first-pass metabolism, which accounts for their low potency after oral administration. Heroin is more potent than morphine, although its effects arise primarily from metabolism to morphine. The potency difference is attributed to heroin's greater membrane permeability and resultant increased absorption into the brain.

Tolerance and Dependence

Tolerance to the unpleasant effects experienced by some individuals at the initiation of opioid use develops readily. Significant tolerance also occurs to the analgesic, respiratory depressant, emetic, and euphoric effects, although it develops somewhat more slowly to respiratory depression. Little tolerance to the GI effects and miosis develops. Cross-tolerance occurs with all known opioid analgesics. Opioid tolerance develops more quickly and to a greater extent than it does for most other drugs of abuse. The lethal opioid dose can be 20-fold higher in a tolerant individual than in a neophyte. Tolerance develops within a few days if potent opioids are given at frequent intervals, such as every 4 to 6 hours. Development of tolerance requires several weeks if the opioid is given only twice a day.

The continued use of opioids results in the development of physical dependence, as demonstrated by the appearance of a characteristic abstinence syndrome upon interruption or cessation of use. The symptoms of withdrawal include hyperactivity, anxiety, restlessness, yawning, diarrhea, vomiting, chills, fever, lacrimation, and runny nose. Piloerection (gooseflesh or cold turkey), mydriasis, increased blood pressure and heart rate, and hyperpyrexia may be observed. Tremors, abdominal cramps, and muscle and joint pain may be present. Drug craving is an important feature of opioid withdrawal. In contrast to some other drugs of abuse, withdrawal is not life threatening.

Treatment of Opioid Dependence

Although the ultimate goal of treatment programs is to achieve drug-free status as quickly as possible, it is rarely achieved without pharmacotherapy. The most commonly used strategy is to switch the patient from a short-acting opioid, such as heroin, to a long-acting ag-

onist, such as methadone. It is easier to withdraw patients from methadone because it produces a protracted withdrawal syndrome that is less intense than that produced by heroin.

Opioid antagonists, such as naltrexone, provide another treatment option in that addicts who are completely withdrawn from an opioid can be maintained on antagonists that will block the pleasurable effects of subsequent injections of heroin. Mixed opioid agonist–antagonists show promise in that they have sufficient agonist effects to reduce craving while at the same time exhibiting antagonist properties.

STIMULANTS

A variety of drugs in distinct pharmacological and chemical classes can be considered under the broad classification as stimulants. Xanthines and methylxanthines constitute a weak class of stimulants that includes caffeine, theophylline (aminophylline), and theobromine. Caffeine is freely available in coffee, colas, and certain over-the-counter pills. A low degree of tolerance develops to some of their effects and a mild withdrawal syndrome is observed following immediate cessation of their repeated use.

The primary class of stimulants for which there is a tremendous addiction problem is the sympathomimetic stimulants, which include cocaine, amphetamine, methamphetamine (*Desoxyn*), methylphenidate (*Ritalin*), and phenmetrazine.

Extent and Pattern of Abuse

Sympathomimetic stimulant drugs have very high abuse potential. They are typically used repeatedly for a short period during which time the user escalates the dose to greater and greater levels to attain the desired degree of euphoria. Extended uninterrupted use of stimulants for 24 to 72 hours is often referred to as a *run* and usually ends in a *crash* (24–36 hours of sleep) once the individual is exhausted physically. Besides illicit sources of stimulants, approximately 5 billion doses of these drugs are prescribed per year, and there appears to be a significant degree of abuse via prescription diversion.

While some stimulants, such as amphetamine and methylphenidate, are taken orally, others are either volatilized for inhalation or snorted as the solid (nasal insufflation). *It is necessary to convert cocaine and methamphetamine to their free base so that they can be volatilized.* Methamphetamine and cocaine are also abused via the intravenous route.

Pharmacological Aspects

Most of the sympathomimetic stimulants exhibit similar pharmacological properties, differing primarily in the magnitude of their effects. Acute drug administration produces feelings of euphoria, elation, and alertness. Intravenous injections of cocaine and amphetamine can produce a very intense *rush* of sensations that resemble sexual orgasm. At small doses cognition increases and mood is elevated. As the dose of drug escalates during a run, the overall activity of the individual changes from task performance to one generally characterized by stereotypical movements. The person starts performing certain behaviors repeatedly. Some grind or gnash their teeth. Many continuously touch or pick at their face or extremities. At this stage the individual becomes suspicious and may develop anxiety or paranoia. Acute toxic paranoid psychosis can develop, but it usually requires a longer period of abuse than a single acute session.

Besides stimulating the CNS, these drugs activate the autonomic nervous system. Individuals have tachycardia, hypertension, and possibly arrhythmias. Autonomic hyperactivity is also expressed as hyperthermia and mydriasis. More serious effects include the possibility of myocardial infarction, cerebrovascular hemorrhage, seizure, and death.

Mechanism of Action

The sympathomimetic drugs are discussed in Chapter 10. In brief, the most commonly abused of these drugs, such as cocaine, work primarily as indirect agonists of the catecholamine neurotransmitter systems via inhibitory actions upon the transmitter reuptake system. Considerable evidence supports a role for dopamine in mediating the rewarding effects of cocaine. There is also evidence that blockade of serotonin uptake may contribute to cocaine's actions.

Tolerance and Dependence

Tolerance to stimulants develops fairly rapidly, even in the therapeutic dose range. It is the rapid development of tolerance that leads to the escalation of dose during drug abuse runs.

Other Adverse Effects of Chronic Abuse

Chronic stimulant abuse alters the personality of the abuser. These and related changes are the result of neurotoxicity and are not characterized as either acute drug effects or withdrawal signs. Individuals have delusions of being pursued or persecuted and therefore become suspicious and paranoid. They become self-occupied and hostile toward others. Long-term abuse can produce toxic psychosis that closely resembles schizophrenia and must be treated with neuroleptic drugs (haloperidol, chlorpromazine). This psychosis can develop even within 1 to 2 weeks if the person is on a run of very high doses of stimulants.

NICOTINE

Pharmacological Actions

The behavioral effects of nicotine have been defined as both stimulant and depressant, effects that are influenced by the present mental status and expectations of the smoker. Smokers may feel alert and relaxed. Nicotine produces myriad effects on the central nervous system (CNS), almost all of which appear to be mediated through nicotinic receptors. Additionally, nicotine influences multiple neuronal systems. One of its most prominent effects is stimulated release of dopamine, particularly in the nucleus accumbens, which is a major component of the reward system. Nicotine also stimulates the release of endogenous opioids and glucocorticoids.

Tolerance and Dependence

Tolerance to nicotine's effects develops rapidly and most likely involves multiple processes, although the pattern and extent of tolerance development is not identical for all of nicotine's effects. It has been proposed that rapid tolerance or desensitization occurs to the behavioral or reinforcing effects of nicotine. These effects are of such a short duration that a smoker continually cycles between a sensitized and desensitized state. This notion is consistent with the fact that drugs with high abuse liability have a rapid onset and short duration of action.

Regardless of the mechanism of tolerance, nicotine is a highly addicting drug. Even though most individuals are unaware of nicotine's reinforcing properties when smoking, many individuals feel intense, long-lasting craving when attempting to stop. Although most smokers wish to quit, only about one-third attempt to do so each year.

SEDATIVE–HYPNOTICS

The CNS depressants include barbiturates, nonbarbiturate sedatives, and the benzodiazepines. As the medical use of barbiturates decreased, primarily because of their high addiction liability and the danger of acute lethality, the use of the benzodiazepine anxiolytics increased. The most commonly abused barbiturates are secobarbital, pentobarbital, and amobarbital. Phenobarbital is not generally abused, because of its slow onset of action. The most commonly abused anxiolytics include diazepam, chlordiazepoxide, midazolam, lorazepam, and flurazepam. These drugs are readily attainable from illicit sources.

Abused nonbarbiturate sedatives include glutethimide and meprobamate.

Pharmacological Aspects

CNS depressants, including barbiturate, benzodiazepine, and ethanol, produce a similar intoxication. These drugs are abused for their euphoric effects and as a means to reduce anxiety and limit insomnia. As the dose of depressant increases, along with the degree of intoxication, the effects progress from anxiety reduction and muscle relaxation to motor impairment and unconsciousness. The difference between the classes of drugs is primarily dose responsiveness. Intoxication progresses from mild to severe over a relatively narrow dose range in the case of the barbiturates. The benzodiazepine dose–response curve is such that great increases in dose are necessary to make such a transition. Thus, the benzodiazepines are a safer class of depressant drugs.

The acute effects of depressants can include euphoria, anxiety reduction, anticonvulsant activity, sedation, ataxia, motor incoordination, impaired judgment, anesthesia, coma, and respiratory depression resulting in death. *The benzodiazepines are rarely involved in lethality, but all CNS depressants enhance the effects of other depressant drugs.* The physiological effects of high-dose depressants include miosis, shallow respiration, and reduction in reflex responses.

Tolerance and Dependence

Tolerance to many of the effects of the depressants develops. Unlike opioids, barbiturate and benzodiazepine tolerance develops slowly. Also, tolerance is incomplete in some instances or does not influence some pharmacological effects. One such exception is the lack of tolerance to barbiturate lethality. The lethal dose in a tolerant individual is not much different from that of the general population. Cross-tolerance develops to some degree between the depressant classes of drugs.

Dependence on benzodiazepines, as evidenced by a withdrawal syndrome, can develop to large doses of drugs. Mild dependence is produced at therapeutic doses.

Individuals report some craving for drug during withdrawal from benzodiazepines, but the level is not as great as among those who abuse alcohol. Once the withdrawal syndrome has dissipated, the abusers of benzodiazepines are not as likely to resume drug consumption as are alcoholics. Withdrawal signs appear to be more likely following chronic exposure to short-acting benzodiazepines, such as alprazolam (half-life of less than 15 hours) or lorazepam than long-acting drugs. Despite gradual dose reduction, individuals may have anxiety attacks, confusion, agitation, restlessness, sweating, clouded sensorium, heightened sensory perception, perceptual disturbances, sleep disruption, muscle cramps, muscle twitches, and tremors; 2% of addicts may have a seizure during withdrawal. Withdrawal signs peak the second day after abrupt withdrawal and last for at least 5 to 7 days. Withdrawal symptoms following long-acting benzodiazepines (diazepam, clorazepate) peak during the second week of abstinence. In contrast to alcohol and the barbiturate sedatives, withdrawal from benzodiazepines is not life threatening.

ETHANOL

Ethanol is the most widely abused drug in the world. There are more than 10 million alcoholics in the United States alone. Excessive consumption of alcoholic beverages has been linked to as many as half of all traffic accidents, two-thirds of homicides, and three-fourths of suicides, and it is a significant factor in other crimes, in family problems, and in personal and industrial accidents. The annual cost to the American economy has been estimated to exceed $100 billion in lost productivity, medical care, and property damage.

Alcoholism has been difficult to define because of its complex nature. A person is generally considered an alcoholic, however, when his or her lifestyle is dominated by the procurement and consumption of alcoholic beverages and when this behavior interferes with personal, professional, social, or family relations.

A *light drinker* generally is defined as one who consumes an average of one drink or less per day, usually with the evening meal; a *moderate drinker* is one who has approximately three drinks per day; and a *heavy drinker* is one who has five or more drinks per day (or in the case of binge drinkers, at least once per week with five or more drinks on each occasion).

Chemistry

Ethanol (ethyl alcohol, alcohol) is a simple organic molecule composed of a single hydroxyl group and a short two-carbon aliphatic chain, CH_3CH_2OH. The hydroxyl and ethyl moieties confer both hydrophilic and lipophilic properties on the molecule. Therefore, ethanol is an *amphophile*, a property important to its pharmacological activity.

Absorption, Distribution, Metabolism, and Excretion

After oral administration, ethanol is almost completely absorbed throughout the gastrointestinal tract. The rate of absorption is largely determined by the quantity consumed, the concentration in the beverage, the rate of consumption, and the composition of the gastric contents. Eating food before or during drinking retards absorption, especially if the food has a high lipid content.

After absorption, ethanol is distributed throughout body water. In organs with high blood flow, such as the brain, liver, lungs, and kidney, equilibrium occurs rapidly. Conversely, in organs with low blood flow, such as muscle, equilibrium occurs more slowly. *Ethanol readily passes through the blood–placenta barrier into the fetal circulation.* Although the concentration of ethanol in the blood can be quite predictable, measurements of blood ethanol, especially when the concentrations are rising, may lead to erroneous conclusions, since the values obtained can underestimate the concentration of ethanol in the brain. This fact can confound legal proceedings in drunk-driving cases where blood ethanol concentrations are considered an accurate and legally acceptable determinant of the amount of ethanol consumed.

Ethanol is metabolized primarily in the liver by at least two enzyme systems. The best-studied and most important enzyme is zinc dependent: alcohol dehydrogenase. Salient features of the reaction can be seen in Fig. 35.1. The *rate* of metabolism catalyzed by alcohol dehydrogenase is generally linear with time except at low ethanol concentrations and is relatively independent of the ethanol concentration (i.e., zero-order kinetics). The rate of metabolism after ingestion of different amounts of ethanol is illustrated in Fig. 35.2.

In adults, ethanol is metabolized at about 10 to 15 mL/hour. Since metabolism of ethanol is slow, ingestion must be controlled to prevent accumulation and intoxication. *There is little evidence* that chronic ingestion of ethanol leads to a significant induction of alcohol dehydrogenase, even in heavy drinkers.

Some populations, most notably East Asians, exhibit an unusual response after drinking ethanol. The symptoms include facial flushing, vasodilation, and tachycardia. These individuals apparently have a genetic deficiency of the enzyme aldehyde dehydrogenase, which leads to an accumulation of acetaldehyde even after they drink relatively small amounts of ethanol. If drugs such as metronidazole, griseofulvin, quinacrine, the hypoglycemic sulfonylureas, phenothiazines, and phenylbutazone are coadministered with ethanol, a similar accumulation of acetaldehyde may occur.

In addition to alcohol dehydrogenase, *ethanol can be oxidized to acetaldehyde by the microsomal mixed-function oxidase system (cytochrome P450 2 EI)*, as illustrated in Figure 35.1. Although this microsomal ethanol-oxidizing system probably has minor impor-

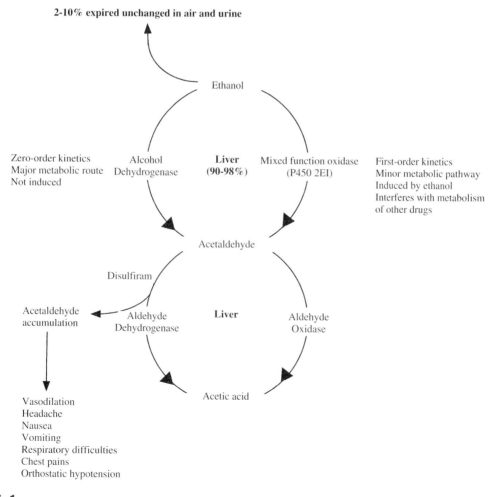

FIGURE 35.1
Metabolism and excretion of ethanol.

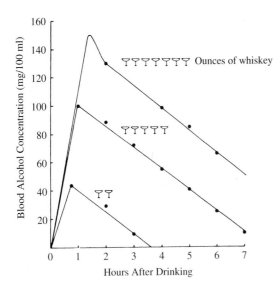

FIGURE 35.2

Blood alcohol concentration (mg/dL) after the consumption of various amounts of alcohol (for an adult of about 150 lb).

tance in the metabolism of ethanol in humans, it may be involved in some of the reported interactions between ethanol and other drugs that are also metabolized by this system. *Microsomal mixed-function oxidases may be induced by chronic ethanol ingestion.* Because ethanol is metabolized in the liver, it can interfere with the metabolism of other drugs by blocking microsomal hydroxylation and demethylation. Drug classes whose metabolism is most affected include the barbiturates, coumarins, and anticonvulsants, such as phenytoin. *Liver damage resulting from chronic abuse of ethanol can impair metabolism of a variety of drugs.*

Normally, 90 to 98% of an ingested dose of ethanol is metabolized by the liver. Most of the remaining 2 to 10% is excreted unchanged in the urine and expired air. The ethanol content in the urine is normally about 130% of the blood concentration and is quite constant; the expired air contains about 0.05% of the blood ethanol level, a concentration that also is remarkably consistent.

Mechanism of Action

A great deal of attention has been focused on a class of proteins termed the *ligand-gated ion channels* as being important to the mechanism of action of alcohol. These integral membrane proteins function as gates or pores that allow the passage of certain ions into and out of neurons upon binding of the appropriate neurotransmitter. This flux of ions largely determines the degree of neuronal activity. Two distinct types of ligand-gated ion channels are particularly sensitive to concentrations of alcohol that produce intoxication and sedation. These are the α-aminobutyric acid (GABA) chloride

ionophore and the *N*-methyl-D-aspartate (NMDA) subtype of glutamate receptor. The GABA–chloride ion channel reduces neuronal activity by hyperpolarizing the neurons, while activation of the NMDA receptor causes neuronal depolarization or excitation. Alcohol has been shown to increase chloride flux through the $GABA_A$ receptor and reduce calcium flux through the NMDA receptor. These actions result in powerful suppression of nerve cell activity, which is consistent with the depressant actions of alcohol in the brain.

Pharmacological Actions
Central Nervous System

Alcohol is primarily a CNS depressant, and the degree of depression is directly proportional to the quantity of ethanol consumed. However, behavioral *stimulation* can be found after ingestion of small amounts of ethanol. This stimulation is expressed as decreased social and psychological inhibition and is most likely the result of a depression of inhibitory pathways in the brain with release of cortical activity. The behavioral and physiological effects are associated with different blood ethanol concentrations. As the blood ethanol concentration begins to increase, behavioral activation, characterized by euphoria, talkativeness, aggressiveness, and loss of behavioral control, generally precedes the overt CNS depression induced by ethanol. At progressively higher blood ethanol concentrations, the stage of relaxation is transformed into decreased social inhibitions, slurred speech, ataxia, decreased mental acuity, decreased reflexive responses, coma, and, finally, death resulting from respiratory arrest. In moderation, however, there is no evidence that the judicious use of small amounts of alcoholic beverages (e.g., a glass of wine with meals) is permanently harmful.

Other Body Systems

In general, ethanol in low to moderate amounts, is relatively benign to most body systems. A moderate amount of ethanol causes peripheral vasodilation, especially of cutaneous vessels, and stimulates the secretion of salivary and gastric fluids; the latter action may aid digestion. On the other hand, ethanol consumption in high concentrations, as found in undiluted spirits, can induce hemorrhagic lesions in the duodenum, inhibit intestinal brush border enzymes, inhibit the uptake of amino acids, and limit the absorption of vitamins and minerals. In addition, ethanol can reduce blood testosterone levels, resulting in sexual dysfunction.

Ethanol is a diuretic. This effect may be caused by its ability to inhibit secretion of antidiuretic hormone from the posterior pituitary, which leads to a reduction in renal tubular water reabsorption. The large amount of fluid normally consumed with ethanol also contributes to increased urine production.

Adverse Effects
Acute Ethanol Intoxication and Hangover

Ethanol intoxication is probably the best-known form of drug toxicity. Intoxicated individuals are a threat to themselves and others, particularly if they attempt to drive or operate machinery. Although death can result from ethanol overdose, usually the patient lapses into a coma before ingesting lethal quantities. Ethanol intoxication is sometimes mistakenly diagnosed as diabetic coma, schizophrenia, overdosage of other CNS depressant drugs, or skull fracture. An additional feature commonly associated with excessive ethanol consumption is difficulty in regulating body temperature. *Hypothermia* frequently results, with body temperature falling toward that of the ambient environment. This problem can be particularly severe in the elderly, who normally have difficulty regulating their body temperature.

One of the consequences of ethanol intoxication is the hangover, a condition characterized by headache, nausea, sweating, and tremor. Although unpleasant, a hangover is not dangerous, even though the person having one may feel otherwise.

Treatment for Acute Intoxication

Generally, no treatment is required for acute ethanol intoxication. Allowing the individual to sleep off the effects of ethanol ingestion is the usual procedure. Hangovers are treated similarly; that is, no effective remedy exists for a hangover, except for controlling the amount of ethanol consumed. Sometimes ethanol overdose is a medical emergency. For example, prompt treatment is required if the patient is in danger of dying of respiratory arrest, is comatose, has dilated pupils, is hypothermic, or displays tachycardia.

Treatment for severe ethanol overdose is generally supportive. Increased intracranial pressure can be relieved by intravenous administration of hypertonic mannitol. Hemodialysis can accelerate the removal of ethanol from the body. Stimulants of ethanol metabolism, such as fructose, are not sufficiently effective, and *use of analeptics is not recommended because of the possibility of precipitating convulsions.*

Alcoholism

Alcoholism is among the major health problems in most countries. *Dependence on ethanol, as with other addictive drugs, is expressed as drug-seeking behavior and is associated with a withdrawal syndrome that occurs after abrupt cessation of drinking.* The ethanol withdrawal syndrome is characterized by tremors, seizures, hyperthermia, hallucinations, and autonomic hyperactivity.

A number of organs are affected adversely by chronic ethanol use, the result of a *direct cytotoxic action.* Hepatic fatty infiltration and cirrhosis are common

in alcoholics; cancer may develop in advanced stages of hepatic disease.

Ethanol produces a number of depressant effects on the myocardium. Atrial arrhythmias and ventricular tachycardia may arise from chronic ethanol use. A serious clinical entity, *alcoholic cardiomyopathy,* has also been described.

A high rate of ethanol consumption can lead to inhibition of gastric secretion and irritation of the gastric mucosa. Ethanol irritates the entire gastrointestinal tract, which may lead to constipation and diminished absorption of nutrients. Other pathological effects include pancreatitis and peripheral neuropathy. Severe gonadal failure is often found in both men and women, accompanied by low blood levels of sex hormones.

A variety of pathological problems involving the CNS have been described in chronic alcoholics, the main ones being *Wernicke's encephalopathy* and *Korsakoff's psychosis.* Brain damage from chronic ethanol consumption can be especially severe in the elderly and may accelerate aging.

Ethanol readily passes across the placenta and into the fetal circulation. *The fetal alcohol syndrome has three primary features: microcephaly, prenatal growth deficiency, and short palpebral fissures.* Other characteristics include postnatal growth deficiency, fine motor dysfunction, cardiac defects, and anomalies of the external genitalia and inner ear. A definite risk of producing fetal abnormalities occurs when ethanol consumption by the mother exceeds 3 oz daily, the equivalent of about six drinks.

Treatment for Alcoholism

The immediate concern in the treatment of alcoholics is detoxification and management of the ethanol withdrawal syndrome. Once the patient is detoxified, long-term treatment requires complete abstinence, psychiatric treatment, family involvement, and frequently support from lay organizations such as Alcoholics Anonymous.

One pharmacological approach is aversion therapy using drugs such as disulfiram to associate drinking ethanol with unpleasant consequences. If ethanol is taken after disulfiram administration, blood acetaldehyde concentrations increase 5 to 10 times, resulting in vasodilation, pulsating headache, nausea, vomiting, severe thirst, respiratory difficulties, chest pains, orthostatic hypotension, syncope, and blurred vision. In certain cases, marked respiratory depression, cardiac arrhythmias, cardiovascular collapse, myocardial infarction, acute congestive heart failure, unconsciousness, convulsions, and sudden death have been reported. Despite these potentially severe consequences, disulfiram is prescribed for some alcoholic patients.

Another pharmacological approach is the use of anticraving drugs, for example serotonin uptake inhibitors, dopaminergic agonists, and opioid antagonists. The only treatment that has shown considerable promise is one that uses the opioid antagonist naltrexone.

MARIJUANA

The hemp plant, or cannabis (*Cannabis sativa*), continues to be the most frequently abused illicit substance in America. The dried leaves and flowering tops of the plant are referred to as marijuana, and it is typically smoked in pipes or rolled as cigarettes. It also may be consumed in baked goods. *Hashish* is a solid black resinous material obtained from the leaves of the plant and is usually smoked in a pipe.

Chemistry

The major psychoactive constituent in marijuana use is Δ^9-tetrahydrocannabinol (THC), the prototypical cannabinoid. Although marijuana contains a large number of cannabinoids, they lack behavioral activity with the exception of cannabinol, which is approximately one-tenth as potent as THC. The THC content in hashish is more than double that in marijuana.

Pharmacokinetic Aspects

Δ^9-THC is readily absorbed when marijuana is smoked. Pharmacological effects are produced rapidly and generally peak within 30 minutes of the onset of smoking. The dynamics of smoking (number of puffs, spacing, hold time, and lung capacity) substantially influence how much drug is absorbed. Although oral ingestion of marijuana produces similar pharmacological effects, Δ^9-THC is absorbed more slowly than by smoking. Impairment on various performance measures related to driving skills has been demonstrated immediately following marijuana smoking and up to 24 hours thereafter. Generally, behavioral and physiological effects return to baseline levels 4 to 6 hours after usage. Blood concentrations of Δ^9-THC peak prior to drug-induced effects. This time discordance between blood concentrations of Δ^9-THC and effects has made it difficult to establish a meaningful relationship between blood concentrations and effects.

Δ^9-THC is rapidly distributed to all tissues despite being tightly bound by plasma proteins. Δ^9-THC is a highly lipophilic substance and so accumulates in tissue high in lipid content. Traces of Δ^9-THC have been found in adipose tissue more than 30 days after the subject smoked a single joint. The terminal half-life of Δ^9-THC in plasma ranges from 18 hours to 4 days.

Mechanism of Action

A cannabinoid receptor identified in the brain of several species, including humans, is termed *CB1*. It is one of the most abundant receptors in the CNS, and its distribution within the brain reflects the pharmacological effects produced by Δ^9-THC. High receptor densities in the extrapyramidal motor system and the cerebellum are consistent with the actions of cannabinoids on many forms of movement. The effects of cannabinoids on cognition and memory may be due to the relatively dense receptor populations in the hippocampus and cortex. The presence of cannabinoid receptors in the ventromedial striatum and nucleus accumbens suggests an association with dopamine neurons hypothesized to mediate brain reward.

Pharmacological Actions
Central Nervous System

Marijuana produces a distinctive behavioral syndrome that is easily distinguished from that of most other drugs. The most prominent feature is the initial period of euphoria, or high, which has been described as a sense of well-being and happiness. Euphoria is frequently followed by a period of drowsiness or sedation. Perception of time is altered, along with distortions in both hearing and vision. However, illusions and hallucinations occur infrequently. The subjective effects also include dissociation of ideas.

The subjective effects of marijuana vary from individual to individual as a function of dose, route of administration, the experience and expectation of the subjects, and individual vulnerability to certain psychoactive substances. Motor coordination also may decrease, especially in situations requiring highly complex motor skills, such as flying an airplane and driving an automobile.

Increased appetite is frequently attributed to smoking marijuana. Cannabinoids are effective antiemetics, particularly in treating emesis arising during chemotherapy. Δ^9-THC has been reported to be as effective as codeine as an analgesic, although pronounced behavioral effects occur with analgesic doses.

Other Organ Systems

The most consistent pharmacological effect produced by marijuana is tachycardia, which is closely associated with the blood levels of Δ^9-THC. There is relatively little effect on blood pressure unless large quantities of marijuana are smoked, in which case there can be marked orthostatic hypotension. Cannabinoids are also vasodilatory, which results in the characteristic conjunctival reddening following marijuana smoking. They also reduce intraocular pressure and are capable of producing bronchodilation.

Adverse Effects

Marijuana is unique among drugs of abuse in that there have been no credible reports of fatal overdose. The most prominent effect of acute marijuana use is intoxication, which can impair the cognitive and motor skills needed to complete complex tasks. Anxiety and panic reactions are occasionally reported in inexperienced users or following use of large quantities of marijuana. Δ^9-THC causes its greatest effects on short-term memory, as measured in free-recall tasks. Marijuana does not affect the retrieval of previously learned facts. In contrast to alcohol, there is no residual hangover from a single use of high quantities of marijuana.

Heavy marijuana smoking produces bronchitis, and some individuals have evidence of precancerous lung conditions. However, definitive evidence of the relationship between marijuana smoking and the incidence of lung cancer is lacking.

Tolerance develops to many of Δ^9-THC's effects in heavy marijuana users. Although chronic cannabis use does not result in severe withdrawal symptoms, numerous case reports attest to development of dependence in subjects taking high doses of THC for several weeks. The most prominent symptoms were irritability and restlessness; others included insomnia, anorexia, increased sweating, and mild nausea. Cessation of mild or moderate use of marijuana, however, does not produce a withdrawal syndrome.

HALLUCINOGENS

The term *hallucinogen* is often used to describe a drug that produces a change in sensory perception, usually either visual or auditory. Drugs commonly assigned to this class include lysergic acid diethylamide (LSD), mescaline (derived from the peyote cactus), and psilocybin (derived from a mushroom). However, this rather limited definition fails to include the other prominent property of this class of drugs, which is a change in thought and mood. For this reason the term is sometimes used interchangeably with *psychedelic* or *psychotomimetic*, the latter term representing the CNS effects beyond the hallucination itself. Most literal definitions of the term *hallucinogen* are inadequate, but it should be used to signify substances that consistently produce changes in sensory perception, thought, and mood. An hallucinogen is a drug that *reliably* produces alterations in perceptions as a primary effect. Drugs that should not be included are those that produce alterations in sensory perception only at toxic doses (e.g., antimuscarinic agents, antimalarials, and opioids) and fail to produce these effects in all individuals. This does not preclude a drug's being classified as an hallucinogen if it has other properties as well. Several drugs that reliably alter mood at low doses and produce altered sensory perceptions at slightly higher doses are close chemical analogues to the CNS stimulant class of drugs. These drugs that also reliably produce differing degrees of CNS stimulation in a dose-

responsive fashion include phencyclidine (PCP), methylenedioxymethamphetamine (MDMA), and methylenedioxyamphetamine (MDA).

The hallucinogens generally fall into two chemical classes. The indole alkylamines include LSD, psilocybin, psilocin, dimethyltryptamine (DMT), and diethyltryptamine (DET), all of which are structurally similar to serotonin. The other chemical subclass of hallucinogens contains phenylethylamine derivatives such as mescaline, MDMA, MDA, and DOM (dimethoxymethyl amphetamine). A related stimulatory hallucinogen, PCP, is a piperidine analogue that produces unique effects.

Extent and Pattern of Abuse

LSD is very potent and produces both CNS and peripheral effects. Because of the rapid tolerance produced with these drugs, the typical abuser does not use the drug on a daily basis. Generally, an hallucinogen is abused approximately once per month.

Illicit PCP abuse began in the 1960s, primarily by oral ingestion. However, its use was limited because PCP frequently produced dysphoria, which was unpredictable.

Pharmacological Aspects

The effects of LSD may be observed for 8 hours. The specific acute effects of a drug like LSD include euphoria, depersonalization, enhanced awareness of sensory input, alterations in the perception of time or space or body image, and to some extent, minor stimulant effects. Sometimes the dreamlike quality of the experience produces relaxation, good humor, and a sense of wonder or euphoria.

Often the effect is a function of expectation and environmental conditions. Someone who is anxious about the use of the hallucinogen may have drug-induced anxiety, panic, or even paranoid ideation. The loss of individuality can be perceived as a disintegration of the person and can lead to a panic attack. Even if the drug experience initially is euphoric, tremendous mood swings can occur and suddenly plunge the abuser into emotions of great anxiety or terror. These negative phenomena are not always precipitated by an unexpected or sudden frightful event but can be a function of the labile mood induced by the drug.

The visual hallucinations are often composed of extremely vivid colors of geometric patterns, such as cones, spirals, or cobweb-like structures. Other types of hallucinations are possible. A true hallucination involves the belief by the individual that the (altered) sensations and perceptions actually represent reality. However, generally the person abusing LSD and related drugs retains the ability to test reality versus illusion and knows that the experience is not real. Thus, the typical drug-induced hallucinatory state would be more appropriately termed a *pseudohallucination,* though real hallucinations are possible. The subjective or psychotomimetic changes are those considered to be changes in mood. These effects are somewhat more variable than the hallucinatory effects or changes in sensory perception. Though these effects can occur with LSD, they seem to be more common with other specific hallucinogens, such as MDMA and MDA.

MDMA (XTC, or *ecstasy*) possesses hallucinogenic activity similar to that of mescaline but also produces stimulant activity similar to that of amphetamine. Initially MDMA produces euphoria, increases the ability to communicate with others, increases the degree of intimacy one feels toward others in the surroundings, increases self-esteem and mood, and generally appears reduce perceived intensity of psychological problems. Hallucinatory activity occurs at higher doses. One residual effect of abuse is the MDMA hangover, which is the occurrence on the second day after abuse of drowsiness and sore jaw muscles along with other possible side effects due to the stimulant properties of the drug.

MDA, which is similar to MDMA, has been termed the *love drug* because it produces a feeling of closeness to others. Typically, a dose of 75 mg produces the primary psychotomimetic effects, while a dose of 150 mg produces LSD-like effects, and a dose of 300 mg produces amphetaminelike CNS stimulation. The amphetaminelike stimulation of the CNS and periphery is prominent with both MDA and MDMA. To a lesser degree this stimulation also occurs with LSD. The effects that can be produced by stimulatory doses of hallucinogens include tachycardia, hypertension, and arrhythmias.

PCP is unique in terms of its hallucinogenic properties and its other pharmacological effects. It possesses CNS stimulatory actions, but it is also a dissociative anesthetic. It induces a wide variety of psychotomimetic and hallucinatory effects during emergence from anesthesia. Because it possesses CNS stimulant properties comparable with those of amphetamine, it does not produce depression of the cardiovascular system like other anesthetics, though it does depress the respiratory system. At a low dose, individuals believe they are thinking and acting rapidly and efficiently. The general mood is happiness, though (especially at higher doses) the individual can vacillate between euphoria and depression. It primarily produces auditory hallucinations. At higher doses the stimulatory effects are more pronounced and the likelihood of tremendous mood swings more likely. At near anesthetic doses, it produces more typical depressant effects, including motor incoordination, catalepsy, vacant stare, or even amnesia. Coma is produced subsequent to respiratory depression.

Tolerance and Dependence

Tolerance to the effects of hallucinogens develops rapidly. In fact, a high degree of tolerance can be produced after as few as three to four daily doses of drug. Generally, the abuser self-imposes the requirement for a 2- to 3-day drug-free period before another drug session. Additionally, there is a tremendous degree of cross-tolerance between the hallucinogens, so other LSD-like hallucinogens cannot be abused during the drug-free period either. One danger with the stimulant subclass of hallucinogens is rapid development of tolerance to some of their effects while the stimulatory properties remain and produce various side effects. Despite the apparent overlap of effects with stimulant drugs, however, there is no cross-tolerance with the CNS stimulants such as amphetamine.

There are no observable physical withdrawal signs during drug abstinence, nor is there a tremendous craving for drug during the drug-free period. Therefore, clearly no dependence is attributed to the hallucinogens. Though there is an abuse potential with this class of drug, and individuals express drug-seeking behavior, there does not seem to be the magnitude of craving found with other drug classes, such as the CNS stimulants.

Treatment Strategies

The difference between the abused and the lethal dose of LSD is very large, so little pharmacological intervention is necessary. Treatment involves limiting external stimuli and placing the individual in a safe environment.

Treatment of PCP intoxication also involves limiting external stimuli, minimizing lighting, noise, and unnecessary physical contact. The life-threatening nature of PCP overdose, however, may require symptomatic treatment of respiratory depression by artificial respiration or use of neuroleptics to control violent rage or panic anxiety.

Mechanism of Action

Hallucinogens disorganize neural function in the CNS. The structural similarities between the indole hallucinogens and the endogenous neurotransmitter serotonin led to the hypothesis that a primary mechanism of action for the hallucinogens is the activation of the 5-HT$_2$-receptor. LSD acts directly on this receptor as an agonist. Other drugs, such as MDMA, induce the release of endogenous serotonin, which activates the serotonin receptor.

INHALANTS

Volatile chemicals and gases that produce behavioral effects are subject to abuse. These agents represent a broad range of chemical classes but in general can be classified as gases, volatile organic solvents, and aliphatic nitrites. Inhalant abuse differs from that of many other drugs in that it is confined primarily to juveniles and young adults. The use of gases is primarily confined to nitrous oxide by young medical professionals who have ready access to this agent. It produces short-lived mild intoxication that typifies the early stages of anesthesia. Deaths occur occasionally by individuals inhaling nitrous oxide alone. Volatile organic solvents are usually aliphatic and aromatic hydrocarbons. They include substances such as gasoline, paint and lacquer thinners, lighter fluid, degreasers (methyl chloride and methylene chloride), and the solvents in airplane glue, typewriter correction fluid, and bathroom deodorizers. These agents produce a sense of exhilaration and light-headedness. Judgment and perception of reality are impaired, and hallucinations may be produced. The mechanism by which inhalants produce their behavioral effects are poorly understood, but there are some indications that their actions are similar to those of other centrally acting depressants, including alcohol. Toxicity depends on the properties of the individual solvents. The consequences of inhaling these substances can be severe, for they have been implicated in producing cancer, cardiotoxicity, neuropathies, and hepatotoxicity.

DESIGNER DRUGS

In an effort to avoid federal regulations, chemists in clandestine laboratories adopted the strategy of synthesizing analogues of controlled substances. Although these drugs are technically not illegal until scheduled, the consequences of their abuse are unpredictable and in some instances lethal. Efforts to make synthetic heroin led to the synthesis of at least six chemicals that are structurally similar to fentanyl. These agents gained considerable attention because their increased potency over fentanyl and heroin led to a rash of overdoses and numerous deaths. The two derivatives are referred to as China White and are 900 and 1,100 times as potent as morphine. Meperidine has also been used as a template for preparing synthetic heroin, the end product being 1-methyl-4-propionoxy-4-phenylpi-peridine (MPPP). However, MPPP is sometimes contaminated with the side reaction product 1-methyl,4-phenyl-1,2,3,6-tetra-hydropyridine (MPTP), which produces a parkinsonian syndrome through nigrostriatal lesions. Several substituted derivatives of amphetamine have also been called designer drugs. The most widely known of this group is the hallucinogen MDMA (*ecstasy*).

ANABOLIC STEROIDS

Historically, drugs used to increase the ability of an athlete to perform in a given sport included the use of stimulants to diminish the onset of fatigue or opiates to diminish the pain of exertion. Recently, abuse of *anabolic–androgenic steroids* (derivatives of testosterone) has increased. They are used to increase muscle size and definition (in the case of body-building competitors) and are sometimes coabused with other growth enhancers, such as human growth hormone. In sports in which mass, physical size, or even total strength (a function of total muscle mass) is important, the abuse of anabolic steroids provides a shortcut to attainment of the physical stature that might otherwise require much more extensive training and exercise. However, it is a misconception to believe that anabolic steroid abuse is limited to professional athletes and body builders. There is clear evidence that these drugs are abused by adult men and women who are not athletes, who are blue-collar and white-collar workers, and by male and female athletes at the college, high school, and junior high school levels. For more details see Chapter 63.

Study QUESTIONS

1. A 28-year-old man, a long-term opioid user, is brought to the emergency department with typical abstinence symptoms and asks for your help in breaking his heroin habit. What do you do?
   (A) You prescribe a 3-day regimen of meperidine.
   (B) You prescribe methadone and indicate it may be for an extended period.
   (C) You prescribe a one-time dose of naltrexone.

2. A patient is brought into the emergency department on Saturday night exhibiting paranoia and hostility and tells you that he is being pursued by strangers. He is emaciated, hungry, and filthy. What is the best solution for this case?
   (A) He has schizophrenia and should be admitted to the psychiatric ward.
   (B) He abuses alcohol and should undergo detoxification.
   (C) He has acutely abused a stimulant and should be treated with a neuroleptic drug.
   (D) He abuses heroin and should be prescribed methadone maintenance.

3. Barbiturate abuse is much less common now than it was 25 years ago. What is the main reason?
   (A) Barbiturate use is much less now than it was 25 years ago.
   (B) Barbiturates available today are much safer than those of 25 years ago.
   (C) People who abuse drugs today choose heroin and cocaine over barbiturates.
   (D) The antidotes to barbiturates prevent the abuse.

4. The most widely abused drug in the world is
   (A) Marijuana
   (B) Cocaine
   (C) Heroin
   (D) Alcohol
   (E) Amphetamine

5. A patient has piloerection, mydriasis, increased blood pressure, and abdominal cramps. Your diagnosis is
   (A) Alcohol abstinence
   (B) Barbiturate abstinence
   (C) Benzodiazepine abstinence
   (D) Opioid abstinence
   (E) Amphetamine abstinence

ANSWERS

1. **B.** The most commonly used treatment and the most effective is to stabilize the patient with methadone and gradually reduce the maintenance dose until the patient is drug free. The administration of meperidine would reverse the abstinence syndrome but it is unlikely to help the patient terminate his opioid habit. The use of naltrexone would likely further precipitate the abstinence syndrome and without additional counseling, would not likely offer long-term benefit.

2. **C.** Abuse of stimulants can produce toxic psychosis that closely resembles schizophrenia. An agent such as haloperidol or a phenothiazine will provide immediate relief of the symptoms. The fact that he is emaciated and hungry is evidence that he has been on a prolonged run with stimulants. The symptoms are very different from those seen with alcohol or with opioids.

3. **A.** Barbiturates are seldom prescribed. The lack of availability is a major reason these compounds are only rarely abused.

4. **D.** There are more than 10 million alcoholics in the United States alone. The numbers of individuals who abuse the other drugs listed are much lower.

5. **D.** These are classic features of opioid abstinence syndrome. The abstinence syndrome in chronic alcohol or barbiturate users consists of hallucinations, tremors, hyperthermia, and autonomic hyperactivity. The abstinence syndrome for users of cocaine and amphetamine is not as stereotyped as for opioids or CNS depressants, such as alcohol and barbiturates.

SUPPLEMENTAL READING

Adams IB and Martin BR. Cannabis: Pharmacology and toxicology in animals and humans. Addiction 1996;91:1585–1614.

Benowitz NL. Nicotine addiction. Prim Care 1999;26:611–631.

Goldstein A and Nestler EJ. Introduction to the neurobiology of addiction. Drug Alc Dep 1998;51:1–3.

Medical Letter. Acute reactions to drugs of abuse. 2002;44:21–24.

Schuckit MA. Drug and Alcohol Abuse: Clinical Guide to Diagnosis and Treatment (4th ed.). New York: Plenum, 1995.

Woods JH, Katz JL, and Winger G. Benzodiazepines: Use, abuse and consequences. Pharmacol Rev 1992;44:151–347.

Woodward JJ. Alcohol. In Miller NS (ed.). Principles of Addiction Medicine. Chevy Chase, Md.: American Society of Addiction Medicine, 1994.

CASE Study Alcohol Toxicity

A 24-year-old medical student is brought into the emergency department complaining of vomiting, light-headedness, chest pains, and difficulty breathing. You discover that he fell ill at a party following the block examinations midway during the first semester. Initially he and his friends deny any drugs other than a couple of beers at the party. You are at a loss to explain the symptoms until his girlfriend states that the only drug she is aware he is taking is something for his athlete's foot. You continue checking and discover that he has been taking metronidazole for about the past 10 days to alleviate the symptoms of athlete's foot. What might be the cause of his symptoms?

ANSWER: Metronidazole shares the ability of disulfiram to block the metabolism of alcohol and cause an accumulation of acetaldehyde. The student's symptoms are consistent with an accumulation of this agent.

SECTION

THERAPEUTIC ASPECTS OF INFLAMMATORY AND SELECTED OTHER CLINICAL DISORDERS

36

Antiinflammatory and Antirheumatic Drugs

Karen A. Woodfork and Knox Van Dyke

 DRUG LIST

The classical signs of inflammation are redness, swelling, heat, pain, and loss of function. The actual expression of these processes depends on the site of inflammation. For example, a skin abscess may result in the appearance of all of these features. In contrast, pneumonia, because of the inaccessibility of the lung to examination, may manifest only as loss of function (shortness of breath and hypoxia). Nevertheless, similar pathological processes occur in both sites.

Inflammation is characterized by the orderly occurrence of several processes: *initiation* of the event by a foreign substance or physical injury, *recruitment and chemoattraction* of inflammatory cells, and activation of these cells to *release inflammatory mediators* capable of damaging or killing an invading microbe or tumor. In some instances, the inflammatory response is initiated by an otherwise harmless foreign material (e.g., pollen). Inflammation can also result from an autoimmune response to the host's own tissue, as occurs in rheumatoid arthritis.

As the result of an inflammatory response, the host tissue may undergo collateral injury, since many of the inflammatory mediators are not specific for a particular tissue target. For example, many of the clinical signs (fever and labored breathing) and symptoms (shortness of breath and cough) of pneumococcal pneumonia are the result of inflammation rather than the invading microorganism. In most cases, the inflammatory response eventually subsides, but if such a self-limiting regulation does not occur, the inflammatory response will require pharmacological intervention. *The need for anti-inflammatory drugs arises when the inflammatory response is inappropriate, aberrant, sustained, or causes destruction of tissue.*

THE INFLAMMATORY PROCESS

Inflammation begins when a stimulus, such as infection, physical stress, or chemical stress, produces cellular damage (Fig. 36.1). This damage initiates the activation of transcription factors that control the expression of many inflammatory mediators. *Among the more important inflammatory mediators are the eicosanoids, biological oxidants, cytokines, adhesion factors, and digestive enzymes* (proteases, hyaluronidase, collagenase, and elastase). Only the first three of these are therapeutic targets for anti-inflammatory drugs.

The inflammatory response changes with time and can be divided into phases. The rapid phase occurs within seconds to minutes and consists of vasodilation, increased blood flow, edema, and pain. The acute phase is characterized by induction of inflammatory genes by NF-κB and other transcription factors. During this phase, moderate amounts of inflammatory mediators are produced. The chronic phase occurs over months to years and is marked by dramatically increased production of inflammatory mediators. The secondary chronic phase of inflammation occurs after years of oxidative damage has degraded blood vessels and tissues. Such chronic inflammation appears to play a role in many disease states, such as arteriosclerosis and cancer.

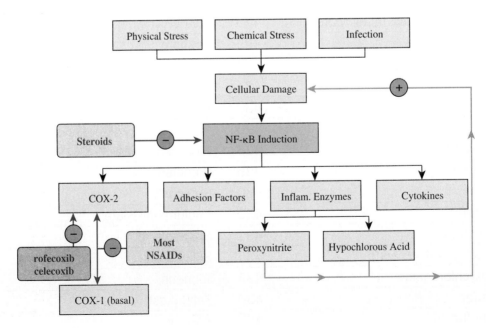

FIGURE 36.1
Overview of inflammatory processes.

Eicosanoids

The eicosanoids, so called because of their derivation from a 20-carbon unsaturated fatty acid, arachidonic acid (eicosatetraenoic acid), are obtained from membrane phospholipids and synthesized de novo at the time of cellular stimulation. Arachidonic acid is cleaved from membrane-bound phosphatidylcholine by the enzyme phospholipase A_2. Alternatively, arachidonic acid may be derived by the sequential actions of phospholipase C and diacylglyceryl lipase. Arachidonic acid can then follow either of two enzymatic pathways that result in the production of inflammatory mediators. The pathway initiated by cyclooxygenase (COX) produces prostaglandins; the lipoxygenase pathway generates leukotrienes (Fig. 36.2).

The COX enzyme exists in at least two isoforms. COX-1 is a constitutive or "housekeeping" isoform that is responsible for the basal production of prostaglandins, prostacyclins, and thromboxanes. *COX-2 is inducible by cytokines and other inflammatory stimuli and is believed to predominate during chronic inflammation.* The final product of the COX pathway is tissue specific. For example, platelets produce thromboxane A_2 (TxA_2); vascular endothelial cells produce prostacyclin (PGI_2); mast cells produce prostaglandin D_2 (PGD_2);

and the vasculature, gastrointestinal (GI) tract, lung, and other tissues produce prostaglandin E_2 (PGE_2).

The biological effects of the more important eicosanoids are listed in Table 36.1. *The production of inflammatory eicosanoids is an important target of many anti-inflammatory drugs. In addition, the side effects of these drugs frequently result from their inhibition of eicosanoid production.*

A number of eicosanoids are used as therapeutic agents. In infants with congenital heart anomalies, a patent ductus arteriosus can be temporarily maintained by the PGE_1 analogue alprostadil (*Prostin VR Pediatric*) until surgical correction can be performed. In patients undergoing treatment with nonsteroidal anti-inflammatory drugs, the PGE_1 analogue misoprostol (*Cytotec*) is often used to decrease gastric acid secretion, thereby inhibiting the ulceration caused by these agents. Misoprostol is also used in several non-FDA–approved applications, including the induction of labor by enhancing cervical ripening, and the induction of abortion in combination with mifepristone (RU-486). These uses of misoprostol are associated with an increased risk of uterine rupture or perforation. Dinoprostone (*Prostin E_2*), a synthetic PGE_2, causes uterine contraction and is used clinically to induce abortion during the second trimester and to empty the

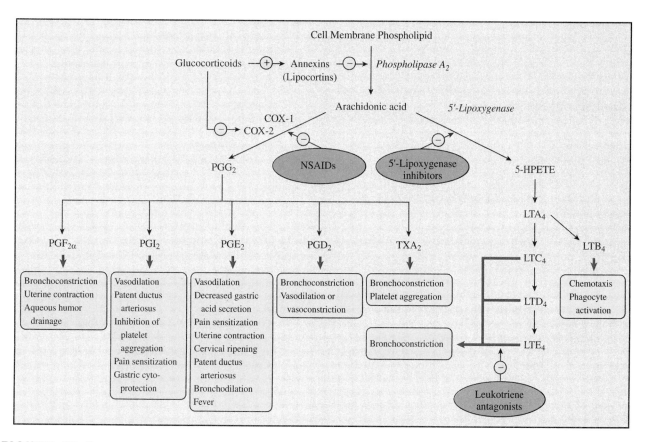

FIGURE 36.2
Eicosanoid synthesis pathway.

TABLE 36.1   Biological Effects of Eicosanoids

Eicosanoid	Primary Biological Effects
PGE_1	Vasodilation, decreased gastric acid secretion, bronchodilation
PGE_2	Vasodilation, decreased gastric acid secretion, pain sensitization, uterine contraction, cervical ripening, maintenance of patent ductus arteriosus, bronchodilation, fever
$PGF_{2\alpha}$	Bronchoconstriction, uterine contraction, increases drainage from aqueous humor
PGI_2	Vasodilation, maintenance of patent ductus arteriosus, inhibition of platelet aggregation, pain sensitization, gastric cytoprotection
TXA_2	Platelet aggregation, bronchoconstriction
LTC_4, D_4, E_4	Bronchoconstriction
LTB_4	Chemoattraction and activation of polymorphonuclear leukocytes

uterus following fetal death, missed abortion, or benign hydatidiform mole. Carboprost (*Hemabate*) is a PGF_2 analogue that can be used to terminate pregnancy or to control refractory postpartum bleeding by stimulating uterine contraction. Primary pulmonary hypertension can be treated by the synthetic PGI epoprostenol (*Flolan*). Elevated intraocular pressure may be treated with latanoprost (*Xalatan*), an analogue of PGF_2. Zafirlukast (*Accolate*) is an oral leukotriene receptor antagonist for control of the inflammatory process of asthma (see Chapter 39). Zileuton (*Zyflo*) inhibits the first enzyme in the lipoxygenase pathway and is used for the treatment of asthma.

Biological Oxidants

The biologically derived oxidants are potent bacterial killers but are also a major contributing factor in tissue injury that results from the inflammatory response. These oxidants include the superoxide anion ($\cdot O_2^-$), hydrogen peroxide (H_2O_2), nitric oxide ($\cdot NO$), peroxynitrite ($\cdot OONO^-$), hypochlorous acid (HOCl), peroxidase-generated oxidants of undefined character, probably the hydroxyl radical ($\cdot OH$), and possibly singlet oxygen ($^1O_2$). These oxidants, largely generated by phagocytic cells such as neutrophils and macrophages, induce tissue injury beyond that produced by digestive enzymes and eicosanoids. *Inhibition of production of these oxidants or inactivation of these substances by antioxidants is an important strategy for the treatment of inflammatory disorders.*

Cytokines

Numerous cytokines participate in inflammation; among the most important regulators of this process

are *tumor necrosis factor-α* (TNF-α) and *interleukin 1* (IL-1). TNF-α and IL-1 are produced primarily by cells of the monocyte–macrophage lineage. They work in concert to stimulate inflammatory responses such as pain, fever, and the recruitment of lymphocytes. In addition, they induce production of many other inflammatory mediators and contribute to the tissue damage seen in chronic inflammation.

TNF-α and IL-1 are current targets of antiinflammatory drug therapy. A homotrimer of 17-kDa protein subunits whose effects include the activation of neutrophils and eosinophils, induction of COX-2, induction of proinflammatory cytokines (e.g., IL-1, IL-6), enhancement of endothelial layer permeability, induction of adhesion molecules by endothelial cells and leukocytes, stimulation of fibroblast proliferation, degradation of cartilage, and stimulation of bone reabsorption. Two receptors mediate these effects: a 55-kDa receptor (p55) and a 75-kDa receptor (p75). Each of these receptors is found in both cell surface and soluble forms. The binding of two or three cell surface receptors to TNF-α initiates an inflammatory response. Soluble p55 also acts as a signaling receptor for inflammatory responses, whereas soluble p75 acts as an antagonist.

IL-1 occurs as two polypeptides, IL-1α and IL-1β, and produces many of the same effects as TNF-α. An 80-kDa type 1 IL-1 receptor and a 68-kDa type 2 IL-1 receptor found on the surface of some cell types bind both forms of IL-1. An endogenous 17-kDa IL-1 receptor antagonist (IL-1ra) competes for binding with IL-1 and counterbalances the inflammatory response.

NONSTEROIDAL ANTIINFLAMMATORY DRUGS

The nonsteroidal anti-inflammatory drugs (NSAIDs) have a variety of clinical uses as antipyretics, analgesics, and anti-inflammatory agents. They reduce body temperature in febrile states and thus are effective antipyretics. They are also useful as analgesics, relieving mild to moderate pain (see Chapter 26) such as myalgia, dental pain, dysmenorrhea, and headache. Unlike the opioid analgesics, they do not cause neurological depression or dependence. As anti-inflammatory agents, NSAIDs are used to treat conditions such as muscle strain, tendinitis, and bursitis. They are also used to treat the chronic pain and inflammation of rheumatoid arthritis (adult onset and juvenile), osteoarthritis, and arthritic variants such as gouty arthritis and ankylosing spondylitis. While NSAIDs used to be the sole agent of choice for mild to moderate rheumatoid disease, they are now frequently used in conjunction with the *disease-modifying antirheumatic drugs (DMARDs)* early in the treatment of these disorders. This is because the *NSAIDs reduce pain and inflammation associated with rheumatoid diseases but do not delay or reverse the disease's progress.*

Mechanism of Action

The anti-inflammatory actions of the NSAIDs are most likely explained by their inhibition of prostaglandin synthesis by COX-2. The COX-2 isoform is the predominant COX involved in the production of prostaglandins during inflammatory processes. Prostaglandins of the E and F series evoke some of the local and systemic manifestations of inflammation, such as vasodilation, hyperemia, increased vascular permeability, swelling, pain, and increased leukocyte migration. In addition, they intensify the effects of inflammatory mediators, such as histamine, bradykinin, and 5-hydroxytryptamine. All NSAIDs except the COX-2-selective agents inhibit both COX isoforms; the degree of inhibition of COX-1 varies from drug to drug. *No one NSAID is empirically superior for the treatment of inflammatory diseases; instead, each individual's response to and tolerance of a drug determines its therapeutic utility.*

Adverse Effects

A number of the toxicities commonly caused by the NSAIDs result from the inhibition of prostaglandin synthesis (Table 36.2). *The ability of NSAIDs to increase gastric acid secretion and inhibit blood clotting can lead to GI toxicity.* Mild reactions, such as heartburn and indigestion, may be decreased by adjusting the dosage, using antacids, or administering the drugs after meals. Occult loss of blood from the GI tract and iron deficiency anemia are also possible. More serious toxicity can result from prolonged NSAID therapy, including peptic ulceration and rarely, GI hemorrhage.

NSAIDs can impair renal function, cause fluid retention, and provoke hypersensitivity reactions, including bronchospasm, aggravation of asthma, urticaria, nasal polyps, and rarely, anaphylactoid reactions. These reactions may occur even in those who have previously used NSAIDs without any ill effects. NSAIDs inhibit uterine contraction and can cause premature closure of the fetal ductus arteriosus.

The spectrum of toxicity produced by each NSAID is related to its inhibition of specific COX isoforms. The earliest NSAIDs inhibit both isoforms of COX. Certain of these drugs are more specific for COX-1, whereas others inhibit COX-1 and COX-2 with roughly equal potency. *More recently developed drugs selectively inhibit COX-2 and therefore do not elicit the GI and antiplatelet side effects common to drugs that inhibit COX-1.*

Adverse effects that are not unequivocally related to inhibition of prostaglandin synthesis include hepatic effects (hepatitis, hepatic necrosis, cholestatic jaundice, increased serum aminotransferases), dermal effects (photosensitivities, Stevens-Johnson syndrome, toxic epidermal necrolysis, onycholysis), central nervous system (CNS) effects (headaches, dizziness, tinnitus, deafness, drowsiness, confusion, nervousness, increased sweating, aseptic meningitis), ocular effects (toxic amblyopia, retinal disturbances), and certain renal effects (acute interstitial nephritis, acute papillary necrosis).

Contraindications and Drug Interactions

Co-morbid factors that increase the risk of NSAID-induced GI bleeding include history of ulcer disease, advanced age, poor health status, treatment with certain drugs (discussed later), long duration of NSAID therapy, smoking, and heavy alcohol use. Because of their renal effects, NSAIDs must be used with caution in

TABLE 36.2 **Adverse Effects of NSAIDs – Relationship to Prostaglandin Synthesis Inhibition and Cyclooxygenase Isoforms**

System Affected	Adverse Effects	Prostaglandin Effects Inhibited by NSAIDs	COX Isoforms Involved
Gastrointestinal	Erosive gastritis, peptic ulceration	PGE_2-mediated suppression of gastric acid secretion, which helps maintain mucosal barrier and regulate microcirculation	COX-1
Platelet	Prolonged bleeding time, GI blood loss	TXA_2-mediated platelet aggregation	COX-1
Renal	Decreased Na$^+$ and H_2O excretion, renal failure, decreased effectiveness of diuretics and antihypertensives	PGE_2- and PGI_2-induced vasodilation in juxtamedullary apparatus (increases renal blood flow, antagonizes renin, inhibits reabsorption of Na$^+$ and H_2O)	COX-1 COX-2
Lungs, hypersensitivity, allergic reactions	Bronchospasm, urticaria, rhinitis, nasal polyposis	All prostaglandin synthesis – when inhibited, leukotriene formation is favored	COX-1 COX-2
Uterine	Delayed parturition, dystocia	PGE_2, $PGF_{2\alpha}$, and other prostaglandins are involved cervical ripening, uterine contractions	COX-2

patients with renal impairment, heart failure, hypertension, and edema. The use of NSAIDs is contraindicated in persons who have had a hypersensitivity reaction to salicylates or any other NSAID. Asthmatics are at particular risk for these reactions. NSAIDs should be used during pregnancy only if the potential benefit justifies the risk to the fetus.

A significant number of drug interactions are common to most of the NSAIDs. The likelihood of NSAID-induced GI toxicity is increased by concomitant treatment with corticosteroids (long term), other NSAIDs, bisphosphonates, or anticoagulants. Certain NSAIDs can also compete for protein binding sites with warfarin, compounding the risk of GI bleeding if these drugs are coprescribed. Agents that cause thrombocytopenia (e.g., myelosuppressive antineoplastic drugs) can also increase the likelihood that NSAIDs will cause bleeding. NSAIDs can decrease the clearance of methotrexate, resulting in severe hematological and GI toxicity. This does not appear to be a significant problem with low-dose methotrexate used in the treatment of rheumatoid arthritis; however, higher methotrexate doses used in the treatment of psoriasis or cancer may produce this toxicity. NSAIDs, when used in conjunction with immunosuppressive agents, can mask fever and other signs of infection.

Because NSAIDs decrease prostaglandin synthesis in the kidney, these drugs can increase the nephrotoxicity of agents such as aminoglycosides, amphotericin B, cidofovir, cisplatin, cyclosporine, foscarnet, ganciclovir, pentamidine, and vancomycin. NSAIDs can decrease the renal excretion of drugs such as lithium. NSAIDs can decrease the effectiveness of antihypertensive drugs such as β-blockers and diuretics. The elderly and those with decreased renal function are at particular risk for this interaction. Elevated hepatic enzymes and hepatic toxicity can occur with some drugs.

Specific Nonsteroidal Antiinflammatory Drugs

The acidic NSAIDs include the salicylates and an increasing number of other compounds. The latter agents, as a group, share many common properties: they may have toxicities, are highly protein bound and have the potential for interacting with other protein-bound drugs. The choice of a particular agent often depends on the reaction of the patient. Table 36.3 illustrates pharmacokinetic properties of selected NSAIDs.

Salicylates

The salicylates are also discussed in Chapter 26. Only observations that are relevant to their use as antiinflammatory agents are discussed in this chapter.

TABLE 36.3   **Pharmacokinetic Properties of Selected NSAIDs**

Drug	Time to Peak Plasma Level (fasting) (hr)	Plasma Half-Life (hr)	Protein Binding (%)	Urinary Excretion (%)	Notes
Celecoxib	2–4	11	97	57	H, R
Diclofenac	2–3	1–2	99	65	F
Etodolac	1.3	7	99	84	E, H
Fenoprofen	2	2.5–3	99	95	h
Flurbiprofen	0.5–4	6	99	95	h R
Ibuprofen	1	2r	90–99	90	H
Indomethacin	1–2	1.8–2.5	90–99	60	E, h
Ketoprofen	0.5–2	2–4	99	90	h, R
Ketorolac	0.5–1	4–6	99	91	h R
Meclofenamate sodium	0.5–2	2–4	Extensive	70	h
Meloxicam	4–5	15–20	99	40	E[b]
Nabumetone[a]	2.5	24	99	80	h, R
Naproxen	2–4	14	99	90+	h, R
Oxaprozin	3–6	36–92	99.9	65	h R
Piroxicam	2–4	30–86	99	66	E, h
Rofecoxib	2–3	17	87	72	H, R
Sulindac[a]	2	16–18	98	80	E, h
Tolmetin	0.5–1	5	99	100	h

[a]Properties of the active metabolite of this drug are given.
[b]Not recommended for those with severe renal and hepatic disease. E, enterohepatic cycling; F, extensive first pass metabolism; h, dosage adjustment may be necessary in patients with hepatic impairment; H, dosage adjustment recommended for patients with hepatic impairment; R, dosage adjustment necessary for patients with renal impairment.

Among the salicylates, aspirin and sodium salicylate are by far the most commonly used.

The salicylates are useful in the treatment of minor musculoskeletal disorders such as bursitis, synovitis, tendinitis, myositis, and myalgia. They may also be used to relieve fever and headache. They can be used in the treatment of inflammatory disease, such as acute rheumatic fever, rheumatoid arthritis, osteoarthritis, and certain rheumatoid variants, such as ankylosing spondylitis, Reiter's syndrome, and psoriatic arthritis. However, other NSAIDs are usually favored for the treatment of these chronic conditions because of their lower incidence of GI side effects. Aspirin is used in the treatment and prophylaxis of myocardial infarction and ischemic stroke.

Basic Pharmacology

Aspirin is available as capsules, tablets, enteric-coated tablets (*Ecotrin*), timed-release tablets (*ZORprin*), buffered tablets (*Ascriptin, Bufferin*), and as rectal suppositories. Sodium salicylate is available generically. Other salicylates include choline salicylate (*Arthropan*), choline magnesium trisalicylate (*Trilisate*), and magnesium salicylate (*Momentum*).

Although aspirin itself is pharmacologically active, it is rapidly hydrolyzed to salicylic acid after its absorption, and *it is the salicylate anion that accounts for most of the anti-inflammatory activity* of the drug. The superior analgesic activity of aspirin compared with sodium salicylate implies that aspirin has an intrinsic activity that is not totally explainable by its conversion to salicylic acid. Aspirin inhibits COX-1 to a much greater extent than COX-2; sodium salicylate is more selective for COX-1. This, combined with the ability of aspirin to acetylate proteins, might account for some of the therapeutic and toxicological differences between aspirin and the other salicylates.

The binding of salicylic acid to plasma proteins varies with its plasma concentrations. At serum salicylic acid concentrations of less than 100 μg/mL, 90 to 95% is protein bound; at 100 to 400 μg/mL, 70 to 85% is protein bound; and at concentrations greater than 400 μg/mL, 20 to 60% is protein bound. *The plasma concentration of salicylate that is associated with anti-inflammatory activity (200–300 μg/mL) is about six times that needed to produce analgesia.* At these higher concentrations, salicylate metabolism is reduced, resulting in a longer half-life for the drug. This reaction is a consequence of the saturable enzyme systems that metabolize salicylates. The plasma half-life for salicylate has been estimated to be 3 to 6 hours at the lower (analgesic) dosage and 15 to 30 hours at the higher (anti-inflammatory) dosages. The rate of hydrolysis of aspirin to salicylic acid is not dose limited, and no differences in the absorption of aspirin have been observed between arthritic patients and normal individuals.

Adverse Effects

The most common adverse effects produced by the salicylates are GI disturbances. Occult blood loss from the GI tract, peptic ulceration, and rarely, severe GI hemorrhage can occur. Because salicylic acid is highly bound to plasma proteins, it may be displaced by other highly protein-bound drugs such as oral anticoagulants, sulfonylureas, phenytoin, penicillins, and sulfonamides. The nonacetylated salicylates have greatly reduced effects on blood loss and produce fewer adverse GI effects. In addition, they may be somewhat kidney sparing. Salicylates may provoke hypersensitivity reactions and prolonged bleeding time in some individuals. Tinnitus, hearing impairment, blurred vision, and light-headedness are indicators of toxic dosages. *The use of aspirin in conjunction with any other NSAID is not recommended* because of the lack of evidence that such combinations increase efficacy and because of the increased potential for an adverse reaction. Salicylates are contraindicated in children with febrile viral illnesses because of a possible increased risk of Reye's syndrome.

Aryl and Heteroarylakanoic Acid–Type Drugs

The prototypes of this large class of NSAIDs are indomethacin and ibuprofen. These drugs are indicated for the relief of acute and chronic rheumatoid arthritis and osteoarthritis. In addition, a number of drugs of this class are also useful in ankylosing spondylitis, acute gouty arthritis, bursitis, and tendinitis.

Adverse reactions are common with the use of these drugs but usually do not result in serious morbidity. GI and CNS effects and prolonged bleeding may occur. Fluid retention, skin rashes, and ocular toxicity also occur, but with much lower frequency than with the salicylates. The selectivity for COX-1 and COX-2 varies from drug to drug and accounts for some of the differences in toxicity. *None of the agents seems to be clearly more efficacious than the others; however, they generally cause less GI blood loss and fewer other adverse reactions than does aspirin*, and the overall incidence of adverse reactions may be lower with these drugs.

Indomethacin

Indomethacin (*Indocin*) is used in the treatment of acute gouty arthritis, rheumatoid arthritis, ankylosing spondylitis, and osteoarthritis. It is not recommended for use as a simple analgesic or antipyretic because of its potential for toxicity. While indomethacin inhibits both COX-1 and COX-2, it is moderately selective for COX-1. It produces more CNS side effects than most of the other NSAIDs. Severe headache occurs in 25 to 50% of patients; vertigo, confusion, and psychological disturbances occur with some regularity. GI symptoms also are more frequent and severe than with most other

NSAIDs. Hematopoietic side effects (e.g., leukopenia, hemolytic anemia, aplastic anemia, purpura, thrombocytopenia, and agranulocytosis) also may occur. Ocular effects (blurred vision, corneal deposits) have been observed in patients receiving indomethacin, and regular ophthalmological examinations are necessary when the drug is used for long periods. Hepatitis, jaundice, pancreatitis, and hypersensitivity reactions also have been noted.

Sulindac

Sulindac (*Clinoril*) is chemically related to indomethacin and is generally used for the same indications. It is a prodrug that is metabolized to an active sulfide metabolite and an inactive metabolite. The most frequently reported side effects are GI pain, nausea, diarrhea, and constipation. The incidence of these effects is lower than for indomethacin, presumably because sulindac is a prodrug and thus the active metabolite is not highly concentrated at the gastric mucosa. As with indomethacin, a rather high incidence of CNS side effects (dizziness, headache) also occurs.

Tolmetin

Tolmetin (*Tolectin*) is indicated for the relief of osteoarthritis, rheumatoid arthritis, ankylosing spondylitis, and moderate pain. It is ineffective in gouty arthritis for unknown reasons. Tolmetin can inhibit both COX-1 and COX-2 but has a moderate selectivity for COX-1. The most frequently reported side effects are GI disturbance and CNS reactions (e.g., headache, asthenia, and dizziness). These effects are less frequently observed than after aspirin or indomethacin use. Blood pressure elevation, edema, and weight gain or loss have been associated with tolmetin administration. Tolmetin metabolites in urine have been found to produce pseudoproteinuria in some laboratory tests.

Ketorolac

Ketorolac (*Toradol*), an NSAID chemically related to indomethacin and tolmetin, is mainly used as an analgesic, not for the treatment of inflammatory disease. It is available in oral, parenteral, and topical formulations.

Etodolac

Etodolac (*Lodine*) is indicated for the treatment of osteoarthritis, rheumatoid arthritis, and acute pain. It inhibits COX-2 with slightly more selectivity than COX-1 and therefore produces less GI toxicity than many other NSAIDs. Common adverse effects include skin rashes and CNS effects.

Diclofenac

Diclofenac (*Voltaren, Cataflam*) is approved for use in rheumatoid arthritis, osteoarthritis, ankylosing spondylitis, dysmenorrhea, and topically for the treatment of ocular inflammation and actinic keratosis. Diclofenac exhibits approximately equal selectivity for COX-1 and COX-2. The most common adverse reactions are GI disturbances and headache. A reversible elevation of serum transaminases occurs in 15% of patients.

Ibuprofen

Ibuprofen (*Advil, Motrin*) is used as an analgesic and antipyretic as well as a treatment for rheumatoid arthritis and degenerative joint disease. The most frequently observed side effects are nausea, heartburn, epigastric pain, rash, and dizziness. Incidence of GI side effects is lower than with indomethacin. Visual changes and cross-sensitivity to aspirin have been reported. Ibuprofen inhibits COX-1 and COX-2 about equally. It decreases platelet aggregation, but the duration is shorter and the effect quantitatively lower than with aspirin. Ibuprofen prolongs bleeding times toward high normal value and should be used with caution in patients who have coagulation deficits or are receiving anticoagulant therapy.

Fenoprofen

Fenoprofen (*Nalfon*) is chemically and pharmacologically similar to ibuprofen and is used in the treatment of rheumatoid arthritis, osteoarthritis, and mild to moderate pain. GI effects such as dyspepsia and pain are most common, although dizziness, pruritus, and palpitations may occur. GI bleeding, sometimes severe, has been reported, and interstitial nephritis has been rarely associated with this drug. Concomitant administration of aspirin decreases the biological half-life of fenoprofen by increasing the metabolic clearance of hydroxylated fenoprofen. Chronic administration of phenobarbital also decreases the drug's half-life.

Naproxen

Naproxen (*Naprosyn*) also has pharmacological properties and clinical uses similar to those of ibuprofen. It exhibits approximately equal selectivity for COX-1 and COX-2 and is better tolerated than certain NSAIDs, such as indomethacin. Adverse reactions related to the GI tract occur in about 14% of all patients, and severe GI bleeding has been reported. CNS complaints (headache, dizziness, drowsiness), dermatological effects (pruritus, skin eruptions, echinoses), tinnitus, edema, and dyspnea also occur.

Ketoprofen

Ketoprofen (*Orudis*) is indicated for use in rheumatoid and osteoarthritis, for mild to moderate pain, and in dysmenorrhea. The most frequently reported side effects are GI (dyspepsia, nausea, abdominal pain, diarrhea, constipation, and flatulence) and CNS related (headache, excitation). Edema and increased blood urea nitrogen have also been noted in more than 3% of patients. Ketoprofen can cause fluid retention and increases in plasma creatinine, particularly in the elderly and in patients taking diuretics.

Flurbiprofen

Flurbiprofen (*Ansaid*) is indicated for the treatment of rheumatoid arthritis and osteoarthritis. Its half-life, longer than that of many of the NSAIDs, allows for twice daily dosing. The most common adverse effects of flurbiprofen are similar to those of the other acidic NSAIDs. Flurbiprofen inhibits both COX isoforms about equally.

Oxaprozin

Oxaprozin (*Daypro*) is approved for the treatment of osteoarthritis and rheumatoid arthritis. Its long half-life allows for once daily dosing. The most frequently reported adverse effects of this drug are nausea, vomiting, and dyspepsia.

Nabumetone

Nabumetone (*Relafen*) is approved for rheumatoid arthritis, osteoarthritis, and pain management. Its long half-life allows for once-daily dosing. Although this drug is a weak inhibitor of COX, it is metabolized in the liver to 6-methoxy-2-naphthylacetic acid (6-MNA), a strong COX inhibitor that is chemically similar to naproxen. As with most NSAIDs, GI side effects are most commonly reported. The incidence of gastric ulceration is lower with nabumetone than with many other NSAIDs. This is due to its nature as a prodrug, not to COX-2 selectivity. Lower-bowel complaints, rashes, and CNS disturbances are common adverse effects.

Sulfonylphenyl Derivatives

Celecoxib (*Celebrex*) and rofecoxib (*Vioxx*) are highly selective COX-2 inhibitors. *Because of this, they produce less erosion of the GI mucosa and cause less inhibition of platelet aggregation than do the nonselective COX inhibitors.* Short-term (6 months-to a year) clinical trials have shown that celecoxib and rofecoxib produce less GI toxicity than nonselective NSAIDs. However, serious GI bleeding and ulceration have occurred in patients taking these drugs, and long-term prospective studies of their safety have yet to be completed. *Like the nonselective NSAIDs, the selective COX-2 inhibitors can produce renal side effects such as hypertension and edema.*

Celecoxib is indicated for the treatment of osteoarthritis and rheumatoid arthritis. Its use is contraindicated in individuals with hypersensitivity to sulfonamides or other NSAIDs. It should be used with caution in persons with hepatic disease. Interactions occur with other drugs that induce CYP2C9 (e.g. ri-

fampin) or compete for metabolism by this enzyme (e.g. fluconazole, leflunomide). The most common adverse reactions to celecoxib are mild to moderate GI effects such as dyspepsia, diarrhea, and abdominal pain. Serious GI and renal effects have occurred rarely.

Rofecoxib is approved for the treatment of osteoarthritis, dysmenorrhea, and acute pain. The most common adverse reactions to rofecoxib are mild to moderate GI irritation (diarrhea, nausea, vomiting, dyspepsia, abdominal pain). Lower extremity edema and hypertension occur relatively frequently (about 3.5%). It is not metabolized by CYP2C9, so rofecoxib should not be subject to some of the interactions seen with celecoxib. However, its metabolism is increased by the coadministration of rifampin, which acts as a nonspecific inducer of hepatic metabolism.

Oxicam-Type Drugs

The oxicams are as effective as indomethacin, and their long half-life allows for once-daily dosing. Piroxicam (*Feldene*) is indicated for the treatment of rheumatoid arthritis and osteoarthritis. Piroxicam is a nonspecific COX inhibitor that has a much higher affinity for COX-1 than COX-2. This may account for the large proportion (over 30%) of patients receiving long-term therapy who have reported side effects. Adverse GI reactions have been the most frequently reported side effect, but edema, dizziness, headache, rash, and changes in hematological parameters have also occurred in 1 to 6% of patients. *Piroxicam can cause serious GI bleeding, ulceration, and perforation, particularly in the elderly,* if the recommended dosage is exceeded or if aspirin is being taken concurrently.

Meloxicam (*Mobic*), recently introduced for the treatment of osteoarthritis, is also used for rheumatoid arthritis and certain acute conditions. Although meloxicam is sometimes reported to be a selective COX-2 inhibitor, it is considerably less selective than celecoxib or rofecoxib. Its adverse effects are similar to those of piroxicam and other NSAIDs; however, the frequency of GI side effects is lower for meloxicam than for piroxicam and several other NSAIDs.

Fenamate-Type Drugs

Two compounds of the fenamate class of antiinflammatory drugs are marketed in the United States. Mefenamic acid (*Ponstel*) is indicated only for analgesia and primary dysmenorrhea when therapy will not exceed 1 week. Meclofenamate sodium (*Meclomen*) is prescribed for rheumatoid arthritis and osteoarthritis.

The fenamates show no clear superiority in antiinflammatory activity and may produce more adverse effects than other NSAIDs. Diarrhea may be severe enough to necessitate discontinuation of drug use. Other adverse GI reactions include nausea, vomiting, abdominal pain, bleeding, and peptic ulceration. Decreases in the hematocrit or hemoglobin values occur in approximately one-sixth of patients taking meclofenamic acid, but these do not usually require discontinuation of therapy. Because of the rare possibility of drug-induced hemolytic anemia, hematological analyses should be performed on patients receiving long-term therapy if anemia is suspected.

Phenylbutazone-Type Drugs

The phenylbutazone-type drugs include phenylbutazone, oxyphenbutazone, antipyrine, dipyrone, and aminopyrine. The use of these drugs has decreased because of their propensity to cause blood dyscrasias. Only antipyrine, used in as otic drops with benzocaine (*Otocalm*), is available in the United States today; phenylbutazone is used in Canada, and dipyrone is used in some European countries.

Acetaminophen

Acetaminophen (*Tylenol*) is an effective antipyretic and analgesic that is well tolerated at therapeutic doses. It has only weak antiinflammatory activity; thus, it is not useful in the treatment of rheumatoid arthritis and other inflammatory conditions. The properties of acetaminophen are described in Chapter 26.

DISEASE-MODIFYING ANTIRHEUMATIC DRUGS

While NSAIDs alleviate the pain and inflammation of rheumatoid arthritis, they do nothing to halt the loss of bone associated with this disease. The DMARDs are a chemically diverse class of agents, all of which have varying capacities to slow the progression of joint erosion. Their actions manifest over the course of weeks to months; they are usually employed in combination with NSAIDs and sometimes other DMARDs. Until the mid-1990s, DMARDs were reserved for treatment of the later stages of the disease in which significant joint erosion had already occurred. These agents were added individually, in slow succession (more than 6 months), as the disease progressed. More recent therapies employ certain DMARDs early in the treatment of disease, since they are effective in slowing the joint deterioration that occurs at this stage.

Methotrexate

Of the DMARDs, methotrexate (*Rheumatrex*) is the most widely prescribed. It is indicated for the treatment of rheumatoid arthritis and psoriasis; it is also used for psoriatic arthritis, systemic lupus erythematosus, and

sarcoidosis. It is generally as efficacious as the other agents, with a low incidence of serious side effects when prescribed on a low-dose weekly schedule. Additional uses of methotrexate as an anticancer and immunosuppressive agent are described in Chapters 56 and 57, respectively.

Basic Pharmacology

Methotrexate is a folate antimetabolite that inhibits dihydrofolate reductase and other folate-dependent enzymes in cells. The absorption, metabolism, and excretion of methotrexate are fully described in Chapter 56. When given in high doses, methotrexate exerts potent suppressing action on cellular and humoral immunity (see Chapter 57). At the low doses used in the therapy of rheumatoid arthritis, methotrexate appears to be acting more as an antiinflammatory agent than as an immunosuppressant. Methotrexate inhibits folate-dependent enzymes involved in adenosine degradation, increasing concentrations of extracellular adenosine. Adenosine acts via cell surface receptors to inhibit the production of inflammatory cytokines such as TNF-α and IFN-γ. Methotrexate also decreases the production of inflammatory prostaglandins and proteases, though a direct action on the COX enzymes has not been noted.

Adverse Effects

In the low-dose regimen used for rheumatoid arthritis, most side effects of methotrexate are mild and can be managed by temporarily stopping the drug or reducing the dose. These include nausea, stomatitis, GI discomfort, rash, diarrhea, and headaches. Changes in liver aminotransferases and mild to moderate immunosuppression have been reported in rheumatoid arthritis patients taking methotrexate. Severe toxicity is possible but rare and may be a function of drug accumulation. These effects include hepatotoxicity progressing to cirrhosis, pneumonitis progressing to pulmonary fibrosis, and bone marrow depression with anemia, leukopenia, and thrombocytopenia. Folic acid supplementation is often used to alleviate certain side effects of methotrexate therapy (stomatitis, GI irritation, hematopoietic effects) but may also contribute to resistance to this therapy.

Contraindications and Drug Interactions

Methotrexate is teratogenic and is contraindicated during pregnancy and breast-feeding. Prior to attempting pregnancy, women should wait at least one menstrual cycle and men at least 3 months after discontinuing this drug. Additional contraindications to methotrexate administration include kidney, liver, and lung disease; moderate to high alcohol use; immunodeficiency; blood dyscrasias; and hypersensitivity. Elderly persons may be at increased risk for toxicity because of decreased renal and hepatic function.

Methotrexate clearance can be decreased by the coadministration of NSAIDs; however, this not usually a problem with the low doses of methotrexate used to treat arthritis. Methotrexate can be displaced from plasma protein binding sites by phenylbutazone, phenytoin, sulfonylureas, and sulfonamides and certain other antibiotics. The antifolate effects of methotrexate are additive with those of other folate-inhibitory drugs, such as trimethoprim.

Sulfasalazine

Sulfasalazine (*Azulfidine*) is approved for the treatment of rheumatoid arthritis and ulcerative colitis. It is also used to treat ankylosing spondylitis and Crohn's disease. Comparisons of sulfasalazine with other DMARDs suggest that it is more effective than hydroxychloroquine, azathioprine, and oral gold compounds. It is at least as effective as intramuscular gold and penicillamine. It has a greater degree of toxicity than hydroxychloroquine but less than gold compounds and penicillamine. After 5 years, approximately 75% of patients have discontinued sulfasalazine therapy, primarily because of a lack of efficacy as opposed to intolerable side effects.

Basic Pharmacology

Sulfasalazine is a prodrug of which 70% is converted by colon bacteria to two active metabolites, sulfapyridine and 5-aminosalicylic acid (mesalamine). Sulfapyridine has antibacterial activities, and 5-aminosalicylic acid is antiinflammatory; however, these effects do not account for the ability of this drug to slow the processes of rheumatoid arthritis. Recent research suggests additional activities of sulfasalazine that may be relevant to these effects: its ability to increase adenosine levels, its inhibitory effects on IL-1 and TNF-α release, and its inhibition of NF-κB. The pharmacokinetic data for this and other DMARDs are provided in Table 36.4.

Adverse Effects

Mild to moderate side effects, including nausea, vomiting, abdominal pain, diarrhea, anorexia, and headache, occur in up to 33% of patients taking this drug. Skin rash and discoloration, fever, reversible male infertility, and liver enzyme elevation occur less frequently. Rare hematological abnormalities, such as agranulocytosis, aplastic anemia, hemolytic anemia, neutropenia, or other blood dyscrasias, can be fatal. Hypersensitivity reactions occur rarely.

Contraindications and Drug Interactions

Sulfasalazine is contraindicated in individuals with hypersensitivity to salicylates, sulfonamides, sulfonylureas, and certain diuretics (furosemide, thiazides, and carbonic anhydrase inhibitors). Because it can cause kernicterus, sulfasalazine is contraindicated in infants and children under 2 years of age. Sulfasalazine passes into breast milk and is therefore contraindicated for nursing mothers. Similarly, pregnant women near term should not use this drug, although it appears to be the safest of the DMARDs during early pregnancy.

TABLE 36.4 Pharmacokinetic Properties of Selected DMARDs

Drug	Time to Peak Plasma Level (fasting) (hr)	Plasma Half-Life	Protein Binding (%)	Urinary Excretion (%)	Notes
Anakinra	3–7	4–6 (hr)	–	–	–
Auranofin	2	26 d[a] 80 d[b]	60	60	–
Aurothioglucose	2–6	160 d–1 yr[b]	98	70	–
Etanercept	72	115	–	–	–
Hydroxychloroquine	3	32 d	45	Predominant	–
Infliximab	–	8–9.5 d	–	–	–
Leflunomide (M1 metabolite)	6–12	15 d	99	Minor	E, H, R
Sulfasalazine	SZ: 1.5–6 SP: 6–24	SZ: 5–7 (hr) SP: 6–14 (hr)	99%+ –	SP: 75 Mes: 67	R –

[a]Blood
[b]Tissues
E, enterohepatic cycling; H, not recommended for patients with hepatic impairment; R, dosage adjustment necessary for patients with renal impairment; SZ, sulfasalazine; SP, sulfapyridine; Me, mesalamine.

Sulfasalazine can precipitate attacks of porphyria and should not be used by individuals with bowel or urinary obstruction.

Sulfasalazine can inhibit the absorption of cardiac glycosides and folic acid. It may displace certain drugs, including warfarin, phenytoin, methotrexate, tolbutamide, chlorpropamide, and oral sulfonylureas, from their protein binding sites. Sulfasalazine can diminish the effectiveness of penicillins and estrogen-containing oral contraceptives.

Antimalarials

Hydroxychloroquine (*Plaquenil*) and chloroquine (*Aralen*) are 4-aminoquinoline antimalarial drugs that possess modest DMARD activity. They are indicated for the treatment of rheumatoid arthritis and systemic lupus erythematosus; their use as antimalarials is detailed in Chapter 53. The onset of action of these drugs is longer than that of other DMARDs, and their side effects are relatively mild. Because of this, these agents show promise as ingredients of combination therapies for rheumatoid arthritis.

Basic Pharmacology

Hydroxychloroquine and chloroquine are similar in activity; however, hydroxychloroquine has a lower incidence of ocular side effects and is used more frequently. These drugs are weak bases that enter and interfere with the functioning of lysosomes and other subcellular compartments of T- and B-lymphocytes, monocytes, and macrophages. This in turn inhibits the ability of these cells to produce and release inflammatory cytokines and hydrolytic enzymes.

Adverse Effects

Skin rashes and pruritus are common adverse effects of the 4-aminoquinoline antimalarials, as are GI effects. The incidence of the most serious toxic reaction, irreversible retinopathy with resultant blindness, is dose related and can be minimized by maintaining a daily dose of hydroxychloroquine less than 6.5 mg/kg or chloroquine less than 4 mg/kg. Eye examinations should be performed regularly during treatment with these drugs. Severe hematological toxicity (neutropenia, thrombocytopenia, aplastic anemia) is rare. Reversible side effects observed during high-dose, long-term therapy with the aminoquinolines include lichenoid skin lesions, leukopenia, neuromyopathy, hair loss, sensitivity to sunburn, and changes in the electrocardiogram.

Contraindications and Drug Interactions

The aminoquinolines accumulate in lung, kidney, and liver; thus, any preexisting pathology in these tissues contraindicates their use. Similarly, any ocular pathology precludes their use. Psoriasis and porphyria are frequently exacerbated by the administration of the aminoquinolines.

Aminoquinolines can increase plasma concentrations of penicillamine, hence the potential for serious hematological or renal toxicity. Similarly, aminoquinolines can increase digoxin levels. Gold and an aminoquinoline probably should not be administered concurrently because of the propensity of each to produce dermatitis.

Leflunomide

Leflunomide (*Arava*) is an isoxazole derivative approved for the treatment of rheumatoid arthritis in 1998. Limited data suggest that it is comparable in efficacy to sulfasalazine and produces fewer adverse effects. It has a faster onset of action (4 weeks) than other DMARDs.

Basic Pharmacology

Leflunomide is a prodrug that is converted to an active malonitrilamide metabolite, A77 1726 (M1). M1 inhibits T-cell proliferation by blocking de novo pyrimidine synthesis and inhibiting the tyrosine kinases that are associated with certain cytokine and growth factor receptors.

Adverse Effects

Diarrhea occurs in approximately one-third of patients taking this drug; indigestion, nausea, and vomiting occur in about 10%. Other common adverse effects include weight changes, headache, skin rashes, pruritus, and reversible alopecia and hepatic enzyme elevation. Although leflunomide acts as an immunosuppressive, it does not appear to cause significant bone marrow depression.

Contraindications and Drug Interactions

Leflunomide is teratogenic in animal models; it is absolutely contraindicated in pregnancy, in women who may become pregnant, and in breast-feeding women. Because of its long half-life, the M1 metabolite of leflunomide may remain in the body for up to 2 years; therefore, a drug elimination procedure using cholestyramine should be used before any attempt at pregnancy. This drug is not recommended for use in children. Caution should be used when administering this drug to individuals with renal or hepatic disease, heavy alcohol use, or immunosuppression.

The long half-life of leflunomide must be taken into account to prevent drug interactions. Hepatotoxicity is possible if leflunomide is given in conjunction with a hepatotoxic agent such as methotrexate or certain NSAIDs. Leflunomide inhibits CYP2C9, the enzyme responsible for the metabolism of numerous drugs. Rifampin induces the P450 enzyme responsible for converting leflunomide to its M1 metabolite. Cholestyramine enhances the clearance of leflunomide and its M1 metabolite.

TNF-α Inhibitors

Two recently introduced biological therapies were designed to interfere with the inflammatory cascade initiate by TNF-α. Etanercept (*Enbrel*) is indicated for the treatment of moderate to severe rheumatoid arthritis in individuals over age 4. Infliximab in conjunction with methotrexate (*Remicade*) is approved for use by adults in the treatment of rheumatoid arthritis. It is also indicated for therapy of Crohn's disease. Over the short term, the efficacy of these drugs in the treatment of rheumatoid arthritis appears to be superior to that of methotrexate alone; however, their ability to prevent bone erosion for longer than 24 months must be further studied. The cost of both drugs is significantly higher than that of the other DMARDs.

Basic Pharmacology

Etanercept is a recombinant fusion protein produced in Chinese hamster ovary cells. It consists of the intracellular ligand-binding portion of the human p75 TNF receptor linked to the Fc portion of human immunoglobulin (Ig) G_1. Two p75 molecules are attached to each Fc molecule. Etanercept binds to soluble TNF-α and TNF-β and forms inactive complexes, effectively lowering circulating levels of these cytokines. It is administered subcutaneously, generally twice weekly.

Infliximab is a chimeric monoclonal antibody targeted against TNF-α. It consists of a human IgG_1 Fc heavy chain and partial κ-light chain fused to a murine hypervariable region. Infliximab binds to both soluble and transmembrane forms of TNF-α and inhibits their ability to bind to TNF receptors. It does not inhibit TNF-β, which binds to the same receptors as TNF-α. Infliximab is administered intravenously, usually at 4- to 8-week intervals.

Adverse Effects

The most common adverse reaction to etanercept is mild to moderate erythema, pain, or pruritus at the injection site (37%). Headaches and abdominal pain can also occur. New positive autoantibodies, such as antinuclear antibodies (ANA), anti-dsDNA antibodies, and anticardiolipin antibodies, can develop in patients treated with etanercept. Although there is so far no association between this and the development of autoimmune diseases or malignancies, long-term studies have yet to be done. Rare cases of pancytopenia may be associated with this drug. Although clinical trials showed no increased risk of infection with etanercept treatment, postmarketing reports of serious infections, sepsis, and associated fatalities exist.

Infliximab produces an acute infusion-related reaction consisting of fever and chills in approximately 20% of patients. Other common side effects include headache, nausea, and diarrhea. Persons given infliximab with methotrexate may have a greater elevation of hepatic enzyme levels than those given methotrexate alone. Because it is a human–mouse fusion protein, infliximab seems to be more immunogenic than etanercept. During infliximab treatment, autoantibodies (anti-dsDNA, ANA) and antibodies to the drug itself (human antichimeric antibodies) can develop. Concomitant therapy with methotrexate or immunosuppressive drugs decreases this risk somewhat. It is possible that infliximab may increase the incidence of autoimmune diseases and malignancies; however, long-term data are needed to determine whether this is the case. As with etanercept, a low risk of serious infection was seen in clinical trials of infliximab; however, sepsis, disseminated tuberculosis, and other potentially fatal infections have been reported in patients taking this drug.

Contraindications and Drug Interactions

Etanercept therapy should not be initiated in patients with active infection. If an infection develops in a person taking etanercept, he or she should be closely monitored. If a serious infection or sepsis occurs, the drug should be discontinued. Etanercept should be used with caution in individuals who have conditions predisposing them to serious infection (e.g., uncontrolled diabetes, hematological abnormalities). Data on drug interactions are limited. Live virus vaccines are contraindicated because of the potential for secondary transmission of the infection by the vaccine. Myelosuppressive antirheumatic agents have been associated with pancytopenia in some patients treated with etanercept.

Infliximab should not be given to individuals with known hypersensitivity to murine proteins. As with etanercept, precautions for the prevention of serious infections must be taken, and live virus vaccines are contraindicated.

Interleukin-1 Antagonists

Anakinra (*Kineret*) is the first antirheumatic agent that acts by blocking the action of IL-1. This drug was recently approved for the treatment of moderately to severely active rheumatoid arthritis in adults who have not responded to therapy with one or more DMARDs. Anakinra may be used alone or in combination with DMARDs other than the TNF antagonists. Clinical trials have shown anakinra to be more effective than placebo, either alone or in conjunction with methotrexate.

Basic Pharmacology

Anakinra is a nonglycosylated form of the human IL-1 receptor antagonist (IL-1ra). It is produced in a recombinant *Escherichia coli* expression system and has an additional methionine residue at its amino terminus. In rheumatoid arthritis patients, the amount of naturally occurring IL-1ra in the synovial fluid is not sufficient to counteract the high levels of locally produced IL-1. Anakinra acts as a competitive antagonist of the type 1 IL-1 receptor and decreases the pain and inflammation produced by IL-1. It is administered as a daily subcutaneous injection.

Adverse Effects

The most common adverse reactions to anakinra are redness, bruising, pain, and inflammation at the injection site. Neutropenia may occur, and the risk of serious infection is somewhat elevated, particularly in asthmatic patients. Antibodies to anakinra can develop with long-term therapy, but no correlation between antibody development and clinical response or adverse effects has been observed.

Contraindications and Drug Interactions

No drug interaction studies have been conducted in humans. Animal studies indicate no change in the clearance or toxicity of either methotrexate or anakinra when the two agents are administered together. Concomitant administration of a TNF blocker appears to increase the risk of serious infection. The response to vaccines may be diminished in patients taking anakinra.

Gold Compounds

Gold compounds (chrysotherapy) are the oldest of the DMARDs in use to treat rheumatoid arthritis. Parentally administered gold is generally believed to be somewhat less effective than methotrexate; oral gold is less effective than parenteral preparations. Gold compounds take several months to produce a measurable effect. Among patients who can tolerate this therapy, some benefit will be obtained in about 80%, and complete remission will be induced in 20% of cases. Remissions are maintained for varying periods after discontinuing therapy, with a relapse rate as high as 80%. Relapse is usually less severe in such patients, and a second course of gold therapy usually produces beneficial effects.

Basic Pharmacology

The gold preparations available in the United States include two preparations administered via intramuscular injection: gold sodium thiomalate (GSTM, *Myochrysine, Aurolate*) and aurothioglucose (gold sodium thioglucose, GSTG, *Solganal*), and an oral preparation, aura-

nofin (*Ridaura*). Although called gold salts, these compounds contain monovalent gold bound to sulfur, a bond that is at least partly covalent. For this reason, these complexes are termed gold preparations or gold compounds in this chapter.

The mechanism by which gold compounds produce their antiarthritic effects is not known. Since gold therapy can suppress the increased phagocytic activity that occurs in rheumatoid arthritis, the antirheumatic activity of gold preparations may involve the inhibition of either antigen processing by macrophages or lysosomal enzyme release in the joint. Gold preparations also directly inhibit certain lysosomal enzymes found in polymorphonuclear leukocytes and macrophages.

Generally, 2 months of multiple dosing of gold compounds is required to reach steady-state levels. Auranofin therapy produces lower steady-state blood gold concentrations than does treatment with parenteral gold compounds, but it also produces a lower incidence of adverse effects.

Adverse Effects

Toxic manifestations of gold therapy are most common after a minimal total amount (200–300 mg) of gold has been administered. Serious reactions necessitating discontinuance of therapy or antidotal therapy are encountered in perhaps 5% of the patients.

Both oral and parenteral gold therapy frequently produces dermatitis, usually preceded and accompanied by pruritus. Stomatitis may accompany dermatitis, which may be preceded by a metallic taste in the mouth of the patient. Blue or gray skin discoloration can arise from gold deposition in that tissue, and photosensitivity may also occur. Unlike parenteral gold compounds, auranofin does not accumulate appreciably in the skin. Auranofin, but not the parenteral gold preparations, most frequently causes diarrhea (about 50%), abdominal pain, nausea, and anorexia.

Mild proteinuria is fairly common and does not always require discontinuance of therapy; however, severe proteinuria may indicate a toxic nephritis. The proteinuria is usually reversible when gold administration is stopped. Hepatotoxicity has also been reported. Fatalities from gold therapy have been reported, usually a consequence of a blood dyscrasia. The most common hematological abnormality is eosinophilia. Serious blood dyscrasias, such as thrombocytopenia, agranulocytosis, and hypoplastic or aplastic anemia, are rare.

To complement steroidal and other measures used in treating gold toxicity, it may be necessary to hasten the elimination of gold from the body. Appropriate chelating agents include dimercaprol and penicillamine (see Chapter 2). The proper administration of either of these agents markedly increases the excretion of gold and alleviates the signs and symptoms of gold toxicity.

Contraindications and Drug Interactions

Gold compounds are contraindicated for use in patients with systemic lupus erythematosus, Sjögren's syndrome, severe debilitation, or uncontrolled congestive heart failure or hypertension. Caution must be used in administering gold compounds to individuals who have conditions that might increase their susceptibility to gold toxicity: blood dyscrasias, immunosuppression, renal disease, hepatic disease, skin diseases, or inflammatory bowel disease. Animal studies have shown adverse effects on reproduction; gold compounds may distribute to breast milk and are therefore contraindicated for women who are breast-feeding.

Gold should be used cautiously in patients receiving drugs that can also cause nephrotoxicity. Interactions between gold compounds and penicillamine may result in severe hematological and renal side effects.

Other Drugs for Rheumatoid Arthritis Therapy

The following drugs are not commonly used as first-line treatments of rheumatoid arthritis, either because they lack the efficacy of other drugs or because they produce more serious side effects or both. They do, however, remain useful in specific clinical situations and in individuals in whom more conservative therapies have failed.

Corticosteroids

Serious adverse effects are produced by long-term, high-dose exposure to the corticosteroids; therefore, these drugs are not agents of choice for the treatment of rheumatic disease. In general, the use of low-dose corticosteroids avoids significant side effects (e.g. fluid retention, osteoporosis, GI bleeding, immunosuppression) but does not completely control the disease. However, for patients whose disease is refractory to other agents or who cannot tolerate the side effects of other DMARDs, a corticosteroid such as prednisone may be used to control symptoms. Low-dose corticosteroids may also be used as an alternative to more toxic DMARDs in pregnant, elderly, or debilitated individuals. Intraarticular injection of corticosteroids can control acute inflammation of a specific joint without causing systemic side effects. High-dose steroids can control severe systemic manifestations of autoimmune disease, such as iritis, pericarditis, nephritis, or vasculitis. Following discontinuation of corticosteroid treatment, rebound joint deterioration is common.

A detailed discussion of the pharmacodynamics, mechanism of action, and adverse effects of the corticosteroids and their role in therapeutics can be found in Chapter 60.

Immunosuppressive Drugs

The immunosuppressive drugs are used in rheumatoid arthritis and certain other autoimmune conditions that are refractory to less toxic treatments. Their pharmacology and additional clinical uses are described in Chapter 57. Azathioprine (*Imuran*) is a prodrug that is metabolized to a purine antimetabolite. Its disease-modifying activity results from the inhibition of lymphocyte proliferation and secretion of certain cytokines. This drug is used in the treatment of rheumatoid arthritis, lupus nephritis, and psoriatic arthritis. Cyclosporine (*Sandimmune, Neoral*) is used in refractory rheumatoid arthritis, psoriasis, and inflammatory bowel disease. It acts by blocking the transcriptional activation of many genes involved in the first phase of T cell activation. Cyclophosphamide (*Cytoxan*) is an alkylating agent that was used in severe rheumatoid in the past but is seldom used today because of its severe bladder toxicity, bone marrow toxicity, and carcinogenicity.

Minocycline

The tetracycline antibiotic minocycline (*Minocin*) is modestly effective in the treatment of rheumatoid arthritis and is generally well tolerated. Radiographic evidence of its efficacy as a DMARD is lacking, although clinical symptoms do abate. It can be useful in the treatment of early, mild disease. A more detailed description of the pharmacology and clinical uses of minocycline is found in Chapter 47.

Penicillamine

Penicillamine (*Cuprimine*) can be used to treat acute, severe rheumatoid arthritis, producing reductions in joint pain, edema, and stiffness. The response to penicillamine is usually delayed (4–12 weeks), and remissions can last several months after withdrawal of treatment. Radiographic evidence of this drug's efficacy is limited; thus, penicillamine is seldom used to treat rheumatoid arthritis. The mechanism of action of penicillamine is unknown, but some evidence suggests that it may involve the inhibition of angiogenesis, synovial fibroblast proliferation, or transcriptional activation. Because penicillamine can chelate copper and promote its excretion, it is used to treat Wilson's disease (hepatolenticular degeneration) and has also been used in mercury and lead intoxication.

Penicillamine is readily absorbed from the GI tract and is rapidly excreted in the urine, largely as the intact molecule. Gradually increasing its dose minimizes side effects, which necessitate discontinuance of penicillamine therapy in perhaps one-third of patients. The most common side effects are maculopapular pruritic dermatitis, GI upset, loss of taste sensation, mild to occasionally severe thrombocytopenia and leukopenia, and mild proteinuria, which at times may progress to the nephritic syndrome. Discontinuance of therapy usually results in a rapid disappearance of side effects.

NEW APPROACHES TO THE TREATMENT OF RHEUMATOID ARTHRITIS

In previous decades, a pyramid model dominated the treatment of rheumatoid arthritis. Early in the course of the disease, salicylates were used to control pain and stiffness. If salicylates were poorly tolerated or began to lose efficacy, they were discontinued and a different NSAID was used. As the efficacy of NSAID therapy waned and joint deterioration progressed, treatment with a DMARD was added. DMARDs were employed singly and sequentially for periods of up to 6 months before clinicians could determine their efficacy and switch to a new drug if necessary.

The most recent treatment paradigm calls for earlier, more aggressive treatment of rheumatoid arthritis. DMARDs are frequently employed along with NSAIDs in the initial treatment of the disease. The COX-2 inhibitors are often used because they are less likely to cause serious GI toxicity than are the nonspecific COX inhibitors. The usual DMARD of choice for patients with mild rheumatoid arthritis is hydroxychloroquine or sulfasalazine; methotrexate is used for those with moderate to serious disease. Other DMARDs are used if these agents are poorly tolerated or do not produce sufficient response. Combination therapy of methotrexate and another agent is also used to treat disease that is not responsive to individual DMARDs.

Study QUESTIONS

1. A man aged 74 has moderate hypertension controlled with hydrochlorothiazide 12.5 mg once daily and losartan 50 mg once daily. He is prescribed rofecoxib 50 mg once daily to control osteoarthritis pain. After 3 months of this therapy, his blood pressure begins to rise. This increase in blood pressure is most likely due to
   (A) Inhibition of COX-2 by rofecoxib, which leads to decreased renal blood flow
   (B) Increased metabolism of losartan due to induction of CYP2C9 by rofecoxib
   (C) Increased excretion of hydrochlorothiazide due to increased renal blood flow caused by rofecoxib
   (D) Arteriolar contraction in the peripheral circulation caused by inhibition of COX-1 by rofecoxib
   (E) Weight gain caused by rofecoxib's ability to decrease basal metabolic rate.

2. The use of low-dose methotrexate in the treatment of rheumatoid arthritis is most frequently
   (A) Reserved for cases in which NSAIDs no longer adequately control pain and stiffness
   (B) Initiated only after significant joint destruction
   (C) Contraindicated in individuals being treated with NSAIDs
   (D) Used for pregnant women, since it is the DMARD with the least fetal toxicity
   (E) Initiated early in the course of moderate to severe forms of the disease

3. A 52-year-old woman with a history of eczema and heavy alcohol use begins taking ibuprofen to control hip and knee pain due to osteoarthritis. Over the course of 6 months, as the pain worsens, she increases her dosage to a high level (600 mg four times daily). What toxicity is most likely to occur, and why?
   (A) Abnormal heart rhythms; alcohol induces cytochrome P450 isozymes that convert ibuprofen to a cardiotoxic free radical metabolite
   (B) Necrotizing fasciitis; eczema predisposes an individual to this toxicity of ibuprofen
   (C) Gastric ulceration; heavy alcohol use increases the susceptibility of an individual to ibuprofen-induced GI toxicity
   (D) Confusion and ataxia; these CNS toxicities of ibuprofen are additive with those of ethanol
   (E) Eosinophilia; this rare complication of ibuprofen therapy is exacerbated by the immunosuppression frequently seen in alcoholics

4. Etanercept produces its antirheumatic effects by direct
   (A) Inhibition of cAMP phosphodiesterase in monocytic lineage leukocytes
   (B) Selective inhibition of COX-2
   (C) Enhancement of leukotriene synthesis at the expense of prostaglandin synthesis
   (D) Reduction of circulating active TNF-α levels
   (E) Inhibition of the production of autoantibodies

5. An advantage of celecoxib over most other NSAIDs is
   (A) Less inhibition of PGE$_2$ effects on the gastric mucosal
   (B) Less risk of bronchospasm and hypersensitivity reactions

(C) Once-daily dosing allows the patient convenience

(D) Less risk of harm to the developing fetus in the third trimester

(E) Greater degree of efficacy in the treatment of rheumatoid arthritis

ANSWERS

1. **A.** By blocking renal prostaglandin synthesis, COX-2 inhibitors, such as rofecoxib, decrease the blood flow to the juxtaglomerular apparatus, thus stimulating the release of renin and subsequent Na^+ retention and blood pressure elevation. Rofecoxib is neither metabolized nor induced by CYP2C9. It decreases rather than increases renal blood flow and does not increase the excretion of hydrochlorothiazide. Item D is incorrect because rofecoxib has very little effect on COX-1 and prostaglandins are not a major controlling factor of peripheral vascular tone. Rofecoxib does not decrease basal metabolic rate.

2. **E.** Treatment guidelines suggest the use of DMARDs early in the course of rheumatoid arthritis to slow the joint deterioration associated with the disease. Methotrexate is the DMARD of choice for people with moderate to severe forms of rheumatoid arthritis. Although NSAIDs can decrease methotrexate clearance, NSAIDs can be safely used with the low doses of methotrexate used in the therapy of rheumatoid arthritis. Methotrexate is highly teratogenic and should not be used by women who are or may become pregnant.

3. **C.** The likelihood of gastric ulceration and GI bleeding is increased by heavy alcohol use, poor health, advanced age, long-term NSAID use, and use of drugs such as corticosteroids and anticoagulants. Ibuprofen is not converted to a cardiotoxic metabolite. Dermal toxicities, such as epidermal necrolysis, are rare complications of ibuprofen therapy, but necrotizing fasciitis is not one of them. Confusion and ataxia are not side effects associated with ibuprofen, nor is eosinophilia.

4. **D.** Etanercept is a recombinant fusion protein consisting of two TNF receptor domains linked to one IgG Fc molecule. It binds to soluble TNF-α and TNF-β and forms inactive complexes. It does not directly affect cAMP phosphodiesterase, leukotriene synthesis, or autoantibody production.

5. **A.** Celecoxib selectively inhibits COX-2, so it does not inhibit the constitutive activity of COX-1 in the regulation of gastric acid secretion. When prostaglandin synthesis by COX-1 or COX-2 is blocked, eicosanoids are shifted into the leukotriene pathway, so bronchospasm and hypersensitivity reactions are favored. The shorter half-life of celecoxib does not allow once-daily dosing. This drug is no less able than other NSAIDs to close the ductus arteriosus during the third trimester. None of the NSAIDs is empirically more efficacious than the others; a patient's own response and side effects determine the best drug for him or her.

SUPPLEMENTAL READING

Beehrle DM and Evans D. A review of NSAID complications: Gastrointestinal and more. Prim Care Pract 1999;3:305–315.

Case JP. Old and new drugs used in rheumatoid arthritis: A historical perspective. Part 1: The older drugs. Am J Ther 2001;8:123–143.

Case JP. Old and new drugs used in rheumatoid arthritis: A historical perspective. Part 2: The newer drugs and drug strategies. Am J Ther 2001;8:163–179.

Kremer JM. Rational use of new and existing disease-modifying agents in rheumatoid arthritis. Ann Intern Med 2001;134:695–706.

Lee DM and Weinblatt ME. Rheumatoid arthritis. Lancet 2001;358:903–911.

McCarberg BH and Herr KA. Osteoarthritis: How to manage pain and improve patient function. Geriatrics 2001;56:14–17, 20–22, 24.

Mitchell JA, Larkin S, and Williams TJ. Cyclooxygenase-2 regulation and relevance in inflammation. Biochem Pharmacol 1995;50:1535–1542.

CASE **Study**   **A Visit to University Student Health**

A 21-year-old college student presented to her university's student health center with an acute exacerbation of asthma. Her respiratory rate was increased, and she was in obvious respiratory distress, with wheezes audible on both sides of the chest. The examination of the nasal passages revealed mucosal edema and a polyp on the right. There was marked swelling about the eyes, and her upper lip was swollen (angioedema). Her fingertips were slightly cyanotic. Her peak expiratory flow rate was 25% of the predicted normal value. Oxygen was given by face mask. She was given 1:1000 aqueous epinephrine 0.3 mL subcutaneously, diphenhydramine HCl 50 mg intramuscularly, and prednisone 40 mg by mouth. Subsequently she was given nebulized albuterol, and the peak flow rate improved to 75% of predicted. When questioned further, she said she had taken a friend's ibuprofen for menstrual cramps.

The case in context: Dysmenorrhea is a common condition caused by uterine contraction during menses. $PGF_{2\alpha}$ may be the uterine contractant.

NSAIDs, such as ibuprofen, relieve dysmenorrhea by inhibiting the biosynthesis of $PGF_{2\alpha}$. This allows for enhanced production of the leukotrienes by a 5-lipoxygenase. The leukotrienes are potent bronchoconstrictors, and patients with asthma and nasal polyps are often much more sensitive to them than are other asthmatics and normal individuals. The logic of her therapy is as follows: Oxygen is needed in patients with peak flow rates less than 30% of their predicted value; epinephrine is a bronchodilator (β-adrenergic effect) and vasoconstrictor that prevents further angioedema (α-adrenergic effect); diphenhydramine is an H_1 antihistamine; albuterol is a β_2-adrenergic agonist; prednisone (a glucocorticoid) is the most effective drug for asthma. Although its onset of action is slow (about 4 hours), many patients with an acute attack of asthma have a late response several hours later due to the influx and activation of lymphocytes, eosinophils, and perhaps neutrophils, which release further mediators of inflammation, such as the leukotriene-5. The patient should be warned to avoid NSAIDs in the future.

37 Drugs Used in Gout

Knox Van Dyke

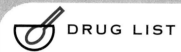

DRUG LIST

GENERIC NAME	PAGE	GENERIC NAME	PAGE
Allopurinol	445	Oxypurinol	446
Colchicine	443	Phenylbutazone	446
Indomethacin	446	Probenecid	445
Oxyphenbutazone	446	Sulfinpyrazone	445

Gout is characterized biochemically as a disorder of uric acid metabolism and clinically by hyperuricemia and recurrent attacks of acute arthritis. Gouty arthritis is most frequently seen as an acute inflammation primarily in the large toe, instep, ankle, or heel. Less often the initial symptoms appear in the knee or elbow; occasionally they are seen in the wrist. If the condition remains untreated over years, sodium urate crystals may form in the subcutaneous tissue, joints, renal parenchyma, and renal pelvis. Uric acid stones may form in the lumen of the urinary tract, and progressive renal failure often occurs in the later stages of untreated gout. Also, microcrystalline deposits of sodium urate frequently result in inflammatory bulges or bumps, termed *tophi,* appearing in the subcutaneous tissue of the earlobes, elbows, and hands and at the base of the large toe.

The elevated blood uric acid concentration in gout is an easily identified and readily treated abnormality. However, it is essential to identify the condition and institute therapy early to avoid the complications that result from a prolonged elevated uricemia. Complications include arthritis, tophi, urinary calculi, and gouty nephropathy.

Although all forms of gout have the common trait of hyperuricemia, their causes can be manifold. *Primary, or genetic, gout results from either increased synthesis of uric acid or decreased renal excretion of the substance.* Some gout patients have an unusual shunt mechanism that converts glycine directly to uric acid rather than to its normal metabolic products. *Secondary gout may result from either overproduction or impaired elimination of uric acid.* Overproduction is usually secondary to some other disorder, most frequently of hematological origin. For instance, in leukemia, myeloid metaplasia, lymphoma, polycythemia vera, and rapid weight loss (dieting), breakdown of cellular nucleoprotein is increased, which can lead to excess formation of uric acid.

In secondary gout, diminished elimination of uric acid can be due to lead nephropathy, glycogen storage disease, or sickle cell anemia. In addition, several drugs, including salicylates, pyrazinamide, alcohol, ethambutol, nicotinic acid, cyclosporine, fructose, cytotoxic agents, and certain diuretics (e.g., thiazides, furosemide, bumetanide) will impair the renal elimination of uric acid. These drugs competitively inhibit the active secretion of uric acid (see Chapter 4) into the urine, with resulting hyperuricemia.

CHEMISTRY OF URIC ACID

Humans excrete approximately 0.7 g uric acid daily. Most of this is derived from the metabolic breakdown of the purine bases adenine and guanine. Uric acid is less ionized and less water soluble at most acidic pH's. It exists mostly as the monovalent salt *sodium urate*. However, uric acid itself may be the predominant form found in an acid urine. Because the urine becomes more acidic as it moves through the renal tubular system, filtered urate is increasingly converted to uric acid. The relatively limited solubility of urate at a urinary pH of 5 is clinically significant in patients with gout because of the possibility of the formation of uric acid stones.

RENAL URATE HOMEOSTASIS

The binding of uric acid to plasma proteins is relatively small and probably does not have great physiological significance. However, even this limited binding may be affected by administration of drugs, such as salicylates, phenylbutazone, probenecid, and sulfinpyrazone. These drugs probably affect urate protein binding only secondarily; that is, their principal action is to interfere with renal transport of uric acid, which in turn leads to alterations in plasma urate binding.

The renal mechanisms involved in the handling of uric acid are complex and involve filtration, reabsorption, secretion, and possibly postsecretory reabsorption. The proximal tubule is the principal site of both carrier-mediated reabsorption and secretion of urate. Urate is believed to be transported from the ultrafiltrate to the intracellular space by an anion (hydroxyl, bicarbonate, chloride, or lactate) exchange mechanism in the *luminal membrane*. This active transport system can be inhibited by drugs, such as probenecid, sulfinpyrazone, and salicylate. The urate accumulated in the cell moves passively across the basolateral membrane and into the peritubular fluid down its electrochemical gradient. Conversely, active tubular secretion of urate occurs as a consequence of carrier-mediated transport across the *basolateral membrane* of the proximal tubule. The urate accumulated in the cell moves passively across the luminal membrane into the ultrafiltrate along its concentration gradient. The carrier-mediated secretion of urate can be inhibited by a variety of organic anions, including the thiazide and loop diuretics.

The intracellular concentration of urate in the proximal tubule will ultimately be determined by the balance of influx and efflux. When the transport of urate from the *peritubular fluid* is high, there is a net elimination of urate across the luminal membrane. In contrast, when the transport of urate from *luminal fluid* is high, there is a net reabsorption across the basolateral membrane.

Urate excretion is subject to modification by a variety of organic anions, including uricosuric agents, phenylbutazone, diuretics, radiographic contrast agents, and certain anticancer compounds. A further complicating feature is that drug effects may be biphasic; that is, small amounts may depress urate excretion, while larger doses have uricosuric effects.

RELATIONSHIP OF URIC ACID LEVELS TO GOUT

The degree of risk of acquiring gouty arthritis is related primarily to the extent and duration of the hyperuricemia. The risk is essentially zero at serum urate concentration below 7 mg/dL, whereas at concentrations of 10 to 11 mg/dL, the likelihood of having the disorder is relatively high. Gouty arthritis due to impaired renal excretion of uric acid may be diagnosed through a quantification of the patient's uric acid excretion. If a patient on a purine-restricted diet for 1 week excretes more than 600 mg uric acid per 24 hours, the individual is probably an overproducer. If, however, less than 350 mg of uric acid is eliminated in 24 hours, suspect impaired renal function.

ROLE OF PHAGOCYTOSIS IN ACUTE GOUTY ARTHRITIS

The mere presence of urate crystals in the joint cannot be correlated with the appearance of acute gouty arthritic symptoms. Individuals who have never had any gouty arthritic problems have nonetheless been found to have uric acid deposited on their articular cartilage. Acute attacks are generally the result of granulocytic phagocytosis of the urate crystals. This engulfing of the crystals is accompanied by cellular release of chemotactic lipids, lysosomal enzymes, and acidic substances into the synovial tissues. The lipids appear to trigger further phagocytosis, whereas the acidic compounds decrease local pH to the point that increased urate crystal formation is favored.

In addition to the phagocytic activity of the leukocytes, small peptide substances, such as the kinins, which are thought to be partially responsible for the local inflammatory response in gouty arthritis, accumulate in the joint space. The inflammation is associated with local vasodilation, increased vascular permeability, and pain.

PRINCIPLES OF GOUT MANAGEMENT

Initial treatment of gout and its associated hyperuricemia must involve therapy directed toward terminating the painful inflammatory process that is a prominent feature of acute gouty arthritis. A variety of nonsteroidal antiinflammatory compounds (e.g., indomethacin, oxyphenbutazone, ibuprofen, naproxen, sulindac) can be administered either alone or in combination with *colchicine,* a relatively specific agent for use in acute gouty attacks. Glucocorticosteroids, such as prednisone, can be given as a tapered dose over 10 days to replace colchicine. These steroids cause fewer side effects than does colchicine. If the diagnosis is uncertain, colchicine should be used, since a response to this drug is generally taken as establishing the diagnosis of acute gouty arthritis.

Although the treatment of the hyperuricemia of gout depends upon lowering blood uric acid levels, most physicians caution against employing drugs such as *allopurinol, probenecid,* or *sulfinpyrazone* during an acute attack, since the therapy itself, at least during the initial stages, may exacerbate the condition. Once the acute symptoms are under control and the patient is asymptomatic, appropriate treatment should include not only drug therapy but also management of body weight and control of dietary purine intake. *Long-term treatment is directed toward decreasing uric acid production from nucleoprotein, increasing excretion, or both.*

Uric acid production is more easily controlled by drug therapy than by dietary restriction, because only a small portion of blood uric acid is derived from the dietary intake of purines. Excretion of uric acid may be increased by increasing the rate of urine flow or by using uricosuric agents. Since uric acid is filtered at the glomerulus and both actively secreted and reabsorbed by the proximal tubule cells, both approaches are effective.

Since overproducers are already excreting large quantities of uric acid in their urine, drugs that further increase the rate of excretion (i.e., uricosuric compounds) increase the likelihood of renal stone formation. In these patients, the use of a compound that inhibits uric acid synthesis is preferable. Although at first glance the use of a combination of drugs—a drug that reduces production along with one that is uricosuric—would seem to be a rational therapeutic approach, in practice this has not worked well. Apparently the effectiveness of a drug that inhibits uric acid synthesis can be diminished by uricosuric agents, and therefore the combination has less value than each drug used separately. Furthermore, side effects appear to occur more frequently during combination drug therapy.

COLCHICINE

Gouty inflammation of the tissues or joints is associated with local accumulation of urate microcrystals by the phagocytic neutrophils. After sufficient amounts of these crystals have been taken up into the phagolysosomes of the neutrophil, these organelles disrupt and release their degradative enzymes, accumulated microcrystals (which may be rephagocytized), and chemotac-

tic factors. It is these released substances that are responsible for much of the local inflammation and pain associated with acute attacks of gout.

Colchicine, an alkaloid obtained from the autumn crocus, has long been used and is relatively selective for the treatment of acute gouty arthritis. Unlike many of the newer agents for use in gout, *colchicine has minimal effects on uric acid synthesis and excretion;* it decreases inflammation associated with this disorder. *It is thought that colchicine somehow prevents the release of the chemotactic factors and/or inflammatory cytokines from the neutrophils, and this in turn decreases the attraction of more neutrophils into the affected area* (Fig. 37.1). The ability of colchicine to bind to leukocyte microtubules in a reversible covalent complex and cause their depolymerization also may be a factor in decreasing the attraction of the motile leukocytes into the inflamed area.

Colchicine is rapidly absorbed after oral administration and tends to concentrate in the spleen, kidney, liver, and gastrointestinal tract. Leukocytes also avidly accumulate and store colchicine even after a single intravenous injection. Since colchicine can accumulate in cells against a concentration gradient, it is postulated that an active transport process may be involved in its cellular uptake. The drug is metabolized, primarily in the liver, by deacetylation. Fecal excretion plays a major role in colchicine elimination, since it and its metabolites are readily secreted into the bile. Only about 15 to 30% of the drug is eliminated in the urine except in patients with liver disease; urinary excretion is more important in these individuals.

The major use of colchicine is as an antiinflammatory agent in the treatment of acute gouty arthritis; it is not effective in reducing inflammation in other disorders. It also can be used to prevent attacks. Since colchicine is so rapidly effective in relieving the acute symptoms of gout (substantial improvement is achieved within hours), it has been used as a diagnostic aid in this disorder.

Therapy with colchicine is usually begun at the first sign of an attack and is continued until symptoms subside, adverse gastrointestinal reactions appear, or a maximum dose of 6 to 7 mg has been reached. The drug can be given intravenously as well as orally, but care must be exercised, since extravasated drug may result in local sloughing of skin and subcutaneous tissues. Relief of pain and inflammation usually occurs within 48 hours. Small doses of colchicine can be used during asymptomatic periods to minimize the reappearance or severity of acute attacks. It should be used with caution in patients with preexisting compromised heart, kidney, gastrointestinal tract, and liver disease.

Diarrhea, nausea, vomiting, and abdominal pain are the major limiting side effects that ultimately determine the tolerated dosage. These symptoms occur in approximately 80% of patients who take colchicine, especially

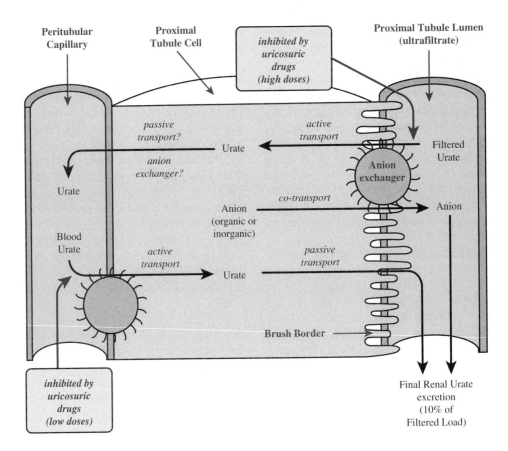

FIGURE 37.1
Renal handling of uric acid. Uric acid may be actively reabsorbed from the ultrafiltrate following its glomerular filtration or it may be secreted from the blood across the basolateral membrane into the proximal tubular cell. Both passive and active transport mechanisms are involved in the handling of urate. Uricosuric drugs at appropriate doses interfere with these processes.

in those taking high dosages. The hepatobiliary recycling of colchicine and its antimitotic effect on cells that are rapidly turning over, such as those of the intestinal epithelium, account for its gastrointestinal toxicity. Gastrointestinal symptoms generally intervene before the appearance of more serious toxicity and thereby provide a margin of safety in drug administration. Ingestion of large doses of colchicine may be followed by a burning sensation in the throat, bloody diarrhea, shock, hematuria, oliguria, and central nervous system (CNS) depression.

URICOSURIC AGENTS

The uricosuric drugs (or urate diuretics) are anions that are somewhat similar to urate in structure; therefore, they can compete with uric acid for transport sites. Small doses of uricosuric agents will actually decrease the total excretion of urate by inhibiting its tubular secretion. *The quantitative importance of the secretory mechanism is relatively minor, however, and at high dosages these same drugs increase uric acid elimination by inhibiting its proximal tubular reabsorption.* Thus, uricosuric drugs have a seemingly paradoxical effect on both serum and urinary uric acid levels: at low doses, they increase serum levels while decreasing the urinary levels; they have the opposite effect on these two levels at high dosages.

The two most clinically important uricosuric drugs, probenecid and sulfinpyrazone, are organic acids. *The initial phase of therapy with uricosuric drugs is the most dangerous period.* Until uricosuric drug levels build up sufficiently to fully inhibit uric acid reabsorption as well as secretion, there may be a temporary increase in uric acid blood levels that significantly increases the risk of an acute gouty attack. Therefore, *it is wise to begin therapy with the administration of small amounts of colchicine before adding a uricosuric drug to the therapeutic regimen.* In addition, the initial rise in urinary uric acid concentrations during uricosuric drug therapy may result in renal stone formation.

Probenecid

When probenecid (*ColBENEMID*) is given in sufficient amounts, *it will block the active reabsorption of uric acid in the proximal tubules following its glomerular filtration,* thereby increasing the amount of urate eliminated. In contrast, low dosages of probenecid appear to compete preferentially with plasma uric acid for the proximal tubule anionic transport system and thereby block its access to this active secretory system. The uricosuric action of probenecid, however, is accounted for by the drug's ability to inhibit the active reabsorption of *filtered* urate.

Probenecid is rapidly absorbed after oral administration, with peak plasma levels usually reached in 2 to 4 hours. Its half-life is somewhat variable (6–12 hours) because of both its extensive plasma protein binding and its active proximal tubular secretion. Since tubular back-diffusion is decreased at alkaline urinary pH ranges, probenecid excretion increases with increasing urinary pH. Probenecid is rapidly metabolized, with less than 5% of an administered dose being eliminated in 24 hours. The major metabolite is an acyl monoglucuronide.

Probenecid is an effective and relatively safe agent for controlling hyperuricemia and preventing tophi deposition in tissues. Chronic administration will decrease the incidence of acute gouty attacks as well as diminish the complications usually associated with hyperuricemia, such as renal damage and tophi deposition. Probenecid is still used by some physicians to maintain high blood levels of penicillin, cephalosporin, acyclovir, and cyclosporine. It is not useful in treating acute attacks of gouty arthritis. If the total amount of uric acid excreted is greater than 800 mg/day, the urine should be alkalinized to prevent kidney stone formation and promote uric acid.

Probenecid can impair the renal active secretion of a variety of acidic compounds, including sulfinpyrazone, sulfonylureas, indomethacin, penicillin, sulfonamides, and 17-ketosteroids. If these agents are to be given concomitantly with probenecid, their dosage should be modified appropriately. *Salicylates interfere with the clinical effects of both sulfinpyrazone and probenecid and should be avoided in patients treated with uricosuric agents.* Uricosuric agents also can influence the volume of distribution and hepatic metabolism of a number of drugs.

Adverse reactions associated with probenecid therapy include occasional rashes, allergic dermatitis, upper gastrointestinal tract irritation, and drowsiness. The drug is contraindicated in patients with a history of renal calculi.

Sulfinpyrazone

Sulfinpyrazone (*Anturane*), another uricosuric agent, is chemically related to the antiinflammatory and uricosuric compound phenylbutazone. However, it lacks the antiinflammatory, analgesic, and sodium-retaining properties of phenylbutazone and possesses a number of undesirable side effects that limit its therapeutic usefulness. The mechanism of sulfinpyrazone's uricosuric activity is similar to that of probenecid.

Sulfinpyrazone is readily absorbed after oral administration, with peak blood levels reached 1 to 2 hours after ingestion. It is more highly bound to plasma protein (98–99%) than is probenecid (84–94%) and is a more potent uricosuric agent. Most of the drug (90%) is eliminated through active proximal tubular secretion of the intact parent compound. Sulfinpyrazone also undergoes *p*-hydroxylation to form a uricosuric metabolite, the formation of which undoubtedly contributes to the drug's prolonged activity (about 10 hours) and potency relative to probenecid. In contrast to probenecid, the rate of excretion of sulfinpyrazone is not enhanced by alkalinization of the urine, since the drug is largely ionized at all urinary pH ranges and therefore not a candidate for passive back-diffusion.

Sulfinpyrazone, although less effective than allopurinol in reducing serum uric acid levels, remains useful for the prevention or reduction of the joint changes and tophus deposition that would otherwise occur in chronic gout; it has no antiinflammatory properties. During the initial period of sulfinpyrazone use, acute attacks of gout may increase in frequency and severity. It is recommended, therefore, that either colchicine or a nonsteroidal antiinflammatory agent be coadministered during early sulfinpyrazone therapy.

Abdominal pain, nausea, and possible reactivation of peptic ulcer have been reported. The drug should be used with caution in patients with compromised renal function, and adequate fluid intake should always accompany sulfinpyrazone administration to minimize the possibility of renal calculus formation.

Allopurinol

Allopurinol (Zyloprim) *is the drug of choice in the treatment of chronic tophaceous gout* and is especially useful in patients whose treatment is complicated by renal insufficiency.

Mechanism of Action

Allopurinol, in contrast to the uricosuric drugs, *reduces serum urate levels through a competitive inhibition of uric acid synthesis* rather than by impairing renal urate reabsorption. This action is accomplished by inhibiting *xanthine oxidase,* the enzyme involved in the metabolism of hypoxanthine and xanthine to uric acid. After enzyme inhibition, the urinary and blood concentrations of uric acid are greatly reduced and there is a simultaneous increase in the excretion of the more soluble uric acid precursors, xanthine and hypoxanthine.

Allopurinol itself is metabolized by xanthine oxidase to form the active metabolite oxypurinol, which tends to accumulate after chronic administration of the parent drug. This phenomenon contributes to the therapeutic effectiveness of allopurinol in long-term use. *Oxypurinol is probably responsible for the antigout effects of allopurinol.* Oxypurinol itself is not administered because it is not well absorbed orally.

Absorption, Metabolism, and Excretion

Allopurinol is largely absorbed after oral ingestion, reaching peak blood levels in about 1 hour. In contrast to the uricosuric drugs, allopurinol is not appreciably bound to plasma proteins and is only a minor substrate for renal secretory mechanisms. The formation of oxypurinol and the finding that this metabolite is in part actively reabsorbed in the proximal tubule account for the long half-life of the metabolite (18–20 hours) and permits once-a-day drug administration.

Clinical Uses

Allopurinol is especially indicated in the treatment of chronic tophaceous gout, since patients receiving it show a pronounced decrease in their serum *and* urinary uric acid levels. Because it does not depend on renal mechanisms for its efficacy, allopurinol is particularly beneficial for patients who already have developed renal uric acid stones, patients with excessively high urate excretion (e.g., above 1,200 mg in 24 hours), patients with a variety of blood disorders (e.g., leukemia, polycythemia vera), patients with excessive tophus deposition, and patients who fail to respond well to the uricosuric drugs.

Allopurinol also inhibits reperfusion injury. This injury occurs when organs that either have been transplanted or have had their usual blood perfusion blocked are reperfused with blood or an appropriate buffer solution. The cause of this injury is local formation of free radicals, such as the superoxide anion, the hydroxyl free radical, or peroxynitrite. These substances are strong oxidants and are quite damaging to tissues.

Adverse Effects

Common toxicities associated with allopurinol administration include a variety of skin rashes, gastrointestinal upset, hepatotoxicity, and fever. These reactions are often sufficiently severe to dictate termination of drug therapy. It is advised that therapy not be initiated during an acute attack of gouty arthritis. As with the uricosuric drugs, *therapy with allopurinol should be accompanied both by a sufficient increase in fluid intake to ensure water diuresis and by alkalinization of the urine.* Prophylactic use of colchicine also helps to prevent acute attacks of gout that may be brought on during the initial period of allopurinol ingestion.

Drug Interactions

Since allopurinol is metabolized by the hepatic microsomal drug-metabolizing enzymes, coadministration of drugs also metabolized by this system should be done with caution. Because allopurinol inhibits the oxidation of mercaptopurine and azathioprine, their individual administered doses must be decreased by as much as 75% when they are given together with allopurinol. Allopurinol may also increase the toxicity of other cytotoxic drugs (e.g., vidarabine). The actions of allopurinol are not antagonized by the coadministration of salicylates.

OTHER DRUGS

A number of drugs other than those discussed in detail in this chapter have been used to control the symptoms of acute gouty arthritis. Since the principal aspects of their pharmacology have been described elsewhere, they are mentioned only briefly here.

Indomethacin (*Indocin*) (see Chapter 36) exerts antiinflammatory, antipyretic, and analgesic properties. These qualities make it useful for the short-term management of the symptoms of acute gouty arthritis, although it has little effect on serum uric acid levels. Its antiinflammatory activity and ability to inhibit leukocytic phagocytosis make it particularly valuable in treating the early stages of gout, because a decrease in the leukocytic phagocytosis of urate crystals results in a decrease in the amount of peptides, prostaglandins, and other substances released from leukocyte lysosome organelles.

Phenylbutazone (*Butazolidin, Tandearil*) (see Chapter 36) also displays antipyretic, analgesic, and antiinflammatory activity. In addition, it possesses some uricosuric potency and therefore is widely used for the treatment of acute attacks of gouty arthritis, in which it is about equal to colchicine in effectiveness. Although the drug does promote the renal excretion of uric acid, its usefulness is generally attributed to its antiinflammatory actions.

Oxyphenbutazone (*Oxalid, Tandearil*) is the principal uricosuric metabolite of phenylbutazone. It has the same indications and toxicities as phenylbutazone.

Corticosteroids

The use of corticosteroids is often suggested for elderly patients with chronic tophaceous gout, since gout in the older individual often displays symptoms similar to those of rheumatoid arthritis. Patients can be given short-term administration of corticosteroids, especially for acute flare-ups. The concomitant use of alcohol, nonsteroidal antiinflammatory drugs, and most diuretics should be avoided.

Study QUESTIONS

1. The most widely used agent for the treatment of acute gouty arthritis is
   (A) Probenecid
   (B) Allopurinol
   (C) Colchicine
   (D) Indomethacin
   (E) Phenylbutazone

2. The mechanism by which probenecid lowers plasma levels of uric acid is
   (A) By inhibiting proximal tubular reabsorption of uric acid
   (B) By inhibiting production of uric acid in the liver
   (C) By promoting tubular secretion of uric acid
   (D) By inhibiting breakdown of purines to uric acid

3. Allopurinol reduces serum urate levels by
   (A) Promoting the active secretion of uric acid in kidneys
   (B) Inhibiting uric acid synthesis
   (C) Impairing renal urate reabsorption
   (D) Decreasing metabolism of uric acid

4. The primary location in the kidney where both carrier-mediated reabsorption and secretion of urate occurs is the
   (A) Ascending loop of Henle
   (B) Distal tubules
   (C) Collecting duct
   (D) Proximal tubule
   (E) Descending loop of Henle

5. Drug therapy is more effective in controlling uric acid production than is dietary restriction because
   (A) Dietary restriction does not affect production of uric acid
   (B) Drug therapy is more specific to the site of action
   (C) Only a small portion of blood uric acid is derived from the diet
   (D) The source of uric acid cannot be established

ANSWERS

1. **C.** Colchicine is relatively selective for the treatment of acute gouty arthritis because it appears to prevent the release of inflammatory cytokines and chemotactic factors. Probenecid (A) blocks renal uric acid reabsorption but is generally not used alone during the acute phase of gout. Allopurinol (B) is the drug of choice in chronic tophaceous gout. Indomethacin (D) and phenylbutazone (E) have antiinflammatory activity and are useful in treating acute gouty arthritis but are not used nearly as widely as colchicine for initial treatment.

2. **A.** Probenecid blocks active reabsorption of uric acid in the proximal tubules following glomerular filtration. It does not inhibit uric acid synthesis (B), stimulate tubular secretion (C), or inhibit the metabolism of purines (D).

3. **B.** Allopurinol inhibits xanthine oxidase, the enzyme involved in the conversion of hypoxanthine and xanthine to uric acid. It has no known ability to increase uric acid synthesis markedly (A), inhibit reabsorption (C), or impair uric acid breakdown (D).

4. **D.** While the other parts of the renal tubular system do contain active transport systems, these systems do not have an affinity of urate transport.

5. **C.** The dietary intake of purines is not a major contributing factor to uric acid blood levels. Therefore, pharmacological reduction of uric acid synthesis or increased excretion is required. Dietary restriction (A) can affect uric acid production if precursor molecules are lowered sufficiently, but this usually is not feasible. The question of drug specificity (B) is not germane to the question. Pathways of uric acid synthesis in the body (D) are well known.

SUPPLEMENTAL READING

Emmerson BT. The management of gout. N Engl J Med 1996;334:445–451.

Gonzalex EB, Miller SB, and Agudelo CaA. Optimal management of gout in older patients. Drug Ther 1994;4:128–134.

Grantham JJ and Chonko AM. Renal handling of organic anions and cations: Excretion of uric acid. In Brenner BM and Rector FC (eds.). *The Kidney* (4th ed.). Philadelphia: Saunders, 1991.

Molad Y. Update on colchicine and its mechanism of action. Curr Rheumatol Rep 2002;4:252–256.

Schlesinger N and Schumacher HR Jr. Gout: Can management be improved? Curr Opin Rheumatol 2001;13:240–244.

Taylor CT, Brooks NC, and Kelley KW. Corticotropin for acute management of gout. Ann Pharmacother 2001;35:365–368.

Star VL and Hochberg MC. Prevention and management of gout. Drugs 1993; 45:212–222.

Terkeltaub RA. Gout and mechanisms of crystal-induced inflammation. Curr Opin Rheumatol 1993;5:510–516.

CASE Study   Injudicious Food Intake Can Lead to Pain

T. D. arrives in your office complaining of pain in his toe. He woke up in the middle of the night with the feeling that his large toe had been set on fire. He has inflammation over the ankle and toes of his right foot and complains of severe pain when you put slight pressure on the ankle. The patient is about 60 lb overweight. He consumes red meat at least 6 times a week, always with three or more glasses of red wine. You suspect that T. D. may be having an attack of acute gout. What do you do?

ANSWER: You first take a blood sample for determination of serum urate levels to substantiate your preliminary diagnosis. Pending the results of the serum urate determination, you prescribe an NSAID. Upon finding a serum urate level of 12 mg/dL and continuing pain, you prescribe colchicine. You tell your patient that he must strongly consider dietary restriction, particularly of meat and meat products. Furthermore, he should decrease his alcohol intake. Inform him that if his attacks return in spite of changes in lifestyle, you are likely going to institute other drug measures. Point out the long-term consequences of gout.

38

Histamine and Histamine Antagonists

Knox Van Dyke and Karen A. Woodfork

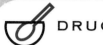 DRUG LIST

GENERIC NAME	PAGE	GENERIC NAME	PAGE
Brompheniramine	454	Diphenhydramine	454
Carbinoxamine	454	Famotidine	455
Cetirizine	453	Fexofenadine	453
Chlorpheniramine	454	Hydroxyzine	454
Cimetidine	455	Loratadine	453
Clemastine	454	Meclizine	455
Cromolyn sodium	455	Nedocromil	455
Cyclizine	455	Promethazine	455
Cyproheptadine	454	Pyrilamine	455
Desloratadine	453	Ranitidine	455
Dimenhydrinate	455	Tripelennamine	454

HISTAMINE

Sinus problems, hay fever, bronchial asthma, hives, eczema, contact dermatitis, food allergies, and reactions to drugs are all allergic reactions associated with the release of histamine and other autocoids, such as serotonin, leukotrienes, and prostaglandins. Histamine release is frequently associated with various inflammatory states and may be increased in urticarial reactions, mastocytosis, and basophilia. Histamine also acts as a neurotransmitter in the central nervous system (CNS). Upon release from its storage sites, histamine exerts effects ranging from mild irritation and itching to anaphylactic shock and eventual death.

Histamine is found in animal tissues and venoms and in many bacteria and plants. Within the human body, the largest histamine concentrations are in the skin, lungs, and gastrointestinal mucosa, while concentrations are smaller in almost all other organs and tissues. Histamine is present in human plasma at relatively low concentrations (usually less than 0.5 ng/mL); in contrast, whole-blood levels can be as high as 30-fold greater. Substantial quantities of histamine are present in urine, with excretion rates varying from 10 to 40 μg per 24 hours.

Synthesis and Storage

Virtually all of the histamine found in individual organs and tissues is synthesized locally and stored in subcellular secretory granules. *Within the tissues, the mast cells are the principal sites of storage; in the blood, the ba-*

449

sophils serve this function. Histamine is also present in neurons of the CNS, where it acts as a neurotransmitter.

Histamine is synthesized from the amino acid histidine by an action of the enzyme *histidine decarboxylase* (Fig. 38.1). Following synthesis, histamine is either rapidly inactivated or stored in the secretory granules of mast cells and basophils as an inactive complex with proteases and heparin sulfate or chondroitin sulfate.

Release from Storage Sites

Histamine can be released from mast cell granules in two ways, both of which have pharmacological impor-

tance. Endogenous or exogenous compounds can promote an exocytotic release of histamine without cell destruction or lysis. Alternatively, histamine can be released from mast cells by a variety of nonexocytotic processes, including mast cell lysis, modification of mast cell membranes, and physical displacement of histamine.

Both *exocytotic* and *nonexocytotic* mechanisms can contribute to adverse drug reactions that involve histamine release. Histamine is only one of several potent physiological mediators that are released from mast cells; the other substances can also contribute to the overall immediate hypersensitivity reaction.

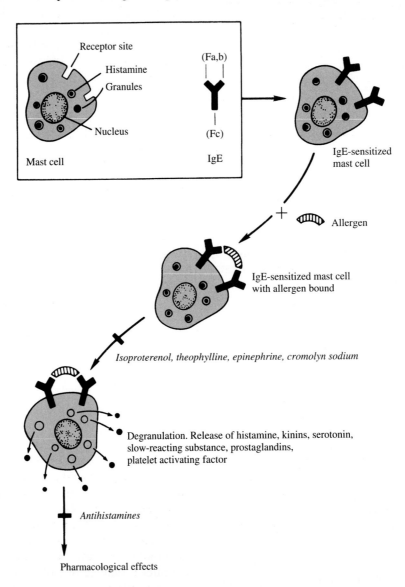

FIGURE 38.1

IgE-mediated release of mast cell contents. *Inset,* Intact mast cell with histamine stored in granules. An IgE antibody molecule is depicted adjacent to the mast cell. Two IgE molecules combine with a mast cell (sensitization). The attachment of an antigen (allergen) to the sensitized mast cell initiates release of histamine (and other substances) from the mast cell. This degranulation can be prevented by such agents as isoproterenol, theophylline, epinephrine, and cromolyn sodium. H_1 antihistamines do not interfere with degranulation but instead prevent actions of histamine at various pharmacological receptors.

Antigen-Mediated Histamine Release

Specific antigen–antibody interactions initiate the degranulation of tissue mast cells and blood basophils as part of the immediate hypersensitivity reaction. Immunoglobulin E (IgE) antibodies (reaginic antibodies) directed against an allergenic substance attach to the outer surface of the cell membrane and initiate a series of biochemical events that culminate in the release of the secretory granule contents (Fig. 38.1). Although allergens are the most frequent initiators of immediate hypersensitivity reactions, certain drugs, particularly in association with endogenous high-molecular-weight molecules, may also promote the sensitization process and mast cell degranulation on subsequent drug exposure.

Certain endogenous and exogenous compounds modulate the antigen-mediated release of histamine from sensitized tissues. Histamine inhibits its own release in skin mast cells and blood basophils by binding to H_2 histamine receptors, which when activated, inhibit degranulation. This feedback inhibition does not appear to occur in lung mast cells. Agonists of β_2-adrenoceptors inhibit antigen-induced histamine release from mast cells, whereas muscarinic and α-adrenergic agonists enhance mast cell degranulation.

Non–Antigen-Mediated Release of Histamine

Histamine may be released from mast cells by mechanisms that do not require prior sensitization of the immune system. Drugs, high-molecular-weight proteins, venoms, and other substances that damage or disrupt cell membranes can induce the release of histamine. Any thermal or mechanical stress of sufficient intensity also will result in histamine release. Cytotoxic compounds, may release histamine as the result of disruption of cell membranes.

Drugs, particularly organic bases, may release histamine from mast cells by physically displacing the amine from its storage sites. Morphine, codeine, d-tubocurarine, guanethidine, and radiocontrast media can release histamine from mast cells. Basic polypeptides, such as bradykinin, neurotensin, substance P, somatostatin, polymyxin B, and the anaphylatoxins resulting from complement activation, also stimulate histamine release. Venoms often contain basic polypeptides as well as the histamine-releasing enzyme phospholipase A.

Inactivation of Released Histamine

The inactivation of histamine is achieved both by enzymatic metabolism of the amine and by transport processes that reduce the concentration of the compound in the region of its receptors. Histamine metabolism occurs primarily through two pathways (Fig. 38.1). The most important of these involves *histamine N-methyltransferase*, which catalyzes the transfer of a methyl group from S-adenosyl-1-methionine to one of the imidazole nitrogen substitutions, forming 1-methylhistamine. This enzyme is present in tissues but not in blood. 1-Methylhistamine is converted by monoamine oxidase (MAO) to 1-methylimidazoleacetic acid.

An alternative pathway of histamine metabolism involves oxidative deamination by the enzyme *diamine oxidase (histaminase)* to form 5-imidazoleacetic acid. Diamine oxidase is present in both tissues and blood and plays a particular role in metabolizing the large concentrations of histamine that may be present in food. An additional metabolite, N-acetyl histamine (a conjugate of acetic acid and histamine), can be produced if histamine is ingested orally. This product may result from metabolism of histamine by gastrointestinal tract bacteria. Because of its rapid breakdown after oral administration, histamine produces few systemic effects when given by this route.

Physiological Effects of Histamine

Histamine mediates a diverse group of processes ranging from vasodilation to gastric acid secretion. It produces its effects by binding to and activating receptors on the surface of cardiac, smooth muscle, endothelial, neuronal, and other cells. There are at least four receptor populations, H_1, H_2, H_3, and H_4. All four receptor subtypes have been cloned and belong to the G protein–coupled receptor superfamily. The histamine receptors can be distinguished on the basis of their post–receptor signal transduction mechanisms, tissue distribution, and sensitivities to various agonists and antagonists (Table 38.1). Currently, only the H_1- and H_2-receptors are targets of clinical drug therapy.

Cardiovascular System

A slow intravenous injection of histamine produces marked vasodilation of the arterioles, capillaries, and venules. This causes a fall in blood pressure whose magnitude depends on the concentration of histamine injected, the degree of baroreceptor reflex compensation, and the extent of histamine-induced release of adrenal catecholamines. Vasodilation of cutaneous blood vessels reddens the skin of the face, while a throbbing headache can result from vasodilation of brain arterioles. Vasodilation is mediated through both H_1- and H_2-receptors on vascular smooth muscle. Stimulation of H_1-receptors produces a rapid and short-lived response, whereas stimulation of H_2-receptors produces a more sustained response that is slower in onset. Stimulation of H_3-receptors on sympathetic nerve terminals inhibits the release of norepinephrine and its associated vasoconstriction.

Histamine increases the permeability of capillaries and postcapillary vessels, resulting in passage of fluid

TABLE 38.1   Histamine Receptors

Receptor	G Protein	Intracellular Signaling	Tissue Distribution	Selective Agonists	Selective Antagonists
H_1	$G_{q/11}$	Phospholipase C–mediated Ca^{++} mobilization	Brain, smooth muscle, heart, endothelium	2-(3-trifluoromethyl) phenyl histamine	Mepyramine, chlorpheniramine, triplodine
H_2	G_s	Adenylyl cyclase–catalyzed cAMP production	Brain, stomach, smooth muscle, heart, mast cells	Arpromidine, impromidine, amthamine, dimaprit	Cimetidine, ranitidine, famotidine
H_3	$G_{i/o}$	Decreased Ca^{++} influx through G protein–coupled N-type Ca^{++} channels	Brain, autonomic nerve endings, some endothelia	Imetit, immepip, R-α-methylhistamine	Thioperamide, iodophenpropit, clobenpropit
H_4	$G_{i/o}$	Decreased Ca^{++} influx through G protein coupled N-type Ca^{++} channels	Bone marrow, brain, peripheral leukocytes, lung	–	–

and protein into the extracellular space and eventually edema. This H_1-receptor–mediated process is responsible for the urticarial effect of histamine on the skin (hives).

In addition to its effects on the vasculature, histamine exerts direct positive inotropic and chronotropic effects on the heart through the stimulation of H_2-receptors. H_3-receptors on sympathetic nerve terminals in the heart decrease norepinephrine release; however, this effect appears to be significant only during stress states such as ischemia.

Extravascular Smooth Muscle

Histamine stimulates bronchiolar smooth muscle contraction through activation of H_1-receptors. A much smaller bronchodilatory response is evoked by stimulation of H_2-receptors. Asthmatics are generally more sensitive to the bronchoconstrictor actions of histamine than are nonasthmatics.

Histamine is able to cause uterine contraction. Although the magnitude of this effect in humans is normally small, the large amounts of histamine released during anaphylactic reactions can initiate abortion in pregnant women. Histamine can also stimulate contraction of gastrointestinal smooth muscle, with large doses able to produce diarrhea.

Glandular Tissue

Histamine stimulates the secretion of gastric acid and pepsin through an effect on the H_2-receptors of the parietal cells of the gastric mucosa. Secretion of acid is a complex process that is stimulated by histamine, acetylcholine, and gastrin and inhibited by somatostatin. The ability of H_2-receptor antagonists to inhibit the enhanced gastric acid secretion caused by acetylcholine and gastrin suggests that histamine release is of primary importance in this process. Histamine also stimulates secretion by the salivary glands and glands in the small and large intestines. High concentrations of histamine promote the release of catecholamines from the adrenal gland.

Nervous System

Postsynaptic H_1- and H_2-receptors are responsible for a variety of processes in the CNS. H_1-receptors mediate the maintenance of wakeful states, while H_1- and H_2-receptors participate in the regulation of blood pressure, body temperature, fluid homeostasis, and pain sensation. Presynaptic H_3-receptors serve as feedback inhibitors of the release of histamine, norepinephrine, and other neurotransmitters.

In the periphery, H_1-receptors on sensory neurons in the epidermis and dermis mediate itch and pain, respectively. Autonomic afferent nerve endings may be similarly stimulated by histamine. As in the CNS, presynaptic H_3-receptors act in a feedback inhibitory capacity.

Lewis Triple Response

The *Lewis triple response* illustrates the effects of histamine on vascular smooth muscle, vascular endothelium, and sensory nerve endings. Intradermal injection of as little as 10 μg histamine produces three distinct effects:

1. Dilation of capillaries in the immediate vicinity of the injection results in a local red or blue region (*flush*).
2. Dilation of arterioles results in an irregular red *flare* over an area that is generally wider than that due to the capillary dilation. The flare probably results from an axon reflex in which histamine stimulates autonomic nerve endings, causing release of vasodilatory mediators.

3. Swelling (*wheal*) appears in the area of capillary dilation. The increased permeability of the blood vessels in this region is responsible for the edema.

In addition to the flush, wheal, and flare, transient pain and itching result from the effects of histamine on sensory nerve endings. In sensitized individuals, intradermal injection of specific antigens produces a wheal; this reaction is the basis for a skin test to quantify the extent of the allergic response.

Anaphylaxis

During an anaphylactic reaction, large quantities of inflammatory mediators are rapidly released. The resultant reaction is severe and may threaten the life of the individual. The introduction of a specific antigen—usually in food or in injected material—into a sensitized individual can cause the rapid release of mast cell contents, producing a decrease in blood pressure, impaired respiratory function, abdominal cramps, and urticaria. Extreme and severe anaphylaxis is life threatening and requires prompt medical intervention.

Clinical Uses of Histamine

Histamine has only minor uses in clinical medicine. In the past it was used to diagnose pernicious anemia, in which histamine fails to evoke the usual secretion of gastric acid. Histamine has been used to assess bronchial hyperreactivity, although this test may be quite hazardous for asthmatics. Today the main clinical use of histamine is as a positive control injection for allergy skin testing.

HISTAMINE ANTAGONISM AND HISTAMINE ANTAGONISTS

The effects of histamine on body tissues and organs can be diminished in four ways: inhibition of histamine synthesis, inhibition of histamine release from storage granules, blockade of histamine receptors, and physiological antagonism of histamine's effects. Of these approaches, only the inhibition of histamine synthesis has not been employed clinically. The focus of this chapter is on H_1 histamine receptor antagonists; it provides a brief overview of the H_2 blockers and the inhibitors of histamine release. More details can be found in Chapters 39 and 40.

H_1-Receptor Antagonists

The most common use of the H_1-receptor antagonists is for the relief of allergic reactions such as rhinitis and urticaria. These compounds are also used to prevent motion sickness, to treat vestibular disturbances, such as Ménière's syndrome, and as over-the-counter sleep aids.

Chemistry

The H_1-receptor antagonists for the most part are substituted ethylamine compounds. In comparison with histamine, the H_1-antagonists contain no imidazole ring and have substituents on the side chain amino group.

The H_1-antagonists are classified as either first- or second-generation compounds. Second-generation antihistamines have lipophilicity and ionization profiles that make them less able to cross the blood-brain barrier; thus they produce dramatically less sedation than do the first-generation drugs.

Pharmacokinetics

First-generation antihistamines are well absorbed after oral administration, with peak blood levels occurring within 1 to 2 hours; the therapeutic effect usually lasts 4 to 6 hours, although some drugs are much longer acting (Table 38.2). These antagonists are generally metabolized in the liver through hydroxylation. The metabolites and a small amount of parent compound are excreted in the urine.

The second-generation H_1-receptor antagonists are also rapidly absorbed, with peak plasma concentrations being reached within 1 to 3 hours. Their duration of action generally varies between 4 and 24 hours (Table 38.2). Loratadine (*Claritin*) and its active metabolite, desloratadine (*Clarinex*), undergoes extensive first-pass metabolism and is converted by CYP3A4 isozymes to an active metabolite. A number of drug interactions result from the ability of various compounds to induce, inhibit, or compete for metabolism by this cytochrome P450 system. In contrast, cetirizine (*Zyrtec*) and fexofenadine (*Allegra*) undergo little hepatic metabolism and are eliminated mainly as unchanged compounds in the urine and feces, respectively.

The reduction in therapeutic effectiveness that can occur when antihistamines are given for long periods is probably related to an induction of hepatic drug-metabolizing enzymes. Children tend to eliminate antihistamines more rapidly than adults, while individuals with hepatic impairment may eliminate them more slowly.

Mechanism of Action

At therapeutic doses, the first- and second-generation antihistamines are equilibrium-competitive inhibitors of H_1-receptor–mediated responses. Certain second-generation drugs are noncompetitive inhibitors at high concentrations. Both first- and second-generation compounds have negligible abilities to block the H_2-, H_3-, or H_4-receptors. The therapeutic effectiveness of these

TABLE 38.2   Representative H₁Receptor Antagonists

Drug	Trade Name	Duration of Action (hr)	Sedative Activity	Anti–Motion Sickness Activity	Anticholinergic Activity
First-Generation Antihistamines					
Ethanolamines					
Carbinoxamine	Rondec	3–6	++		+++
Clemastine	Tavist	12	++		+++
Diphenhydramine	Benadryl	4–6	+++	++	+++
Dimenhydrinate	Dramamine	4–6	+++	++	+++
Ethylenediamines					
Pyrilamine	Ryna	4–6	++		+
Tripelennamine	PBZ	4–6	++		+
Alkylamines					
Chlorpheniramine	Chlor-Trimeton	4–6	+		+
Brompheniramine	Dimetane	4–6	+		+
Piperazines					
Cyclizine	Marezine	4–6	+	++	++
Hydroxyzine	Atarax		+++	+++	+++
Meclizine	Antivert	12–24	+	++	++
Phenothiazines					
Promethazine	Phenergan	4–6	+++	+++	+++
Piperidines					
Cyproheptadine	Periactin	4–6	++		++
Second-Generation Antihistamines					
Piperidines					
Loratadine	Claritin	24			
Fexofenadine	Allegra	12			
Piperazines					
Cetirizine	Zyrtec	12–24			

+, slight activity, ++, moderate activity, +++, marked activity

drugs arises from their capacity to block histamine-mediated vasoconstriction, microvascular permeability enhancement, and sensory nerve terminal stimulation. H₁-antagonists generally produce sedation through an effect on the CNS; however, excitation can occur when toxic dosages are ingested.

Many of these drugs have effects that are not mediated by H₁-receptors (Table 38.2). The antimuscarinic activity of several first-generation H₁-blockers may account for their effectiveness in combating motion sickness and their limited ability to suppress parkinsonian symptoms. The phenothiazines have some capacity to block α-adrenoceptors, whereas cyproheptadine (*Periactin*) is an antagonist at serotonin receptors. Diphenhydramine (*Benadryl*), pyrilamine (*Ryna*), and promethazine (*Phenergan*) are effective local anesthetics. Many second-generation antihistamines also have been found to inhibit the non–histamine-mediated release of various inflammatory substances; this may account for some of their effectiveness in allergic conditions.

Adverse Effects

Sedation is the most frequent adverse reaction to the first-generation antihistamines. An additive effect on alertness and motor skills will result if alcohol or another depressant is taken with these drugs. Antimuscarinic effects caused by these drugs include dry mouth and respiratory passages, urinary retention, and dysuria. Nausea, vomiting, constipation or diarrhea, dizziness, insomnia, nervousness, and fatigue also have been reported. Drug allergy, especially after topical application, is fairly common. Tolerance to certain antihistamines may develop after prolonged administration. Teratogenic effects of the piperazine antihistamines have been shown in animal studies. Epidemiological studies have not shown such an association in humans. The effects of toxic doses of first-generation antihistamines, similar to those seen following atropine administration, include excitement, hallucinations, dry mouth, dilated pupils, flushing, convulsions, urinary retention, sinus tachycardia, coma, and death.

The second-generation H_1-antagonists are often referred to as nonsedating antihistamines; however, doses above the usual therapeutic level can cause sleepiness in certain individuals. A more serious adverse effect of some earlier second-generation antihistamines is cardiotoxicity. Terfenadine (*Seldane*) and astemizole (*Hismanal*) were withdrawn from the U. S. market after they were found, in rare cases, to induce a potentially fatal ventricular arrhythmia, *torsades de pointes*. These drugs block the cardiac K^+ channels responsible for the repolarizing current (I_{Kr}) of the action potential (see Chapter 16) and therefore prolong the QT interval. Arrhythmias result when these drugs accumulate to toxic levels, such as when their metabolism is impaired, as in liver disease or following coadministration of drugs that inhibit the CYP3A family of enzymes. Fexofenadine, the active antihistaminic metabolite of terfenadine, does not produce *torsades de pointes*.

Clinical Uses

The H_1-receptor blocking drugs find their greatest use in the symptomatic treatment of allergic conditions. The second-generation antihistamines and the first-generation alkylamines are most frequently used to treat allergic rhinitis. Allergic conjunctivitis and the acute form of urticaria are also effectively treated with antihistamines. The allergic responses seen in susceptible individuals after intradermal injections of allergens (e.g., skin testing) can be prevented for several hours by prior administration of H_1-antagonists. However, the H_1-antagonists are not drugs of choice in acute anaphylactic emergencies or the viral-caused common cold.

Although the antihistamines are not useful as primary agents in the treatment of asthma, a number of studies have shown that the second-generation compounds are effective as adjunctive therapies in asthmatic patients with concomitant rhinitis, urticaria, or dermatitis. Cetirizine has been used to prevent the progression from atopic dermatitis to asthma in young children.

Another important use of H_1-antagonists is in the treatment of motion sickness. Diphenhydramine (*Benadryl*), dimenhydrinate (*Dramamine*), cyclizine (*Marezine*), and meclizine (*Antivert*) have anticholinergic activity and are the preferred antihistaminic agents for reducing the symptoms of motion sickness.

Diphenhydramine is known to be at least partially effective in Parkinson's disease, perhaps because of its anticholinergic properties.

Many H_1-receptor blocking drugs have sedative properties, and some have been used in over-the-counter sleep aids. The most widely used H_1-blocking drugs for sleep induction are diphenhydramine, promethazine, and pyrilamine.

H_2-Receptor Antagonists

The H_2-receptor blockers include cimetidine, famotidine, and ranitidine. These drugs are used to decrease gastric acid secretion in the treatment of peptic ulcer, gastroesophageal reflux disorder, and hypersecretory conditions, such as Zollinger-Ellison syndrome. The pharmacodynamics and clinical uses of these drugs are discussed in Chapter 40.

Cromolyn and Nedocromil

Although cromolyn sodium (*Intal*) and nedocromil sodium (*Tilade*) are widely known for their ability to prevent the release of histamine and other inflammatory mediators by mast cells during the early response to antigen challenge, these drugs have a wide variety of inhibitory effects on many cell types, including eosinophils, neutrophils, monocytes, and neurons. Cromolyn sodium and nedocromil sodium are used as pulmonary inhalants in the treatment of asthma. Nasal (*Nasalcrom*) and ophthalmic (*Opticrom*) preparations of cromolyn sodium can be used to reduce the symptoms of allergic rhinitis and conjunctivitis. More detailed information on these compounds may be found in Chapter 39.

New Directions in Antihistamine Therapy

None of the selective agonists and antagonists of H_3-receptors are available for clinical use. Antagonists of H_3-mediated inhibition of neurotransmission may have potential in the treatment of CNS disorders, since animal studies have found that these compounds may enhance learning, ameliorate learning deficits, and decrease seizure activity. H_3-receptor agonists have been shown to inhibit gastric acid release and block certain inflammatory processes. In cardiac ischemia, they can prevent the arrhythmia and cardiac damage that may result from norepinephrine overflow and thus may be useful in the treatment of myocardial infarction. Selective agonists and antagonists of H_4-receptors are not yet available.

Study QUESTIONS

1. The antigen-mediated release of histamine can
   (A) Be inhibited by the binding of histamine to H_3-receptors on mast cells
   (B) Be stimulated by β_2-adrenoceptor agonists
   (C) Be initiated by organic bases such as morphine without prior sensitization
   (D) Occur only in the tissues, not in the blood
   (E) Produce pain and itching through an effect on sensory nerve endings

2. Effects mediated by the H_1 histamine receptor include
   (A) Inhibition of gastric acid secretion
   (B) Induction of hepatic cytochrome P450 enzymes
   (C) Maintenance of a wakeful state
   (D) Bronchodilation
   (E) Vasoconstriction of arterioles

3. All four types of histamine receptors
   (A) Are found on the surface of mast cells and basophils
   (B) Are G protein–coupled
   (C) Modulate adenylyl cyclase activity
   (D) Are involved in the release of multiple neurotransmitters

4. Ms. Jones takes fexofenadine 60 mg twice a day for seasonal allergies. She comes to her physician with a sinus infection and receives a prescription for erythromycin, a drug known to inhibit CYP3A4. As a result of this drug interaction, you would expect Ms. Jones to
   (A) Exhibit no changes in fexofenadine elimination
   (B) Exhibit decreased metabolism of erythromycin, with potential toxicity
   (C) Be at risk for development of torsades de pointes, due to decreased metabolism of fexofenadine
   (D) Exhibit decreased elimination of fexofenadine without risk of torsades de pointes
   (E) Exhibit moderate anticholinergic effects commonly seen with fexofenadine

5. Mr. Smith has severe motion sickness during air travel. He will be flying to Brazil next week, and you, his physician, would like to prescribe an antihistamine to prevent motion sickness. Which of the following would be most effective?
   (A) Scopolamine
   (B) Dimenhydrinate
   (C) Chlorpheniramine
   (D) Fexofenadine
   (E) Tripelennamine

ANSWERS

1. **E.** Histamine inhibits its own release through an effect on H_2-receptors on mast cells. Its release is inhibited, not stimulated, by β_2-adrenoceptor agonists. Organic bases can displace histamine from its storage granules and cause non–antigen-mediated release of histamine; antigen-mediated release requires prior sensitization. Antigen-mediated histamine release occurs in both tissues and blood. Histamine stimulates sensory nerve endings, resulting in pain and itching.

2. **C.** Histamine stimulates gastric acid secretion through an effect on H_2-receptors of gastric parietal cells. Although certain antihistamines are metabolized by cytochrome P450 enzymes, histamine does not induce their production. Histamine helps to maintain a wakeful state through an effect on H_1-receptors. Histamine-mediated broncho*constriction* is mediated by H_1-receptors, while histamine-mediated vaso*dilation* occurs as a result of stimulation of H_1- and H_2-receptors.

3. **B.** H_2-receptors are found on the surface of mast cells and basophils. All four types of histamine receptors belong to the G protein–coupled receptor superfamily. Only H_2-receptors are coupled to adenylyl cyclase through the G protein G_s.

4. **A.** Fexofenadine undergoes little or no hepatic metabolism and is excreted primarily as unchanged drug. Therefore, administering an inhibitor of CYP3A4 would not affect fexofenadine elimination. Fexofenadine does not inhibit erythromycin metabolism, nor does it produce *torsades de pointes*. Unlike many first-generation antihistamines, fexofenadine does not have anticholinergic side effects.

5. **B.** Although scopolamine effectively combats motion sickness, it is an antimuscarinic agent, not an antihistamine. Dimenhydrinate is an antihistamine with significant antimuscarinic properties that are likely to contribute to its anti–motion sickness activity. Chlorpheniramine, fexofenadine, and tripelennamine are antihistamines without significant efficacy in the treatment of motion sickness.

SUPPLEMENTAL READING
Hough LB. Genomics meets histamine receptors: New subtypes, new receptors. Mol Pharmacol 2001;59:415–424.

Marshall GD Jr. Therapeutic options in allergic disease: Antihistamines as systemic antiallergic agents. J Allergy Clin Immunol 2000;106:S303–S309.

Nicolas JM. The metabolic profile of second-generation antihistamines. Allergy 2000;55:46–52.

Taglialatela M and Annunziato L. Evaluation of the cardiac safety of second-generation antihistamines. Allergy 2000;55 Suppl 60:22–30.

Walsh GM et al. New insights into the second-generation antihistamines. Drugs 2001;61:207–236.

CASE Study   Behavior Changes and the Bladder

Anisette Doe, a 28-year old woman, went to the emergency department with abdominal bloating and inability to void her bladder; she had been unable to urinate for 16 hours. A urinary catheter was inserted and 2.5 L of urine was withdrawn. Subsequent testing revealed no calculi or masses in the bladder, urethra, ureters, or kidneys. Ms. Doe's medical records indicated that she was being treated with clozapine for paranoid schizophrenia. She reported no significant side effects as a result of this treatment. For 2 days prior to admission to the hospital, Ms. Doe complained of a cold and was taking diphenhydramine (*Benadryl*) 50 mg every 6 to 8 hours. What is a possible explanation for the sudden onset of her inability to void her bladder?

The case in context: Clozapine is a newer antipsychotic that can, like other agents in its class, produce antimuscarinic side effects. Although Ms. Doe had not complained of anticholinergic effects prior to beginning treatment with a moderate dose of diphenhydramine, it is likely that the additive anticholinergic effects of clozapine and diphenhydramine resulted in urinary retention.

39 Drugs Used in Asthma

Theodore J. Torphy and Douglas W. P. Hay

DRUG LIST

GENERIC NAME	PAGE	GENERIC NAME	PAGE
Albuterol	460	Metaproterenol	461
Beclomethasone	465	Nedocromil sodium	467
Bitolterol	460	Pirbuterol	460
Cromolyn sodium	467	Prednisone	465
Epinephrine	462	Salmeterol	462
Flunisolide	465	Terbutaline	462
Fluticasone	465	Theophylline	463
Ipratropium	464	Triamcinolone	465
Isoproterenol	462	Zafirlukast	465
Montelukast	465	Zileuton	466

The word *asthma* is derived from a Greek word meaning difficulty in breathing. The clinical expression of asthma varies from a mild intermittent wheeze or cough to severe chronic obstruction that can restrict normal activity. Acute asthma attacks are triggered by a variety of stimuli, including exposure to allergens or cold air, exercise, and upper respiratory tract infections. Recently, a number of genetic polymorphisms have been associated with an increased risk of developing asthma. Thus, genetic factors probably contribute to the exaggerated response of the asthmatic airway to various environmental challenges. The most severe exacerbation of asthma, *status asthmaticus,* is a life-threatening condition that requires hospitalization and must be treated aggressively. Unlike most exacerbations of the disease, status asthmaticus is by definition unresponsive to standard therapy.

The most important outcomes for successful therapy of asthma are as follows:

- Prevent chronic and troublesome symptoms
- Maintain (near) normal pulmonary function
- Maintain normal activity levels
- Prevent recurrent exacerbations of asthma and minimize the need for emergency department visits or hospitalizations
- Provide optimal pharmacotherapy with minimal or no adverse effects

Pathophysiology

Asthma symptoms are produced by reversible narrowing of the airway, which increases resistance to airflow and consequently reduces the efficiency of movement of air to and from the alveoli. In addition to airway obstruction, cardinal features of asthma include inflammation and hyperreactivity of the airway. In contrast to *chronic obstructive pulmonary disease* (emphysema and chronic bronchitis), the airway obstruction associated with asthma is generally reversible. However, severe long-standing asthma changes the architecture of the airway. These changes, including smooth muscle hypertrophy and bronchofibrosis, can lead to an irreversible decrement in pulmonary function. These structural changes are limited to the airways. The lung parenchyma is generally spared.

An aberrant immune response associated with allergy appears to underlie asthma in most children over age 3 years and in most young adults; allergy-induced asthma is also known as *extrinsic asthma.* In contrast, a large number of patients, especially those who acquire asthma as older adults, have no discernible immunological basis for their condition, although airway inflammation remains a characteristic of the disease; this type of asthma is termed *intrinsic asthma.* Other patients may have both allergic and nonallergic forms of asthma.

Airway Obstruction

Three factors contribute to airway obstruction in asthma: (1) contraction of the smooth muscle that surrounds the airways; (2) excessive secretion of mucus and in some, secretion of thick, tenacious mucus that adheres to the walls of the airways; and (3) edema of the respiratory mucosa. Spasm of the bronchial smooth muscle can occur rapidly in response to a provocative stimulus and likewise can be reversed rapidly by drug therapy. In contrast, respiratory mucus accumulation and edema formation are likely to require more time to develop and are only slowly reversible.

Airway Inflammation

The recognition that asthma is a disease of airway inflammation (Fig. 39.1) *has fundamentally changed the*

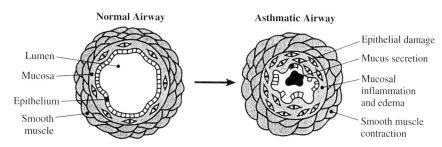

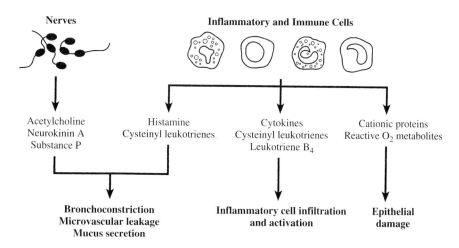

FIGURE 39.1

Cellular pathophysiology of asthma. *Top,* Cross-section of the normal airway and the asthmatic airway. Mediators released during the inflammatory process associated with asthma cause bronchoconstriction, mucus secretion, and mucosal inflammation and edema. These changes reduce the size of the airway lumen and increase resistance to airflow, which leads to wheezing and shortness of breath. *Bottom,* The multitude of inflammatory cells (macrophages, eosinophils, mast cells, neutrophils) and neurotransmitters implicated in asthma pathophysiology.

manner in which the disease is treated. Thus, it is useful to discuss the involvement of various mediators and inflammatory cells in antigen-induced asthma, an extensively studied, albeit simplistic, model of the disease. In this model, antigens, such as ragweed pollen or house mite dust, sensitize individuals by eliciting the production of antibodies of the immunoglobulin (Ig) E type. These antibodies attach themselves to the surface of *mast cells* and *basophils.* If the individual is reexposed to the same antigen days to months later, the resulting antigen–antibody reaction on lung mast cells will trigger the release of *histamine* and the *cysteinyl leukotrienes,* agents that produce bronchoconstriction, mucus secretion, and pulmonary edema. Mast cells also release a variety of chemotactic mediators, such as *leukotriene B₄* and *cytokines.* These agents recruit and activate additional inflammatory cells, particularly eosinophils and alveolar macrophages, both of which are also rich sources of leukotrienes and cytokines. *Ultimately, repeated exposure to antigen establishes a chronic inflammatory state in the asthmatic airway.*

TREATMENT STRATEGY

Clinical symptoms alone cannot be used as an accurate assessment of the severity of physiological impairment in the asthmatic patient, because a substantial degree of impairment may persist even after symptoms are relieved by treatment. Consequently, the overall objectives of antiasthma therapy are to return lung function to as near normal as possible and to prevent acute exacerbations of the disease. For quality of life, the ideal regimen permits normal activities, including exercise, with minimal or no side effects.

The primary classes of drugs used to treat asthma are bronchodilators and antiinflammatory agents. Bronchodilators include theophylline, a variety of adrenomimetic amines, and ipratropium bromide. Antiinflammatory therapy consists of the corticosteroids. A growing collection of drugs called *alternative therapies* cannot be classified clearly as either bronchodilators or antiinflammatory agents. These agents include the leukotriene modulators, cromolyn sodium, and nedocromil sodium.

Bronchodilators are used both in maintenance therapy and as needed to reverse acute attacks. These agents are often referred to as *relievers* because they provide rapid symptomatic relief but do not affect the fundamental disease process. Based on the underlying pathophysiology of the disease, *antiinflammatory therapy must be used in conjunction with bronchodilators in all but the mildest asthmatics.* Antiinflammatory agents are also called *controllers* because they provide long-term stabilization of symptoms. In addition to drug therapy, all treatment regimens should include patient education

focused on three key behaviors: (1) the appropriate use of medications to control symptoms (e.g., proper technique for use of metered-dose inhalers), (2) recognition of the signs of a deteriorating disease status (e.g., a progressive increase in the use of bronchodilators), and (3) prevention strategies (e.g., avoidance of antigenic material; influenza vaccination to forestall virus-induced exacerbations).

Pharmacotherapy of asthma is managed in a stepwise fashion according to the severity of the disease. Recommendations for the stepwise treatment of asthma in adults and children older than 5 years of age are shown in Table 39.1.

BRONCHODILATORS

When administered in sufficient quantities by an appropriate route, bronchodilators will usually reduce the work of breathing, relieve asthmatic symptoms, and improve ventilation. Bronchodilators can produce a substantial increase in pulmonary function by relaxing bronchial smooth muscle, thus dilating the airways. Commonly used bronchodilators are discussed next.

Adrenomimetic Agents

Adrenergic drugs (Table 39.2) used for the management of acute and chronic asthma are epinephrine (*Primatene*), isoproterenol (*Isuprel*), and a group of adrenoceptor agonists, including albuterol (*Proventil, Ventolin, Salbutamol*), terbutaline (*Brethine, Brethaire*), and salmeterol (*Serevent*), that are relatively selective for β₂-adrenoceptors (see Chapter 10). *This class of agents has become the mainstay of modern bronchodilator therapy.* These agents are used both as needed to reverse acute episodes of bronchospasm and prophylactically to maintain airway patency over the long term.

Basic Pharmacology

The general pharmacological actions of adrenomimetics are described in detail in Chapter 10. The principal pharmacological effects that may be observed in humans treated for bronchospasm are bronchodilation, tachycardia, anxiety, and tremor. Stimulating β₂-adrenoceptors produces all of these effects either directly or indirectly.

Epinephrine activates both α- and β-adrenoceptors, whereas isoproterenol is selective for β-adrenoceptors but does not discriminate between β₁- and β₂-adrenoceptors. Much-improved selectivity is offered by agents such as albuterol, terbutaline, and salmeterol. These compounds have a higher affinity for β₂-adrenoceptors, the predominant subtype in the airway, than for β₁-adrenoceptors. Other β₂-selective adrenomimetics used as bronchodilators are bitolterol (*Tornalate*) and pir-

TABLE 39.1 Guidelines for the Treatment of Asthma

Step	Status	Symptoms	Lung Function (FEV$_1$ or PEF)	Drug Therapy
1	Mild intermittent	≤twice a week	≥80% predicted	Short-acting inhaled β$_2$-agonists as needed
2	Mild persistent	> twice a week but < once a day Exacerbations may affect activity	≥80% predicted PEF variability 20–30%	Step 1 and ONE of the following: Antiinflammatory therapy (low dose of inhaled corticosteroid) Cromolyn or nedocromil Theophylline Leukotriene modulator
3	Moderate persistent	Daily Daily use of β$_2$-agonists Exacerbations may affect activity Exacerbations ≥ twice a week	60–80% predicted PEF variability > 30%	Step 2 with medium dose of inhaled corticosteroid If needed, ADD a long-acting bronchodilator (inhaled salmeterol, oral β$_2$-agonist, or theophylline)
4	Severe persistent	Continual symptoms Limited physical activity Frequent exacerbations	≤60% PEF variability > 30%	Step 3 with high dose of inhaled corticosteroid and long-acting bronchodilator Oral corticosteroid long term (2 mg/kg/day, not to exceed 60 mg/day)

From U. S. Department of Health and Human Service, National Institutes of Health, National Heart, Lung and Blood Institute; July 1997. FEV$_1$, forced expiratory volume in 1 second (values < 100% indicate increased airway obstruction); PEF, peak expiratory flow (greater variability indicates less control of disease).

TABLE 39.2 Adrenomimetics and Anticholinergics Used as Bronchodilators

Class	Agent	Trade name	Route
α-, β-Adrenoceptor agonists	Epinephrine	–	Subcutaneous
		Primatene	Inhalation
β-Adrenoceptor agonists	Isoproterenol	Isuprel Mistometer	Inhalation
	Metaproterenol	Alupent	Oral Inhalation
Selective β2-adrenoceptor agonists	Albuterol	Proventil Ventolin	Oral
	Bitolterol	Tornalate	Inhalation
	Pirbuterol	Maxair	Inhalation
	Salmeterol	Serevent	Inhalation
	Terbutaline	Brethine	Subcutaneous
		Brethine	Oral
		Brethaire	Inhalation
Anticholinergics	Ipratropium bromide	Atrovent	Inhalation

buterol (*Maxair*). Metaproterenol (*Alupent*), another β-adrenomimetic used as a bronchodilator, is less selective for β$_2$-adrenoceptors than is albuterol or terbutaline.

Epinephrine administered subcutaneously is used to manage severe acute episodes of bronchospasm and status asthmaticus. In addition to its bronchodilator activity through β-adrenoceptor stimulation, a portion of the therapeutic utility of epinephrine in these acute settings may be due to a reduction in pulmonary edema as a result of pulmonary vasoconstriction, the latter effect resulting from α-adrenoceptor stimulation. The effects on pulmonary function are quite rapid, with peak effects occurring within 5 to 15 minutes. Measurable improvement in pulmonary function is maintained for up to 4 hours. The characteristic cardiovascular effects seen at therapeutic doses of epinephrine include increased heart rate, increased cardiac output, increased stroke volume, an elevation of systolic pressure and decrease in diastolic pressure, and a decrease in systemic vascular resistance. *The cardiovascular response to epinephrine represents the algebraic sum of both α- and β-adrenoceptor stimulation.* A decrease in diastolic blood pressure and a decrease in systemic vascular resistance are reflections of vasodilation, a β_2-adrenoceptor response. The increase in heart rate and systolic pressure is the result of either a direct effect of epinephrine on the myocardium, primarily a β_1 effect, or a reflex action provoked by a decrease in peripheral resistance, mean arterial pressure, or both. Overt α-adrenoceptor effects, such as systemic vasoconstriction, are not obvious unless large doses are used.

Isoproterenol is administered almost exclusively by inhalation from metered-dose inhalers or from nebulizers. The response to inhaled isoproterenol and other inhaled adrenomimetics is instantaneous. The action of isoproterenol is short-lived, although an objective measurement of pulmonary function has shown an effective duration of up to 3 hours. When it is administered by inhalation, the cardiac effects of isoproterenol are relatively mild, although in some cases a substantial increase in heart rate occurs.

Terbutaline and albuterol are administered either orally or by inhalation, whereas salmeterol is given by inhalation only. All three agents are *relatively selective* for β_2-adrenoceptors and theoretically are capable of producing bronchodilation with minimal cardiac stimulation. However, the term β_2-*selectivity* is a pharmacological classification based primarily on the relative potency of an individual adrenomimetic to stimulate the pulmonary or the cardiovascular system. Indeed, β_2-agonists invariably produce a degree of tachycardia at large doses, either by activating sympathetic reflex pathways as a consequence of systemic vasodilation or by directly stimulating cardiac β_1-adrenoceptors. In addition, a significant number of β_2-adrenoceptors are present in the human heart, and stimulation of these receptors may contribute to the cardiac effects of β_2-adrenoceptor agonists.

Inhaled salmeterol has a pharmacological half-life in excess of 12 hours, much longer than either albuterol or terbutaline. The likely basis for this long half-life is that the long lipophilic tail of salmeterol promotes retention of the molecule in the cell membrane. Its long duration of action makes salmeterol particularly suitable for prophylactic use, such as in preventing nocturnal symptoms of asthma. Because of its relatively slow onset of action, *salmeterol should not be used to treat acute symptoms.*

The second messenger, cyclic adenosine monophosphate (cAMP), is thought to mediate the bronchodilator effects of the adrenomimetics. Adrenomimetics enhance the production of cAMP by activating adenylyl cyclase, the enzyme that converts adenosine triphosphate (ATP) to cAMP. *This process is triggered by the interaction of the adrenomimetics with β_2-adrenoceptors on airway smooth muscle.*

Clinical Uses

Epinephrine is used in a variety of clinical situations, and although concern has been expressed about the use of epinephrine in asthma, it is still used extensively for the management of acute attacks.

Isoproterenol is used principally by inhalation for the management of bronchospasm. It is also used intravenously for asthma and as a stimulant in cardiac arrest.

Terbutaline, albuterol, salmeterol and other β_2-adrenoceptor agonists are used primarily in the management of asthma. Terbutaline and albuterol have very rapid onset of action and are indicated for acute symptom relief. Salmeterol, in contrast, has a slow onset of action but a long duration of action. Salmeterol is thus used as prophylactic therapy only, not to reverse acute symptoms.

In addition to its use as a bronchodilator, terbutaline is used extensively to control premature labor, since contractions of uterine smooth muscle are abolished by adrenomimetics (see Chapter 62).

Adverse Effects

Patients treated with recommended dosages of epinephrine will complain of feeling nervous or anxious. Some will have tremor of the hand or upper extremity and many will complain of palpitations. Epinephrine is dangerous if recommended dosages are exceeded or if the drug is used in patients with coronary artery disease, arrhythmias, or hypertension. The inappropriate use of epinephrine has resulted in extreme hypertension and cerebrovascular accidents, pulmonary edema, angina, and ventricular arrhythmias, including ventricular fibrillation.

At recommended dosages, adverse effects from inhaled isoproterenol are infrequent and not serious. When excessive dosages are used, tachycardia, dizziness, and nervousness may occur, and some patients may have arrhythmias.

The limiting side effect associated with orally administered β_2-adrenoceptor agonists is *muscle tremor,* which results from a direct stimulation of β_2-adrenoceptors in skeletal muscle. This effect is most notable on the initiation of therapy and gradually improves on continued use. β_2-Agonists also cause tachycardia and palpitations in some patients. When used by intravenous infusion for premature labor, β_2-agonists have been reported to produce tachycardia and pulmonary edema in the mother and hypoglycemia in the baby. When administered by inhalation, the β_2-agonists produce only minor side effects.

A few epidemiological studies suggest that the overuse of β-adrenoceptor agonists is associated with an overall deterioration in disease control and a slight increase in asthma mortality. This apparent trend may be caused by several factors, the most likely of which is that patients rely too heavily on bronchodilator therapy to control acute symptoms at the expense of antiinflammatory therapy to control the underlying disease process.

Theophylline

Twenty years ago theophylline (*Theo-Dur, Slo-bid, Uniphyl, Theo-24*) and its more soluble ethylenediamine salt, aminophylline, were the bronchodilators of choice in the United States. Although the β_2-adrenoceptor agonists now fill this primary role, theophylline continues to have an important place in the therapy of asthma because it appears to have antiinflammatory as well as bronchodilator activity.

Basic Pharmacology

Smooth muscle relaxation, central nervous system (CNS) excitation, and cardiac stimulation are the principal pharmacological effects observed in patients treated with theophylline. The action of theophylline on the respiratory system is easily seen in the asthmatic by the resolution of obstruction and improvement in pulmonary function. Other mechanisms that may contribute to the action of theophylline in asthma include antagonism of adenosine, inhibition of mediator release, increased sympathetic activity, alteration in immune cell function, and reduction in respiratory muscle fatigue. Theophylline also may exert an antiinflammatory effect through its ability to modulate inflammatory mediator release and immune cell function.

Inhibition of cyclic nucleotide phosphodiesterases is widely accepted as the predominant mechanism by which theophylline produces bronchodilation. Phosphodiesterases are enzymes that inactivate cAMP and cyclic guanosine monophosphate (GMP), second messengers that mediate bronchial smooth muscle relaxation.

Clinical Uses

The principal use of theophylline is in the management of asthma. It is also used to treat the reversible component of airway obstruction associated with chronic obstructive pulmonary disease and to relieve dyspnea associated with pulmonary edema that develops from congestive heart failure.

Adverse Effects, Drug Interactions, and Contraindications

Theophylline has a narrow therapeutic index and produces side effects that can be severe, even life threatening. Importantly, the plasma concentration of theophylline cannot be predicted reliably from the dose. In one study, the oral dosage of theophylline required to produce therapeutic plasma levels (i.e., between 10 and 20 μg/mL) varied between 400 and 3,200 mg/day. *Heterogeneity among individuals in the rate at which they metabolize theophylline appears to be the principal factor responsible for the variability in plasma levels.* Such conditions as heart failure, liver disease, and severe respiratory obstruction will slow the metabolism of theophylline.

The most frequent complaints of patients taking theophylline are nausea and vomiting, which occur most frequently in patients receiving theophylline for the first time and when the plasma level approaches 20 μg/mL but rarely occur at plasma concentrations below 15 μg/mL. The fact that patients who receive the drug intravenously also have the same complaint suggests that the nausea and vomiting result from an action in the CNS.

When serum concentrations exceed 40 μg/mL, there is a high probability of seizures. Nausea will not always be a premonitory sign of impending toxicity. For instance, in children, restlessness, agitation, diuresis, or fever can occur even when nausea does not. A rapid intravenous injection of theophylline can cause arrhythmias, hypotension, and cardiac arrest. Thus, extreme caution should be used when giving the drug by this route. Since *it is not possible to predict blood levels on the basis of dosage,* toxicity is fairly common by any route of administration. Consequently, plasma concentrations of theophylline should be determined when a patient begins therapy and then at regular intervals of 6 to 12 months thereafter.

Theophylline should be used with caution in patients with myocardial disease, liver disease, and acute myocardial infarction. The half-life of theophylline is prolonged in patients with congestive heart failure. Because of its narrow margin of safety, extreme caution is warranted when coadministering drugs, such as cimetidine or zileuton, that may interfere with the metabolism of theophylline. Indeed, coadministration of zileuton with theophylline is contraindicated. It is also prudent to be careful when using theophylline in patients with a history of seizures.

Anticholinergics

The parasympathetic cholinergic pathway emanating from the vagus nerve exerts the main neuronal control in human airways. The cholinergic efferent nerves synapse in ganglia within the airways, and from there, short postganglionic fibers innervate the end organs, including the airway smooth muscle and mucous glands. *Stimulation of these nerve fibers, with the resultant release of acetylcholine and activation of muscarinic cholinoreceptors, elicits bronchoconstriction, mucous secretion, and bronchial vasodilation.* Thus, the cholinergic pathways play a key role in the maintenance of the caliber of the airways and contribute to the airway obstruction in both asthma and chronic obstructive pulmonary disease.

Basic Pharmacology

The airway effects of released acetylcholine are mediated via activation of three distinct muscarinic receptor subtypes: M_1, in parasympathetic ganglia, mucous glands and alveolar walls; autoinhibitory M_2, in parasympathetic nerve terminals; and M_3, in airway smooth muscle, mucus glands, and airway epithelium.

Although atropine and related compounds possess bronchodilator activity, their use is associated with the typical spectrum of anticholinergic side effects (see Chapter 13), and they are no longer used in the treatment of asthma. To improve the clinical utility of anticholinergics, quaternary amine derivatives of atropine were developed. By virtue of their positive charge, these drugs are absorbed poorly across mucosal surfaces and thus produce fewer side effects than atropine, especially when given by inhalation.

Clinical Uses

Ipratropium bromide (*Atrovent*) is a quaternary amine derivative that is used via inhalation in the treatment of chronic obstructive pulmonary disease and to a lesser extent, asthma. Ipratropium has a slower onset of action (1–2 hours for peak activity) than β_2-adrenoceptor agonists and thus may be more suitable for prophylactic use. Compared with β_2-adrenoceptor agonists, ipratropium is generally at least as effective in chronic obstructive pulmonary disease but less effective in asthma.

Ipratropium has greater effectiveness than β_2-adrenoceptor agonists in two settings: in psychogenic asthma and in patients taking β_2-adrenoceptor antagonists. A fixed combination of ipratropium and albuterol (*Combivent*) is approved for use in chronic obstructive pulmonary disease.

Adverse Effects

Ipratropium is virtually devoid of the CNS side effects associated with atropine. The most prevalent peripheral side effects are dry mouth, headache, nervousness, dizziness, nausea, and cough. Unlike atropine, ipratropium does not inhibit mucociliary clearance and thus does not promote the accumulation of secretions in the lower airways.

ANTIINFLAMMATORY AGENTS

The medical and scientific communities have recognized that *asthma is not simply a disease marked by acute bronchospasm but rather a complex chronic inflammatory disorder of the airways.* On the basis of this knowledge, antiinflammatory agents, particularly corticosteroids, are now included in the treatment regimens of an ever-increasing proportion of asthmatic patients.

Corticosteroids

A major breakthrough in asthma therapy was the introduction in the 1970s of *aerosol corticosteroids.* These agents (Table 39.3) maintain much of the impressive therapeutic efficacy of parenteral and oral corticosteroids, but by virtue of their local administration and markedly reduced systemic absorption, they are associated with a greatly reduced incidence and severity of side effects. The success of inhaled steroids has led to a substantial reduction in the use of systemic corticosteroids. *Inhaled corticosteroids, along with β_2-adrenoceptor agonists, are front-line therapy of chronic asthma.*

TABLE 39.3   Corticosteroids Used in Asthma

Class	Agent	Trade Name	Route
Oral corticosteroids	Prednisone	Deltasone	Oral
	Methylprednisolone	Medrol	Oral
Parenteral corticosteroids	Methylprednisolone	Depo-Medrol	Intramuscular
		Solu-Medrol	Intravenous
	Hydrocortisone	Hydrocortone	Intravenous
Inhaled corticosteroids	Triamcinolone acetonide	Azmacort	Inhalation
	Beclomethasone dipropionate	Beclovent	Inhalation
		Vanceril	
	Flunisolide	AeroBid	Inhalation
	Fluticasone	Flovent	Inhalation

Basic Pharmacology

All corticosteroids have the same general mechanism of action; they traverse cell membranes and bind to a specific cytoplasmic receptor. The steroid-receptor complex translocates to the cell nucleus, where it attaches to nuclear binding sites and initiates synthesis of messenger ribonucleic acid (mRNA). The novel proteins that are formed may exert a variety of effects on cellular functions. The precise mechanisms whereby the corticosteroids exert their therapeutic benefit in asthma remain unclear, although the benefit is likely to be due to several actions rather than one specific action and is related to their ability to inhibit inflammatory processes. At the molecular level, corticosteroids regulate the transcription of a number of genes, including those for several cytokines.

The corticosteroids have an array of actions in several systems that may be relevant to their effectiveness in asthma. These include inhibition of cytokine and mediator release, attenuation of mucus secretion, upregulation of β-adrenoceptor numbers, inhibition of IgE synthesis, attenuation of eicosanoid generation, decreased microvascular permeability, and suppression of inflammatory cell influx and inflammatory processes. The effects of the steroids take several hours to days to develop, so they cannot be used for quick relief of acute episodes of bronchospasm.

Clinical Uses

The corticosteroids are effective in most children and adults with asthma. They are beneficial for the treatment of both acute and chronic aspects of the disease. Inhaled corticosteroids, including triamcinolone acetonide (*Azmacort*), beclomethasone dipropionate (*Beclovent, Vanceril*), flunisolide (*AeroBid*), and fluticasone (*Flovent*), are indicated for maintenance treatment of asthma as prophylactic therapy. *Inhaled corticosteroids are not effective for relief of acute episodes of severe bronchospasm.* Systemic corticosteroids, including prednisone and prednisolone, are used for the short-term treatment of asthma exacerbations that do not respond to β$_2$-adrenoceptor agonists and aerosol corticosteroids. Systemic corticosteroids, along with other treatments, are also used to control status asthmaticus. *Because of the side effects produced by systemically administered corticosteroids, they should not be used for maintenance therapy unless all other treatment options have been exhausted.*

A fixed combination of inhaled fluticasone and salmeterol (*Advair*) is available for maintenance antiinflammatory and bronchodilator treatment of asthma.

Adverse Effects and Contraindications

The side effects of corticosteroids range from minor to severe and life threatening. The nature and severity of side effects depend on the route, dose, and frequency of administration, as well as the specific agent used. Side effects are much more prevalent with systemic administration than with inhalant administration. The potential consequences of systemic administration of the corticosteroids include adrenal suppression, cushingoid changes, growth retardation, cataracts, osteoporosis, CNS effects and behavioral disturbances, and increased susceptibility to infection. The severity of all of these side effects can be reduced markedly by alternate-day therapy.

Inhaled corticosteroids are generally well tolerated. In contrast to systemically administered corticosteroids, inhaled agents are either poorly absorbed or rapidly metabolized and inactivated and thus have greatly diminished systemic effects relative to oral agents. The most frequent side effects are local; they include oral candidiasis, dysphonia, sore throat and throat irritation, and coughing. Special delivery systems (e.g., devices with spacers) can minimize these side effects. Some studies have associated slowing of growth in children with the use of high-dose inhaled corticosteroids, although the results are controversial. Regardless, the purported effect is small and is likely outweighed by the benefit of control of the symptoms of asthma.

Care should be taken in transferring patients from systemic to aerosol corticosteroids, as deaths due to adrenal insufficiency have been reported. In addition, allergic conditions, such as rhinitis, conjunctivitis, and eczema, previously controlled by systemic corticosteroids, may be unmasked when asthmatic patients are switched from systemic to inhaled corticosteroids. Caution should be exercised when taking corticosteroids during pregnancy, as glucocorticoids are teratogenic. Systemic corticosteroids are contraindicated in patients with systemic fungal infections.

ALTERNATIVE THERAPIES

A number of medications useful in the treatment of asthma are neither strictly bronchodilators nor antiinflammatory agents. They are classified as alternative asthma therapies (Table 39.4). These drugs, used prophylactically to decrease the frequency and severity of asthma attacks, are not indicated for monotherapy. They are used along with adrenomimetic bronchodilators, corticosteroids, or both.

Leukotriene Modulators

Until the late 1990s, nearly 3 decades had passed since the introduction of a truly new class of antiasthma drugs having a novel mechanism of action. This situation changed with the introduction of zafirlukast (*Accolate*) and montelukast (*Singulair*), *cysteinyl leukotriene (CysLT)*

TABLE 39.4   Alternative Asthma Therapies

Class	Agent	Trade name	Route
Chromones	Cromolyn Sodium	Intal	Inhalation
	Nedocromil Sodium	Tilade	Inhalation
Leukotriene modulators			
Synthesis inhibitor	Zileuton	Zyflo	Oral
Receptor antagonists	Montelukast	Singulair	Oral
	Zafirlukast	Accolate	Oral

receptor antagonists, and zileuton (*Zyflo*), a *leukotriene synthesis inhibitor.* CysLTs include leukotrienes C_4, D_4, and E_4. These mediators are products of arachidonic acid metabolism and make up the components of *slow-reacting substance of anaphylaxis.*

Basic Pharmacology

The cysteinyl leukotrienes are generated in mast cells, basophils, macrophages, and eosinophils. These mediators have long been suspected of being key participants in the pathophysiology of asthma. In particular, the powerful bronchoconstrictor activity of these leukotrienes has implicated them as major contributors to the reversible component of airway obstruction. Additional evidence suggests that their pathophysiologic role extends beyond their ability to elicit bronchoconstriction. Thus, it is now believed that these substances stimulate mucus secretion and microvascular leakage, both of which contribute to airway obstruction. The relative importance of the various actions of the cysteinyl leukotrienes in the complex pathophysiology of asthma is not clear.

The biological actions of the cysteinyl leukotrienes are mediated via stimulation of $CysLT_1$ receptors. Montelukast and zafirlukast are competitive antagonists of these receptors. In contrast, zileuton suppresses synthesis of the leukotrienes by inhibiting 5-lipoxygenase, a key enzyme in the bioconversion of arachidonic acid to the leukotrienes. Zileuton also blocks the production of leukotriene B_4, another arachidonic acid metabolite with proinflammatory activity. The $CysLT_1$-receptor antagonists alter neither the production nor the actions of leukotriene B_4.

Clinical Uses

Montelukast, zafirlukast, and zileuton are indicated for the prophylaxis and chronic treatment of asthma. They should not be used to treat acute asthmatic episodes. All three agents are administered orally.

Adverse Effects, Drug Interactions, and Contraindications

Dyspepsia is the most common side effect of zileuton. Liver transaminase levels are elevated in a small percentage of patients taking zileuton. Serum liver transaminase levels should be monitored and treatment halted if significant elevations occur. *Zileuton inhibits the metabolism of theophylline.* Thus, when these agents are used concomitantly, the dose of theophylline should be reduced by approximately one-half, and plasma concentrations of theophylline should be monitored closely. Caution should also be exercised when using zileuton concomitantly with warfarin, terfenadine, or propranolol, as zileuton inhibits the metabolism of these agents. *Zileuton is contraindicated in patients with acute liver disease* and should be used with caution in patients who consume substantial quantities of alcohol or have a history of liver disease.

Zafirlukast and montelukast are well tolerated. Zafirlukast increases plasma concentrations of warfarin and decreases the concentrations of theophylline and erythromycin. In rare cases, treatment of patients with CysLT receptor antagonists is associated with the development of Churg-Strauss syndrome, a condition marked by acute vasculitis, eosinophilia, and a worsening of pulmonary symptoms. Because these symptoms often appear when patients are given the leukotriene receptor antagonists when they are being weaned from oral corticosteroid therapy, it is not clear whether they are related to the action of the antagonists or are due to a sudden reduction in corticosteroid therapy.

Cromolyn Sodium and Nedocromil Sodium

Cromolyn sodium (*Intal*) and nedocromil sodium (*Tilade*) are chemically related drugs called chromones that are used for the prophylaxis of mild or moderate asthma. Both are administered by inhalation and have very good safety profiles, making them particularly useful in treating children.

Basic Pharmacology

The precise mechanism or mechanisms whereby cromolyn sodium and nedocromil sodium exert their antiasthmatic activities is unknown. Early work suggested that these agents act by "stabilizing" mast cells, preventing mediator release. However, several other compounds exhibit greater potency for stabilization of mast cells yet possess no clinical efficacy in asthma. This suggests that the therapeutic activity of cromolyn sodium and nedocromil sodium in asthma is related to one or more other pharmacological mechanisms. Postulates include inhibitory effects on irritant receptors, nerves, plasma exudation, and inflammatory cells in general.

Cromolyn sodium and nedocromil sodium attenuate bronchospasm induced by various stimuli, including antigen, exercise, cold dry air, and sulfur dioxide. They suppress inflammatory cell influx and chemotactic activity along with antigen-induced bronchial hyperreactivity. Also inhibited is C-fiber sensory nerve activation in animal models, which may in turn suppress reflex-induced bronchospasm.

Clinical Uses

Cromolyn sodium and nedocromil sodium are used almost exclusively for the prophylactic treatment of mild to moderate asthma and should not be used for the control of acute bronchospasm. These agents are effective in about 60 to 70% of children and adolescents with asthma. Unfortunately, there is no reliable means to predict which patients will respond. They are less effective in older patients and in patients with severe asthma. It may take up to 4 to 6 weeks of treatment for cromolyn sodium to be effective in chronic asthma, but it is effective after a single dose in exercise-induced asthma. With respect to clinical efficacy, cromolyn sodium and nedocromil sodium do not differ in a substantial way.

Adverse Effects

Cromolyn sodium and nedocromil sodium are the least toxic of available therapies for asthma. Adverse reactions are rare and generally minor. Those occurring in fewer than 1 in 10,000 patients include transient bronchospasm, cough or wheezing, dryness of throat, laryngeal edema, swollen parotid gland, angioedema, joint swelling and pain, dizziness, dysuria, nausea, headache, nasal congestion, rash, and urticaria.

STATUS ASTHMATICUS

Status asthmaticus is a life-threatening exacerbation of asthma symptoms that is unresponsive to standard therapy. It must be treated very aggressively, and hospitalization may be necessary. A provocative factor such as prolonged allergen exposure or a respiratory infection often precedes status asthmaticus. A rapid increase in the daily use of bronchodilators to control acute symptoms is a danger sign of an impending crisis. Treatment includes oxygen, inhaled short-acting β_2-agonists, and oral or parenteral corticosteroids. Subcutaneous β-agonists can be given to those who respond poorly to inhaled adrenomimetics. Inhaled ipratropium may be effective in some patients.

Study QUESTIONS

1. The underlying pathophysiology of asthma is best described by which of the following statements?
   (A) Asthma is a psychosomatic disorder.
   (B) Asthma is caused by an aberrant response to vaccinations.
   (C) Asthma is a disease of airway inflammation.
   (D) Asthma is a disorder of the lung parenchyma.
   (E) Asthma is an infectious disease.
2. Status asthmaticus is best described by which of the following statements?
   (A) Status asthmaticus is well-controlled asthma.
   (B) Status asthmaticus is a life-threatening exacerbation of asthma.

   (C) Status asthmaticus is best treated with inhaled controller medication, such as cromolyn sodium or a leukotriene modulator.
   (D) Status asthmaticus always resolves without drug treatment.
   (E) Status asthmaticus occurs without warning in patients whose asthma symptoms are stable and well controlled.
3. Which one of the following β-adrenoceptor agonists has such a slow onset of action that it is not indicated for the relief of acute asthma symptoms?
   (A) Salmeterol
   (B) Albuterol

(C) Epinephrine
(D) Terbutaline
(E) Isoproterenol

4. The standard treatment regimen for asthma is best described by which of the following?
(A) Theophylline and exercise
(B) Inhaled β_2-adrenoceptor agonists only
(C) Inhaled corticosteroids only
(D) A combination of inhaled bronchodilators and inhaled corticosteroids
(E) Oral corticosteroids

5. Symptoms typically produced by inhaled β-adrenoceptor agonists include which of the following?
(A) Tachycardia, dizziness, and nervousness
(B) Dysphonia, candidiasis, and sore throat
(C) Dyspepsia and Churg-Strauss syndrome
(D) Nausea, agitation, and convulsions
(E) Muscle tremor, tachycardia, and palpitations

ANSWERS

1. **C.** Inflammation of the airway is a hallmark of asthma. The use of antiinflammatory drugs, such as inhaled corticosteroids, is critical to the long-term control of asthma. No credible data indicate either that asthma is psychosomatic or that it develops in response to vaccinations against childhood diseases. Asthma is a disease limited to the airways. It does not involve the lung parenchyma. Although upper respiratory tract infections can exacerbate asthma symptoms, asthma is not caused by infection, nor is it communicable.

2. **B.** Status asthmaticus is a dangerous exacerbation of asthma symptoms. It requires immediate and aggressive treatment with oxygen, inhaled bronchodilators, and systemic corticosteroids. Hospitalization of the patient is often indicated. By definition, status asthmaticus is not a condition in which symptoms are well controlled. Neither cromolyn sodium nor a leukotriene modulator is indicated for the treatment of status asthmaticus, as their onset of action is too slow. Status asthmaticus often does not resolve without aggressive intervention. Indeed, the patient's condition can deteriorate rapidly to death. Upper respiratory tract infection or excessive exposure to an allergen often precedes status asthmaticus, as does increased use of inhaled bronchodilators.

3. **A.** The other agents have rapid onset and are appropriate for acute symptomatic relief of asthma.

4. **D.** In all asthma treatment regimens, inhaled β_2-adrenoceptor agonists are used as bronchodilators as needed to relieve acute symptoms. As asthma is an inflammatory disease of the airway, inhaled corticosteroids are also used as standard therapy to control symptoms in all but the mildest cases. The potential for dangerous side effects and drug interactions has relegated theophylline, once a mainstay of asthma treatment, to add-on therapy for hard to control symptoms. Inhaled β_2-adrenoceptor agonists or inhaled corticosteroids are not typically used as monotherapy, although the former class of agent can be used alone for patients with very mild symptoms. Because of extensive systemic side effects, oral corticosteroids are not typically used to treat asthma except when symptoms cannot be controlled by standard therapy.

5. **A.** Tachycardia, dizziness, and nervousness are often produced by larger doses of inhaled β-agonists. Dysphonia, candidiasis, and sore throat are associated with the use of inhaled corticosteroids. The emergence of Churg-Strauss syndrome, though uncommon, is associated with the use of oral leukotriene modulators. Theophylline produces a range of side effects, including nausea, agitation, and life-threatening convulsions. Muscle tremor and palpitations are frequently observed with oral β-adrenoceptor agonists but rarely occur when these agents are administered via inhalation.

SUPPLEMENTAL READING

Bisgaard H. Pathophysiology of the cysteinyl leukotrienes and effects of leukotriene receptor antagonists in asthma. Allergy 2001;56 Suppl 66:7–11.

Bryan SA, Leckie MJ, Hansel TT, and Barnes PJ. Novel therapy for asthma. Expert Opin Invest Drugs 2000;9:25–42.

Fahy JV, Corry DB, and Boushey HA. Airway inflammation and remodeling in asthma. Curr Opin Pulmon Med 2000;6:15–20.

Hall IP. Genetics and pulmonary medicine. 8: Asthma. Thorax 1999;54:65–69.

Kelly HW. Asthma pharmacotherapy: Current practices and outlook. Pharmacotherapy 1997;17:13S–21S.

Kips JC and Pauwels RA. Long-acting inhaled beta$_2$-agonist therapy in asthma. Am J Respir Crit Care Med 2001;64:923–932.

Kips JC, Peleman RA, and Pauwels RA. The role of theophylline in asthma management. Current Opin Pulmon Med 1999;5:88–92.

Levy BD, Kitch B, and Fanta CH. Medical and ventilatory management of status asthmaticus. Intensive Care Med 1998;24:105–117.

Second Expert Panel on Management of Asthma. Guidelines for the diagnosis and management of asthma. Bethesda, MD: U.S. Department of Health and Human Services, Public Health Service, National Institutes of Health, National Heart, Lung and Blood Institute, 1997.

Williams DM. Clinical considerations in the use of inhaled corticosteroids for asthma. Pharmacotherapy 2001;21:38S–48S.

CASE **Study** Drug Interactions

A 67-year-old man arrives at the emergency department complaining of excessive bleeding from minor shaving cuts and bruising for no apparent reason. Although the signs are alarming to the patient, the intern on duty does not view them as particularly serious. Upon taking the patient's history, the intern learns that for the last 5 years the patient has been taking warfarin for atrial fibrillation. In addition, the patient has had asthma since childhood. About 3 weeks ago the asthma symptoms were increasing in frequency and severity, prompting his pulmonologist to prescribe oral theophylline on top of the inhaled corticosteroid and β-adrenoceptor agonist that the patient was already taking. This new regimen seems to be controlling the asthma well. What is the most appropriate treatment for this patient?

ANSWER: The key event in this patient's recent history is the addition of theophylline to his asthma regimen. Theophylline interferes with the metabolism of warfarin, and elevated warfarin levels can cause bleeding. Moreover, orally administered theophylline is notorious for producing widely variable plasma concentrations. Warfarin levels should be monitored in this patient, and his warfarin dosages should be adjusted accordingly. Withdrawing warfarin completely or administering vitamin K is not necessary, as the bleeding complications are not severe. Moreover, these actions could precipitate adverse clotting events (e.g., transient ischemic attack). Withdrawing asthma medication could impair asthma control. Pulmonary function tests are not necessary, as the patient's asthma symptoms are adequately controlled.

40 | Drugs Used in Gastrointestinal Disorders

Lisa M. Gangarosa and Donald G. Seibert

 DRUG LIST

INTRODUCTION TO NORMAL PHYSIOLOGY

The gastrointestinal (GI) tract consists of the esophagus, stomach, small intestine, and colon. It processes ingested boluses of food and drink and expels waste material. Intervention by disease or pharmacological therapy may alter function of the GI tract. This chapter discusses drugs employed in the treatment of several GI disorders, emphasizing disease pathophysiology and drug mechanisms of action.

From the mid esophagus to the anus, smooth muscle surrounds the alimentary canal and is responsible for active movement and segmentation of intestinal contents. This smooth muscle, which lies in the muscularis propria, consists of a circular and a longitudinal layer of muscle.

From the gastric body to the colon, repetitive spontaneous depolarizations originate in the interstitial cells of Cajal, from which they spread to the circular muscle layer and then to the longitudinal muscle layer. The rate of slow-wave contraction varies in different regions of the gastrointestinal tract, occurring approximately 3 per minute in the stomach, 12 per minute in the proximal intestine, and 8 per minute in the distal intestine. The increased frequency of contraction in the proximal intestine forms a gradient of contraction, and intestinal contents are therefore propelled distally. Though the stomach has fewer spontaneous contractions than does the small intestine, there is normally no retrograde spread of a depolarization wave from duodenum to stomach.

The underlying intrinsic smooth muscle motility is modulated by neurohormonal influences. Afferent sensory neurons, extrinsic motor neurons, and intramural neurons innervate the gut. It also has mucosal sensory receptors for monitoring chemical, osmotic, or painful stimuli and muscle receptors to monitor degrees of stretch.

Both the parasympathetic and sympathetic nervous systems provide extrinsic gastrointestinal innervation. Parasympathetic stimulation increases muscle contraction of the gut, while sympathetic stimulation inhibits contractions. Stimulation of either α- or β-adrenoceptors will result in inhibition of contractions. The intramural nervous system consists of a myenteric (Auerbach's) plexus between the circular and longitudinal muscle areas and a submucosal (Meissner's) plexus between the muscularis mucosa and the circular muscle layers. *These two plexuses contain stimulatory cholinergic neurons.*

Ingested liquids are rapidly emptied from the stomach into the intestine, while digestible solids are first mechanically broken down in the stomach by peristaltic contractions. Stimulation of osmotic, carbohydrate, and fat receptors in the small bowel inhibits gastric peristaltic contractions and retards gastric emptying.

The small intestinal motility in the fed state consists of random slow-wave contractions that result in slow transit and long contact of food with enzymes and absorptive surfaces. With fasting, an organized peristaltic wave, termed the interdigestive *migrating motor complex,* begins to cycle every 84 to 112 minutes. During the migrating motor complex, a peristaltic contraction ring travels from the stomach to the cecum at 6 to 8 cm per minute. In the stomach the contractions sweep against a widely patent pylorus, permitting the passage of undigestible solids. In the small intestine this is to clear the intestine of undigested material: it functions as an intestinal housekeeper. The migrating motor complex appears to correlate with *motilin* hormonal levels and is modulated by vagal innervation. Motilin is a 22–amino acid polypeptide released from the duodenal mucosa as a regulator of normal GI motor activity. Exogenous motilin is a potent inducer of gastric motor activity.

Colonic motor function also has cyclic slow waves in the proximal colon. These contractions are primarily retrograde in the proximal colon, allowing segmentation and liquid reabsorption. In the distal colon a propulsive mass movement occurs intermittently. This may be stimulated by food ingestion and is termed the *gastrocolonic reflex.*

Approximately 1 to 1.5 L of fluid is ingested per day, and coupled with secretions from the stomach, pancreas, and proximal duodenum, approximately 8 L of chyme enters the jejunum per day. Reabsorption of 6 to 7 L occurs within the small bowel, leaving a residual of 1.5 L fluid, 90% of which is reabsorbed in the colon. This pattern of liquid reabsorption permits the elimination of fecal waste containing an average of 0.1 to 0.2 L fluid per day. *Diarrhea* occurs if there is an altered rate of intestinal motility, if mucosal function or permeability is altered, or if the fluid load entering the colon overwhelms colonic reabsorption. *Constipation* may occur if intestinal movement is inhibited or if there is a fixed obstruction.

DRUGS THAT INCREASE GI MOTILITY

Decreased GI motility can affect one or more parts of the GI tract and can be the result of a systemic disease, intrinsic GI disorder, or medication. *Gastroparesis* is the term for delayed gastric emptying. Symptoms may range from postprandial bloating and fullness to nausea and vomiting. Half of ingested liquid should be emptied within 30 minutes, and half of a digestible solid should be emptied within 2 hours. Emptying time can be prolonged as a result of autonomic neuropathy seen with long-standing diabetes mellitus. Pseudoobstruction due to an idiopathic intestinal muscle disease or intestinal neuropathy may also cause delays in gastric emptying and intestinal transit. Rarer causes of delayed GI motility include Chagas' disease, muscular dystrophy, scleroderma, and infiltrative diseases, such as amyloidosis. Decreased GI transit can occur acutely following electrolyte disorders and gastroenteritis. In addition, many medications, including anticholinergic medications, tricyclic antidepressants, levodopa, and β-adrenergic agonists, inhibit GI motility.

Drugs that enhance GI motility are often called *prokinetics*. Their goal is to increase contractile force and accelerate intraluminal transit. Most of these drugs act either by enhancing the effect of acetylcholine or by blocking the effect of an inhibitory neurotransmitter such as dopamine. The prokinetics discussed in this chapter are metoclopramide, cisapride and tegaserod, and erythromycin.

Metoclopramide Hydrochloride

Metoclopramide (*Reglan*) stimulates upper GI tract motility and has both central and peripheral actions. Centrally, it is a dopamine antagonist, an action that is important both for its often desirable *antiemetic* effect and other less desirable effects. Peripherally, it stimulates the release of intrinsic postganglionic stores of acetylcholine and sensitizes the gastric smooth muscle to muscarinic stimulation. The ability of metoclopramide to antagonize the inhibitory neurotransmitter effect of dopamine on the GI tract results in increased gastric contraction and enhanced gastric emptying and small bowel transit.

Metoclopramide is rapidly absorbed following an oral dose in a patient with intact gastric emptying. Peak plasma concentration is achieved within 40 to 120 minutes. With normal renal function, plasma half-life is about 4 hours. About 20% of an oral dose is eliminated unchanged in the urine, while 60% is eliminated as sulfate or glucuronide conjugates.

Improved gastric emptying will frequently alleviate symptoms in patients with diabetic, postoperative, or idiopathic gastroparesis. Since metoclopramide also can decrease the acid reflux into the esophagus that results from slowed gastric emptying or lower esophageal sphincter pressure, the drug can be used as an adjunct in the treatment of reflux esophagitis.

Side effects include fatigue, insomnia, and altered motor coordination. Parkinsonian side effects and acute dystonic reactions also have been reported. Metoclopramide stimulates prolactin secretion, which can cause galactorrhea and menstrual disorders. Extrapyramidal side effects seen following administration of the phenothiazines, thioxanthenes, and butyrophenones may be accentuated by metoclopramide.

Cisapride and Tegaserod

Cisapride (*Propulsid*) and tegaserod (*Zelnorm*) are both serotonin-4 ($5\text{-}HT_4$) receptor agonists that stimulate GI motility. Cisapride appears to act by facilitating the release of acetylcholine from the myenteric plexus. It has no antiadrenergic, antidopaminergic, or cholinergic side effects. Following oral administration, peak plasma levels occur in 1.5 to 2 hours; the drug's half-life is 10 hours. Cisapride has been successfully used to treat gastroparesis and mild gastroesophageal reflux disease. The most frequent side effect has been diarrhea. A few patients had seizure activity that was reversible after medication was discontinued. Cisapride was pulled from the U.S. market after deaths from drug-associated cardiac arrhythmias, including ventricular tachycardia, ventricular fibrillation, torsades de pointes, and QT prolongation.

Tegaserod is being developed as a treatment for constipation-predominant irritable bowel syndrome (IBS). Within the first week, patients treated with tegaserod had significant improvements in abdominal pain and discomfort, constipation, and overall well-being. Efficacy was maintained throughout the treatment period. Tegaserod also demonstrated significant improvements in the three bowel-related assessments (stool frequency, stool consistency, and straining) within the first week, and these improvements were sustained throughout the treatment period. The most common adverse events reported thus far are headache and diarrhea.

Erythromycin

Erythromycin is an antibiotic in the macrolide family (see Chapter 47) that also has promotility effects because it is a motilin agonist. Erythromycin is used (off-label indication) to accelerate gastric emptying in diabetic gastroparesis and postoperative gastroparesis. Tachyphylaxis will occur, so it cannot be used uninterruptedly for long periods.

DRUGS THAT DECREASE GI MOTILITY

Diarrhea is the frequent passage of watery, unformed stools. Its many causes include IBS, infectious disorders, thyrotoxicosis, malabsorption, medication side effect, and laxative abuse. Attempts to treat diarrhea should first focus on the patient's list of medications followed by a search for an underlying systemic disorder. Opioids and $5\text{-}HT_3$ receptor antagonists, such as alosetron, slow motility and can therefore decrease or eliminate diarrhea.

Opioids

Most of the opioids have a constipating action; morphine was used in the treatment of diarrhea before it was used as an analgesic. Unfortunately, many of the opium preparations, while relieving diarrhea and dysentery, also produce such objectionable side effects as respiratory depression and habituation (see Chapter 26). *The opioids are capable of altering the motility pattern in all parts of the GI tract.* These compounds usually produce an increase in segmentation and a decrease in the rate of propulsive movement. The feces become dehydrated as a result of their longer stay in the GI tract. The tone of the internal anal sphincter is increased, and the subjective response to the stimulus of a full rectum is reduced by the central action of the opioids. All of these actions produce constipation. Opioids should not be used indiscriminately in bloody diarrhea, since their use in inflammatory bowel disease involving the colon may increase the risk of megacolon and their use in infectious enterocolitis may promote intestinal perforation.

The dangers of dependency and addiction clearly preclude the use of such compounds as morphine, meperidine, and methadone as treatment for diarrhea. Antidiarrheal specificity therefore is of paramount importance in choosing among the synthetic opioids and their analogues (e.g., diphenoxylate and loperamide).

Diphenoxylate (marketed in combination with atropine as *Lomotil* in the United States) is chemically related to both analgesic and anticholinergic compounds. It is as effective in the treatment of diarrhea as the opium derivatives, and at the doses usually employed, it has a low incidence of central opioid actions. Diphenoxylate is rapidly metabolized by ester hydrolysis to the biologically active metabolite difenoxylic acid. Lomotil is recommended as adjunctive therapy in the management of diarrhea. It is contraindicated in children under 2 years old and in patients with obstructive jaundice. Adverse reactions often caused by the atropine in the preparation include anorexia, nausea, pruritus, dizziness, and numbness of the extremities.

Loperamide hydrochloride (*Imodium*) structurally resembles both haloperidol and meperidine. In equal doses, loperamide protects against diarrhea longer than does diphenoxylate. It reduces the daily fecal volume and decreases intestinal fluid and electrolyte loss. Loperamide produces rapid and sustained inhibition of the peristaltic reflex through depression of longitudinal and circular muscle activity. The drug also possesses antisecretory activity, presumably through an effect on intestinal opioid receptors. Loperamide is effective against a wide range of secretory stimuli and can be used in the control and symptomatic relief of acute diarrhea that is not secondary to bacterial infection. Adverse effects associated with its use include abdominal pain and distention, constipation, dry mouth, hypersensitivity, and nausea and vomiting.

Tincture of opium (10% opium) is a rapidly acting preparation for the symptomatic treatment of diarrhea.

The more widely used paregoric (camphorated opium tincture) is equally effective and is frequently used in combination with other antidiarrheal agents. Codeine also has been used for short-term symptomatic treatment.

Alosetron

Alosetron (*Lotronex*) is a 5-HT$_3$ receptor antagonist. Blocking this receptor results in decreased GI motility. Alosetron received FDA approval in February 2000 for the treatment of women with diarrhea-predominant IBS. In November 2000, at the request of the FDA, the drug was voluntarily withdrawn due to reported cases of ischemic colitis, including some fatalities.

PHARMACOLOGICAL MODULATION OF DIARRHEA AND CONSTIPATION BY MECHANISMS THAT DO NOT DIRECTLY AFFECT MOTILITY

Drugs Useful for Treating Diarrhea: Adsorbents and Bulking Agents

Kaolin powder and other hydrated aluminum silicate clays, often combined with pectin (a complex carbohydrate), are the most widely used adsorbent powders (e.g., *Kaopectate*). Kaolin is a naturally occurring hydrated aluminum silicate that is prepared for medicinal use as a very finely divided powder. The rationale behind its use in acute nonspecific diarrhea stems from its ability to adsorb some of the bacterial toxins that often cause the condition. It is almost harmless and is effective in many cases of diarrhea if taken in large enough doses (2–10 g initially, followed by the same amount after every bowel movement). The adsorbents are generally safe, but they may interfere with the absorption of some drugs from the GI tract.

Bismuth subsalicylate (*Pepto-Bismol*) also binds intestinal toxins and may coat irritated mucosal surfaces. This compound is a salicylate and may therefore produce signs of salicylate toxicity (e.g., ringing of the ears) if taken chronically, especially with aspirin. Bismuth is radiopaque and may interfere with radiological examinations. Its use may cause temporary gray-black discoloration of the stool and brown pigmentation of the tongue. High dose Pepto-Bismol (8 tablets/day) has been efficacious in some patients with diarrhea secondary to collagenous or lymphocytic colitis.

Hydrophilic substances such as calcium polycarbophil (*FiberCon, Equalactin*), methylcellulose (*Citrucel*), and various psyllium seed derivatives (*Metamucil*) are natural or synthetic fiber supplements that bind water and bile salts and may be useful in controlling diarrhea associated with the passing of excessively watery stools.

Drugs Useful for Treating Constipation

There is a great deal of variability in bowel habits from person to person; a normal stool frequency may vary from three stools per week up to three stools per day. Constipation is defined as the infrequent passage of stool. It may be secondary to sluggish colonic motility, in which soft stool is seen throughout the colon, or to difficulties with evacuation in which firm stool is seen primarily in the sigmoid and rectum.

The dangers of excessive purging are salt and fluid loss and gradually increasing desensitization of the bowel to normal stimuli; the latter effect forces the cathartic user to employ larger and larger doses.

Laxatives are used to increase stool frequency and reduce stool viscosity. Even with long-term use, bulk laxatives and pure osmolar laxatives do not predispose patients to formation of a cathartic-type colon and should be the initial agents used for chronic constipation after a structural obstructing lesion has been excluded. Laxatives are also used before radiological, endoscopic, and abdominal surgical procedures; such preparations quickly empty the colon of fecal material. Nonabsorbable hyperosmolar solutions or saline laxatives are used for this purpose. Classification and comparison of representative laxatives are provided in Table 40.1.

Stool Softeners

Fecal softeners are substances that are not absorbed from the alimentary canal and act by increasing the bulk of the feces and softening the stool so that it is easier to pass. Mineral oil has been in use for many years, either as the oil or as a white emulsion; it is a mixture of liquid hydrocarbons. Its use has been criticized for many reasons. It dissolves the fat-soluble vitamins and prevents their absorption. It is itself absorbed slightly and appears in the mesenteric lymph nodes, and if it is inhaled into the lungs (which it may be in elderly or debilitated patients), it may produce inflammatory responses such as lipoid pneumonia. Its continual use, therefore, is contraindicated, although its occasional administration in otherwise well patients is not harmful. It is employed primarily in patients who must avoid straining at stool, including persons with hemorrhoids and other painful anal lesions. Leakage of mineral oil past the anal sphincter may lead to soiling of clothing.

Docusate dioctyl sodium sulfosuccinate (*Colace*), dioctyl calcium sulfosuccinate (*Surfak*), and dioctyl potassium sulfosuccinate (*Diocto-K*) are surface-active agents that produce fecal softening in 1 or 2 days. By means of its detergent properties, docusate allows water to penetrate and soften colonic contents when it is administered as a retention enema. Orally ingested docusate may also act as a stool softener by stimulating the secretion of water and electrolytes into the intestinal lumen. Docusate has been used both alone and in combination with other laxatives. Although by itself it appears to be relatively nontoxic, it may, when taken in combination with other laxatives, increase their absorption and lead to liver toxicity. Caution is necessary when docusate is prescribed together with mineral oil, since the detergent increases the absorption of the oil.

Bulk Forming Laxatives

The bulk-forming laxative group includes the hydrophilic substances described previously: calcium polycarbophil (*FiberCon, Equalactin*), methylcellulose (*Citrucel*), and various psyllium seed derivatives (*Metamucil*). All act by increasing the bulk of the feces, part of this action being due to their capacity to attract water and form a hydrogel. The increased volume of feces stretches the walls of the GI tract and stimulates peristalsis. Their action may not be evident for 2 to 3 days after starting treatment. Because their use results

---

TABLE 40.1   Classification and Comparison of Representative Laxatives: Type, Cathartic Effect, and Latency

Softening of Formed Stool (1–3 d)	Soft, Semifluid Stool (6–12 hr)	Watery Stool (2–6 hr)
Bulk-forming agents	Saline laxatives (low dose)	Saline laxatives (high dose)
Dietary fiber	Milk of magnesia	Magnesium citrate
Methylcellulose	Magnesium sulfate	Magnesium sulfate
Psyllium	Diphenylmethane derivatives	Sodium phosphates
Calcium polycarbophil	Phenolphthalein	Castor oil
Docusate salts	Bisacodyl	Polyethylene glycol–electrolyte preparations
Sodium, potassium, or calcium salts	Anthraquinone derivatives	
of dioctyl sulfosuccinate	Senna	
Lactulose	Cascara sagrada	
Sorbitol		
Polyethylene glycol		

Adapted with permission from AMA Drug Evaluations (6th Ed.). Chicago: American Medical Association, 1986.

in increased water content in the feces, the patient should be advised to drink adequate amounts of water; otherwise dehydration may result.

The use of *high-fiber diets* has recently received a great deal of publicity, and many claims have been made for the value of such diets. Fiber in the diet is derived entirely from plant material, either from fruit and vegetables or from cereals, the latter being known as *bran*. The fiber content in each case is a complex carbohydrate in the form of cellulose, pectin, and lignin. These fibers pass through the human GI tract relatively unaltered by enzymes.

A high-fiber diet is effective in the prevention of constipation and diverticulitis. Claims also have been made that such diets prevent cancer of the colon. Such allegations require further study.

Since clear advantages accrue from a high-bran diet (a reduction in both constipation and diverticulitis) and since there is no associated toxicity, *a bulk-forming laxative is the laxative of choice for constipated patients.*

Osmotic Laxatives

Osmotic laxatives (e.g., lactulose, sorbitol) are poorly absorbed or nonabsorbable compounds that draw additional fluid into the GI tract. Lumen osmolality increases, and fluid movement occurs secondary to osmotic pressure. Lactulose is a synthetic disaccharide that is poorly absorbed from the GI tract, since no mammalian enzyme is capable of hydrolyzing it to its monosaccharide components. It therefore reaches the colon unchanged and is metabolized by colonic bacteria to lactic acid and to small quantities of formic and acetic acids. Since lactulose does contain galactose, it is contraindicated in patients who require a galactose-free diet. Metabolism of lactulose by intestinal bacteria may result in increased formation of intraluminal gas and abdominal distention. Lactulose is also used in the treatment of hepatic encephalopathy.

Polyethylene glycol (*Miralax*) is another osmotic laxative that is colorless and tasteless once it is mixed.

Saline Laxatives

Saline laxatives are soluble inorganic salts that contain multivalent cations or anions (milk of magnesia, magnesium citrate, and sodium phosphate [*Fleet Phospho Soda*]). These charged particles do not readily cross the intestinal mucosa and therefore tend to remain in the lumen of the GI tract, where they help retain fluid through the osmotic effect exerted by the unabsorbed ions. The volume in the GI tract is increased, distending the colon and producing a physiological stimulus for peristalsis through activation of stretch receptors. This explanation of the mechanism by which the saline laxatives exert their effects, however, may be too simplistic, since active secretion of fluid into the gut lumen has

been documented following the administration of magnesium-containing agents.

These salts should always be given with substantial amounts of water; otherwise the patient may be purged at the expense of body water, resulting in dehydration. Sodium-containing laxatives should not be used in patients with congestive heart failure, since the patient may absorb excessive sodium. Similarly, in cases of renal failure, magnesium or phosphate-containing products should not be used, since the loss of a renal clearance of these ions may result in cumulative toxic levels despite their minimal absorption.

Enemas may contain water, salts, soap, mineral detergent (docusate potassium), or hypertonic (sorbitol, sodium phosphate–biphosphate) fluids. These are convenient and generally safe for short-term use. Many of these solutions irritate the mucosa and may produce excessive mucus in the stool. Excessive use of these enema products may result in water intoxication and hyponatremia.

A new formulation of a saline laxative, *Visicol*, that is useful to prepare patients for procedures, was approved for use in 2001. Each 2-g tablet contains 1.102 g sodium phosphate monobasic monohydrate and 0.398 g sodium phosphate dibasic anhydrous, for a total of 1.5 g sodium phosphate. Visicol tablets, taken in two doses of 30 g approximately 12 hours apart, induce diarrhea that rapidly and effectively cleanses the entire colon. Each administration has a purgative effect for approximately 1 to 3 hours.

Stimulant Cathartics

The stimulant cathartics contain a variety of drugs whose exact mode of action is not known, although it is thought that they act on the mucosa of the intestine to stimulate peristalsis either by irritation or by exciting reflexes in the myenteric plexuses. All act in the lumen of the GI tract and are inactive if given parenterally. They produce irritation of the mucosa if given in large doses, and this irritation affects water and ion transport. However, a direct local irritation may not be essential to their action. It has been suggested that these drugs may act by stimulating afferent nerves to initiate a reflex increase in gut motility.

Anthraquinone derivatives (e.g., cascara, aloe, senna, and rhubarb) are among the oldest laxatives known. They act on the colon rather than on the ileum and produce evacuation 8 to 10 hours after administration. This makes them particularly suitable for dosage overnight. Cascara sagrada is one of the mildest of the anthraquinone-containing laxatives.

Phenolphthalein is partially absorbed (about 15% of a given dose) and excreted into the bile; hence, if it is taken constantly, it will accumulate and exert too drastic an action. It inhibits active sodium and glucose absorption in the bowel. Once widely available in many over-the-counter products, it was pulled from the market when it was linked to cancer.

Castor oil is a bland oil that is hydrolyzed in the gut to yield ricinoleic acid, the active purging agent. This hydrolysis requires bile, a fact that is sometimes overlooked when castor oil is given as a laxative before radiography in biliary obstruction. The ricinoleic acid acts on the ileum and colon to induce an increased fluid secretion and colonic contraction.

Bisacodyl (*Dulcolax*) causes colonic contraction and inhibits water absorption in the small and large intestine.

Isoosmotic Electrolyte Colonic Lavage Solutions

Electrolyte colonic lavage solutions (e.g., *GoLYTELY, Colyte, Nulytely*) contain polyethylene glycol and salts such as sodium sulfate, sodium bicarbonate, sodium chloride, and potassium chloride in an isoosmotic solution. The dose is 4 L ingested over 2 to 4 hours either orally or through a nasogastric tube. There is minimal net absorption or excretion of fluid or electrolytes, and thus these are safe to use in patients with renal insufficiency. The patient has repeated liquid stools until the administered solution has been expelled. If gastric emptying is slow, patients may have abdominal distention with vomiting. This preparation should not be used if a bowel obstruction or impaired gag reflex is present. It is used primarily to clear the bowel before radiological or endoscopic procedures and occasionally to assist with evacuation in a patient who has a sluggish colon.

PHARMACOLOGICAL MODULATION OF VOMITING

Vomiting is a complex series of integrated events culminating in the forceful expulsion of gastric contents through the mouth. The sequence of events frequently begins with nausea, which may be accompanied by increased salivation, pupillary dilation, sweating, and pallor. Duodenal and jejunal tone is increased, while gastric tone and peristalsis are diminished, tending to cause a reflux of duodenal contents into the stomach. Retching follows nausea, during which the abdominal muscles contract with simultaneous attempts at inspiration against a closed glottis. The gastric antrum contents and gastric contents begin to move into the esophagus. During vomiting, which is the third and final stage, there is sustained contraction of the diaphragm and abdominal musculature. The resultant high intragastric pressure moves more gastric contents into the esophagus, and with continued force, contents are expelled through the mouth.

These events are coordinated by the *emetic center,* which lies within the lateral reticular formation of the medulla oblongata close to the respiratory and salivary centers. Stimulation of the emetic center may occur from peripheral sites, the cortex, or the *chemoreceptor trigger zone* (CTZ). Peripheral stimulation, which is mediated by vagal and sympathetic nerves, may originate from the vestibular system (motion sickness), from the coronary arteries (cardiac ischemia), or from distention and inflammation of sites in the GI tract.

The CTZ, which is responsive to chemical (particularly dopamine) stimulation, is connected to the emetic center through the fasciculus solitarius. Most drug-induced emesis, including emesis induced by apomorphine, levodopa, cardiac glycosides, most cancer chemotherapeutic agents, and nicotine, appears to be mediated by this route. Cytotoxic chemotherapy also stimulates the release of serotonin from enterochromaffin cells of the upper GI tract. Vomiting may then be induced through serotonergic stimulation of enteric vagal afferents or possibly through direct central nervous system stimulation.

Emetics

The most commonly used emetics are ipecac and apomorphine. Induced emesis is the preferred means of emptying the stomach in awake patients who have ingested a toxic substance or have recently taken a drug overdose. Emesis should not be induced if the patient has central nervous system depression or has ingested certain volatile hydrocarbons and caustic substances.

Ipecac syrup is prepared from the dried rhizome and roots of *Cephaelis ipecacuanha* or *Cephaelis acuminata,* plants from Brazil and Central America that have the alkaloid *emetine* as their active principal ingredient. It acts directly on the CTZ and also indirectly by irritating the gastric mucosa. Ipecac is cardiotoxic if absorbed and can cause cardiac conduction disturbances, atrial fibrillation, or fatal myocarditis. If emesis does not occur, gastric lavage using a nasogastric tube must be performed.

Apomorphine, a derivative of morphine, acts directly on the CTZ. It also is more effective if water is first administered before oral or subcutaneous dosing. Excessive dosage may cause respiratory depression and circulatory collapse. Opioid antagonists such as naloxone usually reverse the depressant actions of apomorphine. Because of the possibility of respiratory depression, apomorphine is infrequently used as an emetic.

Antiemetics

Antiemetics may prevent emesis by blocking the CTZ or by preventing peripheral or cortical stimulation of the emetic center.

Antihistamines

The antihistamines appear to block peripheral stimulation of the emetic center. They are therefore most effective in motion sickness and inner ear dysfunction, as is seen in Ménière's syndrome, labyrinthitis, and streptomycin ototoxicity. Dimenhydrinate, diphenhydramine, and meclizine hydrochloride are the three antihistamines primarily used in the prevention of nausea from inner ear stimulation. A more complete discussion of the H_1 antihistamines can be found in Chapter 38.

Anticholinergics

The transdermal adhesive form of scopolamine (*Transderm Scop*) provides up to 72 hours of antiemetic protection when applied to the postauricular area. Side effects are similar to those of oral scopolamine (see Chapter 13) but milder.

Benzodiazepines

Benzodiazepines and their congeners may help prevent central cortical-induced vomiting. A prominent side effect is drowsiness. They are frequently used in combination with other antiemetics for treating chemotherapy-related nausea and vomiting. Discussion of these agents is found in Chapter 30.

Cannabinoids

The antiemetic site of action of tetrahydrocannabinol (THC) (*Marinol*) is unknown, although it appears to affect the central cerebral cortex axis. Relief may occur in individuals refractory to other antiemetics. It is less effective in the elderly, primarily because of its side effects. The antiemetic effect is associated with a high, and this appears to be better tolerated in the young. Sedation is seen in approximately 30% of patients. Ataxia, drowsiness, dry mouth, or orthostatic hypotension may be seen in up to 35% of the older patient population. GI absorption is variable, though blood levels correlate with efficacy. The bioavailability is not as variable if the agent is smoked. The coadministration of prochlorperazine may prevent some of the central nervous system side effects seen with the use of tetrahydrocannabinol.

Dopamine Antagonists

Metoclopramide is a dopamine antagonist that centrally inhibits stimulation of the CTZ. By improving gastric emptying, it can decompress the stomach, thereby decreasing a peripherally associated stimulation of the emetic center. Metoclopramide may precipitate extrapyramidal reactions and sedation. For further details, see earlier section, Drugs that Increase GI Motility.

Phenothiazine Derivatives

Phenothiazine derivatives, which include prochlorperazine (*Compazine*) and promethazine (*Phenergan*), act at the CTZ by inhibiting dopaminergic transmission. They also decrease vomiting caused by gastric irritants, suggesting that they inhibit stimulation of peripheral vagal and sympathetic afferents. Sedation will frequently occur following their administration. Patients also may have problems with acute dystonic reactions, orthostatic hypotension, cholestatic hepatitis, and blood dyscrasias.

5-HT₃ Receptor Antagonists

Ondansetron (*Zofran*) and granisetron (*Kytril*) are potent antagonists of 5-HT₃ receptors, which are found peripherally on vagal nerve terminals and centrally in the CTZ. During chemotherapy that induces vomiting, mucosal enterochromaffin cells in the GI tract release serotonin, which stimulates 5-HT₃ receptors. This causes vagal afferent discharge, inducing vomiting. In binding to 5-HT₃ receptors, ondansetron and granisetron block serotonin stimulation, hence vomiting, after emetogenic stimuli such as cisplatin. Headache is the most frequently reported adverse effect of these medications.

DRUGS THAT DECREASE OR NEUTRALIZE GASTRIC ACID SECRETION

Functionally, the gastric mucosa is divided into three areas of secretion. The *cardiac gland area* secretes mucus and pepsinogen. The *oxyntic (parietal) gland area*, which corresponds to the fundus and body of the stomach, secretes hydrogen ions, pepsinogen, and bicarbonate. The *pyloric gland area* in the antrum secretes gastrin and mucus.

The parietal cells secrete H^+ in response to gastrin, cholinergic, and histamine stimulation (Fig. 40.1). Both cholinergic- and gastrin-induced types of stimulation bring about a receptor-mediated rise in intracellular calcium, an activation of intracellular protein kinases, and eventually an increased activity of the H^+–K^+ pump leading to acid secretion into the gastric lumen. Following histamine stimulation, a guanine nucleotide–binding protein (G_s) activates adenylyl cyclase, leading to an increase in intracellular levels of the second messenger, cyclic adenosine monophosphate (cAMP). Activation of cAMP-dependent protein kinases initiates the stimulation of the H^+–K^+ pump.

The cephalic–vagal axis, gastric distention, and local mucosal chemical receptors can modulate acid secretion by the stomach. The smell, taste, sight, or discussion of food may result in cephalic–vagal postganglionic cholinergic stimulation of target parietal cells and enhanced antral gastrin release. After food is ingested, gastric distention initiates vagal stimulation and short intragastric neural reflexes, both of which increase acid secretion. Proteins in ingested meals also stimulate acid

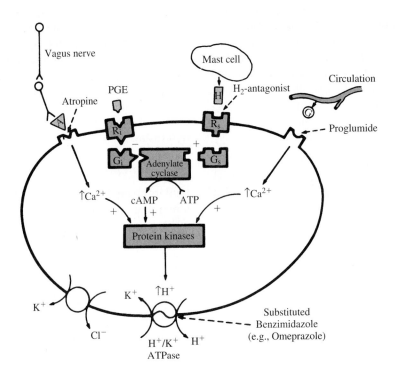

FIGURE 40.1

Influences on parietal cell acid secretion. The pathways by which secretagogues are believed to stimulate hydrogen ion production and secretion are shown. In addition, the sites of action (broken arrows) of various acid suppressive medications are shown. A, atropine; PGE, prostaglandin E; H, histamine; G, gastrin, R_i and R_s, inhibitory and stimulatory receptor-binding sites; G_i and G_s, inhibitory and stimulatory catalytic subunits; ATP, adenosine triphosphate; ATPase, adenosine triphosphatase. (Reprinted with permission from Wolfe MM and Soll AH. The physiology of gastric acid secretion. N Engl J Med 1988;319:1707.)

secretion. Evidence from animal studies suggests that after protein amino acids are converted to amines, gastrin is released.

Gastric acid secretion is inhibited in the presence of acid itself. A negative feedback occurs when the pH approaches 2.5 such that further secretion of gastrin is inhibited until the pH rises. Ingested carbohydrates and fat also inhibit acid secretion after they reach the intestines; several hormonal mediators for this effect have been proposed. The secretion of pepsinogen appears to parallel the secretion of H^+, while the patterns of secretion of mucus and bicarbonate have not been well characterized.

The integrity of the mucosal lining of the stomach and proximal small bowel is in large part determined by the mucosal cytoprotection provided by mucus and bicarbonate secretion from the gastric and small bowel mucosa. Mucus retards diffusion of the H^+ from the gastric lumen back into the gastric mucosal surface. In addition, the bicarbonate that is secreted into the layer between the mucus and epithelium permits a relatively high pH to be maintained in the region next to the mucosal surface. If any H^+ does diffuse back to the level of the mucosal surface, both the local blood supply and the ability of the local cells to buffer this ion will ultimately determine whether peptic ulceration will occur. With duodenal and gastric peptic ulcer disease, a major causative cofactor is the presence of gastric *Helicobacter pylori* infection.

Medications that raise intragastric pH are used to treat peptic ulcer disease and gastroesophageal reflux disease. In addition, agents that enhance mucosal cytoprotection are used to decrease ulcer risk.

Antacids

The rationale for the use of antacids in peptic ulcer disease lies in the assumption that buffering of H^+ in the stomach permits healing. The use of both low and high doses of antacids is effective in healing peptic ulcers as compared with placebo. Healing rates are comparable with those observed after the use of histamine (H_2) blocking agents. The buffering agents in the various antacid preparations consist of combinations of ingredients that include sodium bicarbonate, calcium carbonate, magnesium hydroxide, and aluminum hydroxide. If diarrhea occurs or if there is renal failure, a magnesium-based preparation should be discontinued. The agents are generally safe, but some patients resist because some of the formulations are unpalatable and expensive.

A variety of adverse effects have been reported following the use of antacids. If sodium bicarbonate is absorbed, it can cause systemic alkalization and sodium overload. Calcium carbonate may induce hypercalcemia and a rebound increase in gastric secretion secondary to the elevation in circulating calcium levels. Magnesium hydroxide may produce osmotic diarrhea, and the excessive absorption of Mg^{++} in patients with renal failure may result in central nervous system toxicity. Aluminum hydroxide is associated with constipation; serum phosphate levels also may become depressed because of phosphate binding within the gut. The use of antacids in general may interfere with the absorption of a number of antibiotics and other medications.

H₂-Receptor Antagonists

The histamine receptor antagonists (H_2 blockers) marketed in the United States are cimetidine (*Tagamet*), ranitidine (*Zantac*), famotidine (*Pepcid*), and nizatidine (*Axid*). These agents bind to the H_2-receptors on the cell membranes of parietal cells and prevent histamine-induced stimulation of gastric acid secretion. After prolonged use, down-regulation of receptor production occurs, resulting in tolerance to these agents. H_2-blockers are approved for the treatment of gastroesophageal reflux disease, acute ulcer healing, and post–ulcer healing maintenance therapy. Although there are substantial differences in their relative potency, 70 to 85% of duodenal ulcers are healed during 4 to 6 weeks of therapy with any of these agents. The incidence of healing of gastric ulceration after 6 to 8 weeks of therapy approaches 60 to 80% with the use of cimetidine or ranitidine. Since nocturnal suppression of acid secretion is particularly important in healing, nighttime-only dosing can be used. Most are available in low-dose over-the-counter formulations.

Cimetidine, the first released H_2-blocker, like histamine, contains an imidazole ring structure. It is well absorbed following oral administration, with peak blood levels 45 to 90 minutes after drug ingestion. Blood levels remain within therapeutic concentrations for approximately 4 hours after a 300-mg dose. Following oral administration, 50 to 75% of the parent compound is excreted unchanged in the urine; the rest appears primarily as the sulfoxide metabolite.

Cimetidine may infrequently cause diarrhea, nausea, vomiting, or mental confusion. A rare association with granulocytopenia, thrombocytopenia, and pancytopenia has been reported. Gynecomastia has been demonstrated in patients receiving either high-dose or long-term therapy. This occurs because cimetidine has a weak antiestrogen effect. Since cimetidine is partly metabolized by the cytochrome P450 system, coadministered drugs such as the benzodiazepines, theophylline, and warfarin, which are also metabolized by this system, may accumulate if their dosage is not adjusted.

Ranitidine is well absorbed after oral administration, with a peak plasma level achieved 1 to 3 hours after ingestion. Elimination is by renal (25%) and hepatic (50%) routes. The half-life of elimination is 2.5 to 3.0 hours. Nizatidine is the newest H_2-receptor antagonist. Similar to ranitidine, it has a relative potency twice that of cimetidine. About 90% of an oral dose is absorbed, with a peak plasma concentration occurring after 0.5 to 3 hours; inhibition of gastric secretion is present for up to 10 hours. The elimination half-life is 1 to 2 hours, and more than 90% of an oral dose is excreted in the urine. Famotidine has an onset of effect within 1 hour after oral administration, and inhibition of gastric secretion is present for the next 10 to 12 hours. It is the most potent H_2-blocker. Elimination is by renal (65–70%) and hepatic (30–35%) routes. Ranitidine, famotidine, and nizatidine do not alter the microsomal cytochrome P450 metabolism of other drugs, nor do they cause gynecomastia. A reduction in dosage of any of the H_2-blockers is recommended in the presence of renal insufficiency.

Proton Pump Inhibitors

The proton pump inhibitors available in the United States are omeprazole (*Prilosec*), lansoprazole (*Prevacid*), pantoprazole (*Protonix*), rabeprazole (*Aciphex*), and esomeprazole (*Nexium*). These are substituted benzimidazole prodrugs, which accumulate on the luminal side of parietal cells' secretory canaliculi. They become activated by acid transport and then bind covalently to the actual H^+–K^+ ATPase enzymes (proton pumps) irreversibly blocking them. *These drugs markedly inhibit gastric acid secretion.* New proton pumps are continuously formed, and thus no tolerance develops. Peptic ulcers and erosive esophagitis that are resistant to other therapies will frequently heal when these agents are used. The proton pump inhibitors are also used to treat patients with *Zollinger-Ellison syndrome,* which is the result of a gastrin-hypersecreting neuroendocrine tumor.

The prodrugs are unstable in the presence of acid and therefore must be administered as an enteric-coated preparation or as a buffered suspension. Pantoprazole is also available in an intravenous formulation. The most commonly reported side effects are diarrhea and headache. Hypergastrinemia has been noted as a reaction to the marked reduction in acid secretion. Gastric carcinoid tumors have developed in rats but not in mice or in human volunteers, even after long-term use.

TREATMENT OF INFLAMMATORY BOWEL DISEASE

Inflammatory bowel disease mainly refers to *ulcerative colitis* and *Crohn's disease.* Ulcerative colitis is characterized by a relapsing inflammatory condition involving the mucosa of variable lengths of the colon resulting in bleeding, urgency, diarrhea, and tenesmus. The endoscopic and radiographic appearance may demonstrate multiple diffuse erosions or ulcerations. Biopsy reveals distorted crypt abscesses and diminished goblet cells. When involvement is limited to the rectum, it is termed ulcerative proctitis. Crohn's disease may involve the gut from esophagus to anus; however, the small bowel or colon or both are the major areas of involvement. Inflammation is transmural. If the colon is predominantly involved, the symptoms and presentation are quite similar to those of ulcerative colitis. Small bowel involvement may result in large-volume bloodless diarrhea or obstruction. Normal areas of gut may be found between areas of inflamed mucosa. Fistulas, strictures, and abscess formation are fairly common in Crohn's disease.

The present primary mode of therapy for these diseases involves the use 5-amino-salicylate (5-ASA) products. Often patients require additional medications, including corticosteroids, to help induce remission and various immune modulators, such as azathioprine, 6-mercaptopurine or methotrexate, to maintain remission. In Crohn's disease certain antibiotics, such as metronidazole and ciprofloxacin, and infliximab (*Remicade*), an anti–tumor necrosis factor-α(TNFα) antibody, also have been used. The pharmacology of antibiotics, immunosuppressive drugs, and corticosteroids is discussed in Chapters 43, 57, and 60, respectively.

5-Aminosalicylates

Sulfasalazine (*Azulfidine*) was first introduced in 1940 as a treatment for rheumatoid arthritis. It was found that a number of patients with coexistent inflammatory bowel disease showed improvement of their GI symptoms, and the drug has subsequently been used for the treatment of patients with inflammatory bowel disease.

Sulfasalazine is composed of sulfapyridine and 5-ASA molecules linked by an azo bond. Sulfapyridine has no effect on the inflammatory bowel disease, and instillation of this agent into the colon does not heal colonic mucosa. It is, however, responsible for most of sulfasalazine's side effects, including sulfa allergic reactions. 5-ASA, the active metabolite, may inhibit the synthesis of mediators of inflammation.

Following oral administration, 30% of the sulfasalazine is absorbed from the small intestine. Because most of the compound that is absorbed is later excreted into the bowel, 75 to 85% of the administered oral dose eventually reaches the colon intact. Bacteria in the colon then split the azo linkage, liberating sulfapyridine and 5-ASA. The sulfapyridine is absorbed, acetylated, hydroxylated, and conjugated to glucuronic acid in the liver. The major portion of the sulfapyridine molecule and its metabolites are excreted in the urine. The 5-ASA remains in the colon, eventually reaching high fecal levels.

Sulfasalazine treatment results in an 85% remission rate in mild to moderate ulcerative colitis. Termination of therapy leads to an 80% relapse within the next year. In Crohn's disease, sulfasalazine acts primarily on involved colonic mucosa, although remission of ileal disease also has been reported. The National Cooperative Crohn's Disease Study found sulfasalazine to be better in the treatment of colonic disease, while corticosteroids were judged better in the treatment of small bowel disease. Since sulfasalazine does not prevent relapse of Crohn's disease once remission is achieved, maintenance therapy is not characteristically used.

Nausea, vomiting, and headaches, the most common side effects, are related to the blood level of sulfapyridine. If the dose is reduced, symptoms frequently improve. Fever, rash, aplastic anemia, and autoimmune hemolysis are hypersensitivity reactions to the medication. These occur less commonly and are not dose related. Sulfasalazine should not be used in patients with hypersensitivity agranulocytosis or aplastic anemia.

Since sulfasalazine inhibits the absorption of folic acid, patients may become folate deficient during long-term therapy. Sulfasalazine decreases the bioavailability of digoxin. Cholestyramine reduces the metabolism of sulfasalazine. Sulfasalazine causes a reversible decrease in sperm counts. Sulfasalazine is safe in pregnancy.

To avoid the side effects of sulfapyridine, various preparations to target 5-ASA directly to sites of disease have been formulated. Also known as mesalamine, 5-ASA has been formulated in oral forms (*Pentasa, Asacol*). Pentasa is a time-release capsule that releases the drug throughout the GI tract. Asacol is a pH-dependent–release preparation that delivers drug to the distal small bowel and colon. The response of ulcerative colitis to this formulation appears to be identical to that seen with sulfasalazine. Mesalamine can also be administered as a suppository (*Canasa*) or enema (*Rowasa*) for distal colonic disease.

Olsalazine sodium (*Dipentum*) links two 5-ASA molecules with an azo linkage. Following cleavage of the azo linkage in the colon, two 5-ASA molecules are released. Olsalazine is approved for maintenance of remission of ulcerative colitis, but a commonly reported side effect is a paradoxical increase in diarrhea. The U. S. Food and Drug Administration (FDA) has approved balsalazide disodium (*Colazal*) as a treatment of mild to moderately active ulcerative colitis. Balsalazide disodium is delivered intact to the colon, where it is cleaved by bacterial azoreduction to release equimolar quantities of mesalamine, the therapeutically active portion of the molecule, and 4-aminobenzoyl-β-alanine; the latter compound is only minimally absorbed and is largely inert.

Infliximab

TNF-α is an inflammatory cytokine thought to have a contributory role in producing chronic inflammation in various diseases, including Crohn's disease and rheumatoid arthritis (see Chapter 36). Infliximab (*Remicade*) is a mouse–human chimeric monoclonal *neutralizing* antibody to human TNF-α and is considered a biological drug. Specific indications are for the reduction of signs and symptoms in patients with moderately to severely active Crohn's disease who have had an inadequate response to conventional therapies (single infusion) and for reduction of the number of draining enterocutaneous fistulas in patients with fistulizing Crohn's disease (three-infusion regimen). Responses occur within 2 weeks of an infusion, and significant clinical responses were reported in 50 to 80% of patients in initial trials with infliximab. This antibody is being studied as maintenance therapy for Crohn's disease and to determine the best induction regimen to achieve remission.

The most common side effects, which are related to the intravenous infusion itself, include rash, low blood pressure, chills, and chest pain. These symptoms are generally temporary and often respond to a decrease in infusion rate. In addition, some patients develop antibodies, which have been associated in rare cases with symptoms similar to those of patients with systemic lupus erythematosus. These symptoms were also temporary. Another side effect is increased risk of infections. Fatal cases of tuberculosis have been reported following infliximab therapy. Another potential side effect is an increased risk of lymphoma. Its occurrence remains controversial.

Budesonide

Recently, budesonide (*Entecort EC*) has been approved for the treatment of mildly to moderately active Crohn's disease involving the ileum and/or ascending colon. Budesonide is a synthetic corticosteroid having a potent glucocorticoid and weak mineralocorticoid activity. In standard in vitro and animal models, budesonide has an approximately 200-fold higher affinity for the glucocorticoid receptor and a 1000-fold higher topical antiinflammatory potency than cortisol. While budesonide is well absorbed from the GI tract, its oral bioavailability is low (about 10%), primarily because of extensive first-pass metabolism in the liver. Two major metabolites (16α-hydroxyprednisolone and 6β-

hydroxybudesonide) are formed via the cytochrome P450 3A enzyme. In vitro studies on the binding of the two primary metabolites to the corticosteroid receptor indicate that their affinity for the receptor is less than 1% of that of the parent compound. It is hoped that use of this drug will avoid the long-term adverse reactions seen with systemically active corticosteroids.

MISCELLANEOUS GI DRUGS

Additional drugs in classes of their own are also used in the treatment and/or prevention of various GI conditions. They include misoprostol, sucralfate, and octreotide.

Misoprostol

Prostaglandins of the A, E, and I type inhibit gastric acid secretion. The prostaglandins also stimulate increased mucus and bicarbonate secretion by gastric mucosa. Misoprostol (*Cytotec*), which is an analogue of prostaglandin E_1, has been approved for use in the prevention of nonsteroidal antiinflammatory drug–induced ulceration. It also is approved in other countries for the treatment of peptic ulcer disease. Misoprostol is absorbed rapidly after oral administration and is hydrolyzed to the active compound. It is metabolized by the liver and excreted mainly in the urine. Adverse effects include crampy abdominal pain, dose-related diarrhea, and uterine contractions. The last-named effect has led to its use in the control of postpartum bleeding (see Chapter 62).

Sucralfate

Sucralfate (*Carafate*) is an aluminum hydroxide–sulfated sucrose complex that is only minimally absorbed from the GI tract. After exposure to gastric acid, the compound becomes negatively charged, creating a viscous adherent complex. This complex is believed to inhibit back-diffusion of H^+. Other effects are a direct reduction in pepsin activity and a slight rise in tissue prostaglandin levels. Stimulation of a cytoprotection mechanism may therefore assist mucosal healing. The drug has no acid-buffering capacity.

Sucralfate is frequently used for prophylaxis of stress-induced gastritis in patients in intensive care units. It has also been successfully used in small numbers of patients as a suspension enema to treat radiation proctitis.

Constipation is the main side effect associated with its oral use. As with other aluminum compounds, the drug may bind phosphorus, resulting in secondary hypophosphatemia. Binding to a number of other coadministered medications may result in a significant reduction in their bioavailability.

Octreotide

Octreotide (*Sandostatin*) is a synthetic somatostatin analogue. It is used in a variety of situations and must be given subcutaneously or intravenously. Most commonly, it is used as a continuous intravenous infusion in patients hospitalized with bleeding varices, because it decreases splanchnic circulation and therefore reduces portal pressures. A long-acting depot form is approved for the suppression of severe diarrhea and flushing associated with malignant carcinoid syndrome and for the treatment of the profuse watery diarrhea associated with vasoactive intestinal peptide tumor.

Study QUESTIONS

1. A 36-year-old woman with severe erosive esophagitis is prescribed pantoprazole. One of the most common adverse side effects of such therapy is which of the following?
   (A) Vomiting
   (B) Constipation
   (C) Headache
   (D) Heartburn
   (E) Paresthesias

2. While taking a NSAID for arthritis, a 65-year-old man developed a gastric ulcer. He was prescribed ranitidine for 8 weeks. This drug binds a receptor located where?
   (A) Nucleus
   (B) Nucleolus
   (C) Cytoplasm
   (D) Cell membrane
   (E) Cell wall

3. A 20-year-old woman goes to the emergency department, stating that within the past hour she ingested "a handful of sleeping pills." She is still awake. Which of the following drugs can be given to induce vomiting?
   (A) Metoclopramide
   (B) Ipecac
   (C) Morphine
   (D) Promethazine
   (E) Ondansetron

4. A 17-year-old boy with a history of sulfa allergy is diagnosed with left-side ulcerative colitis after a 3-week history of bloody diarrhea and tenesmus. On examination he is afebrile and has no abdominal tenderness. The appropriate drug therapy to institute initially is which of the following?
   (A) Metronidazole
   (B) Sulfasalazine
   (C) Mesalamine
   (D) Cyclosporine
   (E) Prednisone

5. A 62-year-old woman on hemodialysis is scheduled for a screening colonoscopy. Which should be prescribed for her colonic preparation?
   (A) Visicol
   (B) Fleet Phospho soda
   (C) Magnesium citrate
   (D) Dulcolax
   (E) GoLYTELY

6. Gastric acid secretion is stimulated by the presence of
   (A) Gastrin and acetylcholine
   (B) Histamine and motilin
   (C) Norepinephrine and gastrin
   (D) Norepinephrine and histamine
   (E) Acetylcholine and pepsin

ANSWERS

1. **C.** The most commonly reported side effects for all of the proton pump inhibitors are headache, diarrhea, and abdominal pain. Heartburn is improved by these agents. Vomiting, constipation, and paresthesias are not typical side effects of proton pump inhibitors.

2. **D.** Ranitidine is an H_2-receptor antagonist. H_2-receptors are found in the cell membrane of parietal cells, not in the nucleus, nucleolus, or cytoplasm. Mammalian cells do not have cell walls.

3. **B.** Two medicines, ipecac and apomorphine, induce vomiting. Metoclopramide is a prokinetic with antiemetic properties and therefore would have the opposite of the desired effect. Morphine is an opioid with analgesic and sedating properties. Promethazine and ondansetron are also antiemetics, not emetics.

4. **C.** The information provided suggests the patient has mild to moderate disease. Initial therapy should be a 5-ASA containing product, which includes sulfasalazine and mesalamine. However, the patient has a sulfa allergy, precluding the use of sulfasalazine. Metronidazole is useful in the treatment of some patients with Crohn's disease. Cyclosporine has been used in patients with fulminant ulcerative colitis. Prednisone may have to be added to this patient's therapy, but only if he fails to respond to the mesalamine. It should not be used initially.

5. E. A patient on hemodialysis has end-stage renal disease and therefore cannot tolerate excess magnesium and phosphorus. Visicol and Fleet Phospho soda have phosphates, and magnesium citrate has magnesium. GoLYTELY is an isosmotic unabsorbable electrolyte–polyethylene glycol colonic lavage solution that is safe for patients with end-stage renal disease. Dulcolax is a stimulant cathartic but is not sufficient for colonoscopy preparation.

6. A. Gastrin, histamine, and acetylcholine stimulate gastric acid secretion. Pepsin is a digestive protein secreted by the stomach in response to a meal. Norepinephrine is a neurotransmitter that does not affect gastric acid secretion.

SUPPLEMENTAL READING

Borum ML. Irritable bowel syndrome. Prim Care 2001;28:523–538.

Hatlebakk JG. Medical therapy. Management of the refractory patient. Gastroenterol Clin North Am 1999;28:847–860.

Huang JQ. Pharmacological and pharmacodynamic essentials of H(2)-receptor antagonists and proton pump inhibitors for the practicing physician. Ballieres Best Pract Res Clin Gastroenterol 2001;15:355–370.

Kromer W. Endogenous and exogenous opioids in the control of gastrointestinal motility and secretion. Pharmacol Rev 1988;40:121–162.

Smoot DT. Peptic ulcer disease. Prim Care 2001;28:487–503.

Stein RB. Medical therapy for inflammatory bowel disease. Gastroenterol Clin North Am 1999;28:297–321.

Stotland BR. Advances in inflammatory bowel disease. Med Clin North Am 2000;84:1107–1124.

Wald A. Constipation. Med Clin North Am 2000;84:1231–1246.

CASE Study Peptic Ulcer Disease

JK is a 32-year-old white woman who works as the administrative assistant to the chief executive officer of a large firm. She has two small children and describes her life as stressful. She smokes 1 pack of cigarettes per day. She frequently takes naproxen for headaches. For the past 5 weeks she has noticed significant epigastric discomfort. This morning she went to the emergency department complaining of hematemesis. She was admitted, and the gastroenterologist performed an upper endoscopy that revealed a 1-cm ulcer. Is further evaluation necessary, and what recommendations would you make to this patient?

ANSWER: Peptic ulcer disease is most frequently secondary to either *Helicobacter pylori* infection or use of NSAIDs. The patient does admit to NSAID use (naproxen), but should also be checked for concomitant *H. pylori* infection at time of endoscopy or by a serology test. If the patient was found to have *H. pylori*, an appropriate eradication regimen should be prescribed. The patient should also be counseled to avoid NSAIDs. The patient should be prescribed a proton pump inhibitor for 8 weeks to heal the ulcer. A repeat endoscopy should be done at that time to document ulcer healing and rule out gastric cancer. In addition, the patient should be counseled to stop smoking, which is a risk factor for more severe peptic ulcer disease.

41 Drugs Used in Dermatological Disorders

Eric L. Carter, Mary-Margaret Chren, and David R. Bickers

 DRUG LIST

Although skin diseases only infrequently affect longevity, they significantly influence one's sense of well-being. The skin functions not simply as a passive barrier but also as an important organ intimately connected to the immune and nervous systems. Furthermore, transdermal drug delivery for systemic therapy and the recognition of the skin as a potential target for gene replacement have enhanced awareness of the skin's importance.

SKIN STRUCTURE

The skin consists of two main compartments, the *epidermis*, a stratified squamous epithelium, and the underlying *dermis*, a richly vascularized tissue embedded in a connective tissue matrix (Fig. 41.1). The epidermis consists of multiple layers of keratinocytes, which differentiate into the outermost layer, the stratum corneum. This layer contains the hydrophilic structural

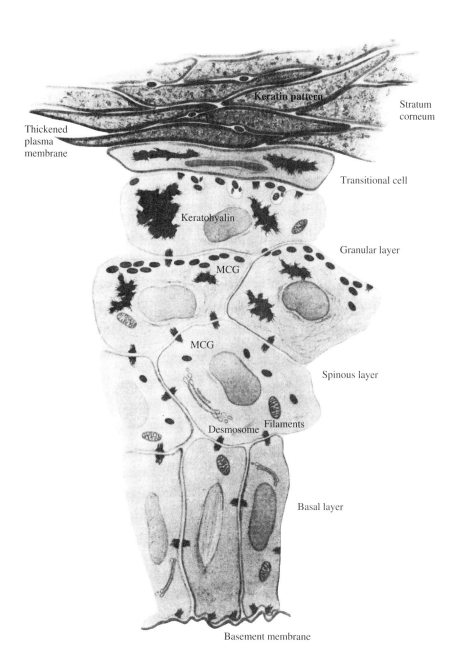

FIGURE 41.1

The layers of the epidermis. (Adapted with permission from Montagna W and Parakkal PF. The Structure and Function of Skin [3rd ed.]. New York: Academic, 1974.)

protein *keratin* surrounded by hydrophobic intercellular lipids, a remarkably effective barrier to many topically applied agents. The differentiation of keratinocytes in the basal layer from proliferative cells to highly differentiated nondividing cells in the stratum corneum is tightly regulated by a variety of intrinsic and extrinsic factors, including cytokines and calcium. The epidermis also contains *melanocytes,* which synthesize the photoprotective pigment melanin, and *Langerhans cells,* the dendritic antigen-presenting cells that compose the farthest outpost of the body's immune system.

The dermis provides a base for the epidermis and contains *fibroblasts* that elaborate proteins, such as collagens and elastin, which are crucial for the skin's structural integrity. In addition, *mast* cells, enriched in a variety of proinflammatory substances, play an important role in tissue remodeling, wound healing, and fibrosis.

PERCUTANEOUS ABSORPTION

The rate of diffusion of a chemical across the skin is related to these, among other features:

- Its concentration when applied
- The surface area to which it is applied
- Its movement through the epidermis (the *diffusion constant*)
- The relative tenacity with which it binds to its vehicle compared with epidermis (the *partition coefficient*)
- The thickness of the stratum corneum (barrier)

The amount of drug absorbed can be enhanced by increasing its applied concentration, increasing the size of the area to which it is applied, decreasing the barrier to its mobility through the layers (generally by hydrating the skin), and increasing its affinity for the skin (usually by increasing its hydrophobic component). Drug absorption is also greater in regions in which the skin is thinner.

PRACTICAL CONSIDERATIONS IN TOPICAL DRUG THERAPY

For designing effective topical drug therapy it is important to understand the principles of transmembrane transport and the unique structure of the stratum corneum. Some practical factors:

- *Dosage–surface area relationships:* In general, about 2 g of a topical product is required to cover the scalp, face, or hand; 3 g to cover an arm; 4 g to cover a leg; and 30 to 60 g to cover the entire body.

- *Hydration of the stratum corneum:* Hydration enhances the drug's solubility in and mobility through the skin (and its absorption) as much as tenfold. Hydration is usually achieved by using an occlusive vehicle or covering the treated skin with impermeable plastic film.
- *Type of vehicle:* In addition to their importance for hydration of the skin, vehicles vary in their partition coefficients (i.e., oil–water solubility ratio) for a given drug with respect to the stratum corneum. For example, a lipophilic drug moves more readily into the epidermis if it is in an aqueous vehicle, to which it is less tightly bound. Also, certain vehicles are soothing in various types of skin eruptions; dry, chronic inflammation often improves with drugs administered in lipophilic vehicles, whereas moist acute inflammation is best treated with aqueous preparations. Chemical constituents of vehicles can occasionally cause irritation or allergic sensitization that in turn may enhance penetration of drugs. Remember that for most topical drugs the vehicle constitutes more than 99% of the formulation.
- *Variation in penetration at different anatomic sites:* Drug penetration is inversely related to thickness of the stratum corneum. Thus, permeability (and often toxicity) is greater in areas of thinner skin, such as the face or scrotum.
- *Inflammation:* Permeability to most drugs is greater in inflamed skin.
- *Age:* Systemic toxicity from topically applied drugs is most likely in infants and small children because of their high ratio of surface area to body weight

TOPICAL GLUCOCORTICOSTEROIDS

Topical glucocorticosteroids are the most widely prescribed drugs for skin diseases. Like systemic glucocorticosteroids (Chapter 60), topical glucocorticosteroids bind to cytoplasmic receptors that transport the drug to the nucleus, where the complex binds to particular regions of DNA known as the glucocorticoid response element (GRE) and alters gene expression. Such receptors have been identified in both epidermis and dermis.

Drug absorption is enhanced by the use of agents with lipophilic side chains; by application of the drug to larger areas of skin, to inflamed areas, and/or for long periods; and by the use of occlusive dressings. Like their systemic counterparts, topical glucocorticosteroids have myriad pharmacological effects. Especially important in skin diseases are their antiinflammatory and immunosuppressive effects and their catabolic characteristics (hence their usefulness in eczematous dermatitis and their toxicity of dermal atrophy, respectively).

Although their exact mechanism of action is unclear, they are known to inhibit the expression of various cytokines and adhesion molecules and to antagonize the activity of transcription factors, including NF-κB, NF-AT, and AP-1.

Topical corticosteroids are most useful in inflammatory dermatoses, such as eczematous dermatitis and psoriasis; they may also be helpful in other skin diseases that have a prominent inflammatory component, such as autoimmune blistering diseases (e.g., bullous pemphigoid and pemphigus vulgaris) and lupus erythematosus.

Many compounds are available in both proprietary and generic forms, and their bioequivalence is difficult to document. Nonetheless, the drugs are classified into seven categories according to their relative potencies (Table 41.1).

Systemic toxicity from topical corticosteroids can occur, particularly from the more potent agents. Cushing's syndrome, although rare, has been reported.

Milder suppression of the hypothalamic–pituitary–adrenal axis is more common. Local toxicity is relatively frequent and may not be reversible. Dermal atrophy, appearing as striae or telangiectasias, is especially likely in intertriginous areas, where occlusion occurs naturally and the skin is likely to be thin. Less commonly, steroid-induced acneiform eruptions, rosacea, and perioral dermatitis can occur. Glaucoma and cataracts have been reported from chronic application around the eye. The normal inflammatory response to local infections may be masked by corticosteroids, complicating diagnosis and therapy. Contact allergy to the glucocorticosteroid preparations has been recognized with increasing frequency. This may present as diagnostically confusing eczematous dermatitis or unresponsiveness of the original dermatosis to treatment because the steroid–allergen maintains partial antiinflammatory properties.

RETINOIDS

Retinoids are a family of naturally occurring and synthetic analogues of vitamin A. The skin of subjects deficient in vitamin A becomes hyperplastic and keratotic (phrynoderma, or toad skin). While natural vitamin A is occasionally employed therapeutically, synthetic retinoids are more effective and represent a major advance in dermatological pharmacotherapy. Retinoids have myriad effects on cellular differentiation and proliferation; it is likely that nuclear retinoic acid receptors mediate these effects by activating gene expression in a manner analogous to receptors for steroid hormones and thyroid hormones. Despite a common mechanism of action, however, retinoids vary widely in their physiological effects.

Retinoid action depends on binding to both cytosolic and nuclear retinoic acid receptors (RARs). RARs have distinct DNA and retinoid-binding domains, and they function as pairs and bind to the retinoic acid receptor element (RARE) to regulate transcriptional activity.

Isotretinoin

Isotretinoin (*Accutane*) alters keratinization in the acroinfundibulum of sebaceous glands and shrinks them, thereby reducing sebum excretion and comedogenesis. These features underlie its usefulness in acne vulgaris, since sebum secretion is a hallmark of acne-prone skin. Furthermore, the drug has antiinflammatory activity.

Isotretinoin is rapidly absorbed orally, with peak blood concentrations 3 hours after ingestion. It is not stored in tissue, and the elimination half-life is 10 to 20 hours, either after a single dose or during chronic therapy.

Isotretinoin is most useful for the treatment of severe recalcitrant nodular acne vulgaris. It may also be

TABLE 41.1   **Selected Topical Corticosteroid Preparations**

Potency class[a]	Drug
1	Betamethasone dipropionate cream, ointment 0.05%
	Clobetasol propionate cream, ointment 0.05%
	Diflorasone diacetate 0.05%
2	Amcinonide ointment 0.1%
	Desoximetasone cream or ointment 0.25%, gel 0.05%
	Fluocinonide cream, ointment, gel 0.05%
	Halcinonide cream 0.1%
3	Betamethasone valerate ointment 0.1%
	Diflorasone diacetate cream 0.05%
	Triamcinolone acetonide ointment 0.1%, cream 0.5%
4	Amcinonide cream 0.1%
	Desoximetasone cream 0.05%
	Fluocinolone acetonide cream 0.2%
	Fluocinonide acetonide ointment 0.025%
	Hydrocortisone valerate ointment 0.2%
5	Betamethasone dipropionate lotion 0.05%
	Betamethasone valerate cream, lotion 0.1%
	Fluocinolone acetonide cream 0.025%
	Hydrocortisone valerate cream 0.2%
	Triamcinolone acetonide cream, lotion 0.1%
	Triamcinolone acetonide cream 0.025%
6	Aclometasone dipropionate cream 0.05%
	Desonide cream 0.05%
7	Hydrocortisone 0.5%, 1.0%, 2.5%

[a]Using the vasoconstrictor bioassay, class 1 is most potent; class 7 is least potent.
Adapted with permission from Arndt KA. Manual of Dermatologic Theraputics. Boston: Little, Brown, 1989.

helpful in other disorders of keratinization, but it is not useful for psoriasis. High doses of isotretinoin (2mg/kg/day) are effective as cancer chemoprevention agents to reduce the frequency of cutaneous malignancies in patients at increased risk, such as those with xeroderma pigmentosum, an inherited disorder in which DNA repair is deficient, or in immunosuppressed patients.

The most serious toxicity of isotretinoin is teratogenicity. Pregnant women should never receive the drug, and women should not conceive for at least 1 month after its discontinuation. Other toxicities:

- *Skin complaints,* particularly xerosis, conjunctivitis, and cheilitis.
- *Hypertriglyceridemia* in about a quarter of patients.
- *Elevation of liver function test findings,* which is usually reversible.
- *Headache,* which rarely may be attributable to pseudotumor cerebri.
- *Arthralgias,* including skeletal changes such as hyperostoses, tendinous calcifications, premature epiphysial closure, and pathological fractures.
- *Depression and suicidal ideation* may occur, but no mechanism of action for these events has been established.

Acitretin

Unlike isotretinoin, acitretin (*Soriatane*) is not primarily sebosuppressive. Rather, it promotes normalization of dysregulated keratinocyte proliferative activity in the epidermis and is also antiinflammatory. Oral absorption is optimal when acitretin is taken with a fatty meal; peak levels are reached approximately 3 hours after ingestion, while steady-state plasma levels are achieved after approximately 3 weeks of daily dosing. The mean terminal elimination half-life of the parent compound is 49 hours. However, when consumed with ethanol, acitretin may be transesterified to form etretinate, a retinoid that is stored in adipose tissue, resulting in a much longer half-life (3–4 months or longer).

Acitretin is most useful for the treatment of severe psoriasis, particularly the pustular and erythrodermic variants. Psoriatic nail changes and arthritis also may respond. Combining the drug with ultraviolet light therapy (Re-UVB, in the case of ultraviolet B radiation, or Re-PUVA, with psoralen plus ultraviolet A radiation) permits the use of lower doses of both acitretin and ultraviolet radiation. Other conditions for which the drug may be especially useful include congenital and acquired hyperkeratotic disorders, such as the ichthyoses and palmoplantar keratodermas, and severe lichen planus.

Like other systemic retinoids, acitretin is a serious teratogen and should not be prescribed for women of childbearing potential unless no acceptable alternative is available and the patient has acknowledged in writing that she understands the need to use two effective forms of contraception during therapy and for 3 years following discontinuation of therapy. Because of the much longer half-life of etretinate, which may be formed when ethanol is ingested with acitretin, female patients of childbearing potential must also agree not to ingest alcohol during treatment and for 2 months following its discontinuation. Other toxicities are similar to those of isotretinoin; they include cutaneous irritation and inflammation, bone and joint pain, hyperlipidemia, hepatic enzyme elevation, and tendinous and ligamentous calcifications. Alopecia (hair loss) may also occur in some patients.

Tretinoin

Topical tretinoin (*Retin-A, Renova, Avita*), like isotretinoin, alters keratinization in the acroinfundibulum. In addition, it reverses certain premalignant and other histological changes associated with the photoaging changes that accompany chronic exposure to ultraviolet radiation. Topically applied tretinoin is indicated in comedogenic and papulopustular acne vulgaris, and its mild exfoliative effects make it sometimes useful in molluscum contagiosum, flat warts, and some ichthyotic disorders. It is often prescribed to lessen the clinical signs of photoaging (wrinkling and hyperpigmented macules).

The major toxic effect of tretinoin is erythema and irritation of the skin to which it is applied, especially if the skin is moist. This toxicity often decreases with continued therapy.

Adapalene

Adapalene (*Differin*) is a polyaromatic retinoidlike compound that binds to specific retinoic acid nuclear receptors and is thought to normalize the differentiation of keratinocytes in the sebaceous acroinfundibulum. Adapelene is indicated for topical treatment of acne. Minor local irritation is a common, usually tolerable side effect. In contrast to other drugs of the retinoid group, adapalene has not been shown to be teratogenic in rodents. However, since adequate human studies are lacking, its use in pregnant women should be discouraged until further information is available.

Tazarotene

Like other retinoids, tazarotene (*Tazorac*) acts by binding to RARs and altering gene expression. Tazarotene appears to be particularly selective for the retinoid receptors RAR-β and RAR-γ, but the clinical significance of this observation is unknown.

In the United States, tazarotene has been approved for topical treatment of psoriasis (involving up to 20% body surface area) and mild to moderate facial acne. Application site burning, stinging, and desquamation are common side effects, especially with acne. Tazarotene is contraindicated in women who are pregnant.

Bexarotene

Bexarotene (*Targretin*) belongs to a subclass of retinoids that selectively bind to and activates retinoid X receptors (RXRs), which have biological properties distinct from those of RARs. In vitro, bexarotene exerts antiproliferative effects on some tumor lines of hematopoietic and squamous cell origin.

Bexarotene is available in oral and topical formulations. Peak plasma levels are achieved within 2 hours of oral administration, although higher levels are obtained when the drug is ingested with a fatty meal. It is thought to be metabolized primarily by the hepatobiliary system, with a terminal half-life of approximately 7 hours.

Topical and oral bexarotene are approved for early-stage (patch and plaque) cutaneous T-cell lymphoma that is refractory to at least one other therapy. Oral bexarotene is also approved for refractory cases of advanced disease; however, the best response has been noted in early disease.

Local irritation, such as burning, pruritus, and irritant contact dermatitis, is common following topical application. Major side effects seen after systemic administration include dyslipidemia, leukopenia, liver function test abnormalities, and possibly development of cataracts. Unlike other systemic retinoids, oral bexarotene causes thyroid abnormalities in approximately half of patients, which may necessitate treatment for hypothyroidism. Bexarotene is teratogenic and should not be prescribed in topical or oral form to women of childbearing potential unless a negative serum pregnancy test has been obtained and the patient agrees in writing to use two effective forms of contraception from 1 month before to 1 month after treatment.

Alitretinoin

Alitretinoin (*Panretin*) is a naturally occurring endogenous retinoid that binds to and activates all known retinoid receptors (both RARs and RXRs). It is approved for the topical treatment of cutaneous lesions of Kaposi's sarcoma. Most patients have local irritation while using alitretinoin gel; however, the irritation rarely necessitates discontinuation of therapy.

β-Carotene

This naturally occurring retinoid (*Solatene*), a dimer of vitamin A, reduces free radical formation induced by photosensitizing porphyrins and light. Its major use in dermatology is for decreasing skin photosensitivity in patients with erythropoietic protoporphyria. Its major side effect is a yellow-orange discoloration of skin.

PHOTOCHEMOTHERAPY

Photochemotherapy is exposure of the patient to light of an appropriate wavelength after topical application or oral ingestion of a photosensitizing drug. The most common photosensitizing drugs used in dermatology are synthetic psoralens; psoralens also occur naturally in many plants, such as citrus fruits and celery).

Psoralen and Ultraviolet A Therapy

Psoralens form covalent linkages with pyrimidine bases in DNA when exposed to light of the appropriate wavelength, and if oxygen is present, reactive oxygen species also are generated. Although inhibition of DNA replication may account for some of the beneficial effects of PUVA therapy in certain hyperproliferative disorders such as psoriasis, PUVA has other important biological effects. It suppresses contact hypersensitivity and may evoke other immunological changes by affecting T lymphocytes and epidermal Langerhans cells. It increases melanin pigmentation in the skin and is useful in treating vitiligo. PUVA also inhibits mast cell release of inflammatory mediators.

Orally administered psoralens are rapidly absorbed (maximum photosensitivity for the most common preparation, 8-methoxypsoralen [*Oxsoralen Ultra*], is 1–1.5 hours). Although the elimination half-life is 2.2 hours, the skin remains photosensitive for 8 to 12 hours. Most excretion is renal, and the drug does not accumulate. It can be absorbed if applied topically, and after application to the entire body, therapeutic plasma levels can be detected.

PUVA is most useful for the treatment of severe psoriasis. Early (patch and plaque) stage cutaneous T-cell lymphoma (CTCL) also responds to PUVA therapy. In addition, patients in advanced stages of CTCL have been treated with a modification of PUVA known as *extracorporeal photopheresis*. In this therapy, blood from a CTCL patient who has taken psoralen is exposed to UVA light and returned to the patient. Lymphocytes are altered or destroyed by the treatment, and theoretically, the return of these abnormal cells triggers an immune response directed against certain lymphocyte surface antigens. The effectiveness of this modality appears to be variable.

Both topical and systemic PUVA are useful in some patients with vitiligo, although repigmentation is rarely complete. Other skin diseases for which PUVA may be helpful include atopic dermatitis, dyshidrotic eczema, and polymorphous light eruption.

Nausea is the most common acute side effect. About 36 to 48 hours after therapy, erythema and blistering can occur, especially if the UVA dose is too high or if the patient is exposed to other sources of UVA (such as sunlight). Long-term toxicities include the following:

- *Squamous cell carcinoma of the skin* (especially of the male genitalia). This risk is increased in patients already at risk because of fair skin, a history of skin cancer, and a history of exposure to other cutaneous carcinogens.
- *Melanoma.* After 15 years or more of PUVA (>200 treatments) the risk of melanoma increases approximately fivefold in patients treated with higher doses in the United States.
- *Cataracts.* Patients should wear UVA-absorbing wraparound sunglasses when exposed to ultraviolet light during the 24 hours after taking the drug.
- *Hyperpigmentation and development of discreet dark macules* called PUVA lentigines.

PHOTODYNAMIC THERAPY

Porphyrins are potent photosensitizing intermediates in heme synthesis and are thought to accumulate in malignant cells. This feature is used in *photodynamic therapy,* in which a synthetic porphyrin is administered and the patient is exposed to visible light. This modality has been shown to be effective in treating basal cell and squamous cell skin cancers, although a limiting toxicity has been that patients remain extremely photosensitive for weeks after treatment because of the long elimination half-life of the porphyrin analogues.

AMINOLEVULINIC ACID

Aminolevulinic acid (ALA HCl, *Levulan Kerastick*) is indicated for the treatment of nonhyperkeratotic actinic keratosis of the face and scalp. It has two components, an alcohol solution vehicle and ALA HCl as a dry solid. The two are mixed prior to application to the skin. When applied to human skin, ALA is metabolized to protoporphyrin, which accumulates and on exposure to visible light produces a photodynamic reaction that generates reactive oxygen species (ROS). The ROS produce cytotoxic effects that may explain therapeutic efficacy. Local burning and stinging of treated areas of skin due to photosensitization can occur.

DAPSONE

Although dapsone (*Avlosulfon*) is most often used as an antimicrobial agent, it has important antiinflammatory properties in many noninfectious skin diseases. Its pharmacology and toxicities are discussed in Chapter 49. The mechanism of action of dapsone in skin disease is not clear. Most of the cutaneous diseases for which it is effective manifest inflammation and are characterized by an infiltration of neutrophils; the drug's antiinflammatory effect may arise from its inhibition of intracellular neutrophil reactions mediated by myeloperoxidase and hydrogen peroxide or from its scavenging of reactive oxygen species, which inhibits inflammation.

Dapsone is approved for the treatment of an autoimmune blistering skin disease, dermatitis herpetiformis. This intensely pruritic eruption is characterized histologically by a dense dermal infiltration of neutrophils and subepidermal blisters. Other skin diseases in which dapsone is helpful are linear immunoglobulin A (IgA) dermatosis, subcorneal pustular dermatosis, leukocytoclastic vasculitis, and a variety of rarer eruptions in which neutrophils predominate, including some forms of cutaneous lupus erythematosus.

THALIDOMIDE

Thalidomide (*Thalomid*) is a derivative of glutamic acid that is chemically related to glutethimide. It exerts a number of biological effects as an immunosuppressive, antiinflammatory, and antiangiogenic agent, yet its mechanisms of action have not been fully elucidated. Thalidomide potently inhibits production of tumor necrosis factor (TNF) α and interleukin (IL) 12, and its effect on these and other cytokines may account for some of its clinical effects.

Its absorption from the gastrointestinal tract is slow, with peak plasma levels being reached after 3 to 6 hours. It appears to undergo nonenzymatic hydrolysis in the plasma to a large number of metabolites. The elimination half-life is approximately 9 hours.

Thalidomide is approved for use in the United States for the treatment of cutaneous manifestations of erythema nodosum leprosum, a potentially life-threatening systemic vasculitis that occurs in some patients with leprosy. Although not approved for other indications, thalidomide has also been shown to be very effective in the management of Behçet's disease, HIV-related mucosal ulceration (aphthosis), and select cases of lupus erythematosus.

Thalidomide is a highly teratogenic drug, characteristically causing phocomelia (aplasia of the midportions of the limbs). Even a single dose may cause fetal malformation. Thalidomide should be prescribed to women of childbearing potential only when no acceptable alternative exists. Because it is not known whether thalidomide is present in the ejaculate of males receiving the drug, male patients must use a latex condom when engaging in sexual activity with women of childbearing potential.

Other side effects of thalidomide may include sedation (in fact, thalidomide was originally marketed in Europe as a sleeping aid), constipation, and peripheral neuropathy, which may be permanent.

ANTIMALARIAL DRUGS

Like dapsone, the antimalarial drugs chloroquine, hydroxychloroquine, and quinacrine are useful in some noninfectious skin diseases, although the mechanism of their therapeutic effect is unknown. Their pharmacology is discussed in Chapter 53.

Antimalarial drugs have many effects, including impairment of lysosomal phagosomal activity, inhibition of neutrophilic iodination and locomotion, and diminution of macrophage and T-cell responsiveness in vitro. Chloroquine (*Aralen*) and hydroxychloroquine (*Plaquenil*) also form complexes with hepatic porphyrins and can chelate iron, thereby enhancing their urinary excretion. Both drugs have an affinity for melanin, which may at least partially explain their ophthalmological toxicities (retinopathy).

Hydroxychloroquine is approved for the treatment of both systemic and cutaneous lupus erythematosus. Both chloroquine and quinacrine (*Atabrine*) are also effective in this skin disease. Low-dose chloroquine is used for the therapy of porphyria cutanea tarda in patients in whom phlebotomy has failed or is contraindicated. Other skin diseases in which the drugs are useful (after sunscreens and avoidance of sun exposure) include polymorphous light eruption and solar urticaria.

The duration of treatment for skin diseases is often longer than it is for malaria, and therefore, dose-related toxicities are important. The most serious toxicities are ophthalmological. Reversible alterations include ciliary body dysfunction and corneal changes with edema and deposits. Irreversible retinopathy also occurs; however, it is less common with quinacrine than with the other two drugs. Toxicity may be asymptomatic, but the earliest symptoms are night blindness, scotoma, or tunnel vision.

ANTIMICROBIAL AGENTS

Systemic Antibiotics

Antibiotics are used in dermatology for both infectious and noninfectious skin eruptions. Noninfectious skin eruptions, such as acne vulgaris and acne rosacea, are often treated with systemic antibiotics. The mechanism of action is not clear, although tetracycline inhibits lipases derived from resident flora in the sebaceous follicle (*Staphylococcus epidermidis, Propionibacterium acnes*). These lipases cleave irritating fatty acids from triglycerides in sebum, presumably contributing to cutaneous inflammation.

Topical Antibiotics

Topical antibiotics are helpful in acne vulgaris and acne rosacea and probably in reducing the frequency of infections related to intravenous catheters. One drug, mupirocin (*Bactroban*), is effective in treating impetigo contagiosa. Mupirocin binds to bacterial isoleucyl-transfer RNA synthetase and prevents the incorporation of isoleucine into protein sequences. Mupirocin is most effective against gram-positive bacteria. Toxicity is uncommon.

Another topical antibiotic, metronidazole, is effective in the treatment of acne rosacea. Metronidazole is a synthetic nitroimidazole derivative that reduces inflammation by an unknown mechanism. Other selected topical antibiotics are listed in Table 41.2.

DRUGS FOR CUTANEOUS FUNGAL INFECTIONS

Like bacterial infections of skin, cutaneous fungal infections are treated with either topical or systemic agents. The pharmacology and toxicities of these agents are discussed in Chapter 52.

Systemic Agents
Griseofulvin

Griseofulvin (*Fulvicin, Grifulvin V*) has been used safely and effectively for decades for dermatophyte infections of scalp and nails and for more widespread skin eruptions. However, infections in certain sites (e.g.. toenails) respond poorly. The drug is generally well tolerated, even in the long-term courses necessary for nail disease.

Ketoconazole

Ketoconazole (*Nizoral*) is approved for treating dermatophyte infections unresponsive to griseofulvin and for patients unable to tolerate that drug. A single oral

T A B L E 41.2 **Selected Topical Antibiotics**

Drug	Major Use
Clindamycin	Acne vulgaris
Erythromycin	Acne vulgaris
Metronidazole	Acne rosacea
Bacitracin	Superficial infection (gram-positive bacteria)
Polymixin B	Superficial infection (gram-negative bacteria)
Neomycin	Superficial infection (mainly gram-negative bacteria)

dose is also effective for the treatment of pityriasis versicolor. Other effective drugs that are less hepatotoxic may be preferred, however.

Fluconazole

Fluconazole (*Diflucan*) may be better absorbed and is possibly less hepatotoxic than ketoconazole, but it is considerably more expensive, an important consideration given the required length of therapy for most cutaneous fungal diseases.

Itraconazole

Itraconazole (*Sporanox*), a triazole, is highly lipophilic and concentrates in skin. It is approved for both cutaneous deep fungal infections and dermatophyte nail disease, for which shorter courses of therapy are probably effective. Pulse therapy, whereby the drug is administered for 1 week and then the patient is off treatment for 3 weeks between pulses, may reduce toxicity without compromising antifungal efficacy.

Terbinafine

Terbinafine (*Lamisil*), an antifungal drug, is highly lipophilic and concentrates in stratum corneum and nail plate. It is very effective for many dermatophyte infections, especially those of the nails, with which it may permit shorter courses of therapy than other drugs. Meta-analysis suggests that long-term efficacy of terbinafine is superior to that of the other antifungal drugs used in treating onychomycosis.

Potassium Iodide

Potassium iodide is used to treat the cutaneous lymphatic form of sporotrichosis, although newer agents are also effective in this disorder and may be better tolerated. The drug is also used for erythema nodosum and nodular vasculitis.

Topical Agents

Many effective topical agents are available both with and without a prescription for treating cutaneous dermatophyte infections and seborrheic dermatitis (Table 41.3); the azole drugs are also active against superficial candidal infections.

DRUGS FOR CUTANEOUS VIRAL INFECTIONS

The specific antiviral agents used to treat cutaneous infections caused by herpes simplex and varicella zoster viruses are discussed in Chapter 50.

Interferons

Interferons α-2b (*Intron-A*), α-nl, and α-n3 (*Alferon N*) have both intrinsic antiviral effects and antiproliferative and immunomodulatory actions. These interferons are approved for intralesional therapy of refractory or recurrent condylomata (genital warts). Toxicities include flulike symptoms, nausea, depression of the white blood cell count, and mild diminution in hematocrit.

Podophyllotoxin

Podophyllotoxin (*Podofilox*) is available alone and as the main cytotoxic ingredient in podophyllin (25% podophyllum resin), a mixture of toxic chemicals derived from May apple plants. The active ingredients inhibit cell mitosis. The drugs are used to treat condylomata acuminata. The most common toxic effects are skin irritation and less commonly, ulceration. Systemic

T A B L E 41.3 Topical Antifungal Drugs and Characteristic Courses of Treatment for Tinea Pedis

Drug	Availability	Frequency of application	Duration of course to treat tinea pedis (weeks)
Ciclopirox	Rx	bid	4
Clotrimazole	OTC	bid	4
Econazole	Rx	qd	4
Ketoconazole	Rx	qd	6
Miconazole	OTC	bid	4
Naftifine	Rx	qd	4
Oxiconazole	Rx	qd	4
Terbinafine	Rx	bid	1-4
Tolnaftate	OTC	bid	4

Durations of therapy and frequency of application are those recommended in the package insert. The weekly dose for drugs applied twice a day is 30 g.
OTC, available over the counter; Rx, available only with a prescription.
Data from 1995 Red Book. Montvale, NJ: Medical Economics Data Inc. 1995.

absorption of podophyllin can occur (especially if applied to large, inflamed areas or mucosal surfaces), with gastrointestinal, hematological, renal, and hepatotoxic effects. In addition, seizures and peripheral neuropathy have been reported.

DRUGS USED TO TREAT SCABIES AND LICE

Pyrethrins and Pyrethroids

Pyrethrins are naturally occurring pesticides derived from chrysanthemum plants. They are active against many insects and mites. Over-the-counter liquid and gel preparations of pyrethrins with piperonyl butoxide are available for the treatment of pediculosis (piperonyl butoxide inhibits the hydrolytic enzymes that metabolize the pyrethrins in the arthropod). A synthetic pyrethroid, permethrin (*Elimite*), is available by prescription. A lower concentration of permethrin (*Nix*) is available without prescription. Pyrethrins and permethrin are quite safe.

CYTOTOXIC AND IMMUNOSUPPRESSIVE AGENTS

Cytotoxic and immunosuppressive drugs, which inhibit the synthesis or action of crucial cellular macromolecules, such as nucleic acids, are used in three broad categories of skin disease: hyperproliferative disorders, such as psoriasis; immunological disorders, such as autoimmune bullous diseases; and skin neoplasms. The pharmacology of these drugs is discussed in Chapter 57.

Methotrexate

Methotrexate is approved for use in severe disabling psoriasis recalcitrant to other less toxic treatments. The standard regimen is similar to low-dose therapy used for the treatment of rheumatoid arthritis (see Chapter 36). Although toxicities are similar to those described in the treatment of other diseases, hepatic cirrhosis and unexpected pancytopenia are of special concern given the chronicity of treatment.

Mycophenolate Mofetil

Mycophenolate mofetil (MMF, *CellCept*) is an ester prodrug of mycophenolic acid (MPA), a *Penicillium*-derived immunosuppressive agent (see Chapter 57) that blocks de novo purine synthesis by noncompetitively inhibiting the enzyme inosine monophosphate dehydrogenase. MPA preferentially suppresses the proliferation of cells, such as T and B lymphocytes, that lack the purine salvage pathway and must synthesize de novo

the guanosine nucleotides required for DNA and RNA synthesis. MPA has been used for decades as a systemic treatment for moderate to severe psoriasis. MMF was developed to increase the bioavailability of MPA.

MMF is rapidly and completely cleaved to form MPA, the active metabolite, after oral administration. MPA is converted in the liver and kidney to an inactive glucuronide. However, certain tissues, such as the epidermis, express a glucuronidase that converts the inactive glucuronide back to the active agent. The half-life of MPA is approximately 18 hours; 90 to 95% of the mycophenolate dose is excreted in the urine.

MMF is indicated for the prophylaxis of organ rejection in patients receiving renal, hepatic, and cardiac transplants; it is often used in combination with other immunosuppressive agents for this indication. In dermatology, MMF is particularly useful as monotherapy, or as a steroid-sparing agent, for treatment of autoimmune blistering diseases (bullous pemphigoid and pemphigus). It may also be useful for the treatment of inflammatory skin diseases mediated by neutrophilic infiltration, such as pyoderma gangrenosum, and psoriasis.

The principal advantage of MMF over alternative systemic immunosuppressive agents (e.g., methotrexate, cyclosporine) is its relative lack of hepatotoxicity and nephrotoxicity. Adverse effects produced by MMF most commonly include nausea, abdominal cramps, diarrhea, and possibly an increased incidence of viral and bacterial infections. Whether MMF may be associated with an increased long-term risk of lymphoma or other malignancies is controversial; however, any such risk is likely to be lower in patients treated for skin disease with MMF monotherapy than in transplant patients treated with combination immunosuppressive therapy.

6-Thioguanine

6-Thioguanine is a purine analogue structurally related to 6-mercaptopurine and azathioprine. Thioguanine interferes with several enzymes required for de novo purine synthesis, and its metabolites are incorporated into DNA and RNA, further impeding nucleic acid synthesis. The mechanism of action of thioguanine in psoriasis is not clearly understood; it has been hypothesized to affect the proliferation and trafficking of lymphocytes as well as the proliferation of keratinocytes.

Absorption of orally administered 6-thioguanine is slow and incomplete; only approximately 30% of the oral dose is achieved in the plasma, peak levels being reached after 8 hours. Thioguanine is extensively metabolized prior to excretion. The elimination half-life is on the order of 80 minutes.

Although 6-thioguanine is chiefly used in chemotherapy for acute myelocytic leukemia and other marrow-based malignancies, lower doses are very effective for moderate to severe psoriasis, particularly in patients who cannot tolerate alternative systemic agents such as methotrexate and cyclosporine.

Dose-related myelosuppression is the major adverse effect produced by 6-thioguanine. Patients deficient in thiopurine methyltransferase (TPMT), a cytosolic enzyme required for metabolism of 6-thioguanine, are at heightened risk. Other adverse effects include gastrointestinal complaints and elevations of liver transaminases. There have been rare reports of more serious hepatotoxicity, including acute hepatitis, acute cholestasis, and hepatic venoocclusive disease.

TOPICAL IMMUNE-MODULATING AGENTS

Tacrolimus

Tacrolimus is a macrolide lactone originally derived from *Streptomyces tsukubaensis*. Although structurally unrelated to cyclosporine, tacrolimus has a very similar mechanism of action; that is, it blocks the production of proinflammatory cytokines by T lymphocytes by inhibiting calcineurin. Tacrolimus, however, appears to be 10 to 100 times as potent as an immunosuppressive. Oral tacrolimus (FK506) is used for prevention of organ rejection in recipients of renal and hepatic transplants. A topical formulation (*Protopic*) has recently been approved for treatment of moderate to severe atopic dermatitis in children and adults who have not responded to other therapies. Levels of systemic absorption are low even when applied to a relatively large body surface area. Local irritant reactions (burning, stinging, erythema) are a common side effect, but these usually resolve within the first few days of treatment. The major benefit of topical tacrolimus over topical corticosteroids is that tacrolimus does not cause atrophy, striae, or telangiectasia, even with chronic use.

Pimecrolimus

Pimecrolimus (SDZ ASM 981, *Elidel*) is another recently approved macrolide immunosuppressant that acts by inhibiting calcineurin and blocking the release of proinflammatory cytokines from T lymphocytes. The parent compound, ascomycin, was originally isolated from *Streptomyces hygroscopicus* var *ascomyceticus*. Like tacrolimus, pimecrolimus is approved for the topical treatment of moderate to severe atopic dermatitis that is refractory to other therapies. Transient local irritation is a common side effect.

Imiquimod

Imiquimod (*Aldara*) is a topical immune response modifier approved for the treatment of anogenital warts (condylomata acuminata). The exact mechanism of action is unknown; it has no direct antiviral activity in vitro. It is thought to work in vivo by inducing the production of tumor necrosis factor (TNF α), interferons (IFN) αand γ, and other cytokines with antiviral activity. It may also be useful for treatment of other types of warts, molluscum contagiosum, and certain forms of skin cancer. Local irritant reactions related to the frequency of application are common.

5-Fluorouracil

5-Fluorouracil (*Efudex, Fluoroplex*) is an antimetabolite used for the topical treatment of actinic keratoses. It is also useful for the treatment of superficial basal cell carcinomas when conventional surgical modalities are impractical. Local inflammatory reactions characterized by erythema, edema, crusting, burning, and pain are common (and, some would argue, desirable) but may be minimized by reduced frequency of application or use in combination with a topical corticosteroid.

Mechlorethamine

Mechlorethamine (*Mustargen*) is a cytotoxic alkylating agent. Topical application of freshly prepared aqueous solutions are used in patients with early stages of cutaneous T-cell lymphoma. A major disadvantage to the use of this drug is the rapid induction of allergic contact dermatitis in some patients.

ANTIHISTAMINES

A large number of oral H_1-receptor antagonists (see Chapter 38) are available with and without prescription for the treatment of mast cell–mediated diseases, such as acute and chronic urticaria, angioedema, and cutaneous mastocytosis. Until relatively recently, two major limitations of the available antihistamines, such as diphenhydramine (*Benadryl*), hydroxyzine (*Atarax*), promethazine (*Phenergan*), and cyproheptadine (*Periactin*), were their short half-lives and sedative effects. New-generation long-acting antihistamines pass the blood-brain barrier much less readily and are theoretically less likely to cause somnolence. Examples of these relatively nonsedating drugs are fexofenadine (*Allegra*), cetirizine (*Zyrtec*), and loratadine (*Claritin*).

DOXEPIN

The tricyclic tertiary amine doxepin (*Zonalon, Prudox*), a potent H_1- and H_2-receptor antagonist, is indicated for the short-term relief of pruritus associated with topical eczematous dermatitis. Systemic absorption occurs, and the drug may potentiate or alter the metabolism of a variety of other systemic agents. Drowsiness is the most common adverse side effect.

DRUGS USED TO TREAT DISORDERS OF PIGMENTATION

Hydroquinone

Hydroquinone interferes with the production of the pigment melanin by epidermal melanocytes through at least two mechanisms: it competitively inhibits tyrosinase, one of the principal enzymes responsible for converting tyrosine to melanin, and it selectively damages melanocytes and melanosomes (the organelles within which melanin is stored).

Hydroquinone is applied topically to treat disorders characterized by excessive melanin in the epidermis, such as melasma. In the United States, nonprescription skin-lightening products contain hydroquinone at concentrations of 2% or less; higher concentrations are available by prescription.

The incidence of adverse effects with hydroquinone increases in proportion to its concentration. A relatively common side effect is local irritation, which may actually exacerbate the discoloration of the skin being treated. Allergic contact dermatitis occurs less commonly. A rare but more serious complication is exogenous ochronosis, in which a yellow-brown pigment deposited in the dermis results in blue-black pigmentation of the skin that may be permanent.

Monobenzone

Monobenzone (*Benoquin*) potently inhibits melanin production and destroys melanocytes. Like hydroquinone, monobenzone was originally introduced for the topical treatment of disorders of excess melanin pigmentation, including melasma. It is now used only to permanently depigment the remaining normally pigmented skin in patients with extensive vitiligo. Irritant and allergic contact dermatitis are common side effects.

RECOMBINANT PROTEINS AND OTHER BIOLOGICALS

Becaplermin

Becaplermin (*Regranex*) is a recombinant human platelet–derived growth factor (rhPDGF-BB) which is thought to enhance wound healing by stimulating granulation tissue. It is approved for the treatment of lower extremity neuropathic ulcers extending to the subcutaneous tissue in diabetic patients with an adequate blood supply. Local irritant reactions (erythema, burning, pain) occur in a minority of patients.

Etanercept

Etanercept (*Enbrel*) is a recombinant fusion protein designed to block the action of TNF-α (see Chapter 40). The drug is composed of the extracellular ligand-binding portion of the 75-kilodalton human TNF receptor linked to the Fc portion of human IgG$_1$. TNF-α is a cytokine thought to play a major role in the pathogenesis of a number of inflammatory skin diseases, including psoriasis. Etanercept binds soluble TNF-α, preventing it from binding to and activating receptors for TNF that are present on cell membranes.

Etanercept is administered by subcutaneous injection. The maximum serum concentration is reached after approximately 72 hours. The half-life is approximately 115 hours.

Etanercept is approved in the United States for the treatment of psoriatic arthritis and rheumatoid arthritis. Although etanercept has not been specifically approved for the treatment of the cutaneous manifestations of psoriasis, it significantly improves the skin lesions of patients with moderate to severe cutaneous psoriasis who have used it for psoriatic joint disease.

Injection site reactions characterized by mild to moderate erythema, itching, burning, and/or pain occur in approximately one-third of patients but rarely necessitate drug discontinuation. The impact of etanercept on the host's response to new or chronic infections is not fully understood. Serious infections and sepsis, including fatalities, have been reported in patients treated with etanercept. Increased levels of autoantibodies, including antinuclear antibodies and anti-double-stranded DNA antibodies, have also been reported, but the clinical significance of this observation is unknown.

Denileukin Diftitox

Denileukin diftitox (DAB$_{389}$ IL-2, *Ontak*) is indicated for treatment of patients with cutaneous T-cell lymphoma whose malignant cells express the CD25 component of the IL-2 receptor. Denileukin diftitox is a recombinant fusion protein composed of IL-2 amino acid sequences joined to sequences of diphtheria toxin. The drug targets and destroys cells expressing the high-affinity (CD25/CD122/CD132) IL-2 receptor, including the malignant cells of cutaneous T-cell lymphoma.

The half-life of the drug is approximately 75 minutes after intravenous infusion. Antibodies directed against the diphtheria domain decrease mean systemic exposure by approximately 75%. Approximately 85% of patients develop such antibodies after a single course of treatment, and nearly all do after 3 cycles.

Most patients using denileukin diftitox have flulike symptoms (fever, chills, myalgias, nausea, diarrhea) within a few hours to days of treatment. Another common adverse effect is an immediate hypersensitivity syndrome in which hypotension, back pain, dyspnea, chest pain or tightness, and rash may occur. Other notable side effects include a vascular leak syndrome (edema, hypoalbuminemia, hypotension), infections, and elevations of transaminases.

Botulinum Toxin

Botulinum toxin purified neurotoxin complex (*Botox*) is a purified form of botulinum toxin type A, produced from a culture of *Clostridium botulinum*. Injection of botulinum toxin into muscle induces paralysis by inhibiting the release of acetylcholine from motor neurons, thereby blocking neuromuscular conduction. It is approved for the treatment of blepharospasm, strabismus, and excessive sweating. *Botox* is also approved for use in dermatology to induce paralysis of the muscles of facial expression to reverse deep wrinkles. The effect of an individual treatment usually becomes apparent within 3 days and lasts approximately 3 months. The effect may persist for a longer period after a series of treatments because the muscles atrophy. The major adverse effect is temporary loss of function of a muscle required for normal social functioning, as may occur after inadvertent injection of muscles required for smiling or raising the upper eyelids.

MISCELLANEOUS TOPICAL AGENTS

Azelaic Acid

Azelaic acid (*Azelex*) is a naturally occurring dicarboxylic acid produced by the yeast *Malassezia furfur*. Azelaic acid inhibits tyrosinase, a rate-limiting enzyme in the synthesis of the pigment melanin. This may explain why diminution of melanin pigmentation occurs in the skin of some patients with pityriasis versicolor, a disease caused by *M. furfur*. Azelaic acid is bacteriostatic against a number of species thought to participate in the pathogenesis of acne, including *Propionibacterium acnes*. The drug may also reduce microcomedo formation by promoting normalization of epidermal keratinocytes. Azelaic acid is used for the treatment of mild to moderate acne, particularly in cases characterized by marked inflammation-associated hyperpigmentation.

Analgesia Anesthetics

Topically administered local anesthetics are useful in dermatology for preparation of the skin prior to minor surgical procedures, such as skin biopsies, laser treatment of vascular malformations, and curettage of molluscum contagiosum lesions, particularly in young children and needle-phobic adults. The topical anesthetic may be used alone or may be applied prior to intradermal injection of a local anesthetic to reduce the pain caused by the needle. Two recently approved drugs in

this group are *ELA-Max*, a topical formulation of lidocaine, and *EMLA*, which contains a mixture of lidocaine and prilocaine.

Capsaicin

Capsaicin (*Zostrix*) is approved for the relief of pain following herpes zoster infection (postherpetic neuralgia). The drug depletes neurons of substance P, an endogenous neuropeptide that may mediate cutaneous pain. It is applied to affected skin after open lesions have healed. Local irritation is common.

Anthralin

Anthralin (*Anthra-Derm*) is a potent reducing agent whose mechanism of action is unknown. It is approved for the treatment of psoriasis and also may be helpful in alopecia areata. The major toxicities are discoloration of skin, hair, and nails and irritant dermatitis.

Benzoyl Peroxide

Benzoyl peroxide is a potent oxidizing agent that has both antimicrobial and comedolytic properties; its primary use is in treating acne vulgaris. It is converted in the skin to benzoic acid; clearance of absorbed drug is rapid, and no systemic toxicity has been observed. The major toxicities are irritation and contact allergy. Outgrowth of bacteria resistant to topical antibiotics used to treat acne can be reduced by the addition of benzoyl peroxide in combination products such as erythromycin (*Benzamycin*) and clindamycin (*Benzaclin*).

Calcipotriene

Calcipotriene (*Dovonex*), a synthetic vitamin D_3 derivative, is indicated for the treatment of moderate plaque psoriasis. Its mechanism of action is unknown, although it competes for calcitriol receptors on keratinocytes and normalizes differentiation. It also has a variety of immunomodulatory effects in the skin. Although the drug can cause local irritation, the most serious toxicities are hypercalciuria and hypercalcemia, which are usually reversible.

KERATOLYTICS

Drugs that are used to treat hyperkeratosis, a thickening of the stratum corneum, are called keratolytics. Examples of these agents are salicylic acid, urea, lactic acid, and colloidal or precipitated sulfur. The precise mechanisms by which these agents treat hyperkeratosis are not known. Presumably, a common property is the ability to denature keratin, the major structural protein of the epidermis. Other beneficial effects vary among the different drugs. All of them have antimicrobial or antiparasitic properties. Salicylic acid is a potent antiin-flammatory agent. Urea is highly hygroscopic, enhancing the ability of tissue to absorb and retain water. Keratolytics are especially useful for treatment of corns and calluses, warts, palmoplantar keratodermas, ichthyoses, and psoriasis. When used in conjunction with topical steroids for treatment of psoriasis, keratolytics enhance the steroid's penetration. Urea may also be used for chemical avulsion of dystrophic nails.

Selenium Sulfide

Selenium sulfide is a cytostatic and sporicidal agent available without prescription in a variety of shampoos and lotions for treatment of scalp seborrheic dermatitis. Higher concentrations are available by prescription for the treatment of pityriasis versicolor, which is caused by the yeast *M. furfur,* and tinea capitis.

SUNSCREENS

Sunscreens absorb ultraviolet radiation before it can be absorbed in the skin. They are recommended to protect the skin from the major toxicities of sun exposure: sunburn and skin cancer. Most available agents primarily absorb UVB, although newer preparations also provide protection against UVA. Physical sunscreens (which are generally opaque, like titanium dioxide and zinc oxide) block all ultraviolet radiation.

The frequency of application of sunscreen is guided by the SPF (sun protection factor) of the preparation. This derived value is the ratio of the time of ultraviolet exposure that causes erythema with the sunscreen to the time that causes erythema without the sunscreen. The higher the SPF, the less frequent the needed application of sunscreen. SPFs of available preparations vary from 2 to 50.

Study QUESTIONS

1. Botulinum toxin is used in dermatology to reverse deep wrinkles. Its pharmacological mechanism of action in this use is
   (A) Blockade of acetylcholine esterase
   (B) Inhibition of release of acetylcholine from motor neurons
   (C) Inhibition of synthesis of acetylcholine by inhibiting choline acetyl transferase
   (D) Inhibition of acetylcholine binding to muscarinic receptors
2. Which one of the following agents is known to be a potent teratogen in humans?
   (A) Levulan Kerastick
   (B) Dapsone
   (C) Thalidomide
   (D) Mupirocin
3. Several very useful dermatological agents are derived directly from plants. A compound occurring in the May apple is
   (A) Interferonα-2b
   (B) Mycophenolate mofetil
   (C) Methotrexate
   (D) 6-Thioguanine
   (E) Podophyllotoxin
4. Melasma is a condition characterized by excess melanin in the epidermis. A topical agent that is frequently successful in this condition is
   (A) Becaplermin
   (B) Etanercept
   (C) Hydroquinone
   (D) Botulinum toxin

ANSWERS
1. **B.** Botulinum toxin has no ability to inhibit esterase (A) or inhibit enzymes involved in the acetylcholine synthetic pathways (C), nor does it possess muscarinic receptor blocking properties (D).
2. **C.** Thalidomide caused a high incidence of phocomelia, particularly in Europe, where it was approved as a sedative agent. There is no definitive evidence associating teratogenic activity with the other compounds.
3. **E.** Interferon-α-2b is a recombinant product (A). Mycophenolate mofetil is derived from a *Penicillium* sp. (B). Methotrexate and 6-thioguanine (C and D) are totally synthesized.
4. **C.** Hydroquinone inhibits the enzyme tyrosine kinase, which converts tyrosine to melanin. It also damages melanocytes. Becaplermin (A) is a recombinant human platelet–derived growth factor that is useful in enhancing wound healing. Etanercept (B) is a recombinant fusion protein approved for treatment of psoriatic arthritis and rheumatoid arthritis. Botulinum toxin (D) is a purified form of botulinum toxin type A approved for therapy of blepharospasm and strabismus.

SUPPLEMENTAL READING
Chren MM and Landefeld CS. A cost analysis of topical drug regimens for dermatophyte infections. JAMA 1994;272:1992–1925.

Foss FM. DAB (389) IL-2 (ONTAK): A novel fusion therapy for lymphoma. Clin Lymphoma 2000;1:110–116.

Huang W and Vidimos A. Topical anesthetics in dermatology. J Am Acad Dermatol 2000;43:286–298.

Mukhtar H (ed.). Pharmacology of the Skin. Boca Raton, FL: CRC, 1992.

Ngheim P, Pearson G, and Langley RG. Tacrolimus and pimecrolimus: From clever prokaryotes to inhibiting calcineurin and treating atopic dermatitis. J Am Acad Dermatol 2002;46:228–241.

Perry CM and Lamb HM. Topical imiquimod: A review of its use in genital warts. Drugs 1999;58:375–390.

Tseng S et al. Rediscovering thalidomide: A review of its mechanism of action, side effects, and potential uses. J Am Acad Dermatol 1996;35:969–979.

Wolverton SE. (ed.). Comprehensive Dermatologic Drug Therapy. Philadelphia: Saunders, 2001.

Zhu YI and Stiller MJ. Dapsone and sulfones in dermatology: Overview and update. J Am Acad Dermatol 2001;45:420–434.

CASE Study   Treatment May Be Worse Than the Condition

A 35-year-old mother of two has moderate psoriasis. She tells you that her mother had a similar condition 3 years ago and was successfully treated with the agent acitretin. She has come to you because her regular physician refused to write her a prescription for acitretin, and she is very uncomfortable with her skin condition. You tell her that there is a serious risk of teratogenicity if she should become pregnant. She informs you that she is taking oral contraceptives and that the possibility of pregnancy is very low. Do you prescribe the drug she has requested anyway?

ANSWER: Acitretin should not be prescribed for women of childbearing potential unless no acceptable alternative is available and the patient has acknowledged in writing that she understands the need to use two effective forms of contraception during therapy and for 3 years after she discontinues the drug. She has not yet been treated with PUVA. You convince her that this is a more appropriate therapy, considering her age and her childbearing potential. She grudgingly accepts your suggestions and begins a course of PUVA treatment. She responds well to the treatment, and after 6 months the psoriasis is greatly improved and treatment is terminated.

42 Drugs for the Control of Supragingival Plaque

Angelo Mariotti and Arthur F. Hefti

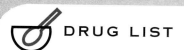

DRUG LIST

GENERIC NAME	PAGE	GENERIC NAME	PAGE
Chlorhexidine	501	Triclosan	502
Fluorides	504	Sodium lauryl sulfate	504

The periodontium, which is responsible for the retention of teeth in the maxilla and mandible, consists of four tissue types. Cementum and alveolar bone are the hard tissues to which the fibrous periodontal ligament anchors the tooth into the skeleton, and the gingiva is the covering tissue of the periodontium (Fig. 42.1). The gingiva is a unique body tissue in that it allows the penetration of calcified tissue (i.e., teeth) into an intact mucosa while protecting the underlying periodontal tissues. The accumulation of microorganisms on the tooth surface along the gingival margin can alter the structure and function of the gingiva, inducing an oral inflammatory reaction. Its clinical expression is called *gingivitis*.

During adolescence gingivitis is almost universal, and in adulthood it affects approximately 50% of the population. Because of the frequent appearance of gingivitis, this disease remains a principal concern for the dentist, since it can convert to other more destructive forms of periodontal disease. Hence, the prevention or cure of gingivitis is of particular interest.

The most common method of eliminating gingivitis is by the mechanical removal of the microorganisms found in dental plaque via toothbrush and floss. However, effective mechanical removal of plaque is a tedious, time-consuming process that is affected by an individual's gingival architecture, tooth position, dexterity, and motivation. Consequently, incomplete removal of dental plaque by mechanical means allows for the induction, continued progression, or both of gingivitis. Therefore, pharmacological agents that prevent or reduce plaque can aid the dentist by effectively preventing or eliminating gingival inflammation. Accordingly, the development of safe and effective topical liquid antimicrobial agents will help in the maintenance of healthy gingival tissues. This chapter examines the relationship of supragingival dental plaque to gingivitis and the unique pharmacokinetic characteristics of common antiplaque agents.

THE ROLE OF SUPRAGINGIVAL DENTAL PLAQUE IN THE INITIATION OF GINGIVITIS

Many types of materials accumulate on teeth. By far the most widespread and important deposit is dental plaque. *Plaque consists primarily of microorganisms in an organized matrix of organic and inorganic components.* Bacteria account for at least 70% of the mass of plaque. In fact, one cubic millimeter of dental plaque contains more than 100 million bacteria consisting of more than 400 species. The organic matrix of plaque consists of polysaccharide, protein, and lipid components, while the inorganic matrix is composed primarily of calcium and phosphorous ions.

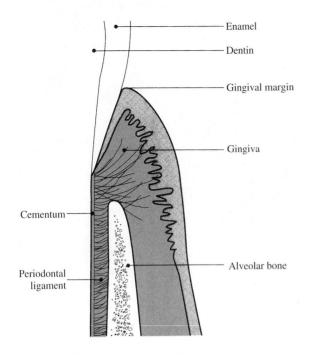

FIGURE 42.1
Anatomical landmarks in the periodontium.

The dental plaque above the gingival margin of the tooth is designated as supragingival, and the dental plaque below the gingival margin (i.e., in the gingival sulcus or pocket) is called subgingival. Gingivitis can be experimentally induced in an uninflamed periodontium by allowing the unimpeded accumulation of supragingival plaque and is reversed completely by the thorough and complete removal of supragingival plaque.

Gingivitis is due principally to the accumulation and retention of plaque at or near the gingival margin. The accumulation of supragingival plaque is also a prime influence in the development of subgingival plaque. As undisturbed plaque matures, it changes in composition and becomes more complex. A bacterial succession occurs whereby microorganisms associated with gingival health, that is, gram-positive rods and cocci, are replaced by microorganisms associated with gingivitis, that is, gram-negative rods and cocci, as well as spiral organisms and spirochetes. As a consequence of the change in microflora, the inflammation-induced changes in the gingiva cause an increase in epithelial cell turnover and connective tissue degradation, resulting in anatomical changes that tend to deepen the gingival sulcus, causing a gingival pocket to form. This change in gingival architecture and the subgingival environment provides a new and better protected niche for bacteria to grow. Here they are continually bathed by exudate from the gingival crevice and end products from the supragingival plaque. Hence, control of supragingival plaque will also have a profound influence on the developing composition of periodontitis-associated subgingival plaque.

PHARMACOKINETICS OF THE ORAL CAVITY

The therapeutic outcome of topically applied agents used to control oral infections will depend on the characteristics of drugs that take advantage of the unique physiological and anatomical circumstances in the oral cavity. This section is a broad overview of important oral pharmacokinetic principles.

Absorption

The vascularity of the oral cavity, combined with a thin epithelial lining in some areas, allows for the absorption of drugs at a rapid rate. Un-ionized drugs, such as nitroglycerin, take advantage of these tissue characteristics and diffuse rapidly across the oral mucosa into the bloodstream. Unlike most drugs, for which the principal objective is to introduce the agent into the bloodstream rapidly, the goal of oral topical agents is to be retained in the oral cavity for as long as possible. Absorption can lead to toxic effects elsewhere in the body and a significant reduction of the free drug in the oral cavity. In most instances, the drugs used to restrain plaque levels are highly ionized and therefore are generally unable to penetrate the oral mucosa.

Distribution

Once an agent is topically applied in the oral cavity, the free drug can act at the primary site (i.e., bacteria in the plaque), or it can be partitioned to compartments where the drug binds nonspecifically. These drug reservoirs include the enamel, dentin, and/or cementum of the tooth, the oral mucosa, the organic and inorganic components of plaque, and salivary proteins.

The fraction of the administered dose that is nonspecifically bound to oral reservoirs is highly dependent on the drug's concentration and chemical nature and the amount of time it remains at the site. For example, a 1-minute rinse with 0.2% chlorhexidine will result in approximately 30% of the total amount dispensed being retained, whereas a 3-minute rinse with 0.1% sodium fluoride will result in less than 1% of the administered dose being found in the oral cavity after an hour. The ability of oral agents to bind to oral reservoirs nonspecifically and reversibly is an important quality for sustained release of drugs.

Metabolism

In the oral cavity, drug metabolism occurs in mucosal epithelial cells, microorganisms, and enzymes in the saliva; metabolism also takes place in renal and hepatic tissue once the drug is swallowed. Although biotransformation of agents in the oral cavity is potentially an important aspect of reducing effective drug concentra-

The labels on the figure: Enamel, Dentin, Gingival margin, Gingiva, Cementum, Alveolar bone, Periodontal ligament

tions, quantitatively it accounts for only a small percentage of drug inactivation.

Excretion

Salivary flow is extremely important in the removal of many agents from the oral cavity. Human saliva has a diurnal flow that varies between 500 and 1,500 mL in the daytime to less than 10 mL of secretion at night. The rate of clearance of a drug from the oral cavity therefore is profoundly important in determining the amount of time a drug is in contact with the tooth surface.

Substantivity

The period that a drug is in contact with a particular substrate in the oral cavity is *substantivity*. Drugs that have a prolonged duration of contact are considered to have high substantivity. In the oral cavity, substantivity depends on two important pharmacokinetic features: the degree of reversible nonspecific binding to oral reservoirs and the rate of clearance by salivary flow (Fig. 42.2).

Oral reservoirs are an important source for the continued release of drugs. The oral compartments that accumulate a drug must reversibly bind large portions of the administered dose and release therapeutic concentrations of free drug to the site of action over long periods. Therefore, effective agents with high substantivity ideally would not bind irreversibly, nor would they bind with high affinity to oral reservoirs.

Salivary flow also will significantly affect the substantivity of topically applied liquid agents. The clearance of an agent from the oral cavity is directly proportional to the rate of salivary flow. Hence, during periods of high salivary flow, a greater release of drug from oral

reservoirs is necessary to maintain therapeutic concentrations. Strategies that use natural or drug-induced periods of low salivary flow can increase the substantivity of an oral agent.

ANTIPLAQUE AGENTS

Bisbiguanides

Chlorhexidine is a symmetrical cationic molecule that is most stable as a salt; the highly water-soluble digluconate is the most commonly used preparation. Because of its cationic properties, it binds strongly to hydroxyapatite (the mineral component of tooth enamel), the organic pellicle on the tooth surface, salivary proteins, and bacteria. Much of the chlorhexidine binding in the mouth occurs on the mucous membranes, such as the alveolar and gingival mucosa, from which sites it is slowly released in active form.

Pharmacokinetics

The rate of clearance of chlorhexidine from the mouth after one mouth rinse with 10 mL of a 0.2% aqueous solution follows approximately first-order kinetics, with a half-life of 60 minutes. This means that following application of a single rinse with a 0.2% chlorhexidine solution, the concentration of the compound exceeds the minimum inhibitory concentration (MIC) for oral streptococci (5 mg/mL) for almost 5 hours. The pronounced substantivity, along with the relative susceptibility of oral streptococci, may account for the great effectiveness of chlorhexidine in inhibiting supragingival plaque formation.

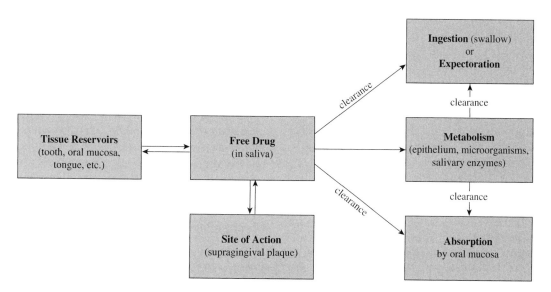

FIGURE 42.2
Pharmacokinetic factors that affect substantivity of rinsing agents.

Mechanisms of Action

Although chlorhexidine affects virtually all bacteria, gram-positive bacteria are more susceptible than are gram-negative organisms. Furthermore, *Streptococcus mutans* and *Antinomies viscosus* seem to be particularly sensitive. *S. mutans* has been associated with the formation of carious lesions in fissures and on interproximal tooth surfaces and has been identified in large numbers in plaque and saliva samples of subjects with high caries activity.

Low concentrations of chlorhexidine are bacteriostatic, while high concentrations are bactericidal. Bacteriostasis is the result of chlorhexidine binding to the negatively charged bacterial cell wall (e.g., lipopolysaccharides), where it interferes with membrane transport systems. Oral streptococci take up sugars via the phosphoenolpyruvate-mediated phosphotransferase (PEP-PTS) system. The PEP-PTS is a carrier-mediated group translocating process in which a number of soluble and membrane-bound enzymes catalyze the transfer of the phosphoryl moiety of PEP to the sugar substrate with the formation of sugar phosphate and pyruvate. Chlorhexidine is known to abolish the activity of the PTS at bactericidal concentrations. High chlorhexidine concentrations cause intracellular protein precipitation and cell death. Despite its pronounced effect on plaque formation, no detectable changes in resistance of plaque bacteria were found in a 6-month longitudinal study of mouth rinses.

Clinical Uses

The previous routine treatment for cases of severe gingival disease consisted of calculus and plaque removal and oral hygiene instructions. Subsequent resolution of the gingival inflammation was largely dependent on daily plaque control by the patient. However, the use of a 0.1 to 0.2% chlorhexidine mouthwash supplementing daily plaque control will facilitate the patient's effort to fight new plaque formation and to resolve gingivitis. Consequently, use of chlorhexidine is indicated in the following situations: in disinfection of the oral cavity before dental treatment; as an adjunct during initial therapy, especially in cases of local and general aggressive periodontitis; and in handicapped patients.

Adverse Effects and Toxicity

The most conspicuous side effect of chlorhexidine is the development of a yellow to brownish extrinsic stain on the teeth and soft tissues of some patients. The discoloration on tooth surfaces is extremely tenacious, and a professional tooth cleaning using abrasives is necessary to remove it completely. The staining is dose dependent, and variation in severity is pronounced between individuals. This side effect is attributed to the cationic nature of the antiseptic. Desquamative soft tissue lesions have also been reported with use of drug concentrations exceeding 0.2% or after prolonged application. A frequently observed side effect is impaired taste sensation. It was reported that rinsing with a 0.2% aqueous solution of chlorhexidine digluconate resulted in a significant and selective change in taste perception for salt but not for sweet, bitter, and sour.

In vitro, chlorhexidine can adversely affect gingival fibroblast attachment to root surfaces. Furthermore, protein production in human gingival fibroblasts is reduced at chlorhexidine concentrations that would not affect cell proliferation. Such findings corroborate earlier studies showing delayed wound healing in standardized mucosal wounds after rinsing with 0.5% chlorhexidine solution.

As an oral rinsing agent, to date chlorhexidine has not been reported to produce any toxic systemic effects. Since chlorhexidine is poorly absorbed in the oral cavity and gastrointestinal tract, little if any enters the bloodstream. A summary of chlorhexidine oral rinses is given in Table 42.1.

Nonionic Bisphenols

Triclosan is a broad-spectrum antimicrobial compound. It was originally used in soaps, antiperspirants, and cosmetic toiletries as a germicide. Today, triclosan is incorporated into toothpaste because of its wide spectrum of antimicrobial activities and low toxicity.

Pharmacokinetics

Triclosan is retained in dental plaque for at least 8 hours, which in addition to its broad antibacterial property could make it suitable for use as an antiplaque agent in oral care preparations. However, the compound is rapidly released from oral tissues, resulting in relatively poor antiplaque properties as assessed in clinical studies of plaque formation. This observation is further corroborated by a poor correlation between minimal inhibitory concentration values generated in vitro and clinical plaque inhibitory properties of triclosan. Improvement of substantivity was accomplished by incorporation of triclosan in a polyvinyl methyl ether maleic acid copolymer (PVM/MA, *Gantrez*). With the combination of PVM/MA copolymer and triclosan, the substantivity of the triclosan was increased to 12 hours in the oral cavity.

Mechanism of Action

Triclosan is active against a broad range of oral gram-positive and gram-negative bacteria. The primary target of its antibacterial activity is the bacterial cell membrane. High concentrations cause membrane leakage and ultimately lysis of the bacterial cell. Effects at lower

TABLE 42.1 Comparison of Antiplaque Agents in Oral Rinses

Rinse	Active Agent	Concentration (%)	Pharmacological Actions	Effect on Plaque	Effect on Gingivitis	Dispensed	Side Effects
PerioGard[a] Peridex[a]	Chlorhexidine	0.12	Interferes with sugar transport Disrupts cell membranes Precipitates intracellular proteins	↓↓↓	↓↓↓	P	Extrinsic tooth staining Altered taste sensation Enhanced calculus formation Oral ulcers
Viadent	Sanguinarine	0.01	Suppresses bacterial enzymes	↓	↓	OTC	Burning sensation Bitter taste
Listerine[a]	Essential oils[b] Alcohol	0.25 26.90	Inhibits bacterial enzymes Reduces amount of endotoxin Denatures bacterial cell walls	↓	↓/o	OTC	Bitter taste Burning sensation Desiccation of mucous membranes
Act[c]	Fluoride	0.23	Inhibits bacterial glycolysis	o	o	OTC	Mild tooth staining
Plax[a]	Sodium benzoate Sodium lauryl sulfate	Unknown Unknown	Dissolves plaque?	o	o	OTC	None reported

↓, decrease; o, no change; P, prescription; OTC, over the counter.
[a]PerioGard, Peridex, Listerine, and Plax are trade name examples; other similar generic rinsing agents are commercially available.
[b]Essential oils contain eucalyptol, methyl salicylate, thymol, and menthol.
[c]Suggested use of fluoride rinses at these concentrations is for control of carious lesions.

concentration are more subtle. Triclosan has been shown to bind to cell membrane targets and inhibit enzymes associated with the phosphotransferase and proton motive force systems.

Clinical Effects

Triclosan plus copolymer is available in toothpaste. Commercially available dentifrice concentrations contain 0.3% triclosan and 2.0% PVM/MA copolymer. This product (*Total*) was tested in a large number of short-term controlled clinical trials, from which a statistically significant but clinically modest 15 to 20% plaque reduction was reported. The same toothpaste composition also exhibited significant anticalculus properties. Typically, the reported reductions in calculus formation ranged from 25 to 35%. Finally, of considerable interest is the observation that triclosan inhibits gingivitis by a mechanism independent of its antiplaque activity. In a clinical study, minimal plaque effects accompanied an average 50% reduction in gingivitis. An explanation of this surprising effect stems from research conducted using a gingival fibroblast cell culture model. These experiments revealed that triclosan could inhibit the IL-1-induced production of prostaglandin E_2.

Essential Oils

A mixture of essential oils consisting of thymol 0.06%, eucalyptol 0.09%, methyl salicylate 0.06%, and menthol 0.04% in an alcohol-based vehicle (26.9%) provides the plaque-inhibiting properties of rinsing agents such as *Listerine.*

Essential oils may reduce plaque levels by inhibiting bacterial enzymes and by reducing pathogenicity of plaque via reduction of the amount of endotoxin; the alcohol is probably responsible for denaturing bacterial cell walls. The substantivity of Listerine appears to be quite low, and therefore, it must be used at least twice a day to be effective. A variety of clinical studies have demonstrated that Listerine is capable of reducing plaque and gingivitis over extended periods; however, the degree of reduction is variable. Listerine will reduce plaque and gingivitis anywhere from 14.9 to 20.8% and 6.5 to 27.7%, respectively (Table 42.1). Adverse reactions include a bitter taste and burning sensation in the oral cavity. Regular use of high-alcohol rinses can aggravate existing oral lesions and desiccate mucous membranes. In addition to Listerine, a huge number of American Dental Society (ADA) approved generic equivalents available over the counter.

Fluorides

Fluorides are widely used in caries prevention, for which they have been highly effective. Systemic administration of fluorides for caries prevention is available via drinking water (1 mg/L), tablets (0.25–1 mg), drops (0.125–0.5 mg), topical application by mouthwashes (200–1,000 mg/L), gels for home use (900 mg/kg) and professional use (9,000–19,000 mg/kg), and dentifrices (1,000 mg/kg). In contrast to the efficacy of fluorides in preventing carious lesions, these formulations have relatively poor antibacterial properties (Table 42.1). The weak therapeutic benefit of fluorides on gingivitis is due to a modest inhibition of glycolysis in plaque bacteria. Sodium fluoride, monofluorophosphate, and stannous fluoride are the compounds used in topically applied agents.

A few well-controlled clinical studies suggested a potential plaque-inhibiting effect for dentifrices containing stannous fluoride. However, these results were most likely due to the stannous ion rather than to fluoride; the positive charge of the stannous ion may interfere with bacterial membrane function, bacterial adhesion, and glucose uptake, thereby inhibiting the formation of plaque.

Mild tooth staining has been observed after use of stannous fluoride products. The ADA Council on Dental Therapeutics endorses fluorides for their caries-inhibiting effect but not for plaque inhibition.

Prebrushing Rinses

The topical application of a liquid rinse before brushing as an aid in the mechanical removal of supragingival plaque is a novel idea. Since the introduction of the first prebrushing rinse there has been a rapid increase in the number of generic products that claim to physically loosen or remove plaque. Prebrushing rinses usually contain a plethora of ingredients, and it is not known which constituent is the active chemical. It has been suggested that sodium lauryl sulfate acts as a detergent to dislodge or loosen the plaque on teeth (Table 42.1). When prebrushing rinses were tested against placebo rinses, prebrushing rinses appeared to have no effect on plaque reduction.

FUTURE DIRECTIONS

Today gingivitis and periodontitis are prevented principally through mechanical plaque control; however, dentition free of supragingival and subgingival plaque is extremely difficult to accomplish and maintain. On an annual basis, Americans spend more than $750 million on oral rinsing agents, although few effective plaque-inhibiting oral rinses are available and many are associated with side effects that prohibit long-term use.

The goal of future product development is not so much an improvement in the antiplaque performance of the existing effective compounds but rather lessening of their side effects and development of better delivery systems. Products that combine various known compounds with well-established plaque-inhibiting properties are under investigation. Among the most promising products are amine fluoride plus stannous fluoride and copper sulfate plus hexetidine. In the future, chemoprevention of supragingival plaque will depend on products that are effective, substantive, and safe.

Study QUESTIONS

1. The period during which a drug is in contact with a substrate in the oral cavity is
   (A) Excretion
   (B) Absorption
   (C) Distribution
   (D) Substantivity
   (E) Drug clearance
2. Yellow or brownish extrinsic stain of teeth is a frequently observed side effect of
   (A) Fluoride
   (B) Triclosan
   (C) Essential oils
   (D) Chlorhexidine
   (E) Sodium lauryl sulfate
3. The LEAST effective chemical agent for reduction of dental plaque is
   (A) Triclosan
   (B) Essential oils
   (C) Chlorhexidine
   (D) Stannous fluoride
   (E) Sodium lauryl sulfate
4. Which of the following agents was combined with the PVM/MA polymer to improve substantivity?
   (A) Fluoride
   (B) Triclosan
   (C) Essential oils
   (D) Chlorhexidine
   (E) Sodium lauryl sulfate
5. Which commercial product would you prescribe for a recovering alcoholic?
   (A) Act
   (B) Plax
   (C) Total
   (D) Peridex
   (E) Listerine

ANSWERS

1. **D.** Excretion (A) and drug clearance (E) are factors involved in drug elimination, while absorption (B) describes the ability of a drug to cross membranes and enter the blood stream. Distribution (C) describes the ability of a drug to enter a variety of body compartments during its circulation in the blood.
2. **D.** It is due to the ability of this cation to strongly bind to tooth surfaces, requiring strong abrasives to remove the stain. The other four compounds are not cationic and do not bind strongly to tissues.
3. **E.** Triclosan (A) is active against a broad range of oral gram-positive and gram-negative bacteria. Essential oils (B) are effective in reducing plaque levels by inhibiting bacterial enzymes. Chlorhexidine (C) is generally effective against all bacteria, but *Streptococcus mutans* and *Actinomyces viscosus,* two bacteria particularly associated with dental lesions, are especially susceptible to its action. Stannous fluoride (D) is widely used in caries prevention, and many studies have proven its effectiveness.
4. **B.** None of the other compounds listed has been shown to decrease supragingival plaque in combination with the polymer in a commercial preparation.
5. **C.** All of the other preparations contain alcohol.

SUPPLEMENTAL READING
Addy M and Renton-Harper P. The role of antiseptics in secondary prevention. In NP Lang, T Karring, J Lindhe (Eds.). Proceedings of the 2nd European Workshop on Periodontology. London: Quintessenz Verlag, 1997:152–173.

Adriaens PA and Gjermo P. Anti-plaque and anti-gingivitis efficacy of toothpastes. In NP Lang, T Karring, J Lindhe (Eds.). Proceedings of the 2nd European Workshop on Periodontology. London: Quintessenz Verlag, 1997:204–220.

Goodson JM. Pharmacokinetic principles controlling efficacy of oral therapy. J Dent Res 1989;68(Special issue);1625–1632.

Mariotti A and Burrell KH. Mouthrinses and Dentifrices. In Ciancio SG (Ed.). ADA Guide to Dental Therapeutics. Chicago: ADA, 2000:211–229.

Rölla G, Kjaerheim V, and Waaler SM. The role of antiseptics in primary prevention. In NP Lang, T Karring, J Lindhe (Eds.). Proceedings of the 2nd European Workshop on Periodontology. London: Quintessenz Verlag, 1997:120–130.

Wennström JL. Rinsing, irrigation and sustained local delivery. In NP Lang, T Karring, J Lindhe (Eds.). Proceedings of the 2nd European Workshop on Periodontology. London: Quintessenz Verlag, 1997:131–151.

CASE Study   Drug Research and Periodontal Disease

A 21-year old white woman who works as a research analyst for the Food and Drug Administration was evaluating the results of a new drug for the treatment of periodontal disease. Her review of the phase III clinical data caused her to visit her dentist, since she was concerned that her oral cavity exhibited many of the signs of the subjects who were participants in the clinical study. A review of her periodontium by her dentist revealed swollen and tender gingiva that were accompanied by erythema and bleeding upon mild provocation. Her dental radiographs revealed no abnormalities, and her physician found her to be healthy at her last physical examination. She reports taking no medications and denies allergies to any medicine. She is concerned about her health because her gingiva will bleed when she eats fibrous foods (e.g., apples) and affects her appearance.

1. What do you think is the most likely cause of her periodontal disease?
2. Should she be referred to a physician for further physical examination for a systemic alteration that was overlooked at her last physical examination? If so, what problem should be considered, and what tests should be ordered?
3. Should an oral chemotherapeutic agent be prescribed for her periodontal disease? If so, which one would you prescribe and what would be the benefit and disadvantage of using this agent for this patient?

ANSWER:

1. In most instances, dental plaque can cause erythema and gingival bleeding, but the gingival response can also be exacerbated by a variety of systemic conditions, including diabetes mellitus, leukemia, malnutrition, puberty and pregnancy.
2. An examination by the dentist should eliminate many of the potential systemic issues that can affect the periodontium of this patient. For example, the age of the patient, her appearance, and questions about her diet should be enough to rule in or out issues concerning puberty and malnutrition. However, if systemic conditions cannot be ruled out, an additional physical examination by a physician may be necessary. Additional tests to be requested could include oral glucose tolerance test for diabetes mellitus, human chorionic gonadotropin levels for pregnancy, and/or qualitative and quantitative evaluation of bone marrow cells and blood cells for leukemia.
3. If the patient's periodontal disease is the result of a leukemia or diabetes mellitus, the first response should be to treat the disease that is exacerbating the oral response to plaque. In these cases, an intensive oral physiotherapy program using over-the-counter toothpastes with triclosan would be warranted for home care. If the patient is pregnant, a thorough review of oral hygiene combined with over-the-counter toothpaste with triclosan would be appropriate. If persistent inflammation and gingival enlargement continue, the use of a prescription antiplaque rinse, such as chlorhexidine, would be warranted.

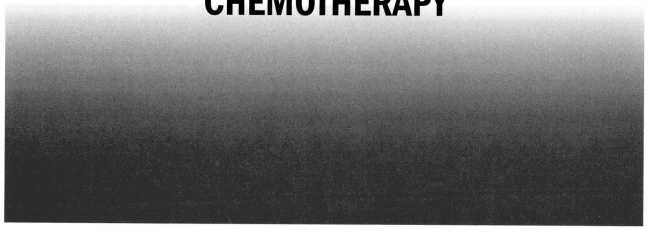

43 | Introduction to Chemotherapy

Steven M. Belknap

Paul Ehrlich introduced the term *chemotherapy* in 1907 to describe his important early studies of *Trypanosoma brucei,* the tsetse fly–borne parasite that causes African trypanosomiasis (sleeping sickness). The term *chemotherapy,* initially referring to antiparasitic therapy, now refers more broadly to the use of any chemical compound that selectively acts on microbes or cancer. Ehrlich had previously developed selective chemical stains for the microscopic examination of *Mycobacterium tuberculosis* and other microorganisms, using the coal-tar derivative dyes. He tested many of these organic compounds for their selective toxicity against trypanosomes but failed to find an effective nontoxic antischistosomal agent. Turning to the chemotherapy of syphilis, Ehrlich eventually discovered the arsenical compound salvarsan, which was both remarkably nontoxic to humans and remarkably toxic against a number of treponemal diseases, including syphilis and yaws. Ehrlich called salvarsan the magic bullet.

The search for safe, effective chemotherapeutic drugs is hindered by the common evolutionary legacy humans share with all living organisms; success requires exploitation of metabolic or structural differences between normal human cells and disease-producing cells. The more closely related the undesirable cells are to normal human cells, the more difficult the task of finding a magic bullet. For example, it is easier to cure malaria than cancer. Since viruses commandeer human cells to provide the necessary structural and metabolic apparatus for their functioning, they also are difficult to kill; transformed virus-infected human cells are only slightly altered normal human cells.

Humans were not the first to exploit the *selective toxicity* of chemicals. Many fungi and bacteria make toxic substances that kill or suppress the growth of competing microorganisms or facilitate infection of a host. Plants make a vast array of toxins for their self-defense. Exploitation of the selective toxicity of chemicals is an ancient and widely employed technique.

Humans first discovered this process in 1928 with Alexander Fleming's chance observation of the antibacterial effect of a substance secreted by *Penicillium notatum* mold. Howard Florey subsequently had the insight that this substance could be purified and injected into patients so as to provide systemic treatment of infection. Once scientists had learned of penicillin, they found many other naturally synthesized antibiotics, including tetracycline, streptomycin, and the cephalosporins. When the structures of these natural antibiotics were elucidated, chemists began to experiment with semisynthetic derivatives of the natural products and invented entire classes of related drugs that were safer or more effective than the naturally produced drug. The new semisynthetic or wholly synthetic drugs had improved pharmacokinetic properties, greater stability, and extended spectrums of action.

The emergence of microbial antibiotic drug resistance was speeded by the indiscriminate use of antibiotics in humans and livestock. Exposure to very low concentrations of antibiotic in meat or milk may have provided a path whereby human pathogens could eventually evolve high-level antibiotic drug resistance. Recently some strains of enterococcus and tuberculosis have developed resistance to all known antibiotic drugs. *Inappropriate use of antibiotics is very common, and it accelerates the development of resistance in pathogens.*

THE PATIENT–DRUG–PATHOGEN INTERACTION

In the laboratory the strain of pathogen, the number of infecting organisms, the culture medium, the antibiotic concentration, and the duration of antibiotic exposure can be precisely specified. This precision cannot be obtained in patients. In addition, chemotherapy of human disease is complex, as it depends on a complex patient–drug–pathogen interaction. This interaction has six components:

- *Pharmacokinetics:* What the patient does to the drug. For example, a patient with renal failure will have diminished renal clearance of gentamicin.
- *Pharmacodynamics:* What the drug does to the patient. For example, erythromycin stimulates gut motilin receptors and may induce nausea. The patient may stop taking the erythromycin.
- *Immunity:* What the patient does to the pathogen. For example, a patient with AIDS who is exposed to tuberculosis may develop the disease in spite of receiving a course of postexposure prophylactic antituberculosis chemotherapy, which would be effective in a patient with an intact immune system. Immunity includes both nonspecific complement-mediated opsonization and specific antibody- and cell-mediated immunity.
- *Sepsis:* What the pathogen does to the patient. For example, a patient with gram-negative bacillary pneumonia may receive a perfectly adequate course of antibiotic chemotherapy, only to succumb to systemic inflammatory response syndrome (SIRS), an exaggerated and counterproductive release of inflammatory cytokines.
- *Resistance:* What the pathogen does to the drug. For example, some strains of *Pseudomonas aeruginosa* produce a plasmid-mediated adenylase that inactivates gentamicin by chemically altering its structure.
- *Selective toxicity:* What the drug does to the pathogen. For example, acyclovir triphosphate, the phosphorylated derivative of acyclovir, lacks the 3'-hydroxy group necessary for adding the next nucleotide to the chain and terminates DNA elongation. This effect is selective, since herpes simplex DNA elongation is inhibited by markedly lower concentrations than is mammalian DNA elongation.

Pharmacokinetics

To be clinically useful, a chemotherapeutic drug must have both selective toxicity against pathogens and favorable pharmacokinetics. The processes of absorption, distribution, metabolism, and elimination compose a drug's pharmacokinetics. The concentration of the drug in a patient's body as a function of time is determined by the dose administered and the drug's pharmacokinetics in that patient.

Absorption from the gastrointestinal tract can be affected by other drugs and by food. Aluminum, calcium, and magnesium ions in antacids or dairy products form insoluble chelates with all tetracyclines and inhibit their absorption. Food inhibits tetracycline absorption but enhances doxycycline absorption; food delays but does not diminish metronidazole absorption; fatty food enhances griseofulvin absorption.

The chemical structure of a drug determines which enzymes metabolize it; a drug that fails to cross the cell membrane because of its polarity or size will be unmetabolized even if biochemically active degradative enzymes are present in the cytosol. Systemic use of drugs that are poorly absorbed or are destroyed by the gastrointestinal environment requires parenteral administration. Of course, if the goal is to attack pathogens in the gastrointestinal tract, then poor gastrointestinal absorption may be an advantage.

An antibiotic drug that is itself nontoxic may have metabolites that are toxic, diminishing its usefulness. For example, imipenem is hydrolyzed by renal dipeptidase to a metabolite that is inactive against bacteria but is toxic to humans. Coadministration of cilastatin inhibits the renal dipeptidase, which both prevents the formation of the toxic metabolite and decreases imipenem clearance, prolonging the half-life of the drug.

Partitioning of some drugs into cells occurs. Red blood cells parasitized by malaria selectively take up chloroquine, which accounts in part for the efficacy of this antimalarial against intracellular malarial forms. The intrahepatocellular concentration of chloroquine is 500 times that of the blood plasma concentration. Macrolides and fluoroquinolones are also selectively partitioned into cells, which accounts in part for their efficacy against mycoplasma and chlamydia, both intracellular pathogens.

Extensive protein binding of a drug decreases its free level and decreases the compound's glomerular filtration. Because protein binding is reversible, bound drug and free drug are in dynamic equilibrium; thus protein binding determines the optimal dose and dosing interval of the drug. A drug's pharmacokinetic properties are an important source of variation in the clinical response of patients to chemotherapy.

As mentioned earlier, pharmacokinetics is not solely the property of a drug but instead is the consequence of interactions between the drug and the physiology of the patient. Thus, statements like "the half-life of gentamicin is 2 hours" are not very useful, as the half-life is likely be longer or shorter in a given individual patient.

Individualization of dosing of chemotherapeutic drugs with a low therapeutic index is essential to effective, safe chemotherapy.

The concentrations of chemotherapeutic drugs in blood plasma, cerebrospinal fluid, urine, or ascites fluid can be measured to determine whether sufficient drug is present to inhibit or kill a given pathogen and to ensure that the concentration is not so high as to be toxic to the patient.

In severe bacterial infections that are difficult to eradicate, such as endocarditis or osteomyelitis, it may be important to ensure that the patient's serum remains bactericidal at the lowest, or trough, concentration in the dosing interval. Dilutions of patient's serum can be incubated with the organism isolated from the patient and the minimum bactericidal concentration determined through serial dilutions. Treatment is considered adequate if the serum remains bactericidal at a dilution of 1:8.

Pharmacodynamics

In the case of antibiotic chemotherapy, the ideal pharmacodynamic response is usually *no* pharmacodynamic response; the pharmacological target is not normal human cells but rather a parasite, a virus-infected human cell, or a cancerous cell. *The less selective the chemotherapeutic drug, the greater the severity of adverse effects.* Cancer chemotherapy is often severely toxic, even life threatening. Suppression of a viral infection, such as occurs in the treatment of HIV with antiviral drugs, is often complicated by serious drug-associated toxicity, such as hepatotoxicity or bone marrow suppression.

Compared with other pharmacological agents, antibacterial chemotherapeutic drugs are remarkably safe. Toxicity is common mainly in patients who are given inappropriately high doses or who develop high drug levels because of decreased drug clearance. Most antibiotics are renally cleared, so renal failure is a common cause of diminished antibiotic drug clearance.

The adverse reactions associated with the use of antibacterial chemotherapy include allergic reactions, toxic reactions resulting from inappropriately high drug doses, interactions with other drugs, reactions related to alterations in normal body flora, and idiosyncratic reactions. Several types of allergic responses occur, including immediate hypersensitivity reactions (hives, anaphylaxis), delayed sensitivity reactions (interstitial nephritis), and hapten-mediated serum sickness. Allergic cross-reactions to structurally related antibiotics can occur. Although an alternative non–cross-reacting antibiotic is generally preferred, desensitization protocols are available for situations in which there is no good alternative.

There is heterogeneity in human populations for the hepatic microsomal cytochrome P450 enzyme (see Chapter 4). Possession of an unfavorable phenotype may place a patient at risk for drug toxicity. For example, some patients who are slow acetylators of isoniazid may develop peripheral neuropathy with standard-dose isoniazid therapy.

Toxicity is most likely in tissues that interact with the drug. For example, gentamicin is polycationic and binds to anionic phospholipids in the cell membranes of renal proximal tubular cells, where it inhibits phospholipases and damages intracellular organelles.

Some adverse reactions are unrelated to either allergy or overdose; these are termed *idiosyncratic.* For instance, sulfonamides may precipitate acute hemolysis in some people having a glucose-6-phosphate dehydrogenase deficiency.

Many antibiotics alter the enteric microbial flora, particularly if high concentrations reach the colon. Antibiotic-sensitive bacteria are suppressed or killed, thereby removing their inhibitory effects on potentially pathogenic organisms. Overgrowth of pathogenic microbes can then occur. Unlike anaerobes, *Clostridium difficile* is resistant to clindamycin and some β-lactams. Use of such an antibiotic permits the proliferation of *C. difficile,* which then elaborates its toxin in high concentration. This toxin can cause pseudomembranous colitis, which can be fatal if not recognized and treated.

The effectiveness of chemotherapy is enhanced by adequate immune function; however, some antibiotics suppress immune function. For example, tetracyclines can decrease leukocyte chemotaxis and complement activation. Rifampin decreases the number of T lymphocytes and depresses cutaneous hypersensitivity. Antibiotics such as the sulfonamides may induce granulocytopenia or bone marrow aplasia. These effects are not well understood but may be due to enteric bacterial metabolic byproducts of these antibiotics.

Immunity

In the absence of antibiotic therapy, many patients survive infection, even infection by highly virulent pathogens. Thus, immunity may be due to factors such as a high functional reserve of organs or to an enhanced nonspecific opsonization of pathogens by complement. In other cases, specific partial immunoglobulin (Ig) G–mediated immunity was produced during prior exposure to the pathogen or a new IgM-mediated immunity develops during the course of the infection. Specific immunity can be either cell mediated or antibody mediated and may be enhanced by endogenously produced cytokines. Exogenously administered cytokines also may prove clinically useful as adjuncts to antibiotic chemotherapy.

Sepsis

Sepsis, or SIRS, is a maladaptive reaction to severe infection in which a variety of inflammatory mediators are released. Some of these mediators are bacterial metabolic products, while others are cytokines produced by humans during infection or other inflammatory disease. These mediators can induce failure of several organ systems. Cardiac function can be suppressed; acute respiratory distress syndrome can occur; renal failure is common; and disseminated intravascular coagulation can occur.

Through their ability to cause cell lysis, antibiotics such as the β-lactams or aminoglycosides may increase the release of bacterial inflammatory mediators (e.g., gram-negative bacillary endotoxin). Antibiotics also may induce the release of endogenous cytokines, such as interleukin (IL) 1-β, IL-6, and tumor necrosis factor (TNF-α) from monocytes and IL-4 and IFN-γ from lymphocytes. These cytokines are important in inflammatory and immunological responses and may contribute to the development of SIRS. Alternatively, these cytokines also may enhance immune function and enhance antimicrobial activity. Although many drugs have been examined for their ability to reverse SIRS, no clinical studies of interventions in sepsis have yet been shown to significantly lessen mortality.

Resistance

Some pathogens are naturally resistant to certain chemotherapeutic drugs. Resistance can occur through mutation, adaptation, or gene transfer. The mechanisms accounting for innate and acquired resistance are essentially the same. Spontaneous mutation in bacterial cells occurs at a frequency of approximately one per million cells. Such mutations may confer resistance to the chemotherapeutic drug. Spontaneous mutation is not a major concern unless the use of the drug results in selection and proliferation of resistant mutant pathogens in the patient.

Resistance to an antibiotic can be the result of one or more mechanisms. Alterations in the lipopolysaccharide structure of gram-negative bacilli can affect the uptake of lipophilic drugs. Similarly, changes in porins can affect the uptake of hydrophilic drugs. Once the drug enters the cell, it may be enzymatically inactivated. Some bacteria possess pumps that remove drugs from the bacterial cytosol. The antibiotic also may be ineffective as a result of mutation of genes coding for the target site (e.g., penicillin-binding proteins, DNA gyrase, or ribosomal proteins).

It is clinically important to understand the nature of the mechanism of resistance to an antibiotic drug. For example, the β-lactam resistance of *Streptococcus pneumoniae* is due to the appearance of altered penicillin-binding proteins. Thus, the use of a combination of a β-lactam and a penicillinase inhibitor, such as clavulanate, will not overcome streptococcal β-lactam resistance, because the mechanism of resistance is not due to the production of a penicillinase.

Multiple resistance may occur. Such resistance is recognized as a major problem in controlling bacterial infections and may be either chromosome or plasmid mediated. *Plasmids* (extrachromosomal genetic elements), which code for enzymes that inactivate antimicrobials, can be transferred by conjugation and transduction from resistant bacteria to previously sensitive bacteria. Such a transfer can also occur between unrelated species of bacteria. Enzymes coded by plasmids (e.g., penicillinase, cephalosporinase, and acetylases) that are specific for a given antimicrobial inactivate the drug either by removal or addition of a chemical group from the molecule or by breaking a chemical bond. *Transposons* are segments of genetic material with insertion sequences at the end of the gene; these sequences allow genes from one organism to be easily inserted into the genetic material of another organism. Some of these transposons code for antibiotic resistance.

In vitro laboratory tests of sensitivity of a microorganism to specific antimicrobial agents are used to predict efficacy in vivo. Often, it is enough to identify the causative pathogen in culture; the general resistance pattern of the pathogen and local patterns of resistance of the pathogen may then allow proper choice of chemotherapy. It is sometimes helpful to measure the antibiotic sensitivity of the specific isolated pathogen. Generally, a battery of tests against a selection of possible antibiotic drugs is employed.

Some organisms, such as *Staphylococcus aureus*, *Neisseria gonorrhoeae*, and *Haemophilus influenzae*, may produce β-lactamase and therefore be resistant to penicillin and its congeners. Testing for β-lactamase production by isolates enables an early decision on the use of penicillin and congeners in treatment of the disease.

Lethal Versus Inhibitory Effects

Antibiotics can be classified according to their effects on the biochemistry or molecular biology of pathogens. There are ribosomal inhibitors (macrolides), cell wall disrupters (β-lactams), DNA disturbers (fluoroquinolones), and metabolic poisons (trimethoprim-sulfamethoxazole). Antibiotics also can be classified according to whether they are *static* (inhibitory) or *cidal* (lethal). The classification of drugs as either static or cidal is based on laboratory assessment of the interaction of pathogen and antibiotic drug.

Cidal effects can be a result of the disruption of the cell wall or membrane. Cell lysis may occur when water diffuses into the high-osmolarity bacterial cytosol through the antibiotic-induced holes in the membrane, causing the bacteria to swell and burst. Cidal effects also can occur as a consequence of inhibition of bacterial DNA replication or transcription.

Static effects occur when the toxic effects of a chemotherapeutic drug are reversible. For example, inhibition of folate synthesis interferes with methylation, an important biochemical synthetic process. Reversal of this static effect can occur when the antibiotic concentration falls or if a compensatory increase in the synthesis of the inhibited enzymes occurs. The static versus cidal designation is a false dichotomy, since there is a continuous spectrum of activity between the two categories. The place of a drug along this spectrum will depend on both the pharmacological properties of the drug and such clinical factors as immune system function, inoculum size, drug concentration in tissue, and duration of therapy. A cidal drug may prove to be merely static if an inappropriately low dose or short treatment course is prescribed. A static drug may be cidal if given in high doses for prolonged courses to exquisitely sensitive pathogens.

MANAGING CHEMOTHERAPY

Initial therapy is usually empirical; and the regimen is adjusted according to the results of culture and sensitivity testing. Physicians must select a drug, administration route, dosage, and dosing interval. These may be changed several times during therapy. For example, severe nausea and high severity of illness may necessitate initial parenteral antibiotic administration. Several days later, when the nausea has abated and the patient is clinically stable, the patient may be switched to oral chemotherapy. Such an adjustment of therapy reduces the length of hospital stay while providing effective, safe treatment.

Once a chemotherapy regimen has been selected, the next step in managing chemotherapy is to define the outcome measures that will define therapeutic success and those that will define unacceptable toxicity and necessitate discontinuation of the chosen drugs. For example, resolution of fever and purulent sputum production, normalization of the white blood cell count, reversal of tachypnea and hypoxia, and improvement of constitutional signs and symptoms may be selected as measures that will be used to evaluate whether treatment of pneumonia is successful.

Often treatment must be continued for several days after objective signs and symptoms of infection have resolved. Patients should be instructed to continue antibiotics for the full duration indicated, even if they feel better. If the patient's recovery is delayed from what is reasonably expectable, the diagnosis should be reconsidered.

Many patients receive lengthy courses of antibiotics that probably should not have been started. *More than half of courses of antimicrobial chemotherapy are inappropriate.* Influenza pneumonia and viral upper respiratory infections, for example, are impervious to assault by antibiotics, although many patients with these illnesses receive such antibiotics. Of course, influenza may be complicated by postinfluenzal staphylococcal pneumonia, for which antibiotics *are* indicated. Careful sequential evaluation of seriously ill patients for whom antibiotics are deferred is as important as in patients for whom antibiotics are prescribed.

Study QUESTIONS

1. Choose the best answer. Selective toxicity is
   (A) What the drug does to the patient
   (B) What the patient does to the drug
   (C) What the pathogen does to the patient
   (D) What the drug does to the pathogen
   (E) What the pathogen does to the drug
2. A 60-year-old patient with AIDS presents to the emergency department with a temperature of 102°F, confused, and is going in and out of consciousness. He exhibits rapid respiration and a blood pressure of 80/40. You determine that both the sputum and urine are negative by Gram staining. Which of the following is the best choice?
   (A) Administer penicillin G intravenously.
   (B) Administer vancomycin.
   (C) Administer clindamycin and amikacin.
   (D) Send a clinical sample to laboratory to find out what the organism is before treating.

3. The term magic bullet was coined for
   (A) Ehrlich discovering the drug salvarsan for the treatment of syphilis
   (B) Fleming discovering the antibacterial effect of penicillium notatum
   (C) Florey showing the effectiveness of penicillin in patients
   (D) Wilson discovering the broad spectrum antibiotic streptomycin
4. Choose the best answer for the following. The emergence of microbial antibiotic drug resistance
   (A) Requires the concurrent administration of more than one antibiotic
   (B) Is a direct result of the use of antibiotics in livestock
   (C) Is a problem that was overcome by the development of vancomycin
   (D) Is due in large part to the indiscriminate use of antibiotics in humans

5. A patient refuses to continue to take erythromycin because it makes him vomit. This is an example of which patient–drug–pathogen interaction?
   (A) Pharmacokinetics
   (B) Pharmacodynamics
   (C) Immunity
   (D) Resistance
   (E) Selective toxicity

ANSWERS

1. **D.** A drug may be selective to a particular enzyme system that is found only in the microbe and have no harmful effect on the patient. An example is sulfonamides blocking the enzyme dihydropteroate synthesis. This is a necessary step in the synthesis of dihydrofolic acid. Humans can use preformed dihydrofolic acid and do not need this enzymatic step to produce purines. Pharmacodynamics describes what the drug does to the patient. Pharmacokinetics describes what the patient does to the drug. Sepsis describes what the pathogen does to the patient. Resistance is what the pathogen does to the drug.

2. **C.** The patient is very ill, and you cannot afford to wait for the diagnosis. You administer a combination of clindamycin and amikacin to ensure that you have coverage for gram-negative and gram-positive organisms and anaerobes. Vancomycin and penicillin G are effective against Gram-positive organisms only.

3. **A.** Ehrlich called salvarsan the magic bullet for its nontoxic effect to humans and to its toxicity against the organism responsible for syphilis.

4. **D.** The indiscriminate use of antibiotics in humans is the major reason for the emergence of microbial antibiotic resistance. Such resistance, which is most apparent in hospitals, has developed to all antibiotics, including vancomycin. The use of antibiotics in livestock has compounded the problem.

5. **B.** Pharmacodynamics describes what the drug does to the patient. Erythromycin stimulates gut motilin receptors and may induce nausea; this leads to the patient refusing to continue therapy. Pharmacokinetics describes what the patient does to the drug. Immunity is what the patient does to the pathogen; resistance is what the pathogen does to the drug; and selective toxicity is what the drug does to the pathogen.

SUPPLEMENTAL READING

Lewis K et al. (eds.). Bacterial Resistance to Antimicrobials. New York: Marcel Dekker, 2001.

Levy SB. The challenge of antibiotic resistance. Sci Am 1998;278:46–53.

Nightingale Ch, Morakawa T, and Ambrose PG (eds.). Antimicrobial Pharmacodynamics in Theory and Clinical Practice. New York: Marcel Dekker, 2001.

Tufano MA et al. Antimicrobial agents induce monocytes to release IL-1 β, IL-6, and TNFα and induce lymphocytes to release IL-4 and IFN-γ Immunopharmacol Immunotoxicol 1992;14:769–782.

Rosenblatt JE. Laboratory tests used to guide antimicrobial therapy. Mayo Gin Proc 1991;66:942.

CASE Study   A Beneficial Example of Pharmacokinetics

A patient is being treated with the compound imipenem for penicillin-resistant pneumococcal infection and is responding well. After several days of treatment, the patient begins vomiting and has diarrhea. You observe a slight seizure at the same time. The infection is very severe, and you do not wish to terminate the imipenem but you fear that the adverse effects will make this a necessity. What do you do?

ANSWER: You decide that a metabolite of imipenem is responsible for the sudden toxicity. You add a second drug, cilastatin, to the patient's regimen. Coadministration of cilastatin inhibits renal dipeptidase, the enzyme responsible for the metabolism of imipenem. This prevents the formation of the toxic metabolite and decreases the clearance of imipenem. The side effect disappears within 12 hours and the patient recovers from the infection.

Synthetic Organic Antimicrobials: Sulfonamides, Trimethoprim, Nitrofurans, Quinolones, Methenamine

44

Marcia A. Miller-Hjelle, Vijaya Somaraju, and J. Thomas Hjelle

 DRUG LIST

GENERIC NAME	PAGE	GENERIC NAME	PAGE
Cinoxacin	519	Ofloxacin	519
Ciprofloxacin	519	Sparfloxacin	521
Enoxacin	519	Sulfacetamide	515
Gatifloxacin	521	Sulfadiazine (silver)	515
Levofloxacin	519	Sulfamerazine	517
Lomefloxacin	519	Sulfamethazine	517
Mafenide	517	Sulfamethoxazole	516
Methenamine	522	Sulfisoxazole	517
Moxifloxacin	519	Trimethoprim	517
Nalidixic acid	519	Trimethoprim–sulfamethoxazole	518
Nitrofurantoin	521	Trisulfapyrimidine	517
Nitrofurazone	521	Trovafloxacin	519
Norfloxacin	519		

SULFONAMIDES

Chemistry, Structure, and Function

The sulfonamides are a large group of compounds that are structural analogues of *p*-aminobenzoic acid (PABA). They differ primarily in the substituents on either the amido group (SO_2-NH-R) or the amino group (-NH_2) of the sulfanilamide nucleus. Substitutions on the sulfonamide group modify the drug's solubility characteristics, resulting in congeners with different rates of absorption and excretion. One group of sulfonamides remains largely unabsorbed in the gastrointestinal (GI) tract following oral administration. Sulfadiazine, for example, produces changes only on local gut bacterial flora and finds wide use in presurgical bowel sterilization. Other sulfonamides, such as sulfisoxazole, are rapidly absorbed and highly soluble, and they undergo rapid urinary excretion, mainly in the unaltered form. A third group are rapidly absorbed and slowly excreted and maintain adequate blood levels for up to 24 hours (e.g., sulfamethoxazole). These drugs are useful in treating chronic urinary infections. Finally, some sulfonamides (e.g., sulfacetamide and sulfadiazine [silver salt]) are designed for topical use such as in infection of the eye and in burn patients.

515

Mechanism of Action and Resistance

Both sulfonamides and trimethoprim (not a sulfonamide) sequentially interfere with folic acid synthesis by bacteria. Folic acid functions as a coenzyme in the transfer of one-carbon units required for the synthesis of thymidine, purines, and some amino acids and consists of three components: a pteridine moiety, PABA, and glutamate (Fig. 44.1). The sulfonamides, as structural analogues, competitively block PABA incorporation; sulfonamides inhibit the enzyme dihydropteroate synthase, which is necessary for PABA to be incorporated into dihydropteroic acid, an intermediate compound in the formation of folinic acid. Since the sulfonamides *reversibly block* the synthesis of folic acid, *they are bacteriostatic drugs. Humans cannot synthesize folic acid and must acquire it in the diet; thus, the sulfonamides selectively inhibit microbial growth.*

Resistance to the sulfonamides can be the result of decreased bacterial permeability to the drug, increased production of PABA, or production of an altered dihydropteroate synthetase that exhibits low affinity for sulfonamides. The latter mechanism of resistance is plasmid mediated. Active efflux of the sulfonamides has also been reported to play a role in resistance. The inhibitory effect of the sulfonamides also can be reversed by the presence of pus, tissue fluids, and drugs that contain releasable PABA.

Antibacterial Spectrum and Resistance

The sulfonamides are broad-spectrum antimicrobials that are effective against gram-positive and some gram-negative organisms of the Enterobacteriaceae. There is good activity against *Escherichia coli,* moderate activity against *Proteus mirabilis* and *Enterobacter* spp.; poor activity against indole-positive *Proteus* and *Klebsiella* spp., and no inhibitory activity against *Pseudomonas aeruginosa* and *Serratia* spp. They are also effective against *Chlamydia* spp., but superior drugs are now available. Sulfonamides are used in treating infections caused by *Toxoplasma gondii* and occasionally chloroquine-resistant *Plasmodium falciparum.*

Resistance occurs as the result of one or more alterations in the cellular metabolism of the bacteria; both mutation and plasmid-mediated resistance occurs. These changes, which can be irreversible, include alterations in the physical or enzymatic characteristics of the enzyme or enzymes that metabolize PABA and participate in the cellular synthesis of tetrahydrofolic acid. The appearance of alternative pathways for PABA synthesis within the bacteria or the development of an increased capacity to inactivate or eliminate the sulfonamide also may contribute to bacterial cell resistance. Bacteria that can use preformed folate are not inhibited by sulfonamides.

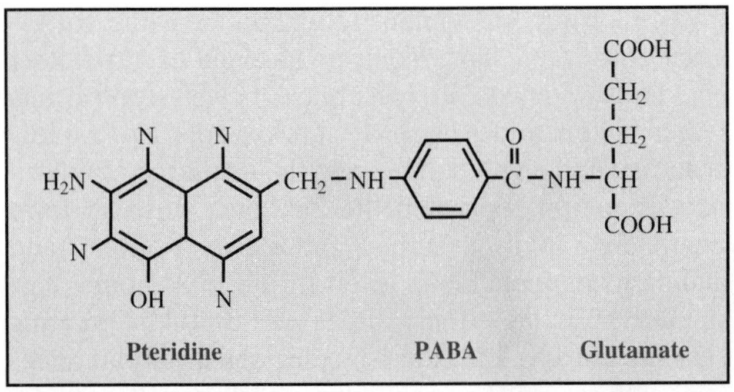

Pharmacokinetic Properties
Absorption

Sulfonamides are usually given orally, although the soluble sodium salts can be given parenterally, a route that is infrequently used. Except for compounds designed for local gut effects, the sulfonamides are rapidly absorbed from the intestinal tract, primarily from the small intestine. They can usually be found in serum and urine within 30 minutes after ingestion. Peak serum levels are obtained in 2 to 6 hours; urine levels can reach above 500 μg/mL. Although absorption can occur via other routes (e.g., burned and/or abraded skin, stomach), the amounts absorbed are usually low and unpredictable. A burn area larger than 20% of total body surface can absorb enough drug to result in toxicity, especially if accompanied by renal dysfunction.

Distribution

Systemically absorbed sulfonamides readily distribute throughout body fluids. They pass the placental barrier and enter the cerebrospinal fluid (CSF) even in the absence of inflammation. The degree of protein binding, the half-life, and the drug's solubility in urine will vary considerably from one sulfonamide to another. Half-lives range from 2.5 to 17 hours, the latter exhibited by sulfadiazine. Sulfadiazine and sulfacetamide tend to have lower protein binding (about 20–30%) than the other major systemic sulfonamides, whose binding ranges from 80 to 90% (e.g., sulfamethoxazole, sulfisoxazole). The effects of high protein binding by a sulfonamide become almost negligible in body fluids with a paucity of protein (e.g., synovial, peritoneal, ocular); thus, the drug in these sites is primarily in the active unbound form. Most drugs with protein binding above 30% do not cross the placenta; while this reduces toxic potential, it concomitantly lowers drug antibacterial activity.

FIGURE 44.1
Folic acid and its component molecules.

Metabolism and Excretion

The sulfonamides are degraded in the liver by acetylation and oxidation; metabolites have reduced bacteriological activity. The parent compound and the metabolites are excreted in the urine, primarily by glomerular filtration followed by tubular reabsorption. Some sulfonamides exhibit diurnal variations in excretion, being three times greater at night than during the day.

Clinical Uses

Sulfonamides have a long record of successful use in the treatment of a wide range of both gram-positive and gram-negative bacterial infections. They are also active against some of the less frequently encountered infections, such as leprosy, malaria, toxoplasmosis, and nocardiosis. Current indications are more limited, especially to the treatment of urinary tract and ear infections, because of frequently encountered resistance and the availability of better and safer agents for infections such as shigellosis, salmonellosis, and meningococcal meningitis. In contrast, the growth of rickettsial organisms is actually stimulated.

Acute uncomplicated urinary tract infections caused by *E. coli* and other pathogens generally respond promptly to one of the short-acting sulfonamides. Recurrent urinary tract infections (UTIs), when related to some structural abnormality in the tract, are frequently caused by sulfonamide-resistant bacteria.

Sulfadiazine and sulfisoxazole still play a useful role in the prophylaxis of group A streptococcal infections in patients with rheumatic fever who are hypersensitive to penicillin. This is tempered with the potential for toxicity and infection with resistant *Streptococcus pyogenes*.

Trisulfapyrimidine (a combination of sulfadiazine, sulfamerazine, and sulfamethazine), trimethoprim–sulfamethoxazole, or sulfisoxazole can be used as an alternative drug for the treatment of melioidosis caused by *Pseudomonas pseudomallei* and for infections produced by *Nocardia* spp.

A number of infections caused by *Chlamydia trachomatis*, such as trachoma, inclusion conjunctivitis, pneumonia, and urethritis, can be treated with topical or systemic sulfonamides, although tetracycline or erythromycin is preferred.

Sulfonamides, such as sulfadiazine, in combination with pyrimethamine, are considered the treatment of choice of symptomatic toxoplasmosis. Patients should be well hydrated to prevent crystalluria; this problem may be reduced with the use of triple sulfas (trisulfapyrimidine). Some regimens have included a sulfonamide (sulfadoxine) in combination with pyrimethamine (*Fansidar*) for the treatment of chloroquine-resistant malaria caused by *P. falciparum*.

Topically active sulfonamides are useful in preventing infections in burn patients. Mafenide acetate

(*Sulfamylon Cream*), the most widely used compound, is effective against *P. aeruginosa*, an organism that frequently colonizes burns. It is less effective against staphylococci, which also colonize burns. Local absorption of the acetate preparation, which is acidic, can result in respiratory alkalosis. Silver sulfadiazine in a 1% cream can be used as an alternative to mafenide and has good activity against gram-negative bacteria.

Sulfacetamide is used topically for treatment of ocular infections.

Adverse Effects and Drug Interactions

If the concentration of the sulfonamide is sufficiently high and its aqueous solubility is sufficiently low, the free drug or its metabolites may form crystals and cause bleeding or complete obstruction of the kidneys. Combinations of sulfa compounds have been developed for the purpose of lowering the dosage of individual components to reduce the chance of crystalluria (e.g., triple sulfas, such as the trisulfapyrimidines).

The sulfonamides do cause hypersensitivity reactions (e.g., rashes, eosinophilia, and drug fever) in a small number of patients. Other rare allergic reactions include vasculitis, photosensitivity, agranulocytosis, and thrombocytopenia. Stevens-Johnson syndrome is also associated with sulfonamide use; it is characterized by fever, malaise, erythema multiforme, and ulceration of the mucous membranes of the mouth and genitalia. Hemolytic anemia may develop in persons with a genetic deficiency of red blood cell glucose-6-phosphate dehydrogenase (G6PD).

Sulfonamides compete for sites on plasma proteins that are responsible for the binding of bilirubin. As a result, less bilirubin is bound, and in the newborn, the unbound bilirubin can be deposited in the basal ganglia and subthalamic nuclei, causing *kernicterus*, a toxic encephalopathy. For this reason, *sulfonamides should not be administered to newborns or to women during the last 2 months of pregnancy*.

Significant drug–drug interactions are those that potentiate the effects of other agents and require dosage modification. These include certain anticoagulants, hypoglycemic sulfonylureas, and hydantoin anticonvulsants.

TRIMETHOPRIM

Chemistry, Structure, and Mechanism of Action

Trimethoprim (*Trimpex, Proloprim*) is a structural analogue of the *pteridine portion* of dihydrofolic acid. It differs from the sulfonamides in that it acts at a second step in the folic acid synthetic pathway; that is, it competitively inhibits dihydrofolate reductase. This is the enzyme that catalyzes the reduction of dihydrofolic acid to tetrahydrofolic acid, the active form of folate. Dihydrofolate reductase is present in both mammalian tissue and bacteria, but 20,000 to 60,000 times more drug is required to inhibit the mammalian enzyme; this accounts for its *selective toxicity* against bacteria.

Trimethoprim–sulfamethoxazole (TMP-SMX) was introduced as a fixed dose combination in 1968. Trimethoprim was added to sulfamethoxazole to synergistically and sequentially inhibit bacterial synthesis of tetrahydrofolic acid. The combination was also designed to delay development of bacterial resistance. Sulfamethoxazole was selected in part because it is a congener of the frequently used sulfisoxazole but exhibits slower enteric absorption and urinary excretion. Sulfamethoxazole has a half-life similar to that of trimethoprim.

Antibacterial Spectrum and Resistance

Trimethoprim exhibits broad-spectrum activity. It is most commonly used in combination with sulfamethoxazole and is active against most gram-positive and gram-negative organisms, especially the Enterobacteriaceae. There is little activity against *anaerobic* bacteria; *P. aeruginosa*, enterococci, and methicillin-resistant staphylococci should be considered resistant to trimethoprim.

Resistance can develop from alterations in dihydrofolate reductase, bacterial impermeability to the drug, and by overproduction of the dihydrofolate reductase. The most important mechanism of bacterial resistance to trimethoprim clinically is the production of plasmid-encoded trimethoprim-resistant forms of dihydrofolate reductase.

Because trimethoprim and sulfamethoxazole have their effects at different points in the folic acid synthetic pathway, a synergistic effect results when the two are administered together. The incidence of bacterial resistance to the combination is less than that observed when the drugs are used individually. Resistance is an increasing problem in a number of bacteria, but is especially problematic in the Enterobacteriaceae, against which the combination is used in AIDS patients for *Pneumocystis carinii* pneumonia prophylaxis.

Absorption, Metabolism, and Excretion

Trimethoprim is well absorbed from the GI tract, and peak blood levels are achieved in about 2 hours. Tissue levels often exceed those of plasma, and the urine concentration of trimethoprim may be 100 times that of the plasma. Trimethoprim readily enters the CSF if inflammation is present. The half-life of the drug is approximately 11 hours. Sulfamethoxazole ($t_{1/2}$ = 10 hours) is frequently coadministered with trimethoprim in a fixed dose ratio of 1:5 (trimethoprim to sulfamethoxazole).

Peak drug levels in plasma are achieved in 1 to 4 hours following oral administration and 1 to 1.5 hours after IV infusion. At this time, the TMP-SMX plasma ratio is 1:20, which is the ratio most effective for producing a synergistic effect against most susceptible pathogens. The ratio is also influenced by the greater lipid solubility of trimethoprim, which results in its larger volume of distribution. Both trimethoprim and sulfamethoxazole bind to plasma protein (45 and 66% respectively) and both are metabolized in the liver. Approximately 40 to 60% of both parent drugs and their metabolites is excreted by the kidney within 24 hours; in moderate to severe renal dysfunction the dose should be reduced by approximately one-half. Only the parent compounds are excreted in the bile. Both drugs cross the placenta and are found in breast milk (see adverse effects).

Clinical Use of Trimethoprim–Sulfamethoxazole

TMP-SMX (*Septra, Bactrim*) is used in the treatment of genitourinary, GI, and respiratory tract infections caused by susceptible bacteria. *E. coli*, enterococci, *P. mirabilis*, some indole-positive strains of *Proteus* spp., and *Klebsiella pneumoniae* are usually sensitive to this combination therapy for both chronic and recurrent UTIs. Trimethoprim is present in vaginal secretions in high enough levels to be active against many of the organisms found in the introital area that are often responsible for recurrent UTIs. In some patients with recurrent UTIs, most notably women of childbearing age, the long-term use of one tablet taken at night is an effective form of chemoprophylaxis. The drug is approved for use by the U. S. Food and Drug Administration (FDA) for treating UTIs in both children and adults.

TMP-SMX is also used in the treatment of infection caused by ampicillin-resistant *Shigella* spp. and for antibiotic-resistant *Salmonella* spp.. The combination is also effective for covering the carrier state of *Salmonella typhi,* the agent of typhoid fever, and other *Salmonella* spp.. Successful treatment of traveler's diarrhea due to susceptible *E. coli* is another advantage of the use of this combination. The combination is not indicated in the therapy of enterohemorrhagic *E. coli* strains such as O157:H7 because of the risk of developing hemolytic–uremic syndrome associated with the release of the cytotoxic enterotoxin by the drugs.

Because trimethoprim accumulates in the prostate, TMP-SMX is used to treat prostatitis caused by sensitive organisms. Therapy can be prolonged (4–6 weeks) and repeat courses of therapy may be necessary. Trimethoprim alone, because of its lipid solubility, can be effectively used when patients exhibit an allergic response to the sulfonamide component.

Otitis media in children and purulent exacerbations of chronic bronchitis respond well to TMP-SMX because of its activity against both susceptible *Streptococcus pneumoniae* and *Haemophilus influenzae type b* (*Hib*); the latter organism is now a much less frequent pathogen in otitis because of the use of the Hib vaccine.

Gonorrhea, typhoid fever, and brucellosis have been treated with TMP-SMX with cure rates comparable to those attained by standard therapy. It also has been used in the treatment of nocardial infections.

TMP-SMX remains the antimicrobial therapy of choice in both the treatment and prevention of infections caused by *P. carinii*, a protozoan that produces serious pneumonitis in patients with hematological malignancies and AIDS. In those with AIDS, treatment is more prolonged and relapse is common. These patients are at increased risk for untoward effects such as fever, hepatitis, rash, and leukopenia.

Adverse Effects and Drug Interactions

Serious adverse effects are rare except in AIDS patients. TMP-SMX can cause the same adverse effects as those associated with sulfonamide administration, including skin rashes, central nervous system (CNS) disturbances, and blood dyscrasias. Blood dyscrasias, hepatotoxicity, and skin rashes are particularly common in patients with AIDS. Most of the adverse effects of this combination are due to the sulfamethoxazole component. Trimethoprim may increase the hematological toxicity of sulfamethoxazole. Long-term use of trimethoprim in persons with borderline folic acid deficiency, such as alcoholics and the malnourished, may result in megaloblastic anemia, thrombocytopenia, and granulocytopenia.

Trimethoprim has been reported to decrease the therapeutic effect of cyclosporine with a concomitant increased risk of nephrotoxicity. Increased levels of dapsone, warfarin, methotrexate, zidovudine, and sulfonylureas may occur when given together with trimethoprim; dosages of these drugs should be modified and the patient monitored accordingly.

Because both drugs may interfere with folic acid metabolism, their use during pregnancy is usually contraindicated by the potential for effects on the fetus, such as the development of neural tube defects associated with folate deficiency. The use of trimethoprim is contraindicated in patients with blood dyscrasias, hepatic damage, and renal impairment.

QUINOLONES: NALIDIXIC ACID AND FLUOROQUINOLONES

Chemistry, Mechanism of Action, and Classification

All clinically approved quinolones in use in the United States contain a carboxylic acid moiety in the 3-position of the basic ring structure (the 4-quinolones). The 4-quinolones inhibit DNA synthesis through their specific action on DNA gyrases, which are composed of two A and two B subunits. DNA subunits A (gyrase A gene) have a strand-cutting function to prevent overwinding (supercoiling) of the DNA strands during separation and eventual replication of the mirror strand. The A subunits are the site of action for the 4-quinolones. Recently a second target, unique to the fluoroquinolones, has been identified as topoisomerase type IV. This enzyme is responsible for separating the daughter cells following replication.

The DNA gyrases and type IV topoisomerase both belong to the general class of DNA enzymes called topoisomerases. The effect of quinolones on these DNA enzymes is initially bacteriostatic but becomes bactericidal when bacteria are unable to repair the DNA lesions. These drug targets may be primary or secondary depending upon the organism; this observation can affect the bacterial potential for the development of drug resistance; this may require the use of another drug with a different specificity and spectrum of activity.

The quinolones are now often classified into generations, much like the cephalosporins. Each generation (first through fourth) has spectrum specificity and unique pharmacological properties, although there is considerable overlap: First, nalidixic acid and cinoxacin; second, norfloxacin, ciprofloxacin, ofloxacin, enoxacin, and lomefloxacin; third. levofloxacin, sparfloxacin, gatifloxacin; and fourth, trovafloxacin and moxifloxacin. Several of the newer quinolones have been recently removed from the market as a result of QT prolongation and serious hematological and renal problems.

Antibacterial Spectrum and Resistance

The first-generation and oldest quinolones exhibit limited gram-negative activity. Nalidixic acid and cinoxacin do not achieve systemic antibacterial levels and are thus restricted to therapy of bladder infections caused by urinary pathogens, such as *E. coli* and *Klebsiella* and *Proteus* spp. Although they are bactericidal agents, their use is restricted by resistance.

The second-generation drugs demonstrate their most reliable activity against gram-negative organisms, including Enterobacteriaceae. *Haemophilus* spp. and sexually transmitted disease (STD) agents, such as *Neisseria gonorrhoeae, Chlamydia trachomatis, Ureaplasma urealyticum,* and *Moraxella catarrhalis* (formerly *Neisseria catarrhalis;* causes otitis media) are also susceptible. The antipseudomonal activity of ciprofloxacin, norfloxacin, ofloxacin, and lomefloxacin is due to their piperazine moiety; resistance to these agents, however, is becoming more prevalent.

Significantly greater activity against gram-positive organisms, such as *S. pneumoniae,* is demonstrated by the third and fourth generations. Methicillin-resistant *Staphylococcus aureus* and *Enterococcus faecium* are resistant. The fourth-generation quinolones also possess activity against anaerobes.

With the exception of the first generation, the quinolones are active against a variety of pathogens associated with respiratory tract infections, such as *Chlamydia pneumoniae, Mycoplasma pneumoniae, Legionella pneumophila,* and *Mycobacterial* spp., although these drugs are not FDA-approved for the latter. *Recently, ciprofloxacin has gained popular attention in providing coverage for Bacillus anthracis, a major bioterrorism agent.*

Resistance is related to mutations in the DNA gyrase, with the gyrase gene A (gyrA) being the predominant site. The primary mutation sites affected by organisms are topoisomerase IV and gyrA. Mutations at these points influence the degree of resistance, with lower levels of resistance associated with topoisomerase IV and higher levels with gyrA. Alterations in porins (gram-negative bacteria) that result in a decreased uptake of the drug and the appearance of an active efflux system for transport of the drug out of the cell also contribute to resistance. Resistance is chromosomally mediated; plasmid-associated resistance has not been reported. Killing by quinolones is concentration dependent, while that for the β-lactams is time dependent; thus the quinolones demonstrate a long postantibiotic effect. Cross-resistance between the quinolones can occur, particularly if resistance is strong. Moxifloxacin appears less susceptible to the appearance of cross-resistance.

Absorption, Metabolism, and Excretion

The quinolones are rapidly and almost completely absorbed after oral administration and are widely distributed in body tissues. Levels in extravascular spaces can often exceed serum levels. Levels lower than those found in serum occur in CSF, bone, and prostatic fluids. Ciprofloxacin and ofloxacin have been detected in breast milk and ofloxacin levels in ascites fluid are close to serum levels. Food ingestion does not affect bioavailability, which ranges from 50 to 95%. The half-life for most quinolones is 3 to 4 hours.

Elimination of the fluoroquinolones is through glomerular filtration and tubular secretion. In patients with moderate to severe renal insufficiency, quinolone dosages should be modified. The fluoroquinolones are also metabolized by hepatic conjugation and glucuronidation. Caution should be observed with administration of trovafloxacin because of its potential to induce hepatic toxicity. Dosage, peak serum levels, percent protein binding, urine concentrations, and degree of metabolism differ to varying degrees among the quinolones.

Clinical Uses

Therapeutic uses of the quinolones include urinary and respiratory tract infections, GI and abdominal infections, STDs, and bone, joint, and soft tissue infections. Nalidixic acid is effective for urinary tract infections; however, bacteria can become resistant, particularly if the drug is used for long periods. The second-generation fluoroquinolones are all equally efficacious in UTIs, and their activity is comparable to that of TMP-SMX. These drugs have shown efficacy in treating prostatitis and can serve as an alternative therapy for patients not responding to TMP-SMX.

The fluoroquinolones have a variety of indications in the treatment of respiratory infections, although they may not be the drugs of choice; these infections include acute and chronic bacterial sinusitis. A second-generation cephalosporin, such as cefuroxime, is usually the drug of choice in acute sinusitis associated with *M. catarrhalis, H. influenzae,* and *S. pneumoniae.* The second-generation quinolones usually have poor activity in treating community-acquired pneumonia (CAP) because of their poor activity against *S. pneumoniae.* The third- and fourth-generation fluoroquinolones are significantly more effective in treating CAP because of their activity against *S. pneumoniae.* The fluoroquinolones are also indicated for nosocomial pneumonia, chronic bronchitis (acute exacerbations), and chronic otitis media.

The fluoroquinolones have indications for a variety of GI infections, including traveler's diarrhea due to *E. coli,* shigellosis, and typhoid fever. In the AIDS patient these drugs are effective in treating bacteremias and eradicating the carrier state due to nontyphoidal organisms. *Importantly, the fluoroquinolones are contraindicated in the treatment of enterohemorrhagic* E. coli *because they can induce the cytotoxic Shiga-like toxin.*

Primary cervicitis, urethritis, and extended infections, such as pelvic inflammatory disease due to the STD agents *N. gonorrhoeae* and *C. trachomatis,* are successfully treated with fluoroquinolones. Both ciprofloxacin and ofloxacin appear to be more effective than other fluoroquinolones, although resistance has been reported to be emerging. Because coinfections in patients treated with ciprofloxacin and ofloxacin are frequent, especially in women (≥50%), caution should be observed in using these agents if resistance becomes predominant in either infecting organism. Ciprofloxacin and ofloxacin are ineffective against *Treponema pallidum* but are active against the less common *Haemophilus ducreyi.*

The use of fluoroquinolones in bone and joint infections is influenced by the causative agent and the rate of resistance development. The use of the oral route for administration of the fluoroquinolones is especially advantageous in treating chronic infections that often require long-term therapy.

Adverse Effects and Drug Interactions

In general, the quinolones and fluoroquinolones are well tolerated. The most frequently reported side effects are associated with the GI tract (2–13%); these include nausea, vomiting, diarrhea, and abdominal pain. CNS effects (1–8%), such as drowsiness, weakness, headache, dizziness, and in severe cases, convulsions and toxic psychosis, have been reported. Some side effects, such as photosensitivity, correlate with specific chemical structures, including the halogen substitution on the eighth position, as found in sparfloxacin and lomefloxacin. Adverse cardiovascular effects (6–7%; vascular embolism, cardiac insufficiency, hypotension) also occur with sparfloxacin. Sparfloxacin, moxifloxacin, and gatifloxacin can exacerbate QT prolongations. Fulminant hepatotoxicity associated with trovafloxacin has resulted in acute liver failure, and the FDA has recommended limiting therapy to life-threatening infections.

The use of the quinolones in pregnant or breast-feeding women and children whose epiphysial plates have not closed is generally contraindicated. Their use for treating young cystic fibrosis children infected with *Pseudomonas* spp. is an exception; the patient should be monitored carefully for untoward effects.

All quinolones interact with multivalent cations, forming chelation complexes resulting in reduced absorption. Major offenders are antacids; vitamins containing calcium and iron can also be problematic. All fluoroquinolones interact with warfarin, didanosine (ddi), and phenytoin, resulting in decreased absorption or metabolism. Ciprofloxacin and other second-generation drugs interact with theophylline by decreasing its clearance, which leads to theophylline toxicity.

Allergic reactions (e.g., rashes, urticaria, and eosinophilia) have been observed. These drugs have occasionally been associated with cholestatic jaundice, blood dyscrasias, hemolytic anemia, hypoglycemia, and nephrotoxicity. Recently the use of ciprofloxacin for prophylaxis protection against anthrax infection has been associated with damage to muscle ligaments.

URINARY ANTISEPTICS

Urinary antiseptics are drugs that exert their antimicrobial effect in the urine and are devoid of virtually any significant systemic effect. Prolonged use for prophylaxis and/or suppression is common in recurrent or chronic UTIs where other antimicrobials can be used only for short durations because they do not sustain sterility.

Nitrofurans (Nitrofurantoin)
Chemistry and Mechanism of Action

A number of 5-nitro-2-furaldehyde derivatives, called *nitrofurans*, are used in the treatment and/or prophylaxis of microbial infections, primarily in the urinary tract. Recent evidence suggests that the reduction of the 5-nitro group to the nitro anion results in bacterial toxicity. Intermediate metabolites modify various bacterial macromolecules that affect a variety of biochemical processes (e.g., DNA and RNA synthesis, protein synthesis); this observation may explain the lack of resistance development to these drugs. Evidence also indicates that the nitro anion undergoes recycling with the production of superoxide and other toxic oxygen compounds. It is presumed that the nitrofurans are selectively toxic to microbial cells because in humans, the slower reduction by mammalian cells prevents high serum concentrations.

Antibacterial Spectrum and Resistance

Nitrofurantoin (*Furadantin, Macrodantin*) is primarily active against gram-negative bacteria (*E. coli, P. mirabilis* is variable) and some susceptible gram-positive organisms, such as *S. aureus* and *Enterococcus faecalis*. In vitro activity is demonstrated against *Staphylococcus saprophyticus* and *Staphylococcus epidermidis*, but it may not be helpful in predicting patient response; the same applies for certain species of *Klebsiella* and *Citrobacter*. Most *Proteus* (indole positive), *Serratia*, and *Pseudomonas* spp. are resistant. Development of resistant strains is virtually unknown, and cross-resistance with other antimicrobials has not been reported.

Absorption, Metabolism, and Excretion

Nitrofurantoin is administered orally and is rapidly and almost completely absorbed from the small intestine; only low levels of activity are achieved in serum because the drug is rapidly metabolized. Relatively high protein binding (about 70%) also affects serum levels, reducing potential for systemic toxicity and alteration of intestinal flora. Relative tissue penetration is much lower than other antimicrobials for UTIs, and therefore, nitrofurantoin is not indicated in the therapy of infections such as pyelonephritis and renal cortical or perinephric abscesses. Nitrofurantoin is rapidly excreted by glomerular filtration and tubular secretion to yield effective urinary levels. In moderate to severe renal dysfunction, toxic blood levels may occur while urinary levels may be inadequate. The drug is inactivated in the liver.

Nitrofurazone (*Furacin*) is used topically and is not readily absorbed from the skin.

Clinical Use

The singular indication for nitrofurantoin is the treatment and long-term prophylaxis of lower UTIs caused by susceptible bacteria; it is not used as a bacterial suppressant. It is often used prophylactically post intercourse in women with chronic UTIs. Although serum drug concentrations are low, concentrations (100–200 μg/mL) are found in urine that are well above the minimum inhibitory concentration for susceptible bacteria. The bacteriostatic or bactericidal activity of nitrofurantoin is concentration dependent; a urinary concentration greater than 100 μg/mL ensures bactericidal activity. Because nitrofurantoin lacks the broad tissue distribution of other antimicrobial agents, urine cultures should be obtained before and after therapy. Alkalinization of the urine increases urinary concentrations of the drug but decreases its antibacterial efficacy; acidifying agents, including cranberry juice, can be useful.

Nitrofurazone, a topical antibiotic, is occasionally used in the treatment of burns or skin grafts in which bacterial contamination may cause tissue rejection.

Adverse Effects and Drug Interactions

Nausea and vomiting are the most commonly observed adverse effects. Pulmonary hypersensitivity reactions can result in chronic morbidity, usually after therapy lasting at least 6 months. Findings can include *chronic desquamative interstitial pneumonia with fibrosis*. Resolution may not occur with discontinuation of therapy; fever is absent. Reactions may also be acute or subacute. Patients may present acutely with findings resembling acute respiratory distress syndrome. Infiltrates (especially at the base of the lung) and/or effusions may develop but are usually reversible when the drug is stopped; fever is a common finding. In contrast, resolution of pulmonary disease may require several months, especially in subacute reactions, with which fever is not frequent. These reaction types have all been reported as contributing factors in mortality. *When a patient taking nitrofurantoin develops pulmonary symptoms, a suspicion of drug-associated toxicity must be entertained.*

Intrahepatic cholestasis and hepatitis similar to that seen in chronic active hepatitis can rarely occur; fatalities have been reported. Nitrofurantoin can interfere with immature red blood cell enzyme systems found in babies less than 1 month of age and in nursing infants. This leads to cellular damage and anemia. Nitrofurantoin use is also contraindicated in pregnant women near term.

In vitro antagonism between nitrofurantoin and the quinolones has been shown, but a demonstration of clinical relevance warrants further study. Certain drugs used in treating gout, which inhibit tubular secretion, can affect UTI therapy by raising serum levels of nitrofurantoin with concomitant diminished urinary levels.

Nitrofurazone is a relatively safe topical agent. Skin sensitization has been reported.

Methenamine

Methenamine (hexamethylenetetramine) is an aromatic acid that is hydrolyzed at an acid pH (<6) to liberate ammonia and the active alkylating agent formaldehyde, which denatures protein and is bactericidal. Methenamine is usually administered as a salt of either mandelic (*Mandelamine*) or hippuric (*Hiprex, Urex*) acid. Not only do these acids acidify the urine, which is necessary to generate formaldehyde, but also, the resulting low urine pH is by itself bacteriostatic for some organisms.

Methenamine is administered orally and is well absorbed from the intestinal tract. However, 10 to 30% decomposes in the stomach unless the tablets are protected by an enteric coating. The inactive form (methenamine) is distributed to virtually every body fluid. Almost all of the methenamine moiety is excreted into the urine by 24 hours, having reached the urine by both glomerular filtration and tubular secretion.

Methenamine is primarily used for the long-term prophylactic or suppressive therapy of recurring UTIs. *It is not a primary drug for therapy of acute infections.* It should be used to maintain sterile urine after appropriate antimicrobial agents have been employed to eradicate the infection.

Gastric distress (nausea and vomiting) is one of the most frequently reported adverse reactions. Bladder irritation (e.g., dysuria, polyuria, hematuria, and urgency) may occur. The mandelic salt can crystallize in urine if there is inadequate urine flow and should not be given to patients with renal failure. Patients with preexisting hepatic insufficiency may develop acute hepatic failure due to the small quantities of ammonia formed during methenamine hydrolysis.

The coadministration of methenamine with certain sulfonamides (sulfamethizole or sulfathiazole) can form a urine precipitate resulting in drug antagonism.

Study QUESTIONS

1. A 24-year-old AIDS patient is interested in starting chemoprophylaxis for *Pneumocystis* pneumonia (PCP) and cerebral toxoplasmosis. He has no drug allergies. Which of the following prophylactic agents is appropriate for the prevention of both PCP and cerebral toxoplasmosis?
(A) Nitrofurantoin
(B) Trimethoprim–sulfamethoxazole
(C) Norfloxacin
(D) Methenamine
(E) Nalidixic acid

2. Urinalysis of a 38-year-old woman with recurrent UTIs revealed pH 6.8, 30 to 50 WBC per high-power field, and gram-negative bacilli identified as *Proteus mirabilis*. Which of the following produces a bacteriostatic urinary environment for *P. mirabilis*?
(A) Urease enzyme
(B) Hippuric acid
(C) Catalase enzyme
(D) Folic acid
(E) Coagulase enzyme

3. A 3-day-old baby is given a presumptive diagnosis of kernicterus. Which of the following mechanisms is involved in sulfonamide-induced kernicterus?
(A) Competes for the bilirubin-binding sites on plasma proteins
(B) Defective bilirubin hepatic conjugation and metabolism
(C) Physiological jaundice due to destruction of fetal red blood mass
(D) Pregnancy-induced hepatic congestion and cholestasis
(E) Primary biliary cirrhosis of the liver

4. A 6-year-old relatively healthy boy is diagnosed with external otitis and was prescribed a 7-day course of TMP-SMX. Which of the following is the basic mechanism of action of the sulfonamides?
(A) Selective inhibition of incorporation of PABA into human cell folic acid synthesis.
(B) Competitive inhibition of incorporation of PABA into microbial folic acid.
(C) Inhibition of transpeptidation reaction in bacterial cell wall synthesis.
(D) Changes in DNA gyrases and active efflux transport system resulting in decreased permeability of drug.
(E) Structural changes in dihydropteroate synthase and overproduction of PABA.

5. Evaluation of a yearly chest radiograph of a 73-year-old patient taking nitrofurantoin prophylactically for recurrent UTIs revealed new findings of bilateral interstitial fibrosis. What is the possible explanation for the patient's pulmonary presentation and what is the next step?
(A) Acute urosepsis; add a broad-spectrum antibiotic to nitrofurantoin.
(B) Possible allergic reaction to nitrofurantoin; stop it immediately.
(C) Nitrofurantoin-resistant *E. coli* infection; stop it immediately.
(D) Acute community-acquired streptococcal pneumonia; treat accordingly.
(E) Nitrofurantoin-induced hemolysis; requires permanent urinary catheter.

6. A 16-year-old girl, a cystic fibrosis patient, is diagnosed with a ciprofloxacin-resistant *Pseudomonas aeruginosa* lower respiratory tract infection. Bacteria acquire quinolone resistance by which of the following mechanisms?
(A) Overproduction of PABA
(B) Changes in the synthesis of DNA gyrases
(C) Plasmid-mediated changes in efflux transport system
(D) Inhibition of synthesis of peptidoglycan subunits in bacterial cell walls
(E) Inhibition of folic acid synthesis by blocking different steps

ANSWERS
1. **B.** Nitrofurantoin (A) is a urinary antiseptic agent active against many of the Enterobacteriaceae. Nitrofurantoin has no effect on *Toxoplasma* or *P. carinii*, as both are protozoans. TMP-SMX (B) daily or three times a week has proved to prevent both PCP and toxoplasmosis in AIDS patients. Norfloxacin (C) and other second-generation fluoroquinolones are known for their antipseudomonal and Enterobacteriaceae activity. The antimicrobial activity is exerted through inhibition of DNA *gyrase* A and type IV topoisomerase. Methenamine (D) is active against various Enterobacteriaceae; it has no activity against protozoa. Formaldehyde denatures proteins and is bactericidal. Nalidixic acid (E) is used in urinary tract infections caused by Enterobacteriaceae (e.g., *E. coli, Klebsiella,* and *Proteus*). It has no activity against protozoa.

2. **B.** Proteus species produce urease (A) that produces ammonia and urea, alkalizing urine. Urine requires acidification for effective therapy. Hippuric (B), mandelic, or ascorbic acids or methionine are urinary acidifying agents. The normal acidic urinary environment is disturbed by recurrent *Proteus* in-

fections. Catalase (C) is produced by staphylococcal spp. The catalase test differentiates Staphylococci from Streptococci. It has no urinary activity. Folic acid (D) is a water-soluble vitamin and has no effect on urinary pH or acidification. Humans cannot synthesize folic acid, which must be obtained from the diet. A coagulase enzyme (E) is produced by *Staphylococcus aureus*. Coagulase test differentiates *S. aureus* from other staphylococci .It has no urinary antimicrobial activity.

3. **A.** Sulfonamides (A) compete for bilirubin binding sites on plasma albumin and increase fetal blood levels of unconjugated bilirubin. Unbound bilirubin crosses the blood-brain barrier and can be deposited in the basal ganglia and subthalamic nuclei causing kernicterus, a toxic encephalopathy. Defective bilirubin hepatic conjugation (B) is due to glucuronyl transferase deficiency resulting in Gilbert's syndrome. When seen in adults it usually presents with jaundice that is precipitated by fasting. Physiological jaundice (C) usually occurs in the newborn within a week of birth. It is due to the immature fetal acetyltransferase system resulting in peripheral destruction of a large fetal red cell mass. Pregnancy-induced hepatic congestion (D), cholestasis, and acute cholecystitis are seen in pregnant women, not in the newborn. Primary biliary cirrhosis (E) is commonly seen in middle-aged women. It is a chronic progressive autoimmune disorder requiring steroids and sometimes liver transplant.

4. **B.** Humans cannot synthesize folic acid (A); diet is their main source. Sulfonamides selectively inhibit microbially synthesized folic acid. Incorporation (B) of PABA into microbial folic acid is competitively inhibited by sulfonamides. The TMP-SMX combination is synergistic because it acts at different steps in microbial folic acid synthesis. All sulfonamides are bacteriostatic. Inhibition of the transpeptidation reaction (C) involved in the synthesis of the bacterial cell wall is the basic mechanism of action of β-lactam antibiotics Changes in DNA gyrases (D) and active efflux transport system are mechanisms for resistance to quinolones. Structural changes (E) in dihydropteroate synthetase and overproduction of PABA are mechanisms of resistance to the sulfonamides.

5. **B.** Acute urosepsis (A) is possible, but the patient's physical examination produced benign findings. Adding a broad-spectrum antibiotic has no benefit without evidence of active disease. Possible allergic reaction (B) to nitrofurantoin; it is appropriate to stop the drug immediately to guard against one of three potential pulmonary reactions: (1) acute pres-

entation with basilar infiltrate and pleural effusion, (2) chronic progressive bilateral interstitial fibrosis; (3) a subacute presentation. Nitrofurantoin-resistant *E. coli* infection (C) and urosepsis are possible in patients who are taking chronic prophylaxis, but his examination produced benign findings. Acute community-acquired streptococcal pneumonia (D) shows one or more lobar infiltrates on radiography. The patient described has bilateral interstitial fibrosis. Nitrofurantoin-induced hemolysis (E) is possible in G6PD patients, but physical examination produced benign findings; G6PD patients usually present with hematuria.

6. **B.** Overproduction (A) of PABA is one of the resistance mechanisms of sulfonamides. Changes in the synthesis of DNA gyrases (B) is a well-described mechanism for quinolone resistance. Plasmid-mediated resistance (C) does not occur with quinolones. An active efflux system for transport of drug out of the cell has been described for quinolone resistance, but it is not plasmid mediated. Inhibition of structural blocks (D) in bacterial cell wall synthesis is a basic mechanism of action of β-lactam antibiotics. Inhibition of folic acid synthesis (E) by blocking different steps is the basic mechanism of action of sulfonamides.

SUPPLEMENTAL READING

Guay DR. An update on the role of nitrofurans in the management of urinary tract infections. [Review]. Drugs 2001;61:353–364.

Hooper DC. New uses for new and old fluoroquinolones and the challenge of resistance. Infect Dis 2000;30:243–254.

Hooper DC. Urinary tract agents: Nitrofurantoin and methenamine. In Mandell GL, Dolin R, and Bennet JE (Eds.). Mandell, Douglas, and Bennett's Principles and Practice of Infectious Diseases, 5th ed. New York: Churchill Livingstone, 2000.

Lipsky BA and Baker CA. Fluoroquinolone toxicity profiles: A review focusing on newer agents. Clin Infect Dis 1999;28:352–364.

Martin JN et al. Emergence of trimethoprim-sulfamethoxazole resistance in the AIDS era. J Infect Dis 1999;180:1809–1818.

Smith JM, Curi AL, and Pavesio CE. Crystalluria with sulphadiazine. Br J Ophthalmol 2001;85:1265–1269.

Walker RC. The fluoroquinolones. Mayo Clin Proc 1999;74:1030–1037.

Wright SW, Wrenn KD, and Haynes ML. Trimethoprim-sulfamethoxazole resistance among urinary coliform isolates. J Gen Intern Med 1999;14: 606–609.

A 62-year-old man with a history of benign hypertrophic prostate (BPH) has deep pelvic pain and a low-grade fever. He has a history of chronic bilateral osteoarthritis of the knees and was recently diagnosed with diet-controllable diabetes mellitus. The patient denies any drug allergy but is an active smoker and drinks three or four cans of beers daily.

Physical examination: elderly man is not in acute distress. His oral temperature is 37.7°C (100.1°F); blood pressure is 110/70 and heart rate is 90/minute. His prostate gland was enlarged and very tender, consistent with acute prostatitis. His routine blood work and liver function test findings were within normal limits. A urine sample was sent for analysis and cultures; ciprofloxacin 750 mg twice a day was started.

About a week later, the patient was admitted to the hospital with acute onset of confusion and possible seizurelike activity. His wife states that he is compliant with medications and even felt well after initiation of antibiotics. Possible ciprofloxacin-induced acute CNS toxicity or drug interaction was suspected, and all his medications were discontinued. Which of the following is the possible explanation for the patient's acute onset of CNS toxicity?

(A) Ciprofloxacin can displace GABA from its receptors resulting in neuroexcitation.
(B) Acute alcohol withdrawal was precipitated by ciprofloxacin due to an alcohol-drug interaction.
(C) He has fulminant gram-negative urosepsis with possible ciprofloxacin-resistant bacteria.
(D) He has cumulative CNS toxicity of ciprofloxacin secondary to poor urinary and prostatic tissue penetration.
(E) He has delayed stomach absorption and metabolism of the drug secondary to diabetic gastroparesis.

ANSWER: A. Ciprofloxacin can significantly interfere with the normal physiology of GABA. Displacement of GABA from its receptors by ciprofloxacin results in increased levels of the neuroexcitatory transmitter and acute CNS toxicity. The neuroexcitation can range from irritability, confusion, and agitation to seizures and toxic psychosis. Ciprofloxacin has no interaction with alcohol. A disulfiramlike reaction (flushing, nausea, vomiting, and profuse sweating) is associated with alcohol and metronidazole. Avoid alcohol and metronidazole coadministration.

Cumulative CNS toxicity secondary to poor tissue concentration is incorrect. In fact, high tissue concentrations are achieved with oral ciprofloxacin, especially in the prostate and urinary tract. For this reason, it is widely used for prostatitis and UTIs. Diabetic gastroparesis is seen in long-standing severe diabetes. Drug absorption problems are seen in these patients secondary to delayed gastric emptying and frequent vomiting. The patient described has newly diagnosed diet-controlled diabetes mellitus, so this does not explain his symptoms.

45

β-Lactam Antibiotics

James F. Graumlich

 DRUG LIST

INTRODUCTION

A number of antibiotics produced by fungi of the genus *Cephalosporium* have been identified. These antibiotics called cephalosporins contain, in common with the penicillins, a β-lactam ring. In addition to the numerous penicillins and cephalosporins in use, three other classes of β-lactam antibiotics are available for clinical use. These are the carbapenems, the carbacephems, and the monobactams. All β-lactam antibiotics have the same bactericidal mechanism of action. They block a critical step in bacterial cell wall synthesis.

MECHANISM OF ACTION

The final reaction in bacterial cell wall synthesis is a cross-linking of adjacent peptidoglycan (murein) strands by a transpeptidation reaction. In this reaction, bacterial transpeptidases cleave the terminal D-alanine from a pentapeptide on one peptidoglycan strand and then cross-link it with the pentapeptide of another peptidoglycan strand. The cross-linked peptidoglycan (murein) strands give structural integrity to cell walls and permit bacteria to survive environments that do not match the organism's internal osmotic pressure.

The β-lactam antibiotics structurally resemble the terminal D-alanyl-D-alanine (D-Ala-D-Ala) in the pentapeptides on peptidoglycan (murein) (Fig. 45.1). Bacterial transpeptidases covalently bind the β-lactam antibiotics at the enzyme active site, and the resultant acyl enzyme molecule is stable and inactive. The intact β-lactam ring is required for antibiotic action. The β-lactam ring modifies the active serine site on transpeptidases and blocks further enzyme function.

In addition to transpeptidases, other penicillin-binding proteins (PBPs) function as transglycosylases and carboxypeptidases. All of the PBPs are involved with assembly, maintenance, or regulation of peptidoglycan cell wall synthesis. When β-lactam antibiotics inactivate PBPs, the consequence to the bacterium is a structurally weakened cell wall, aberrant morphological form, cell lysis, and death.

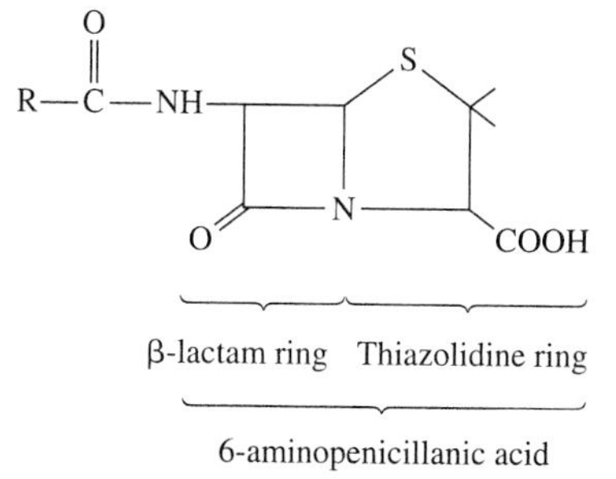

β-lactam ring   Thiazolidine ring

6-aminopenicillanic acid

FIGURE 45.1
The structure of penicillins.

MECHANISMS OF RESISTANCE

A number of microorganisms have evolved mechanisms to overcome the inhibitory actions of the β-lactam antibiotics. There are four major mechanisms of resistance: inactivation of the β-lactam ring, alteration of PBPs, reduction of antibiotic access to PBPs, and elaboration of antibiotic efflux mechanisms. Bacterial resistance may arise from one or more than one of these mechanisms.

The most important mechanism of resistance is hydrolysis of the β-lactam ring by β-lactamases (penicillinases and cephalosporinases). Many bacteria (*Staphylococcus aureus*, *Moraxella* [*Branhamella*] *catarrhalis*, *Neisseria gonorrhoeae*, Enterobacteriaceae, *Haemophilus influenzae*, and *Bacteroides* spp.) possess β-lactamases that hydrolyze penicillins and cephalosporins. The β-lactamases evolved from PBPs and acquired the capacity to bind β-lactam antibiotics, form an acyl enzyme molecule, then deacylate and hydrolyze the β-lactam ring. Some bacteria have chromosomal (inducible) genes for β-lactamases. Other bacteria acquire β-lactamase genes via plasmids or transposons. Transfer of β-lactamase genes between bacterial species has contributed to the proliferation of resistant organisms resulting in the appearance of clinically important adverse consequences.

Efforts to overcome the actions of the β-lactamases have led to the development of such β-lactamase inhibitors as clavulanic acid, sulbactam, and tazobactam. They are called suicide inhibitors because they permanently bind when they inactivate β-lactamases. Among the β-lactamase inhibitors, only clavulanic acid is available for oral use. Chemical inhibition of β-lactamases, however, is not a permanent solution to antibiotic resistance, since some β-lactamases are resistant to clavulanic acid, tazobactam, or sulbactam. Enzymes resistant to clavulanic acid include the cephalosporinases produced by *Citrobacter* spp., *Enterobacter* spp., and *Pseudomonas aeruginosa*.

An additional mechanism of antibiotic resistance involves an alteration of PBPs. Resistant bacteria, usually gram-positive organisms, produce PBPs with low affinity for β-lactam antibiotics. The development of mutations of bacterial PBPs is involved in the mechanism for β-lactam resistance in *Streptococcus pneumoniae*, *Enterococcus faecium*, and methicillin-resistant *S. aureus* (MRSA).

Some gram-negative bacteria employ a third mechanism of resistance, namely, one that reduces antibiotic access to PBPs. Gram-positive organisms have an exposed peptidoglycan layer easily accessible to β-lactam antibiotics (Fig. 45.2). In contrast, gram-negative organisms have an outer membrane surrounding the peptidoglycan layer. The gram-negative outer membrane hinders ingress of large molecules and helps bacteria resist the actions of antibiotics. In susceptible gram-negative

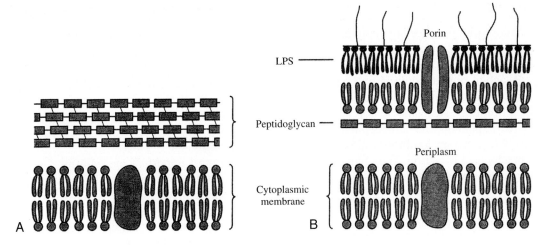

FIGURE 45.2

Differences between gram-positive and gram-negative bacteria that affect antibiotic access. **A.** The cell wall structure of a gram-positive organism. The exposed porous peptidoglycan (murein) layer allows easy antibiotic access. **B.** The cell wall structure of a gram-negative organism. The outer membrane contains lipopolysaccharides (LPS) and porins with narrow, restrictive channels that function as barriers to antibiotic permeability. (Modified with permission from Nikaido H. Prevention of drug access to bacterial targets: Permeability barriers and active efflux. Science 1994;264:382–388.)

bacteria, protein channels (porins) allow β-lactam antibiotics to traverse the outer membrane and interact with PBPs in the periplasmic space. In resistant bacteria like *P. aeruginosa*, porin mutants impede the β-lactam transfer across the outer membrane.

Finally, some gram-negative organisms demonstrate a fourth mechanism of resistance. For example, strains of *P. aeruginosa* produce xenobiotic efflux pumps to eject antibiotics. Drug efflux mechanisms are associated with multiple drug resistance, including resistance to β-lactam antibiotics.

Widespread use of β-lactam antibiotics exerts selective pressure on bacteria and permits the proliferation of resistant organisms. A comparison of current antibiograms with those from previous decades shows an alarming increase in bacterial resistance to β-lactam antibiotics.

PENICILLINS

The penicillins are a large group of bactericidal compounds. They can be subdivided and classified by their chemical structure and spectrum of activity. The structure common to all penicillins is a β-lactam ring fused with a thiazolidine nucleus (Fig. 45.1). The antimicrobial activity of penicillin resides in the β-lactam ring. Splitting of the β-lactam ring by either acid hydrolysis or β-lactamases results in the formation of penicilloic acid, a product without antibiotic activity. Addition of various side chains (R) to the basic penicillin molecule

creates classes of compounds with the same mechanism of action as penicillin but with different chemical and biological properties. For example, some analogues are resistant to hydrolysis by acid or β-lactamase; some have an extended the spectrum of antibacterial activity; and others show improved absorption from the intestinal tract.

Penicillins may be classified into four groups: natural penicillins (G and V), antistaphylococcal (penicillinase-resistant) penicillins, aminopenicillins, and antipseudomonal penicillins. Natural penicillins have therapeutic effects limited to streptococci and a few gram-negative organisms. The antistaphylococcal (penicillinase-resistant) penicillins treat infections caused by streptococci and staphylococci but do not affect MRSA. The aminopenicillins are effective against streptococci, enterococci, and some gram-negative organisms but have variable activity against staphylococci and are ineffective against *P. aeruginosa*. The antipseudomonal penicillins retain activity against streptococci and possess additional effects against gram-negative organisms, including various Enterobacteriaceae and *Pseudomonas*.

Natural Penicillins

Penicillin G (benzylpenicillin) is an acid-labile compound having variable bioavailability after oral administration. Consequently, penicillin G is most appropriate for intramuscular or intravenous therapy. The drug distributes to most tissues and serosa-lined cavities, although low concentrations appear in breast milk and cerebrospinal fluid. When the meninges are inflamed, cerebrospinal fluid concentrations of penicillin G approximate 5% of the serum concentration. In inflamed joints, concentrations of the drug approach serum levels.

Penicillin G is excreted by the kidneys, with 90% of renal elimination occurring via tubular secretion and 10% by glomerular filtration. Probenecid blocks tubular secretion and has been used to increase the serum concentration and prolong the half-life of penicillin G and other penicillins. Additional pharmacokinetic information can be found in Table 45.1.

The clinical uses of penicillin G include endocarditis caused by *S. viridans* (or *Streptococcus bovis*), pharyngitis (group A β-hemolytic streptococci), cat bite cellulitis (*Pasteurella multocida*), and syphilis (*Treponema pallidum*).

Depot intramuscular formulations of penicillin G, including procaine penicillin and benzathine penicillin, have decreased solubility, delayed absorption, and a prolonged half-life. Drug concentrations are detectable 24 hours after injection of procaine penicillin, and low levels of benzathine penicillin (0.003 units/mL) are detectable 4 weeks after injection.

When prescribing one of the penicillin G depot formulations, practitioners must individualize treatment to clinical and microbial conditions. Some long-acting formulations may not maintain adequate plasma and tissue concentrations to treat specific organisms or infections. For acute streptococcal meningitis, the goal is rapid achievement of high antibiotic concentrations in the cerebrospinal fluid. Consequently, depot formulations are inappropriate for meningitis. Intravenous penicillin G is among the antibiotics of first choice for therapy of meningitis caused by susceptible *S. pneumoniae*. In contrast, a depot formulation of benzathine penicillin G suffices for rheumatic fever prophylaxis.

Penicillin V is an orally administered phenoxymethyl congener of penicillin G having an antibacterial spectrum of activity that is similar to that of penicillin G. Penicillin V is used to treat streptococcal infections when oral therapy is appropriate and desirable.

Antistaphylococcal (penicillinase-resistant) Penicillins

Nafcillin, oxacillin, cloxacillin, and dicloxacillin are more resistant to bacterial β-lactamases than is penicillin G. Consequently, these antibiotics are effective against streptococci and most community-acquired penicillinase-producing staphylococci. Methicillin, which is no longer marketed in the United States, is another penicillinase-resistant antibiotic similar to nafcillin and oxacillin. For historical reasons, staphylococci resistant to oxacillin or nafcillin are labeled methicillin resistant. Many hospitals are reservoirs for MRSA and methicillin-resistant *Staphylococcus epidermidis* (MRSE). These nosocomial pathogens are resistant in vitro to all β-lactam antibiotics.

TABLE 45.1 **Pharmacokinetic Parameters of Selected Penicillins**

Drug	Route	Half-life (hr)	Renal Excretion (%)	Dose Adjustment in Renal Failure
Natural penicillins				
Penicillin G	IM, IV	0.5	79–85	Yes
Penicillin V	Oral	0.5	20–40	Yes
Antistaphylococcal penicillins (penicillinase resistant)				
Nafcillin	IM, IV	0.8–1.2	31–38	No
Oxacillin	IM, IV	0.4–0.7	39–66	No
Cloxacillin	Oral	0.5–0.6	40–70	No
Dicloxacillin	Oral	0.6–0.8	35–90	No
Aminopenicillins				
Ampicillin	Oral, IM, IV	1.1–1.5	40–92	Yes
Amoxicillin	Oral	1.4–2.0	86	Yes
Antipseudomonal penicillins				
Carbenicillin	Oral	0.8–1.2	85	Yes
Mezlocillin	IM, IV	0.9–1.7	61–69	Yes
Piperacillin	IM, IV	0.8–1.1	74–89	Yes
Ticarcillin	IM, IV	1.0–1.4	95	Yes

IM, intramuscular; IV, intravenous.

For parenteral therapy, nafcillin and oxacillin offer comparable efficacy and antimicrobial spectra of activity. Although both drugs undergo hepatic metabolism, only nafcillin requires dose adjustment in patients with combined hepatic and renal insufficiency. Other pharmacokinetic data for nafcillin and oxacillin appear in Table 45.1. Indications for nafcillin or oxacillin include severe staphylococcal infections like cellulitis, empyema, endocarditis, osteomyelitis, pneumonia, septic arthritis, and toxic shock syndrome.

For oral therapy, cloxacillin and dicloxacillin are comparable alternatives. Both undergo hepatic metabolism, and neither drug requires dose adjustment in patients with hepatic insufficiency. Additional pharmacokinetic data are in Table 45.1. Indications for cloxacillin or dicloxacillin include clinically mild staphylococcal infections like impetigo.

Aminopenicillins

The pharmacokinetics of ampicillin and amoxicillin are similar (Table 45.1). Both have good oral bioavailability; ampicillin is also bioavailable after intramuscular injection. Concomitant ingestion of food decreases the bioavailability of ampicillin but not amoxicillin. Consequently, oral doses of ampicillin should be given on an empty stomach. Ampicillin achieves therapeutic concentrations in the cerebrospinal fluid only during inflammation. Therefore, ampicillin is effective treatment for meningitis caused by *Listeria monocytogenes*. Amoxicillin does not reach adequate concentrations in the central nervous system and is not appropriate for meningitis therapy. Other indications for ampicillin include serious infections like enterococcal endocarditis and pneumonia caused by β-lactamase-negative *H. influenzae*. Amoxicillin oral therapy is appropriate for clinically acute nonserious bacterial infections like otitis media and sinusitis. Amoxicillin also has use in multidrug regimens for the eradication of *Helicobacter pylori* in duodenal and gastric ulcers.

Antipseudomonal Penicillins

Mezlocillin, piperacillin, and ticarcillin are parenteral antibiotics formulated as sodium salts, so prescribers must consider the sodium content of these antibiotics when administering them to patients with congestive heart failure. During their distribution phase, antipseudomonal penicillins achieve only low concentrations in the cerebrospinal fluid. Consequently, antipseudomonal penicillins are not among the drugs of first choice for meningitis therapy.

The antipseudomonal penicillins undergo renal elimination (Table 45.1). Piperacillin and ticarcillin have minimal hepatic metabolism. In contrast, mezlocillin has significant hepatic metabolism and requires dose adjustment in patients with hepatic insufficiency.

The antipseudomonal penicillins have comparable spectra of activity against many gram-positive and gram-negative pathogens, including most anaerobes. Mezlocillin, piperacillin, and ticarcillin have similar clinical outcomes in patients with known or suspected *P. aeruginosa* infections. Antipseudomonal penicillins are used to treat pneumonias associated with cystic fibrosis or mechanical ventilation.

Carbenicillin indanyl sodium is an antipseudomonal penicillin formulated for oral administration. The drug achieves negligible carbenicillin concentrations in the urine of patients with renal failure. Consequently, carbenicillin is not appropriate for patients with renal failure. In patients with normal renal function, however, carbenicillin indanyl sodium is used to treat urinary tract infections caused by *P. aeruginosa, Proteus* spp., and *Escherichia coli*.

β-Lactamase Inhibitor Combinations

Several formulations combine a β-lactam antibiotic with a β-lactamase inhibitor (ampicillin-sulbactam [*Unasyn*], ticarcillin-clavulanic acid [*Timentin*], piperacillin-tazobactam [*Zosyn*], and amoxicillin–clavulanic acid [*Augmentin*]). All of the β-lactamase inhibitor combinations except amoxicillin-clavulanic acid are parenteral formulations. Amoxicillin–clavulanic acid is the only combination drug with oral bioavailability. Elimination of the combination drugs occurs primarily by renal excretion. Therefore, all of the β-lactamase inhibitor combinations require dose adjustments in patients with renal insufficiency. The addition of the β-lactamase inhibitor significantly broadens the spectrum of antibacterial activity against β-lactamase-producing organisms. Consequently, these drugs have clinical use in treating infections with known or suspected mixed bacterial flora, such as biliary infections, diabetic foot ulcers, endomyometritis, and peritonitis.

β-Lactam Antibiotics in Pregnancy

All of the penicillin antibiotics are classified by the U.S. Food and Drug Administration (FDA) in pregnancy category B, that is, as drugs having either no fetal risk in animal studies but human trials are inadequate, or animal studies show adverse fetal effects but well-controlled human trials reveal no fetal damage. Obstetricians frequently prescribe ampicillin, penicillin G, and penicillin V because they are effective against the infections most frequently encountered in caring for pregnant women (e.g., upper respiratory and lower urinary tract infections).

Adverse Effects

While being associated with a low percentage of adverse reactions, the β-lactams are the most frequent source of troublesome allergic reactions among the antibiotics. The overall frequency of adverse effects associated with penicillin use is less than 10%, including allergic and other reactions. Anaphylaxis is a serious, rare allergic response with an occurrence rate between 0.004% and 0.015% of penicillin courses. Allergic reactions to penicillin are immediate immunoglobulin (Ig) E–mediated type I immune responses. Symptoms and signs of IgE-mediated reactions may include urticaria, pruritus, bronchospasm, angioedema, laryngeal edema, and hypotension. Late onset immune-mediated reactions to β-lactam antibiotics may manifest as eosinophilia, hemolytic anemia, interstitial nephritis, or serum sickness. In contrast to the rare allergic reactions, nonallergic β-lactam rashes are common. For example, ampicillin is associated with nonurticarial rashes in 5 to 10% of recipients.

The incidence of nonallergic ampicillin eruptions is 40 to 100% in patients with concomitant Epstein-Barr virus (mononucleosis), cytomegalovirus, acute lymphocytic leukemia, lymphoma, or reticulosarcoma. Nonallergic penicillin-associated rashes are characteristically morbilliform (symmetrical, erythematous, confluent, maculopapular) eruptions on the extremities. The onset of typical nonallergic eruptions is more than 72 hours after β-lactam exposure. The mechanism for the nonurticarial ampicillin rash is not known and is not related to IgE or type I hypersensitivity. Penicillin skin tests are not useful in the evaluation of nonurticarial ampicillin rashes. Patients with a history of nonurticarial ampicillin rashes may receive other β-lactam antibiotics without greater risk of subsequent serious allergic reactions.

Allergic cross-reactivity between β-lactam antibiotics is significant. The frequency of allergic reactions to another β-lactam antibiotic is 5.6% among patients with a history of IgE-mediated hypersensitivity to one β-lactam antibiotic plus positive results from a penicillin skin test. In general, patients with a convincing history of type I reaction to one β-lactam antibiotic should avoid all other β-lactam antibiotics except aztreonam. However, most patients give unreliable histories of penicillin allergy because of confusion with nonallergic penicillin rashes. Among patients who report penicillin allergies, 80 to 90% have negative results from penicillin skin tests, and 98% tolerate subsequent β-lactam antibiotic treatments. A careful history may discriminate between nonallergic reactions and true penicillin allergy and permit safe β-lactam therapy.

CEPHALOSPORINS

The cephalosporins are semisynthetic antibiotics derived from products of various microorganisms, including *Cephalosporium* and *Streptomyces*. All cephalosporins have a 7-aminocephalosporanic acid composed of a dihydrothiazine ring fused to a β-lactam ring (Fig. 45.3). As with the penicillins, the cephalosporin β-lactam ring is the chemical group associated with antibacterial activity. The different pharmacological, pharmacokinetic, and antibacterial properties of individual cephalosporins result from substitution of various groups on the basic molecule. Cephalosporins also vary in acid stability and β-lactamase susceptibility. Table 45.2 shows the large number of available cephalosporins.

The β-lactamases (penicillinases) inactivate some cephalosporins but are much less efficient than are the cephalosporinases (β-lactamases specific for the cephalosporins). Resistance to cephalosporins also results from modification of microbial PBPs.

Antibacterial Spectrum

The cephalosporins are classified into generations (Table 45.2) according to their antibacterial spectrum and stability to β-lactamases. The first-generation cephalosporins have in vitro antimicrobial activity against streptococci, methicillin-sensitive *S. aureus*, and a few gram-negative bacilli. The second-generation cephalosporins have greater stability against β-lactamase inactivation and possess a broader spectrum of activity to include gram-positive cocci, gram-negative organisms, and anaerobes. Among the second-generation cephalosporins, the cephamycins (cefoxitin [Mefoxin], cefotetan [Cefotan], and cefmetazole [Zefazone]) have the most activity against *Bacteroides fragilis*. The extended-spectrum, or third-generation, cephalosporins possess a high degree of in vitro potency and β-lactamase stability and a broader spectrum of action against many common gram-negative bacteria and anaerobes while retaining good activity against streptococci. Third-generation cephalosporins are less active against staphylococci than the earlier generations. The agents with the greatest activity against *P. aeruginosa* are cefepime, cefoperazone, and ceftazidime. Cefepime has been called a fourth-generation cephalosporin because of its great in vitro activity against several gram-positive and gram-negative organisms. The distinction between third and fourth

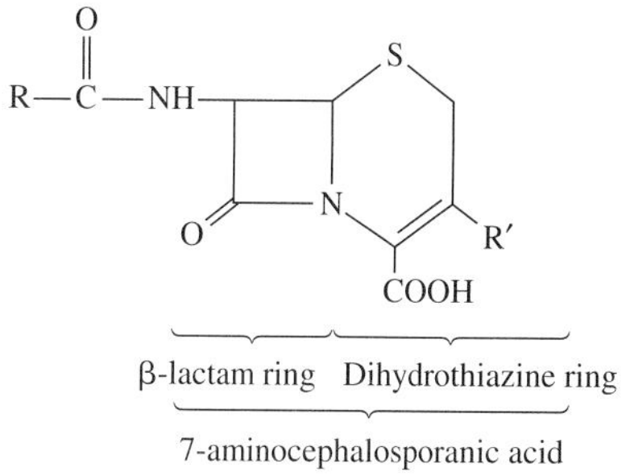

FIGURE 45.3
The structure of cephalosporins.

TABLE 45.2 Pharmacokinetic Parameters of Selected Cephalosporins

Drug	Route	Half-life (hr)	Renal Excretion (%)	Dose Adjustment in Renal Failure
First generation				
Cefadroxil	Oral	1.2–2.5	70–90	Yes
Cefazolin	IM, IV	1.5–2.5	70–95	Yes
Cephalexin	Oral	1.0	95	Yes
Cephapirin	IM, IV	0.6	50–70	Yes
Cephradine	Oral	0.7	75–100	Yes
Second generation				
Cefaclor	Oral	0.6–0.9	60–85	Yes
Cefamandole	IM, IV	0.5–1.2	100	Yes
Cefmetazole	IV	1.2–1.5	85	Yes
Cefonicid	IM, IV	3.5–4.5	95–99	Yes
Cefotetan	IM, IV	2.8–4.6	60–91	Yes
Cefoxitin	IM, IV	0.7–1.0	85	Yes
Cefprozil	Oral	1.2–1.4	64	Yes
Cefuroxime	IM, IV	1.1–1.3	95	Yes
Cefuroxime axetil	Oral	1.1–1.3	52	Yes
Loracarbef[a]	Oral	1.0	87–97	Yes
Third generation				
Cefdinir	Oral	1.7	18	Yes
Cefepime	IM, IV	2.0	70–99	Yes
Cefixime	Oral	2.3–3.7	50	Yes
Cefoperazone	IM, IV	2.0	20–30	No
Cefotaxime	IM, IV	1.0	40–60	Yes
Cefpodoxime proxetil	Oral	1.9–3.7	40	Yes
Ceftazidime	IM, IV	1.9	80–90	Yes
Ceftibuten	Oral	1.5–2.8	57–75	Yes
Ceftizoxime	IM, IV	1.4–1.8	57–100	Yes
Ceftriaxone	IM, IV	5.8–8.7	33–67	No
Carbapenems				
Imipenem-cilastatin	IM, IV	1.0	50–70	Yes
Meropenem	IV	1.0	79	Yes
Monobactam				
Aztreonam	IM, IV	2.0	75	Yes

[a]Loracarbef is in the carbacephem class. IM, intramuscular; IV, intravenous.

generation may be irrelevant, however, since clinical outcomes are similar in human trials comparing cefepime and other third-generation cephalosporins. None of the cephalosporins adequately treats infections caused by *Enterococcus faecalis, E. faecium,* MRSA, or *L. monocytogenes.*

Absorption, Distribution, Metabolism, and Excretion

Most parenteral cephalosporins have good bioavailability after intramuscular injection, and a few members of each cephalosporin generation have good oral bioavailability (Table 45.2). The ester prodrugs cefuroxime axetil (*Ceftin*) and cefpodoxime proxetil (*Vantin*) are oral formulations in which the ester is hydrolyzed during drug passage through the intestinal mucosa; the free cephalosporin enters the systemic circulation. Concomitant ingestion of food reduces the bioavailability of some cephalosporins, e.g., cefaclor (*Ceclor*), and therefore, these compounds should be administered on an empty stomach.

The cephalosporins distribute in satisfactory concentrations to most tissues except the central nervous system. Only cefepime, cefuroxime (*Zinacef*), cefotaxime (*Claforan*), ceftriaxone (*Rocephin*), and ceftazidime (*Fortaz*) achieve therapeutic concentrations in cerebrospinal fluid. Cefotaxime and ceftriaxone are antibiotics of first choice for the empirical treatment of brain abscess and meningitis.

There is considerable variation in the protein binding among the cephalosporins. Drugs like ceftriaxone that have extensive protein binding (85–95%) may displace bilirubin from serum albumin. Consequently, ceftriaxone may increase the risk of kernicterus in jaundiced neonates.

Urinary excretion is the major elimination path for most cephalosporins. When prescribing cephalosporins to patients with renal failure, practitioners must consider dose reduction or dose interval extension (Table 45.2). Renal tubular secretion contributes to the elimination of some cephalosporins, and an increase in cephalosporin plasma concentrations may occur when probenecid blocks renal tubular secretion of cephalosporins. Biliary elimination is important for some cephalosporins. Cefmetazole, cefoperazone (*Cefobid*), cefoxitin, and ceftriaxone achieve biliary concentrations greater than those in plasma. After parenteral administration of cefoperazone, 70% of the dose appears in the bile within 24 hours. Practitioners should decrease the dose of cefoperazone when prescribing for patients with hepatic failure or biliary obstruction. Metabolism is not a major elimination path for most cephalosporins. Cefotaxime is one of the few cephalosporins having an active metabolite, desacetyl cefotaxime.

Clinical Uses

The first-generation cephalosporins have activity against most of the bacterial pathogens that colonize skin and infect wounds. Consequently, first-generation cephalosporins are useful in antimicrobial prophylaxis before surgery. Second-generation cephalosporins are used to treat infections caused by susceptible organisms. For example, cefoxitin and cefotetan have good anaerobic activity, and they have utility in the treatment and prophylaxis of lower abdominal and gynecological infection. A broad spectrum of antibacterial activity makes third-generation cephalosporins important in the treatment of a wide range of infections, including Lyme disease, pneumonia, peritonitis, and sepsis syndrome.

Adverse Effects

The cephalosporins have good safety profiles. The overall incidence of adverse events attributed to cephalosporins is between 1 and 10%. The most common adverse drug reactions are rashes (1–5%), eosinophilia (3–10%), gastrointestinal symptoms (3%), hematological abnormalities (1–2%), phlebitis (2%), and fever (<1%). Anaphylactic reactions to cephalosporins are rare (<0.02%).

Because of cross-reactions between cephalosporins and penicillins, caution should be used when prescribing cephalosporins to patients with penicillin allergy. If a patient had anaphylaxis, angioedema, or urticaria following penicillin use, cephalosporins should be avoided. Among patients with morbilliform rashes (resembling measles) after penicillin, the majority (95%) will tolerate cephalosporins without adverse effects and with no increased risk of anaphylaxis. When evaluating patients with histories of allergic penicillin reactions, practitioners may order penicillin skin tests to screen potential cephalosporin recipients. The frequency of allergic reactions to cephalosporins is 1.7% in patients with histories of type I penicillin reactions and negative penicillin skin tests. Most patients with negative penicillin skin tests may receive cephalosporins safely.

The cephalosporins are valuable because of their broad spectrum of antimicrobial activity. However, their bactericidal action alters gut flora and selects for overgrowth of resistant organisms. Cephalosporins have been associated with superinfections with *Clostridium difficile*, enterococci, MRSA, coagulase-negative staphylococci, *P. aeruginosa*, and *Candida albicans*. Overgrowth by toxigenic *C. difficile* occasionally causes pseudomembranous colitis in patients treated with cephalosporins. Some third-generation cephalosporins induce production of extended-spectrum β-lactamases (ESBLs) in *P. aeruginosa*. The ESBLs can transfer to various Enterobacteriaceae and produce organisms resistant to almost all β-lactam antibiotics.

Bleeding is an uncommon but serious side effect of some cephalosporins. The *N*-methylthiotetrazole (MTT) side chain on the R′ substituent inhibits production of active vitamin K. Cephalosporins with the MTT side chain (cefamandole, cefmetazole, cefoperazone, cefotetan) are associated with hypoprothrombinemia, coagulation abnormalities, and bleeding. In addition, the MTT cephalosporins increase the effect of oral anticoagulants. Bleeding or coagulation abnormalities caused by MTT cephalosporins can be treated or prevented with supplemental vitamin K. Additional bleeding problems may result from antiplatelet effects. The MTT side chain confers a structure and activity similar to that of disulfiram, so patients taking MTT cephalosporins who also ingest alcohol may develop symptoms similar to the disulfiram reaction.

Children and adults receiving high doses of ceftriaxone may develop gallbladder sludge (pseudolithiasis). While most patients with sludge have no symptoms, occasionally the sludge identified by abdominal ultrasonography has led to laparotomy. Biliary sludge usually disappears after discontinuation of ceftriaxone.

CARBAPENEMS AND CARBACEPHEMS

The newest classes of β-lactam antibiotics are the carbapenems and carbacephems. Their mechanism of action is the same as those of the other β-lactam antibiotics.

Imipenem

The first carbapenem, imipenem–cilastatin (Primaxin), is a chemically stable analogue of thienamycin produced by *Streptomyces cattleya*. The antibacterial spectrum of imipenem is among the broadest of all of the β-lactam antibiotics. Imipenem is active against most gram-positive, gram-negative, and anaerobic bacteria. When compared with the in vitro activities of third-generation cephalosporins, imipenem is more potent against *E. faecalis, B. fragilis,* and *P. aeruginosa*. Imipenem's stability against β-lactamases is attributable to the trans position of the 6-hydroxyethyl side chain on the β-lactam ring. Organisms resistant to imipenem include *E. faecium, Stenotrophomonas maltophilia,* and MRSA.

Imipenem–cilastatin is only available for intramuscular or intravenous administration because oral bioavailability is poor. The enzyme, dehydropeptidase I, present in renal tubules, converts imipenem to an inactive metabolite. To decrease metabolic clearance, imipenem is combined with cilastatin, an inhibitor of dehydropeptidase I. Additional pharmacokinetic information appears in Table 45.2.

Imipenem–cilastatin is one of the drugs of first choice for the empirical therapy of many polymicrobial pulmonary, intraabdominal, and soft tissue infections. The notable adverse effect of imipenem–cilastatin is seizures affecting 1% of patients. Risk factors for seizures are old age, head trauma, previous seizure disorder, cerebrovascular accident, and renal failure. Among patients with a history of penicillin allergy, 10% are cross-sensitive to imipenem–cilastatin.

Meropenem

Meropenem (*Merrem*) is another carbapenem antibiotic with a broad spectrum of activity comparable to that of imipenem. A methyl group attached at the one-position on the five-member ring confers stability to dehydropeptidase I. Consequently, meropenem does not require administration with cilastatin. When compared in human trials, imipenem–cilastatin and meropenem achieve similar clinical outcomes in patients with serious intraabdominal and soft tissue infections. Both imipenem–cilastatin and meropenem are used to treat infections caused by highly resistant *Klebsiella pneumoniae* producing ESBLs. The major clinically relevant distinction between imipenem–cilastatin and meropenem is the lower likelihood of seizures associated with meropenem.

Loracarbef

Loracarbef (*Lorabid*) is a synthetic β-lactam antibiotic of the carbacephem class. The chemical structure of loracarbef is similar to that of cefaclor. Selected pharmacokinetic information appears in Table 45.2. Loracarbef's spectrum of antibacterial activity resembles those of the second-generation cephalosporins. Comparative clinical trials reveal similar outcomes in patients treated with cefaclor, cefprozil, and loracarbef.

MONOBACTAMS

Another interesting group of compounds produced by several bacterial genera are the monocyclic β-lactams (monobactams). The natural monobactams have little antimicrobial activity. A synthetic derivative, aztreonam (*Azactam*), has excellent activity against gram-negative organisms, including *P. aeruginosa*. Aztreonam has low affinity for penicillin-binding proteins in streptococci, staphylococci, and anaerobes and therefore has no significant activity against gram-positive bacteria or anaerobes. Specific activity against gram-negative organisms relates to the aminothiazolyl oxime moiety on the acyl side chain. Addition of two methyl groups and a carboxylic acid group on the oxime side chain enhances activity against *P. aeruginosa*. Aztreonam is stable to most β-lactamases (chromosomal and plasmid).

The pharmacokinetic properties of aztreonam are similar to those of the parenteral cephalosporins (Table 45.2). Aztreonam is not bioavailable after oral administration. During its distribution phase, the drug can achieve therapeutic concentrations in cerebrospinal fluid in the presence of inflamed meninges. Consequently, aztreonam is an alternative antibiotic to the cephalosporins for the therapy of meningitis caused by gram-negative bacilli.

Aztreonam may be used as a substitute for an aminoglycoside in the treatment of infections caused by susceptible gram-negative organisms. Most of the adverse effects of aztreonam are local reactions at the site of injection. Interestingly, aztreonam rarely causes allergic reactions in patients with a history of type I hypersensitivity to other β-lactam antibiotics.

Study Questions

1. A 32-year-old man with quadriplegia and neurogenic bladder was admitted to the hospital from a long-term care facility. The patient had vomiting, fever, and cloudy urine. A year ago, the patient developed urticaria, wheezing, and hypotension within an hour after his first dose of nafcillin. Subsequently his penicillin skin test was positive. During the current admission, the physician examiner noted fever, quadriplegia, and chronic indwelling bladder catheter. Laboratory tests revealed leukocytosis in blood and urine. Urine stain showed gram-negative rods, and urine culture grew *P. aeruginosa*. Which of the following drugs would be most appropriate for this patient?
   (A) Ampicillin–sulbactam
   (B) Aztreonam
   (C) Cefazolin
   (D) Imipenem–cilastatin
   (E) Piperacillin–tazobactam

2. A 22-year-old woman had her first prenatal visit. Her physical examination was normal for a woman at 12 weeks' gestation. Both the nontreponemal (Venereal Disease Research Laboratory) and fluorescent treponemal antibody tests were positive. She denied previous treatment for syphilis. She could not recall signs or symptoms of primary or secondary syphilis in the past year. She had no previous syphilis serology tests for purposes of comparison. Which of the following would be the best treatment for the patient?
   (A) Benzathine penicillin G
   (B) Doxycycline
   (C) Spectinomycin
   (D) Streptomycin
   (E) Tetracycline

3. A 26-year-old woman, a kindergarten teacher, had pharyngitis last year treated with ampicillin for 3 days. She stopped the ampicillin when she learned her throat culture was negative. Three days after she stopped the ampicillin, she developed a rash. Her physician noted symmetrical erythematous confluent macular–papular eruptions on her extremities with no urticaria. The physician diagnosed non–IgE-mediated ampicillin eruption. Now the patient returns with new fever and sore throat. She has no cough or rash. Her physical examination is normal except for fever, tender anterior cervical lymphadenopathy, and tonsillar exudate. Her rapid streptococcal test of a pharyngeal specimen is positive. Which of the following would be the most appropriate treatment for this patient?

   (A) Amikacin
   (B) Lomefloxacin
   (C) Metronidazole
   (D) Netilmicin
   (E) Penicillin V

4. A 24-year-old man came to the public health clinic because of a urethral discharge. He had had unprotected intercourse with multiple partners. Physical examination revealed a purulent urethral discharge with no penile ulcers or vesicles. There was no inguinal adenopathy. Gram stain of the discharge revealed gram-negative diplococci inside leukocytes. The antibiotic used to treat the patient's infection has which of the following mechanisms of action?
   (A) Inhibits cell membrane integrity by binding to ergosterols to create pores
   (B) Inhibits dihydrofolate reductase, thereby blocking formation of tetrahydrofolate required for purine synthesis
   (C) Inhibits KasA, a β-ketoacyl carrier protein synthetase, thereby blocking mycolic acid synthesis
   (D) Inhibits RNA synthesis by binding to the β-subunit of DNA-dependent RNA polymerase
   (E) Inhibits transpeptidase, thereby blocking cross-linking of peptides in cell wall murein (peptidoglycan)

5. Parents brought their 3-year-old boy to the outpatient clinic because of a facial rash. Today the patient was one of several children sent home from day care because of similar rashes. Physical examination revealed a normal, healthy boy with discrete erythematous papular eruptions on his cheeks. There were no vesicles or bullae. The rash was covered with a honey crust, suggesting impetigo. Which of the following treatments would be most appropriate?
   (A) Dapsone
   (B) Dicloxacillin
   (C) Doxycycline
   (D) Ketoconazole
   (E) Penciclovir

ANSWERS

1. **B.** The patient has complicated urinary tract infection and nonsevere sepsis syndrome caused by *P. aeruginosa*. Effective antibiotics for *Pseudomonas* spp. include mezlocillin, piperacillin, piperacillin–tazobactam, ticarcillin, and ticarcillin–clavulanate. The carbapenems (imipenem and meropenem) and the monobactam (aztreonam) are also active against *P. aeruginosa*. Ampicillin–sulbactam and cefazolin are ineffective against *P.*

aeruginosa. The history defines a patient with type I allergic hypersensitivity to penicillin. The patient should avoid drugs in the penicillin class, including penicillin, nafcillin, oxacillin, cloxacillin, dicloxacillin, ampicillin, amoxicillin, ticarcillin, piperacillin, and mezlocillin. In addition, carbapenems (imipenem, meropenem) should not be administered to patients with a history of type I allergic response to penicillin or positive penicillin skin test. Cefazolin is a cephalosporin. Patients with type I allergy to penicillin and positive penicillin skin test have a 5.6% rate of allergic reactions to cephalosporins. Aztreonam may be used safely in patients with history of type I allergic response to penicillin.

2. **B.** The patient is pregnant and has latent syphilis of indeterminate duration. The pathogenic organism is *T. pallidum.* Benzathine penicillin G is the drug of first choice for treating latent syphilis. Doxycycline and tetracycline are alternatives treatments for non-pregnant patients with latent syphilis. Spectinomycin is not effective against syphilis; it is a treatment for disseminated gonorrhea in patients who are allergic to cephalosporins. Streptomycin is not effective against syphilis.

3. **E.** The patient has exudative pharyngitis, presumably secondary to group A streptococcus. Antibiotic treatment is indicated to reduce the duration and severity of symptoms and to prevent acute rheumatic fever. The antibiotic of first choice is penicillin V. Other reasonable alternatives are benzathine penicillin G, erythromycin, cephalosporin, clindamycin, azithromycin, and clarithromycin. Amikacin, lomefloxacin, metronidazole, and netilmicin are not active against group A streptococcus.

4. **E.** The patient has uncomplicated urethritis caused by *N. gonorrhoeae.* Effective antibiotics for gonorrhea include cephalosporins (ceftriaxone, cefixime, ceftizoxime, cefotaxime, cefotetan, cefoxitin), fluoroquinolones (ciprofloxacin, ofloxacin, enoxacin, lomefloxacin, gatifloxacin), and spectinomycin. Gonorrhea is resistant to trimethoprim and rifampin. Amphotericin B is an antifungal drug, and isoniazid is an antimycobacterial drug. Neither has antigonococcal activity. Cephalosporins and other β-lactam antibiotics act to inhibit bacterial transpeptidase and block cross-linking of peptides in cell wall murein (peptidoglycan). Fluoroquinolone antibiotics inhibit DNA gyrase (topoisomerase) and interfere with bacterial DNA transcription and replication. Spectinomycin and doxycycline inhibit bacterial protein synthesis and act at the 30S ribosome subunit. Azithromycin inhibits bacterial protein synthesis and acts at the 50S ribosome subunit. Trimethoprim inhibits dihydrofolate reductase and blocks formation of tetrahydrofolate required for purine synthesis. Rifampin in-

hibits RNA synthesis by binding to the βsubunit of DNA-dependent RNA polymerase. Amphotericin B inhibits fungal cell membrane integrity by binding to ergosterols to create pores. Isoniazid inhibits KasA, a β-ketoacyl carrier protein synthetase, and blocks mycolic acid synthesis.

5. **B.** The patient has impetigo. The causative organism is either *Streptococcus pyogenes* (group A) or *S. aureus.* Recommended antibiotic treatment is dicloxacillin or cloxacillin. Dapsone is used to treat skin infections with *Mycobacterium leprae* (leprosy) and to treat brown recluse spider (*Loxosceles*) bites. Doxycycline is used to treat skin infections with *Bacillus anthracis* (anthrax), *Bartonella henselae* (bacillary angiomatosis), *Borrelia burgdorferi* (Lyme disease, erythema migrans), *Propionibacterium acnes* (acne vulgaris), *Vibrio vulnificus* and *Vibrio damsela* (hemorrhagic bullous cellulitis). The question does not provide historical or epidemiological information to support these diagnoses. Ketoconazole is used to treat fungal infections of the skin (tinea capitis, tinea cruris, tinea corporis, tinea pedis, tinea versicolor). Dermatophyte infections are usually erythematous, with vesicles, fissures, and scaling. Penciclovir is a treatment for herpes simplex virus infections including herpes labialis fever blisters.

SUPPLEMENTAL READING

Bush LM and Johnson CC. Ureidopenicillins and beta-lactam/beta-lactamase inhibitor combinations. Infect Dis Clin North Am 2000;14:409–433.

Dancer SJ. The problem with cephalosporins. J Antimicrob Chemother 2001;48:463–478.

Kaye KS et al. Risk factors for emergence of resistance to broad-spectrum cephalosporins among *Enterobacter* spp. Antimicrob Agents Chemother 2001;45:2628–2630.

Lowe MN and Lamb HM. Meropenem: An updated review of its use in the management of intra-abdominal infections. Drugs 2000;60:619–646.

Massova I and Mobashery S. Kinship and diversification of bacterial penicillin-binding proteins and beta-lactamases. Antimicrob Agents Chemother 1998;42:1–17.

Nikaido H. Prevention of drug access to bacterial targets: Permeability barriers and active efflux. Science 1994;264:382–388.

Perry CM and Markham A. Piperacillin/tazobactam: An updated review of its use in the treatment of bacterial infections. Drugs 1999;57:805–843.

Salkind AR, Cuddy PG, and Foxworth JW. Is this patient allergic to penicillin? An evidence-based analysis of the likelihood of penicillin allergy. JAMA 2001;285:2498–2505.

Wright AJ. The penicillins. Mayo Clin Proc 1999;74:290–307.

CASE Study   Choosing an Antibiotic Therapy

A 65-year-old man came to the emergency department via ambulance after a generalized seizure. Relatives accompanied the patient and described a 1-day history of fever and intermittent confusion. The patient had a 10-year history of chronic lymphocytic leukemia; 2 months ago, he had a trial of oral chlorambucil because of progressive fatigue, anemia, thrombocytopenia, and splenomegaly. Then, 3 weeks ago, the patient attended a family reunion at a cousin's dairy farm. He enjoyed eating homemade soft cheese, sausage, and fresh vegetables from the garden. Several family members who attended the reunion reported transient febrile gastroenteritis. The patient's physical examination in the emergency department revealed a stuporous man with temperature 103.3°F (39.6°C), blood pressure 122/68 mm Hg, pulse 112 beats per minute, and respirations 26 per minute. He had nuchal rigidity, diffuse adenopathy, and hepatosplenomegaly. Passive flexion of the neck caused flexion at hips and knees (Brudzinski's sign). The patient resisted passive extension of the flexed knee and hip (Kernig's sign). Papilledema was absent. There were no focal neurological deficits. Skin examination revealed no eruption. Peripheral blood tests showed 36,000 leukocytes (66% lymphocytes), hemoglobin 9.0 g/dL, platelet count 99,000. A lumbar puncture was performed. The opening pressure of cerebrospinal fluid was 220 mm of water. Cerebrospinal fluid tests revealed no organisms on Gram stain, glucose 60 mg/dL, protein 200 mg/dL, lactate 50 mg/dL, leukocytes 2000 per mm^3 (10% neutrophils, 60% lymphocytes, 30% monocytes). Bacterial antigen tests on cerebrospinal fluid were negative for *H. influenzae* type B, *S. pneumoniae*, *Neisseria meningitidis*, *E. coli* K1, and group B streptococci. What is the best empirical antibiotic therapy for this patient?

ANSWER: The emergency department physician suspected acute bacterial meningitis in a patient with impaired immunity secondary to hematologic malignancy. The physician also noted the exposure to a food-borne pathogen associated with dairy products. The epidemiological risk assessment suggested the need for empirical antibiotic therapy to cover potential gram-negative enteric pathogens and *L. monocytogenes*. Immediately after obtaining blood and spinal fluid specimens, the emergency department personnel initiated therapy with ampicillin 2 g intravenously every 4 hours and ceftazidime 2 g intravenously every 8 hours. On the next day, the clinical microbiology laboratory reported diphtheroids growing in the patient's blood culture bottles. On the second hospital day, the laboratory identified *L. monocytogenes* growing in blood and spinal fluid specimens. Ceftazidime was discontinued. The patient completed a 21-day course of ampicillin and gentamicin 1.7 mg/kg intravenously every 8 hours.

46

Aminoglycoside Antibiotics

Steven M. Belknap

 DRUG LIST

GENERIC NAME	PAGE	GENERIC NAME	PAGE
Amikacin	538	Netilmicin	538
Gentamicin	538	Streptomycin	538
Kanamycin	538	Tobramycin	538
Neomycin	538		

CHEMISTRY

Aminoglycosides are hydrophilic, polycationic, amine-containing carbohydrates that are usually composed of three to five rings. Most aminoglycosides are either natural products or derivatives of soil actinomycetes. They are often secreted by these actinomycetes as mixtures of closely related compounds. The polycationic aminoglycoside chemical structure results in a binding both to the anionic outer bacterial membrane and to anionic phospholipids in the cell membranes of mammalian renal proximal tubular cells. The former contributes to the bactericidal effects of these compounds, while the latter binding accounts for their toxicity. Because of their hydrophilicity, the transport of aminoglycosides across the hydrophobic lipid bilayer of eukaryotic cell membranes is impeded.

The major clinically important aminoglycosides are amikacin (*Amikin*), gentamicin (*Garamycin*), kanamycin (*Kantrex*), netilmicin (*Netromycin*), neomycin (*Mycifradin*), streptomycin, and tobramycin (*Nebcin*). Their pharmacokinetic characteristics are shown in Table 46.1.

MECHANISM OF ANTIBACTERIAL ACTION

The antibacterial actions of the aminoglycosides involve two possibly synergistic effects. First, the positively charged aminoglycoside binds to negatively charged sites on the outer bacterial membrane, thereby disrupting membrane integrity. It is likely that the aminoglycoside-induced bacterial outer membrane degradation accounts for the rapid concentration-dependent bactericidal effect of these compounds. Second, aminoglycosides bind to various sites on bacterial 30S ribosomal subunits, disrupting the initiation of protein synthesis and inducing errors in the translation of messenger RNA to peptides. They also bind to sites on bacterial 50S ribosomal subunits, although the significance of this binding is uncertain. In addition, they have a postantibiotic effect; that is, they continue to suppress bacterial regrowth even after removal of the antibiotic from the bacterial microenvironment. It is likely that ribosome disruption accounts for this postantibiotic activity.

TABLE 46.1 Characteristics of the Aminoglycosides

Drug	Half-life (hr)	Therapeutic Serum Level (μg/ml)	Toxic Serum Level (μg/ml)
Streptomycin	2–3	25	50
Neomycin	3	5–10	10
Kanamycin	2.0–2.5	8–16	35
Gentamicin	1.2–5.0	4–10	12
Tobramycin	2.0–3.0	4–8	12
Amikacin	0.8–2.8	8–16	35
Netilmicin	2.0–2.5	0.5–10	16

Adapted with permission from Drug Facts and Comparisons. St. Louis: Lippincott, 1985:1372.

The postantibiotic effect is characterized by prolonged suppression of bacterial regrowth after the initially high aminoglycoside concentration has fallen to a subinhibitory level. Perhaps resumption of bacterial ribosomal function requires the time-consuming synthesis of new ribosomes after their disruption by aminoglycosides. The postantibiotic effect explains why aminoglycosides can be given in single daily doses despite their short half-life.

Penetration of aminoglycosides through the outer bacterial membrane occurs both by outer membrane disruption and by diffusion through outer membrane porins. Penetration through the inner bacterial membrane occurs in two phases. The first requires that the cytosol have a negative electron potential and therefore be inhibited by the presence of a low pH. The second phase depends on aerobic bacterial metabolism and therefore will be inhibited by low oxygen tension. The latter two observations are of considerable clinical relevance, since both a low pH and a low oxygen tension frequently occur in bacterial abscesses. Administration of β-lactam antibiotics will reverse the negative effects of both low pH and low oxygen tension on the ability of aminoglycosides to penetrate into bacteria; this ability accounts in part for the synergism that occurs between aminoglycoside and β-lactam antibiotic drugs.

MECHANISM OF ANTIBACTERIAL RESISTANCE

The frequency of bacterial aminoglycoside resistance encountered in clinical practice has remained nearly constant over the past 2 decades. Of the three recognized mechanisms of resistance that occur in aerobic gram-negative bacteria, plasmid-mediated expression of enzymes that acetylate, adenylate, or phosphorylate the aminoglycosides is the most important. Ring one is the primary target of these enzymes.

Two other common mechanisms of resistance are known. Some cases of resistance of aerobic gram-negative bacilli to streptomycin are due to mutations in the proteins of the bacterial ribosomes. Streptococci, staphylococci, and Pseudomonadaceae resist aminoglycosides as a result of decreased transport of the aminoglycosides into the bacterial cytosol.

Anaerobes also are resistant to aminoglycosides because of decreased transport into the bacterial cytosol. Combining an aminoglycoside with an antibiotic that disrupts the bacterial cell wall can overcome this natural resistance.

PHARMACOKINETICS

The blood plasma drug concentrations achieved during multiple daily dose therapy with aminoglycosides usually correlates with clinical outcome in patients with bacteremia and in patients with pneumonia. Raising the aminoglycoside plasma concentration to its in vitro minimum inhibitory concentration against the isolated pathogen is a useful indicator of the adequacy of aminoglycoside dosing.

Both the rate and extent of gastrointestinal absorption of individual aminoglycosides are generally quite low. For example, more than 95% of an oral dose of neomycin is excreted unchanged in the feces. The systemic bioavailability of the aminoglycosides is low across other membranes as well. For example, gentamicin is poorly absorbed from a topical ophthalmic preparation, and there is little systemic absorption of either inhaled tobramycin or aminoglycosides instilled into the urinary bladder. Neomycin bioavailability across intact skin is also low, although absorption across damaged skin can be significant: nephrotoxicity can occur in burn patients treated with topical neomycin.

Because of their aqueous solubility and modest binding to plasma and tissue proteins, the distribution of the aminoglycosides corresponds to that of the extracellular fluid. Four compartments can be distinguished. The central compartment corresponds to the intravascular space; the rapidly equilibrating compartment corresponds to the extracellular visceral space; the slowly equilibrating compartment largely corresponds to that of skeletal muscle; and the extremely slowly equilibrating compartment presumably corresponds to that of bone, proximal renal tubules, otolymph, and other tissue where binding to phospholipids or mineral matrix occurs. Gentamicin fails to reach intraocular fluid or cerebrospinal fluid in significant concentrations after intravenous injection, although it may reach bactericidal levels in cerebrospinal fluid in patients with meningeal inflammation, such as occurs in meningitis. However, direct intrathecal injection of gentamicin may still be required for reliable bactericidal levels.

Most of the enzymes that catalyze the metabolism of foreign compounds are found inside cells. As aminoglycosides do not penetrate most cells, they do not undergo any significant metabolism. Nearly all of an intravenous dose is cleared by the kidneys and can be recovered in the urine. Aminoglycoside clearance is approximately equal to that of the glomerular filtration rate, resulting in fairly high urine concentrations; the latter contributes to the efficacy of the aminoglycosides in urinary tract infections.

CLINICAL USES

Serious Gram-Negative Bacillary Infections

Gentamicin is the aminoglycoside antibiotic most commonly used to treat serious infections due to gram-negative aerobic bacilli, such as *Escherichia coli* and *Klebsiella pneumoniae,* and *Proteus, Serratia, Acinetobacter, Citrobacter,* and *Enterobacter* spp. Gentamicin also has significant activity against *Staphylococcus aureus.* The aminoglycosides are often used in combination with β-lactams in the initial empirical therapy of sepsis and of fever in immunocompromised patients. The combination is used both to ensure adequate antibiotic coverage in these seriously ill patients and to exploit the synergistic antibiotic activity that β-lactams and aminoglycosides have against many species. These drugs should not, however, be injected simultaneously, since the β-lactams can chemically inactivate the aminoglycosides.

Aminoglycosides are often used in patients with gram-negative bacillary pneumonia. Single daily dosing may be of particular importance in patients with pneumonia, since this regimen can increase the peak concentration of the aminoglycosides in bronchial secretions.

Acute salpingitis (pelvic inflammatory disease) due to *Neisseria gonorrhoeae, Chlamydia trachomatis,* or both is often complicated by superinfection with gram-negative bacilli and anaerobes. A combination of gentamicin, clindamycin, and doxycycline has been shown to be an effective treatment for this polymicrobial infection.

The combination of gentamicin and clindamycin is useful in patients with an intraabdominal infection or an abscess secondary to penetrating trauma, diverticulitis, cholangitis, appendicitis, peritonitis, or postsurgical wound infection. These infections are often polymicrobial, including gram-negative bacilli and anaerobes. Definitive treatment of these conditions may also require surgical or other intervention to drain the abscess.

Choice of one aminoglycoside over another for the treatment of serious infections should be guided both by assessment of the antibiotic sensitivities of the specific bacterial strain causing the patient's infection and by familiarity with local patterns of bacterial resistance. *Pseudomonas aeruginosa* is more likely than other gram-negative bacilli to exhibit resistance to gentamicin. However, *Pseudomonas* spp. resistant to gentamicin may be susceptible to amikacin or tobramycin. Streptomycin is the drug of choice for patients with pneumonia due to *Yersinia pestis* (plague) or *Francisella tularensis* (tularemia).

Eradication of Facultative Gut Flora

A combination of neomycin and nonabsorbable erythromycin base given orally prior to colorectal surgery can markedly reduce the incidence of postoperative wound infection. Orally administered neomycin is sometimes used to suppress the facultative flora of the gut in patients with hepatic encephalopathy. It is unclear how this improves coma, but one theory is that it reduces systemic absorption of the bacterial metabolites that allegedly cause hepatic encephalopathy. Although more than 95% of an oral dose of neomycin is excreted unchanged in the stool of normal subjects, the bioavailability of neomycin may be much higher in patients with an abnormal gastrointestinal mucosa.

Neomycin is often combined with other antibiotics, such as polymyxin B and bacitracin, and applied as an ointment to prevent any infection of minor skin abrasions, burns, and cuts.

Cystic Fibrosis

P. aeruginosa is commonly found in the bronchial secretions of patients with cystic fibrosis. In one study, daily inhalation of large doses of tobramycin decreased the colonization by this organism 100-fold and significantly improved pulmonary function.

Endocarditis

A combination of gentamicin and ampicillin is recommended as prophylaxis of endocarditis prior to surgery or instrumentation of the gastrointestinal or genitourinary tracts for patients at high risk for endocarditis. Gentamicin plus vancomycin is recommended as prophylaxis of endocarditis for high-risk patients with a history of β-lactam allergy. Gentamicin or streptomycin will act synergistically with penicillin for the treatment of enterococcal endocarditis.

Meningitis

The degree of penetration of the aminoglycosides into cerebrospinal fluid is proportional to the degree of inflammation of the meninges. However, aminoglycosides are best combined with the β-lactams or other antibiotics in the treatment of meningitis.

Tuberculosis

In response to the increasing prevalence of mycobacterial resistance to standard antibiotic chemotherapy, the use of aminoglycosides is increasing in patients at high risk for having resistant infections. Inhaled aminoglycosides may also have a role in patients with persistently positive sputum despite therapy. Streptomycin is useful in the initial therapy of severe or disseminated tuberculosis, which is most common in immunocompromised patients.

Ophthalmological Infection

Because of the very high concentrations of gentamicin achieved in the conjunctival sac, it is effective against nearly all of the typical bacterial pathogens that cause conjunctivitis. Special high-dose formulations of gentamicin are necessary for treating bacterial ophthalmic keratitis. Gentamicin is not active against viral conjunctivitis, although it may prevent a secondary bacterial infection. Bacterial endophthalmitis, an infection of the vitreous humor, usually requires both vitreous aspiration and intravitreal instillation of gentamicin and cefazolin.

Gonococcal Urethritis

Spectinomycin (*Trobicin*), an aminocyclitol antibiotic chemically related to the aminoglycosides, is occasionally used to treat uncomplicated gonococcal urethritis in patients who are allergic to β-lactam. Treatment failures have occurred, however, when spectinomycin was used in gonococcal pharyngitis or systemic gonococcal infection.

SINGLE DAILY DOSING

Single daily doses of aminoglycosides are at least as effective as and no more toxic than multiple daily doses. Some studies suggest that single daily dosing may actually be less nephrotoxic than more frequent dosing. Since aminoglycoside uptake across the brush border of proximal renal cortical tubular cells is saturable, giving a single large dose should result in less renal accumulation; this has now been shown in patients receiving a single bolus injection of gentamicin compared with those administered a continuous 24-hour intravenous infusion. One clinical trial recently demonstrated that ototoxicity was also reduced when single daily dosing was used.

The magnitude of the rapid-killing effect and the duration of the postantibiotic effect of the aminoglycosides are proportional to their peak concentration at the site of the infection; that is, the higher the peak concentration, the more pronounced these effects. Giving aminoglycosides as a single daily dose results in a higher peak tissue concentration than if the total daily dose were divided and given more frequently. Single daily dosing with amikacin results in higher drug concentrations in the bronchial secretions of patients with pneumonia.

Clinical trials of single daily dosing of aminoglycosides have been done in adults, pregnant women, and children for a variety of indications, including serious infections, pelvic inflammatory disease, abdominal sepsis, cystic fibrosis, and the empirical treatment of neutropenic patients with fever. While single daily dosing of aminoglycosides is justified in most patients, it may be inadequate when given to provide synergism with β-lactam antibiotics in enterococcal endocarditis.

TOXICITY

Aminoglycosides cause nephrotoxicity, and the relative toxicity of the various aminoglycosides can be correlated with the number of constituent amine groups that each contains; neomycin is the most nephrotoxic and streptomycin is the least. Although their polycationic structure prevents their entry into most cells, aminoglycosides can diffuse from the tubular lumen across the apical membrane of proximal renal tubular cells following drug filtration through the glomerulus. Passage of the aminoglycosides across the apical membrane occurs via a saturable process of adsorption of polycationic aminoglycoside molecules to the proximal renal tubular lumen's anionic brush border and subsequent endocytosis and accumulation in lysosomes.

Once the drug is within the lysosomes, it will bind to anionic phospholipids, inhibiting lysosomal phospholipase A_2. This leads to lysosomal distension, rupture, and release of acid hydrolases and the aminoglycoside into the cytosol. Free aminoglycoside then binds to other cellular organelles. Gentamicin accumulation in mitochondria displaces Ca^{++}, leading to mitochondrial degeneration and cell necrosis. The necrotic cellular debris then sloughs off and is passed in the urine, leaving a denuded basement membrane. The development of toxicity depends upon the duration of aminoglycoside therapy and the mean trough blood plasma drug concentration. Nephrotoxicity is more likely in aminoglycoside-treated patients with gram-negative bacillary bacteremia than in those with staphylococcal bacteremia. Nephrotoxicity is most common and most severe in patients with extrahepatic biliary obstruction, hepatitis, or cirrhosis.

The severity of aminoglycoside nephrotoxicity is additive with that of vancomycin, polymixin, gallium, furosemide, enflurane, cisplatin, and cephalosporins. Aminoglycoside nephrotoxicity is synergistic with that of amphotericin B and cyclosporine.

Even quite severe aminoglycoside-induced nephrotoxicity is nearly always reversible upon prompt discontinuation of the drug. Verapamil and Ca^{++} can lessen the nephrotoxicity, but the latter may also inhibit the antibacterial effect of the aminoglycosides. Polyaspartic acid is a promising new agent that lessens aminoglycoside nephrotoxicity, although it also may partially inhibit the drug's antibacterial activity.

Aminoglycosides accumulate in otolymph and can cause both vestibular and auditory ototoxicity, both of which can be irreversible. Uptake is driven by the concentration gradient between blood and the otolymph; this process is saturable. Sustained high concentrations in otolymph first destroy hair cells that are sensitive to high-frequency sounds. Streptomycin is more likely to cause vestibular toxicity than ototoxicity. The severity of aminoglycoside-induced ototoxicity is worsened by the coadministration of vancomycin, furosemide, bumetanide, and ethacrynic acid. Ca^{++} may lessen the ototoxic effect.

Aminoglycosides can cause neuromuscular junction blockade by displacing Ca^{++} from the neuromuscular junction, inhibiting the Ca^{++}-dependent prejunctional release of acetylcholine and blocking postsynaptic acetylcholine receptor binding. This is usually clinically significant only in patients with myasthenia gravis, hypocalcemia, or hypermagnesemia or when the aminoglycoside is given shortly after the use of a neuromuscular blocking agent. The neuromuscular blockade can be reversed by administration of intravenous calcium.

Study QUESTIONS

1. Many antibiotics appear to have as their mechanism of action the capacity to inhibit bacterial cell wall synthesis. This does NOT appear to be a mechanism of
   (A) Aminoglycosides
   (B) Penicillins
   (C) Bacitracin
   (D) Cephalosporins

2. Many antibiotics are not useful in treating infections in the central nervous system because they do not readily penetrate the blood-brain barrier. Which one of the following agents does get into the brain in reasonable concentrations?
   (A) Penicillin G
   (B) Ampicillin
   (C) Cefotaxime
   (D) Kanamycin
   (E) Neomycin

3. Aminoglycoside antibiotics are frequently used in combination with the β-lactam antibiotics. Which of the following choices best explains the rationale for this use?
   (A) The combination provides for a much greater spectrum of activity.
   (B) A synergistic effect is often seen when the combination is employed.
   (C) The β-lactam antibiotics prevent toxic effects of the aminoglycoside antibiotics.
   (D) The combination decreases incidence of superinfections.

4. Patients with myasthenia gravis may exhibit greater toxicity to aminoglycosides than do patients without this condition. The most likely explanation is
   (A) Aminoglycosides have muscarinic blocking properties.

(B) Aminoglycosides cause an increased metabolism of acetylcholine.
(C) Aminoglycosides cause a neuromuscular block by displacing Ca^{++} from the neuromuscular junction.
(D) Aminoglycosides inhibit second messenger activity at the neuromuscular junction.

5. As a class, the aminoglycoside antibiotics do not exhibit significant metabolism in the patient. The most likely reason is that
   (A) Their chemical structure is unique and not prone to chemical reactions commonly seen in drug metabolism.
   (B) The liver does not contain appropriate enzymes to break down the compounds.
   (C) The body apparently lacks a necessary cofactor for the metabolism of aminoglycosides.
   (D) Aminoglycosides do not readily get to the site of degradative enzymes.

ANSWERS

1. **A.** The aminoglycosides appear to act by binding to various sites on bacterial 30S ribosomal subunits and disrupting the initiation of protein synthesis. The other agents appear to have the capacity to directly inhibit bacterial cell-wall synthesis.

2. **C.** The selection of agents to treat brain infections is quite limited because most agents do not penetrate into cerebrospinal fluid or the brain itself.

3. **B.** A synergistic effect when the combination of an aminoglycoside and β-lactam antibiotic are administered concurrently is well documented. The reasons for the synergistic response are not well documented but may be related to the actions of the β-lactam antibiotic to raise pH and oxygen tension

in areas of abscess and thereby increase the penetrability of the aminoglycoside.

4. **C.** Aminoglycosides can cause neuromuscular junction blockade by the mechanism of displacing Ca^{++} from the neuromuscular junction and thus leading to the Ca^{++}-dependent prejunctional release of acetylcholine. This is of clinical significance only in patients with myasthenia gravis, hypocalcemia, and hypermagnesemia.

5. **D.** Aminoglycosides do not penetrate most cells, and most drug-metabolizing enzymes are found on the inside of the cells. Therefore, aminoglycosides are poorly metabolized, and nearly all of an intravenous dose can be recovered in the urine.

SUPPLEMENTAL READING

Clancy JP et al. Evidence that systemic gentamicin suppresses premature stop mutations in patients with cystic fibrosis. Am J Respir Crit Care Med 2001;163:1683–1692.

Gaillard J et al. Cerebrospinal fluid penetration of amikacin in children with community-acquired bacterial meningitis. Antimicrob Agents Chemother 1995;39:253–255.

Lortholary O et al. Aminoglycosides. Med Clin North Am 1995;79:761787.

Moore R, Lietman P, and Smith C. Clinical response to aminoglycosides: Importance of the ratio of peak concentration to minimal inhibitory concentration. J Infect Dis 1987;155:93–99.

Santre C et al. Amikacin levels in bronchia secretions of 10 pneumonia patients with respiratory support treated once daily versus twice daily. Antimicrob Agents Chemother 1995;39:264–267.

CASE Study   Neomycin in Hepatic Encephalopathy

A 50-year-old man diagnosed with hepatic coma was successfully treated with a daily oral dose of neomycin 2 weeks prior to coming to your clinic. The patient complains that he can't hear as well now as he could prior to his recent hospitalization. You suspect that this may be due to the patient's treatment during his episode with hepatic coma. What is your next response?

ANSWER: Ototoxicity and nephrotoxicity are common adverse effects of aminoglycoside therapy, particularly when administered orally. You immediately arrange to check renal function and fortunately discover that renal function is not significantly impaired in this patient. You inform the patient that the hearing loss is probably permanent and that he should carefully check with pharmacists and physicians in the future to be certain that any prescriptions drugs that he might receive do not further aggravate this condition.

47 Tetracyclines, Chloramphenicol, Macrolides, and Lincosamides

Richard P. O'Connor

DRUG LIST

TETRACYCLINES

Structure and Mechanism of Action

Although all tetracyclines have a similar mechanism of action, they have different chemical structures and are produced by different species of *Streptomyces*. In addition, structural analogues of these compounds have been synthesized to improve pharmacokinetic properties and antimicrobial activity. While several biological processes in the bacterial cells are modified by the tetracyclines, their *primary mode of action is inhibition of protein synthesis*. Tetracyclines bind to the 30S ribosome and thereby prevent the binding of aminoacyl transfer RNA (tRNA) to the A site (acceptor site) on the 50S ribosomal unit. The tetracyclines affect both eukaryotic and prokaryotic cells but are *selectively toxic for bacteria, because they readily penetrate microbial membranes and accumulate in the cytoplasm through an energy-dependent tetracycline transport system that is absent from mammalian cells.*

Resistance is related largely to changes in cell permeability and a resultant decreased accumulation of drug due to increased efflux from the cell by an energy-dependent mechanism. Other mechanisms, such as production of a protein that alters the interaction of tetracycline with the ribosome and enzymatic inactivation of the drug, have been reported.

Antibacterial Spectrum

The tetracyclines display broad-spectrum activity and are effective against both gram-positive and gram-negative bacteria, including *Rickettsia, Coxiella, Mycoplasma,* and *Chlamydia* spp.. Tetracycline resistance has increased among pneumococci and gonococci, which limits their use in the treatment of infections caused by these organisms.

Although several congeners of the tetracyclines are available, they all have a similar spectrum of in vitro activity. Minocycline is somewhat more active and oxytetracycline and tetracycline are somewhat less active than other members of this group.

Absorption, Distribution, Metabolism, and Excretion

These antibiotics are partially absorbed from the stomach and upper gastrointestinal tract. *Food impairs absorption of all tetracyclines except doxycycline and minocycline.* Absorption of doxycycline and minocycline is improved with food. Since *the tetracyclines form insoluble chelates with calcium (such as are found in many antacids), magnesium, and other metal ions,* their simultaneous administration with milk (calcium), magnesium hydroxide, aluminum hydroxide, or iron will interfere with absorption. Because some of the tetracyclines are not completely absorbed, any drug remaining in the intestine may inhibit sensitive intestinal microorganisms and alter the normal intestinal flora.

The tetracyclines are distributed throughout body tissues and fluids in concentrations that reflect the lipid solubility of each individual agent. Minocycline and doxycycline are the most lipid soluble, while oxytetracycline is the least lipid soluble. The tetracyclines penetrate (but somewhat unpredictably) the uninflamed meninges and cross the placental barrier. Peak serum levels are reached approximately 2 hours after oral administration; cerebrospinal fluid (CSF) levels are only one-fourth those of plasma.

The various congeners differ in their half-lives and their protein binding ability (Table 47.1). Significant differences in serum half-life allow the grouping of the tetracyclines into subclasses: *short acting* (tetracycline, chlortetracycline, and oxytetracycline), *intermediate acting* (demeclocycline and methacycline), and *long acting* (minocycline and doxycycline).

The tetracyclines are metabolized in the liver and are concentrated in the bile. Bile concentrations can be up to five times those of the plasma. Doxycycline, minocycline, and chlortetracycline are excreted primarily in the feces. The other tetracyclines are eliminated primarily in the urine by glomerular filtration. Obviously, these tetracyclines have greater urinary antibacterial activity than those (e.g., doxycycline) that are excreted by nonrenal mechanisms.

Clinical Uses

There is little difference in clinical response among the various tetracyclines. The selection of an agent, therefore, is based on tolerance, ease of administration, and cost. The restriction of their use in pregnancy and in patients under the age of 8 years applies to all preparations.

Two tetracyclines have sufficiently distinctive features to warrant separate mention. Doxycycline, with its longer half-life and lack of nephrotoxicity, is a popular choice for patients with preexisting renal disease or those who are at risk for developing renal insufficiency. The lack of nephrotoxicity is related mainly to biliary excretion, which is the primary route of doxycycline elimination. *Doxycycline is the preferred parenteral tetracycline.* Doxycycline is a potential first-line agent in the prophylaxis of anthrax after exposure. Doxycycline is the treatment of choice for the primary stage of Lyme disease in adults and children older than 8 years.

Minocycline is an effective alternative to rifampin for eradication of meningococci, including sulfonamide-resistant strains, from the nasopharynx. However, the high incidence of dose-related vestibular side effects renders it less acceptable. Although minocycline has good in vitro activity against *Nocardia* spp., further studies are necessary to confirm its clinical efficacy.

The tetracyclines are still the *drugs of choice* for treatment of cholera, diseases caused by *Rickettsia* and *Coxiella,* granuloma inguinale, relapsing fever, the chlamydial diseases (trachoma, lymphogranuloma

TABLE 47.1 Some Properties of Tetracycline and Its Congeners

Drug, *Trade Name*	Preferred Route	Serum half-life (hr)	Serum protein binding (%)
Tetracycline hydrochloride *Achromycin, Panamycin, Hydrochloride*	Oral, IV	8	25–60
Chlortetracycline hydrochloride *Aureomycin*	Oral, IV	6	40–70
Oxytetracycline hydrochloride *Terramycin Hydrochloride*	Oral, IV	9	20–35
Demeclocycline hydrochloride *Declomycin*	Oral	12	40–90
Methacycline hydrochloride *Rondomycin*	Oral	13	75–90
Doxycycline *Vibramycin*	Oral, IV	18	25–90
Minocycline hydrochloride *Minocin, Vectrin*	Oral, IV	16	70–75

venereum, and psittacosis), and nonspecific urethritis. They are also effective in the treatment of brucellosis, tularemia, and infections caused by *Pasteurella* and *Mycoplasma* spp., although other agents may be equally effective. Tetracyclines are clinically effective in acne because of their antioxidant effect on the degranulated neutrophils in the comedone acidic contents (in which long-term low-dose therapy is popular). Mild to moderate attacks of pelvic inflammatory disease often respond to tetracycline, probably as a result of the drug's action on anaerobic bacteria and chlamydia.

Tetracyclines no longer can be entirely relied on in the treatment of streptococcal infections; up to 40% of *Streptococcus pyogenes* and 10% of *Streptococcus pneumoniae* are resistant.

Adverse Effects

Oral administration can cause nausea, vomiting, epigastric burning, stomatitis, and glossitis, and an intravenous injection can cause phlebitis. When given over long periods, use of these agents can result in a negative nitrogen balance, which may lead to elevated blood urea nitrogen. Hepatotoxicity occurs infrequently but is particularly severe during pregnancy, when the combination of uremia and increasing jaundice can be fatal. In addition, these antibiotics are occasionally nephrotoxic and should not be administered with other potentially nephrotoxic drugs. Staining of both the deciduous and permanent teeth and retardation of bone growth can occur if tetracyclines are administered after the fourth month of gestation or if they are given to children less than 8 years of age.

Photosensitivity, observed as abnormal sunburn reaction, is particularly associated with demeclocycline and doxycycline administration. Superinfection may result in oral, anogenital, and intestinal *Candida albicans* infections, whereas *Staphylococcus aureus* or *Clostridium difficile* overgrowth may cause enterocolitis. Minocycline can produce vertigo.

Minocycline is frequently used in the treatment of chronic facial dermatoses. Increased usage has resulted in local skin pigmentation, particularly at sites of previous tissue trauma that is unrelated to the photosensitization phenomenon characteristic of this class of drug. This effect does not appear to be dose dependent and usually resolves in months to years following drug discontinuation.

Other significant side effects of minocycline may make it unsuitable for some light-skinned patients. In particular, dark bone pigmentation is severe enough to be visible through the mucosae of the alveolar ridges in the mouth and other areas where bone directly adheres to skin (black bone disease). Thyroid staining is visible through the overlying skin of the neck but does not affect the endocrine function of the gland.

Pulmonary eosinophilic syndrome, characterized by extreme hypoxemia, eosinophilia, interstitial pneumonitis, hilar lymphadenopathy, and pleural effusions, can be severe and can occur with as little as 7 to 9 days of therapy with the tetracyclines. In severe cases steroid therapy is required, but the outcome following drug discontinuation is nearly always good.

Pseudotumor cerebri is another potential complication of chronic use of these agents, particularly in individuals treated for severe cystic acne with simultaneous use of isotretinoin. This complication can be induced within several days of initiation of therapy and usually resolves with cessation of treatment.

Chronic use always predisposes to the development of fungal esophagitis, which may be so severe as to require treatment with antifungal therapy. Prompt recognition of dysphagia and cessation of treatment are usually curative.

CHLORAMPHENICOL

Mechanism of Action

Chloramphenicol (*Chloromycetin*) is a nitrobenzene derivative that affects protein synthesis by binding to the 50S ribosomal subunit and preventing peptide bond formation. It prevents the attachment of the amino acid end of aminoacyl-tRNA to the A site, hence the association of peptidyltransferase with the amino acid substrate. Resistance due to changes in the ribosome-binding site results in a decreased affinity for the drug, decreased permeability, and plasmids that code for enzymes that degrade the antibiotic.

The drug-induced inhibition of mitochondrial protein synthesis is probably responsible for the associated toxicity.

Antibacterial Spectrum

Chloramphenicol is a broad-spectrum antibiotic that is effective against gram-positive and gram-negative bacteria, including *Rickettsia*, *Mycoplasma*, and *Chlamydia* spp. Chloramphenicol is also effective against most anaerobic bacteria, including *Bacteroides fragilis*.

Absorption, Distribution, Metabolism, and Excretion

Chloramphenicol is rapidly and completely absorbed from the gastrointestinal tract and is not affected by food ingestion or metal ions. Parenteral administration is generally reserved for situations in which oral therapy is contraindicated, as in the treatment of meningitis and septicemia or when vomiting prohibits oral administration. The biological half-life of chloramphenicol is 1.5 to

3.5 hours. Although up to 60% of the drug is bound to serum albumin, it penetrates the brain and CSF and crosses the placental barrier.

Chloramphenicol is inactivated in the liver by glucuronosyltransferase and is rapidly excreted (80–90% of dose) in the urine. About 5 to 10% of the administered drug is excreted unchanged. Renal elimination is by tubular secretion and glomerular filtration. Other degradation pathways are known to exist and may account for some of the toxicity seen in neonates and children.

Clinical Uses

The potentially fatal nature of chloramphenicol-induced bone marrow suppression restricts its use to a few life-threatening infections in which the benefits outweigh the risks. *There is no justification for its use in treating minor infections.*

Chloramphenicol is no longer recognized as the treatment of choice for any bacterial infection. In almost all instances, other effective antimicrobial agents are available. Since effective CSF levels are obtained, it used to be a choice for treatment of specific bacterial causes of meningitis: *Haemophilus influenzae, Neisseria meningitidis,* and *S. pneumoniae.* Additionally, it was effective against *H. influenzae*–related arthritis, osteomyelitis, and epiglottitis. The development of β-lactamase-producing strains of *H. influenzae* increased the use of chloramphenicol. However, with the advent of third-generation cephalosporins such as ceftriaxone and cefotaxime, chloramphenicol use has significantly decreased. If the patient is hypersensitive to β-lactams, chloramphenicol administration is appropriate therapy for meningitis caused by *N. meningitidis* and *S. pneumoniae.*

Chloramphenicol remains a major treatment of typhoid and paratyphoid fever in developing countries. However, with increasing resistance to ampicillin, trimethoprim-sulfamethoxazole and, to some extent, chloramphenicol, fluoroquinolones and some third-generation cephalosporins (e.g., ceftriaxone) have become the drugs of choice. Salmonella infections, such as osteomyelitis, meningitis and septicemia, have also been indications for chloramphenicol use. Nevertheless, antibiotic resistance patterns can be a problem. As noted previously, nontyphoidal salmonella enteritis is not benefited by treatment with chloramphenicol or other antibiotics.

Chloramphenicol also is widely used for the topical treatment of eye infections. It is a very effective agent because of its extremely broad spectrum of activity and its ability to penetrate ocular tissue. The availability of safer, less irritating instilled ophthalmic antibiotics and the increase in fatal aplastic anemia associated with the use of this dosage form suggest that this agent might best be withdrawn.

Chloramphenicol is an alternative to tetracycline for rickettsial diseases, especially in children younger than 8 years, and alone or in combination with other antibiotics, it has been used to treat vancomycin-resistant enterococci. Another indication for chloramphenicol is in the treatment of serious anaerobic infections caused by penicillin-resistant bacteria, such as *B. fragilis.* Clindamycin and metronidazole are now preferred for treatment of anaerobic infections. Chloramphenicol, in combination with surgical drainage, is useful in treating cerebral abscesses caused by anaerobic bacteria, particularly those that are resistant to penicillin.

Adverse Effects

Newborn infants, especially those born prematurely, cannot adequately conjugate chloramphenicol to form the glucuronide; they also have depressed rates of glomerular and tubular secretion. Because of these metabolic deficiencies, high levels of free chloramphenicol may accumulate and cause a potentially fatal toxic reaction, the *gray baby syndrome.* This syndrome is characterized by abdominal distention, vomiting, progressive cyanosis, irregular respiration, hypothermia, and vasomotor collapse. The mortality rate is high. The syndrome also has been observed in older children and is associated with high serum levels of chloramphenicol.

The presence of multiple metabolites in the serum of neonates treated with chloramphenicol suggests that the biotransformation of chloramphenicol takes place by multiple routes to include oxidation, reduction, and conjugation. The presence of particular metabolites does not appear to correlate with toxicity.

The most publicized adverse affects are those involving the hematopoietic system; they are manifested by toxic bone marrow depression or idiosyncratic aplastic anemia. The bone marrow depression is dose related and is seen most frequently when daily doses exceed 4 g and plasma concentrations exceed 25 μg/mL. The bone marrow depression is characterized by anemia, sometimes with leukopenia or thrombocytopenia, but it is reversible on discontinuation of chloramphenicol.

Aplastic anemia occurs in only about 1 in 24,000 to 40,000 cases of treatment. It is not a dose-related response and can occur either while the patient is taking chloramphenicol for days to months after completion of therapy. The aplastic or hypoplastic response involves all cellular elements of the marrow and is usually fatal. The mechanism is not known, but it occurs most frequently with oral or ocular administration.

MACROLIDE ANTIBIOTICS

Structure

The *macrolide antibiotics* are those that consist of a large lactone ring to which sugars are attached. Antibiotics in this group include erythromycin (*Ilotycin, E-mycin,*

Robimycin), clarithromycin (*Biaxin*), azithromycin (*Zithromax*), and oleandomycin (*Matromycin*). Erythromycin and its derivatives (clarithromycin, azithromycin) are the only macrolides in common use, although the acetylated derivative of oleandomycin (troleandomycin, *TAO*) is available for oral use.

Mechanism of Action

Macrolides bind to the 50S ribosomal subunit of bacteria but not to the 80S mammalian ribosome; this accounts for its selective toxicity. Binding to the ribosome occurs at a site near peptidyltransferase, with a resultant inhibition of translocation, peptide bond formation, and release of oligopeptidyl tRNA. However, unlike chloramphenicol, the macrolides do not inhibit protein synthesis by intact mitochondria, and this suggests that the mitochondrial membrane is not permeable to erythromycin.

Antibacterial Spectrum

The macrolides are effective against a number of organisms, including *Mycoplasma* spp., *H. influenzae*, *Streptococcus* spp. (including *S. pyogenes* and *S. pneumoniae*), staphylococci, gonococci, *Legionella pneumophila,* and other *Legionella* spp. There has been increasing resistance of *S. pneumoniae* to macrolides worldwide. This is true especially if the strain is resistant to penicillin. This resistance includes not only erythromycin but also clarithromycin and azithromycin. Approximately 10 to 15% of *S. pneumoniae* in the United States show complete resistance to macrolides. Staphylococci resistant to erythromycin are resistant to all macrolides. The hemolytic streptococci also exhibit varying degrees of cross-resistance to the macrolides and to lincomycin and clindamycin, although the macrolides are chemically unrelated to the last two agents. There are only minor variations in the antibacterial spectrum of the newer macrolides. Clarithromycin is very active against *H. influenzae*, *Legionella*, and *Mycobacterium avium-intracellulare*, whereas azithromycin is superior against *Branhamella*, *Neisseria*, and *H. influenzae* but less active against mycobacterial species. Clarithromycin and azithromycin have significant activity against *Mycobacterium avium* complex (MAC), and it is one of the drugs of choice in treating disseminated MAC. Both azithromycin and clarithromycin can be used prophylactically in HIV and AIDS patients to help prevent disseminated MAC.

Absorption, Distribution, Metabolism, and Excretion

The macrolides are absorbed from the intestinal tract, although the presence of food interferes with absorption and part of the dose is destroyed because of the relative acid lability of these antimicrobials. To minimize destruction and enhance absorption, erythromycin is administered as a stearate or oleate salt or is enteric coated. Because stearate and estolate erythromycins are not acid labile, the administration of these formulations results in higher blood levels. The *O*-methyl substitution of erythromycin that results in clarithromycin also confers acid stability and better absorption with food.

The macrolides diffuse readily into tissues and cross placental membranes. CSF levels are about 20% of plasma levels, while biliary concentrations are about 10 times plasma levels. Although the serum levels of clarithromycin and azithromycin are low, these antibiotics concentrate in tissue and reach high levels.

Erythromycin and azithromycin are excreted primarily in active form in bile, with only low levels found in urine. Clarithromycin is metabolized to the biologically active 14-OH metabolite and is eliminated largely by the kidney. The half-life of erythromycin is approximately 1.4 hours, whereas the half-life of clarithromycin is 3 to 7 hours and that of azithromycin approaches 68 hours.

Clinical Uses

Although erythromycin is a well-established antibiotic, there are relatively few primary indications for its use. These indications include the treatment of *Mycoplasma pneumoniae* infections, eradication of *Corynebacterium diphtheriae* from pharyngeal carriers, the early preparoxysmal stage of pertussis, chlamydial infections, and more recently, the treatment of Legionnaires' disease, *Campylobacter* enteritis, and chlamydial conjunctivitis, and the prevention of secondary pneumonia in neonates.

Erythromycin is effective in the treatment and prevention of *S. pyogenes* and other streptococcal infections, but not those caused by the more resistant fecal streptococci. Staphylococci are generally susceptible to erythromycin, so this antibiotic is a suitable alternative drug for the penicillin-hypersensitive individual. It is a second-line drug for the treatment of gonorrhea and syphilis. Although erythromycin is popular for the treatment of middle ear and sinus infections, including *H. influenzae*, possible erythromycin-resistant *S. pneumoniae* is a concern.

The new macrolides have similar indications for use as erythromycin but with some additional areas of potential value. Clarithromycin has activity against *Toxoplasma gondii* and *Mycobacterium avium-intracellulare*, and it has expanded coverage against untypable *H. influenzae* strains that predominate in exacerbations of chronic bronchitis. Azithromycin has less coverage against these organisms, and because of its lower peak serum concentrations and prolonged protein binding, it partitions less well across bronchial membranes. The prolonged half-life and protein binding and the use of an abbreviated one-time dose of azithromycin appear to be extremely beneficial in the treatment of sexually transmitted diseases.

Adverse Effects

The incidence of side effects associated with erythromycin therapy is very low. Mild gastrointestinal upset with nausea, diarrhea, and abdominal pain are reported to occur more commonly when the propionate and estolate salts are used. Rashes are seen infrequently but may be a part of a general hypersensitivity reaction that includes fever and eosinophilia. Thrombophlebitis may follow intravenous administration, as may transient impairment of hearing.

Cholestatic hepatitis may occur when drug therapy lasts longer than 10 days or repeated courses are prescribed. The hepatitis is characterized by fever, enlarged and tender liver, hyperbilirubinemia, dark urine, eosinophilia, elevated serum bilirubin, and elevated transaminase levels. Hepatitis has been associated with the estolate salt of erythromycin but not with other formulations. Although the hepatitis usually occurs 10 to 20 days after the initiation of therapy, it can occur within hours in a patient who has had such a reaction in the past. The hepatitis is believed to be the result of both a hepatotoxic effect and a hypersensitivity reaction; this latter effect is reversible on withdrawal of the drug. Erythromycin and derivatives induce hepatic microsomal enzymes and interfere with the actions of various drugs, including theophylline and carbamazepine.

LINCOSAMIDES

Mechanism of Action

The lincosamide family of antibiotics includes lincomycin (*Lincocin*) and clindamycin (*Cleocin*), both of which inhibit protein synthesis. They bind to the 50S ribosomal subunit at a binding site close to or overlapping the binding sites for chloramphenicol and erythromycin. They block peptide bond formation by interference at either the A or P site on the ribosome. Lincomycin is no longer available for human use in the United States.

Absorption, Distribution, Metabolism, and Excretion

Food in the stomach does not interfere with the absorption of either clindamycin or lincomycin. Peak serum levels can be obtained 1 hour after intravenous administration of clindamycin, and approximately 90% of the antibiotic is protein bound.

Lincomycin and clindamycin penetrate most tissues well, including bone. Therefore, bone and joint infections caused by susceptible organisms respond well to treatment with clindamycin. These drugs also concentrate within phagocytic cells, which may offer a therapeutic advantage. Lincomycin and clindamycin do not readily penetrate the normal or inflamed meninges. They do, however, pass readily through the placental barrier. Their half-life is 2 to 2.5 hours.

Both clindamycin and lincomycin are metabolized by the liver, and 90% of the inactivated drug is excreted in the urine. If renal function is impaired, the amount of drug excreted in the feces will be increased.

Clinical Uses

Clindamycin is highly active against staphylococci and streptococci other than enterococci. Also, clindamycin has significant antibacterial activity against *S. pyogenes* (group A strep). However, the adverse reaction of pseudomembranous colitis has limited its use to individuals who are unable to tolerate other antibiotics and to the treatment of penicillin-resistant anaerobic bacterial infections. Clindamycin has shown excellent activity topically against *Corynebacterium acnes* in patients with recalcitrant cystic facial acne who cannot tolerate tetracyclines. Precautions should be given to all patients using the topical preparations, since the development of colitis is possible.

Both clindamycin and choramphenicol have excellent activity against anaerobic bacteria but have potentially life-threatening adverse reactions and should not be used without good justification.

Adverse Effects

The major adverse reactions reported are hypersensitivity rashes and diarrhea. The rash is usually itchy, morbilliform, and general. Gastrointestinal intolerance with abdominal pain, nausea, and vomiting occurs infrequently. Hepatotoxicity and bone marrow suppression have been noted.

It is important to differentiate between gastrointestinal irritation and pseudomembranous colitis. In its most extreme form, the colitis results in mucosal ulceration and bleeding and infrequently may necessitate colectomy. On rare occasions it has been fatal.

Study QUESTIONS

1. Which of the following best treats the initial stage of Lyme disease *in adults*?
   (A) Penicillin V
   (B) Erythromycin
   (C) Clarithromycin
   (D) Doxycycline
   (E) Clindamycin

2. Chloramphenicol is the drug of choice for which of the following?
   (A) *S. pneumoniae* meningitis
   (B) *B. fragilis* in abdominal abscess infection
   (C) *H. influenzae* epiglottitis
   (D) Typhoid fever in the United States
   (E) Typhoid fever in some developing countries

3. A 39-year-old man has AIDS and a CD_4 count less than 50. Recently he has had chills and fever. Several blood cultures drawn especially for acid-fast bacilli are positive. Which antibiotic should be included in a treatment regimen for this disease?
   (A) Tetracycline
   (B) Amoxicillin
   (C) Cephalexin
   (D) Clarithromycin
   (E) Doxycycline

4. A 37-year-old postal worker has a job at a mail sort facility. An envelope that passed through the facility and was delivered to a governmental office was noted upon opening to have anthrax spores. One of the postal worker's fellow employees subsequently developed inhalation anthrax. Because of this, medical authorities recommended that other employees working at the same facility be tested and receive prophylactic antimicrobial therapy. The drug of choice is a quinolone. However, this employee has a history of allergy to ciprofloxacin. Which of the following antibiotics is also recognized as being effective prophylactic therapy for potential anthrax exposure?
   (A) Amoxicillin
   (B) Erythromycin
   (C) Clarithromycin
   (D) Doxycycline
   (E) Clindamycin

5. An 18-year-old man sustains a minor laceration of his right forearm. Approximately 2 days later the laceration site becomes red and swollen. He also begins to develop fever and chills. The patient eventually goes to the local hospital's emergency department. By this point his forearm is swollen and the skin is light brown. Cultures of his wound and two blood cultures 15 minutes apart are obtained. Intravenous cephalosporin is begun. However, over 3 days the discoloration of his forearm begins to ascend to the upper arm and shoulder. Blood cultures are positive in approximately 12 hours for gram-positive cocci in chains. Wound cultures of the laceration also grow similar organisms, and high-dose penicillin G is prescribed. What other antibiotic would be extremely useful in treating this condition?
   (A) Gentamicin
   (B) Clindamycin
   (C) Ciprofloxacin
   (D) Clarithromycin
   (E) Chloramphenicol

ANSWERS

1. **D.** Doxycycline is the preferred parenteral tetracycline for the primary state of Lyme disease in adults and children older than 8 years of age. Penicillin V (A) would be ineffective. Erythromycin (B) and clarithromycin (C) also are not effective against *Borrelia burgdorferi,* the gram-negative anaerobe organism responsible for Lyme disease.

2. **E.** Chloramphenicol is no longer the treatment of choice for any bacterial infection because of the potentially fatal chloramphenicol-induced bone marrow suppression. In the past it has been used against the infections indicated in choices A, B, C, and D. It remains a major treatment for typhoid and paratyphoid fever in some developing countries, since alternative drugs are much more expensive.

3. **D.** Clarithromycin is one of the recommended antimicrobials for use in combination with other antimicrobials in treating disseminated *Mycobacterium avium* complex.

4. **D.** Although ciprofloxacin is the primary agent recommended for prophylaxis against anthrax, doxycycline is an equally effective agent. Amoxicillin (A) is not as effective. The macrolides (B) and (C) also are not as effective. Clindamycin (E) is not indicated for this use.

5. **B.** This individual most likely has a group A streptococcal infection due to a minor wound. Now it appears he is developing necrotizing fascitis, a serious complication. Sometimes when a large amount of group A streptococcal organisms are present, penicillin is not effective. Clindamycin is usually very active against streptococcal infections because the size of the bacterial inoculum will not affect its efficacy. Actually, the treatment of choice for this condition is immediate and possibly repeated surgical debridement of the involved area. Antibiotics are supportive therapy.

SUPPLEMENTAL READING

Boswell FG and Wise R. Advances in the macrolides and quinolones. Infect Dis Clin North Am 1998;12:647–670.

Alvarez-Elleoro S and Enzler MJ. Symposium on antimicrobial agents: Part IX. The macrolides: Erythromycin, clarithromycin, and azithromycin. Mayo Clin Proc 1999;74:613–634.

Kasten MJ. Symposium on antimicrobial agents: Part XI. The macrolides: Clindamycin, metronidazole, and chloramphenicol. Mayo Clin Proc 1999;74:825–833.

Similak JD. Symposium on antimicrobial agents: Part X. The tetracyclines. Mayo Clin Proc 1999;74:727–729.

Standiford HC. Tetracyclines and chloramphenicol. In Mandell GL, Bennett JE, and Dolin R (eds.). Principles and Practice of Infectious Diseases (5th ed.). Philadelphia: Churchill Livingstone, 2000.

Steigbigel NH. Macrolides and clindamycin. In Mandell GL, Bennett JE, and Dolin R (eds.). Principles and Practice of Infectious Diseases (5th ed.). Philadelphia: Churchill Livingstone, 2000.

CASE Study   The Dangers of Vacations

A 28-year-old white man was on vacation for 2 weeks in northern Minnesota in July. He was fishing and hiking in the forest for a number of days. He was healthy, with no known underlying disease or illness. Approximately 3 weeks after returning from his vacation, a red macule–papule developed on his right anterior thigh. Increasing redness developed around the initial site. The central area of this lesion showed some clearing. Several other similar lesions developed on his right leg and trunk. The patient did not note any arthropod bites. Which of the following antimicrobials would be the drug of choice for this patient?

(A) Chloramphenicol

(B) Cephalexin

(C) Doxycycline

(D) Gentamicin

(E) Ampicillin

ANSWER: **C.** The primary stage of Lyme disease is readily treatable with oral antibiotics. Doxycycline is considered to have the best activity against Lyme disease, so it the drug of choice for treatment in adults unless there is a history of allergy or intolerance to doxycycline.

48 Bacitracin, Glycopeptide Antibiotics, and the Polymyxins

Mir Abid Husain

DRUG LIST

GENERIC NAME	PAGE	GENERIC NAME	PAGE
Bacitracin	552	Teicoplanin	553
Colistin sulfate	554	Vancomycin	553
Polymyxin B	554		

Bacitracin and the polymyxins are polypeptide antibiotics. They are relatively toxic drugs and have had only limited use in chemotherapy until recently. Vancomycin, a glycopeptide, although not without side effects, is widely used. Teicoplanin is a new glycopeptide antibiotic that may be beneficial against certain infections caused by gram-positive organisms. The mechanisms of action of this group vary. Bacitracin and the glycopeptides affect cell wall synthesis, whereas the polymyxins affect the cell membrane. Bacitracin and the glycopeptides are used for the treatment of infections caused by gram-positive bacteria; the polymyxins are used for treating gram-negative infections and are active against *Pseudomonas aeruginosa*.

BACITRACIN

Structure and Mechanism of Action

Bacitracin is a mixture of polypeptide antibiotics produced by *Bacillus subtilis*. As with penicillin, it contains a thiazolidine nucleus attached through L-leucine to a peptide composed of both D- and L-amino acids. However, it does not contain a β-lactam ring. *Bacitracin prevents cell wall synthesis by binding to a lipid pyrophosphate carrier that transports cell wall precursors to the growing cell wall.*

Bacitracin inhibits the dephosphorylation of this lipid carrier, a step essential to the carrier molecule's ability to accept cell wall constituents for transport.

Antimicrobial Spectrum

Bacitracin inhibits gram-positive cocci, including *Staphylococcus aureus,* streptococci, a few gram-negative organisms, and one anaerobe, *Clostridium difficile.*

Absorption, Distribution, and Excretion

Bacitracin is primarily a *topical* antibiotic. Previously, it was administered intramuscularly, but the toxicity associated with its parenteral administration has precluded systemic use. The bacitracins are not absorbed from the gastrointestinal tract following oral administration.

Clinical Uses

Bacitracin is highly active against staphylococci, *Streptococcus pyogenes,* and *C. difficile.* Its high degree of activity against the group A streptococci is used in the laboratory as a means of differentiating between the Lancefield group A streptococci and other streptococci.

Bacitracin is well tolerated topically and orally and is frequently used in combination with other agents (notably polymyxin B and neomycin) in the form of creams, ointments, and aerosol preparations. Hydrocortisone has been added to the combination for its antiinflammatory effects. Bacitracin preparations are effective in the treatment of impetigo and other superficial skin infections. However, poststreptococcal nephritis has followed the topical treatment of impetigo, and therefore oral penicillin therapy is preferred. Bacitracin has been used with limited success for eradication of *S. aureus* in the nares. Because of the risk of serious nephrotoxicity, the *parenteral use of bacitracin is not justified.*

GLYCOPEPTIDES: VANCOMYCIN AND TEICOPLANIN

Structure and Mechanism of Action

Vancomycin (*Vancocin*) is a complex tricyclic glycopeptide antibiotic produced by *Streptomyces orientalis,* while teicoplanin (*Targocid*) is derived from *Actinoplanes* (*Actinomyces*) *teichomyceticus.* Teicoplanin has two major components: a phosphoglycolipid (A$_1$) and five chlorine-containing glycopeptides (A$_2$). It is available as an investigational drug.

The glycopeptides are inhibitors of cell wall synthesis. They bind to the terminal carboxyl group on the D-alanyl-D-alanine terminus of the *N*-acetylglucosamine-*N*-acetylmuramic acid peptide and *prevent polymerization* of the linear peptidoglycan by peptidoglycan synthase. They are bactericidal in vitro.

Antimicrobial Spectrum

The glycopeptides are narrow-spectrum agents that are active against gram-positive organisms. Like vancomycin, teicoplanin is bacteriostatic against staphylococci, streptococci, and enterococci. Gram-positive rods, such as *Bacillus anthracis, Corynebacterium diphtheriae, Clostridium tetani,* and *Clostridium perfringens,* are also sensitive to the glycopeptides. The glycopeptides are not effective against gram-negative rods, mycobacteria, or fungi.

Absorption, Distribution, and Excretion

Vancomycin is poorly absorbed from the gastrointestinal tract, resulting in high concentrations in the feces. In neutropenic patients and others with altered gastrointestinal mucosa with denudation, significant oral absorption of vancomycin may occur and may be accompanied by additive toxicity if rapid infusion or large parenteral doses of the drug are given concomitantly. Except for the treatment of staphylococcal enterocolitis and pseudomembranous colitis, it is administered intra-

venously. Peak serum levels are achieved 2 hours after intravenous (IV) administration, and about 55% is bound to serum protein. The therapeutic range is a trough concentration between 5 and 15 µg/mL, and the peak should stay below 60 µg/mL to avoid side effects. In normal adults the serum half-life is 5 to 11 hours. With impaired renal function, the half-life is 7 to 9 days. The dose of vancomycin must be carefully adjusted to avoid toxicity or ineffective treatment, especially in patients undergoing hemodialysis. Pediatric oncology patients with normal renal function may require vancomycin dosage regimens that are substantially greater than predicted. Similar studies in adult patients with hematological malignancies have suggested a larger dosage requirement as well, owing to an increased volume of distribution.

After IV administration, vancomycin diffuses into serous cavities and across inflamed but not normal meninges. It can be used in the treatment of meningitis with susceptible organisms. It is also given via ventriculoatrial or ventriculoperitoneal shunts when these become infected.

Renal excretion is predominant, with 80 to 90% of an administered dose eliminated in 24 hours. Only small amounts appear in the stool and bile after intravenous administration.

Teicoplanin, like vancomycin, is not absorbed from the intestinal tract. Peak plasma levels are achieved about 2 hours after intramuscular administration. The drug distributes widely in tissues; plasma protein binding is about 90%. The half-life approximates 50 hours, which is considerably longer than that of vancomycin, and may make it useful for outpatient administration. Like vancomycin, teicoplanin is excreted by the kidneys.

Clinical Uses

Vancomycin and teicoplanin display excellent activity against staphylococci and streptococci, but because of the wide availability of equally effective and less toxic drugs, they are *second-line drugs in the treatment of most infections.* As antistaphylococcal agents they are less effective than β-lactam cephalosporin antibiotics, such as nafcillin and cefazolin. They have attained much wider use in recent years as a consequence of the emergence of methicillin-resistant *S. aureus* (MRSA) infections, in particular the growing importance of *Staphylococcus epidermidis* infections associated with the use of intravascular catheters and in patients with peritonitis who are on continuous ambulatory peritoneal dialysis.

Vancomycin is also an effective alternative therapy for the treatment of staphylococcal enterocolitis and endocarditis. The combination of vancomycin and either streptomycin or gentamicin acts synergistically against enterococci and is used effectively for the treatment or prevention of enterococcal endocarditis. Teicoplanin demonstrates similar synergy.

Staphylococcal vascular shunt infections in persons undergoing renal dialysis have been successfully treated with vancomycin. Vancomycin in oral form can also be used in patients in whom *C. difficile* colitis is not responding to metronidazole.

Teicoplanin, although not available in the United States, has been used to treat a wide range of gram-positive infections, including endocarditis and peritonitis. It is not as effective as the β-lactams, but its actions are similar to those of vancomycin against staphylococcal infections.

An increased prevalence of MRSA has resulted in a greater use of vancomycin for this disorder. High-grade resistance of pneumococci to penicillin may also necessitate vancomycin therapy. Enterococci that are resistant to vancomycin are emerging as major nosocomial pathogens. These strains are generally resistant to a number of other antibiotics, such as penicillin, ampicillin, and gentamicin, which limits treatment options. The possibility of transferring these resistance determinants to other gram-positive organisms, like *S. aureus,* is a valid concern. It is therefore necessary to limit the use of vancomycin to treatment of serious infections caused by methicillin-resistant staphylococci and situations in which allergies preclude the use of other antibiotics.

Adverse Effects

The major adverse effect associated with vancomycin therapy is ototoxicity, which may result in tinnitus, high-tone hearing loss, and deafness in extreme instances. More commonly, the intravenous infusion of vancomycin can result in chills, fever, and a maculopapular skin rash often involving the head and upper thorax (red man syndrome). Red man syndrome is associated with increased levels of serum histamine. Vancomycin is rarely nephrotoxic when used alone. Teicoplanin rarely causes red man syndrome or nephrotoxicity.

THE POLYMYXINS

The polymyxins are a group of antibiotics produced by *Bacillus polymyxa.* Polymyxin B (*Aerosporin*) and colistin (polymyxin E, *Coly-Mycin*) are used in the treatment of bacterial diseases.

Structure and Mechanism of Action

The polymyxins are polypeptide antibiotics that contain both hydrophilic and lipophilic regions. These antibiotics accumulate in the cell membrane and probably interact with membrane phospholipids. Most likely the fatty acid portion of the antibiotic penetrates the hydrophobic portion of the membrane phospholipid and the polypeptide ring binds to the exposed phosphate groups of the membrane. Such an interaction would distort the membrane, impair its selective permeability, produce leakage of metabolites, and inhibit cellular processes. In the laboratory polymyxin B can neutralize the effects of bacterial lipopolysaccharide (LPS) of gram-negative organisms and may stimulate the biosynthesis of complement component C_3, factor B, interleukin (IL) 6, and granulocyte-macrophage colony stimulating factor (GM-CSF). Its clinical use in gram-negative sepsis has not been established. These antibiotics also are toxic to mammalian cells.

Antimicrobial Spectrum

The polymyxins are active against facultative gram-negative bacteria, *P. aeruginosa* in particular.

Absorption, Distribution, and Excretion

Polymyxin B and colistin are not well absorbed from the gastrointestinal tract. An intramuscular injection of the polymyxins results in high drug concentrations in the liver and kidneys, but the antibiotic does not enter the cerebrospinal fluid (CSF), even in the presence of inflammation.

The polymyxins are slowly excreted by glomerular filtration; the slow elimination rate is due to binding in tissues. Elimination is decreased in patients with renal disease, and drug accumulation can lead to toxicity. Sodium colistimethate, the parenteral preparation, binds less to tissue and is excreted faster than the free base.

Clinical Uses

With the advent of potent broad-spectrum antibiotics, such as the quinolones and third-generation cephalosporins, *the indications for the use of the polymyxins, with their serious potential for toxicity, are few.* Their only justifiable use may be as topical agents.

In combination with neomycin, polymyxin B can be used as a bladder irrigant to reduce the risk of catheter-associated infections, although this use remains controversial. It also can be used as topical therapy in external otitis caused by *P. aeruginosa.*

Adverse Effects

Colistin and polymyxin B can cause extreme nephrotoxicity when used parenterally, and any preexisting renal insufficiency will potentiate the nephrotoxicity caused by these antibiotics.

Neurotoxicity is a rare adverse reaction that can be recognized by perioral paresthesia, numbness, weakness, ataxia, and blurred vision. These drugs may precipitate respiratory arrest both in patients given muscle relaxants during anesthesia and in persons with myasthenia gravis.

Study QUESTIONS

1. A pediatric nurse is found to be colonized with MRSA in her nares during an outbreak investigation in the pediatric intensive care unit. The best strategies to eradicate her nasal carriage could be
   (A) Parenteral therapy with IV vancomycin
   (B) Oral vancomycin
   (C) Bacitracin ointment application to her nasal passages
   (D) Polymyxins
   (E) A month-long furlough from patient care

2. In the treatment of uncomplicated urinary tract infection caused by gram-negative bacteria, the therapy of choice would be
   (A) Teicoplanin
   (B) Bacitracin
   (C) IV vancomycin
   (D) IV polymyxin B
   (E) Trimethoprim-sulfamethoxazole

3. Effective interventions for treating a minor surgical suture site infection should definitely include one of the following choices:
   (A) Polymyxins
   (B) Bacitracin
   (C) Triple antibiotics (bacitracin, Polymyxin B, and neomycin) ointment
   (D) IV vancomycin
   (E) Observation

4. A urine culture in an asymptomatic female patient with an indwelling Foley catheter comes back with more than 50,000 colonies of enterococci. The urinalysis is unremarkable. The best course of action would be to
   (A) Start IV vancomycin to cover enterococci
   (B) Seek the newly approved drug linezolid for possibility of vancomycin-resistant enterococci (VRE)
   (C) Initiate a quinolone like levofloxacin with broad-spectrum coverage for UTIs
   (D) Discontinue use of the Foley catheter if possible and obtain follow-up cultures if she develops symptoms
   (E) Watchful waiting

5. Which glycopeptide or polypeptide antibiotic is still investigational and not used in the United States for parenteral therapy?
   (A) Polymyxins
   (B) Vancomycin
   (C) Teicoplanin
   (D) Bacitracin
   (E) Linezolid

ANSWERS

1. **C.** In an outbreak setting, involved hospital staff may undergo culture investigation of their skin flora and orifices to determine the source of infection. Oral vancomycin is not usually absorbed from the GI tract to be effective, and IV vancomycin is not indicated to eradicate colonization. Bacitracin ointment has been used with limited success and may be an option, along with strict handwashing and isolation precautions. Polymyxins are effective topical agents for gram-negative infections. A furlough from patient care responsibilities is unlikely to eradicate her nasal colony.

2. **E.** Trimethoprim, which exhibits broad-spectrum activity, with sulfamethoxazole is active against most aerobic and facultative gram-positive and gram-negative organisms. It is very effective in UTIs caused by gram-negative bacteria. Teicoplanin, bacitracin, and vancomycin are antibiotics with limited spectra of gram-positive coverage. Although polymyxins are active against gram-negative organisms, their only use is topical because of severe nephrotoxicity associated with IV therapy. Alternative therapy would be to use quinolone.

3. **C.** Minor suture irritation and superficial infection can be treated topically. Effective agents in the absence of culture results would be an ointment such as triple antibiotic, which has gram-positive and gram-negative spectra. Generally, polymyxins are active only against gram-negative organisms, and bacitracin works only against gram-positive organisms. Intravenous antibiotics are not indicated unless this evolves into a deeper soft tissue infection. Observation without any active management is unlikely to be successful.

4. **D.** It is not unusual to get colonized by hospital flora, especially with an indwelling Foley catheter. If the patient does not have any clinical evidence of infection, it is not necessary to start therapy with vancomycin or for that matter, any antibiotic. Enterococcal UTI can still be treated with penicillins, but they are increasingly resistant to penicillins and even vancomycin. Since susceptibility data are still pending, neither vancomycin nor the new drug linezolid is yet indicated. Levofloxacin, although a good drug for UTIs, does not have enterococcal coverage. Discontinuation of the Foley catheter if possible and follow-up appear to be the best option. Watchful waiting may not be effective because these patients may go on to develop complicated UTIs.

5. **C.** Teicoplanin, although used in Europe, is not approved for use in the United States. It can be used to treat a variety of gram-positive infections and should be considered in resistant gram-positive infections as well. Bacitracin and polymyxins are topical agents with potential for serious nephrotoxicity when used parenterally. Linezolid is recently approved for resistant gram-positive infections (VRE and MRSA) and is available in the United States.

SUPPLEMENTAL READING

Garrett DO et al. The emergence of decreased susceptibility to vancomycin in *Staphylococcus epidermidis.* Infect Control Hosp Epidemiol1999;20:167–170.

Healy DP et al. Vancomycin-induced histamine release and "red man syndrome": Comparison of 1- and 2-hour infusion. Antimicrob Agents Chemother 1990;34:550–554.

Hogasen AK and Abrahamsen TG. Polymyxin B stimulates production of complement components and cytokines in human monocytes. Antimicrob Agents Chemother 1995;39:529–532.

McMaster P et al. The emergence of resistant pneumococcal meningitis: implications for empiric therapy. Arch Dis Child 2002;87:207–210.

Murray BE. Vancomycin-resistant enterococcal infections. N Engl J Med 2000;342:710–721.

Robinson-Dunn B et al. Emergence of vancomycin resistance in *Staph aureus.* Glycopeptide-Intermediate *S. aureus* Working Group. N Engl J Med 1999;340:493–501.

Schaison G, Graninger W, and Bouza E. Teicoplanin in the treatment of serious infection. J Chemother 2000;12(Suppl 5):26–33.

Srinivasan A, Dick JD, and Perl TM. Vancomycin resistance in staphylococci. Clin Microbiol Rev 2002;15:430–438.

Yoshikawa TT. Antimicrobial resistance and aging: Beginning of the end of the antibiotic era? J Am Geriatr Soc 2002;50:S226–S229.

CASE **Study**　Endovascular Infection

A 72-year-old male nursing home resident is brought to the emergency department with change in mental status, fever, and shortness of breath. Last year he underwent partial resection of his colon to treat ischemic bowel disease. He receives total parenteral nutrition (TPN) via a central line. His examination revealed temperature 104°F (40°C), heart rate 110 beats/minute, respiratory rate 32/minute, blood pressure 90/50 mm Hg. He was lethargic but arousable. He denied any cough or headache, abdominal pain, or change in bowel or bladder function except that his urinary output has fallen over the past few shifts. Pertinent points in his examination included a supple neck and a central venous catheter in place without any evidence of infection. Heart sounds were normal, without any murmurs, and he reported diffuse nonspecific vague abdominal discomfort without any localization or rebound tenderness. His laboratory findings were WBC 29,000/mm², hemoglobin 13 g/dL, platelets 300,000.

　　Urinalysis showed 2 to 5 WBC with a negative-gram stain and nitrite test. He had clear lung fields with a few old calcific deposits. An abdominal series showed no evidence of obstruction or perforation. You get a call from the nursing home that three of four bottles of blood cultures drawn the day before were positive for gram-positive cocci in clusters. A correct statement with regard to his management is

Because of recent surgery, perforation of the bowels should be considered and an emergency laparotomy performed.

With a chronic indwelling Foley catheter, he most likely has urosepsis.

His central line should be immediately discontinued, and specific therapy with vancomycin should be initiated.

He has aspiration pneumonia. The lung fields were clear because findings on chest radiographs take time to evolve, and film may remain negative at initial presentation.

Discontinue his central line and initiate treatment with IV nafcillin.

ANSWER: This patient has line sepsis. The causation of his infection is not clear initially, and his presentation, without any localizing features, gives rise to the possibility of a line infection. The catheter sites frequently do not reveal any evidence of infection, but high-grade bacteremia (3 of 4 bottles) with gram-positive cocci strongly suggests an endovascular infection. With a high prevalence of methicillin resistance in staphylococcal infections in hospital and nursing home settings, vancomycin therapy should be initiated along with discontinuation of the line. Indeed, the organisms later prove to be MRSA, and neither nafcillin nor any other β-lactam or cephalosporin would be effective in management of his infection.

49 | Drugs Used in Tuberculosis and Leprosy

Vijaya Somaraju

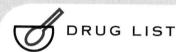

DRUG LIST

GENERIC NAME	PAGE	GENERIC NAME	PAGE
Amikacin	562	Levofloxacin	562
Azithromycin	562	Ofloxacin	562
Capreomycin	562	Para-aminosalicyclic acid	560
Ciprofloxacin	562	Pyrazinamide	559
Clarithromycin	562	Rifabutin	561
Clofazimine	564	Rifampin	559
Cycloserine	561	Rifapentine	562
Dapsone	563	Streptomycin	560
Ethambutol	560	Sulfoxone	564
Ethionamide	561	Thiacetazone	562
Isoniazid	558	Viomycin	562
Kanamycin	562		

Tuberculosis remains the most important communicable disease in the world. The World Health organization (WHO) estimates that one-third of the world's population is infected with *Mycobacterium tuberculosis*. Groups that are at high risk for tuberculosis infection include HIV-infected persons, immigrants from countries with high rates of tuberculosis, the homeless, health care professionals, intravenous drug users, persons taking immunosuppressive agents, and those in institutional settings, such as nursing homes and correctional facilities. Along with the recent increase in cases of tuberculosis, there is a progressive increase in multidrug-resistant (MDR) tuberculosis. Some of the MDR isolates are resistant to as many as seven of the commonly employed antimycobacterial drugs.

KEY CONCEPTS IN THE TREATMENT OF TUBERCULOSIS

The ability of the tubercle bacillus to remain dormant but viable and capable of causing disease is a major therapeutic challenge. The mycobacteria are slow-growing intracellular organisms that require the administration of a combination of drugs for extended periods to achieve effective therapy and to prevent the emergence of resistance. The risk of adverse reactions therefore must be a major consideration in drug selection.

The three basic concepts in tuberculosis treatment are as follows: (1) Regimens must contain multiple drugs to which the organism is susceptible. (2) Drugs must be taken regularly. (3) Drug therapy must continue for a sufficient time. Traditionally, antituberculosis drugs that are classified as *first-line* drugs are superior in efficacy and possess an acceptable degree of toxicity. These agents include isoniazid, rifampin, pyrazinamide, ethambutol, and streptomycin. Most patients with tuberculosis can be treated successfully with these drugs.

Second-line drugs are more toxic and less effective, and they are indicated only when the *M. tuberculosis* organisms are resistant to the first-line agents. Therapy with second-line agents may have to be prolonged beyond the standard period of treatment, depending on the clinical, radiographic, and microbiological response to therapy. The second-line agents include cycloserine, ethionamide, aminosalicylic acid, rifabutin, quinolones, capreomycin, viomycin, and thiacetazone.

FIRST-LINE ANTITUBERCULOSIS DRUGS

Isoniazid

Isoniazid (isonicotinic acid hydrazide, or INH) is the most active drug for the treatment of tuberculosis caused by susceptible strains. It is a synthetic agent with a structural similarity to that of pyridoxine.

Mechanism of Action

Isoniazid is active against susceptible bacteria only when they are undergoing cell division. Susceptible bacteria may continue to undergo one or two divisions before multiplication is arrested. Isoniazid can inhibit the synthesis of mycolic acids, which are essential components of mycobacterial cell walls. The mycobacterial enzyme catalase–peroxidase *KatG* activates the administered isoniazid to its biologically active form. The target sites for the activated isoniazid action are acyl carrier protein AcpM and Kas A, a β-ketoaceyl carrier protein synthetase that blocks mycolic acid synthesis. Isoniazid exerts its lethal effects at the target sites by forming covalent complexes.

Antimicrobial Activity

Isoniazid is bactericidal against actively growing *M. tuberculosis* and bacteriostatic against nonreplicating organisms. The minimal tuberculostatic inhibitory concentration (MIC) of isoniazid is 0.025 to 0.05 μg/mL.

Resistance

The most common mechanism of isoniazid resistance is the mycobacteria's formation of mutations in catalase–peroxidase KatG, the enzyme that is responsible for activation of isoniazid. Another resistance mechanism is through a missense mutation related to the inhA gene involved in mycolic acid biosynthesis.

An active tuberculosis cavity may contain as many as 10^7 to 10^{10} microorganisms. The frequency of isoniazid-resistant mutants in a susceptible mycobacterial population is about 1 bacillus in 10^6, and this organism is readily selected out if isoniazid is given as the sole agent. If a second drug having a similar drug resistance (1 in 10^6) is combined with isoniazid, the odds that a bacillus is resistant to both drugs become 1 in 10^{12}. *Therefore, it is vital to combine at least two antitubercular agents to which the organism is susceptible.*

Pharmacokinetic Properties

Isoniazid is water soluble and is well absorbed when administered either orally or parenterally. Oral absorption is decreased by concurrent administration of aluminum-containing antacids.

Isoniazid does not bind to serum proteins; it diffuses readily into all body fluids and cells, including the caseous tuberculous lesions. The drug is detectable in significant quantities in pleural and ascitic fluids, as well as in saliva and skin. The concentrations in the central nervous system (CNS) and cerebrospinal fluid are generally about 20% of plasma levels but may reach close to 100% in the presence of meningeal inflammation.

Isoniazid is acetylated to acetyl isoniazid by *N*-acetyltransferase, an enzyme in liver, bowel, and kidney. Individuals who are genetically rapid acetylators will have a higher ratio of acetyl isoniazid to isoniazid than will slow acetylators. Rapid acetylators were once thought to be more prone to hepatotoxicity, but this is not proved. The slow or rapid acetylation of isoniazid is rarely important clinically, although slow inactivators tend to develop peripheral neuropathy more readily. Metabolites of isoniazid and small amounts of unaltered drug are excreted in the urine within 24 hours of administration.

Clinical Uses

Isoniazid is among the safest and most active mycobactericidal agents. It is considered the primary drug for use in all therapeutic and prophylactic regimens for susceptible tuberculosis infections. It is also included in the first-line drug combinations for use in all types of tuberculous infections. Isoniazid is preferred as a single agent in the treatment of latent tuberculosis infections in high-risk persons having a positive tuberculin skin reaction with no radiological or other clinical evidence of tuberculosis. *Mycobacterium kansasii* is usually susceptible to isoniazid, and it is included in the standard multidrug treatment regimen.

Adverse Effects

The incidence and severity of adverse reactions to isoniazid are related to dosage and duration of therapy. Isoniazid-induced hepatitis and peripheral neuropathy are two major untoward effects.

A minor asymptomatic increase in liver aminotransferase is seen in 10 to 20% of patients, whereas fatal hepatitis is seen in fewer than 1% of isoniazid recipients. Risk factors for hepatitis include underlying liver disease, advanced age, pregnancy, and combination therapy with acetaminophen. Early recognition and prompt discontinuation of the drug is recommended to prevent further damage to the liver.

Peripheral neuropathy is observed in 10 to 20% of patients taking more than 5 mg/kg/day of isoniazid. Patients with underlying chronic disorders such as alcoholism, malnutrition, diabetes, and AIDS are at particular risk for neurotoxicity; compared with fast acetylators, neurotoxicity is more frequent in slow acetylators because slow acetylators achieve higher drug plasma levels. Isoniazid promotes renal excretion of pyridoxine, resulting in a relative deficiency and neuropathy. CNS toxicity may range from excitability and seizures to psychosis. The neurotoxic effects are reversed without altering the antimycobacterial action by the administration of 10 to 50 mg/day of pyridoxine. Other adverse reactions include gastrointestinal (GI) intolerance, anemia, rash, tinnitus, and urinary retention.

Drug Interactions

High isoniazid plasma levels inhibit phenytoin metabolism and potentiate phenytoin toxicity when the two drugs are coadministered. The serum concentrations of phenytoin should be monitored, and the dose should be adjusted if necessary.

Rifampin
Mechanism of Action

Rifampin is a semisynthetic macrocyclic antibiotic produced from *Streptomyces mediterranei.* It is a large lipid-soluble molecule that is bactericidal for both intracellular and extracellular microorganisms. Rifampin binds strongly to the β-subunit of bacterial DNA-dependent RNA polymerase and thereby inhibits RNA synthesis. Rifampin does not affect mammalian polymerases.

Antibacterial Activity and Resistance

In addition to *M. tuberculosis,* rifampin is active against *Staphylococcus aureus, Neisseria meningitidis, Haemophilus influenzae,* Chlamydiae, and certain viruses. Rifampin resistance results from a point mutation or deletion in rpoB, the gene for the β-subunit of RNA polymerase, thereby preventing the binding of RNA polymerase.

Pharmacokinetic Properties

Rifampin is well absorbed orally, and a peak serum concentration is usually seen within 2 to 4 hours. Drug absorption is impaired if rifampin is given concurrently with aminosalicylic acid or is taken immediately after a meal. It is widely distributed throughout the body, and therapeutic levels are achieved in all body fluids, including cerebrospinal fluid. Rifampin is capable of inducing its own metabolism, so its half-life can be reduced to 2 hours within a week of continued therapy. The deacetylated form of rifampin is active and undergoes biliary excretion and enterohepatic recirculation. Most of the drug is excreted into the GI tract and a small amount in the urine. Moderate dose adjustment is required in patients with underlying liver disease.

Clinical Uses

Rifampin is a first-line antitubercular drug used in the treatment of all forms of pulmonary and extrapulmonary tuberculosis. Rifampin is an alternative to isoniazid in the treatment of latent tuberculosis infection. Rifampin also may be combined with an antileprosy agent for the treatment of leprosy and to protect those in close contact with patients having *H. influenza* type b and *N. meningitidis* infection; rifampin is also used in methicillin-resistant staphylococcal infections, such as osteomyelitis and prosthetic valve endocarditis.

Adverse Reactions

The most commonly observed side effects are GI disturbances and nervous system symptoms, such as nausea, vomiting, headache, dizziness, and fatigue. Hepatitis is a major adverse effect, and the risk is highest in patients with underlying liver diseases and in slow isoniazid acetylators; the rate of hepatotoxicity is increased if isoniazid and rifampin are combined.

Other major untoward reactions are the result of rifampin's ability to induce hepatic cytochrome P-450 enzymes, leading to an increased metabolism of many drugs; this action has especially complicated the treatment of tuberculosis in HIV-infected patients whose regimen includes protease inhibitors and nonnucleoside reverse transcriptase. Since rifabutin has relatively little of these effects, it is commonly substituted for rifampin in the treatment of tuberculosis in HIV-infected patients.

Hypersensitivity reactions, such as pruritus, cutaneous vasculitis, and thrombocytopenia, are seen in some patients, and an immune-mediated systemic flulike syndrome with thrombocytopenia also has been described. Rifampin imparts a harmless red-orange color to urine, feces, saliva, sweat, tears, and contact lenses. Patients should be advised of such discoloration of body fluids.

Pyrazinamide

Pyrazinamide is a synthetic analogue of nicotinamide. Its exact mechanism of action is not known, although its target appears to be the mycobacterial fatty acid synthetase involved in mycolic acid biosynthesis. Pyrazinamide requires an acidic environment, such as that found in the phagolysosomes, to express its tuberculocidal activity. Thus, pyrazinamide is highly effective on intracellular mycobacteria. The mycobacterial enzyme pyrazinamidase converts pyrazinamide to pyrazinoic acid, the active form of the drug. A mutation in the gene (pncA) that encodes pyrazinamidase is responsible for drug resistance; resistance can be delayed through the use of drug combination therapy.

Pyrazinamide is well absorbed from the GI tract and is widely distributed throughout the body. It penetrates tissues, macrophages, and tuberculous cavities and has excellent activity on the intracellular organisms; its plasma half-life is 9 to 10 hours in patients with normal renal function. The drug and its metabolites are excreted primarily by renal glomerular filtration.

Clinical Uses

Pyrazinamide is an essential component of the multidrug short-term therapy of tuberculosis. In combination with isoniazid and rifampin, it is active against the intracellular organisms that may cause relapse.

Adverse Reactions

Hepatotoxicity is the major concern in 15% of pyrazinamide recipients. It also can inhibit excretion of urates, resulting in hyperuricemia. Nearly all patients taking pyrazinamide develop hyperuricemia and possibly acute gouty arthritis. Other adverse effects include nausea, vomiting, anorexia, drug fever, and malaise. Pyrazinamide is not recommended for use during pregnancy.

Ethambutol

Ethambutol is a water-soluble, heat-stable compound that acts by inhibition of arabinosyl transferase enzymes that are involved in cell wall biosynthesis. Nearly all strains of M. tuberculosis and M. kansasii and most strains of Mycobacterium avium-intracellulare are sensitive to ethambutol. Drug resistance relates to point mutations in the gene (EmbB) that encodes the arabinosyl transferases that are involved in mycobacterial cell wall synthesis.

Orally administered ethambutol is well absorbed (70–80%) from the gut, and peak serum concentrations are obtained within 2 to 4 hours of drug administration; it has a half-life of 3 to 4 hours. Ethambutol is widely distributed in all body fluids, including the cerebrospinal fluid, even in the absence of inflammation. A majority of the unchanged drug is excreted in the urine within 24 hours of ingestion. Up to 15% is excreted in the urine as an aldehyde and a dicarboxylic acid metabolite. Ethambutol doses may have to be modified in patients with renal failure.

Ethambutol has replaced aminosalicylic acid as a first-line antitubercular drug. It is commonly included as a fourth drug, along with isoniazid, pyrazinamide, and rifampin, in patients infected with MDR strains. It also is used in combination in the treatment of M. avium-intracellulare infection in AIDS patients.

The major toxicity associated with ethambutol use is retrobulbar neuritis impairing visual acuity and red-green color discrimination; this side effect is dose related and reverses slowly once the drug is discontinued. Mild GI intolerance, allergic reaction, fever, dizziness, and mental confusion are also possible. Hyperuricemia is associated with ethambutol use due to a decreased renal excretion of urates; gouty arthritis may result.

Streptomycin

Streptomycin, an aminoglycoside antibiotic (see Chapter 46), was the first drug shown to reduce tuberculosis mortality. Streptomycin is bactericidal against M. tuberculosis in vitro but is inactive against intracellular organisms. Most M. tuberculosis strains and nontuberculosis species, such as M. kansasii and M. avium-intracellulare, are sensitive. Spontaneous resistance to streptomycin, seen in approximately 1 in 10^6 tubercle bacilli, is related to a point mutation that involves the gene (rpsl or rrs) that encodes for ribosomal proteins and binding sites. About 80% of strains that are resistant to isoniazid and rifampin are also resistant to streptomycin.

Streptomycin is indicated as a fourth drug in combination with isoniazid, rifampin, and pyrazinamide in patients at high risk for drug resistance. It is also used in the treatment of streptomycin-susceptible MDR tuberculosis.

Ototoxicity and nephrotoxicity are the major concerns during administration of streptomycin and other aminoglycosides. The toxic effects are dose related and increase with age and underlying renal insufficiency. All aminoglycosides require dose adjustment in renal failure patients. Ototoxicity is severe when aminoglycosides are combined with other potentially ototoxic agents.

SECOND-LINE ANTITUBERCULOUS DRUGS

Para-aminosalicyclic Acid

Para-aminosalicyclic Acid (PAS), like the sulfonamides (see Chapter 44), is a structural analogue of p-aminobenzoic acid (PABA). It is a folate synthesis antagonist that interferes with the incorporation of PABA into folic acid. PAS is bacteriostatic, and in vitro, most strains of M. tuberculosis are sensitive to a concentration of 1μg/mL. The antibacterial activity of PAS is highly specific for *M. tuberculosis;* it is not effective against other mycobacterium species.

PAS is readily absorbed from the GI tract and is widely distributed throughout body fluids except cerebrospinal fluid. It penetrates tissues and reaches high concentrations in the tuberculous cavities and caseous tissue. Peak plasma levels are reached within 1 to 2 hours of drug administration, and the drug has a half-life of about an hour. PAS is primarily metabolized by hepatic acetylation. When combined with isoniazid, PAS can function as an alternative substrate and block hepatic acetylation of isoniazid, thereby increasing free isoniazid levels. Both the acetylated and unaltered drug are rapidly excreted in the urine. The concentration of PAS in urine is high and may result in crystalluria.

Use of PAS has diminished over the years following the introduction of more effective drugs, such as rifampin and ethambutol. At present, therapy with PAS is limited to the treatment of MDR tuberculosis. Problems with primary resistance, poor compliance due to GI intolerance, and lupuslike reactions have further discouraged its use.

Ethionamide

Ethionamide (*Trecator*) is a derivative of isonicotinic acid and is chemically related to isoniazid. It is a secondary agent used in combination when primary agents are ineffective or contraindicated; it is a bacteriostatic antituberculosis agent. Its exact mechanism of action is unknown but is believed to involve inhibition of oxygen-dependent mycolic acid synthesis. It is thought that mutations in the region of the (inhA) gene that are involved in mycolic acid synthesis can cause both isoniazid and ethionamide resistance.

Ethionamide is well absorbed following oral administration. It is rapidly and widely distributed to all body tissues and fluids, including the cerebrospinal fluid. Metabolism of ethionamide is extensive, and several dihydropyridine metabolites are produced. Less than 1% of the drug is eliminated in the urine unchanged.

GI disturbances, including nausea, vomiting, and intense gastric irritation, are frequent. In addition, ethionamide may cause a wide range of neurological side effects, such as confusion, peripheral neuropathy, psychosis, and seizures. Neurological effects can be minimized by pyridoxine supplementation. Other rare side effects include gynecomastia, impotence, postural hypotension, and menorrhagia.

Cycloserine

Cycloserine is a broad-spectrum antibiotic produced by *Streptomyces orchidaceus.* It is structural analogue of D-alanine and acts through a competitive inhibition of the D-alanine that is involved in bacterial cell wall synthesis. Cycloserine is inhibitory to *M. tuberculosis* and active against *Escherichia coli, S. aureus,* and *Enterococcus, Nocardia,* and *Chlamydia* spp. It is used in the treatment of MDR tuberculosis and is useful in renal tuberculosis, since most of the drug is excreted unchanged in the urine.

Cycloserine is readily absorbed orally and distributes throughout body fluids including the cerebrospinal fluid. The concentrations of cycloserine in tissues, body fluids, and the cerebrospinal fluid are approximately equal to the plasma level. Cycloserine is partially metabolized, and 60 to 80% is excreted unchanged by the kidney.

Neurological symptoms, which tend to appear in the first week of therapy, consist of dizziness, confusion, irritability, psychotic behavioral changes, and even suicidal ideation. Cycloserine is contraindicated in patients with underlying psychiatric and seizure disorders. Other side effects include occasional peripheral neuropathy and low magnesium levels.

Rifabutin

Rifabutin (*Mycobutin*), an antibiotic related to rifampin, shares its mechanism of action, that is, inhibition of RNA polymerase. Rifabutin has significant activity in vitro and in vivo against *M. avium-intracellular* complex (MAC) isolates from both HIV-infected and non–HIV-infected individuals. It has better activity against MAC organisms than rifampin. Rifabutin is active against *M. tuberculosis,* including some rifampin-resistant strains, such as *M. leprae* and *M. fortuitum.* It has a spectrum of activity against gram-positive and gram-negative organisms similar to that of rifampin. The molecular basis for resistance to rifabutin is shared by both rifampin and rifabutin; this explains the virtually complete cross-resistance that occurs between these drugs.

Rifabutin is well absorbed orally, and peak plasma concentrations are reached in 2 to 3 hours. Because of its lipophilicity, rifabutin achieves a 5- to 10-fold higher concentration in tissues than in plasma. The drug has a half-life range of 16 to 96 hours and is eliminated in urine and bile.

Rifabutin appears as effective as rifampin in the treatment of drug-susceptible tuberculosis and is used in the treatment of latent tuberculosis infection either alone or in combination with pyrazinamide. Clinical use of rifabutin has increased in recent years, especially in the treatment of HIV infection. It is a less potent inducer of cytochrome 450 enzymes pathways than rifampin and results in less drug interaction with the protease inhibitors and nonnucleoside reverse transcriptase inhibitors. Rifabutin is therefore commonly substituted for rifampin in the treatment of tuberculosis in HIV-infected patients. Another important use of rifabutin in the HIV-infected population is prevention and treatment of disseminated MAC.

The adverse effects that most frequently result in discontinuation of rifabutin include GI intolerance, rash, and neutropenia. Rifabutin levels will be increased with concurrent administration of fluconazole and clarithromycin, resulting in anterior uveitis, polymyalgia syndrome, and a yellowish-tan discoloration of the skin (pseudojaundice). Other adverse reactions are similar to those of rifampin, such as hepatitis, red-orange discoloration of body fluids, and drug interactions due to effects on the hepatic P450 cytochrome enzyme system.

Rifapentine

Rifapentine is an analogue of rifampin that is active against *M. tuberculosis* and *M. avium*. Rifapentine's mechanism of action, cross-resistance, hepatic induction of P450 enzymes, drug interactions, and toxic profile are similar to those of rifampin. It has been used in the treatment of tuberculosis caused by rifampin-susceptible strains.

Capreomycin

Capreomycin (*Capastat*) is a polypeptide antibiotic derived from *Streptomyces capreolus*. It is bacteriostatic against most strains of *M. tuberculosis,* including the MDR strain. In addition, it is active against *M. kansasii, M. avium,* and in high concentrations, some gram-positive and gram-negative bacteria. Like other antitubercular drugs, resistance to capreomycin occurs rapidly if the drug is used alone. There is no cross-resistance between streptomycin and capreomycin, but some isolates resistant to capreomycin are resistant to viomycin.

Capreomycin is poorly absorbed from GI tract and so must be given parenterally. It is excreted mainly unchanged in the urine following glomerular filtration. Capreomycin is a used as a second-line agent in combination with other drugs. It appears to be particularly useful in multidrug regimens for the treatment of drug-resistant tuberculosis, especially with streptomycin resistance. Capreomycin is associated with ototoxicity and nephrotoxicity, and these adverse effects can be severe in patients with preexisting renal insufficiency.

Amikacin and Kanamycin

Amikacin and kanamycin (see Chapter 46) have been used in the treatment of tuberculosis. Amikacin is very active against several mycobacterium species; however, it is expensive and has significant toxicity. It is considered in the treatment of MDR tuberculosis after streptomycin and capreomycin. An additional use of amikacin is in the treatment of disseminated MAC in AIDS patients. There is no cross-resistance between streptomycin and other aminoglycosides; most *M. tuberculosis* strains that are resistant to streptomycin are sensitive to kanamycin. The latter drug may be preferred over viomycin due to its lower toxicity.

Viomycin

Viomycin is a complex polypeptide antibiotic that is active against MDR strains of tuberculosis. Cross-resistance between viomycin and kanamycin is less frequent than between viomycin and capreomycin.

Clofazimine

Clofazimine has some activity against *M. tuberculosis* and is used as a last resort drug for the treatment of MDR tuberculosis. It is primarily used in the treatment of *M. leprae* and *M. avium-intracellulare*. Further details are discussed later, under the treatment of leprosy.

Macrolides

The macrolide antibiotics (see Chapter 47) clarithromycin and azithromycin have demonstrated in vitro activity against mycobacteria, although they have limited activity against *M. tuberculosis*. Clarithromycin is four times as active as azithromycin against *M. avium-intracellulare* in vitro. Azithromycin's lower potency may be compensated for by its greater intracellular penetration and its two-fold higher tissue levels than plasma levels. Clarithromycin with azithromycin, in combination with other drugs, has gained an important role in the prevention and treatment of MAC in HIV-infected patients.

Thiacetazone

Thiacetazone is active against many strains of *M. tuberculosis*. It is not marketed in the United States. However, because of its low cost, it is used as a first-line agent in East Africa, especially in combination with compounds such as isoniazid. The most common side effects of thiacetazone include GI intolerance and development of rashes. It causes significant ototoxicity, especially when coadministered with streptomycin. *Life-threatening hypersensitivity reactions, such as hepatitis, transient marrow aplastic syndromes, neutropenia, and thrombocytopenia, have been reported.*

Quinolones: Ciprofloxacin, Levofloxacin and Ofloxacin

Most of the fluoroquinolones antibiotics (see Chapter 44) have activity against *M. tuberculosis* and *M. avium-intracellulare*. Ciprofloxacin, ofloxacin, and levofloxacin inhibit 90% of the strains of susceptible tubercula bacilli at concentrations of less than 2 μg/mL. Levofloxacin is preferred because it is the active L-optical isomer of ofloxacin and is approved for once-daily use. The quinolones act by inhibition of bacterial DNA gyrase. Resistance is the result of spontaneous mutations in genes that either change the DNA gyrase or decrease the ability of the drug to cross the cell membrane.

Quinolones are important recent additions to the therapeutic agents used against *M. tuberculosis,* especially in MDR strains. Clinical trials of ofloxacin in combination with isoniazid and rifampin have indicated activity comparable to that of ethambutol. In addition, quinolones, particularly ciprofloxacin, are used as part of a combined regimen in HIV-infected patients.

β-Lactam and Clavulanate Antibiotics

All mycobacteria produce β-lactamase. In vitro, several β-lactamase-resistant antibiotics or a combination of a β-lactam with β-lactamase inhibitors, such as clavulanic acid, are active against *M. tuberculosis* and nontuberculous mycobacteria. However, the activity of β-lactam agents against intracellular mycobacteria is generally poor. The β-lactam agents may be useful in the treatment of MDR tuberculosis in combination with other antitubercular drugs but never as monotherapy.

RECOMMENDATION FOR THE TREATMENT OF LATENT TUBERCULOSIS INFECTION

Recently revised recommendations for the treatment of latent tuberculosis infection (LTBI) include new therapeutic regimens as follows:

Isoniazid for 9 months daily or twice weekly is preferred for all adults.
Or
Isoniazid for 6 months daily or twice weekly is acceptable for HIV-negative patients and is cost effective.
Or
Rifampin and pyrazinamide daily for 2 months is appropriate for isoniazid-resistant tuberculosis.
Or
Rifampin daily for 4 months may be given to individuals who cannot tolerate pyrazinamide.

RECOMMENDATIONS FOR TREATMENT OF ACTIVE TUBERCULOSIS

The most commonly used regimen for drug-susceptible tuberculosis consists of isoniazid, rifampin, and pyrazinamide daily for 2 months, followed by isoniazid and rifampin daily or two to three times a week for 4 months. If isoniazid resistance is suspected, ethambutol or streptomycin should be added to the regimen until the susceptibility of the mycobacterium is determined. This regimen will provide at least two drugs to which the *M. tuberculosis* isolate is susceptible in more than 95% of patients in the United States.

Alternative regimens include isoniazid, rifampin, pyrazinamide, and either streptomycin or ethambutol for 2 weeks followed biweekly with the same regimen for 6 weeks, and subsequently with biweekly administration of isoniazid and rifampin for 16 weeks. In HIV-infected patients the treatment should be prolonged 9 to 12 months or sometimes even longer if the response is slow. Treatment of tuberculosis is more challenging in an HIV-infected population taking highly active anti-retroviral therapy because of drug interactions.

TREATMENT OF LEPROSY

Leprosy is a chronic infectious disease caused by *Mycobacterium leprae.* Host defenses are crucial in determining the patient's response to the disease, the clinical presentation, and the bacillary load. These factors also influence the length of therapy and the risk of adverse reactions to medication. *M. leprae* cannot be grown on routine laboratory culture media, so drug sensitivity testing in vitro is not possible. Growth and drug susceptibility testing are done by injecting into animal models.

One description of a clinical picture that results from *tuberculoid leprosy* is characterized by intact cell-mediated immunity, a positive lepromin skin reaction, granuloma formation, and a relative paucity of bacilli. At the other extreme, *lepromatous leprosy* is characterized by depressed cell-mediated immunity, numerous bacilli within the tissues, no granulomas, and a negative skin test for lepromin. Within these two extremes are the patients with an intermediate or borderline form of leprosy who show a variable lepromin reaction and few bacilli; they may progress to either tuberculoid or lepromatous leprosy.

Current recommendations for the treatment of leprosy suggest multidrug regimens rather than monotherapy because such a regimen has proven to be more effective, delays the emergence of resistance, prevents relapse, and shortens the duration of therapy. Established agents used in the treatment of leprosy are dapsone, clofazimine, and rifampin. Treatment of tuberculoid leprosy is continued for at least 1 to 2 years, while patients with lepromatous leprosy are generally treated for 5 years. In addition to chemotherapy, patients with leprosy need psychosocial support, rehabilitation, and surgical repair of any disfiguration.

Dapsone and Sulfones

The sulfones are structural analogues of PABA and are competitive inhibitors of folic acid synthesis. Sulfones are bacteriostatic and are used only in the treatment of leprosy. Dapsone (*Avlosulfon*) is the most widely used sulfone for the long-term therapy of leprosy. Although the sulfones are highly effective against most strains of *M. leprae*, a small number of organisms, especially those found in lepromatous leprosy patients, are less susceptible and can persist for many years, resulting in relapse. Before the introduction of current multidrug regimens, resistance rates were as high as 20% with dapsone monotherapy.

Sulfones, such as dapsone and sulfoxone (*Diasone*), are well absorbed orally and are widely distributed throughout body fluids and tissues. Peak concentrations of dapsone are reached within 1 to 3 hours of oral administration and have a half-life of 21 to 44 hours; about 50% of administered dapsone is bound to serum proteins. The sulfones tend to remain in the skin, muscle, kidney, and liver up to 3 weeks after therapy is stopped. The concentration in inflamed skin is 10 to 15 times higher than that found in normal skin. The sulfones are retained in the circulation for a long time (12–35 days) because of hepatobiliary drug recirculation. The sulfones are acetylated in the liver, and 70 to 80% of drug is excreted in the urine as metabolites.

Dapsone, combined with other antileprosy agents like rifampin and clofazimine, is used in the treatment of both multibacillary and paucibacillary *M. leprae* infections. Dapsone is also used in the treatment and prevention of *Pneumocystis carinii* pneumonia in AIDS patients who are allergic to or intolerant of trimethoprim–sulfamethoxazole.

Acedapsone is a derivative of dapsone that has little activity against *M. leprae* but is converted to an active dapsone metabolite. It is a long-acting intramuscular repository form of dapsone with a half-life of 46 days. It may prove useful in leprosy patients who cannot tolerate long-term oral dapsone therapy.

The sulfones can produce nonhemolytic anemia, methemoglobinemia, and sometimes acute hemolytic anemia in persons with a glucose-6-phosphate dehydrogenase deficiency. Within a few weeks of therapy some patients may develop acute skin lesions described as sulfone syndrome or dapsone dermatitis. Some rare side effects include fever, pruritus, paresthesia, reversible neuropathy, and hepatotoxicity.

Clofazimine

Clofazimine is a weakly bactericidal dye that has some activity against *M. leprae*. Its precise mechanism of action is unknown but may involve mycobacterial DNA binding. Its oral absorption is quite variable, with 9 to 70% of the drug eliminated in the feces. Clofazimine achieves significant concentrations in tissues, including the phagocytic cells; it has a plasma half-life of 70 days. It is primarily excreted in bile, with less than 1% excretion in urine.

Clofazimine is given to treat sulfone-resistant leprosy or to patients who are intolerant to sulfones. It also exerts an antiinflammatory effect and prevents erythema nodosum leprosum, which can interrupt treatment with dapsone. This is a major advantage of clofazimine over other antileprosy drugs. Ulcerative lesions caused by *Mycobacterium ulcerans* respond well to clofazimine. It also has some activity against *M. tuberculosis* and can be used as last resort therapy for the treatment of MDR tuberculosis.

The most disturbing adverse reaction to clofazimine is a red-brown discoloration of the skin, especially in light-skinned persons. A rare but serious adverse reaction is acute abdominal pain significant enough to warrant exploratory laparotomy or laparoscopy. Other infrequent side effects include splenic infarction, bowel obstruction, paralytic ileus, and upper GI bleeding.

Ethionamide and Prothionamide

Ethionamide and prothionamide are weakly bacteriocidal against *M. leprae* and can be used as alternatives to clofazimine in the treatment of MDR leprosy. Both cause GI intolerance and are expensive.

Study QUESTIONS

1. A 35-year-old man under treatment for pulmonary tuberculosis has acute-onset right big toe pain, swelling, and low- grade fever. His physical examination was consistent with gouty arthritis, and he was found to have high serum uric acid levels. Which of the following antituberculosis drugs is known to cause high uric acid levels?
(A) Cycloserine
(B) Thiacetazone
(C) Pyrazinamide
(D) Rifampin
(E) Aminosalicylic acid

2. A 26-year-old truck driver, a recent immigrant from Mexico, could not obtain a Florida driving license because of his poor performance in red-green color vision discrimination. He denies any family history of color vision–related problems in the past. He is taking a four-drug regimen for pulmonary tubercu-

losis. He does not recall the names of the drugs. Which of the following antituberculosis drugs is responsible for his lack of color vision discrimination?
(A) Ethambutol
(B) Ethionamide
(C) Aminosalicylic acid
(D) Rifampin
(E) Isoniazid

3. A 68-year-old white South African man receiving treatment for lepromatous leprosy has increasing red-brown pigmentation. Which of the following antileprosy drugs is responsible for the patient's skin pigmentation?
(A) Dapsone
(B) Rifampin
(C) Clofazimine
(D) Capreomycin
(E) Thiacetazone

4. A 23 year-old college student is diagnosed with *Neisseria meningitidis* based on his clinical presentation, gram-negative diplococci on Gram stain, and isolation of bacteria from cerebrospinal fluid. Which of the following drugs can be used as a prophylactic agent for roommates and other close contacts?
(A) Amoxicillin
(B) Isoniazid
(C) Dapsone
(D) Clarithromycin
(E) Rifampin

5. A 32-year-old Haitian man has acute-onset confusion and suicidal ideation. Two weeks ago he began combination therapy for multi–drug resistant pulmonary tuberculosis. He has a history of depression that required intermittent treatment in the past. Which of the following antitubercular agents is responsible for the patient's neurological symptoms?
(A) Pyrazinamide
(B) Aminosalicylic acid
(C) Cycloserine
(D) Rifampin
(E) Ethambutol

ANSWERS

1. **C.** Pyrazinamide is known to cause hyperuricemia and precipitate gouty arthritis. Pyrazinamide-induced gouty arthritis does not respond to uricosuric therapy with probenecid but may respond to acetylsalicylic acid. Cycloserine (A) can cause headaches, confusion, tremors, and seizures, possibly secondary to low levels of magnesium in the cerebrospinal fluid; cycloserine should be avoided in patients with epilepsy and mental depression. It is not associated with hyperuricemia. Thiacetazone (B) is an antibiotic that is rarely used in tuberculosis. The most common adverse reactions are general rashes and GI intolerance. Its use is not associated with hy-

peruricemia. Rifampin (D) is associated with hepatitis, GI intolerance, drug interactions and a red-orange discoloration of saliva, tears, and urine. It is not associated with hyperuricemia. Aminosalicylic acid (E) is sometimes associated with sodium overload and fluid retention when large doses of the sodium salt of PAS is administered; it is not associated with hyperuricemia.

2. **A.** Ethambutol is associated with retrobulbar neuritis, resulting in loss of central vision and impaired red-green discrimination. Ethionamide (B) is an analogue of isonicotinic acid and is associated with GI intolerance and peripheral neuropathy, but not the optic neuritis or color vision discrimination problems. Aminosalicylic acid (C) can cause GI irritation and bleeding problems, so caution is required in peptic ulcer patients. It has no neurological side effects. Rifampin (D) is associated with red-orange discoloration of saliva, tears, and urine but not the color vision problems. Isoniazid (E) is associated with peripheral neuritis in chronic alcoholics and malnourished individuals and requires pyridoxine supplements. It is not associated with optic neuritis.

3. **C.** Clofazimine has antilepromatous and antiinflammatory properties. Its most disturbing side effect is red-brown pigmentation of skin, particularly in light-skinned persons. Dapsone (A) can produce rashes and erythema nodosum, including Stevens-Johnson syndrome (dapsone dermatitis), but it is not associated with altered skin pigmentation. Rifampin (B) imparts a harmless red-orange discoloration of saliva, sweat, urine, feces, tears, and contact lenses but is not associated with skin pigmentation changes. Capreomycin (D) is similar to streptomycin and can cause ototoxicity and nephrotoxicity. Its use is not associated with skin discoloration or pigment problems. Thiacetazone (E) is rarely used in the treatment of leprosy. Rashes and GI intolerance are common side effects. It is not associated with any skin discoloration or pigment problem.

4. **E.** Rifampin, commonly used in the prophylaxis of *Neisseriae meningitidis,* is given to individuals who are in close contact with someone having the disease. Other drugs that can be used include ciprofloxacin and sulfonamides. Amoxicillin (A) is used as prophylaxis of endocarditis in patients with a history of endocarditis or a preexisting valvular heart disease. Isoniazid (B) is a commonly used drug for latent tuberculosis infection in high-risk patients who are positive PPD and have a negative chest radiograph. Dapsone (C) is used as a chemoprophylactic agent for *Pneumocystis carinii* pneumonia in AIDS patients who are allergic or intolerant to trimethoprim-sulfamethoxazole. Clarithromycin (D) is used

as a chemoprophylactic agent for MAC in AIDS patients.

5. **C.** Cycloserine is associated with confusion, psychosis, and suicidal ideation; symptoms are usually seen within a week of therapy. Cycloserine should be avoided in patients with psychiatric disorders. Pyrazinamide (A) is associated with a hepatic dysfunction that must be closely monitored. Nearly all patients taking pyrazinamide develop hyperuricemia. It has no neurological side effects. Aminosalicylic acid (B) is associated with GI intolerance, especially acute bleeding, due to severe gastritis. It has no neurological side effects. Rifampin (D) is associated with hepatitis, drug interactions, red-orange discoloration of body fluids, and rarely, a flulike syndrome. It has no neurological side effects. Ethambutol (E) is associated with retrobulbar neuritis and color vision impairment. It may cause peripheral neuritis but is not associated with behavioral problems.

SUPPLEMENTAL READING

Small PM and Fujiwara PI. Medical progress: Management of tuberculosis in the United States. N Engl J Med 2001;345:189–200.

Targeted tuberculin testing and treatment of latent infection. Centers For Disease Control and Prevention MMWR 2000;49:1–54.

Updated Guidelines for the Use of Rifabutin or Rifampin for the Treatment and Prevention of Tuberculosis Among HIV-infected Patients Taking Protease Inhibitors or Non-nucleoside Reverse Transcriptase Inhibitors. Centers For Disease Control and Prevention MMWR 2000;49:185.

Update: fatal and severe liver injuries associated with rifampin and pyrazinamide for latent tuberculosis infection. MMWR 2001;50:733–735.

WHO Expert Committee on Leprosy. World Health Organ Tech Rep Ser 1998,874:1–43.

CASE Study   Genetic Influences on Metabolism

A 36-year-old steroid-dependent man, an asthmatic and injection drug user, presents with a cough, 10-lb weight loss, and general weakness. His recent HIV screening was negative. He is taking oral prednisone 20 mg per day and denies any drug allergies. Upon examination, he appears to be chronically ill with a low-grade temperature of 100°F (38°C). His physical examination produced benign findings except for bilateral rhonchi over the apical lung fields. A presumptive diagnosis of pulmonary tuberculosis is based on the history and the appearance of right apical infiltrates on the chest radiograph. Four-drug therapy with isoniazid, rifampin, pyrazinamide, and ethambutol was ordered along with pyridoxine supplements pending the final culture and susceptibilities.

Metabolism of which ONE of the above-mentioned drugs is genetically predetermined?

(A)   Rifampin
(B)   Isoniazid (INH)
(C)   Pyrazinamide
(D)   Ethambutol

ANSWER: B. Rifampin (A) is known to induce certain cytochrome P-450 enzymes and accelerates the metabolism of coadministered drugs that undergo biotransformation through CYP-450. No genetic predetermination is involved in this process. Isoniazid (B) is acetylated to acetyl isoniazid by *N*-acetyltransferase present in the liver. The human population shows heterogenicity with regard to the rate of acetylation. Rapid acetylators have higher ratios of acetyl isoniazid to isoniazid than do slow acetylators. This genetic determination is rarely important clinically. Pyrazinamide (C) is deaminated by the microsomal drug metabolizing enzyme pyrazinamide deaminase to form pyrazinoic acid. There is no genetic predetermination for this process. Ethambutol (D) is a synthetic antitubercular agent. Orally it is well absorbed and distributed, and about 15% is excreted in the form of two metabolites. This process is not genetically predetermined.

50

Antiviral Drugs

Knox Van Dyke and Karen Woodfork

DRUG LIST

GENERIC NAME	PAGE	GENERIC NAME	PAGE
Acyclovir	569	Lamivudine	580
Amantadine	575	Oseltamivir	575
Cidofovir	570	Palivizumab	581
Docosanol	571	Penciclovir	571
Famciclovir	571	Ribavirin	579
Fomivirsen	572	Rimantadine	575
Foscarnet	572	Trifluridine	574
Ganciclovir	573	Valacyclovir	569
Idoxuridine	574	Valganciclovir	573
Immune globulin	577	Vidarabine	575
Interferons	578	Zanamivir	577

VIRAL INFECTION AND DISEASE

Viruses are obligate intracellular parasites that use many of the host cell's biochemical mechanisms and products to sustain their viability. A mature virus (virion) can exist outside a host cell and still retain its infective properties. However, *to reproduce, the virus must enter the host cell, take over the host cell's mechanisms for nucleic acid and protein synthesis, and direct the host cell to make new viral particles.*

Classification of Viruses

Viruses are composed of one or more strands of a nucleic acid (core) enclosed by a protein coat (capsid). Many viruses possess an outer envelope of protein or lipoprotein. Viral cores can contain either DNA or RNA; thus, viruses may be classified as DNA viruses or RNA viruses. Further classification is usually based on morphology, cellular site of viral multiplication, or other characteristics.

Examples of DNA viruses and the diseases that they produce include adenoviruses (colds, conjunctivitis); hepadnaviruses (hepatitis B); herpesviruses (cytomegalovirus, chickenpox, shingles); papillomaviruses (warts); and poxviruses (smallpox). Pathogenic RNA viruses include arborviruses (tick-borne encephalitis, yellow fever); arenaviruses (Lassa fever, meningitis); orthomyxoviruses (influenza); paramyxoviruses (measles, mumps); picornaviruses (polio, meningitis, colds); rhabdoviruses (rabies); rubella virus (German measles); and retroviruses (AIDS).

Viral Replication

Although the specific details of replication vary among types of viruses, the overall process can be described as consisting of five phases: (1) attachment and penetration, (2) uncoating, (3) synthesis of viral components, (4) assembly of virus particles, and (5) release of the virus. An overview of the viral replication cycle is shown in Figure 50.1.

Infection begins when specific receptor sites on the virus recognize corresponding surface proteins on the host cell. The virus penetrates the host membrane by a mechanism resembling endocytosis and is encapsulated

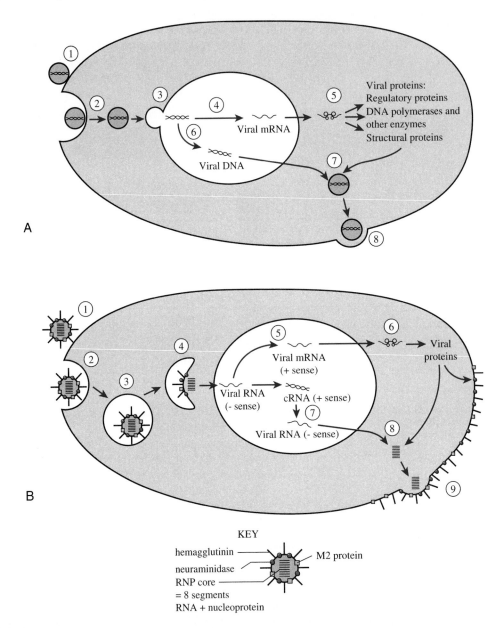

FIGURE 50.1

Replicative cycles of representative DNA and RNA viruses. **A.** Replicative cycle of a herpesvirus, an example of a DNA virus. *1.* Attachment. *2.* Membrane fusion. *3.* Release of viral DNA through nuclear pores. *4.* Transcription of viral mRNA. *5.* Synthesis of viral proteins by host cell's ribosomes. *6.* Replication of viral DNA by viral polymerases. *7.* Assembly of virus particles. *8.* Budding and release of progeny virus. **B.** Replicative cycle of an influenza virus, an example of an RNA virus. *1.* Attachment. *2.* Endocytosis. *3.* Influx of H^+ through M2 protein. *4.* Fusion of the viral envelope with the endosomes membrane, dissociation of the RNP complex, and entry of viral RNA into the nucleus. *5.* Synthesis of viral mRNA by viral RNA polymerase. *6.* Translation of viral mRNA by host cell's ribosomes. *7.* Replication of viral RNA, using viral RNA polymerase, via cRNA replicative form. *8.* Assembly of virus particles. and *9.* Budding and release of progeny virus.

by the host cell's cytoplasm, forming a vacuole. Next, the protein coat dissociates and releases the viral genome, usually into the host cell's nucleus.

Following the release of its genome, the virus synthesizes nucleic acids and proteins in sequence. In DNA viruses, the first genes to be transcribed are the immediate–early genes. These genes code for regulatory proteins that in turn initiate the transcription of the early genes responsible for viral genome replication. After the viral DNA is replicated, the late genes are transcribed and translated, producing proteins required for the assembly of the new virions. RNA viruses have several major strategies for genome replication and protein expression. Certain RNA viruses contain enzymes that synthesize messenger RNA (mRNA) using their RNA as a template; others use their own RNA as mRNA. The retroviruses use viral reverse transcriptase enzymes to produce DNA using viral RNA as a template. The newly synthesized DNA integrates into the host genome and is transcribed into mRNA and genomic RNA for progeny virions.

Following their production, the viral components are assembled to form a mature virus particle. The viral genome is encapsulated by viral protein; in some cases (e.g. adenovirus, poliovirus), it is not encapsulated. In certain viruses, such as the poxviruses, multiple membranes surround the capsid. Release of the virus from the host cell may be rapid and produce cell lysis and death. A slower process resembling budding may allow the host cell to survive.

Overview of Antiviral Therapy

Three basic approaches are used to control viral diseases: vaccination, antiviral chemotherapy, and stimulation of host resistance mechanisms. Vaccination has been used successfully to prevent measles, rubella, mumps, poliomyelitis, yellow fever, smallpox, chickenpox, and hepatitis B. Unfortunately, the usefulness of vaccines appears to be limited when many stereotypes are involved (e.g., rhinoviruses, HIV). Furthermore, vaccines have little or no use once the infection has been established because they cannot prevent the spread of active infections within the host. Passive immunization with human immune globulin, equine antiserum, or antiserum from vaccinated humans can be used to assist the body's own defense mechanisms. Intramuscular preparations of immune globulin may be used to prevent infection following viral exposure and as replacement therapy in individuals with antibody deficiencies. Peak plasma concentrations of intramuscular immune globulins occur in about 2 days. In contrast, intravenously administered immune globulin provides immediate passive immunity.

The chemotherapy of viral infections may involve interference with any or all of the steps in the viral replication cycle. *Because viral replication and host cell processes are so intimately linked, the main problem in the chemotherapy of viruses is finding a drug that is selectively toxic to the virus.* Stimulation of host resistance is the least used of the antiviral intervention strategies.

This chapter focuses on agents used to combat nonretroviral infections. Detailed information on drugs used to treat HIV is found in Chapter 51.

ANTIHERPESVIRUS AGENTS

The following drugs are used primarily in the treatment of herpesviruses. Among these are herpes simplex virus–1 (HSV-1), which typically causes herpes labialis (cold sores) or herpes esophagitis; herpes simplex virus–2 (HSV-2), which is responsible for most cases of genital herpes; varicella zoster virus (VZV), which produces chickenpox and shingles; Epstein-Barr virus (EBV), which is the major cause of infectious mononucleosis; and cytomegalovirus (CMV), which can produce pneumonia, gastroenteritis, retinitis, encephalitis, and mononucleosis in immunocompromised individuals.

Acyclovir and Valacyclovir

Acyclovir (*Zovirax*) is a guanine nucleoside analogue most effective against HSV-1 and HSV-2, but it has some activity against VCV, CMV, and EBV. Valacyclovir (*Valtrex*) is the L-valine ester prodrug of acyclovir. Acyclovir is converted to its active metabolite via three phosphorylation steps. First, viral *thymidine kinase* converts acyclovir to acyclovir monophosphate. Next, host cell enzymes convert the monophosphate to the diphosphate and then to the active compound, acyclovir triphosphate. *Because viral thymidine kinase has a much greater affinity for acyclovir triphosphate than does mammalian thymidine kinase, acyclovir triphosphate accumulates only in virus-infected cells.*

The active metabolite of acyclovir inhibits herpesvirus DNA replication in two ways. Acyclovir triphosphate acts as a competitive inhibitor for the incorporation of deoxyguanosine triphosphate (dGTP) into the viral DNA. In addition, acyclovir that is incorporated into viral DNA acts as a chain terminator because it lacks the 3'-hydroxy group necessary for further chain elongation. Viral DNA polymerase becomes irreversibly bound to an acyclovir-terminated DNA chain and is unavailable for further replicative activity. The effect of acyclovir on host cell DNA synthesis is much smaller than its effect on the viral enzyme. Concentrations of acyclovir significantly beyond the therapeutic range are required to inhibit host cell growth.

In HSV and VZV, the most common mechanism of resistance to acyclovir involves mutations that result in decreased thymidine kinase activity. Therefore, these viral mutants exhibit cross-resistance to other antiviral agents that require thymidine kinase activation, such as famciclovir, ganciclovir, and valacyclovir. Less commonly, thymidine kinase mutations result in altered substrate specificity. A rare mechanism of acyclovir resistance involves decreased affinity of viral DNA polymerase for the drug.

Absorption, Metabolism, and Excretion

Valacyclovir is rapidly and completely converted to acyclovir by intestinal and hepatic first-pass metabolism. The bioavailability of acyclovir following oral valacyclovir dosing is three to five times that resulting from oral acyclovir administration and is comparable to that of intravenous acyclovir.

Acyclovir absorption is variable and incomplete following oral administration. It is about 20% bound to plasma protein and is widely distributed throughout body tissues. Significant amounts may be found in amniotic fluid, placenta, and breast milk. Acyclovir is both filtered at the glomeruli and actively secreted. Most of the dose is excreted in the urine as unchanged drug; a small portion is excreted as an oxidized inactive metabolite. The plasma half-life of acyclovir is 3 to 4 hours in patients with normal kidney function and up to 20 hours in patients with renal impairment.

Clinical Uses

Oral acyclovir is useful in the treatment of HSV-1 and HSV-2 infections, such as genital herpes, herpes encephalitis, herpes keratitis, herpes labialis, and neonatal herpes. In initial episodes of genital herpes, oral acyclovir has been found to reduce viral shedding, increase the speed of healing of lesions, and decrease the duration of pain and new lesion formation. Acyclovir appears to be less effective in the treatment of recurrent herpes genitalis but may be used for the long-term suppression of recurrent HSV.

Intravenous acyclovir is used in the treatment of herpes simplex encephalitis, neonatal HSV infection, and mucocutaneous HSV infection in immunocompromised individuals. Acyclovir ointment is used in the treatment of initial genital herpes but is not effective for recurrent disease. Ophthalmic acyclovir formulations, although not available in the United States, are effective in the treatment of herpes keratoconjunctivitis.

Acyclovir reduces the extent and duration of VZV lesions in adults and children, although higher doses are required than for the treatment of HSV infection. Although not recommended for the routine treatment of uncomplicated varicella in children, acyclovir may be used for chickenpox treatment and prophylaxis in high-risk individuals. Acyclovir accelerates healing in patients with herpes zoster (shingles), but it does not affect postherpetic neuralgia.

Immunocompromised individuals and patients receiving immunosuppressive drugs or cancer chemotherapy have a high incidence of severe reactivated HSV and VZV infections. In these patients, acyclovir has been shown to be effective for the prophylaxis and therapy of HSV and VZV.

Valacyclovir demonstrates efficacy similar to that of acyclovir but requires less frequent oral dosing. While indicated for the treatment of herpes zoster and the treatment and suppression of HSV, it is not approved for use in immunocompromised individuals or for the therapy of disseminated herpes zoster.

Adverse Effects, Contraindications, and Drug Interactions

The adverse effects of valacyclovir and acyclovir are similar. Toxicity is generally minimal, consisting largely of headache, nausea, and diarrhea. Less frequently observed are skin rash, fatigue, fever, hair loss, and depression. Reversible renal dysfunction (azotemia) and neurotoxicity (tremor, seizure, delirium) are dose-limiting toxicities of intravenous acyclovir. Adequate hydration and slow drug infusion can minimize the risk of renal toxicity.

Aside from drug hypersensitivity, there are no absolute contraindications to the use of acyclovir and valacyclovir. Adjustment of drug dosage is required in patients with renal impairment. A potentially fatal disorder, thrombotic thrombocytopenic purpura–hemolytic uremic syndrome (TTP–HUS), has been reported in immunocompromised individuals. Animal studies have demonstrated no teratogenic or embryotoxic effects of valacyclovir and acyclovir. Although there are no large, controlled studies of the safety of these drugs in pregnant women, a prospective epidemiological registry of acyclovir use during pregnancy showed no increase in the incidence of common birth defects.

The potential for drug interactions, particularly with other drugs that are actively secreted by the proximal tubules, should be considered. Probenecid has been shown to inhibit the renal clearance of acyclovir. Cyclosporine and other nephrotoxic agents may increase the risk of renal toxicity of acyclovir.

Cidofovir

Cidofovir (*Vistide*) is an acyclic phosphonate cytosine analogue with activity against herpesviruses including CMV, HSV-1, HSV-2, EBV, and VZV. It also inhibits adenoviruses, papillomaviruses, polyomaviruses, and poxviruses. Activation of cidofovir requires metabolism to a diphosphate by host cellular enzymes. *Because this activation does not depend upon viral enzymes, similar levels of cidofovir diphosphate are seen in infected and uninfected cells.* Cidofovir diphosphate competes with deoxycytidine triphosphate (dCTP) for access to viral

DNA polymerase and also acts as an alternative substrate. The incorporation of one cidofovir molecule into the growing DNA chain slows replication; sequential incorporation of two molecules halts DNA polymerase activity.

Absorption, Metabolism, and Excretion

Cidofovir has extremely low oral bioavailability and so must be administered intravenously. Although the plasma elimination half-life averages 2.6 hours, the diphosphate form of the drug is retained within host cells and has an intracellular half life of 17 to 65 hours. A phosphocholine metabolite has a half-life of approximately 87 hours and may serve as an intracellular reservoir of the drug. Cidofovir is not significantly metabolized and is excreted unchanged by the kidney. Glomerular filtration and probenecid-sensitive tubular secretion are responsible for cidofovir elimination.

Clinical Uses

Cidofovir is approved for the treatment and prophylaxis of CMV retinitis in AIDS patients. It has also been used in the treatment of acyclovir-resistant (viral thymidine kinase-deficient) HSV infections, polyomavirus-associated progressive multifocal leukoencephalopathy, condylomata acuminata (anogenital warts), and molluscum contagiosum.

Adverse Effects, Contraindications, and Drug Interactions

The most immediately serious adverse effect associated with cidofovir therapy is nephrotoxicity. Accumulation of the drug within the proximal tubule epithelial cells can lead to proteinuria, azotemia, glycosuria, elevated serum creatinine, and rarely, Fanconi's syndrome. Probenecid is administered along with cidofovir to block its uptake into the proximal tubule epithelial cells and thereby inhibit its tubular secretion as well as its toxicity. Probenecid carries its own adverse effects, including gastrointestinal upset, hypersensitivity reactions, and a decrease in the elimination of drugs that also undergo active tubular secretion (e.g. nonsteroidal antiinflammatory drugs [NSAIDs], penicillin, acyclovir, zidovudine).

Anterior uveitis and neutropenia are fairly common side effects of cidofovir therapy. Ocular hypotony and metabolic acidosis are rare. Exposure to therapeutic levels of cidofovir causes cancer in rats; therefore, this drug should be considered a potential human carcinogen. Animal studies have also shown cidofovir to produce embryotoxic and teratogenic effects and to impair fertility.

Because of its potential nephrotoxicity, cidofovir should not be used in individuals with renal impairment. Nephrotoxic agents (e.g., aminoglycosides, NSAIDs, amphotericin B, foscarnet) should not be given within 7 days of cidofovir administration.

Docosanol

Docosanol (*Abreva*) is a long-chain saturated alcohol that is clinically effective against HSV. It has in vitro activity against many enveloped viruses, including CMV, influenzavirus, and respiratory syncytial virus.

Docosanol is not directly virucidal; instead, it blocks the entry of the virion into the host cell by inhibiting the fusion of the viral envelope with the host plasma membrane. *Because it does not affect viral replication or protein production, it may be less susceptible to the development of resistance than other antiviral drugs.*

Absorption, Metabolism, and Excretion

Docosanol is topically applied; systemic absorption is minimal.

Clinical Uses

Docosanol cream is approved for the over-the-counter treatment of herpes labialis. It shortens the duration of symptoms of cold sores and fever blisters but does not provide symptomatic relief.

Adverse Effects, Contraindications, and Drug Interactions

Adverse effects of docosanol are minimal. Skin irritation occurs infrequently. Drug interactions are not anticipated.

Famciclovir and Penciclovir

Famciclovir (*Famvir*) is the diacetyl ester prodrug of the acyclic guanosine analogue 6-deoxypenciclovir (*Denavir*). Penciclovir has activity against HSV-1, HSV-2, VZV, and HBV. After oral administration, famciclovir is converted to penciclovir by first-pass metabolism. Penciclovir has a mechanism of action similar to that of acyclovir. It is first monophosphorylated by viral thymidine kinase; then it is converted to a triphosphate by cellular kinases. Penciclovir triphosphate acts as a competitive inhibitor of viral DNA polymerase, but unlike acyclovir, it does not cause chain termination.

Mutations in DNA polymerase or thymidine kinase may result in resistance. *Acyclovir-resistant HSV strains that exhibit thymidine kinase deficiency are also resistant to famciclovir and penciclovir.*

Absorption, Metabolism, and Excretion

Penciclovir is available as a topical cream; its absorption through the skin is undetectable. Famciclovir is well absorbed following oral administration and is rapidly converted to penciclovir by hepatic first-pass metabolism. The bioavailability of penciclovir following oral famciclovir administration is approximately 77%. Penciclovir is less than 20% bound to plasma proteins.

The plasma elimination half-life for penciclovir is 2 to 3 hours; however, the intracellular half-life of penciclovir triphosphate is 7 to 20 hours in infected cells. Most penciclovir is eliminated unchanged by the kidney via glomerular filtration and active tubular secretion. The plasma half-life is increased in individuals with renal insufficiency.

Clinical Uses

Penciclovir is approved as a topical formulation for the treatment of herpes labialis. In immunocompetent individuals, penciclovir shortens the duration of lesion presence and pain by approximately half a day when it is initiated within an hour of lesion development and applied every 2 hours during waking hours for 4 days.

Famciclovir is indicated for the treatment of acute herpes zoster (shingles); it is at least as effective in reducing pain and healing time. Famciclovir is generally as effective as acyclovir in the treatment of HSV. In immunocompetent patients, famciclovir is approved for the treatment and prophylaxis of recurrent genital herpes. For HIV-infected individuals, famciclovir is approved for the treatment of all recurrent mucocutaneous HSV infections.

Adverse Effects, Contraindications, and Drug Interactions

No significant adverse effects to topical penciclovir have been reported. Oral famciclovir is generally well tolerated. Adverse effects include headache, nausea, and diarrhea. Confusion may occur, particularly in the elderly. Hallucinations and urticaria have been reported. Animal studies have indicated that chronic famciclovir administration may be tumorigenic and impair spermatogenesis. Dosage adjustment is necessary in individuals with renal impairment.

Famciclovir may interact with probenecid or other drugs eliminated by renal tubular secretion. This interaction may result in increased blood levels of penciclovir or other agents.

Fomivirsen

Fomivirsen (*Vitravene*), an anti-CMV agent, is the first antisense oligonucleotide to be approved by the U. S. Food and Drug Administration (FDA) as an antiviral therapy. Fomivirsen is an oligonucleotide complementary to the major immediate early region 2 (IE2) of CMV mRNA. *By binding to IE2 mRNA, fomivirsen prevents its translation to protein and thereby blocks viral replication.* Because this mechanism of action is different from that of other antiviral agents, cross-resistance with other drugs used to treat CMV is unlikely.

Absorption, Metabolism, and Excretion

Fomivirsen is injected directly into the vitreous humor of the eye. Animal studies have shown that this drug accumulates in the retina and iris over 3 to 5 days and is cleared from the vitreous humor within 7 to 10 days. Fomivirsen exhibits minimal systemic absorption and is degraded locally by cellular exonucleases.

Clinical Uses

Fomivirsen is used to treat CMV retinitis in patients with AIDS who have not responded to other treatments or in whom other treatments are contraindicated. It appears to be at least as effective as other treatments and produces fewer side effects. Because CMV retinitis is often associated with CMV infection elsewhere in the body, patients undergoing treatment with fomivirsen should be monitored for extraocular CMV disease.

Adverse Effects, Contraindications, and Drug Interactions

Iritis, which affects up to 25% of patients undergoing fomivirsen therapy, can be managed with topical corticosteroids. Vitreitis and increased intraocular pressure may also result from fomivirsen administration. Fomivirsen is contraindicated in patients who have been treated with cidofovir within the previous 2 to 4 weeks because cidofovir increases the risk of ocular inflammation.

Foscarnet

Foscarnet (*Foscavir*) is an inorganic pyrophosphate analogue that acts in vitro against HSV-1, HSV-2, VZV, CMV, EBV, HBV, and HIV. It acts as a noncompetitive inhibitor of viral DNA polymerase and reverse transcriptase by reversibly binding to the pyrophosphate-binding site of the viral enzyme and *preventing the cleavage of pyrophosphate from deoxynucleoside triphosphates.*

Resistance to foscarnet may result from mutation of viral DNA polymerase. Because this drug does not require phosphorylation for activation, thymidine kinase–deficient mutants should not be resistant to foscarnet.

Absorption, Metabolism, and Excretion

Because of its poor oral bioavailability, foscarnet is administered intravenously. Following intravenous infusion, 14 to 17% of foscarnet is bound to plasma proteins. The concentration of this compound in the vitreous humor is approximately the same as its plasma level. Foscarnet accumulates in bone; this property may account for its bimodal initial half-life of 4 to 8 hours and prolonged terminal elimination half-life of 45 to 130 hours. Foscarnet is eliminated primarily as unchanged drug via glomerular filtration and active tubular secretion.

Clinical Uses

Foscarnet is indicated for the treatment of CMV retinitis in AIDS patients. Its effectiveness is comparable to that of ganciclovir; these drugs are synergistic when given to counteract refractory retinitis. A decreased incidence of Kaposi's sarcoma has been observed in AIDS patients who have undergone foscarnet therapy.

Foscarnet is approved for the treatment of acyclovir-resistant mucocutaneous HSV infections in immunocompromised individuals. A clinical study indicated that it is more effective than vidarabine. Foscarnet has also been used for the treatment of acyclovir-resistant VZV and nonretinitis forms of CMV infection, although its efficacy is not so well established.

Adverse Effects, Contraindications, and Drug Interactions

The most clinically significant adverse effect of foscarnet is renal impairment. Nephrotoxicity is most likely to occur during the second week of induction therapy but may occur at any time during induction or maintenance therapy. Serum creatinine levels may be elevated in up to 33 to 50% of patients; this effect is usually reversible upon drug discontinuation. Dehydration, previous renal impairment, and concurrent administration of other nephrotoxic drugs increase the risk of renal toxicity. Infusion of fluids along with foscarnet decreases the likelihood of renal impairment to about 12%. Dosage adjustment is required for patients with renal insufficiency.

Foscarnet is also associated with adverse effects on a variety of other organ systems. It may induce changes in serum electrolytes, including hypocalcemia, hypophosphatemia, hyperphosphatemia, hypomagnesemia, and hypokalemia. Neurological and cardiovascular signs such as paresthesia, tetany, arrhythmias, and seizures may result from these mineral imbalances. Anemia and granulocytopenia occur fairly commonly but seldom require discontinuation of therapy. Headache, vomiting, and diarrhea also occur with regularity. Genital ulceration has been reported and is likely due to high levels of ionized drug in the urine. While studies in rats indicate a lack of carcinogenicity, cell culture studies suggest a mutagenic effect. The safety of foscarnet during childhood, pregnancy, and lactation has not been established.

Foscarnet should not be used in combination with drugs that cause renal toxicity (e.g., acyclovir, aminoglycosides, amphotericin B, NSAIDs). Abnormal renal function has been noted when foscarnet is used with ritonavir or ritonavir and saquinavir. Pentamidine may increase the risk of nephrotoxicity, hypocalcemia, and hypomagnesemia. Caution should be used when foscarnet is given in combination with agents that can cause mineral imbalances.

Ganciclovir and Valganciclovir

Ganciclovir (*Cytovene*) is an acyclic analogue of 2'-deoxyguanosine with inhibitory activity toward all herpesviruses, especially CMV. Valganciclovir (*Valcyte*) is the L-valyl ester prodrug of ganciclovir. Activation of ganciclovir first requires conversion to ganciclovir monophosphate by viral enzymes: protein kinase pUL97 in CMV or thymidine kinase in HSV. Host cell enzymes then perform two additional phosphorylations. The resultant ganciclovir triphosphate competes with dGTP for access to viral DNA polymerase. Its incorporation into the growing DNA strand causes chain termination in a manner similar to that of acyclovir. *Ganciclovir triphosphate is up to 100-fold more concentrated in CMV-infected cells than in normal cells and is preferentially incorporated into DNA by viral polymerase.* However, mammalian bone marrow cells are sensitive to growth inhibition by ganciclovir.

Resistance to ganciclovir has been found in individuals exposed to the drug for long periods and in people who have never been treated with this agent. The principal mechanism of resistance is mutation of the protein kinase gene. Mutations in the DNA polymerase have been seen more rarely.

Absorption, Metabolism, and Excretion

Ganciclovir can be given orally or intravenously; however, its oral absorption is poor (6–9%). Valganciclovir is well absorbed from the gastrointestinal tract and is rapidly metabolized to ganciclovir. The bioavailability of ganciclovir following valganciclovir administration is approximately 60%. Following intravenous administration, ganciclovir is found in the vitreous humor at concentrations approximately equal to plasma levels. Ganciclovir is not metabolized appreciably and is eliminated by glomerular filtration and active tubular secretion. Its rate of elimination is inversely proportional to creatinine clearance. The terminal half-life of ganciclovir is approximately 3.5 hours following intravenous administration and 4.8 hours following oral administration. The half-life of ganciclovir following oral valganciclovir administration is about 4 hours. The intracellular half-life of ganciclovir triphosphate is over 24 hours.

Clinical Uses

Intravenous ganciclovir is indicated for the treatment of CMV retinitis in immunocompromised individuals, including those with AIDS, and for the prevention of CMV infection in organ transplant recipients. Oral ganciclovir is less effective than the intravenous preparation but carries a lower risk of adverse effects. It is approved for the prevention of CMV disease in immunocompromised individuals and transplant patients. It is also indicated as a maintenance therapy for treatment of CMV retinitis in AIDS and other immunocompromised conditions. Ganciclovir is also available as an intravitreal implant (*Vitrasert*) for the treatment of CMV retinitis in AIDS patients.

Oral valganciclovir is comparable to intravenous ganciclovir for the treatment and suppression of CMV retinitis in AIDS patients.

Adverse Effects, Contraindications, and Drug Interactions

Myelosuppression is the most common serious adverse effect of ganciclovir treatment; therefore, patients' blood counts should be closely monitored. Neutropenia and anemia have been reported in 25 to 30% of patients, and thrombocytopenia has been seen in 5 to 10%. Elevated serum creatinine may occur following ganciclovir treatment, and dosage adjustment is required for patients with renal impairment. In animal studies, ganciclovir causes decreased sperm production, teratogenesis, and tumor formation.

Ganciclovir interacts with a number of medications, some of which are used to treat HIV or transplant patients. Ganciclovir may cause severe neutropenia when used in combination with zidovudine. Ganciclovir increases serum levels of didanosine, whereas probenecid decreases ganciclovir elimination. Nephrotoxicity may result if other nephrotoxic agents (e.g., amphotericin B, cyclosporine, NSAIDs) are administered in conjunction with ganciclovir.

Idoxuridine

Idoxuridine (*Herplex*) is a water-soluble iodinated derivative of deoxyuridine that inhibits several DNA viruses including HSV, VZV, vaccinia, and polyoma virus. The triphosphorylated metabolite of idoxuridine inhibits both viral and cellular DNA synthesis and is also incorporated into DNA. Such modified DNA is susceptible to strand breakage and causes aberrant viral protein synthesis. *Because of its significant host cytotoxicity, idoxuridine cannot be used to treat systemic viral infections.* The development of resistance to this drug is common.

Absorption, Metabolism, and Excretion

Idoxuridine is marketed strictly for topical ophthalmic use, and systemic exposure is insignificant. However, after oral dosing, the drug is rapidly metabolized and excreted. It tends not to accumulate in body tissues.

Clinical Uses

The only FDA-approved use of idoxuridine is in the treatment of herpes simplex infections of the eyelid, con-

junctiva, and cornea. It is most effective against surface infections because it has little ability to penetrate the tissues of the eye. intravenous idoxuridine was designated an orphan drug for the treatment of soft tissue sarcoma.

Adverse Effects, Contraindications, and Drug Interactions

Idoxuridine may cause local irritation, mild edema, itching, and photophobia. Corneal clouding and small punctate defects in the corneal epithelium have been reported. Allergic reactions are rare.

Trifluridine

Trifluridine (*Viroptic*) is a fluorinated pyrimidine nucleoside that has in vitro activity against HSV-1 and HSV-2, vaccinia, and to a lesser extent, some adenoviruses. Activation of trifluridine requires its conversion to the 5′monophosphate form by cellular enzymes. Trifluridine monophosphate inhibits the conversion of deoxyuridine monophosphate (dUMP) to deoxythymidine monophosphate (dTMP) by thymidylate synthetase. In addition, it competes with deoxythymidine triphosphate (dTTP) for incorporation by both viral and cellular DNA polymerases. Trifluridine-resistant mutants have been found to have alterations in thymidylate synthetase specificity.

Absorption, Metabolism, and Excretion

No detectable trifluridine is found in the blood following topical instillation of trifluridine into the eyes. Its half-life is approximately 12 minutes.

Clinical Uses

Trifluridine is administered as a topical ophthalmic solution for the treatment of primary keratoconjunctivitis and recurrent keratitis due to HSV-1 or HSV-2. It is not effective in the prophylaxis of these infections; however, it is effective in treating patients who were unresponsive or intolerant to topical idoxuridine or vidarabine.

Adverse Effects, Contraindications, and Drug Interactions

The most frequent adverse reactions to trifluridine administration are transient burning or stinging and palpebral edema. Other adverse reactions include superficial punctate keratopathy, epithelial keratopathy, hypersensitivity, stromal edema, irritation, keratitis sicca, hyperemia, and increased intraocular pressure.

Trifluridine is mutagenic in vitro and carcinogenic and teratogenic when administered subcutaneously to animals. Topical trifluridine was not teratogenic in animal studies. Because it is applied topically in humans, the likelihood of systemic effects is low.

Vidarabine

Vidarabine (adenine arabinoside, *Vira-A*) is an adenine nucleoside analogue containing arabinose in place of ribose. It is obtained from cultures of *Streptomyces antibioticus* and has activity against HSV-1, HSV-2, VZV, CMV, HBV, poxviruses, hepadnaviruses, rhabdoviruses, and certain RNA tumor viruses.

Vidarabine's specific mechanism of action is not fully understood. Cellular enzymes convert this drug to a triphosphate that inhibits DNA polymerase activity. Vidarabine triphosphate competes with deoxyadenosine triphosphate (dATP) for access to DNA polymerase and also acts as a chain terminator. Although vidarabine is incorporated into host DNA to some extent, viral DNA polymerase is much more susceptible to inhibition by vidarabine. Vidarabine also inhibits ribonucleoside reductase and other enzymes. Resistance occurs as a result of DNA polymerase mutation.

Absorption, Metabolism, and Excretion

Vidarabine is administered only as a topical ophthalmic ointment. It has relatively limited solubility and is not significantly absorbed after application to the eye. Within the tissues, it is rapidly deaminated to its principal metabolite, arabinosyl hypoxanthine, which retains some degree of antiviral activity.

Clinical Uses

The principal use of vidarabine is in the treatment of HSV keratoconjunctivitis. It is also used to treat superficial keratitis in patients unresponsive or hypersensitive to topical idoxuridine.

Adverse Effects, Contraindications, and Drug Interactions

The most commonly observed side effects associated with vidarabine are lacrimation, burning, irritation, pain, and photophobia. Vidarabine has oncogenic and mutagenic potential; however, the risk of systemic effects is low because of its limited absorption. It should not be used in conjunction with ophthalmic corticosteroids, since these drugs increase the spread of HSV infection and may produce side effects such as increased intraocular pressure, glaucoma, and cataracts.

ANTIINFLUENZA AGENTS

Influenza is responsible for several thousand deaths each year. Individuals over the age of 65, residents of long-term care facilities, and patients with long-term health problems (i.e., diabetes, HIV or AIDS, heart disease, kidney disease, lung disease, cancer) are at highest risk for severe influenza and complications. Yearly vaccination can prevent influenza infection and minimize the severity of symptoms in those who do contract this disease. However, infection can occur in immunized persons, because influenza viruses mutate rapidly and may not be covered by a particular year's vaccine. The following drugs are used in the treatment of influenza strains A and B and in some cases other viral infections.

Amantadine and Rimantadine

Amantadine (*Symmetrel*) is a synthetic tricyclic amine, and rimantadine (*Flumadine*) is its α-methyl derivative. Both drugs inhibit the replication of the three antigenic subtypes of influenza A (H1N1, H2N2 and H3N2) and have negligible activity against influenza B.

Their mechanism of action involves inhibition of the viral M2 protein, an integral membrane protein that acts as a H^+ channel. Blockade of the M2 protein prevents the acid-mediated dissociation of the ribonucleoprotein complex that occurs early in replication. In certain strains, the pH changes that result from M2 inhibition alter the conformation of hemagglutinin, hence inhibit viral assembly.

Viral resistance develops rapidly in approximately 30% of individuals treated with amantadine or rimantadine. Resistant viruses are associated with the failure of drug prophylaxis in close contacts of infected individuals who have been treated with these antiviral agents. Mutation in the transmembrane domain of the M2 protein is the most frequent cause of resistance to amantadine and rimantadine.

Absorption, Metabolism, and Excretion

Amantadine is rapidly and completely absorbed from the gastrointestinal tract, and peak blood levels are achieved in 2 to 5 hours. The serum half-life of amantadine averages 17 hours in young adults and 29 hours in the elderly. Most of the drug (90%) is eliminated unchanged by glomerular filtration and tubular secretion.

Rimantadine is well absorbed following oral administration, with peak blood levels achieved in 5 to 7 hours. Its elimination half-life averages 25 hours in young adults and 32 hours in the elderly. Less than 25% of the dose is excreted in the urine as unchanged drug; the remainder is eliminated as hydroxylated or conjugated metabolites.

Clinical Uses

Amantadine and rimantadine are used for the treatment of diseases caused by influenza A strains. When these agents are administered within 48 hours of the onset of symptoms, they reduce the duration of fever and systemic complaints by 1 to 2 days and may decrease the duration of viral shedding. Evidence is insufficient to suggest that treatment with these drugs will prevent the development of influenza A virus pneumonitis or other complications in high-risk patients.

The Centers for Disease Control's (CDC) Immunization Practices Advisory Committee recommends annual vaccination as the method of choice in the prevention of influenza infection. However, when vaccination is contraindicated or early vaccination is not possible, amantadine and rimantadine are effective prophylactic agents that have been shown to protect approximately 70 to 90% of patients from influenza A infection. *Since these drugs do not prevent the host immune response to influenza A, they may be used to prevent infection during the 2- to 4-week period required to develop immunity following vaccination.* An additional use of amantadine, unrelated to its antiviral activity, is in the therapy of Parkinson's disease (see Chapter 31).

Adverse Effects, Contraindications, and Drug Interactions

The most frequently reported side effects of amantadine and rimantadine are nausea, anorexia, dizziness, and insomnia. These effects are dose-related and are more common with amantadine than rimantadine. Depression, impaired coordination, confusion, anxiety, light-headedness, urinary retention, and dry mouth are also more frequent with amantadine. High doses of amantadine may produce cardiac arrhythmias, delirium, hallucinations, and suicidal ideation; long-term treatment may cause peripheral edema, orthostatic hypotension, and rarely, congestive heart failure. Abrupt withdrawal of amantadine may produce a neuroleptic malignant syndrome. Both drugs can produce seizures or worsen preexisting seizure disorders. Animal studies have shown that amantadine is teratogenic and rimantadine may be embryotoxic.

Neither drug should be given during pregnancy and lactation. Individuals with congestive heart failure, edema, orthostatic hypotension, seizure disorders, or uncontrolled psychosis should be closely monitored during therapy with amantadine. The dosage of rimantadine must be decreased in cases of renal or hepatic impairment, whereas amantadine requires dosage adjustment only when renal impairment is present. The elderly are more susceptible to the central nervous system (CNS) and gastrointestinal effects of these drugs; rimantadine is generally better tolerated in this population. Individuals over age 65 require half the dose of either drug given to younger adults.

Several drug interactions involving amantadine and rimantadine are clinically significant. Anticholinergic drugs can potentiate the toxicity of amantadine. Thiazide–triamterene, trimethoprim–sulfamethoxazole, quinine, and quinidine increase plasma amantadine levels. Cimetidine decreases rimantadine clearance, and aspirin and acetaminophen decrease rimantadine plasma levels.

Oseltamivir

Oseltamivir phosphate (*Tamiflu*) is the ethyl ester prodrug of oseltamivir carboxylate, an analogue of neuraminic (sialic) acid that is a reversible competitive antagonist of influenza A and B neuraminidase. Neuraminidase, like hemagglutinin, is a viral surface glycoprotein that interacts with host cell receptors containing terminal neuraminic acid residues. The binding of hemagglutinin to its cellular receptors initiates viral penetration and promotes the fusion of the viral envelope to the plasma membrane. Neuraminidase then destroys these hemagglutinin receptors by breaking the bond between the terminal neuraminic acid residue and its adjacent oligosaccharide. The cleavage of hemagglutinin receptors is required for the release of progeny virus from the host cell. It also facilitates the spread of infection by allowing viral particles to penetrate the neuraminic acid–rich respiratory mucus and by preventing the clumping of virus that results from the binding of hemagglutinins to neuraminic acid residues on neighboring viral particles. *Inhibition of neuraminidase activity prevents the release of progeny virus and inhibits viral spread.* The active site of neuraminidase is highly conserved in influenza A and B viruses; thus, oseltamivir and other neuraminidase inhibitors (e.g., zanamivir) are effective against a variety of influenza strains.

Influenza virus resistant to oseltamivir has not been found in naturally acquired isolates but has been isolated from influenza patients who have undergone treatment with this drug. These resistant strains contain mutations in the active site of neuraminidase and are generally less virulent and infective than nonresistant virus. In vitro passage of influenza virus in the presence of oseltamivir carboxylate can produce mutations in hemagglutinin that decrease the overall dependence of viral replication on neuraminidase; however, the clinical relevance of this resistance mechanism is unknown.

Absorption, Metabolism, and Excretion

Orally administered oseltamivir phosphate is rapidly absorbed and converted by hepatic esterases to oseltamivir carboxylate. Approximately 80% of an oral dose reaches the systemic circulation as oseltamivir carboxylate, with peak plasma concentrations achieved within 2.5 to 5 hours. The plasma elimination half-life of oseltamivir carboxylate is 7 to 9 hours. Elimination of the parent drug and its active metabolite occurs primarily by active tubular secretion and glomerular filtration.

Clinical Uses

Oseltamivir is approved for the treatment of uncomplicated acute influenza in patients aged 1 year and older. It decreases the duration of illness by 1 to 1.5 days when treatment is initiated within 48 hours of the onset of symptoms. Oseltamivir is also indicated for the prophylaxis of influenza in individuals aged 13 and older. It reduces infection rates to approximately 10 to 25% of that found in untreated populations; however, it is not intended to substitute for the early vaccination recommended by the CDC. Oseltamivir can be used as post-exposure prophylaxis in household contacts of infected patients, with infection rates of treated patients around 10% of placebo control levels.

Adverse Effects, Contraindications, and Drug Interactions

The most frequently reported adverse effects of oseltamivir are nausea and vomiting. These events are usually mild to moderate, occur during the first 1 to 2 days of treatment, and can be lessened by taking the drug with food. Bronchitis, insomnia, and vertigo may also occur.

Oseltamivir may not be indicated for use in certain individuals. Its efficacy in patients with chronic cardiac or respiratory disease has not been established. In clinical trials, no difference in the incidence of complications was seen between treatment and control groups. The efficacy of oseltamivir has not been demonstrated in immunocompromised patients, patients who begin treatment after 40 hours of symptoms, or patients given repeated prophylactic courses of therapy. Dosage adjustment is recommended for individuals with renal insufficiency; the drug's safety in patients with hepatic insufficiency is unknown.

No formal drug interaction studies of oseltamivir have been performed. Oseltamivir and its carboxylate metabolite do not interact with the cytochrome P450 system. Although probenecid decreases the elimination of oseltamivir, dosage adjustment is not required during coadministration of these drugs because of oseltamivir's margin of safety. Oseltamivir does not interfere with antibody production in response to the influenza vaccine.

Zanamivir

Zanamivir (*Relenza*) is a neuraminidase inhibitor with activity against influenza A and B strains. Like oseltamivir, zanamivir is a reversible competitive antagonist of viral neuraminidase. It inhibits the release of progeny virus, causes viral aggregation at the cell surface, and impairs viral movement through respiratory secretions. Resistant variants with hemagglutinin and/or neuraminidase mutations have been produced in vivo; however, clinical resistance to zanamivir is quite rare at present.

Absorption, Metabolism, and Excretion

Zanamivir has a bioavailability of less than 5% when absorbed through the gastrointestinal tract. It is administered using a breath-actuated inhaler device (*Diskhaler*) that delivers the drug as an aerosol in a lactose carrier. The lactose particles are large, and about 78% deposit in the oropharynx. Following oral inhalation, zanamivir has a bioavailability of 12 to 17%, with peak plasma concentrations being reached within 1.5 hours. It is rapidly eliminated by the kidneys without significant metabolism and has a plasma elimination half-life of 2.5 to 5 hours.

Clinical Uses

Zanamivir is indicated for treatment of uncomplicated acute influenza A and B virus in patients aged 7 and older. Treatment should be initiated no later than 2 days after the onset of symptoms. Zanamivir shortens the duration of illness by 1 to 1.5 days. It is also an effective prophylaxis against influenza; however, the FDA has not approved this indication at the time of publication.

Adverse Effects, Contraindications, and Drug Interactions

Zanamivir is generally well tolerated. Bronchospasm and impaired lung function have been reported in some patients taking this medication, but many of these individuals had serious underlying pulmonary disease. Zanamivir should be discontinued if an individual develops bronchospasm or breathing difficulties; treatment and hospitalization may be required. Allergic reactions, including angioedema, have been rarely reported. The efficacy of zanamivir depends upon the proper use of the inhaler device.

Zanamivir is contraindicated in individuals with severe or decompensated chronic obstructive lung disease or asthma because it has not been shown to be effective in these individuals and can cause serious adverse pulmonary reactions. Individuals with mild to moderate asthma may have a decline in lung function when taking zanamivir. The safety and efficacy of this medication have not been determined in individuals with severe renal insufficiency. No clinically significant drug interactions have been reported. Zanamivir does not decrease the effectiveness of the influenza vaccine.

OTHER ANTIVIRAL AGENTS

The drugs described next are used in the treatment in a variety of viral conditions, including HBV, hepatitis C virus (HCV), respiratory syncytial virus (RSV), human papilloma virus (HPV), and VZV. Some are also used in the therapy of HIV infection; detailed information on the treatment of this disease is found in Chapter 51.

Immune Globulin

Immune globulin (γ-globulin, immunoglobulin [Ig] G) is a fraction obtained from the plasma of normal individuals and is rich in antibodies found in whole blood.

It consists primarily of IgG and contains trace amounts of IgA and IgM. *γ-Globulin provides the patient with passive immunity and does not require time for the development of an antibody response.* It is believed to inhibit viral penetration of host cells, opsonize viral particles, activate complement, and stimulate cell-mediated immunity.

Absorption, Metabolism, and Excretion

γ-Globulin is administered parenterally. Intramuscular or intravenous injections are given during the early infectious stage to alleviate the progression of certain viral disorders. Protection lasts for 2 to 3 weeks after a single injection, although for prolonged infections, injections can be repeated every 2 to 3 weeks.

Clinical Uses

Human immune globulin preparations specifically for the treatment and/or prevention of CMV (*CytoGam*), HBV (*BayHep B*), rabies (*BayRab*), RSV (*RespiGam*), and VZV (*VZIG*) are obtained from individuals with high titers of antibodies against these viruses. A pooled heterogeneous human immune globulin solution (*BayGam, Gamimmune*, others) can be used to lessen the likelihood of measles, varicella, or rubella infection in individuals exposed to these viruses. Immune globulin also can be used as an adjunctive form of therapy with other therapeutic approaches.

Adverse Effects, Contraindications, and Drug Interactions

Hypersensitivity reactions (e.g., anaphylaxis, angioedema) associated with γ-globulin are rare but occur most commonly in individuals with agammaglobulinemia, severe hypogammaglobulinemia, or IgA deficiency. The likelihood of anaphylactoid reaction increases following repeated dosing and for certain preparations, intravenous administration. Immune globulins can also cause urticaria, angioedema, fever, and injection site reactions. Preparations that are administered intravenously (e.g., RSV immune globulin) can produce infusion-related side effects such as flushing, dizziness, blood pressure changes, palpitations, abdominal cramps, and dyspnea; slowing the infusion rate may reduce the severity of these effects. High doses of immune globulins have been associated with rare cases of aseptic meningitis syndrome. A possibility of infection by blood-borne pathogens exists with immune globulin and other human blood products. Although preparations are screened for contamination and viral inactivation processes are used, the risk of transmission of new or undetected pathogens cannot be eliminated.

Treatment with immune globulin can interfere with the response to live virus vaccines (e.g., measles, mumps, rubella). Vaccinations should be deferred until several months after the administration of γ-globulin because the antibodies contained in this preparation may interfere with the development of the host immune response. Individuals who were vaccinated shortly before receiving immune globulin may require revaccination at a later time.

Interferons

The enhanced production of the cytokines called *interferons* is one of the body's earliest responses to a viral infection. These endogenous proteins exert potent antiviral, immunoregulatory, and antiproliferative effects and are classified according to the cell type from which they were initially derived. Interferon-α (type I, leukocyte) and interferon β-β (type I, fibroblast) are synthesized by most types of cells in response to viral infection, certain cytokines, and double-stranded RNA. Interferon-γ (type II, immune) is produced by natural killer (NK) cells and T lymphocytes in response to antigens, mitogens, and certain cytokines. Interferon-α and interferon-β exert the most potent antiviral effects; interferon-γ is antiviral and strongly immunomodulatory.

Although interferons do not directly interact with viral particles, they exert a complex range of effects on virus-infected cells that result in the inhibition of viral penetration, uncoating, mRNA synthesis, translation, and/or virion assembly and release. Interferons bind to cell surface receptors and initiate the JAK-STAT signal transduction pathway. This leads to the induction of numerous proteins, including 2'-5'-oligoadenylate synthetase (2'-5'OAS) and interferon-induced protein kinase. 2'-5'OAS initiates the activation of a cellular ribonuclease that cleaves single-stranded RNAs, and interferon-induced protein kinase phosphorylates and inactivates an elongation factor (eIF-2) involved in translation. Interferons also induce the production of inflammatory cytokines and biological oxidants that further enhance the host immune response. Viral families differ with respect to the step or steps at which interferons exert their effects. Certain viruses are resistant to interferons because they produce proteins that counteract interferon's effects.

Absorption, Metabolism, and Excretion

Natural interferons produced by human leukocytes, recombinant interferons produced in bacteria, and recombinant interferons conjugated to monomethoxy polyethylene glycol (PEG; pegylated interferons) are available in the United States. The various preparations may be administered subcutaneously, intramuscularly, intravenously, or intralesionally (e.g., into genital warts). Natural or recombinant interferons typically achieve peak plasma levels within 4 to 8 hours of subcutaneous or intramuscular injection and are undetectable in the bloodstream within 16 to 36 hours. Maximal plasma concentrations of pegylated interferons are reached 15 to 44 hours after subcutaneous or intramuscular injection and are sustained for much longer than nonpegylated preparations (48 to 72 hours). Intralesional injection of interferons results in negligible systemic absorption. Interferons are eliminated from the bloodstream by a combination of cellular uptake and catabolism in the kidney and liver. Minimal amounts of intact protein are excreted in the urine or feces.

Clinical Uses

Interferon-α-2a (*Roferon-A*) is approved for the treatment of chronic hepatitis C, hairy cell leukemia, AIDS-related Kaposi's sarcoma, and chronic phase Philadelphia chromosome–positive chronic myelogenous leukemia. Interferon-α-2b (*Intron A*) is indicated for hairy cell leukemia, malignant melanoma, follicular lymphoma, condylomata acuminata, AIDS-related Kaposi's sarcoma, and chronic hepatitis B and C. A combination of interferon-α-2b and ribavirin (*Rebetron*) is used for the treatment of chronic hepatitis C. Interferon-α-n3 (*Alferon N*) is a solution of purified natural human interferon-αproteins approved for the treatment of condylomata acuminata by intralesional injection. Interferon alfacon-1 (*Infergen*) is a recombinant interferon constructed from the sequences of several naturally occurring interferon-αsubtypes. This recombinant protein contains the most frequently observed amino acid in each position of the sequence and exhibits in vitro specific activity at least 5 times higher than that of interferon α-2a or -2b. Interferon alfacon-1 and peg interferon-α-2b (*PEG-Intron*) are approved for the treatment of chronic hepatitis C.

Interferon β-1a (*Avonex*) and interferon β-1b (*Betaseron*) are used in the treatment of multiple sclerosis. Interferon γ-1b (*Actimmune*) is used to prevent and diminish the severity of infections associated with chronic granulomatous disease and for delaying the progression of severe, malignant osteopetrosis.

Adverse Effects, Contraindications, and Drug Interactions

Flulike symptoms, including fever, chills, weakness, fatigue, myalgia, and arthralgia, are the most common side effects of interferon therapy. These symptoms occur in more than 50% of patients given injections of interferons either intravenously, intramuscularly, or subcutaneously. Intralesional injection may produce milder flulike symptoms with somewhat less frequency. Tolerance to these symptoms generally develops with repeated dosing.

Interferons are associated with a diverse range of common adverse effects. CNS complaints such as headache, dizziness, impaired memory and concentration, agitation, insomnia, and anxiety occur with regularity. Depression is a common side effect of interferon-α and interferon-β. Suicidal behavior, although rare, can arise in depressed patients; therefore, these individuals should be closely monitored. Myelosuppression occurs frequently and may be dose limiting; potentially fatal aplastic anemia is rare. Gastrointestinal symptoms such as nausea, vomiting, diarrhea, and anorexia are common; however, ulcerative colitis, pancreatitis, hyperglycemia, and diabetes mellitus are rare. Elevation of hepatic enzymes can occur but rarely necessitate discontinuation of treatment. Injection site reaction is common, as is alopecia, for certain interferon preparations. Interferons can decrease fertility and may cause miscarriage at high doses.

Infrequent reactions to interferon therapy include proteinuria, renal toxicity, autoimmune disease, thyroid disease, ophthalmic toxicity, pulmonary dysfunction (pulmonary infiltrates, pneumonitis, and pneumonia), and cardiovascular effects (tachycardia, arrhythmia, hypotension, cardiomyopathy, and myocardial infarction). Rarely, the body may develop antibodies against interferons that inhibit their effectiveness.

Interferons are contraindicated in individuals with autoimmune hepatitis or other autoimmune disease, uncontrolled thyroid disease, severe cardiac disease, severe renal or hepatic impairment, seizure disorders, and CNS dysfunction. Immunosuppressed transplant recipients should not receive interferons. Interferons should be used with caution in persons who have myelosuppression or who are taking myelosuppressive drugs. Preparations containing benzyl alcohol are associated with neurotoxicity, organ failure, and death in neonates and infants and therefore are contraindicated in this population. Interferons should be used during pregnancy only if the potential benefit justifies the potential risk to the fetus.

Interferons reduce the activity of hepatic cytochrome P450 enzymes and decrease the clearance of drugs such as theophylline. Their effects may be additive with other drugs that have neurotoxic, hematotoxic or cardiotoxic activity.

Ribavirin

Ribavirin is a synthetic guanosine analogue that possesses broad antiviral inhibitory activity against many viruses, including influenza A and B, parainfluenza, RSV, HCV, HIV-1, and various herpesviruses, arenaviruses, and paramyxoviruses. Its exact mechanism of action has not been fully elucidated; however, it appears to inhibit the synthesis of viral mRNA through an effect on nucleotide pools. Following absorption, host cell enzymes convert ribavirin to its monophosphate, diphosphate, and triphosphate forms. Ribavirin monophosphate inhibits the guanosine triphosphate (GTP) synthesis pathway and subsequently inhibits many GTP-dependent processes. Ribavirin triphosphate inhibits the 5′capping of viral mRNA with GTP and specifically inhibits influenza virus RNA polymerase. Ribavirin may also act by increasing the mutation rate of RNA viruses, leading to the production of nonviable progeny virions. Ribavirin resistance has not been documented in clinical isolates.

Absorption, Metabolism, and Excretion

Ribavirin can be administered as an aerosol using a small-particle aerosol generator. When administered by this route, the drug has only minimal systemic absorption, with drug concentrations in respiratory tract secretions approximately 100 times as high as those found in plasma. Oral absorption is rapid, and first-pass metabolism is extensive; ribavirin's oral bioavailability is 64% and can be increased by administration with a high-fat meal. Steady-state levels are reached after 4 weeks.

Ribavirin is reversibly phosphorylated by all nucleated cells. It is also metabolized in the liver to a triazole carboxylic acid metabolite that is eliminated in the urine along with the parent compound. The plasma half-life of ribavirin is 9.5 hours when it is administered by aerosol (2.5 hours/day for 3 days), whereas its half-life is around 12.5 days at steady state. The drug accumulates in erythrocytes, with a half-life of 40 days.

Clinical Uses

Ribavirin aerosol (*Virazole*) is indicated in the treatment of high-risk infants and young children with severe bronchiolitis or pneumonia due to RSV infection. Treatment is most effective if begun within 3 days of the onset of symptoms.

Although ribavirin monotherapy is ineffective against HCV, oral ribavirin in combination with interferon-α (*Rebatron*) is approved for this indication and is effective in patients resistant to interferon therapy alone. Intravenous ribavirin may be useful in the therapy of Hantaan virus infection, Crimean or Congo virus hemorrhagic fever, Lassa fever, and severe adenovirus infection.

Adverse Effects, Contraindications, and Drug Interactions

Most adverse effects associated with aerosol ribavirin are local. Pulmonary function may decline if aerosol ribavirin is used in adults with chronic obstructive lung disease or asthma. Deterioration of pulmonary and cardiovascular function has also been seen in severely ill infants given this preparation. Rash, conjunctivitis, and rare cases of anemia have been reported. Health care workers exposed to aerosol ribavirin during its adminis-

tration have reported adverse effects including headache, conjunctivitis, rash, and rarely, bronchospasm.

Oral and intravenous ribavirin are associated with additional adverse effects. When given via these routes, ribavirin can produce hemolytic anemia that is reversible following dosage reduction or cessation of therapy. When given in combination with interferon-α, ribavirin increases the incidence of many of its side effects, such as fatigue, nausea, insomnia, depression, and anemia, and may cause fatal or nonfatal pancreatitis. Ribavirin is mutagenic, teratogenic, and embryotoxic in animals at doses below the therapeutic level in humans. *It is contraindicated in pregnant women and in the male partners of pregnant women.* Women of childbearing potential and male partners of these women must use two effective forms of contraception during ribavirin treatment and for 6 months post therapy. Pregnant women should not directly care for patients receiving ribavirin.

Ribavirin is contraindicated in patients with sickle cell anemia and other hemoglobinopathies because of its propensity to cause anemia. Similarly, persons with coronary disease should not use ribavirin, because anemia may cause deterioration of cardiac function. Oral ribavirin should not be given to individuals with severe renal impairment; no dosage adjustment is necessary for the inhaled formulation. However, patients with hepatic impairment may require dosage adjustment.

Little information on the drug interactions of ribavirin is available. In vitro, ribavirin inhibits the phosphorylation reactions that are required for activation of zidovudine and stavudine.

Lamivudine

Lamivudine is a synthetic cytidine analogue used in the treatment of HIV (see Chapter 51) and HBV. Its activation requires phosphorylation by cellular enzymes. Lamivudine triphosphate competitively inhibits HBV DNA polymerase and HIV reverse transcriptase and causes chain termination. It inhibits the activity of mammalian DNA polymerases with a much lower potency.

HIV-1 frequently acquires mutations in reverse transcriptase that result in resistance to lamivudine within 12 weeks of treatment. Mutations in the DNA polymerase of HBV are associated with decreased lamivudine efficacy and have been documented in patients treated with this agent for 6 months or more.

Absorption, Metabolism, and Excretion

Lamivudine is rapidly absorbed from the gastrointestinal tract and has an oral bioavailability of approximately 85 to 90%. Lamivudine is mainly excreted unchanged by the kidney and has an elimination half-life of 5 to 7 hours.

Clinical Uses

Lamivudine is indicated for the treatment of HIV when used in combination with other antiretroviral agents. A lower dose than that used to treat HIV is approved for the treatment of HBV. Although lamivudine initially improves histological and biochemical measures of hepatic function and reduces HBV DNA to below the limits of detection, withdrawal of the drug usually results in disease recurrence. Resistance appears in up to one-third of patients after 1 year of treatment.

Adverse Effects, Contraindications, and Drug Interactions

The most common adverse effects of lamivudine seen at doses used to treat HBV are mild; they include headache, malaise, fatigue, fever, insomnia, diarrhea, and upper respiratory infections. Elevated alanine aminotransferase (ALT), serum lipase, and creatine kinase may also occur. The safety and efficacy of lamivudine in patients with decompensated liver disease have not been established. Dosage adjustment is required in individuals with renal impairment. Coadministration of trimethoprim–sulfamethoxazole decreases the renal clearance of lamivudine.

Palivizumab

Palivizumab (*Synagis*) is a humanized monoclonal antibody directed against the highly conserved A antigenic site of the F protein on the surface of RSV. It contains 95% human and 5% murine antibody sequences and tends to have little immunogenicity in humans. Palivizumab is composed of the human framework region of the IgG-1 κ-chain joined to the antigen-binding regions of a mouse monoclonal antibody. *Palivizumab neutralizes RSV and inhibits its ability to fuse with host cell membranes.* Resistant strains of RSV have been derived in vitro but have not been found in clinical isolates to date.

Absorption, Metabolism, and Excretion

Palivizumab is administered prophylactically as a monthly intramuscular injection prior to and during RSV season (November to April in the northern hemisphere). The half-life of palivizumab is approximately 20 days.

Clinical Uses

Palivizumab is used to prevent serious lower respiratory tract infection due to RSV. It is used only in high-risk children who are younger than 24 months of age and have bronchopulmonary dysplasia or chronic lung disease that required treatment in the previous 6 months. It is also indicated for premature infants (less than 32 weeks' gestation) until the age of 6 to 12 months. Palivizumab can reduce the incidence of RSV-related hospitalization by approximately half. The safety and efficacy of palivizumab in the treatment of RSV disease have not been established.

Adverse Effects, Contraindications, and Drug Interactions

Serious adverse reactions caused by palivizumab are rare. Mild erythema and pain may occur at the injection site. Although no anaphylactoid reactions have been reported to date, the possibility of this reaction exists because palivizumab is a protein.

Study QUESTIONS

1. Which drug, compared with the rest, would be expected to produce a significantly higher concentration of active metabolite in cells infected with its target virus?
   (A) Cidofovir
   (B) Foscarnet
   (C) Oseltamivir
   (D) Penciclovir
   (E) Lamivudine

2. Which of the following drugs should not be given in combination with zidovudine because of an increased risk of myelosuppression?
   (A) Ganciclovir
   (B) Fomivirsen
   (C) Rimantadine
   (D) Famciclovir
   (E) Zanamivir

3. Caitlyn Doe is a 24-year-old woman in her third month of pregnancy. She has had severe pain, swelling, and redness in both eyes for several days and has been unable to see well enough to go to work. Ms. Doe's physician diagnosed herpes simplex keratoconjunctivitis; the infection has spread deep into the surrounding tissues. Which drug is indicated for HSV keratoconjunctivitis but is least likely to harm the fetus?
   (A) Cidofovir
   (B) Docosanol
   (C) Fomivirsen
   (D) Acyclovir
   (E) Ribavirin

4. Mitchell Jones, a 35-year-old man, began treatment for hepatitis C with interferon-α-2b and ribavirin (*Rebetron*) 4 weeks ago. On returning to his doctor

	Current Values (cells/μL)	Values Before Treatment (cells/μL)	Normal Values (cells/μL)
Erythrocytes	3.3×10^6	5×10^6	$4.3–5.7 \times 10^6$
Platelets	210×10^3	350×10^3	$150–450 \times 10^3$
Myelocytes	0	0	0
Neutrophils, bands	370	350	150–400
Neutrophils, segmented	4800	4200	3000–5800
Lymphocytes	2750	2800	1500–3000
Monocytes	562	480	285–500
Eosinophils	125	100	50–250
Basophils	28	20	15–50
Hemoglobin	9.5 g/dL	16 g/dL	13.5–17.5 g/dL

for routine monitoring of his blood count and liver function, he complained of general fatigue and exertion when walking. His hemoglobin, CBC, differential, and platelet counts are shown in the accompanying table. Which is the most likely explanation of any abnormality?

(A) Ribavirin decreases erythrocyte counts.
(B) Interferon-α-2b decreases erythrocyte counts.
(C) Interferon-α-2b elevates lymphocyte counts.
(D) A and B are true.
(E) A, B, and C are true.

5. Oseltamivir's mechanism of action is generally believed to be

(A) Inhibition of a viral enzyme that aids the spread of virus through respiratory mucus and is required for the release of progeny virus
(B) Competitive inhibition of viral DNA polymerase, which leads to early chain termination of the progeny of viral DNA
(C) Stimulation of the tyrosine kinase activity of the JAK-STAT signal transduction pathway, resulting in enhanced proliferation of immune cells
(D) Inhibition of the synthesis of GTP, which is required for viral genomic replication and is a cofactor for cellular enzymes required for viral replication
(E) Inhibition of the viral protease required for protein processing prior to assembly of progeny virions

ANSWERS

1. **D.** The conversion of penciclovir to its active form requires initial monophosphorylation by viral thymidine kinases, then conversion to its active triphosphate form by cellular enzymes. Thus, the concentration of penciclovir triphosphate is particularly high in cells infected with its target viruses (e.g., HSV, VZV, HBV). Foscarnet is a pyrophosphate analogue that does not require activation. Oseltamivir is a neuraminidase inhibitor that is con-

verted by hepatic esterases to its active form, oseltamivir carboxylate. Lamivudine is converted to its active triphosphate form by host cellular enzymes.

2. **A.** Ganciclovir commonly causes myelosuppression and may produce severe neutropenia when given in combination with zidovudine. Fomivirsen is most commonly associated with iritis and other ocular information; rimantadine with nausea, vomiting, anorexia, and dizziness; famciclovir with headache, nausea, diarrhea, and CNS effects; and zanamivir with bronchospasm.

3. **D.** Acyclovir is in pregnancy category B: animal studies have shown no evidence of harm to the fetus, but no large, controlled studies of human outcomes have been performed. Cidofovir may be used to treat HSV that is resistant to acyclovir; however, it is embryotoxic and teratogenic, and Ms. Doe should avoid it. Docosanol is used for cold sores and is not indicated for ophthalmic use. Fomivirsen is effective against CMV retinitis, not HSV keratitis. Ribavirin is indicated for RSV infection and is also mutagenic, teratogenic, and embryotoxic.

4. **D.** Interferons and ribavirin are both likely to cause anemia; the combination of these two agents increases this possibility. Interferons do not stimulate lymphocyte proliferation.

5. **A.** Oseltamivir inhibits neuraminidase, an enzyme that cleaves neuraminic acid from oligosaccharides. Neuraminidase activity aids the movement of viral particles through neuraminic acid–rich respiratory secretions and is required for the release of progeny virions. Inhibition of viral DNA polymerase is the mechanism of action of nucleoside analogue antiviral drugs. Interferons do stimulate the JAK-STAT signaling pathway but do not stimulate proliferation of immune cells. Ribavirin inhibits GTP synthesis, and the antiretroviral protease inhibitors (e.g., ritonavir) inhibit HIV protease.

SUPPLEMENTAL READING

De Clercq E. Antiviral drugs: Current state of the art. J Clin Virol 2001;22:73–89.

Di Bisceglie AM, McHutchison J, and Rice CM. New therapeutic strategies for hepatitis C. Hepatology 2002;35:224–231.

Gow PJ and Mutimer D. Treatment of chronic hepatitis. BMJ 2001;323:1164–1167.

Gubareva LV, Kaiser L, and Hayden FG. Influenza virus neuraminidase inhibitors. Lancet 2000;355:827–835.

Khare MD and Sharland M. Cytomegalovirus treatment options in immunocompromised patients. Expert Opin Pharmacother 2001;2:1247–1257.

Leung DT and Sacks SL. Current recommendations for the treatment of genital herpes. Drugs 2000;60:1329–1352.

Rajan P and Rivers JK. Varicella zoster virus: Recent advances in management. Can Fam Physician 2001;47:2299–2304.

Sen GC. Viruses and interferons. Annu Rev Microbiol 2001;55:255–281.

CASE Study Picking Up More Than Knowledge in College

Jim Smith had severe herpes labialis while he was in college. At that time, the doctor at the student health service prescribed penciclovir cream to decrease the severity and duration of his many cold sores. After 2 weeks of treatment, Mr. Smith's cold sores had mostly healed. However, he developed itching, redness, and blistering around the mouth in the areas where he had applied penciclovir. The drug was discontinued, Mr. Smith was given antihistamines, and the rash healed within a week. Now, at age 28, Mr. Smith has recently changed jobs and moved to a new city following the breakup of a long-term relationship. He has been under great stress at work and has been getting little sleep. He visited his physician because painful eruptions developed on his chest the previous day. His doctor diagnosed acute herpes zoster (shingles) and prescribed oral famciclovir 500 mg every 8 hours for 7 days. Later that day, after beginning his course of treatment, Mr. Smith went to the emergency department complaining of wheezing and an itchy rash over much of his body. His symptoms were consistent with those of a mild anaphylactoid reaction. What happened?

ANSWER: Famciclovir is a prodrug that is rapidly converted to penciclovir, with a bioavailability of 77%. Maximal plasma concentrations of penciclovir are reached within 45 to 60 minutes of famciclovir administration. Mr. Smith developed an allergy to topical penciclovir when he was treated with this drug during college. This prior contact sensitization to penciclovir allowed him to develop an anaphylactoid reaction following the conversion of oral famciclovir to penciclovir by hepatic first-pass metabolism.

51 Therapy of Human Immunodeficiency Virus

Knox Van Dyke and Karen Woodfork

DRUG LIST

GENERIC NAME	PAGE	GENERIC NAME	PAGE
Abacavir	588	Ritonavir	591
Amprenavir	592	Saquinavir	591
Delavirdine	590	Stavudine	587
Didanosine	587	Tenofovir	588
Efavirenz	589	Zalcitabine	588
Indinavir	592	Zidovudine	586
Lamivudine	588	**Combinations**	
Lopinavir	593	Lopinavir, Ritonavir	593
Nelfinavir	592	Zidovudine, lamivudine	586
Nevirapine	590	Zidovudine, lamivudine, abacavir	586

HUMAN IMMUNODEFICIENCY VIRUS

Human immunodeficiency virus (HIV) is a single-stranded RNA retrovirus that causes acquired immunodeficiency syndrome (AIDS), a condition in which individuals are at increased risk for developing certain infections and malignancies. The virus is found in two major forms: HIV-1, the most prevalent worldwide, and HIV-2, the most common in western Africa. More than 22 million people have died of HIV infection, and 40 million are believed to be infected worldwide. AIDS epidemics threaten populations in sub-Saharan Africa, Southeast Asia, Central and South America, and Russia. In the United States about 450,000 deaths have occurred and another 900,000 people are estimated to carry the virus. Although the development of new drugs, complex multidrug regimens, and behavioral modification have done much to combat the spread of HIV infection, AIDS remains a serious threat because of the expense and inaccessibility of antiretroviral agents in the developing countries in which the disease is most prevalent. In addition, the effectiveness of antiretroviral drugs has been diminished by the emergence of multidrug-resistant virus.

Production of Immunodeficiency by HIV

HIV infects CD4+ T lymphocytes, macrophages, and dendritic cells. Viral entry is initiated when *gp120* (SU), a glycoprotein on the surface of the viral envelope, attaches itself to the *CD4* surface glycoprotein of the target cell (Fig. 51.1). This interaction produces a conformational change in gp120 that allows it to bind to a chemokine coreceptor: *CXCR4* for CD-4 T (helper) cells or *CCR5* for macrophages. Chemokine coreceptor

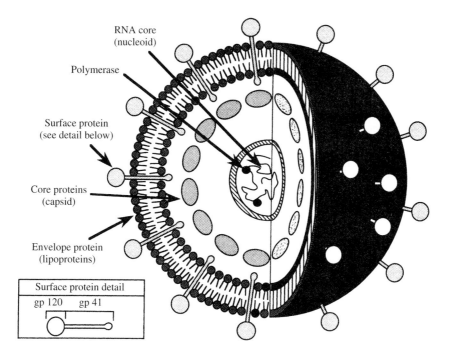

FIGURE 51.1

Exploded view of the human immunodeficiency virus. It is an RNA (retrovirus) virus that contains surface proteins composed of a knoblike glycoprotein (gp120) linked to a transmembrane stalk (gp41). These surface proteins are the infective mechanisms that allow the virus to bind to CD4 proteins of cells, such as T4 lymphocytes and monocytes.

binding is required for viral entry; individuals with genetic defects in these proteins are resistant to HIV infection. The binding of gp120 to CXCR4 or CCR5 causes a rearrangement in the envelope glycoproteins that allows the fusion of a viral transmembrane glycoprotein (*gp41*) with the target cell membrane. Fusion of the viral and cellular membranes follows as the virus enters the target cell.

After entering the host cell and uncoating, viral *reverse transcriptase* synthesizes DNA using viral RNA as a template. This DNA circularizes, enters the nucleus, and is integrated into the host genome by another viral enzyme, *integrase*. The host cell then transcribes the viral genes and produces viral proteins and progeny viral RNA. New virions assemble, bud from the cell membrane, and undergo a maturation process in which the gag-pol polyprotein is cleaved by the viral enzyme *protease*. The resultant mature virus particles spread to infect other susceptible cells.

The majority of viral replication occurs in recently infected CD4+ lymphocytes and depletes them during the first several years of infection. Macrophage populations are depleted or cease to function properly in 3 to 10 years or more. It is during this time that an HIV-infected person becomes immunodeficient and can die of infections that under normal conditions are not life threatening. Eventually the macrophages of the brain

(microglia) may become infected and an inflammation-based dementia may occur.

Several pools of nonreplicating virus serve as reservoirs of infection and limit the effectiveness of antiretroviral therapy. HIV can live and multiply in monocytes and macrophages; these cells are present in all tissues and can live for many months. Infective virus can also reside in long-lived resting CD4+ lymphocytes.

DRUG THERAPY OF HIV INFECTION

The replicative cycle of HIV presents many opportunities for the targeting of antiviral agents. The drugs in clinical use are classified as nucleoside reverse transcriptase inhibitors (NRTIs), nonnucleoside reverse transcriptase inhibitors (NNRTIs), nucleotide reverse transcriptase inhibitors (NTRTIs), and protease inhibitors (PI).

Single agents are seldom used to treat HIV infection. Instead, *multidrug therapy is used to counteract the rapid mutation rate of HIV and to minimize drug toxicity.* Highly active antiretroviral therapy (HAART) uses combinations of reverse transcriptase inhibitors and protease inhibitors (Table 51.1). In this system, drugs working by different mechanisms produce a sequential blockade of steps required for viral reproduction. It is

TABLE 51.1 Antiretroviral Drug Combinations Used in HAART

Combinations of Choice

2 NRTIs and 1 PI
2 NRTIs and 1NNRTI
2 NRTIs and 1 PI with ritonavir
2 NRTIs and abacavir

Secondary Alternatives

1 PI, 1 NRTI, and 1NNRTI
2 PIs, 1 NRTI, and 1 NNRTI

difficult for the HIV to simultaneously develop mutants that provide it with resistance to the multiple drugs that act via different mechanisms. However, even with multidrug regimens, it has been estimated that viruses in 85% of infected people develop resistance to one or more of the antiretroviral agents. Therefore, it is necessary to produce drugs that either inhibit this resistance or find compounds that produce no resistance.

New drugs are being targeted against drug-resistant HIV strains. In addition, a variety of drugs under development act as inhibitors of viral fusion or viral entry into the host cell. New agents designed to inhibit viral integrase have shown promise in early clinical trials. Current therapies do not enhance the host defense system; this may account for their incomplete effectiveness. Protection of the host immune mechanism might increase the efficacy of other drugs that inhibit viral replication.

Nucleoside Reverse Transcriptase Inhibitors

The NRTIs are nucleoside analogues that act as competitive inhibitors of reverse transcriptase. *After conversion to the triphosphate form by host cell kinases, these drugs compete with nucleoside triphosphates for access to reverse transcriptase.* All NRTIs lack a 3'-hydroxyl group; thus, their incorporation into a growing DNA chain results in its termination. These drugs block HIV replication and therefore the infection of new cells, but they have little effect on cells already infected with virus. Combination therapies often include two NRTIs that are analogues of different bases plus a protease inhibitor. The pharmacokinetic properties of the NRTIs are listed in Table 51.2.

The NRTIs inhibit cellular and mitochondrial DNA polymerases and various cellular kinases, resulting in toxicity. Toxicity varies with the state of the immune system; early in the infection there is less toxicity, while late in the infection there is substantially more. *All NRTIs*

can produce a potentially fatal syndrome of lactic acidosis and severe hepatomegaly with hepatic steatosis; this results from the toxic effects of these drugs on mitochondria. Those at highest risk include women, obese individuals, alcoholics, and patients with prolonged exposure to NRTIs. All patients should be monitored for the development of hepatotoxicity; the drug should be discontinued if this occurs.

Resistance to these agents limits their usefulness, particularly as monotherapy. Resistance generally results from the appearance of mutations in reverse transcriptase; cross-resistance to multiple NRTIs also occurs.

Zidouvidine

Zidovudine (AZT, ZDV) was the first antiviral drug used against HIV. It is a thymidine analogue that is effective against HIV-1, HIV-2, and human T-cell lymphotrophic virus (HTLV) I and II. It is available as a single agent (*Retrovir*) or in fixed combinations with lamivudine (*Combivir*) or lamivudine and abacavir (*Trizivir*). Zidovudine, in combination with one or more other antiretroviral agents, is approved for the treatment of HIV infection in adults and children and for postexposure prophylaxis. It is used alone or in combination for the prevention of prenatal and perinatal transmission to the baby by HIV-infected pregnant women.

The most common adverse reactions to zidovudine are headache, nausea, vomiting, and anorexia. Fatigue, confusion, insomnia, malaise, hepatitis, myopathy, and myositis may also occur. Bone marrow toxicity occurs in up to 30% of patients taking zidovudine; anemia, neutropenia, and other hematological abnormalities can necessitate a dosage reduction, drug discontinuation, or therapy with erythropoietin or colony-stimulating factors. Cross-resistance to multiple nucleoside analogues has been documented.

Caution should be exercised when zidovudine is administered to patients with preexisting anemia or neutropenia and to those with advanced cases of AIDS. Dosage adjustment is required for patients with significant renal impairment and may also be necessary in those with hepatic impairment.

Zidovudine should be used cautiously with any other agent that causes bone marrow suppression, such as interferon-α, trimethoprim–sulfamethoxazole, dapsone, foscarnet, flucytosine, ganciclovir, and valganciclovir. Probenecid and interferon-β inhibit the elimination of zidovudine; therefore, a dosage reduction of zidovudine is necessary when the drugs are administered concurrently. Ribavirin inhibits the phosphorylation reactions that activate zidovudine, and zidovudine similarly inhibits the activation of stavudine; thus, the coadministration of zidovudine with ribavirin or stavudine is contraindicated.

TABLE 51.2 Pharmacokinetic Properties of the NRTIs and an NtRTI[a]

Drug	Oral Bioavailability (%)	Plasma Elimination Half-Life (hr)	Protein Binding (%)	Metabolism	Urinary Excretion[b] (%)	Notes
Abacavir	83	1.5	50	ADH, GT	1	H?
Didanosine[c]	42	1.5	<5	Purine elimination pathways	18	F−; H?; R
Lamivudine	86	5–7	<36	Minor	71	H?; R
Stavudine	86	1.4	Negligible	ND	40	R
Tenofovir	25	ND; accumulates in fat	<1	Minor	70–80 32[d]	F+; H?; R
Zalcitabine	>80	2	<4	Minor	60	F−; R
Zidovudine	64	0.5–3	<38	Hepatic non-P450	14	F−; FPM; H?; R

[a]Average values for fasting adult patients following a single oral dose.
[b]Unchanged drug.
[c]Data are given for non–delayed release formulations only.
[d]After multiple dosing.
ADH, alcohol dehydrogenase; F+, food (high-fat meal) increases absorption; F−, food interferes with absorption; FPM, extensive first pass metabolism; GT, glucuronyl transferase; H?, dosage adjustment in patients with hepatic impairment has not been studied; ND, not determined; R, dosage adjustment is necessary in patients with renal impairment.

Stavudine

Stavudine (d4T, *Zerit*) is a thymidine nucleoside analogue that is active against HIV-1 and HIV-2. It is approved for the therapy of HIV infection as part of a multidrug regimen and is also used for postexposure prophylaxis.

The adverse effects with which stavudine is most frequently associated are headache, diarrhea, skin rash, nausea, vomiting, insomnia, anorexia, myalgia, and weakness. Peripheral neuropathy consisting of numbness, tingling, or pain in the hands or feet is also common with higher doses of the drug. Significant elevation of hepatic enzymes may be seen in approximately 10 to 15% of patients. Lactic acidosis occurs more frequently with stavudine than with other NRTIs. Viral resistance to stavudine may develop, and cross-resistance to zidovudine and didanosine may occur.

Stavudine should be used with caution in patients at risk for hepatic disease and those who have had pancreatitis. Persons with peripheral neuropathy, the elderly, and those with advanced HIV disease are at increased risk for neurotoxicity. Dosage adjustment is required for patients with renal insufficiency.

Stavudine possesses several clinically significant interactions with other drugs. Although hydroxyurea enhances the antiviral activity of stavudine and didanosine, combination therapy that includes stavudine and didanosine, with or without hydroxyurea, increases the risk of pancreatitis. Combinations of stavudine and didanosine should not be given to pregnant women because of the increased risk of metabolic acidosis. Zidovudine inhibits the phosphorylation of stavudine; thus, this combination should be avoided.

Didanosine

Didanosine (ddI, *Videx*) is an adenosine analogue with activity against HIV-1, HIV-2, and HTLV-I. It is approved as part of a multidrug regimen for the therapy of HIV infection and is also used as postexposure HIV prophylaxis.

The most common adverse effect produced by didanosine is diarrhea. Abdominal pain, nausea, vomiting, anorexia, and dose-related peripheral neuropathy may occur. Pancreatitis occurs rarely, as do hyperuricemia, bone marrow suppression, retinal depigmentation, and optical neuritis. Resistance to didanosine appears to result from mutations different from those responsible for zidovudine resistance.

Didanosine should be used with great caution in individuals who have a history of pancreatitis. Didanosine tablets contain phenylalanine and should not be taken by phenylketonurics. Didanosine should be used cautiously in patients with gout, peripheral neuropathy, and advanced AIDS.

Buffering agents that are compounded with didanosine to counteract its degradation by gastric acid may interfere with the absorption of other drugs that require acidity (e.g., indinavir, delavirdine, ketoconazole, fluoroquinolones, tetracyclines, dapsone). An enteric-coated formulation (*Videx EC*) that dissolves in the basic pH of the small intestine is not susceptible to these interactions. Ganciclovir and valganciclovir can increase blood levels of didanosine. The use of zalcitabine with didanosine is not recommended because that combination carries an additive risk of peripheral neuropathy. The combination of didanosine with stavudine increases the risk of pancreatitis, hepatotoxicity, and peripheral neuropathy. Stavudine should not be given with didanosine to pregnant women because of the increased risk of metabolic acidosis.

Lamivudine

Lamivudine (3TC, *Epivir*) is a cytosine nucleoside analogue with activity against HIV-1, HIV-2, and hepatitis B virus. It is approved as part of a multidrug regimen for the therapy of HIV infection in adults and children and has been used for HIV postexposure prophylaxis. Combination products contain lamivudine with either zidovudine (*Combivir*) or zidovudine and abacavir (*Trizivir*). The use of low-dose lamivudine in the treatment of chronic hepatitis B is described in Chapter 50.

Lamivudine is the best-tolerated NRTI. Its most common adverse effects include headache, malaise, fatigue, and insomnia. Pancreatitis is rare. Gastrointestinal complaints are common with lamivudine–zidovudine therapy but are probably mainly due to the zidovudine component. Lamivudine resistance sometimes occurs early in treatment. Cross-resistance to zalcitabine, didanosine, and abacavir can occur simultaneously. Withdrawal of lamivudine in patients infected with both hepatitis B virus and HIV can cause a flare-up of hepatitis symptoms.

Lamivudine is associated with an increased risk of pancreatitis in children and should be used with great caution in children who have had pancreatitis or are at high risk for it. Dosage adjustment is necessary in patients with renal impairment. Lamivudine should not be used in combination with zalcitabine, because they inhibit each other's activation by phosphorylation. Trimethoprim inhibits the renal elimination of lamivudine.

Abacavir

Abacavir (*Ziagen*) is a guanosine nucleoside analogue indicated for the therapy of HIV-1 infection in adults and children. It is used as part of a multidrug regimen and is available in a fixed-dose combination with zidovudine and lamivudine (*Trizivir*). It is also used for postexposure HIV infection prophylaxis.

Abacavir is associated with side effects such as anorexia, nausea, vomiting, malaise, headache, and insomnia. *A potentially fatal hypersensitivity reaction develops in approximately 5% of patients, usually early in the course of treatment.* Fever and rash are the most common symptoms of this reaction; malaise, respiratory symptoms, and gastrointestinal complaints may also occur. Resistance to abacavir may be associated with resistance to zidovudine, didanosine, and lamivudine.

Abacavir undergoes extensive hepatic metabolism; therefore, patients with liver disease should be monitored closely if this drug is given. Ethanol inhibits the metabolism of abacavir because it competes for metabolism by alcohol dehydrogenase. Abacavir is not known to inhibit or induce cytochrome P450 isozymes.

Zalcitabine

Zalcitabine (ddC, *Hivid*) is a cytidine analogue active against HIV-1, HIV-2, and hepatitis B virus. It is used for the treatment of HIV infection in adults and asymptomatic children as part of a multidrug regimen. It may be less effective than the other nucleoside inhibitors and is used less frequently.

Peripheral neuropathy occurs in up to 50% of patients taking zalcitabine. Stomatitis, esophageal ulceration, hepatotoxicity, rash, and pancreatitis may occur. Zalcitabine should be used with caution in individuals with a history of pancreatitis, liver disease, or alcohol abuse. Dosage adjustment is necessary for individuals with renal impairment. Zalcitabine should not be used in combination with didanosine, lamivudine, or stavudine.

Nucleotide Reverse Transcriptase Inhibitors
Tenofovir

Tenofovir disoproxil fumarate (*Viread*) is a prodrug of tenofovir, a phosphorylated adenosine nucleoside analogue, and is the only available agent of its class . It is converted by cellular enzymes to tenofovir diphosphate, which competes with deoxyadenosine triphosphate (dATP) for access to reverse transcriptase and causes chain termination following its incorporation. Tenofovir was approved as part of a combination therapy for HIV in adults who failed treatment with other regimens; it appears to be effective against HIV strains that are resistant to NRTIs. The pharmacokinetic properties of tenofovir are provided in Table 51.2.

Tenofovir is taken once daily and is generally well tolerated, perhaps because it produces less mitochondrial toxicity than the NRTIs. Nausea, vomiting, flatulence, and diarrhea occur in 10% or fewer patients. Resistance to tenofovir has been documented, and cross-resistance to NRTIs may occur.

Tenofovir should not be given to patients with renal insufficiency. Its coadministration with didanosine results in increased plasma levels of didanosine that can produce toxicity. Because lactic acidosis and severe hepatomegaly with steatosis have been reported with NRTIs, it is important to monitor patients with known risk factors during treatment with tenofovir.

Nonnucleoside Reverse Transcriptase Inhibitors

The NNRTIs inhibit viral reverse transcriptase by binding adjacent to its active site and inducing a conformational change that causes the enzyme's inactivation. When combined with NRTIs or protease inhibitors,

NNRTIs produce additive and possibly synergistic effects against HIV. The pharmacokinetic parameters of these agents are listed in Table 51.3.

All NNRTIs are active against HIV-1 reverse transcriptase only and do not require phosphorylation for activation. These agents share certain adverse effects (e.g., rash) and are subject to numerous drug interactions due to their metabolism by and induction of hepatic cytochrome P450 enzymes. NNRTIs may modify plasma levels of protease inhibitors, which are also metabolized by cytochrome P450 enzymes (Table 51.4). *The list of drug interactions provided in this text is not all-inclusive; it is necessary to check for all drug interactions when prescribing NNRTIs.* These agents should be used with caution in patients with hepatic disease.

When NNRTIs are used alone, resistance develops rapidly as a result of the development of mutations in reverse transcriptase; therefore, monotherapy with these agents is not recommended. Cross-resistance between NNRTIs occurs frequently but is not seen between NNRTIs and NRTIs or the protease inhibitors.

Efavirenz

Efavirenz (*Sustiva*) is approved for the therapy of HIV infection of adults and children and is also used for postexposure prophylaxis. It is the only NNRTI approved for once-daily dosing. Rash, although rarely severe, is a common adverse effect of efavirenz. Elevated liver enzymes and serum cholesterol also may occur. Central nervous system (CNS) effects in approximately half of patients may include dizziness, headache, insomnia, drowsiness, euphoria, agitation, impaired cognition, nightmares, vivid dreams, and hallucinations. These effects often subside after several weeks to months of therapy.

Efavirenz should be avoided during pregnancy because primate studies have shown it to be teratogenic at doses near therapeutic levels. Women of childbearing

---

T A B L E 51.3 Pharmacokinetic Properties of Selected NNRTIs[a]

Drug	Oral Bioavailability (%)	Plasma Elimination Half-Life (hr)	Protein Binding (%)	Metabolism	Urinary Excretion[b] (%)	Notes
Delavirdine	85	5.8[c]	98	CYP3A4, CYP2D6	<5	H?; R?
Efavirenz	50	40-55	>99	CYP3A4, CYP2B6	<5	F+ (avoid); H?
Nevirapine	>90	25-30	60	CYP3A4	<3	H?; R?

[a]Average values for fed adult patients, following a multiple oral dosing
[b]Unchanged drug
[c]Elimination half-life increases with dose; this value is for dose of 400 mg tid.
F+, food (high-fat meal) increases absorption; H?, dosage adjustment in patients with hepatic impairment has not been studied; R?, dosage adjustment in patients with renal impairment has not been studied.

T A B L E 51.4 Interactions Between NNRTIs and Protease Inhibitors

Drug	Increases Plasma AUC of	Decreases Plasma AUC of	Plasma AUC Increased by	Plasma AUC Decreased by
Delavirdine	Amprenavir Indinavir Lopinavir Nelfinavir Ritonavir Saquinavir			Nelfinavir
Efavirenz	Nelfinavir Ritonavir	Amprenavir Indinavir Lopinavir Saquinavir	Ritonavir	Saquinavir
Nevirapine		Amprenavir Indinavir Lopinavir Saquinavir		

potential should use two methods of birth control to avoid becoming pregnant when taking this drug.

Efavirenz interacts with many drugs via the cytochrome P450 pathways. It induces and is metabolized by CYP3A4 and inhibits CYP2C9 and CYP2C19. It should not be given with cisapride, ergot alkaloids, midazolam, or triazolam because of the potential for life-threatening reactions. Efavirenz has the potential to decrease blood levels of methadone, rifabutin, ketoconazole, and itraconazole. It may inhibit the metabolism of drugs such as alosetron, diazepam, ethinyl estradiol, imipramine, losartan, omeprazole, warfarin, tolbutamide, and topiramate. Efavirenz interacts with cytochrome P450 inducers and substrates (e.g., phenytoin, phenobarbital) in a complex manner; blood levels and side effects should be closely monitored. Patients taking efavirenz should avoid herbal preparations containing St. John's wort because the herb induces CYP3A4 and may cause drug failure or viral resistance. Saquinavir should not be used as the sole protease inhibitor in a regimen containing efavirenz.

Nevirapine

Nevirapine (*Viramune*) is approved for the treatment of HIV infection in adults and children as part of a combination therapy. *During the first 12 weeks of treatment, patients must be closely monitored for the development of potentially fatal hepatic toxicity (i.e., hepatitis, hepatic necrosis, and hepatic failure) and skin reactions (i.e., Stevens-Johnson syndrome, toxic epidermal necrolysis, and hypersensitivity reactions).* Although these toxicities are rare, common side effects include mild to moderate rash, fever, nausea, fatigue, headache, and elevated liver enzymes.

Nevirapine induces and is metabolized by CYP3A4; therefore, coadministration of drugs that induce or are metabolized by this isoenzyme may result in interactions. Nevirapine may decrease the effectiveness of ethinyl estradiol–based contraceptives and can lower plasma concentrations of methadone. Nevirapine should not be administered with ketoconazole, rifampin, or rifabutin.

Delavirdine

Delavirdine (*Rescriptor*) is approved for the treatment of HIV-1 infection in adults and adolescents over age 16 as part of a combination therapy. Rash accompanied by pruritus is the most frequent adverse effect of this agent; however, it usually resolves within several weeks of treatment. Severe skin reactions are rare. Headache, nausea, vomiting, diarrhea, fatigue, and elevated hepatic enzymes also may be associated with delavirdine administration.

Drugs that decrease stomach acidity (e.g., antacids, H_2 receptor blockers, and proton pump inhibitors) decrease the absorption of delavirdine. In vivo and in vitro studies have shown that delavirdine is metabolized by and inhibits CYP3A4. In vitro studies have shown that it also is metabolized by CYP2D6 and inhibits CYP2C9, CYP2D6, and CYP2C19. Delavirdine should not be used in combination with alprazolam, cisapride, ergot alkaloids, midazolam, or triazolam because of the potential for serious adverse reactions. Delavirdine increases serum concentrations of certain protease inhibitors and may reverse the resistance of zidovudine-resistant HIV.

Protease Inhibitors

These drugs inhibit the activity of HIV protease. This enzyme, which is required for the production of a mature infectious virus, cleaves the gag-pol polyprotein into structural proteins and active enzymes. The pharmacokinetic parameters of the protease inhibitors are listed in Table 51.5.

The protease inhibitors are used in the multidrug therapy of HIV infection. Resistance to the HIV protease inhibitors results from mutations in the protease gene and perhaps the cleavage sites of gag-pol. Although different protease mutations tend to be associated with resistance to individual drugs, resistance to one protease inhibitor is often associated with a less than optimal response to other agents of this class. Indinavir, ritonavir, and lopinavir require more mutations to lose their effectiveness than do the other protease inhibitors.

All protease inhibitors can produce nausea, vomiting, diarrhea, and paresthesia. Drug-induced hyperglycemia and insulin resistance may precipitate the onset of diabetes mellitus or worsen existing cases. Protease inhibitors may also cause hypercholesterolemia and hypertriglyceridemia. Liver enzymes may be increased, and hepatic toxicity may occur at high doses. Fat redistribution is common and can manifest as central fat accumulation, peripheral wasting, buffalo hump at the base of the neck, breast enlargement, and/or lipomas.

Protease inhibitors may increase the risk of bleeding in hemophiliacs. These drugs should be used with caution in patients with diabetes, lipid disorders, and hepatic disease. Dosage adjustment may be necessary.

Protease inhibitors interact with a large number of drugs because they are metabolized by and inhibit CYP3A4. Ritonavir is the most potent inhibitor of CYP3A4, with indinavir, amprenavir, and nelfinavir being much less potent and saquinavir the least potent. When given as part of a combination therapy, the protease inhibitors affect plasma levels of NNRTIs as well as each other (Tables 51.4 and 51.6). Many drugs interact with protease inhibitors by inhibiting or inducing their metabolism; similarly, protease inhibitors inhibit or induce the metabolism of numerous drugs (Table 51.7).

TABLE 51.5 Pharmacokinetic Properties of Selected Protease Inhibitors[a]

Drug	Oral Bioavailability (%)	Plasma Elimination Half-Life (hr)	Protein Binding (%)	Metabolism	Urinary Excretion[b] (%)	Notes
Amprenavir	ND	7–11	90	CYP3A4	<2	F−; H; R?
Indinavir	60–65	1.8	60	CYP3A4	10–12	F−; H; R?
Lopinavir, ritonavir	ND	5–6	98–99	CYP3A4	<3	F+; (h); R?
Nelfinavir	ND	3.5–5	>98	CYP3A4[c] CYP2C19	<2	F+; H?; R?
Ritonavir[d]	ND	3–5	>98	CYP3A4[c] CYP2D6	3.5	F+; (h); R?
Saquinavir	13	7–12	97	CYP3A4	<3	F+; FPM; H?; R?
Saquinavir mesylate	4	7–12	97	CYP3A4	<3	F+; FPM; H?; R?

[a]Average values for fed adult patients following multiple oral doses.
[b]Unchanged drug.
[c]Major isoform responsible for drug metabolism.
[d]Capsule formulation.
F+, food (high fat meal) increases absorption; F−, food decreases absorption; FPM, extensive first-pass metabolism; H, dosage adjustment is necessary in patients with hepatic impairment; (h), dosage adjustment may be required in patients with hepatic impairment; H?, dosage adjustment in patients with hepatic impairment has not been studied; R, dosage adjustment is necessary in patients with renal impairment; R?, dosage adjustment in patients with renal impairment has not been studied.

TABLE 51.6 Interactions Among Protease Inhibitors

Drug	Increases Plasma AUC of	Decreases Plasma AUC of	Plasma AUC Increased by	Plasma AUC Decreased by
Amprenavir	Nelfinavir	Indinavir	Indinavir Nelfinavir Ritonavir	
Indinavir	Amprenavir Nelfinavir Saquinavir		Nelfinavir Ritonavir	Amprenavir
Lopinavir[a]			Ritonavir	Amprenavir
Nelfinavir	Amprenavir Indinavir Saquinavir		Amprenavir Indinavir Ritonavir Saquinavir	
Ritonavir	Amprenavir Indinavir Lopinavir Nelfinavir Saquinavir			
Saquinavir	Nelfinavir		Indinavir Nelfinavir Ritonavir	

[a]Coformulation of lopinavir and ritonavir.

Saquinavir

Saquinavir is a potent inhibitor of HIV-1 and HIV-2 protease. *Fortovase*, a soft gel preparation of saquinavir, has largely replaced saquinavir mesylate capsules (*Invirase*) because it has improved bioavailability. Saquinavir is usually well tolerated and most frequently produces mild gastrointestinal side effects.

Ritonavir

Although ritonavir (*Norvir*) is a potent inhibitor of HIV-1 and HIV-2 protease, it is not well tolerated in higher doses. It is mainly used in low doses to increase blood levels of other protease inhibitors and to extend their dosing interval. Ritonavir is more commonly associated with gastrointestinal side effects, altered taste

TABLE 51.7   Drug Interactions Commonly Seen with Protease Inhibitors[a]

Drugs Contraindicated for Use with Protease Inhibitors Because of Risk of Life-Threatening Toxicity

Cisapride (arrhythmias)[b]	Lovastatin (rhabdomyolysis)	Simvastatin (rhabdomyolysis)
Ergot alkaloids (vasospasm)	Midazolam (resp. depression)	Triazolam (resp. depression)

Drugs That May Decrease Plasma Levels of Protease Inhibitors	**Drugs Whose Plasma Levels May Be Decreased by Protease Inhibitors**
Dexamethasone	Ethinyl estradiol
Phenytoin	Phenytoin
Rifampin	
Phenobarbital	**Drugs Whose Plasma Levels May Be Increased by Protease Inhibitors**
Rifabutin	
St. John's wort[c]	Antiarrhythmic agents (some)
Drugs That May Increase Plasma Levels of Protease Inhibitors	Benzodiazepines (some)[d]
	Ketoconazole
	Antidepressants (some)
Clarithromycin	Ca^{++} channel blockers (some)
Itraconazole	Rifabutin
Ketoconazole	β-Blockers (some)
	HMG-CoA reductase inhibitors (some)[c]
	Sildenafil

[a]Interactions may be seen to varying degrees with different protease inhibitors. This list is not all-inclusive; it is important to check individual drug interactions when prescribing protease inhibitors.
[b]Pharmacy sales of this drug have been discontinued in the United States. It is available only via registered prescribers to patients who meet specific eligibility conditions.
[c]The use of St. John's wort is contraindicated in patients taking protease inhibitors because their antiviral activity may be lost and/or drug resistance may result.
[d]Some are absolutely contraindicated for use with protease inhibitors.

sensation, paresthesias, and hypertriglyceridemia than are other protease inhibitors. Pancreatitis may occur in the presence or absence of hypertriglyceridemia.

Of all the protease inhibitors, ritonavir is the most potent inhibitor of CYP3A4; therefore, it tends to produce more frequent and severe interactions with other drugs. It inhibits an additional cytochrome P450 isozyme, CYP2D6, and can increase plasma concentrations of drugs that are metabolized by it (e.g., most antidepressants, some antiarrhythmics, some opioid analgesics, some neuroleptics). For example, ritonavir should not be used in conjunction with amiodarone, bepridil, flecainide, propafenone, quinidine, or pimozide. In addition to CYP3A4, ritonavir induces CYP1A2 and possibly CYP2C9 and may inhibit the breakdown of drugs metabolized by these enzymes.

Indinavir

Indinavir (*Crixivan*) is a potent inhibitor of HIV reverse transcriptase. It produces the side effects common to all protease inhibitors and also may produce nephrolithiasis, urolithiasis, and possibly renal insufficiency or renal failure. *This problem occurs more fre-*

quently in children (approximately 30%) than adults (approximately 10%) and can be minimized by drinking at least 1.5 L of water daily. Additional side effects include asymptomatic hyperbilirubinemia, alopecia, ingrown toenails, and paronychia. Hemolytic anemia rarely occurs. Rifampin should not be given with indinavir.

Nelfinavir

Nelfinavir (*Viracept*) is probably the most commonly used protease inhibitor because of its low incidence of serious adverse effects. Its most common side effects are diarrhea and flatulence; these may resolve with continued use. In addition to the drugs contraindicated for use with all protease inhibitors, amiodarone, rifampin, and quinidine are contraindicated in patients taking nelfinavir.

Amprenavir

Amprenavir (*Agenerase*) is administered twice daily, providing the patient with an advantage over other protease inhibitors that must be taken more frequently (e.g., indinavir, saquinavir). Common side effects of amprenavir include nausea, vomiting, diarrhea, and perioral paraesthesias. Rash occurs in approximately 20 to 30% of patients and can be mild or severe (Stevens-Johnson syndrome).

Amprenavir oral solution contains large amounts of the excipient propylene glycol and should not be given to children under age 4 because it can produce hyperosmolality, lactic acidosis, seizures, and/or respiratory depression. Pregnant women should not take amprenavir oral solution, as fetal toxicity may result. Amprenavir is a sulfonamide and should be used with caution in patients with sulfonamide allergy. Amprenavir oral solution and capsules contain high levels of vitamin E; therefore, patients are advised not to take supplemental vitamin E. In addition to the drugs contraindicated for use with all protease inhibitors, amprenavir should not be given with pimozide or rifampin.

Lopinavir–Ritonavir

Lopinavir is available in the United States only as a fixed-dose combination with ritonavir (*Kaletra*). *In this regimen, a low dose of ritonavir is used to inhibit the rapid inactivation of lopinavir by CYP3A4.* Side effects, which are generally mild, include diarrhea, nausea, asthenia, and headache. Pancreatitis occurs rarely. Ritonavir is a potent inhibitor of CYP3A4 and also inhibits CYP2D6. In addition to the drugs contraindicated for all protease inhibitors, flecainide, propafenone, pimozide, and rifampin should not be given with lopinavir–ritonavir combination therapy.

THE USE OF ANTIRETROVIRAL DRUGS IN PREGNANCY

Zidovudine was the first agent to be used to prevent the transmission of HIV from a pregnant woman to her child. It was given to the mother at 14 to 34 weeks' gestation and to the child for the first 6 weeks of life. Current combination therapies employ zidovudine with another NRTI and a protease inhibitor.

The teratogenic risk associated with administration of antiretroviral drugs during the first trimester of pregnancy is not clear. Women who have not begun therapy prior to becoming pregnant may consider waiting until after 10 to 12 weeks' gestation to begin antiviral treatment. If a woman decides to discontinue antiretroviral therapy during pregnancy, all drugs should be stopped and reintroduced simultaneously to avoid the development of resistance. Pregnant women may be particularly susceptible to hyperglycemia caused by protease inhibitors.

In the United States, the Centers for Disease Control recommend that HIV-infected mothers avoid breast-feeding to prevent the transmission of the virus to their infants. The risk of this type of vertical transmission ranges from 5 to 20%; longer durations of breast-feeding, mastitis, and abscesses are associated with increased risk. In developing countries in which safe infant formula is not readily available, the avoidance of breast-feeding can increase the infant's risk of death from malnutrition and food-borne infection. The World Health Organization recommends that under these circumstances exclusive breast-feeding should be maintained for the first months of life and discontinued when replacement feeding is acceptable, feasible, affordable, sustainable, and safe.

Study QUESTIONS

1. The mechanism of action of lamivudine differs from that of efavirenz in that
(A) Lamivudine inhibits HIV protease; efavirenz inhibits reverse transcriptase.
(B) Lamivudine inhibits reverse transcriptase; efavirenz inhibits HIV protease.
(C) Lamivudine is a cytosine nucleoside analogue; efavirenz is an adenosine nucleotide analogue.
(D) Lamivudine binds to the active site of reverse transcriptase; efavirenz binds adjacent to it.
(E) Lamivudine and efavirenz exhibit the same mechanism of action; there is no difference.
2. Sharon M. is a 35-year-old woman who is approximately 60% above the normal body weight for her height. She has a history of alcohol abuse and has

been taking zidovudine and abacavir for the past 3 years to treat HIV infection. These factors put her at high risk for drug-induced
(A) Lactic acidosis, hepatomegaly, and hepatic steatosis
(B) Peripheral neuropathy
(C) Stevens-Johnson syndrome
(D) Hyperuricemia
(E) Hypersensitivity reaction
3. Mark C. is taking a regimen consisting of zidovudine, lamivudine, and efavirenz for the treatment of HIV infection. To help him fall asleep at night, he took a normal dose of diazepam (10 mg before bed), which he got from a friend. He then had symptoms of diazepam overdose, including grogginess and

difficulty waking and maintaining consciousness. The most likely reason for this is that

(A) Efavirenz inhibits the hepatic metabolism of diazepam

(B) Efavirenz competes with diazepam for renal elimination

(C) Lamivudine potentiates the depressant activity of diazepam

(D) Zidovudine induces the metabolism of diazepam

(E) Lamivudine stimulates conversion of diazepam to its active form

4. Adverse effects commonly associated with NRTIs include

(A) Central fat accumulation and peripheral fat wasting

(B) Drug interactions involving cytochrome P450 enzymes

(C) Myelotoxicity and hemolytic anemia

(D) Hypercholesterolemia and hypertriglyceridemia

(E) Hyperglycemia and insulin resistance

5. A fixed-dose combination of lopinavir and ritonavir is used to treat HIV infection in the United States. This combination is particularly effective because

(A) Ritonavir and lopinavir inhibit HIV reverse transcriptase in different ways

(B) Ritonavir decreases the hepatic metabolism of lopinavir

(C) Ritonavir decreases the renal elimination of lopinavir

(D) Lopinavir inhibits the ability of HIV to mutate in response to ritonavir

(E) Lopinavir inhibits the mutant HIV structural protein that confers viral resistance on ritonavir

ANSWERS

1. **D.** Lamivudine, a cytosine analogue, is a nucleoside reverse transcriptase inhibitor that acts as a competitive inhibitor of reverse transcriptase. Efavirenz is a nonnucleoside reverse transcriptase inhibitor; it acts by binding to a site adjacent to the enzyme's active site. Neither drug exhibits significant activity against HIV protease.

2. **A.** The NRTIs can produce a potentially fatal syndrome of lactic acidosis and severe hepatomegaly with hepatic steatosis. Risk factors associated with the development of this syndrome include female sex, obesity, alcoholism, and prolonged exposure to NRTIs. Peripheral neuropathy is a common side effect of some NRTIs (e.g., stavudine., didanosine, and zalcitabine) but not associated with these risk factors. Stevens-Johnson syndrome is rarely associated with NNRTIs, such as nevirapine, and not with these risk factors. Hyperuricemia is not associated with these risk factors. Hypersensitivity reaction may oc-

cur in the early months of treatment with abacavir but is not associated with this subject's risk factors.

3. **A.** Diazepam is metabolized in the liver by CYP3A4 and CYP2C19; efavirenz inhibits both of these isozymes and is likely to increase plasma levels of diazepam. Diazepam is almost completely converted to inactive metabolites; therefore, renal elimination is not much of a concern. Lamivudine may produce fatigue as a side effect but does not potentiate the depressant activity of diazepam. Zidovudine does not induce cytochrome P450 activity, and diazepam does not have to be converted to an active form for sedative activity.

4. **C.** Myelotoxicity is associated with certain NRTIs such as zidovudine. Fat redistribution, drug interactions involving CYP3A4, dyslipidemia, and diabetic symptoms are all side effects common to the protease inhibitors.

5. **B.** Ritonavir is a potent inhibitor of CYP3A4, the enzyme that rapidly inactivates lopinavir. This combination includes a low dose of ritonavir that is not likely to cause serious side effects but instead inhibits lopinavir metabolism. Ritonavir and lopinavir are HIV protease inhibitors and do not affect reverse transcriptase. Lopinavir is almost completely eliminated by metabolism to inactive metabolites; little is eliminated unchanged by the kidney. Lopinavir is not known to inhibit the ability of HIV to mutate. Lopinavir inhibits the enzyme HIV protease, not a structural protein.

SUPPLEMENTAL READING

Bartlett JA. Addressing the challenges of adherence. J Acquir Immune Defic Syndr 2002;29 Suppl 1:S2–S10.

Campiani G et al. Non-nucleoside HIV-1 reverse transcriptase (RT) inhibitors: Past, present, and future perspectives. Curr Pharm Des 2002;8:615–657.

Greene WC and Peterlin BM. Charting HIV's remarkable voyage through the cell: Basic science as a passport to future therapy. Nat Med 2002;8:673–680.

Jiang S, Zhao Q, and Debnath AK. Peptide and nonpeptide HIV fusion inhibitors. Curr Pharm Des 2002;8:563–580.

Moyle G. Use of HIV protease inhibitors as pharmacoenhancers. AIDS Read 2001;11:87–98.

Pierson T et al. Characterization of chemokine receptor utilization of viruses in the latent reservoir for human immunodeficiency virus type 1. J Virol 2000;74:7824–7833.

Piot P et al. The global impact of HIV/AIDS. Nature 2001;410:968–973.

Sepkowitz KA. AIDS: the first 20 years. N Engl J Med 2001;344:1764–1772.

Setti M et al. Identification of key mutations in HIV reverse transcriptase gene can influence the clinical outcome of HAART. J Med Virol 2001;64:199–206.

Sonza S and Crowe SM. Reservoirs for HIV infection and their persistence in the face of undetectable viral load. AIDS Patient Care STDS. 2001;15:511–518.

Tarrago-Litvak L et al. Inhibitors of HIV-1 reverse transcriptase and integrase: Classical and emerging therapeutical approaches. Curr Pharm Des 2002; 8:595–614.

Tozser J. HIV inhibitors: Problems and reality. Ann N Y Acad Sci 2001;946:145–159.

CASE Study   HIV and Nutriceuticals

Jerome R. is HIV positive and has been taking saquinavir 1200 mg tid and zidovudine 200 mg tid for the past 8 months. During this time, his CD4 count raised from 200 cells/mm³ to 725 cells/mm³. Two months later, Mr. R returned to his physician with a severe herpes outbreak on one side of his face. His CD4 count had fallen to 280 cells/mm³. What happened?

ANSWER: Two months ago, Mr. R. began taking St. John's wort to counteract depression. St. John's wort is a potent inducer of intestinal and hepatic CYP3A4. Saquinavir undergoes extensive first-pass metabolism by intestinal CYP3A4 and is metabolized in the liver by CYP3A4. The use of St. John's wort is contraindicated for individuals taking protease inhibitors because it may decrease protease inhibitor concentrations to subtherapeutic levels, resulting in the loss of virological response and possible resistance to the protease inhibitor. In this case, it appears that saquinavir was no longer present at an effective concentration and the HIV virus became resistant to zidovudine. Discontinuation of St. John's wort and a change in treatment regimen, perhaps to two different NRTIs and an NNRTI, are in order. Mr. R's depression should be treated with a different agent. Many antidepressants are metabolized by cytochrome P450 systems; thus, a reduction in antidepressant dosage may be necessary because NNRTIs and protease inhibitors inhibit cytochrome P450 isoenzymes.

52 Antifungal Drugs

David C. Slagle

DRUG LIST

GENERIC NAME	PAGE	GENERIC NAME	PAGE
Amphotericin B	596	Miconazole	600
Butoconazole	601	Naftifine hydrochloride	602
Capsofungin	601	Nystatin	598
Ciclopirox	602	Oxiconazole nitrate	601
Clotrimazole	600	Sulconazole nitrate	601
Econazole	601	Terbinifine hydrochloride	602
Fluconazole	598	Terconazole	601
Flucytosine	601	Tioconazole	601
Griseofulvin	602	Tolnaftate	602
Itraconazole	599	Undecylenic acid	602
Ketoconazole	599	Voriconazole	600

Fungal infections are usually more difficult to treat than bacterial infections, because fungal organisms grow slowly and because fungal infections often occur in tissues that are poorly penetrated by antimicrobial agents (e.g., devitalized or avascular tissues). Therapy of fungal infections usually requires prolonged treatment. Potentially life-threatening infections caused by dimorphic fungi are becoming more common because increasing numbers of immunocompromised patients are seen in clinical practice; AIDS, organ and bone marrow transplantation, and illnesses associated with neutropenia all predispose individuals to invasive fungal infection.

Superficial fungal infections involve cutaneous surfaces, such as the skin, nails, and hair, and mucous membrane surfaces, such as the oropharynx and vagina. A growing number of topical and systemic agents are available for the treatment of these infections. Deep-seated or disseminated fungal infections caused by dimorphic fungi, the yeasts *Cryptococcus neoformans*, and various *Candida* spp. respond to a limited number of systemic agents: amphotericin B desoxycholate (a polyene), amphotericin B liposomal preparations, flucytosine (a pyrimidine antimetabolite), the newer azoles, including ketoconazole, fluconazole, itraconazole and voriconazole, and capsofungin (an echinocandin).

AMPHOTERICIN B

Chemistry and Mechanism of Action

Amphotericin B (*Fungizone*), a polyene antifungal drug produced by the actinomycete *Streptomyces nodosus*, consists of a large ring structure with both hydrophilic and lipophilic regions. Polyene antifungal drugs bind to the fungal cell membrane component ergosterol, leading to increased fungal cell membrane permeability and the loss of intracellular constituents. Amphotericin has a lesser affinity for the mammalian cell membrane component cholesterol, but this interaction does account for most adverse toxic effects associated with this drug.

Antifungal Spectrum

Amphotericin B is used to treat systemic disseminated fungal infections caused by *Candida* spp., *Cryptococcus neoformans*, and the invasive dimorphic fungi (*Aspergillus* spp., *Histoplasma capsulatum*, *Coccidioides immitis*, *Blastomyces dermatitidis*, and *Sporothrix schenckii*). Intravenous amphotericin B remains the treatment of choice for serious invasive fungal infections unresponsive to other agents.

The development of resistance during amphotericin B therapy is rarely clinically significant but has been reported; relative resistance expressed through alterations in membrane ergosterols has resulted in fungal isolates with reduced growth rates and reduced virulence. Infections with organisms intrinsically resistant to amphotericin B, such as *Candidia lusitaniae* and *Pseudallescheria boydii*, are uncommon but may be increasing in frequency.

Absorption, Distribution, Metabolism, and Excretion

Amphotericin B is primarily an intravenous drug; absorption from the intestinal tract is minimal. After infusion the drug is rapidly taken up by the liver and other organs and is then slowly released back into the circulation, where 90% of the drug is bound to protein. Its initial half-life is about 24 hours; the second elimination phase has a half-life of 15 days. The initial phase comprises elimination from both a central intravascular and a rapidly equilibrating extravascular compartment; the second, longer phase represents elimination from storage sites in a slowly equilibrating extravascular compartment.

Drug concentrations in pleural fluid, peritoneal fluid, synovial fluid, aqueous humor, and vitreous humor approach two-thirds of the serum concentration when local inflammation is present. Meningeal and amniotic fluid penetration, with or without local inflammation, is uniformly poor. Measurement of serum, urine, or cerebrospinal fluid drug levels has not been used clinically.

The major route of elimination of amphotericin B is by metabolism, with little intact drug detected in urine or bile. About 5% of amphotericin B is excreted in the urine as active drug, with drug still detectable in the urine 7 or more weeks after the last dose. Serum levels

are not elevated in renal or hepatic failure, and the drug is not removed by hemodialysis.

Clinical Uses

Amphotericin B is most commonly used to treat serious disseminated yeast and dimorphic fungal infections in immunocompromised hospitalized patients. As additional experience has been gained in the treatment of fungal infections with the newer azoles, the use of amphotericin B has diminished; if azole drugs have equivalent efficacy, they are preferred to amphotericin B because of their reduced toxicity profile and ease of administration. For the unstable neutropenic patient with *Candida albicans* fungemia, amphotericin B is the drug of choice. For the stable nonneutropenic patient with *C. albicans* fungemia, fluconazole appears to be an acceptable alternative. For the AIDS patient with moderate to severe cryptococcal meningitis, amphotericin B appears to be superior to fluconazole for initial treatment; once infection is controlled, fluconazole in a daily oral dose is superior to and more convenient than weekly intravenous amphotericin B in the prevention of clinical relapses. For the AIDS patient with disseminated histoplasmosis, the treatment is similar; amphotericin B is preferred for the initiation of treatment, but once infection is controlled, daily oral itraconazole is preferred to intermittently dosed amphotericin B for suppression of chronic infection. Most forms of blastomycosis and sporotrichosis in normal hosts no longer require amphotericin B treatment.

Amphotericin B remains the drug of choice in the treatment of invasive aspergillosis, locally invasive mucormycosis, and many disseminated fungal infections occurring in immunocompromised hosts (the patient population most at risk for serious fungal infections). For example, the febrile neutropenic oncology patient with persistent fever despite empirical antibacterial therapy is best treated with amphotericin B for possible *Candida* spp. sepsis.

Adverse Effects

Fever, chills, and tachypnea commonly occur shortly after the initial intravenous doses of amphotericin B; this is not generally an allergic hypersensitivity to the drug, which is extremely rare. Continued administration of amphotericin B is accomplished by premedication with acetaminophen, aspirin, and/or diphenhydramine or the addition of hydrocortisone to the infusion bag.

Nephrotoxicity is the most common and the most serious long-term toxicity of amphotericin B administration. This drug reduces glomerular and renal tubular blood flow through a vasoconstrictive effect on afferent renal arterioles, which can lead to destruction of renal tubular cells and disruption of the tubular basement membrane. Wasting of potassium and magnesium in the urine secondary to renal tubular acidosis usually results in hypokalemia and hypomagnesemia and necessitates oral or intravenous replacement of the minerals. Nephrotoxicity can be lessened by avoiding the concomitant administration of other nephrotoxic agents, such as aminoglycosides. Keeping patients well hydrated probably reduces nephrotoxicity; saline infusions prior to amphotericin B dosing have been advocated, and concomitant diuretic therapy should be avoided. Prolonging the infusion rate has been studied as a potential means of decreasing amphotericin B toxicity. Infusing the daily dose over 1 or 4 hours seems to make little difference, but recent data suggest that a continuous infusion of amphotericin B (giving the daily dose over 24 hours) decreases infusion-related adverse effects such as fever and also reduces nephrotoxicity. Increasing the dosing interval for amphotericin B to every other day may lessen nephrotoxicity *only* if the total dose of the drug delivered is reduced.

Normochromic normocytic anemia is the most common hematological side effect of amphotericin B administration; thrombocytopenia and leukopenia are much less common. Infusion of the drug into a peripheral vein usually causes phlebitis or thrombophlebitis. Nausea, vomiting, and anorexia are a persistent problem for some patients.

Lipid Formulations of Amphotericin B

Three lipid formulations of amphotericin B (amphotericin B colloidal dispersion: *Amphocil, Amphotec;* amphotericin B lipid complex: *Ablecet;* and liposomal amphotericin B: *Ambisome*) have been developed in an attempt to reduce the toxicity profile of this drug and to increase efficacy. Formulating amphotericin with lipids alters drug distribution, with lower levels of drug in the kidneys, reducing the incidence of nephrotoxicity. The lipid formulations appear to be equivalent to conventional amphotericin B both in the treatment of documented fungal infections and in the empirical treatment of the febrile neutropenic patient. While less toxic, the lipid formulations are significantly more expensive than conventional amphotericin B.

NYSTATIN

Nystatin (*Mycostatin*) is a polyene antifungal drug with a ring structure similar to that of amphotericin B and a mechanism of action identical to that of amphotericin B. Too toxic for systemic use, nystatin is limited to the topical treatment of superficial infections caused by *C. albicans*. Infections commonly treated by this drug include oral candidiasis (thrush), mild esophageal candidiasis, and vaginitis.

THE AZOLES

Azole antifungal drugs are synthetic compounds with broad-spectrum fungistatic activity. Azoles can be divided into two groups: the older imidazole agents, in which the five-member azole nucleus contains two nitrogens, and the newer triazole compounds, fluconazole and itraconazole, in which the azole nucleus contains three nitrogens.

All azoles exert antifungal activity by binding to cytochrome P450 enzymes responsible for the demethylation of lanosterol to ergosterol. Reduced fungal membrane ergosterol concentrations result in damaged, leaky cell membranes. The toxicity of these drugs depends on their relative affinities for mammalian and fungal cytochrome P450 enzymes. The triazoles tend to have fewer side effects, better absorption, better drug distribution in body tissues, and fewer drug interactions.

FLUCONAZOLE

Absorption, Distribution, Metabolism, and Excretion

Fluconazole (*Diflucan*) does not require an acidic environment, as does ketoconazole, for gastrointestinal absorption. About 80 to 90% of an orally administered dose is absorbed, yielding high serum drug levels. The half-life of the drug is 27 to 37 hours, permitting once-daily dosing in patients with normal renal function. Only 11% of circulating drug is bound to plasma proteins. The drug penetrates widely into most body tissues, including normal and inflamed meninges. Cerebrospinal fluid levels are 60 to 80% of serum levels, permitting effective treatment for fungal meningitis. About 80% of the drug is excreted unchanged in the urine, and 10% is excreted unchanged in the feces. Dosage reductions are required in the presence of renal insufficiency.

Clinical Uses

Fluconazole is very effective in the treatment of infections with most *Candida* spp. Thrush in the end-stage AIDS patient, often refractory to nystatin, clotrimazole, and ketoconazole, can usually be suppressed with oral fluconazole. AIDS patients with esophageal candidiasis also usually respond to fluconazole. A single 150-mg dose has been shown to be effective treatment for vaginal candidiasis. A 3-day course of oral fluconazole is effective treatment for *Candida* urinary tract infection and is more convenient than amphotericin B bladder irrigation. Preliminary findings suggest that *Candida* endophthalmitis can be successfully treated with fluconazole. Stable nonneutropenic patients with candidemia can be adequately treated with fluconazole, but unstable, immunosuppressed patients should initially receive amphotericin B. *Candida krusei* isolates may be resistant to fluconazole.

Fluconazole may be an acceptable alternative to amphotericin B in the initial treatment of mild cryptococcal meningitis, and it has been shown to be superior to amphotericin B in the long-term prevention of relapsing meningitis (such patients require lifelong treatment.). Coccidioidal meningitis, previously treated with both intravenous and intrathecal amphotericin B, appears to respond at least as well to prolonged oral fluconazole therapy. Aspergillosis, mucormycosis, and pseudallescheriasis do not respond to fluconazole treatment. Sporotrichosis, histoplasmosis, and blastomycosis appear to be better treated with itraconazole, although fluconazole does appear to have significant activity against these dimorphic fungi.

A significant decrease in mortality from deep-seated mycoses was noted among bone marrow transplant recipients treated prophylactically with fluconazole, but similar benefits have not been seen in leukemia patients receiving prophylactic fluconazole. Fluconazole taken prophylactically by end-stage AIDS patients can reduce the incidence of cryptococcal meningitis, esophageal candidiasis, and superficial fungal infections.

Adverse Effects

Fluconazole is well tolerated. Nausea, vomiting, abdominal pain, diarrhea, and skin rash have been reported in fewer than 3% of patients. Asymptomatic liver enzyme elevation has been described, and several cases of drug-associated hepatic necrosis have been reported. Alopecia has been reported as a common adverse event in patients receiving prolonged high-dose therapy. Coadministration of fluconazole with phenytoin results in increased serum phenytoin levels.

ITRACONAZOLE

Absorption, Distribution, Metabolism, and Excretion

Although itraconazole and fluconazole are both triazoles, they are chemically and pharmacologically distinct. Itraconazole (*Sporanox*) is lipophilic and water insoluble and requires a low gastric pH for absorption. Oral bioavailability is variable, only 50 to 60% when taken with food and 20% or less when the drug is taken on an empty stomach. Itraconazole is highly protein bound (99%) and is metabolized in the liver and excreted into the bile. With initial dosing, the plasma half-life is 15 to 20 hours; steady-state serum concentrations are reached only after 2 weeks of therapy, when the half-life is extended to 30 to 35 hours. In lipophilic tissues, drug concentration is 2 to 20 times that found in serum. Drug does not appear in significant quantities in the urine and cannot be measured in spinal fluid.

Clinical Uses

Itraconazole is most useful in the long-term suppressive treatment of disseminated histoplasmosis in AIDS and in the oral treatment of nonmeningeal, non–life-threatening blastomycosis. It appears to be the drug of choice for all forms of sporotrichosis except meningitis and may have a lower relapse rate in the treatment of disseminated coccidioidomycosis than does fluconazole.

Itraconazole has replaced ketoconazole as the drug of choice in the treatment of paracoccidioidomycosis and chromomycosis, based on its lower toxicity profile. Efficacy has also been reported in the treatment of invasive aspergillosis.

Despite negligible cerebrospinal fluid concentrations, itraconazole shows promise in the treatment of cryptococcal and coccidioidal meningitis. Additional uses for itraconazole include treatment of vaginal candidiasis, tinea versicolor, dermatophyte infections, and onychomycosis. Fungal nail infections account for most use of this drug in the outpatient setting.

Adverse Effects

Itraconazole is usually well tolerated but can be associated with nausea and epigastric distress. Dizziness and headache also have been reported. High doses may cause hypokalemia, hypertension, and edema. Itraconazole, unlike ketoconazole, is not associated with hormonal suppression. Hepatotoxicity occurs in fewer than 5% of cases and is usually manifested by reversible liver enzyme elevations.

Drug Interactions

Itraconazole has significant interactions with a number of commonly prescribed drugs, such as rifampin, phenytoin, and carbamazepine. Itraconazole raises serum digoxin and cyclosporine levels and may affect the metabolism of oral hypoglycemic agents and coumadin. Absorption of itraconazole is impaired by antacids, H_2 blockers, proton pump inhibitors, and drugs that contain buffers, such as the antiretroviral agent didanosine.

KETOCONAZOLE

Absorption, Distribution, Metabolism, and Excretion

Unlike other imidazoles, ketoconazole (*Nizoral*) can be absorbed orally, but it requires an acidic gastric environment; patients concurrently treated with H_2 blockers or who have achlorhydria have minimal drug absorption. Serum protein binding exceeds 90%. The drug is metabolized in the liver and excreted in the bile. The initial half-life of ketoconazole is 2 hours; 8 to 12 hours after ingestion, the half-life increases to 9 hours.

Reductions in renal and hepatic function do not alter plasma drug concentrations, and ketoconazole is not removed by hemodialysis or peritoneal dialysis. Penetration into cerebrospinal fluid is negligible, so that ketoconazole is ineffective in the treatment of fungal meningitis. Since only small amounts of active drug appear in the urine, ketoconazole is not effective in the treatment of *Candida* cystitis.

Clinical Uses

Ketoconazole remains useful in the treatment of cutaneous and mucous membrane dermatophyte and yeast infections, but it has been replaced by the newer triazoles in the treatment of most serious *Candida* infections and disseminated mycoses. Ketoconazole is usually effective in the treatment of thrush, but fluconazole is superior to ketoconazole for refractory thrush. Widespread dermatophyte infections on skin surfaces can be treated easily with oral ketoconazole when the use of topical antifungal agents would be impractical. Treatment of vulvovaginal candidiasis with topical imidazoles is less expensive.

Blastomycosis, histoplasmosis, sporotrichosis, paracoccidioidomycosis, and chromomycosis are better treated with itraconazole than ketoconazole, although ketoconazole remains an alternative agent. Ketoconazole is ineffective in the treatment of cryptococcosis, aspergillosis, and mucormycosis. Candidemia is best treated with fluconazole or amphotericin B.

Adverse Effects

Nausea, vomiting, and anorexia occur commonly with ketoconazole, especially when high doses are prescribed. Epigastric distress can be reduced by taking ketoconazole with food. Pruritis and/or allergic dermatitis occurs in 10% of patients. Liver enzyme elevations during therapy are not unusual and are usually reversible. Severe ketoconazole-associated hepatitis is rare.

At high doses, ketoconazole causes a clinically significant reduction in testosterone synthesis and blocks the adrenal response to corticotropin. Gynecomastia, impotence, reduced sperm counts, and diminished libido can occur in men, and prolonged drug use can result in irregular menses in women. These hormonal effects have led to the use of ketoconazole as a potential adjunctive treatment for prostatic carcinoma.

Drug Interactions

Both rifampin and isoniazid lower plasma ketoconazole levels, and concomitant administration should be avoided.

Phenytoin serum levels should be monitored closely when ketoconazole is prescribed. Ketoconazole causes increases in serum concentrations of warfarin, cyclosporine, and sulfonylureas. Because of its ability to increase serum cyclosporine levels, ketoconazole has been given to cyclosporine-dependent cardiac transplant recipients to reduce the dose of cyclosporine needed and as a cost-saving measure.

MICONAZOLE

Miconazole (*Monistat*) is a broad-spectrum imidazole antifungal agent used in the topical treatment of cutaneous dermatophyte infections and mucous membrane *Candida* infections, such as vaginitis. Minimal absorption occurs from skin or mucous membrane surfaces. Local irritation to skin and mucous membranes can occur with topical use; headaches, urticaria, and abdominal cramping have been reported with treatment for vaginitis.

CLOTRIMAZOLE

Clotrimazole (*Lotrimin, Gyne-Lotrimin, Mycelex*) is a broad-spectrum fungistatic imidazole drug used in the topical treatment of oral, skin, and vaginal infections with *C. albicans*. It is also employed in the treatment of infections with cutaneous dermatophytes.

Topical use results in therapeutic drug concentrations in the epidermis and mucous membranes; less than 10% of the drug is systemically absorbed. Although clotrimazole is generally well tolerated, local abdominal cramping, increased urination, and transient liver enzyme elevations have been reported.

VORICONAZOLE

Voriconazole (*Vfend*), a derivative of fluconazole, is a second-generation triazole that has improved antifungal activity against *Aspergillus* and *Fusarium* spp., *P. boydii, Penicillium marneffei,* and fluconazole-resistant *Candida* spp. Like fluconazole, voriconazole has high oral bioavailability and good cerebrospinal fluid penetration, but unlike fluconazole, it undergoes extensive hepatic metabolism and is highly protein bound. No significant amount of bioactive drug is excreted into the urine. Dosage reduction is necessary with severe hepatic insufficiency but not with renal insufficiency.

Significant drug interactions include cyclosporins (increased cyclosporine levels), phenytoin, rifampin, and rifabutin (decreased voriconazole levels). Because of its low toxicity profile, this drug may gain importance in the chronic treatment of infections with invasive dimorphic fungi and resistant *Candida* spp.

OTHER IMIDAZOLES

A number of topical imidazoles are available for the treatment of cutaneous and mucous membrane candidiasis, ringworm, and tinea versicolor. Butoconazole (*Femstat*) is an effective topical agent for vaginal candidiasis; terconazole (*Terazol*) is effective in the treatment of vaginal candidiasis; and econazole (*Spectazole*) is useful in the treatment of superficial fungal infections of the skin, achieving high tissue levels in the stratum corneum. Oxiconazole nitrate (*Oxistat*) and sulconazole nitrate (*Exelderm*) are topical imidazole derivatives available for the treatment of dermatophyte infections and pityriasis (tinea versicolor). Tioconazole (*Vagistat*) is available without a prescription for the treatment of dermatophyte infections and candidiasis.

All of these agents have minimal systemic absorption when applied topically, but occasionally use of these drugs can result in systemic toxicity.

FLUCYTOSINE

Chemistry and Mechanism of Action

Flucytosine (5-flucytosine, 5-FC; *Ancoban*) is a fluorinated pyrimidine analogue of cytosine that was originally synthesized for possible use as an antineoplastic agent. 5-FC is converted to 5-fluorouracil inside the cell by the fungal enzyme cytosine deaminase. Subsequently, 5-FC metabolites interfere with fungal DNA synthesis by inhibiting thymidylate synthetase. Incorporation of these metabolites into fungal RNA may inhibit protein synthesis.

Absorption, Distribution, Metabolism, and Excretion

5-FC is well absorbed orally, with greater than 90% bioavailability. The serum half-life is 3 to 5 hours, with serum levels peaking 4 to 6 hours after a single dose. The drug is widely distributed in body fluids, with cerebrospinal fluid levels 60 to 80% of serum levels. The drug also penetrates well into urine, aqueous humor, and bronchial secretions. Minimal serum protein binding allows more than 90% of each dose to be excreted in the urine; significant dosage reductions are required in the presence of renal impairment. 5-FC can be removed by both hemodialysis and peritoneal dialysis. 5-FC conversion to toxic metabolites may occur in mammalian cells to a limited extent, which accounts for 5-FC toxicity.

Clinical Uses

Flucytosine has significant antifungal activity against *C. albicans*, other *Candida* spp., *C. neoformans,* and the fungal organisms responsible for chromomycosis. Not considered the drug of choice for these fungal infections, *5-FC does remain useful as part of combination therapy for systemic candidiasis and cryptococcal meningitis and as an alternative drug for chromomycosis.* When it is used as monotherapy, resistance and clinical failure are common. Potential mechanisms for drug resistance include decreased fungal cell membrane permeability and reduced levels of fungal cytosine deaminase. Combination therapy with amphotericin B and flucytosine in the treatment of cryptococcal meningitis and deep-seated *Candida* infections, such as septic arthritis and meningitis, permits reduced dosing of amphotericin B and prevents the emergence of 5-FC resistance. When higher doses of amphotericin B are used, combination therapy with 5-FC confers no additional clinical benefit except in the treatment of *Candida* endophthalmitis, where tissue penetration remains problematic.

Adverse Effects

When 5-FC is prescribed alone to patients with normal renal function, skin rash, epigastric distress, diarrhea, and liver enzyme elevations can occur. When it is prescribed to patients with renal insufficiency or to patients receiving concurrent amphotericin B therapy, blood levels of 5-FC may rise, and bone marrow toxicity leading to leukopenia and thrombocytopenia is common. 5-FC serum levels should be closely monitored in patients with renal insufficiency. Because of baseline leukopenia, 5-FC is often not tolerated by end-stage HIV-infected patients with disseminated fungal infection.

CAPSOFUNGIN

Capsofungin (*Cancidas*) is a semisynthetic lipopeptide known as an echinocandin, the first representative of a new class of antifungal agents that inhibit the synthesis of β-(1,3)-D-glucan, a cell wall component of filamentous fungi. Capsofungin has in vitro activity against *Aspergillus fumigatus, Aspergillus flavus,* and *Aspergillus terreus;* it is approved for the treatment of invasive aspergillosis in patients not responding to other antifungal agents, such as amphotericin B, lipid formulations of amphotericin B, and itraconazole. Additional indications for the use of this drug await further clinical study.

Capsofungin is not absorbed from the gastrointestinal tract. It is highly protein bound and has a serum half-life of 9 to 11 hours. Capsofungin appears to undergo liver metabolism and is not excreted in the urine. Adverse effects are mediated through histamine release; they include facial flushing, rash, fever, and pruritis. Nausea and vomiting have also been reported. Dose reductions are required in the presence of moderate hepatic insufficiency.

ALLYLAMINES

The allylamines (naftifine hydrochloride and terbinafine hydrochloride) are reversible noncompetitive inhibitors of the fungal enzyme squalene monooxygenase (squalene 2,3-epoxidase), which coverts squalene to lanosterol. With a decrease in lanosterol production, ergosterol production is also diminished, affecting fungal cell membrane synthesis and function. These agents generally exhibit fungicidal activity against dermatophytes and fungistatic activity against yeasts.

Naftifine hydrochloride (*Naftin*) is available for topical use only in the treatment of cutaneous dermatophyte and *Candida* infections; it is as effective as topical azoles for these conditions.

Terbinafine hydrochloride (*Lamisil*) is available for topical and systemic use (oral tablet) in the treatment of dermatophyte skin and nail infections. Terbinafine also exhibits in vitro activity against filamentous and dimorphic fungi, but its clinical utility in treating infections with these organisms has not yet been established. It is used most commonly in the treatment of onychomycosis; in this setting, terbinafine is superior to griseofulvin and at least equivalent to itraconazole. When given systemically, terbinafine is 99% protein bound and accumulates in fat, skin, and nails, persisting for weeks. Cerebrospinal fluid penetration is less than 10%. Dosage reductions are required with renal or hepatic insufficiency. Although terbinafine has little effect on hepatic cytochrome P450 enzyme systems, it does minimally enhance cyclosporine clearance. Oral terbinafine is generally well tolerated but occasionally causes gastric distress and liver enzyme elevation.

GRISEOFULVIN

Griseofulvin (*Gris-PEG, Grifulvin, Grisactin, Fulvicin*) is an oral fungistatic agent used in the long-term treatment of dermatophyte infections caused by *Epidermophyton, Microsporum,* and *Trichophyton* spp. Produced by the mold *Penicillium griseofulvin*, this agent inhibits fungal growth by binding to the microtubules responsible for mitotic spindle formation, leading to defective cell wall development.

Ineffective topically, griseofulvin is administered orally but has poor gastrointestinal absorption; absorption can be improved by microcrystalline processing of the drug and by taking the drug with fatty meals. Peak serum levels occur 4 hours after dosing. Griseofulvin is metabolized in the liver and has a half-life of 24 to 36 hours. The drug binds to keratin precursor cells and newly synthesized keratin in the stratum corneum of the skin, hair, and nails, stopping the progression of dermatophyte infection.

In the treatment of ringworm of the beard, scalp, and other skin surfaces, 4 to 6 weeks of therapy is often required. Therapy failure may be to the result of an incorrect diagnosis; superficial candidiasis, which may resemble a dermatophyte infection, does not respond to griseofulvin treatment. Onychomycosis responds very slowly to griseofulvin (1 year or more of treatment is commonly required) and cure rates are poor; itraconazole and terbinafine hydrochloride are more effective than griseofulvin for onychomycosis.

Griseofulvin is usually well tolerated. Headache is common with initiation of therapy. Hepatotoxicity (especially in patients with acute intermittent porphyria), dermatitis, and gastrointestinal distress also occur. Griseofulvin increases warfarin metabolism, and griseofulvin metabolism is increased by phenobarbital.

MISCELLANEOUS TOPICAL ANTIFUNGAL AGENTS

Ciclopirox olamine (*Loprox*) is a pyridone derivative available for the treatment of cutaneous dermatophyte infections, cutaneous *C. albicans* infections, and tinea versicolor caused by *Malassezia furfur*. It interferes with fungal growth by inhibiting macromolecule synthesis.

Tolnaftate (*Tinactin*, others) is a nonprescription antifungal agent effective in the topical treatment of dermatophyte infections and tinea. The mechanism of action is unknown.

Other older, less effective topical antifungal agents still available include undecylenic acid (*Desenex,* others). Used in the treatment of topical dermatophytes, undecylenic acid is fungistatic, requires prolonged administration, and is associated with a high relapse rate. *Desenex*, containing 5% undecylenic acid and 20% zinc undecylenate, is effective in the prevention of recurrent tinea pedis.

Study QUESTIONS

1. A 65-year-old man with acute leukemia recently underwent induction chemotherapy and subsequently developed neutropenia and fever (with no source of fever identified). Fever persisted despite the use of empirical antibacterial therapy, and amphotericin B has been prescribed for possible fungal sepsis. Which laboratory test is LEAST helpful in monitoring for toxicities associated with amphotericin B?
   (A) Liver function tests
   (B) Serum potassium
   (C) Serum magnesium
   (D) Serum blood urea nitrogen and creatinine
   (E) Hemoglobin and hematocrit

2. A 55-year-old obese woman with adult-onset diabetes mellitus has been receiving amoxicillin for treatment of an acute exacerbation of chronic bronchitis. After a week of therapy, the patient develops dysuria and increased urinary frequency. Urinalysis shows 10 to 50 white blood cells per high-power field, and Gram stain of urine shows many budding yeasts. Which antifungal agent would be best in treating this patient for *Candida* cystitis?
   (A) Oral ketoconazole
   (B) Oral fluconazole
   (C) Topical clotrimazole
   (D) Oral 5-flucytosine
   (E) Oral itraconazole

3. A 43-year-old woman recently underwent allogeneic bone marrow transplantation after chemotherapy failed in the treatment of metastatic breast carcinoma. The patient has had a stormy hospital course after her transplant, with respiratory failure requiring mechanical ventilation. A month into her hospitalization, surveillance sputum cultures reveal *Aspergillus fumigatus*, and a new infiltrate appears on her chest radiograph. Which antifungal agent is recommended for the treatment of invasive pulmonary aspergillosis in this patient?
   (A) Fluconazole
   (B) Amphotericin B
   (C) Amphotericin B with 5-flucytosine
   (D) Capsofungin
   (E) Itraconazole

4. A 57-year-old man with extensive onychomycosis (fungal toenail infection) asks you for an evaluation. He requests a prescription for itraconazole for treatment of this problem after seeing a television advertisement for this drug. He has chronic heartburn attributed to gastroesophageal reflux disease and is treated with the proton pump inhibitor omeprazole. He is taking lovastatin for treatment of hyperlipidemia. Three years ago he underwent cadaveric renal transplantation for end-stage kidney disease secondary to polycystic kidney disease and is taking cyclosporin to prevent transplant rejection. In prescribing itraconazole for this patient, what adjustments in his medication regimen do you recommend?
   (A) Discontinue omeprazole and substitute the H2 blocker ranitidine.
   (B) Discontinue omeprazole and substitute liquid antacids.
   (C) Discontinue omeprazole.
   (D) Continue lovastatin.
   (E) Increase cyclosporin dosing.

ANSWERS

1. **A.** Nephrotoxicity is the most common and most serious toxicity associated with amphotericin B administration. This is manifested by azotemia (elevated serum blood urea nitrogen and creatinine), and by renal tubular acidosis, which results in the wasting of potassium and magnesium in the urine (leading to hypokalemia and hypomagnesemia, requiring oral or intravenous replacement therapy). Normochromic normocytic anemia is also seen with long-term amphotericin B administration. Elevation of liver enzymes is not associated with the use of amphotericin B.

2. **B.** Oral fluconazole is well absorbed from the gastrointestinal tract, and 80% of drug is excreted into the urinary tract, allowing effective treatment of *Candida* cystitis. Subtherapeutic concentrations of itraconazole and ketoconazole are excreted into the urine; these agents are not effective in the treatment of *Candida* cystitis. Topical clotrimazole would be effective in the treatment of *Candida* vaginitis, which can cause dysuria, but would not be an effective treatment for cystitis. While 90% of 5-flucytosine is excreted unchanged in the urine, this more toxic agent is usually used only in combination therapy with a second antifungal agent (usually amphotericin B) in the treatment of systemic candidiasis or cryptococcal meningitis.

3. **B.** Amphotericin B remains the drug of choice in the treatment of disseminated or invasive fungal infections in immunocompromised hosts; bone marrow transplant recipients are the most heavily immunocompromised patients encountered in the hospital setting. 5-Flucytosine has no significant activity against *Aspergillus* spp., and it has bone marrow toxicity as a common adverse effect; it should

not be used in this setting. Fluconazole has not been shown to be effective in the treatment of aspergillosis. Itraconazole has been reported to be effective as salvage treatment in patients with aspergillosis if amphotericin B therapy fails; it should not be used as initial treatment in this setting. Capsofungin, a new echinocandin antifungal agent recently approved by the U. S. Food and Drug Administration for the treatment of refractory aspergillosis when standard therapy with amphotericin B fails, should also not be used to treat invasive aspergillosis until more data showing efficacy are available.

4. **C.** Patients receiving multiple medications may have adverse drug reactions when a new medication is added to the regimen. Itraconazole requires an acidic gastric environment for absorption; any drug reducing gastric acid production (H_2 blockers, proton pump inhibitors) or neutralizing gastric acid (antacids) will significantly reduce itraconazole absorption. Itraconazole inhibits the metabolism of lovastatin and simvastatin and should not be prescribed with these β-hydroxy-β-methyglutaryl–coenzyme A reductase inhibitors. Itraconazole will raise serum cyclosporin levels, resulting in cyclosporin toxicity, unless cyclosporin levels are closely monitored with dose reductions as indicated.

SUPPLEMENTAL READING

Abramowitz M (ed.). Capsofungin (*Cancidas*) for aspergillosis. Med Lett 2001;43:58–59.

Andriole VT. Current and future therapy of invasive fungal infections. In Remington JS and Swartz MN (eds.). Current clinical topics in infectious diseases. Vol. 18. Cambridge, MA: Blackwell Scientific, 1998:19–36.

Edwards JE. Management of severe candidal infections: Integration and review of current guidelines for treatment and prevention. In Remington JS and Swartz MN (eds.). Current clinical topics in infectious diseases. Vol. 21. Cambridge, MA: Blackwell Scientific, 2001:135–147.

Hatem CJ and Kettyle WM (eds.). Infectious Disease Medicine. In Medical knowledge self-assessment program 12. Philadelphia: American College of Physicians, 2000:61–71.

McEvoy GK (ed.). American hospital formulary service drug information 2001. Bethesda, MD: American Society of Health-System Pharmacists, 2001.

Sabo JA and Abdel-Rahman SM. Voriconazole: A new triazole antifungal. Ann Pharmacotherapy 2000;34:1032–1043.

Stevens DA and Bennett JE. Antifungal agents. In Mandell GL, Bennett JE, and Dolin R (eds.). Principles and Practice of Infectious Diseases (5th ed.). New York: Churchill Livingston, 2000:448–459.

Walsh TJ et al. Liposomal amphotericin B for empirical therapy in patients with persistent fever and neutropenia. N Engl J Med 1999;340:764–771.

Wong-Beringer A, Jacobs RA, and Guglielmo BJ. Lipid formulations of amphotericin B: Clinical efficacy and toxicities. Clin Infect Dis 1998;27:603–618.

CASE Study   Chronic Disseminated Candidiasis

A 56-year-old man was admitted to the hospital for initiation of chemotherapy for acute myelogenous leukemia. Several weeks after completing induction chemotherapy, he developed profound neutropenia (absolute granulocyte count of less than 100 cells per milliliter, normal 800–9400), a known complication of chemotherapy. The patient received granulocyte-monocyte colony stimulating factor (GM-CSF), but neutropenia persisted; he then had a temperature elevation to 103°F (39.4°C). The patient received ceftazidime as empirical coverage for gram-negative sepsis. Vancomycin empirical coverage was added 2 days later as high fever persisted. Despite antibacterial coverage, high fevers continued, and 3 days later the patient began empirical therapy with amphotericin B for possible fungal sepsis. With the addition of amphotericin B, the patient appeared to improve clinically, with less fever. However, the patient remained profoundly neutropenic for the next several weeks. He required supplemental intravenous potassium and magnesium to replace electrolytes lost in the urine to amphotericin B–induced renal tubular acidosis. When his serum creatinine rose to 2.5 mg/dL, amphotericin B was discontinued, and a lipid formulation of amphotericin B was substituted; renal function stabilized and then improved slightly. After 4 weeks of profound neutropenia, the patient was noted to have a rapid rebound in granulocyte count. However, the patient once again developed high fever and appeared ill. Liver function tests revealed an elevation in serum transaminases. A computed tomographic scan of the abdomen revealed multiple small low-density lesions in the liver and spleen. Antifungal therapy with a lipid formulation of amphotericin B was continued. The patient had a

CASE **Study**   Chronic Disseminated Candidiasis

stormy course requiring 4 additional weeks of antifungal therapy. Eventually the patient's liver enzymes returned to normal and follow-up abdominal computed tomography showed resolution of hepatic and splenic abscesses. He was discharged home after a 2- month hospitalization. What happened?

ANSWER: Chronic disseminated candidiasis (hepatosplenic candidiasis) occurs in patients with profound neutropenia. This patient was appropriately treated for possible fungal sepsis when antibacterial therapy failed to resolve fever in the setting of neutropenia. Despite therapy, however, the patient did have disseminated candidiasis, which persisted in a subclinical state during the long period of neutrope-

nia. Once neutropenia resolved and the patient could generate an inflammatory response, fever reappeared and the patient worsened clinically. A new elevation in serum transaminases provided the clue that led to abdominal imaging and the detection of abscesses in the liver and spleen. The diagnosis of chronic disseminated candidiasis is often not confirmed by blood culture; the yield of blood cultures in the detection of candidemia is poor, with up to 50% of blood cultures falsely negative in this setting. Chronic disseminated candidiasis in neutropenic leukemia patients is a life-threatening infection with significant morbidity and mortality.

53

Antiprotozoal Drugs

Leonard William Scheibel

DRUG LIST

GENERIC NAME	PAGE	GENERIC NAME	PAGE
Amodiaquine	614	Metronidazole	608
Atovaquone	616	Nifurtimox	610
Chloroguanide	615	Paromomycin	609
Chloroquine	613	Pentamidine	609
Dapsone	615	Primaquine	614
Diloxanide	609	Pyrimethamine	614
Eflornithine	610	Quinine	615
Hydroxychloroquine	614	Sodium stibogluconate	611
Iodoquinol	608	Suramin	609
Mefloquine	616	Trimethoprim	614
Meglumine antimonate	611	Tryparsamide	610
Melarsoprol	610		

Protozoal and helminthic infections are a major cause of disease in many parts of the world. Although some of these diseases are endemic to the United States or can be found in migrant workers or individuals returning from an endemic area, many other such infections are rarely seen in the United States. However, physicians should be aware of these diseases and seek advice from those experienced in their diagnosis and treatment.

Although the mode of action of many antiprotozoals is not well understood, Table 53.1 summarizes the assumed or known modes of action of a number of the agents. The treatment of malaria is discussed at the end of this chapter.

PROTOZOAL DISEASES

Amebiasis and Balantidial Dysentery

The protozoan *Entamoeba histolytica* causes amebiasis, an infection that is endemic in parts of the United States. The parasite can be present in the host as either an encysted or a trophozoite form. Initial ingestion of the cyst may result either in no symptoms or in severe amebic dysentery characterized by the frequent passage of bloodstained stools. The latter symptom occurs after invasion of the intestinal mucosa by the actively motile and phagocytic trophozoite form of the protozoan.

TABLE **53.1** **Chemotherapeutic Agents Used in Treatment of Protozoal Disease**

Drug	Specific Effects	Mode of Action
Arsenicals (melarsoprol, tryparsamide), antimonials	Binds with SH groups; selectively inhibits pyruvate kinase or phosphofructokinase	Affects cellular structure, function, synthesis or energy production
Paromomycin	Interferes with initiation complex; causes misreading of mRNA	Affects protein structure, function, synthesis
Diamidines (pentamidine)	Binds to kinetoplast DNA	Affects synthesis or structure of nucleic acids
Metronidazole	Inhibits DNA replication	Affects synthesis or structure of nucleic acids
Nifurtimox	Generation of toxic oxygen radicals	Unknown
Suramin	Binds to plasma proteins; inhibits glucose utilization	Unknown
Iodoquinol	Steadily liberates inorganic iodine in the lumen	Unknown
Diloxanide furoate	Unknown	Unknown
Eflornithine	Inhibits ornithine decarboxylase and biosynthesis of polyamines	Affects cell division, differentiation

SH, sulfhydryl; mRNA, messenger RNA

Trophozoites may spread to the liver through the portal vein and produce acute amebic hepatitis, or more rarely, the trophozoites may encyst and produce an amebic liver abscess many years later. On rare occasions, amebic abscesses are found in other organs, such as the lungs or the brain.

Many patients continue to excrete cysts for several years after recovery from the acute disease and therefore are a hazard to themselves and other persons; the public health risk is greatest when persons employed as food handlers are affected. More recently, it has been recognized that infection can be transmitted by sexual activities.

Balantidium coli is the largest of the protozoans that infect humans. The trophozoite form is covered with cilia, which impart mobility. Infection is acquired through the ingestion of cyst-contaminated soil, food, or water. The trophozoite causes superficial necrosis or deep ulceration in the mucosa and submucosa of the large intestine. Otherwise healthy persons commonly exhibit nausea, vomiting, abdominal pain, and diarrhea, whereas debilitated or nutritionally stressed patients may develop severe dysentery.

Trichomoniasis and Giardiasis

Trichomoniasis is a genital infection produced by the protozoan *Trichomonas vaginalis.* Infections frequently are asymptomatic in the male, whereas in the female vaginitis characterized by a frothy pale yellow discharge is common. Relapses occur if the infected person's sexual partner is not treated simultaneously.

Giardiasis is caused by the protozoan *Giardia lamblia* and is characterized by gastrointestinal symptoms

ranging from an acute self-limiting watery diarrhea to a chronic condition associated with episodic diarrhea and occasional instances of malabsorption. The parasite is similar to *E. histolytica* in that it exists in two forms, an actively motile trophozoite (usually confined to the upper small bowel) and a cyst (commonly excreted in the feces).

Leishmaniasis and Trypanosomiasis

The flagellate leishmania is transmitted to humans by the bite of the female sandfly of the genus *Phlebotomus.* Three principal diseases result from infection with *Leishmania* spp. *L. donovani* causes visceral leishmaniasis (kala-azar); *L. tropica* and *L. major* produce cutaneous leishmaniasis, and *L. braziliensis* causes South American mucocutaneous leishmaniasis. In visceral leishmaniasis, the protozoan parasitizes the reticuloendothelial cells, and this results in an enlargement of the lymph nodes, liver, and spleen; the spleen can become massive. Cutaneous leishmaniasis remains localized to the site of inoculation, where it forms a raised disfiguring ulcerative lesion. South American leishmaniasis is variable in its presentation. It is characterized by ulceration of the mucous membranes of the nose, mouth, and pharynx; some disfiguring skin involvement also is possible.

African trypanosomiasis follows the bite of *Glossina,* a tsetse fly infected with the protozoan *Trypanosoma brucei.* The ensuing illness (*sleeping sickness*) is initially characterized by the hemolymphatic stage of fever, headache, and lymph node enlargement. These symptoms are followed by meningoencephalopathic involvement, with wasting, mental disturbances, and drowsiness as the disease progresses. This latter more serious stage requires different, more potentially toxic drugs than does the hemolymphatic stage. There are geographical variations of the disease. *Rhodesian sleeping sickness,* acquired in the savannah and woodlands of East Africa from *Glossina morsitans,* is a much more acute and rapidly progressive disease than *Gambian sleeping sickness,* acquired in riverine areas of West Africa from *Glossina palpalis,* in which the incubation period can be more prolonged and the disease more protracted.

Chagas' disease, the South American variety of trypanosomiasis, is caused by *Trypanosoma cruzi.* It is quite different from African trypanosomiasis in its clinical and pathological presentation and in its failure to respond to many agents effective in that disease. It has both an acute and chronic phase. The latter frequently results in gastrointestinal and myocardial disease that ends in death.

ANTIPROTOZOAL DRUGS

Metronidazole

Metronidazole (*Flagyl, Metrogel*) exerts activity against most anaerobic bacteria and several protozoa. The drug freely penetrates protozoal and bacterial cells but not mammalian cells. Metronidazole can function as an electron sink, and because it does so, its 5-nitro group is reduced. The enzyme, pyruvate-ferredoxin oxidoreductase, found only in anaerobic organisms, reduces metronidazole and thereby activates the drug. Reduced metronidazole disrupts replication and transcription and inhibits DNA repair.

Antimicrobial Spectrum

Metronidazole inhibits *E. histolytica, G. lamblia, T. vaginalis, Blastocystis hominis, B. coli,* and the helminth *Dracunculus medinensis.* It is also bactericidal for obligate anaerobic gram-positive and gram-negative bacteria except *Actinomyces* spp. It is not active against aerobes or facultative anaerobes. Drug resistance is infrequent; the mechanism of resistance is not understood. Tinidazole, a 5-nitroimidazole closely related to metronidazole, is effective against vaginal trichomoniasis resistant to metronidazole.

Absorption, Metabolism, and Excretion

Absorption from the intestinal tract is usually good. Food delays but does not reduce absorption. The drug is distributed in body fluids and has a half-life of about 8 hours. High levels are found in plasma and cerebrospinal fluid (CSF). Less than 20% binds to plasma proteins. Metronidazole is metabolized by oxidation and glucuronide formation in the liver and is primarily excreted by the kidneys, although small amounts can be found in saliva and breast milk. Dose reduction is generally unnecessary in renal failure.

Clinical Uses

Metronidazole is the most effective agent available for the treatment of individuals with all forms of amebiasis, with perhaps the exception of the person who is asymptomatic but continues to excrete cysts. That situation calls for an effective intraluminal amebicide, such as diloxanide furoate, paromomycin sulfate, or diiodohydroxyquin. Metronidazole is active against intestinal and extraintestinal cysts and trophozoites.

Although quinacrine hydrochloride has been used for the treatment of giardiasis, many physicians prefer metronidazole. Furazolidone is an alternate choice.

Metronidazole is the drug of choice in Europe for anaerobic bacterial infections; concern about possible carcinogenicity has led to some caution in its use in the United States. Recently it has been found to be effective in treating *D. medinensis* (Guinea worm) infections and *Helicobacter pylori.*

Adverse Effects

The most frequently observed adverse reactions to metronidazole include nausea, vomiting, cramps, diarrhea, and a metallic taste. The urine is often dark or red-brown. Less frequently, unsteadiness, vertigo, ataxia, paresthesias, peripheral neuropathy, encephalopathy, and neutropenia have been reported. Since metronidazole is a weak inhibitor of alcohol dehydrogenase, alcohol ingestion should be avoided during treatment. A psychotic reaction also may be produced. Metronidazole interferes with the metabolism of warfarin and may potentiate its anticoagulant activity. Phenobarbital and corticosteroids lower metronidazole plasma levels by increasing its metabolism, whereas cimetidine raises levels by impairing metronidazole metabolism. The drug is not recommended for use during pregnancy.

Iodoquinol

Iodoquinol (diiodohydroxyquin, *Yodoxin, Moebiquin*) is a halogenated 8-hydroxyquinoline derivative whose precise mechanism of action is not known but is thought to involve an inactivation of essential parasite enzymes. Iodoquinol kills the trophozoite forms of *E. histolytica, B. coli, B. hominis,* and *Dientamoeba fragilis.*

Iodoquinol is absorbed from the gastrointestinal tract and is excreted in the urine as glucuronide and sulfate conjugates. Most of an orally administered dose is excreted in the feces. Iodoquinol has a plasma half-life of about 12 hours.

Iodoquinol is the drug of choice in the treatment of asymptomatic amebiasis and *D. fragilis* infections. It is also used in combination with other drugs in the treatment of other forms of amebiasis and as an alternative to tetracycline in the treatment of balantidiasis.

Adverse reactions are related to the iodine content of the drug; the toxicity is often expressed as skin reactions, thyroid enlargement, and interference with thyroid function studies. Headache and diarrhea also occur. Chronic use of clioquinol, a closely related agent, has been linked to a myelitislike illness and to optic atrophy with permanent loss of vision.

Diloxanide Furoate

Diloxanide furoate (*Furamide*) is an amebicide that is effective against trophozoites in the intestinal tract. In mild or asymptomatic infections, cures of 83 to 95% have been achieved; in patients with dysentery, cure rates may be less impressive. The drug is administered only orally and is rapidly absorbed from the gastrointestinal tract following hydrolysis of the ester group. It is remarkably free of side effects, but occasionally flatulence, abdominal distention, anorexia, nausea, vomiting, diarrhea, pruritus, and urticaria occur. Diloxanide is excreted in the urine, largely as the glucuronide. It is not available in the United States.

Antibiotics

Several antibiotics have been used to treat intestinal protozoal infections. Erythromycin and tetracycline do not have a direct effect on the protozoa; they act by altering intestinal bacterial flora and preventing secondary infection. Tetracycline also reduces the normal gastrointestinal bacterial flora on which the amebas depend for growth.

The aminoglycoside paromomycin (*Humatin*) has a mode of action identical to that of the other aminocyclitols and is directly amebicidal. It is not absorbed from the intestinal tract and thus has its primary effect on bacteria, some amebas (e.g., *E. histolytica*), and some helminths found in the lumen of the intestinal tract. Side effects are limited to diarrhea and gastrointestinal upset.

Amphotericin B, a polyene, is discussed more fully in Chapter 52. It has produced healing of the mucocutaneous lesions of American leishmaniasis, but its potential for nephrotoxicity makes it a drug of second choice. On the other hand, liposomal amphotericin B, approved by the U. S. Food and Drug Administration (FDA) for treatment of visceral leishmaniasis, is considered the drug of choice for that indication and is much less toxic than pentavalent antimonials or amphotericin B.

Pentamidine

Pentamidine (*Pentam 300*) binds to DNA and may inhibit kinetoplast DNA replication and function. It also may act by inhibiting dihydrofolate reductase and interfering with polyamine metabolism. An effect on organism respiration, especially at high doses, also may play a role.

Pentamidine is not well absorbed from the intestinal tract after oral administration and generally is given by intramuscular injection. The drug binds to tissues, particularly the kidney, and is slowly excreted, mostly as the unmodified drug. It does not enter the central nervous system (CNS). Its sequestration in tissues accounts for its prophylactic use in trypanosomiasis.

Pentamidine is active against *Pneumocystis carinii*, trypanosomes, and leishmaniasis unresponsive to pentavalent antimonials. It is an alternative agent for the treatment of *P. carinii* pneumonia. Although it is more toxic than trimethoprim–sulfamethoxazole, it has been widely used in patients with acquired immunodeficiency syndrome (AIDS), in whom *P. carinii* infection is common.

Pentamidine is an alternative drug for visceral leishmaniasis, especially when sodium stibogluconate has failed or is contraindicated. Pentamidine is also a reserve agent for the treatment of trypanosomiasis before the CNS is invaded. This characteristic largely restricts its use to Gambian trypanosomiasis.

Adverse reactions occur frequently. Rapid drug infusion may produce tachycardia, vomiting, shortness of breath, headache, and a fall in blood pressure. Changes in blood sugar (hypoglycemia or hyperglycemia) necessitate caution in its use, particularly in patients with diabetes mellitus. Renal function should be monitored and blood counts checked for dyscrasias.

Suramin

Suramin (*Germanin*) is a derivative of a nonmetallic dye whose antiparasitic mechanism of action is not clear. It appears to act on parasite specific α-glycerophosphate oxidase, thymidylate synthetase, dihydrofolate reductase, and protein kinase but not on host enzymes.

Suramin is not absorbed from the intestinal tract and is administered intravenously. Although the initial high plasma levels drop rapidly, suramin binds tightly to and is slowly released from plasma proteins, and so it persists in the host for up to 3 months. Suramin neither penetrates red blood cells nor enters the CNS. It is taken up by the reticuloendothelial cells and accumulates in the Kupffer cells of the liver and in the epithelial cells of the proximal convoluted tubules of the kidney. It is excreted by glomerular filtration, largely as the intact molecule.

Suramin is used primarily to treat African trypanosomiasis, for which it is the drug of choice. It is effective in treating disease caused by *Trypanosoma gambiense* and *T. rhodesiense* but not *T. cruzi* (Chagas' disease). It can be used alone prophylactically or during the initial hemolymphatic stages of the disease. Later stages, particularly those involving the CNS, are more commonly treated with a combination of suramin and the arsenical melarsoprol.

When CNS involvement occurs, the poor penetration of suramin and pentamidine into the CSF requires alternative forms of chemotherapy, such as melarsoprol in combination with suramin. In treating *Onchocerca volvulus* infections, suramin kills adult worms and is an alternative to ivermectin. Suramin is used after initial treatment with diethylcarbamazine, which is used to kill the microfilariae. It produces favorable results in pemphigus and prolongs the time to disease progression in hormone-refractory prostate cancer.

It is important to test for drug sensitivity by administering a small (200 mg) dose by slow intravenous injection before giving the full amount of suramin. Since adverse reactions occur with greater frequency and severity among the malnourished, greater caution is necessary for patients with advanced trypanosomiasis. An acute reaction in sensitive individuals results in nausea, vomiting, colic, hypotension, urticaria, and even unconsciousness; fortunately, this reaction is rare. Rashes, photophobia, paresthesias, and hyperesthesia may occur later; these symptoms may presage peripheral neuropathy. Mild albuminuria is not uncommon, but hematuria with casts suggests nephrotoxicity and the need to stop treatment.

Eflornithine

Eflornithine (difluoromethyl ornithine, *Ornidyl*) is a unique antiprotozoal agent in that its mode of action involves inhibition of a specific enzyme, ornithine decarboxylase. In eukaryotes, decarboxylation of ornithine is required for biosynthesis of polyamines, which are important in cell division and differentiation.

Eflornithine is given intravenously, and about 80% of the drug is excreted in the urine within 24 hours. It does not bind significantly to plasma proteins and has a terminal plasma half-life of about 3 hours. It crosses the blood-brain barrier and is one of the drugs of choice for treating the hemolymphatic and meningoencephalitic stage of *T. brucei-gambiense*. The most significant side effects are anemia and leukopenia. Oral therapy is associated with considerable gastrointestinal toxicity. Diarrhea, thrombocytopenia, and seizures are occasionally reported.

Arsenicals

Melarsoprol (trivalent) and tryparsamide (pentavalent) are organic compounds containing arsenic that bind to sulfhydryl groups in proteins, thereby affecting cellular structure and function. The action of arsenic is nonspecific, and any selective toxicity achieved is related to differences in drug permeability and sulfhydryl content of the affected structure or enzyme. Melarsoprol shows some selectivity for the trypanosome enzymes phosphopyruvate kinase and trypanothione reductase. These drugs are administered intravenously. Resistance has started to emerge among trypanosomes responsible for African trypanosomiasis.

The arsenicals are trypanocidal. Melarsoprol is highly active against all stages of trypanosomiasis, but its toxicity restricts its application to the meningoencephalitic phase of the disease. Their value lies in their ability to penetrate the CNS; hence, they are useful in treating meningoencephalitis caused by trypanosomes. The drugs are rapidly eliminated.

Vomiting and abdominal cramping occur but may be minimized by slow injection in the supine fasting patient. Great care should be taken to prevent painful drug extravasation into the tissue. The most frequently observed adverse reaction is encephalopathy, which develops on or about the third day of therapy and can be fatal. Other side effects include fever, rashes, proteinuria, peripheral neuropathy, and rarely, agranulocytosis. Since the overall incidence of side effects to tryparsamide is quite high, it largely has been replaced by melarsoprol in the treatment of trypanosome infestation.

Nifurtimox

Nifurtimox (*Lampit*) is a nitrofuran derivative whose likely mechanism of action for killing of trypanosomes is through the production of activated forms of oxygen. Nifurtimox is reduced to the nitro anion radical, which reacts with oxygen to produce superoxide and hydrogen peroxide. The free radical metabolites, an absence of parasite catalase, and a peroxide deficiency lead to lipid peroxidation and cell damage. This production of activated oxygen results in toxicity to the protozoal cells.

The drug is given orally and is well absorbed from the gastrointestinal tract. It is rapidly metabolized, and only low levels are found in blood and tissues. The drug is excreted in the urine, primarily in the form of metabolites.

Nifurtimox is trypanocidal and exerts an effect on the trypomastigote and amastigote forms of *T. cruzi*. It is effective in the treatment of the acute form of Chagas' disease but is less effective once the disease becomes chronic. The drug is moderately well tolerated, and treatment generally lasts 3 to 4 months. Cure rates of 80 to 90% have been reported. Since much of the tissue damage caused by the disease is irreversible, early diagnosis and treatment are important. Nifurtimox has also been used in *T. gambiense* infection with meningoencephalopathic involvement.

Although side effects occur in approximately half the patients treated with nifurtimox, it is necessary to discontinue treatment in only a minority. Nausea, vomiting, abdominal pain, skin rashes, headache, insomnia, convulsions, and myalgia all have been reported.

Antimonials

Sodium stibogluconate (*Pentostam, Triostam*) and meglumine antimonate (*Glucantime*), both pentavalent antimonials, bind to sulfhydryl groups on proteins and may form thio antimonides. Some evidence suggests that the pentavalent form may be reduced in vivo to the trivalent antimonial before binding. Trivalent antimonials inhibit phosphofructokinase, a rate-limiting enzyme in glycolysis, and organisms whose growth is dependent on the anaerobic metabolism of glucose cannot survive without the active enzyme. Whether this is the mechanism by which pentavalent antimonials inhibit protozoa is unclear.

Antimonials are irritating to the intestinal mucosa and therefore are administered by intramuscular or slow intravenous injection. Peak blood concentrations occur in 2 hours. These drugs bind to cells, including erythrocytes, and are found in high concentrations in the liver and spleen. As compared with the trivalent antimonials, which are no longer used, the pentavalent antimonials bind to tissue less strongly. This results in higher blood levels, more rapid excretion, and lowered toxicity. Pentavalent antimonials are rapidly excreted in the urine, with up to one-half of the administered dose excreted in 24 hours.

No pentavalent antimonial is licensed for use, but sodium stibogluconate is available from the Parasitic Disease Drug Service of the Centers for Disease Control (CDC) for treatment of leishmaniasis. While the pentavalent antimony compounds can be given intravenously or intramuscularly, local infiltration of the lesion in cutaneous leishmaniasis is highly effective. Because of the lower toxicity of liposomal amphotericin B, this drug is considered a first-line choice for viscerotropic leishmaniasis rather than the antimonials.

Adverse reactions particularly associated with the trivalent antimonials are coughing, occasional vomiting, myalgia, arthralgia, and changes in the electrocardiogram. Sodium stibogluconate occasionally causes rashes, pruritus, abdominal pain, diarrhea, and anaphylactoid collapse. Liver damage with jaundice is a rare side effect. Toxic reactions are more common with repeated courses of treatment. Biochemical evidence of pancreatitis is usual (97%), but severe or fatal pancreatitis is extremely infrequent.

MALARIA

Malaria is a parasitic disease endemic in parts of the world where moisture and warmth permit the disease

vector, mosquitoes of the genus *Anopheles*, to exist and multiply. The emergence of both drug-resistant strains of malarial parasites and insecticide-resistant strains of *Anopheles* has contributed significantly to the extensive reappearance of this infection. The annual global incidence of malaria is estimated to be approximately 200 million cases, and in tropical Africa alone, malaria is responsible for the yearly deaths of more than 1 million children younger than 14 years. Malaria ranks as a leading cause of mortality in the world today.

Most cases of malaria in the United States result from individuals who have contracted the disease before they entered this country. It is also possible to contract malaria during a blood transfusion if the transfused blood has been taken from a malaria-infected individual. Additionally, hypodermic needles previously contaminated by blood containing malarial parasites can be the source of an infection; this has occurred when needles are shared among drug addicts.

Effective treatment of malaria depends on early diagnosis. Since the patient's symptoms are often relatively nonspecific, it is crucial to examine stained blood smears for the presence of the parasite. Even this procedure may be inconclusive during the early stages of the infection, since the levels of parasitemia can be quite low. Thus, it is important to repeat the blood smear examination several times if malaria is suspected.

Once the presence of malarial parasites has been confirmed, it is vital to identify the particular plasmodial strain involved, since appropriate use of chemotherapy depends on the particular species responsible for the acute attack. Unfortunately, mixed infections, that is, simultaneous infections with more than one species of plasmodia, are often observed. If more than a single species is involved, treatment appropriate for the elimination of all strains must be instituted to avoid delayed attacks or misinterpretations.

Life Cycle of the Malarial Parasite

The malarial parasite is a single-cell protozoan (plasmodium). Although more than 100 species of plasmodia have been identified, only four are capable of infecting humans (*Plasmodium malariae, P. ovale, P. vivax,* and *P. falciparum*); the rest attack a variety of animal hosts. *P. falciparum* and *P. vivax* malaria are the two most common forms.

P. vivax malaria is the most prevalent type of infection and is characterized by periodic acute attacks of chills and fever, profuse sweating, enlarged spleen and liver, anemia, abdominal pain, headaches, and lethargy. Hyperactivity of the reticuloendothelial system and hemolysis are the principal causes of the enlarged spleen and liver; these effects often result in anemia, leukopenia, thrombocytopenia, and hyperbilirubinemia. The cyclical nature of the acute attacks (48 hours for

P. vivax, P. ovale, and *P. falciparum*) is characteristic of malaria and reflects the relatively synchronous passage of the parasites from one red blood cell stage in their life cycle to another. If *P. vivax* malaria is not treated, the symptoms may subside for several weeks or months and then recur. These relapses are due to a latent liver form of the parasite (see the following section), which is not present in *P. falciparum* strains. Although the fatality rate of *P. vivax* malaria is low, it is an exhausting infection and renders the patient more susceptible to other diseases.

Unchecked *P. falciparum* malaria is the most serious and most lethal form of the disease. It is responsible for 90% of the deaths from malaria. The parasitemia achieved can be quite high and will be associated with an increased incidence of serious complications (e.g., hemolytic anemia, encephalopathy). *P. falciparum* malaria produces all of the symptoms listed for *P. vivax* malaria and in addition can cause renal failure and pulmonary and cerebral edema. The tissue anoxia occurring in *P. falciparum* infections results from the unique sequestering of infected erythrocytes deep in the capil-

laries during the last three-fourths of the intraerythrocytic cycle.

Members of the genus *Plasmodium* have a complex life cycle (Fig. 53.1). A sexual stage occurs within the *Anopheles* mosquito, while asexual stages take place in the host. Malaria is actually transmitted from one human to another through the insect vector. Initially, a female mosquito is infected by biting a human with the disease whose blood contains male and female *gamete* forms of the parasite. Fertilization takes place in the mosquito gut, and after differentiation and multiplication, the mature *sporozoite* forms migrate to the insect's salivary glands. At the mosquito's next feeding, the sporozoites are injected into the bloodstream of another human to begin the asexual stages. After a relatively brief residence (less than an hour) in the systemic circulation, the sporozoites invade liver parenchymal cells, where they divide and develop asexually into multinucleated *schizonts*. These are the primary exoerythrocytic tissue forms of the parasite. When this primary stage of development is completed (6–12 days), the schizonts will rupture, releasing *merozoites* into the

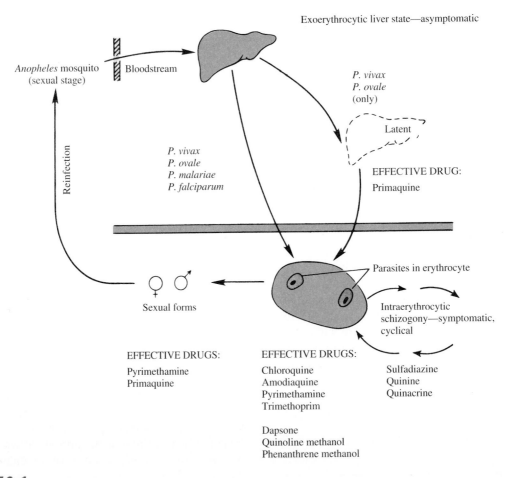

FIGURE 53.1

Life cycle of malaria parasites and locations where specific drugs are effective. The life cycles are not identical for every species.

blood. These latter forms invade host erythrocytes, where they again grow and divide asexually (*erythrocytic schizogony*) and become red cell schizonts. Some of the parasites differentiate into sexual (male and female) forms, or *gametocytes*. If the diseased human is bitten by a mosquito at this time, the gametes will be taken up into the organism's gut to repeat the sexual cycle. The gametocytes and the exoerythrocytic liver forms of *Plasmodium* spp. are not associated with the appearance of clinical symptoms of malaria.

The asexual intraerythrocytic parasites, that is, those that do not differentiate into gametocytes, also multiply and grow until they rupture the cells in which they reside; these new merozoites are released into the bloodstream. This occurrence not only sets up the subsequent cyclical red blood cell stages of the cycle but also gives rise to the symptoms associated with malarial infections. The recurrent chills and fever are thought to be related to the lysis of erythrocytes and the accompanying release of lytic material and parasite toxins into the bloodstream. Although the appearance of a cyclic fever is useful for diagnosis, this symptom may not occur during the early stages of the infection.

In individuals infected with either *P. vivax* or *P. ovale*, the exoerythrocytic tissue (e.g., liver) forms can persist after a latent period and give rise to relapses. In *P. falciparum* and *P. malariae* malaria, however, there do not appear to be any persistent secondary liver forms. Thus, in both of these forms of malaria, the physician must contend only with the asexual erythrocytic forms and the gametes, not with the latent liver forms found in *P. vivax* and *P. ovale*.

Patients who have blood transfusion malaria are infected with the asexual erythrocytic parasites only; exoerythrocytic tissue forms apparently do not develop. *Plasmodium malariae* has been known to produce an infection after transfusion, even when the blood was obtained from a person whose only contact with malaria was 40 years previous to the donation of blood.

Therapeutic Considerations

The main objective in the clinical management of patients suffering from an *acute* malaria attack is the prompt elimination of the parasite form responsible for the symptoms, that is, the asexual erythrocytic form. Drugs that are particularly effective in this regard are called *schizonticidal,* or *suppressive,* agents. They include such compounds as amodiaquine, chloroguanide, chloroquine, hydroxychloroquine, pyrimethamine, quinine, and tetracycline. These drugs have the potential (excluding any drug resistance) for effecting a *clinical cure;* that is, they can reduce the parasitemia to zero. The term *radical cure* also has been used, and it, in contrast to clinical cure, implies the elimination of all parasite forms from the body.

Once the primary therapeutic objective has been achieved, attention can be focused on such additional considerations as elimination of the gametocytes and the tissue forms of the parasite. Success in these areas would help to ensure that relapses do not occur. Since no latent liver forms are associated with mosquito-induced, drug-sensitive *P. falciparum* malaria, administration of chloroquine for up to 3 months after the patient leaves a malarious area will usually bring about a complete or radical cure *unless* the organism is resistant to chloroquine.

The emergence of parasites resistant to chloroquine is an increasingly important problem. Several strains of chloroquine-resistant *P. falciparum* have been identified. This resistance would lead to the reappearance of overt symptoms of *P. falciparum* malaria.

P. falciparum malaria may be accompanied by an infection caused by one of the other three plasmodial forms (*mixed infection*). As long as all of the parasites are drug sensitive, the parasitemia can be eliminated. However, it must be remembered that even though *P. falciparum* malaria may be ameliorated or eliminated, relapses due to *P. vivax* and *P. ovale* still can occur.

Antimalarial Drugs
Chloroquine

Chloroquine (*Aralen*) is one of several 4-aminoquinoline derivatives that display antimalarial activity. Chloroquine is particularly effective against intraerythrocytic forms because it is concentrated within the parasitized erythrocyte. This preferential drug accumulation appears to occur as a result of specific uptake mechanisms in the parasite. Chloroquine appears to work by intercalation with DNA, inhibition of heme polymerase or by interaction with Ca^{++}–calmodulin-mediated mechanisms. It also accumulates in the parasite's food vacuoles, where it inhibits peptide formation and phospholipases, leading to parasite death.

The drug is effective against all four types of malaria with the exception of chloroquine-resistant *P. falciparum*. Chloroquine destroys the blood stages of the infection and therefore ameliorates the clinical symptoms seen in *P. malariae, P. vivax, P. ovale,* and sensitive *P. falciparum* forms of malaria. The disease will return in *P. vivax* and *P. ovale* malaria, however, unless the liver stages are sequentially treated with primaquine after the administration of chloroquine. Chloroquine also can be used prophylactically in areas where resistance does not exist. In addition to its use as an antimalarial, chloroquine has been used in the treatment of rheumatoid arthritis and lupus erythematosus (see Chapter 36), extraintestinal amebiasis, and photoallergic reactions.

The absorption of chloroquine from the gastrointestinal tract is rapid and complete. The drug is distributed widely and is extensively bound to body tissues, with the liver containing 500 times the blood concentration. Such binding is reflected in a large volume of distribution (V_d). Desethylchloroquine is the major metabolite formed following hepatic metabolism, and both the parent compound and its metabolites are slowly eliminated by renal excretion. The half-life of the drug is 6 to 7 days.

Dizziness, headache, itching (especially in dark-skinned people), skin rash, vomiting, and blurring of vision may occur following low doses of chloroquine. In higher dosages these symptoms are more common, and exacerbation or unmasking of lupus erythematosus or discoid lupus, as well as toxic effects in skin, blood, and eyes can occur. Since the drug concentrates in melanin-containing structures, prolonged administration of high doses can lead to blindness. Chloroquine should not be used in the presence of retinal or visual field changes.

Hydroxychloroquine

Hydroxychloroquine (*Plaquenil*), like chloroquine, is a 4-aminoquinoline derivative used for the suppressive and acute treatment of malaria. It also has been used for rheumatoid arthritis and discoid and systemic lupus erythematosus. Hydroxychloroquine has not been proved to be more effective than chloroquine. Adverse reactions associated with its use are similar to those described for chloroquine. The drug should not be used in patients with psoriasis or porphyria, since it may exacerbate these conditions.

Amodiaquine

Amodiaquine (*Camoquin*) is another 4-aminoquinoline derivative whose antimalarial spectrum and adverse reactions are similar to those of chloroquine, although chloroquine-resistant parasites may not be amodiaquine-resistant to the same degree. Prolonged treatment with amodiaquine may result in pigmentation of the palate, nail beds, and skin. There is a 1:2000 risk of agranulocytosis and hepatocellular dysfunction when the drug is used prophylactically.

Primaquine

Primaquine is the least toxic and most effective of the 8-aminoquinoline antimalarial compounds. The mechanism by which 8-aminoquinolines exert their antimalarial effects is thought to be through a quinoline–quinone metabolite that inhibits the coenzyme Q–mediated respiratory chain of the exoerythrocytic parasite.

Primaquine is an important antimalarial because it is essentially the only drug effective against the liver (exoerythrocytic) forms of the malarial parasite. The drug also kills the gametocytes in all four species of human malaria. Primaquine is relatively ineffective against the asexual erythrocyte forms. *Primaquine finds its greatest use in providing a radical cure for* P. vivax *and* P. ovale *malaria.*

Primaquine is readily absorbed from the gastrointestinal tract, and in contrast to chloroquine, it is not bound extensively by tissues. It is rapidly metabolized, and the metabolites are reported to be as active as the parent drug itself. Peak plasma levels are reached in 4 to 6 hours after an oral dose, with almost total drug elimination occurring by 24 hours. The half-life is short, and daily administration is usually required for radical cure and prevention of relapses.

Although primaquine has a good therapeutic index, a number of important side effects are associated with its administration. In individuals with a genetically determined glucose 6-phosphate dehydrogenase deficiency, primaquine can cause lethal hemolysis of red cells. This genetic deficiency occurs in 5 to 10% of black males, in Asians, and in some Mediterranean peoples. With higher dosages or prolonged drug use, gastrointestinal distress, nausea, headache, pruritus, and leukopenia can occur. Occasionally, agranulocytosis also has been observed.

Pyrimethamine

Pyrimethamine (*Daraprim*) is the best of a number of 2,4-diaminopyrimidines that were synthesized as potential antimalarial and antibacterial compounds. Trimethoprim (*Proloprim*) is a closely related compound.

Pyrimethamine is well absorbed after oral administration, with peak plasma levels occurring within 3 to 7 hours. An initial loading dose to saturate nonspecific binding sites is not required, as it is with chloroquine. However, the drug binds to tissues, and therefore, its rate of renal excretion is slow. Pyrimethamine has a half-life of about 4 days. Although the drug does undergo some metabolic alterations, the metabolites formed have not been totally identified.

The only antimalarial drugs whose mechanisms of action are reasonably well understood are the drugs that inhibit the parasite's ability to synthesize folic acid. *Parasites cannot use preformed folic acid and therefore must synthesize this compound* from the following precursors obtained from their host: p-aminobenzoic acid (PABA), pteridine, and glutamic acid. The dihydrofolic acid formed from these precursors must then be hydrogenated to form tetrahydrofolic acid. The latter compound is the coenzyme that acts as an acceptor of a variety of one-carbon units. The transfer of one-carbon units is important in the synthesis of the pyrimidines and purines, which are essential in nucleic acid synthesis.

Whereas the sulfonamides and sulfones inhibit the initial step whereby PABA and the pteridine moiety combine to form dihydropteroic acid (see Chapter 44), *pyrimethamine and trimethoprim inhibit the conversion of dihydrofolic acid to tetrahydrofolic acid, a reaction catalyzed by the enzyme dihydrofolate reductase.* The basis of pyrimethamine selective toxicity resides in the *preferential binding* of the drug to the parasite's reductase enzyme.

The combined use of sulfonamides or sulfones with dihydrofolate reductase inhibitors, such as trimethoprim (*Bactrim, Septra*) or pyrimethamine (*Fansidar*), is a good example of the synergistic possibilities that exist in multiple-drug chemotherapy. This type of impairment of the parasite's metabolism is termed *sequential blockade. Using drugs that inhibit at two different points in the same biochemical pathway produces parasite lethality at lower drug concentrations than are possible when either drug is used alone.*

Pyrimethamine has been recommended for prophylactic use against all susceptible strains of plasmodia; however, it should not be used as the sole therapeutic agent for treating acute malarial attacks. As mentioned previously, *sulfonamides should always be coadministered with pyrimethamine (or trimethoprim)*, since the combined antimalarial activity of the two drugs is significantly greater than when either drug is used alone. Also, resistance develops more slowly when they are used in combination. Sulfonamides exert little or no effect on the blood stages of *P. vivax*, and resistance to the dihydrofolate reductase inhibitors is widespread.

In addition to its antimalarial effects, pyrimethamine is indicated (in combination with a sulfonamide) for the treatment of toxoplasmosis. The dosage required is 10 to 20 times higher than that employed in malarial infections.

Relatively few side effects are associated with the usual antimalarial dosages. However, signs of toxicity are evident at higher dosages, particularly those used in the management of toxoplasmosis. Many of these reactions reflect the interference of pyrimethamine with *host* folic acid metabolism, especially that occurring in rapidly dividing cells. Toxic symptoms include anorexia, vomiting, anemia, leukopenia, thrombocytopenia, and atrophic glossitis. CNS stimulation, including convulsions, may follow an acute overdose. The side effects associated with the pyrimethamine–sulfadoxine combination include those associated with the sulfonamide and pyrimethamine alone. In addition, there is evidence of a greater incidence of allergic reactions, particularly toxic epidermal necrolysis and Stevens-Johnson syndrome, with the combination. This carries an estimated mortality of 1:11,000 to 1:25,000 when used as a chemoprophylactic.

Chloroguanide (Proguanil)

Chloroguanide hydrochloride (*Paludrine*) is activated to a triazine metabolite, cycloguanil, which also interferes with parasite folic acid synthesis. It is a dihydrofolate reductase inhibitor that is used for the prophylaxis of malaria caused by all susceptible strains of plasmodia. Chloroguanide is rapidly absorbed from the gas-

trointestinal tract. Peak plasma levels occur 2 to 4 hours after oral administration, and the drug is excreted in the urine with an elimination half-life of 12 to 21 hours. Its side effects and spectrum of antimalarial activity are quite similar to those of pyrimethamine. The conversion of chloroguanide to the active metabolite is decreased in pregnancy and also as a result of genetic polymorphism in 3% of whites and Africans and 20% of Asians.

Quinine

Quinine is one of several alkaloids derived from the bark of the cinchona tree. The mechanism by which it exerts its antimalarial activity is not known. It does not bind to DNA at antimalarial dosages. It may poison the parasite's feeding mechanism, and it has been termed a general protoplasmic poison, since many organisms are affected by it.

Quinine is rapidly absorbed following oral ingestion, with peak blood levels achieved in 1 to 4 hours. About 70 to 93% of the drug is bound to plasma proteins, depending on the severity of the infection. Quinine is extensively metabolized, with only about 20% of the parent compound eliminated in the urine.

The primary present-day indication for quinine and its isomer, quinidine, is in the intravenous treatment of severe manifestations and complications of chloroquine-resistant malaria caused by *P. falciparum.*

Aside from its use as an antimalarial compound, quinine is used for the prevention and treatment of nocturnal leg muscle cramps, especially those resulting from arthritis, diabetes, thrombophlebitis, arteriosclerosis, and varicose veins.

Cinchonism describes the toxic state induced by excessive plasma levels of free quinine. Symptoms include sweating, ringing in the ears, impaired hearing, blurred vision, nausea, vomiting, and diarrhea. Quinine is a potent stimulus to insulin secretion and irritates the gastrointestinal mucosa. Also, a variety of relatively rare hematological changes occur, including leukopenia and agranulocytosis. Quinine is potentially neurotoxic in high dosages, and severe hypotension may follow its rapid intravenous administration.

Quinacrine

Quinacrine is no longer used extensively as an antimalarial drug and has been largely replaced by the 4-aminoquinolines.

Dapsone

Although dapsone (*Avlosulfon*) was once used in the treatment and prophylaxis of chloroquine-resistant *P. falciparum* malaria, the toxicities associated with its administration (e.g., agranulocytosis, methemoglobinemia, hemolytic anemia) have severely reduced its use.

Occasionally dapsone has been added to the usual chloroquine therapeutic regimen for the prophylaxis of chloroquine-resistant *P. falciparum* malaria. It is also used in combination therapy for leprosy.

Mefloquine

Mefloquine (*Lariam*) is a 4-quinolinemethanol derivative used both prophylactically and acutely against resistant *P. falciparum* malaria. It is ineffective against the liver stage of *P. vivax* malaria.

While its detailed mechanism of action is unknown, it is an effective blood schizonticide; that is, it acts against the form of the parasite responsible for clinical symptoms. Orally administered mefloquine is well absorbed and has an absorption half-life of about 2 hours; the elimination half-life is 2 to 3 weeks. Among its side effects are vertigo, visual alterations, vomiting, and such CNS disturbances as psychosis, hallucinations, confusion, anxiety, and depression. It should not be used concurrently with compounds known to alter cardiac conduction or prophylactically in patients operating dangerous machinery. It should not used to treat severe malaria, as there is no intravenous formulation.

Atovaquone

Atovaquone is a naphthoquinone whose mechanism of action involves inhibition of the mitochondrial electron transport system in the protozoa. Malaria parasites depend on de novo pyrimidine biosynthesis through dihydroorotate dehydrogenase coupled to electron transport. Plasmodia are unable to salvage and recycle pyrimidines as do mammalian cells.

Atovaquone is poorly absorbed from the gastrointestinal tract, but absorption is increased with a fatty meal. Excretion of the drug, mostly unchanged, occurs in the feces. The elimination half-life is 2 to 3 days. Low plasma levels persist for several weeks. Concurrent administration of metoclopramide, tetracycline, or rifampin reduces atovaquone plasma levels by 40 to 50%.

Atovaquone has good initial activity against the blood but not the hepatic stage of *P. vivax* and *P. ovale* malaria parasites. It is effective against erythrocytic and exoerythrocytic *P. falciparum,* and therefore, daily suppressive doses need to be taken for only 1 week upon leaving endemic areas. When used alone, it has an unacceptable (30%) rate of recrudescence and selects for resistant organisms. It and proguanil are synergistic when combined and no atovaquone resistance is seen. This combination (*Malarone*) is significantly more effective than mefloquine, amodiaquine, chloroquine, and combinations of chloroquine, pyrimethamine, and sulfadoxine. In addition to using the combination of atovaquone and proguanil for the treatment and prophylaxis of *P. falciparum* malaria, atovaquone is also used for the treatment and prevention of *P. carinii* pneumonia and babesiosis therapy.

Atovaquone is well tolerated and produces only rare instances of nausea, vomiting, diarrhea, abdominal pain, headache, and rash of mild to moderate intensity.

DRUGS IN DEVELOPMENT

Chinese scientists have isolated several compounds with antimalarial activity from species of *Artemisia*. These include artemisinin (*Qinghaosu*), artesunate, and artemether. These sesquiterpene peroxides are potent and rapidly acting antimalarial drugs that show relatively low human toxicity. They are active against blood stages, especially in patients with severe manifestations, such as cerebral malaria and chloroquine-resistant malarial infections. They possess activity against the erythrocytic stages of human malaria and have no effect on the liver or exoerythrocytic stage of the parasite; their gameticidal activity is not clear. They are most useful in treating life-threatening cerebral edema. At present artemisinin, artesunate, and artemether are available outside the United States.

SELECTION OF DRUGS

The particular agent employed in the treatment of acute malarial infections will depend on the severity of the infection, the strain of the infecting organism, and the degree to which the organism is drug resistant. In addition, *chemoprophylaxis* is considered a valid indication for the use of antimalarial drugs when individuals are traveling in areas where malaria is endemic. The following paragraphs may provide useful guidelines in the therapeutic management and prevention of malarial infections.

Prophylactic Measures for Use in Endemic Areas

Chloroquine may be the drug of choice, but only in areas where chloroquine-sensitive *P. falciparum* organisms are present. Chloroquine prophylaxis is no longer effective for travel to many regions. Daily atovaquone–proguanil appears to be the first choice for chemoprophylaxis for travel to areas of chloroquine resistance. Prophylactic drugs, such as chloroquine or mefloquine, should be started 2 to 4 weeks prior to travel and continued for 6 to 8 weeks after leaving the endemic areas. The atovaquone–proguanil combination is the exception in that it is started 1 to 2 days prior to departure and is continued 1 week after return.

Treatment of an Acute Uncomplicated Attack

Chloroquine phosphate, administered orally, is again the drug of choice unless one suspects the presence of a chloroquine-resistant organism. Oral mefloquine or

Malarone is indicated for uncomplicated infections resistant to chloroquine. For severe infections, parenteral administration of quinidine is indicated with hourly monitoring of serum glucose levels.

Mechanism of Chloroquine Resistance

A particular protein (P_{170} glycoprotein) has been identified in the resistant parasite that appears to function as a drug-transporting pump mechanism to rid the cell of drug. This resistance mechanism is similar to the multidrug resistance system in cancer. Thus, when drug enters the organism, it is rapidly removed before it can exert its toxicity. Drug therapy directed at inhibiting this pump mechanism may be able to reverse this resistance. This is a potentially important new approach to the chemotherapy of malaria.

Treatment of Chloroquine-Resistant P. Falciparum Infection

In areas where chloroquine-resistant *P. falciparum* is common, a combination of a rapidly acting blood schizonticide and pyrimethamine–sulfadoxine may be the treatment of choice. An acute attack of malaria caused by chloroquine-resistant *P. falciparum* complicated by renal failure or cerebral manifestations may be terminated with parenteral quinidine gluconate alone or with oral pyrimethamine and sulfadiazine. Oral mefloquine has been used in place of chloroquine in uncomplicated infections with chloroquine-resistant organisms, but serious CNS side effects (e.g., flashbacks) are frequently seen with its use. Consequently, the atovaquone–proguanil combination is now considered as effective as and better tolerated than mefloquine.

Mixed Infections

Every patient with malaria should be examined for simultaneous infection with more than one species of *Plasmodium.* Infections with both *P. falciparum* and *P. vivax* are among the most commonly encountered mixed infections. In patients with falciparum malaria, attacks of *P. vivax* malaria may later develop; it is important not to misinterpret this delayed *P. vivax* form as a relapse of *P. falciparum* infection. If a mixed infection is identified, a combination of 4-aminoquinoline and primaquine should be administered, since the primaquine helps to eliminate any persisting tissue forms of *P. vivax.*

Study QUESTIONS

1. A 35-year-old medical entomologist comes to the hospital with chief complaints of fever, headache, and photophobia. This illness began about 6 days prior to admission, when he returned from a 2-month visit to the jungles of Central and South America. On his return flight, about 6 days prior to admission, he described having fever and shaking chills. He saw his physician 2 days prior to admission; the physician made a diagnosis of influenza and prescribed tetracycline. On the day of admission, the patient had shaking chills followed by temperature elevation to 104°F (40°C). Physical examination revealed a well-developed man who appeared ill. There is some left upper quadrant tenderness but no organomegaly; blood pressure, 126/90; pulse, 120; and respirations, 22. Laboratory findings were hemoglobin, 14.5 mg/dL (normal, 13.4–17.4 mg/dL); hematocrit, 45% (normal, 40–54%); Giemsa-stained blood smear (thick and thin) revealed *Plasmodium vivax*. What is the oral drug of choice to rid the blood of plasmodia?
   (A) Primaquine
   (B) Chloroquine
   (C) Sulfadiazine
   (D) Quinine
   (E) Mefloquine

2. A 27-year-old ecologist went to his physician with an ulcer on his left wrist 8 weeks after returning from Panama. The patient noted a small pink papule that was pruritic (itchy) and enlarged and developed a crusted appearance. This in time fell off, leaving an oozing shallow ulcer about 2 cm in diameter with indurated margins. He applied over-the-counter topical agents without clinical improvement. No fever or lymphadenopathy was present. Scrapings were taken from the raised margins of the ulcer and stained with Giemsa, revealing intracellular and free small, round and oval bodies measuring 2 to 5 μm in diameter. While this is suggestive of the *Leishmania* amastigote stage in the vertebrate host, culture confirmed it to be *L. braziliensis panamensis*. The patient had New World cutaneous leishmaniasis. What is the drug of choice?
   (A) Praziquantel
   (B) Pyrimethamine–sulfadoxine
   (C) Pentavalent antimonials
   (D) Pyrantel pamoate
   (E) Primaquine phosphate

3. The patient is 43-year-old Agency for International Development worker with chief complaints of fever and headache. He recently returned from a trip to western Kenya and Tanzania. While traveling

cross-country through the woodland and savanna by Land Rover, he indicated that the cab appeared to be filled with tsetse flies of the genus *Glossina*. He was bitten on the forearm and developed a painful chancre with some exudate. Physical examination showed the patient to be febrile, with a temperature of 102°F (38.8°C); he had tachycardia, with a pulse of 120 beats per minute, and appeared acutely ill and lethargic. Low-grade posterior cervical lymphadenopathy was present. There was no edema of the extremities, no organomegaly, and no abnormalities in his neurological examination. Renal and hepatic functions were normal. Giemsa-stained thick and thin blood smears examined to rule out malaria revealed trypomastigotes. Parasites were also found in a drop of exudate from a needle aspiration of the chancre. A lumbar puncture revealed CSF having one white blood cell and two red blood cells with normal glucose and protein levels. No parasites were seen in a centrifuged sample of CSF. What treatment is indicated for this patient?

(A) Sulfadoxine–pyrimethamine
(B) Chloroquine
(C) Suramin
(D) Melarsoprol
(E) Metronidazole

4. A 52-year-old real estate salesperson has a 2-week history of watery diarrhea without blood. The patient states that 4 to 5 weeks ago she and her husband visited Aspen, Colorado, on a backpacking vacation and on occasion drank water from mountain streams. They were sure the water was potable, as the unspoiled, pristine area abounded with fish, beaver, and plant life. She states she has enjoyed perfect health except that she takes antacids for what she describes as gastroesophageal reflux disease. Her physical examination produced unremarkable findings. Examination of liquid stool revealed trophozoites and cysts of *G. lamblia*. Which of the following is the correct treatment for this disease?

(A) Melarsoprol
(B) Mefloquine
(C) Mebendazole
(D) Metronidazole
(E) Meglumine antimonate

5. The patient is a 12-year-old boy with fever and vomiting. The fever began a month prior to admission, spiking to approximately 104°F (40°C) each day. The family physician for a time entertained a presumptive diagnosis of chloroquine-resistant malaria and prescribed mefloquine followed by a week of doxycycline, without effect. Then, 2 days prior to admission, the patient began vomiting after eating. About 4 months earlier the family visited their home of origin in Bihar state in northeast

India. Physical examination revealed a thin, acutely ill child with a temperature of 103°F (39.4°C), pulse of 130, and respirations of 36. Positive finding on physical examination was a nontender distended abdomen with a liver edge palpable 5 finger breadths below the costal margin and a smooth, firm spleen extending to the umbilicus (hepatosplenomegaly). The skin was dry and darkly pigmented. Laboratory findings revealed hemoglobin of 8.5 mg/dL (normal, 13.4–17.4 mg/dL), white blood cell count 3900 cells/mm^3 (normal, 4000–12,000 cells/mm^3), platelet count 99,000 cells/mm^3 (normal, 150,000–400,000 cells/mm^3). A bone marrow aspirate revealed characteristic amastigotes of *L. donovani*. Which of the following is the drug of choice for visceral leishmaniasis?

(A) Liposomal amphotericin B
(B) Albendazole
(C) Atovaquone
(D) Pyrimethamine–sulfadoxine
(E) Proguanil

ANSWERS

1. **B.** The drug of choice for clinical cure of *P. vivax* malaria is oral chloroquine. The only isolated reports of chloroquine-resistant *P. vivax* are from the western Pacific, not Central and South America. The patient should become afebrile in 24 to 48 hours, and parasitemia should decline in 72 hours. Since *P. vivax,* known as benign tertian malaria, responds well to chloroquine, there is no need to resort to parenteral quinine or quinidine or oral mefloquine; these agents have cardiotoxic and neurotoxic side effects. *P. vivax* also does not respond as well to the sulfonamides. In *P. vivax* and *P. ovale* infections, treatment with a blood schizonticide will result only in clinical cure, but radical cure requires additional treatment with a tissue schizonticide, primaquine, to destroy exoerythrocytic stages responsible for relapses. The patient should be checked for glucose 6-phosphate dehydrogenase deficiency before taking primaquine. Also, primaquine is not effective against erythrocytic schizonts at pharmacological levels, so it cannot be used in place of chloroquine.

2. **C.** The first-line drug for cutaneous or mucocutaneous leishmaniasis is sodium stibogluconate (*Pentostam*) or meglumine antimonate (*Glucantime*). Antimonials have not been approved by the U. S. Food and Drug Administration, but sodium stibogluconate is obtained from the Centers for Disease Control and Prevention. Clinical response is determined by species and resistance patterns of *Leishmania* and by host immunity. These drugs are given by intravenous or intramuscular injection. Phlebitis and pain are reduced when these drugs

are given intravenously. In advanced mucocutaneous leishmaniasis amphotericin B may be an alternative, especially in areas of resistance to antimony drugs. Liposomal amphotericin B is the drug of choice for visceral leishmaniasis and has been used successfully in the treatment of cutaneous and mucocutaneous disease. Pentamidine, ketoconazole, and itraconazole have been used effectively to treat the cutaneous but not visceral form of leishmaniasis. Pyrantel pamoate is a roundworm treatment and not indicated here. Primaquine phosphate is used to prevent relapses in tertian malaria, and praziquantel is the drug of choice in treating tapeworm and fluke infections. Pyrimethamine–sulfadoxine is used to treat malaria and is sometimes combined with quinine sulfate in chloroquine resistance. It is also used to treat toxoplasmosis when it is accompanied by leucovorin (folinic acid).

3. **C.** Suramin is the drug of choice for the hemolymphatic stage of *T. rhodesiense* and *T. gambiense* with a normal CSF examination. This drug is almost 100% effective in eliminating trypanosomes from the blood of patients in the early stage of disease. Epidemiologically this patient appears to have East African trypanosomiasis caused by *T. rhodesiense*. Pentamidine isethionate results in lower cure rates in *T. rhodesiense* infections than those with suramin. Suramin does not cross the blood-brain barrier, so it is not effective for patients with meningoencephalopathic involvement. Somnolence, or inability to concentrate, may be seen before the CNS is involved. Treatment for CNS late-stage trypanosomiasis is melarsoprol; however, because of potential toxicity, this drug is reserved for late-stage disease only. Metronidazole is used to treat amebiasis, not trypanosomiasis. Sulfadoxine–pyrimethamine and chloroquine are antimalarial and are not used for this indication. Sulfadoxine–pyrimethamine with leucovorin (folinic acid) can also be used to treat *Toxoplasma gondii*.

4. **D.** Metronidazole is the drug most frequently recommended for treatment of this infection. Quinacrine has been used in the past, but because of toxicity and lack of availability it is not a first choice. Albendazole, not mebendazole, has been used with a good outcome in giardiasis. Mebendazole is used to treat roundworm infections. Melarsoprol is used to treat advanced-stage CNS African trypanosomiasis. Mefloquine is an oral drug used to treat chloroquine-resistant malaria. Meglumine antimonate (*Glucantime*) or sodium stibogluconate (*Pentostam*) is used to treat cutaneous or mucocutaneous leishmaniasis by the IV route. Giardiasis, which may be chronic and the cause of malabsorption, sometimes requires multiple stool examinations or a duodenal aspirate. Infection may be through contaminated food or beverages or may be acquired through surface water contaminated by mammals such as beavers. The risk of human infection appears increased in those with reduced gastric acid production.

5. **A.** Liposomal amphotericin B was approved by the U.S. Food and Drug Administration to treat visceral leishmaniasis. Pentavalent antimony compounds, pentamidine, amphotericin B, and aminosidine (paromomycin) have all been demonstrated efficacious here. The liposomal amphotericin appears to be better taken up by the reticuloendothelial system, where the parasite resides, and partitions less in the kidney, where amphotericin B traditionally manifests its toxicity. In addition to being better tolerated by patients, it has proved to be very effective in India, where resistance to antimony drugs is widespread. This patient appears to have acquired his infection there, where many infected patients develop darkening of the skin, hence the name kala-azar, or black sickness. Albendazole, an anthelmintic, has no role here. Atovaquone, a naphthoquinone, is used to treat malaria, babesiosis, and pneumocystosis. Pyrimethamine–sulfadoxine is used to treat malaria and toxoplasmosis. Proguanil inhibits the dihydrofolate reductase of malaria parasites and is used in combination with atovaquone.

SUPPLEMENTAL READING

Atovaquone/proguanil (Malarone) for malaria. Med Lett Drugs Ther 2000;42:109–111.

Berman JD. Editorial response: U. S. Food and Drug Administration approval of AmBisome (Liposomal Amphotericin B) for treatment of visceral leishmaniasis. Clin Infect Dis 1999;28:49–51.

Cook GC. Manson's tropical diseases (20th ed.). London: Saunders, 1996.

Davidson RN. Practical guide for the treatment of leishmaniasis. Drugs 1998;56:1009–1018.

Drugs for parasitic infections. Med Lett Drugs Ther 2000;42:1–12.

Frayha GJ et al. The mechanisms of action of antiprotozoal and anthelmintic drugs in man. Gen Pharmacol 1997;28:273–299.

Kain KC, Shanks D, and Keystone JS. Malaria chemoprophylaxis in the age of drug resistance. I. Currently recommended drug regimens. Clin Infect Dis 2001;33:226–234.

Looareesuwan S et al. Malarone (atovaquone and proguanil hydrochloride): A review of its clinical development for treatment of malaria. Am J Trop Med Hyg 1999;60:533–541.

Strickland GT. Hunter's tropical medicine and emerging infectious diseases (8th ed.). Philadelphia: Saunders, 2000.

CASE Study   Malaria and Travel

A 57-year-old medical missionary developed fever, diarrhea, headache, vomiting, and dark urine about 10 days after returning to the United States from a month-long trip to East Africa. The patient has been taking chloroquine and proguanil chemoprophylaxis. On physical examination the patient is feverish, agitated, sweating, weak, and in mild distress, with a blood pressure 95/60 (normal, 120/80), a pulse of 120 (normal, 60–100), and temperature of 104°F (40°C) (normal, 98.6°F, 37°C). Laboratory findings are a hematocrit of 25% (normal for male, 40–54%); platelet count 29,000 (normal, 150,000–400,000/mm^3); parasitemia 6% (*P. falciparum*); serum creatinine 3.5 mg/dL (Normal for male, 0.8–1.5 mg/dL); and plasma glucose 39 mg/dL (Normal fasting, 65–110 mg/dL). What is the best choice of drug therapy?

ANSWER: The first and most important step in managing a patient with fever and occasional gastrointestinal symptoms upon return from a malaria-endemic area is to include it prominently in the differential diagnosis. Any delay in the diagnosis and proper treatment places the patient in peril. Untreated *P. falciparum* in a nonimmune individual can quickly overwhelm the patient in a very short time; hence the name malignant tertian malaria. Severe manifestations heralding unfavorable prognosis include hyperparasitemia greater than 5%, hyperpyrexia above 04°F (40°C), unrousable coma or declining neurological status, severe anemia with a hematocrit below 15%, hypoglycemia with blood glucose less than 40 mg/dL, circulatory collapse with systolic blood pressure less than 70 mm Hg in adults or 50 mm Hg in children, renal failure with serum creatinine more than 3 mg/dL, jaundice with serum bilirubin greater than 3 mg/dL. The treatment of choice in this setting is parenteral quinidine gluconate with frequent monitoring of serum glucose. Quinidine and quinine, as well as hyperparasitemia, can depress circulating glucose levels; this must be corrected. Daily determinations of parasitemia are necessary to follow recovery. If this patient was seen while the parasitemia was low and there were no complications, oral atovaquone–proguanil might have been a therapeutic first choice or mefloquine as a second choice. This case underscores the need to avoid inappropriate chemoprophylaxis in countries where known resistance patterns dictate, since the initiation of aggressive therapy with indicated drugs can be lifesaving. *P. falciparum* does not have persistent liver stages to cause relapses, so there is no need to administer primaquine unless one suspects a mixed infection of *P. vivax*.

54

Anthelmintic Drugs

Mir Abid Husain and Leonard William Scheibel

DRUG LIST

GENERIC NAME	PAGE	GENERIC NAME	PAGE
Albendazole	624	Oxamniquine	626
Bithionol	626	Piperazine	622
Diethylcarbamazine	623	Praziquantel	626
Ivermectin	623	Pyrantel pamoate	623
Mebendazole	624	Suramin	623
Metrifonate	626	Thiabendazole	624
Niclosamide	625		

Infection by *helminths* (worms) may be limited solely to the intestinal lumen or may involve a complex process with migration of the adult or immature worm through the body before localization in a particular tissue. Complicating our understanding of the host–parasite relationship and the role of chemotherapy in helminth-induced infections is the complex life cycle of many of these organisms. Whereas some helminths have a simple cycle of egg deposition and development of the egg to produce a mature worm, others must progress through one or more hosts and one or more morphological stages, each metabolically distinct from the other, before emerging as an adult. Furthermore, an infective form may be either an adult worm or an immature worm. Treatment may be further complicated by infection with more than one genus of helminth. Pathogenic helminths can be divided into the following major groups: *cestodes* (flatworms), *nematodes* (roundworms), *trematodes* (flukes) and less frequently, *Acanthocephala* (thorny-headed worms).

The complex life cycle and host–parasite relationship means that treatment is sometimes difficult and may have to be protracted. Most available anthelmintic drugs exert their antiparasitic effects by interference with (1) energy metabolism, (2) neuromuscular coordination, (3) microtubular function, and (4) cellular permeability. The mode of action of most drugs used in the treatment of helminthic infections is summarized in Table 54.1. Some of the drugs used in the treatment of diseases caused by helminths also are used in the treatment of specific protozoal diseases.

TREATMENT FOR INFECTIONS CAUSED BY NEMATODES

Nematodes are long, cylindrical unsegmented worms that are tapered at both ends. Because of their shape, they are commonly referred to as roundworms. Some intestinal nematodes contain a mouth with three lips, and in some the mouth contains cutting plates. Infection occurs after ingestion of embryonated eggs or tissues of another host that contain larval forms of the nematodes.

TABLE 54.1   Mode of Action of Drugs Employed in Chemotherapy of Helminthic Diseases

Drug	Mode of Action	Specific Effect
Piperazine	Paralyzes helminth muscle	Blocks myoneural junction; causes chloride-dependent hyperpolarization, flaccid paralysis
Ivermectin	Paralyzes helminth muscle	Blocks transmission of nerve signals by interactions with glutamate-gated chloride channels
Pyrantel	Paralyzes helminth muscle	Depolarization and spastic paralysis
Niclosamide	Inhibits production of energy	Uncouples anaerobic oxidative phosphorylation in tapeworm mitochondria, causing decreased ATP synthesis
Mebendazole	Inhibits protein function	Binds to tubulin and inhibits polymerization
Diethylcarbamazine	Enhances phagocytosis and killing	Sensitizes microfilaria, entraps them in reticuloendothelial system
Praziquantel	Paralyzes helminth muscle	Increases membrane permeability, unmasks surface proteins
Thiabendazole	Inhibits energy production, protein function	Inhibits fumarate reductase, ATP synthesis; binds to tubulin
Bithionol	Inhibits energy production	Uncouples oxidative phosphorylation
Suramin	Inhibits energy production	Inhibits muscle enzymes of glycolysis and oxygen consumption

Some of the nematodes (filarial worms and guinea worms) live in blood, lymphatics, and other tissues and are referred to as blood and tissue nematodes. Others are found primarily in the intestinal tract. One group, hookworms, undergoes a developmental cycle in soil. The larvae penetrate the skin of humans, enter the venules, and are carried to the lungs, where they enter the alveoli, sometimes causing pneumonitis. The larvae then migrate up the trachea and are swallowed. In the intestine, they attach to the mucosa, and using the cutting plates and a muscular esophagus, feed on host blood and tissue fluid. This may result in vague abdominal pains, diarrhea and, if many worms are present, anemia.

Strongyloides stercoralis infection is acquired, like hookworm, from filariform larvae in contaminated soil that penetrate the skin. This parasite maintains itself for many decades in the small intestine asymptomatically. Persons treated with immunosuppressive drugs or who are debilitated by chronic illness may be at risk for widespread tissue invasion or hyperinfection syndrome. Prompt treatment may be life saving in disseminated disease.

Other intestinal nematodes are acquired by ingestion of eggs from soil. These groups lack cutting plates and may not cause anemia. Still other nematodes, such as pinworms, migrate from the anus to lay eggs, which are transmitted by fingers or through the air. The eggs are ingested and the adult worm develops in the intestinal tract. In some cases, the appendix may be invaded, resulting in symptoms of appendicitis. In most cases, the symptoms are perianal pruritus and a restlessness associated with the migration of the female worm through the anus to the perianal skin. Other nematodes, such as *Ascaris* spp., are ingested in egg form but have a migration similar to that of the hookworm.

The filarial worms differ from other nematodes in that they are threadlike and are found in blood and tissue. The infective larvae enter following the bite of an infected arthropod (fly or mosquito). They then enter the lymphatics and lymph nodes. Fever, lymphangitis, and lymphadenitis are associated with the early stage of the disease. Chronic infections may be characterized by elephantiasis as a result of lymphatic obstruction. Some species of filarial worms migrate in the subcutaneous tissues and produce nodules and blindness (onchocerciasis).

Piperazine

Piperazine (*Vermizine*) contains a heterocyclic ring that lacks a carboxyl group. It acts on the musculature of the helminths to cause reversible flaccid paralysis mediated by chloride-dependent hyperpolarization of the muscle membrane. This results in expulsion of the worm. Piperazine acts as an agonist at gated chloride channels on the parasite muscle.

Piperazine has been used with success to treat *A. lumbricoides* and *E. vermicularis* infections, although mebendazole is now the agent of choice. Piperazine is administered orally and is readily absorbed from the intestinal tract. Most of the drug is excreted in the urine within 24 hours.

Piperazine is an appropriate alternative to mebendazole for the treatment of ascariasis, especially in the presence of intestinal or biliary obstruction. Cure rates of more than 80% are obtained following a 2-day regimen.

Side effects occasionally include gastrointestinal distress, urticaria, and dizziness. Neurological symptoms of ataxia, hypotonia, visual disturbances, and exacerbations of epilepsy can occur in patients with preexisting renal insufficiency. It should not be used in pregnant women because of the formation of a potentially carcinogenic and teratogenic nitrosamine metabolite. Concomitant use of piperazine and chlorpromazine or pyrantel should be avoided.

Diethylcarbamazine

Diethylcarbamazine citrate (*Hetrazan*) is active against several microfilaria and adult filarial worms. It interferes with the metabolism of arachidonic acid and blocks the production of prostaglandins, resulting in capillary vasoconstriction and impairment of the passage of the microfilaria. Diethylcarbamazine also increases the adherence of microfilariae to the vascular wall, platelets, and granulocytes.

Diethylcarbamazine is absorbed from the gastrointestinal tract, and peak blood levels are obtained in 4 hours; the drug disappears from the blood within 48 hours. The intact drug and its metabolites are excreted in the urine.

Diethylcarbamazine is the drug of choice for certain filarial infections, such as *Wuchereria bancrofti, Brugia malayi* and *Loa loa*. Since diethylcarbamazine is not universally active against filarial infections, a specific diagnosis based on blood smears, biopsy samples, and a geographic history is important. Dosage should be adjusted in patients with renal impairment.

Caution is necessary when using this agent, particularly when treating onchocerciasis. The sudden death of the microfilariae can produce mild to severe reactions within hours of drug administration. These are manifested by fever, lymphadenopathy, cutaneous swelling, leukocytosis, and intensification of any preexisting eosinophilia, edema, rashes, tachycardia, and headache. If microfilariae are present in the eye, further ocular damage may result. Other side effects are relatively mild and range from malaise, headache, and arthralgias to gastrointestinal symptoms.

Ivermectin

Ivermectin (*Mectizan*) acts on parasite-specific inhibitory glutamate-gated chloride channels that are phylogenetically related to vertebrate GABA-gated chloride channels. Ivermectin causes hyperpolarization of the parasite cell membrane and muscle paralysis. At higher doses it can potentiate GABA-gated chloride channels. It does not cross the blood-brain barrier and therefore has no paralytic action in mammals, since GABA-regulated transmission occurs only in the central nervous system (CNS). Ivermectin is administered by the oral and subcutaneous routes. It is rapidly absorbed. Most of the drug is excreted unaltered in the feces. The half-life is approximately 12 hours.

Ivermectin has broad-spectrum activity in that it can affect nematodes, insects, and acarine parasites. It is the drug of choice in onchocerciasis and is quite useful in the treatment of other forms of filariasis, strongyloidiasis, ascariasis, loiasis, and cutaneous larva migrans. It is also highly active against various mites. It is the drug of choice in treating humans infected with *Onchocerca volvulus,* acting as a microfilaricidal drug against the skin-dwelling larvae (microfilaria). Annual treatment can prevent blindness from ocular onchocerciasis. Ivermectin is clearly more effective than diethylcarbamazine in bancroftian filariasis, and it reduces microfilaremia to near zero levels. In brugian filariasis diethylcarbamazine-induced clearance may be superior. It also is used to treat cutaneous larva migrans and disseminated strongyloidiasis. Its safe use in pregnancy has not been fully established.

The side effects are minimal, with pruritus, fever, and tender lymph nodes occasionally seen. The side effects are considerably less than those associated with diethylcarbamazine administration.

Suramin

Suramin is widely used as a macrofilaricide in human onchocerciasis, and its action on microfilariae also is considerable. It also is useful in the treatment of the hemolymphatic stage of African trypanosomiasis. Early treatment of the infection with suramin clears trypanosomes from the blood and lymphatics within 30 minutes and keeps them clear for approximately 3 months. Suramin inhibits a number of filarial enzymes involved with carbohydrate metabolism as well as the production of adenosine triphosphate (ATP). It is 35 times more inhibitory to the dihydrofolate reductase of *O. volvulus* than to the same enzyme in human tissue. It is a potent inhibitor of reverse transcriptase, the DNA polymerase of retroviruses, and also has some effects on the infective and cytopathic effects of HIV. It is being evaluated as an anticancer drug, reducing pain and delaying progression in hormone-refractory prostate cancer. Its most significant toxicity has been the development of severe polyradiculoneuropathy.

Pyrantel Pamoate

Pyrantel pamoate (*Antiminth*) is a agonist at the nicotinic acetylcholine receptor, and its actions result in depolarization and spastic paralysis of the helminth muscle. Its selective toxicity occurs primarily because the neuromuscular junction of helminth muscle is more sensitive to the drug than is mammalian muscle. This drug is administered orally, and because very little is absorbed, high levels are achieved in the intestinal tract. Less than 15% of the drug and its metabolites are excreted in urine.

Pyrantel pamoate is active against several round-worms: *A. lumbricoides, Ancylostoma duodenale, Necator americanus*, and *E. vermicularis*. Pyrantel is an alternative drug of choice in treating infections with *A. lumbricoides, E. vermicularis* (pinworms), and hookworms (*N. americanus* and *A. duodenale*). It is not recommended for pregnant patients or for children under age 1 year.

Although most of the drug remains in the intestinal lumen, enough can be absorbed systemically to cause headache, dizziness, and drowsiness. No major adverse effects have been reported on renal, hepatic, or hematological systems.

BENZIMIDAZOLES

Several benzimidazoles are in use for the treatment of helminthic infections. Three of these, mebendazole, thiabendazole and albendazole, are described in this section. They have a broad range of activity against many nematode and cestode parasites, including cutaneous larva migrans, trichinosis, disseminated strongyloidiasis, and visceral larva migrans. A fourth, triclabendazole, is considered as the drug of choice for *Fasciola hepatica* therapy.

Thiabendazole

Thiabendazole (*Mintezol*) inhibits fumarate reductase and electron transport–associated phosphorylation in helminths. Interference with ATP generation decreases glucose uptake and affects the energy available for metabolism. Benzimidazole anthelmintics as a class (e.g., thiabendazole, mebendazole, and albendazole), bind selectively to β-tubulin of nematodes (roundworms), cestodes (tapeworms), and trematodes (flukes). This inhibits microtubule assembly, which is important in a number of helminth cellular processes, such as mitosis, transport, and motility.

Thiabendazole is administered orally and is rapidly absorbed from the intestinal tract, with peak plasma levels achieved in 1 to 2 hours. The drug is metabolized in the liver and excreted in urine within 24 to 48 hours as glucuronide and sulfate esters. Approximately 10% is found in feces.

Thiabendazole shows a broad spectrum of activity against the following nematodes: *A. lumbricoides, N. americanus, A. duodenale, E. vermicularis, S. stercoralis*, and *Trichuris trichiura* (whipworm). It has largely been replaced with safer drugs for all but *Strongyloides* spp. At present, thiabendazole is the drug of choice for the treatment of cutaneous larva migrans (creeping eruption), strongyloidiasis, trichostrongyliasis, and trichinosis.

Anorexia, nausea, vomiting, drowsiness, and vertigo occur in up to one-third of patients. Diarrhea, pruritus, rash, hallucinations, crystalluria, and leukopenia are less common; shock, hyperglycemia, lymphadenopathy, and Stevens-Johnson syndrome are rare. Some patients report that their urine smells like asparagus, a reaction related to excretion of the metabolite asparagine.

Mebendazole

Unlike thiabendazole, mebendazole (*Vermox*) does not inhibit fumarate reductase. While mebendazole binds to both mammalian and nematode tubulin, it exhibits a differential affinity for the latter, possibly explaining the selective action of the drug. The selective binding to nematode tubulin may inhibit glucose absorption, leading to glycogen consumption and ATP depletion.

Mebendazole is given orally; it is poorly soluble, and very little is absorbed from the intestinal tract. About 5 to 10%, principally the decarboxylated derivatives, is recovered in the urine; most of the orally administered drug is found in the feces within 24 hours.

Mebendazole is used primarily for the treatment of *A. lumbricoides, T. trichiura, E. vermicularis*, and hookworm infections, in which it produces high cure rates. It is an alternative agent for the treatment of trichinosis and visceral larva migrans. Owing to its broad-spectrum anthelmintic effect, mixed infections (ascariasis, hookworm infestation, or enterobiasis in association with trichuriasis) frequently respond to therapy. High doses have been used to treat hydatid disease, but albendazole is now thought to be superior.

Abdominal discomfort and diarrhea may occur when the worm load is heavy. Its use is contraindicated during pregnancy.

Albendazole

Albendazole appears to cause cytoplasmic microtubular degeneration, which in turn impairs vital cellular processes and leads to parasite death. There is some evidence that the drug also inhibits helminth-specific ATP generation by fumarate reductase.

Albendazole is given orally and is poorly and variably absorbed (<5%) because of its poor water solubility. Oral bioavailability is increased as much as five times when the drug is given with a fatty meal instead of on an empty stomach. Concurrent treatment with corticosteroids increases plasma concentrations of albendazole. The drug is rapidly metabolized in the liver to an active sulfoxide metabolite. The half life of the metabolites is 8 to 12 hours.

Albendazole has a broad spectrum of activity against intestinal nematodes and cestodes, as well as the liver flukes *Opisthorchis sinensis, Opisthorchis viverrini*, and *Clonorchis sinensis*. It also has been used successfully against Giardia lamblia. Albendazole is an effective treatment of hydatid cyst disease (echinococcosis), especially when accompanied with praziquantel. It also is effective in treating cerebral and spinal neurocysticercosis, particularly when given with dexamethasone. Albendazole is recommended for treatment of gnathostomiasis.

TREATMENT FOR INFECTIONS CAUSED BY CESTODES

Cestodes, or tapeworms, are flattened dorsoventrally and are segmented. The tapeworm has a head with round suckers or sucking grooves. Some tapeworms have a projection (*rostellum*) that bears hooks. This head, or *scolex* (also referred to as the hold-fast organ), is used by the worm to attach to tissues. Drugs that affect the scolex permit expulsion of the organisms from the intestine. Attached to the head is the neck region, which is the region of growth. The rest of the worm consists of a number of segments, called *proglottids,* each of which contains both male and female reproductive units. These segments, after filling with fertilized eggs, are released from the worm and discharged into the environment.

Cestodes that parasitize humans have complex life cycles, usually requiring development in a second or intermediate host. Following their ingestion, the infected larvae develop into adults in the small intestine. Although most patients remain symptom free, some have vague abdominal discomfort, hunger pangs, indigestion, and anorexia, and vitamin B deficiency may develop. In some cestode infections, eggs containing larvae are ingested; the larvae invade the intestinal wall, enter a blood vessel, and lodge in such tissues as muscle, liver, and eye. Symptoms are associated with the particular organ affected.

Niclosamide
Mechanism of Action

For many years, niclosamide (*Niclocide*) was widely used to treat infestations of cestodes. Niclosamide is a chlorinated salicylamide that inhibits the production of energy derived from anaerobic metabolism. It may also have adenosine triphosphatase (ATPase) stimulating properties. Inhibition of anaerobic incorporation of inorganic phosphate into ATP is detrimental to the parasite. Niclosamide can uncouple oxidative phosphorylation in mammalian mitochondria, but this action requires dosages that are higher than those commonly used in treating worm infections.

The drug affects the scolex and proximal segments of the cestodes, resulting in detachment of the scolex from the intestinal wall and eventual evacuation of the cestodes from the intestine by the normal peristaltic action of the host's bowel. Because niclosamide is not absorbed from the intestinal tract, high concentrations can be achieved in the intestinal lumen. The drug is not ovicidal.

Clinical Use

Niclosamide has been used extensively in the treatment of tapeworm infections caused by *Taenia saginata, Taenia solium, Diphyllobothrium latum, Fasciolopsis buski,* and *Hymenolepis nana.* It is an effective alternative to praziquantel for treating infections caused by *T. saginata* (beef tapeworm), *T. solium* (pork tapeworm), and *D. latum* (fish tapeworm) and is active against most other tapeworm infections. It is absorbed by intestinal cestodes but not nematodes. A single dose is usually adequate to produce a cure rate of 95%. With *H. nana* (dwarf tapeworm), a longer treatment course (up to 7 days) is necessary. Niclosamide is administered orally after the patient has fasted overnight and may be followed in 2 hours by purging (magnesium sulfate 15–30 g) to encourage complete expulsion of the cestode, especially *T. solium,* although this is not always considered necessary. Cure is assessed by follow-up stool examination in 3 to 5 months. With the availability of other agents, niclosamide is no longer widely used. The most widely employed agents are praziquantel and the benzimidazoles.

Adverse Effects

No serious side effects are associated with niclosamide use, although some patients report abdominal discomfort and loose stools.

TREATMENT FOR INFECTIONS CAUSED BY TREMATODES

Trematodes (flukes) are nonsegmented flattened helminths that are often leaflike in shape. Most have two suckers, one found around the mouth (oral sucker) and the other on the ventral surface. Most are hermaphroditic. The eggs, which are passed out of the host in sputum, urine, or feces, undergo several stages of maturation in other hosts before the larvae enter humans. The larvae are acquired either through ingestion of food (aquatic vegetation, fish, crayfish) or by direct penetration of the skin. After ingestion, most trematodes mature in the intestinal tract (intestinal flukes); others migrate and mature in the liver and bile duct (liver flukes), whereas still others penetrate the intestinal wall and migrate through the abdominal cavity to the lung (lung flukes). Diarrhea, abdominal pain, and anorexia are common symptoms associated with trematode infestation. Liver flukes may cause bile duct blockage, liver enlargement, upper right quadrant pain, and diarrhea. Liver function tests are usually altered. Lung flukes produce pulmonary symptoms such as cough, hemoptysis, and chest pain.

The *schistosomes* (blood flukes) are a distinct group of trematodes. These helminths are cylindrical at the anterior end and flattened at the posterior end. The sexes are separate. The larvae penetrate skin that is in contact with contaminated water and then migrate through the lymphatics and blood vessels to the liver. After maturing, schistosomes migrate into the mesenteric or vesicular vein, where the adults mate and release eggs. The eggs secrete enzymes that enable them to pass through the wall of the intestine (*Schistosoma mansoni* and *Schistosoma japonicum*) or bladder (*Schistosoma haematobium*). In addition, some eggs may be carried to the liver or the lung by the circulation. Penetration of the skin is associated with petechial hemorrhage, some edema, and pruritus that disappears after about 4 days. Approximately 3 weeks after trematode penetration, patients complain of malaise, fever, and vague intestinal symptoms. With the laying of eggs, acute symptoms of general malaise, fever, urticaria, abdominal pain, and liver tenderness are reported. Diarrhea or dysentery is associated with infestations by S. *mansoni* and S. *japonicum,* whereas hematuria and dysuria are commonly caused by S. *haematobium.* In the chronic form of the disease, fibrosis and hyperplasia can occur in the tissues the eggs inhabit.

Praziquantel

The neuromuscular effects of praziquantel (*Biltricide*) appear to increase parasite motility leading to spastic paralysis. The drug increases calcium permeability through parasite-specific ion channels, so that the tegmental and muscle cells of the parasite accumulate calcium. This action is followed by vacuolization and the exposure of hitherto masked tegmental antigens, lipid-anchored protein, and actin. Insertion of the drug into the fluke's lipid bilayer causes conformational changes, rendering the fluke susceptible to antibody- and complement-mediated assault.

Praziquantel is readily absorbed (80% in 24 hours) after oral administration, with serum concentrations being maximal in 1 to 3 hours; the drug has a half-life of 0.8 to 1.5 hours. Its bioavailability is reduced by phenytoin or carbamazepine and increased by cimetidine. Dexamethasone decreases plasma praziquantel levels by 50%. Praziquantel is excreted by the kidneys.

Praziquantel is an extremely active broad-spectrum anthelmintic that is well tolerated. It is the most effective of the drugs used in the treatment of schistosomiasis, possessing activity against male and female adults and immature stages. Unlike other agents, it is active against all three major species (S. *haematobium*, S. *mansoni,* and S. *japonicum*). In addition, it has activity against other flukes, such as C. *sinensis, Paragonimus westermani*, O. *viverrini*, and the tapeworms (D. *latum, H. nana, T. saginata,* and *T. solium*). It is not as effective against F. *hepatica.* It is used effectively in the treatment of clonorchiasis and paragonimiasis and is an effective alternative agent to niclosamide in the treatment of tapeworm infestations.

Adverse reactions tend to occur within a few hours of administration. They include gastrointestinal intolerance with nausea, vomiting, and abdominal discomfort. This may be due to the liberation of helminth proteins from dead worms rather than any direct effect of the drug.

Oxamniquine

Oxamniquine (*Vansil*) is a tetrahydroquinoline that stimulates parasite muscular activity at low concentrations but causes paralysis at higher concentrations. The drug may act by esterification and binding of DNA, leading to the death of the schistosome by interruption of its nucleic acid and protein synthesis. The fluke may esterify oxamniquine to produce a reactive metabolite that alkylates parasite DNA. Resistance results from absent or defective esterifying activity of the drug. Oxamniquine has a restricted range of efficacy, being active only against S. *mansoni* infections.

Oxamniquine is given orally and is readily absorbed from the intestinal tract. Peak concentrations in plasma are obtained in about 3 hours. The drug is excreted in urine mostly as a 6-carboxyl derivative.

Side effects include CNS toxicity with unsteadiness and occasionally seizures, especially in patients with a history of seizures. It is contraindicated in pregnancy.

Bithionol

Bithionol (*Actamer*) is a phenolic derivative whose mode of action is related to uncoupling of parasite-specific fumarate reductase–mediated oxidative phosphorylation. The drug is administered orally and is absorbed from the intestinal tract. Peak blood levels are achieved in 4 to 8 hours. Excretion is mainly by the kidneys.

Bithionol is used in treatment of F. *hepatica* infections and as an alternative to praziquantel in the treatment of infestation by P. *westermani.* It is highly active against the adult worm but exerts no action against the migratory stages. A second course of treatment is required for complete cure in 20 to 30% of patients.

Side effects are generally mild and transient; they include nausea, vomiting, diarrhea, headache, dizziness, urticaria, and other skin rashes in 50% of patients.

Metrifonate

Metrifonate is an organophosphorous compound that is effective only in the treatment of S. *haematobium.* The active metabolite, dichlorvos, inactivates acetylcholinesterase and potentiates inhibitory cholinergic effects. The schistosomes are swept away from the bladder to the lungs and are trapped. Therapeutic doses produce no untoward side effects except for mild cholinergic symptoms. It is contraindicated in pregnancy, previous insecticide exposure, or with depolarizing neuromuscular blockers. Metrifonate is not available in the United States.

Study QUESTIONS

1. A migrant Mexican worker in Texas has had fever, myalgias, and headache for 10 days. Initially he thought he was recovering from stomach flu; his examination is significant for conjunctival hemorrhage, bilateral periorbital edema, and severe tenderness of neck muscles and jaws. A diagnosis of trichinosis is considered. Which of the following aspects of trichinosis are particularly important?
(A) Eggs in the feces are almost always present.
(B) A negative biopsy of muscle excludes the infection.
(C) Suramin is used in its treatment with considerable success.
(D) Mebendazole plus steroids for severe symptoms may be indicated.
(E) Thiabendazole is not effective.

2. While serving with Doctors Without Borders in Malaysia, you are seeing a patient who has intermittent cough, shortness of breath, and wheezing. Investigation reveals eosinophilia, absence of microfilaria in the blood, and a chest radiograph showing scattered reticulonodular infiltrates. Which of the following points is the most important if your diagnosis is tropical pulmonary eosinophilia (TPE)?
(A) Symptoms get progressively worse and are not fluctuating.
(B) Absence of microfilariae in blood makes the diagnosis unlikely.
(C) Eosinophilia, although commonly seen, is not usually very high.
(D) Ivermectin is the drug of choice.
(E) Diethylcarbamazine is effective therapy.

3. A 10-year-old girl in North Carolina has had abdominal pain and cramps for the past few days. Her examination produced normal findings except for nonspecific abdominal discomfort with a complete blood count showing anemia and 22% eosinophils (elevated). A stool specimen revealed the characteristic eggs of *A. lumbricoides*. The drug of choice in treating this is
(A) Piperazine
(B) Pyrantel pamoate
(C) Mebendazole
(D) Albendazole
(E) Thiabendazole

4. A 15-year-old Hispanic boy is brought in with seizures. No prior history of fever, chills, trauma, or headaches was reported on admission. Computed tomography reveals three ring-enhancing cystic lesions in the brain parenchyma, and a diagnosis of neurocysticercosis is made. Initial therapy in the management of this condition should include

(A) Niclosamide
(B) Praziquantel
(C) Albendazole
(D) Surgery
(E) Thiabendazole

5. A patient with a history of frequenting sushi bars on the West Coast is admitted with abdominal pain, weakness, irritability, and dizziness. His neurological examination produced normal findings even though he had some complaints of paraesthesias. Diphyllobothriasis is diagnosed after stool studies are done. Management of this tapeworm infection is with
(A) Praziquantel or niclosamide
(B) Ivermectin
(C) Albendazole
(D) Vitamin B_{12}
(E) Piperazine

ANSWERS

1. **D.** Trichinosis should be suspected in a patient who has any of the cardinal features of periorbital edema, myositis, fever, and eosinophilia. Infection is acquired after consumption of inadequately cooked pork, bear, or walrus infected with viable larvae. Stool examination does not contain the eggs of the parasite but may contain larvae. Muscle biopsy from a tender, swollen muscle (preferably deltoid or gastrocnemius) may establish the diagnosis, but a negative biopsy does not exclude this infection, especially in light parasitemias. Suramin is not used in trichinosis. Although thiabendazole is effective, mebendazole is the drug of choice, and frequently steroids are also used for severe symptoms.

2. **E.** TPE is caused by microfilariae in the lungs and hyperimmune responsiveness to bancroftian or malayan filariasis. Paroxysmal respiratory symptoms may fluctuate in severity. Eosinophilia, almost always present, is usually very high, and the absence of microfilariae in the blood does not rule out TPE. A presumptive clinical diagnosis can be made by response to therapy without a lung biopsy. Diethylcarbamazine for 14 days is an effective therapy that can be repeated if symptoms persist. The role of ivermectin in TPE has not been established.

3. **D.** In the United States intestinal helminths produce mild disease with nonspecific findings. Piperazine or pyrantel pamoate may be used for the treatment of ascariasis. Mebendazole is an effective drug to be taken for 3 days. Thiabendazole is not used in this condition but is used commonly in strongyloidiasis. Albendazole at a single dose of 400 mg is the preferred mode of therapy. It is a

convenient agent for mass treatment programs that target school children in endemic areas.

4. C. Albendazole (approved by the U. S. Food and Drug Administration for this indication) has a 90% efficacy rate in neurocysticercosis. The initial therapy of parenchymal disease with seizures should focus on symptomatic treatment with anticonvulsants. However, while destroying the cyst, albendazole may result in a profound parenchymal brain reaction and in severe neurological defects or retinal damage (i.e., loss of vision and optic neuritis) in eye lesions. Corticosteroids should be given concomitantly in these situations. In ventricular disease with obstructive hydrocephalus, surgery with shunting can be helpful. Treatment with niclosamide or praziquantel should be considered later to eliminate the adult tapeworm in the gut and prevent further reinfection. Neither piperazine nor thiabendazole is effective in this indication.

5. A. *D. latum,* the fish tapeworm acquired from consumption of raw fish in endemic areas, is best treated with praziquantel or niclosamide. Ivermectin is effective for filarial infections, especially *O. volvulus.* Albendazole, although highly effective in some tapeworm infections, is not used in fish tapeworm infections. Vitamin B_{12} deficiency is due to the parasite competing with the host for the vitamin, sometimes absorbing 80% of ingested amounts. Patients may develop megaloblastic anemia and mild to severe central nervous system manifestations (subacute combined degeneration of spinal cord). Mild B_{12} deficiency should be treated with vitamin injections in addition to specific drug therapy. Piperazine, a roundworm treatment, is not used for this indication.

SUPPLEMENTAL READING

Ammann RW and Eckert J. Cestodes: Echinococcus. Gastroenterol Clin North Am 1996;25:655–689.

Cook GC. Manson's Tropical Diseases (20th ed.). London: Saunders, 1996.

Drugs for parasitic infections. Med Lett Drugs Ther 2000;42:1–12.

Frayha GJ et al. The mechanisms of action of antiprotozoals and anthelmintic drugs in man. Gen Pharmacol 1997;28:273–299.

Gilbert DN, Moellering RC Jr, and Sande MA. The Sanford Guide to Antimicrobial Therapy (32nd ed.). Hyde Park, VT: Antimicrobial Therapy, 2002.

Graham CS, Brodie SB, and Weller PF. Imported *Fasciola hepatica* infection in the United States and treatment with triclabendazole. Clin Infect Dis 2001;33:1–5.

Kohler P. The biochemical basis of anthelmintic action and resistance. Int J Parisitol 2001;31:336–345.

Liu LX and Weller PF. Antiparasitic drugs. N Engl J Med 1996;334:1178–1184.

Martin RJ, Robertson AP, and Bjorn H. Target sites of anthelmintics. Parasitology 1997;114:S111–S124.

Martin RJ. Modes of action of anthelmintic drugs. Vet J 1997;154:11–34.

Strickland GT. Hunter's Tropical Medicine and Emerging Infectious Diseases (8th ed.). Philadelphia: Saunders, 2000.

CASE Study   An Extensive History: Always Useful

The patient is a 64-year-old male resident of a mental institution with a chief complaint of cough and rash. He was a Vietnam veteran with a history of non-Hodgkin's lymphoma treated with combination chemotherapy containing prednisone. Two months later he developed a progressive cough, dyspnea, midepigastric pain, diarrhea, and what he describes as an itchy rash on the lower abdominal wall. The patient's physical examination revealed a thin man in mild distress with a temperature of 100°F (37.8°C), blood pressure 124/70 mmHg, pulse 120, and respiratory rate 25 per minute. Rales were heard throughout his lung fields. His abdomen was soft and flat, with hypoactive bowel sounds. There was marked tenderness without rebound noted on palpation of the epigastric area, with no masses. His skin examination revealed a migratory serpiginous urticarial rash distributed over the lower abdomen, lower trunk, and buttocks (larva currens). Examination of the peripheral blood showed a white count of 16,190/mm³ (normal, 4,000–12,000/mm³) and eosinophils 66% (markedly elevated). His chest radiograph showed diffuse pulmonary infiltrates. A transbronchial lung biopsy showed eosinophilic granulomatous inflammation of the bronchial epithelium. Bronchoalveolar lavage revealed *S. stercoralis* filariform larvae. Microscopic examination of the stool revealed rhabditiform larvae of *S. stercoralis.* Based on the knowledge of *S. stercoralis* hyperinfection syndrome, which agent or agents would be a logical choice for treatment of this life-threatening disease?

CASE Study   An Extensive History: Always Useful

ANSWER: Until recently thiabendazole was the drug of choice to treat strongyloidiasis. Parasite eradication in uncomplicated infections is approximately 90% or higher. However, *S. stercoralis* is a significant health risk in many developing countries and even in parts of eastern Kentucky and rural Tennessee. It presents a serious potential for severe disease in the many military servicemen who were stationed in Southeast Asia during World War II and the Vietnam era. In fact, it was first described in 1876 as "diarrhea of China" in French colonial troops in Indochina by Louis Alexis Norman, physician first class in the French Navy. It is acquired by infective larvae that penetrate the skin and frequently maintain a low level of autoinfection asymptomatically for many decades. Hyperinfection and widespread dissemination may occur following immunosuppression or chronic disease. Prompt treatment can be lifesaving, as hyperinfection syndrome is associated with mortality rates up to 86%. Steroids may suppress the eosinophil response normally seen in this disease, so an appropriate history must be taken and characteristic intestinal and skin findings examined, and a high index of suspicion is needed to make a timely diagnosis of patients who spent time in endemic areas. In immunocompromised hosts, persistent infection and relapse may complicate therapy with thiabendazole (even when given over 7 to 10 days). Alternative therapy with ivermectin appears as effective (64–100% cure rates) as thiabendazole with fewer side effects. Other drug choices are albendazole (cure rates of 38–81%) and mebendazole, but these have not been approved by the FDA for this indication.

55 The Rational Basis for Cancer Chemotherapy

Branimir I. Sikic

Modern cancer chemotherapy originated in the 1940s with the demonstration that nitrogen mustard possessed antitumor activity against human lymphomas and leukemias. Approximately 10 types of human cancer have 40 to 80% "cure" rates using chemotherapy alone or chemotherapy plus surgery or radiation (Table 55.1). For this purpose cure is defined as the disappearance of any evidence of tumor for several years and a high actuarial probability of a normal life span.

Patients with other types of unresectable cancer also may benefit from chemotherapy, as evidenced by prolongation of life, shrinkage of tumor, and improvement in symptoms. Notable among these are ovarian epithelial and breast carcinomas, oat cell (small cell undifferentiated) carcinoma of the lung, and acute myelocytic leukemia. Cancers that are for the most part resistant to today's agents include melanoma, colorectal and renal carcinomas, and non–oat cell cancers of the lung.

CONCEPTS IN TUMOR CELL BIOLOGY

The Normal Cell Cycle

The *normal cell cycle* consists of a definable sequence of events that characterize the growth and division of cells and can be observed by morphological and biochemical means. The cell cycle is depicted in Fig. 55.1. Two of the four phases of the cell cycle can be studied directly: the *M-phase*, or mitosis, is easily visible using light microscopy because of chromosomal condensation, spindle formation, and cell division. The *S-phase* is the period of DNA synthesis and is observed by measuring the incorporation of tritiated thymidine into cell nuclei.

The *mitotic index* is the fraction or percentage of cells in mitosis within a given cell population. The *thymidine labeling index* is the fraction of cells incorporating radioactive thymidine. They represent cells in M-phase and S-phase and define the proliferative characteristics of normal and tumor cells.

The Tumor Cell Cycle

The duration of the S-phase in human tumors is 10 to 20 hours. This period is followed by the G_2-*phase,* or period of preparation for mitosis, in which cells contain a tetraploid number of chromosomes. The G_2-phase lasts only 1 to 3 hours for most cell types, with mitosis itself lasting approximately 1 hour. The two daughter cells then enter the G_1-*phase,* whose duration varies from several hours to days. The G_1-phase also can give rise to a resting state, termed G_0, in which cells are relatively inactive metabolically and are resistant to most chemotherapeutic drugs.

The *generation time,* or T_c, is the time required to complete one cycle of cell growth and division. The T_c will vary with the duration of the G_1-phase. The factors that influence daughter cells to enter the G_0, or resting stage, are not well understood. The ability to cause such resting cells to reenter the cell cycle would be quite useful, since *proliferating cells generally are more sensitive to chemotherapy than are resting cells.*

DRUGS AND THE CELL CYCLE

Various classification schemes have been proposed to describe the effects of drugs on the cell cycle. One such

TABLE 55.1	Cancers with 40 to 80 Percent Cure Rates
Age	**Type of Cancer**
Childhood	Acute lymphocytic leukemia
	Burkitt's sarcoma
	Ewing's sarcoma
	Retinoblastoma
	Rhabdomyosarcoma
	Wilms' tumor
Adult	Hodgkin's disease
	Non-Hodgkin's disease
	Trophoblastic choriocarcinoma
	Testicular and ovarian germ cell cancers

classification divides the anticancer drugs into three categories:

1. *Class 1 agents* (e.g., radiation, mechlorethamine, and carmustine) exert their cytotoxicity in a *nonspecific* (i.e., non–proliferation dependent) manner. They kill both normal and malignant cells to the same extent.

2. *Class 2 agents* are phase specific and reach a plateau in cell kill with increasing dosages. Only a certain *proportion* of cells are sensitive to the toxic effects of these drugs. For example, hydroxyurea and cytarabine kill only cells in the S-phase. Similarly, bleomycin is most toxic to cells in G_2- and early M-phases. Because they affect only a small fraction of the cell population at any one time, it has been suggested that these drugs should be given either by continuous infusion or in frequent small doses. Such a dosage regimen would increase the number of tumor cells exposed to the drug during the sensitive phase of their cell cycle.

3. *Class 3 agents* kill *proliferating* cells in preference to resting cells. It has been recommended

that these proliferation-dependent but non–phase-specific agents be administered in single large doses to take advantage of their sparing effect on normal cells that may be in G_0.

Unfortunately, many human cancers have a large proportion of cells in the resting phase, and these cells are also resistant to the class 3 agents, which include cyclophosphamide, dactinomycin, and fluorouracil.

This classification of anticancer drugs has inherent limitations. For instance, it may be difficult to generalize about the phase specificity of a particular drug, since this may vary among cell types. Several techniques are available to synchronize cell populations in such a way that most cells will be in the same phase of the cell cycle. After synchronization, one can treat cells in each phase and determine their relative sensitivity to drugs throughout the cell cycle.

Some drugs that exert their maximum cytotoxicity during the S-phase of the cycle also prevent cells from progressing through the cell cycle to the S-phase; this is accomplished by sublethal inhibition of RNA and protein synthesis. The antimetabolites methotrexate, fluorouracil, and mercaptopurine all can inhibit RNA synthesis in G_1- and G_2-phases and inhibit DNA synthesis during S-phase. This inhibition of cell cycle progression actually may result in reduced cytotoxicity, and such agents have been termed *S-phase-specific but self-limited.*

TUMOR GROWTH AND GROWTH FRACTION

The rate of growth of human and experimental cancers is initially quite rapid (exponential) and then slows until a plateau is reached. The decrease in growth rate with increasing tumor size is related both to a decrease in the proportion of cancer cells actively proliferating (termed the *growth fraction*) and to an increase in the rate of cell loss due to hypoxic necrosis, poor nutrient supply, immunological defense mechanisms, and other processes.

The rate of spontaneous cell death for some human tumors is thought to be a significant factor in limiting growth. However, the growth fraction, or percentage of cells in the cell cycle, is the most important determinant of overall tumor enlargement. The doubling times of human tumors have been estimated by direct measurement of chest radiographs of lesions or palpable masses to be 1 to 6 months.

The *growth fraction* indicates dividing cells that are potentially sensitive to chemotherapy; thus, it is not surprising that tumors with high growth fractions are the ones most easily curable by drugs. Among human tumors, only Burkitt's lymphoma and trophoblastic choriocarcinoma are readily curable by single-agent chemotherapy; both of these tumors have growth fractions close to 100%.

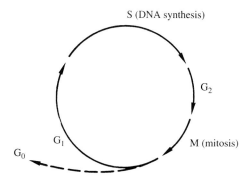

FIGURE 55.1
The cell cycle. S, G_1, G_2, and G_0 are phases of the cell cycle.

As tumors grow larger, the growth fraction within the tumor decreases, and the greater the distance of cells from nutrient blood vessels, the more likely they are to be in the G_0-, or resting, phase. The growth fraction is less than 10% for slow-growing cancers of the colon or lung.

A number of factors must be considered before chemotherapy is instituted for a human cancer that has a low growth fraction. For instance, the larger the tumor, the more cells will be present in the nonproliferating, relatively resistant state. Therefore, the earlier chemotherapy is instituted, the greater the chance of a favorable response. Debulking of tumors by surgery or radiation therapy may be a means of stimulating the remaining cells into active proliferation. Small metastases may respond to drugs more dramatically than will large primary tumors or a larger metastasis in the same patient.

Several cycles of treatment may be necessary to achieve a substantial reduction in tumor size. The chemotherapeutic regimen, especially when one is dealing with large, solid tumors, probably should include agents that have cytotoxic activity against resting cells.

THE LOG CELL KILL HYPOTHESIS

Cytotoxic drugs act by *first-order kinetics;* that is, at a given dose, they kill a *constant fraction* of the tumor cells rather than a fixed number of cells. For example, a drug dose that would result in a three-log cell kill (i.e., 99.9% cytotoxicity) would reduce the tumor burden of an animal that has 10^8 leukemic cells to 10^5 cells. This killing of a fraction of cells rather than an absolute number per dose is called the *log cell kill hypothesis.*

The earliest detectable human cancers usually have a volume of at least 1 cc and contain 10^9 (1 billion) cells. This number reflects the result of at least 30 cycles of cell division, or cell doublings, and represents a kinetically advanced stage in the tumor's growth. Most patients actually have tumor burdens that are greater than 10^9. Since the major limiting factor in chemotherapy is cytotoxicity to normal tissues, only a limited log cell kill can be expected with each individual treatment.

Even in the absence of tumor regrowth, several cycles of therapy would be required for eradication of the tumor, assuming it was sensitive to the drugs employed. When a tumor has decreased in size to approximately 10^8 cells, it is generally no longer detectable clinically and is considered a clinically complete remission. Regrowth of residual cells is the obvious cause of relapse in patients who have achieved clinically complete remissions.

DRUG RESISTANCE

Many patients undergoing chemotherapy fail to respond to treatment from the outset; their cancers are resistant to the available agents. Other patients respond initially, only to relapse.

Cancers can be regarded as populations of cells undergoing spontaneous mutations. The population becomes increasingly heterogeneous as the tumor grows and increasing numbers of mutations occur. Tumors of the same type and size will vary in their responsiveness to therapy because of the chance occurrences of drug-resistant mutations during tumor growth.

Assuming the same initial drug sensitivity, smaller tumors are generally more curable than larger tumors because of the increased probability of drug-resistant mutations in the larger tumors. Therefore, therapy *earlier* in the course of tumor growth should increase the chance for cure. *Combination chemotherapy* is often more effective than treatment with single drugs. Tumors that are resistant to drugs from the outset will always have a largely drug-resistant population and will be refractory to treatment.

Many kinds of biochemical resistance to anticancer drugs have been described. The biochemical and genetic mechanisms of resistance to *methotrexate* are now known in some detail. Three major resistance pathways have been described: (1) decreased drug transport into cells; (2) an alteration in the structure of the target enzyme dihydrofolate reductase (DHFR), resulting in reduced drug affinity; and (3) an increase in DHFR content of tumor cells. The increase in DHFR content occurs through a process of *gene amplification,* that is, a reduplication or increase in the number of copies per cell of the gene coding for DHFR. Amplification of various genes may be a relatively frequent event in tumor cell populations and an important genetic mechanism for generating resistance to drugs.

Tumor cells may become generally resistant to a variety of cytotoxic drugs on the basis of decreased uptake or retention of the drugs. This form of resistance is termed *pleiotropic,* or *multidrug, resistance,* and it is the major form of resistance to anthracyclines, vinca alkaloids, etoposide, paclitaxel, and dactinomycin. The gene that confers multidrug resistance (termed *mdr I*) encodes a high-molecular-weight membrane protein called *P-glycoprotein,* which acts as a drug efflux pump in many tumors and normal tissues.

Possible biochemical mechanisms of resistance to *alkylating agents* include changes in cell DNA repair capability, increases in cell thiol content (which in turn can serve as alternative and benign targets of alkylation), decreases in cell permeability, and increased activity of glutathione transferases. Increased metallothionein content has been associated with tumor cell resistance to cisplatin.

Drugs that require metabolic activation for antitumor activity, such as the *antimetabolites* 5-fluorouracil and 6-mercaptopurine, may be ineffective if a tumor is deficient in the required activating enzymes. Alternatively, a drug may be metabolically inactivated by resistant tumors, which is the case with cytarabine (pyrimidine nucleoside deaminase) and bleomycin (bleomycin hydrolase). Leukemias have been shown to develop resistance to L-asparaginase because of a drug-related induction of the enzyme asparagine synthetase.

Major mechanisms of cellular resistance to anticancer drugs are depicted in Fig. 55.2.

CANCER THERAPY AND THE IMMUNE SYSTEM

Although manipulation of the host immune response in animal tumor models has at times yielded impressive therapeutic results, attempts to extend these results to human cancers generally have been disappointing.

Several proteins that stimulate subsets of lymphocytes involved in various aspects of the immune response are now produced by recombinant DNA techniques. The pharmacology of these "lymphokines" as potential anticancer agents is being investigated. *Interleukin (IL) 2,* originally described as a T-cell growth factor, induces the production of cytotoxic lymphocytes (lymphokine-activated killer cells, or LAK cells). IL-2 produces remissions in 10 to 20% of patients with melanoma or renal cell carcinoma when infused at high doses either alone or with lymphocytes that were previously harvested from the patient and incubated with IL-2 in vitro.

The ability of certain anticancer agents to suppress both humoral and cellular immunity has been exploited in the field of organ transplantation and in diseases thought to be caused by an abnormal or heightened immune response. In particular, the alkylating agents cyclophosphamide and chlorambucil have been used in this context, as have several of the antimetabolites, including methotrexate, mercaptopurine, azathioprine,

and thioguanine. Daily treatment with these agents rather than high-dose intermittent therapy is the preferred schedule for immune suppression.

GENERAL TOXICOLOGICAL PROPERTIES OF ANTICANCER DRUGS

Most of the drugs used in cancer treatment have a therapeutic index that approaches unity, exerting toxic effects on both normal and tumor tissues even at optimal dosages. This *lack of selective toxicity* is the major limiting factor in the chemotherapy of cancer. Rapidly proliferating normal tissues, such as bone marrow, gastrointestinal tract, and hair follicles, are the major sites of acute toxicity of these agents. In addition, chronic and cumulative toxicities may occur. The most commonly encountered toxicities of antineoplastic agents are described in the following section; more detailed information on individual agents is presented in Chapter 56.

Bone Marrow Toxicity

Chemotherapy may result in the destruction of actively proliferating hematopoietic precursor cells. White blood cell and platelet counts may in turn be decreased, resulting in an increased incidence of life-threatening infections and hemorrhage. Maximum toxicity usually is observed 10 to 14 days after initiation of drug treatment, with recovery by 21 to 28 days. In contrast, the nitrosourea drugs exhibit hematological toxicity that is delayed until 4 to 6 weeks after beginning treatment.

The risk of serious infections has been shown to increase greatly when the peripheral blood granulocyte count falls below 1000 cells/mm^3. A chronic bone marrow toxicity or hypoplastic state may develop after long-term treatment with nitrosoureas, other alkylating agents, and mitomycin C. Thus, patients frequently will require a progressive reduction in the dosages of *myelosuppressive* drugs when they are undergoing long-term therapy, since such treatment may result in chronic pancytopenia.

Gastrointestinal Tract Toxicity

The nausea and vomiting frequently observed after anticancer drug administration are actually thought to be caused by a stimulation of the vomiting center or chemoreceptor trigger zone in the central nervous system (CNS) rather than by a direct gastrointestinal effect. These symptoms are ameliorated by treatment with phenothiazines and other centrally acting antiemetics. Commonly, nausea begins 4 to 6 hours after treatment and lasts 1 or 2 days. Although this symptom is distressing to patients, it is rarely severe enough to require cessation of therapy. Anorexia and alterations in taste perception also may be associated with chemotherapy.

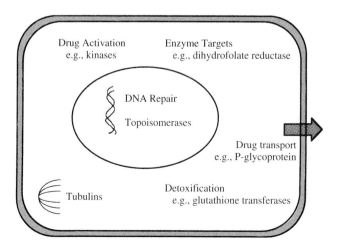

FIGURE 55.2
Mechanisms of cellular resistance to anticancer drugs.

The serotonin antagonist ondansetron (*Zofran*) has proved effective in the prevention of nausea and vomiting due to chemotherapy.

Damage to the normally proliferating mucosa of the gastrointestinal tract may produce stomatitis, dysphagia, and diarrhea several days after treatment. Oral ulcerations, esophagitis, and proctitis may cause pain and bleeding.

Hair Follicle Toxicity

Most anticancer drugs damage hair follicles and produce partial or complete alopecia. Patients should be warned of this reaction, especially if paclitaxel, cyclophosphamide, doxorubicin, vincristine, methotrexate, or dactinomycin is used. Hair usually regrows normally after completion of chemotherapy.

PHARMACOKINETIC CONSIDERATIONS IN CANCER CHEMOTHERAPY

Pharmacokinetic Sanctuaries

The existence of the blood-brain barrier is an important consideration in the chemotherapy of neoplastic diseases of the brain or meninges. Poor drug penetration into the CNS has been a major cause of treatment failure in acute lymphocytic leukemia in children. Treatment programs for this disease now routinely employ craniospinal irradiation and intrathecally administered methotrexate as prophylactic measures for the prevention of relapses. The testes also are organs in which inadequate antitumor drug distribution can be a cause of relapse of an otherwise responsive tumor.

The multidrug transporter P-glycoprotein is expressed in the endothelial lining of the brain and testis but not in other organs and is thought to be a major component of the blood-brain and blood-testis drug barriers.

Schedules of Administration

Although the effects of various schedules are not always predictable, drugs that are rapidly metabolized, excreted, or both, especially if they are phase specific and thus act on only one portion of the cell cycle (e.g., cytarabine), appear to be more effective when administered by continuous infusion or frequent dose fractionation than by high-dose intermittent therapy. On the other hand, intermittent high-dose treatment of Burkitt's lymphoma with cyclophosphamide is more effective than fractionated treatment, since cyclophosphamide acts on all phases of the cell cycle and almost all of the tumor cells in that disease are actively proliferating.

The classic example of *schedule dependency* is cytarabine, a drug that specifically inhibits DNA synthesis and is cytotoxic only to cells in S-phase. Continuous infusion or frequent administration of cytarabine hydrochloride is superior to intermittent injection of the drug. Bleomycin is another drug for which continuous infusion may increase therapeutic efficacy.

Administration of some anticancer drugs by *continuous infusion* has been shown to improve their therapeutic index through selective reduction of toxicity with retained or enhanced antitumor efficacy.

Routes of Administration

In addition to the usual intravenous or oral routes, some anticancer agents have been administered by regional intraarterial perfusion to increase drug delivery to the tumor itself and at the same time diminish systemic toxicity. Thus, patients with metastatic carcinomas of the liver and little or no disease elsewhere (a common occurrence in colorectal cancer) can be treated with a continuous infusion of fluorouracil or floxuridine through a catheter implanted in the hepatic artery.

Intracavitary administration of various agents has been used for patients with malignant pleural or peritoneal effusions. *Intraperitoneal instillations* of cisplatin, etoposide, bleomycin, 5-fluorouracil, and interferon are well tolerated and are being evaluated in patients with ovarian carcinomas, in whom the tumor is frequently restricted to the peritoneal cavity.

Other routes of administration can be employed in certain situations. Methotrexate and cytarabine are given *intrathecally* or *intraventricularly* to prevent relapses in the meninges in acute lymphocytic leukemia and to treat carcinomatous meningitis. Thiotepa and bleomycin have been administered by intravesical instillation to treat early bladder cancers. Fluorouracil can be applied topically for certain skin cancers.

Drug Interactions

Antineoplastic drugs may participate in several types of drug interactions. Methotrexate, for example, is highly bound to serum albumin and can be displaced by salicylates, sulfonamides, phenothiazines, phenytoin, and other organic acids. The induction of hepatic drug-metabolizing enzymes by phenobarbital may alter the metabolism of cyclophosphamide to both active and inactive metabolites. Mercaptopurine metabolism is blocked by allopurinol, an occurrence that may result in lethal toxicity if the dosage of mercaptopurine is not reduced to one-fourth of the usual dosage. Methotrexate is secreted actively by the renal tubules, and its renal clearance may be delayed by salicylates.

Procarbazine exhibits an interesting interaction with ethanol, resulting in headaches, diaphoresis, and facial erythema; patients taking this drug should be fore-warned to abstain from alcohol. Procarbazine is also a monoamine oxidase (MAO) inhibitor and may potentiate the effects of drugs that are substrates for this enzyme.

The biliary and renal excretion of some drugs (e.g., anthracyclines, vinca alkaloids, dactinomycin, etoposide) by the P-glycoprotein multidrug transporter can be inhibited by other drugs that are also transported by P-glycoprotein.

COMBINATION CHEMOTHERAPY

The value of combination chemotherapy has been proved in humans. The combined use of two or more drugs often is superior to single-agent treatment in many cancers, and certain principles have been used in designing such treatments:

1. Each drug used in the combination regimen should have some *individual therapeutic activity* against the particular tumor being treated. A drug that is not active against a tumor when used as a single agent is likely to increase toxicity without increasing the therapeutic efficacy of a combined drug regimen.
2. Drugs that *act by different mechanisms* may have additive or synergistic therapeutic effects. Tumors may contain heterogeneous clones of cells that differ in their susceptibility to drugs. Combination therapy will thus increase log cell kill and diminish the probability of emergence of resistant clones of tumor cells.
3. Drugs with *different dose-limiting toxicities* should be used to avoid cumulative damage to a single organ.

4. Intensive *intermittent schedules* of drug treatment should allow time for recovery from the acute toxic effects of antineoplastic agents, primarily bone marrow toxicity. The use of non-myelosuppressive agents can be considered during the recovery period, especially for treatment of fast-growing cancers.
5. Several *cycles of treatment* should be given, since one or two cycles of therapy are rarely sufficient to eradicate a tumor. *Most curable tumors require at least six to eight cycles of therapy.*

The chemotherapy of advanced Hodgkin's disease is one of the best examples of successful combination chemotherapy. Combination therapy with the MOPP regimen (mechlorethamine, *Oncovin* [vincristine sulfate], procarbazine, prednisone), alternating with ABVD (*Adriamycin* [doxorubicin hydrochloride], bleomycin, vinblastine, dacarbazine), has resulted in cure rates of 50 to 60%.

The treatment of Hodgkin's disease also illustrates the use of combined modalities, that is, radiation plus chemotherapy. The combined modality approach to several childhood tumors (e.g., Ewing's sarcoma, Wilms' tumor, and rhabdomyosarcoma) has dramatically increased the cure rates for these diseases.

Adjuvant chemotherapy involves the use of antineoplastic drugs when surgery or radiation therapy has eradicated the primary tumor but historical experience with similar patients indicates a high risk of relapse due to micrometastases. Adjuvant chemotherapy should employ drugs that are known to be effective in the treatment of advanced stages of the particular tumor being treated. Adjuvant chemotherapy has played a major role in the cure of several types of childhood cancers as well as breast cancer, colorectal cancer, and osteosarcoma in adults.

Study QUESTIONS

1. A patient of yours has been receiving 5-fluorouracil as palliative therapy for adenocarcinoma of the pancreas. You suspect that the patient has become resistant to the treatment. You want to understand the most likely cause of the resistance before you select another agent. Which of the following is the most likely cause?
(A) Drug transport into cells is decreased.
(B) P-glycoprotein is increased.
(C) The tumor can no longer activate the drug.
(D) The tumor is detoxifying the drug more rapidly.

(E) The tumor has developed an increase in metallothionein content.
2. Neurotoxicity is rarely dose limiting in cancer chemotherapy. The only antineoplastic agent that has a dose-limiting neurotoxicity is
(A) Bleomycin
(B) Cisplatin
(C) Vincristine
(D) Doxorubicin
(E) Methotrexate
3. You are asked to devise therapy for a patient with rapidly dividing cancer. You have no additional

information on the nature of the tumor, but you decide that you want to begin by choosing a drug that will kill the tumor cells but spare normal cells. You have the following agents to choose among. Which is your first choice?

(A) Hydroxyurea
(B) Cytarabine
(C) Bleomycin
(D) Mechlorethamine
(E) Dactinomycin

4. To optimize drug therapy, it is necessary to know in what phase of the cell cycle antineoplastic agents are effective. Which one of the following agents is cytotoxic only to cells in the S-phase of the cycle?

(A) Hydroxyurea
(B) Mechlormethamine
(C) Bleomycin
(D) Carmustine
(E) Fluorouracil

5. Combination chemotherapy is frequently used and is often superior to single-agent treatment. All of the following principles have been used in designing combinations EXCEPT which of the following?

(A) Each drug in the combination regimen should have some therapeutic activity individually.
(B) Drugs with different dose-limiting toxicities should be used to avoid damage to a single organ.
(C) Several cycles of treatment should be given.
(D) Intensive intermittent schedules of drug treatment.
(E) Drugs with similar dose-limiting toxicities should be used as initial combination therapy.

ANSWERS

1. **C.** The most likely reason for resistance to 5-fluorouracil or other agents that require activation is that tumors can no longer activate the drug. There is no evidence that 5-fluorouracil becomes unable to penetrate tumor cells. There may be an increase in P-glycoprotein, but this is not usually associated with 5-fluorouracil. There may be an induction in the drug metabolism for some antineoplastic drugs, but this does not appear to be the case for 5-fluorouracil. Increased metallothionein content has been associated with resistance in the case of cisplatin but not 5-fluorouracil.

2. **C.** The dose-limiting toxicity of bleomycin is pulmonary toxicity and that of cisplatin is renal. Doxorubicin produces cardiotoxicity; hematoxicity is dose limiting for methotrexate.

3. **E.** Dactinomycin is a class 3 agent, that is, an agent that kills proliferating cells in preference to resting cells. Hydroxyurea and cytarabine are class 2 agents that specifically kill cells in S-phase. Bleomycin is a class 2 agent that is specific for cells in G_2 and early M-phase. Mechlorethamine (class 1) appears to kills normal and malignant cells to about the same extent.

4. **A.** Carmustine and mechlormethamine kill both normal and malignant cells to the same extent. Hydroxyurea and bleomycin kill cells preferentially in specific phases of the cell cycle. Hydroxyurea is specific for S-phase, while bleomycin is most toxic to cells in G_2- and early M-phase. Flurouracil is cytotoxic in G_1 and G_2 phases.

5. **E.** Intensive intermittent schedules allow time for recovery from the acute toxic effects of the antineoplastic agents. If a drug has no activity by itself, it is not likely to be beneficial in a combination. It is important not to include two drugs with the same dose-limiting toxicity. Most curable tumors require at least six to eight cycles of therapy.

SUPPLEMENTAL READING

Bernal SD (ed.). Drug Resistance in Oncology. New York: Marcel Dekker, 1997.

Brigden M and McKenzie M. Treating cancer patients. Practical monitoring and management of therapy-related complications. Can Fam Physician 2000;46:2258–2268.

Burns EA and Leventhal EA. Aging, immunity, and cancer. Cancer Control 2000;7:513–522.

DeVita VT, Hellman S, and Rosenberg SA (eds.). Cancer: Principles and Practice of Oncology (6th ed.). Philadelphia: Lippincott, 2000.

Lipp HP (ed.). Anticancer Drug Toxicity. Marcel Dekker: New York, 1999.

Roninson IB (ed.). Molecular and Cellular Biology of Multidrug Resistance in Tumor Cells. New York: Plenum, 1990.

Xu XC. COX-2 inhibitors in cancer treatment and prevention, a recent development. Anticancer Drugs 2002;13:127–137.

CASE **Study**   Treatment of Nausea

You are filling in for a colleague who is on vacation when one of her patients makes an appointment to talk with you about his complaint. The patient is a 50-year-old man being treated for Hodgkin's disease using the MOPP regimen. The patient indicates that he was doing quite well until 2 days ago, when he began having nausea and vomiting that were "almost unbearable." The patient indicates that he is ready to terminate his treatment, since the side effects are quite severe, but he wants your opinion first.

You indicate that his regimen is the best available treatment and that the cure rate is excellent, but only if the treatment is continued. You suggest that other agents may help his nausea and vomiting. You prescribe ondansetron. After 2 days, the patient comes back and indicates that the drug decreased the nausea and vomiting but that he was developing severe dermatitis that he attributed to the new agent. You believe he is correct and prescribe chlorpromazine. He calls you the next week to tell you that the new drug worked and he will continue with his chemotherapy.

56 Antineoplastic Agents

Branimir I. Sikic

DRUG LIST

ALKYLATING AGENTS

The alkylating agents are the largest class of anticancer agents, comprising five subgroups: nitrogen mustards, alkyl sulfonates, nitrosoureas, ethyleneimine, and thiazines (Table 56.1). Several other agents, including procarbazine, hexamethylmelamine, dacarbazine, estramustine, and mitomycin C, are thought to act at least in part by alkylation.

By definition, *alkylating agents* are compounds that are capable of introducing alkyl groups into nucleophilic sites on other molecules through the formation of *covalent bonds*. These nucleophilic targets for alkylation include the sulfhydryl, amino, phosphate, hydroxyl, carboxyl, and imidazole groups that are present in macromolecules and low-molecular-weight compounds within cells.

The macromolecular sites of alkylation damage include DNA, RNA, and various enzymes. The inhibition of DNA synthesis occurs at drug concentrations that are lower than those required to inhibit RNA and protein synthesis, and *the degree of DNA alkylation correlates especially well with the cytotoxicity* of these drugs. This interaction also accounts for the mutagenic and carcinogenic properties of the alkylating agents. The reactions of various alkylating agents with DNA have been studied in detail, and the 7-nitrogen (N7) and 6-oxygen (O6) of guanine have been shown to be particularly

TABLE 56.1 Classification of the Anticancer Drugs

I. Alkylating agents
  A. Nitrogen mustards
    1. Mechlorethamine hydrochloride (*Mustargen*, HN$_2$, nitrogen mustard)
    2. Cyclophosphamide (*Cytoxan*)
    3. Chlorambucil (*Leukeran*)
    4. Melphalan (*Alkeran, L-PAM*, L-phenylalanine mustard)
    5. Ifosfamide (*Ifex*)
  B. Alkyl sulfonates
    1. Busulfan (*Myleran*)
  C. Nitrosoureas
    1. Carmustine (BCNU, *BiCNU*)
    2. Lomustine (CCNU, *CeeNU*)
    3. Semustine (methyl-CCNU)
    4. Streptozocin (*Zanosar*, streptozotocin)
  D. Ethylenimines
    1. Thiotepa
  E. Triazenes
    1. Dacarbazine (*DTIC-Dome*)
II. Antimetabolites
  A. Folate antagonist
    1. Methotrexate (*Folex, Mexate*)
  B. Purine analogues
    1. Thioguanine (6-TG, 6-thioguanine)
    2. Mercaptopurine (6-MP, *Purinethol*)
    3. Fludarabine (*Fludara*)
    4. Pentostatin (deoxycoformycin, *Nipent*)
    5. Cladribine (2-chloro-deoxyadenosine, *Leustatin*)
  C. Pyrimidine analogues
    1. Cytarabine (cytosine arabinoside, *Cytosar-U*, ara-C)
    2. Fluorouracil (5-FU, 5-fluorouracil)
III. Antibiotics
  A. Anthracyclines
    1. Doxorubicin hydrochloride (*Adriamycin*)
    2. Daunorubicin (daunomycin, *Cerubidine*)
    3. Idarubicin (*Idamycin*)
  B. Bleomycins
    1. Bleomycin sulfate (*Blenoxane*)
  C. Mitomycin (mitomycin C, *Mutamycin*)
  D. Dactinomycin (actinomycin D, *Cosmegen*)
  E. Plicamycin (*Mithracin*)
IV. Plant-derived products
  A. Vinca alkaloids
    1. Vincristine (*Oncovin*)
    2. Vinblastine (*Velban*)
  B. Epipodophyllotoxins
    1. Etoposide (VP-16, *Vepesid*)
    2. Teniposide (VM-26, *Vumon*)
  C. Taxanes: paclitaxel *Taxol*)
V. Enzymes
  A. L-Asparaginase (*Elspar*)
VI. Hormonal agents
  A. Glucocorticoids
  B. Estrogens, antiestrogens
    1. Tamoxifen citrate (*Nolvadex*)
    2. Estramustine phosphate sodium (*Emcyt*)
  C. Androgens, antiandrogens
    1. Flutamide (*Eulexin*)
  D. Progestins
  E. Luteinizing hormone–releasing hormone (LH-RH) antagonists
    1. Buserelin (*Suprefact*)
    2. Leuprolide (*Lupron*)
  F. Octreotide acetate (*Sandostatin*)
VII. Miscellaneous agents
  A. Hydroxyurea (*Hydrea*)
  B. Procarbazine (*N*-methylhydrazine, *Matulane, Natulan*)
  C. Mitotane (o,p´-DDD, *Lysodren*)
  D. Hexamethylmelamine (HMM)
  E. Cisplatin (*cis*-platinum II; *Platinol*)
  F. Carboplatin (*Paraplatin*)
  G. Mitoxantrone (*Novantrone*)
VIII. Monoclonal antibodies
IX. Immunomodulating agents
  A. Levamisole (*Ergamisol*)
  B. Interferons
    1. Interferon alfa-2a (*Roferon-A*)
    2. Interferon alfa-2b (*Intron A*)
  C. Interleukins: aldesleukin (interleukin-2, IL-2, *Proleukin*)
X. Cellular growth factors
  A. Filgrastim (G-CSF; *Neupogen*)
  B. Sargramostim (GM-CSF, *Leukine, Prokine*)

Proprietary (*italics*) and other names are given in parentheses.

susceptible to attack by electrophilic compounds. There are several possible consequences of N7 guanine alkylation:

1. *Cross-linkage.* Bifunctional alkylating agents, such as the nitrogen mustards, may form covalent bonds with each of two adjacent guanine residues. Such interstrand cross-linkages will inhibit *DNA replication and transcription.* Intrastrand cross-links also may be produced between DNA and a nearby protein.
2. *Mispairing of bases.* Alkylating at N7 changes the O6 of guanine to its enol tautomer, which can then form base pairs with thymine. This may lead to gene miscoding, with adenine–thymine pairs replacing guanine–cytosine. The result is the production of *defective proteins.*
3. *Depurination.* N7 alkylation may cause cleavage of the imidazole ring and excision of the guanine residue, leading to *DNA strand breakage.*

Although all alkylating agents can cause the kinds of genetic damage just discussed, individual drugs differ from one another in their electrophilic reactivity, the structure of their reactive intermediates, and their pharmacokinetic properties. These differences will be reflected in the spectrum of their antitumor activities and in the toxicities they produce in normal tissues.

Nitrogen Mustards
Mechlorethamine

Mechlorethamine (nitrogen mustard; *Mustargen*), a derivative of the war gas sulfur mustard, is considered to be the first modern anticancer drug. In the early 1940s it was discovered to be effective in the treatment of human lymphomas.

Mechlorethamine in aqueous solution loses a chloride atom and forms a cyclic ethylenimmonium ion. This carbonium ion interacts with nucleophilic groups, such as the N7 and O6 of guanine, and leads to an interstrand cross-linking of DNA. Although there is great variation among normal and tumor tissues in their sensitivity to mechlorethamine, the drug is generally more toxic to proliferating cells than to resting or plateau cells. Mechlorethamine has a chemical and biological half-life in plasma of less than 10 minutes after intravenous injection. Little or no intact drug is excreted in urine.

The major indication for mechlorethamine is Hodgkin's disease; the drug is given in the MOPP regimen (mechlorethamine, vincristine, procarbazine, prednisone; see Chapter 55). Other less reactive nitrogen mustards are now preferred for the treatment of non-Hodgkin's lymphomas, leukemias, and various solid tumors.

The dose-limiting toxicity of mechlorethamine is *myelosuppression;* maximal leukopenia and thrombocytopenia occur 10 to 14 days after drug administration, and recovery is generally complete at 21 to 28 days. Lymphopenia and immunosuppression may lead to activation of latent herpes zoster infections, especially in patients with lymphomas. Mechlorethamine will affect rapidly proliferating normal tissues and cause alopecia, diarrhea, and oral ulcerations. *Nausea and vomiting* may occur 1 to 2 hours after injection and can last up to 24 hours. Since mechlorethamine is a potent blistering agent, care should be taken to avoid extravasation into subcutaneous tissues or even spillage onto the skin. Reproductive toxicity includes amenorrhea and inhibition of oogenesis and spermatogenesis. About half of premenopausal women and almost all men treated for 6 months with MOPP chemotherapy become permanently infertile. The drug is teratogenic and carcinogenic in experimental animals.

Cyclophosphamide

Cyclophosphamide (*Cytoxan*) is the most versatile and useful of the nitrogen mustards. Preclinical testing showed it to have a favorable therapeutic index and to possess the broadest spectrum of antitumor activity of all alkylating agents. As with the other nitrogen mustards, cyclophosphamide administration results in the formation of cross-links within DNA due to a reaction of the two chloroethyl moieties of cyclophosphamide with adjacent nucleotide bases. Cyclophosphamide must be activated metabolically by microsomal enzymes of the cytochrome P450 system before ionization of the chloride atoms and formation of the cyclic ethylenimmonium ion can occur. The metabolites phosphoramide mustard and acrolein are thought to be the ultimate active cytotoxic moiety derived from cyclophosphamide.

Cyclophosphamide can be given orally, intramuscularly, or intravenously. The plasma half-life of intact cyclophosphamide is 6.5 hours. Only 10 to 15% of the circulating parent drug is protein bound, whereas 50% of the alkylating metabolites are bound to plasma proteins. Since cyclophosphamide and its metabolites are eliminated primarily by the kidneys, renal failure will greatly prolong their retention.

Cyclophosphamide has a wide spectrum of antitumor activity. In lymphomas, it is frequently used in combination with vincristine and prednisone (CVP [or COP] regimen) or as a substitute for mechlorethamine in the MOPP regimen (C-MOPP). High dosages of intravenously administered cyclophosphamide are often curative in Burkitt's lymphoma, a childhood malignancy with a very fast growth rate. Oral daily dosages are useful for less aggressive tumors, such as nodular lymphomas, myeloma, and chronic leukemias.

Cyclophosphamide is a component of CMF (cyclophosphamide, methotrexate, 5-fluorouracil) and other drug combinations used in the treatment of breast cancer. Cyclophosphamide in combination may produce complete remissions in some patients with ovarian cancer and oat cell (small cell) lung cancer. Other tumors in which beneficial results have been reported include non–oat cell lung cancers, various sarcomas, neuroblastoma, and carcinomas of the testes, cervix, and bladder. Cyclophosphamide also can be employed as an alternative to azathioprine in suppressing immunological rejection of transplant organs.

Bone marrow suppression that affects white blood cells more than platelets is the major dose-limiting toxicity. Maximal suppression of blood cell count occurs 10 to 14 days after drug administration; recovery is generally seen 21 to 28 days after injection. Cyclophosphamide reduces the number of circulating lymphocytes and impairs the function of both humoral and cellular (i.e., B and T cell) aspects of the immune system. Chronic therapy increases the risk of infections. Nausea may occur a few hours after administration. *Alopecia* is more common than with other mustards.

A toxicity that is unique to cyclophosphamide and ifosfamide is cystitis. Dysuria and decreased urinary frequency are the most common symptoms. Rarely, fibrosis and a permanently decreased bladder capacity may ensue. The risk of development of carcinoma of the bladder also is increased. Large intravenous doses have resulted in impairment of renal water excretion, hyponatremia, and increased urine osmolarity and have been associated with hemorrhagic subendocardial necrosis, arrhythmias, and congestive heart failure. Interstitial pulmonary fibrosis may also result from chronic treatment. Other effects of chronic drug treatment include infertility, amenorrhea, and possible mutagenesis and carcinogenesis.

Ifosfamide

Ifosfamide (*Ifex*) is an analogue of cyclophosphamide that requires metabolic activation to form 4-hydroxy-ifosfamide. In general, the metabolism, serum half-life, and excretion of ifosfamide are similar to those of cyclophosphamide.

Ifosfamide is active against a broad spectrum of tumors, including germ cell cancers of the testis, lymphomas, sarcomas, and carcinomas of the lung, breast, and ovary. It is thought to be more active than cyclophosphamide in germ cell cancers and sarcomas.

Ifosfamide is less myelosuppressive than cyclophosphamide but is more toxic to the bladder. It also may produce alopecia, nausea, vomiting, infertility, and second tumors, particularly acute leukemias. Neurological symptoms including confusion, somnolence, and hallucinations have also been reported. It is recommended

that ifosfamide be coadministered with the thiol compound mesna (*Mesnex*) to avoid hemorrhagic cystitis.

Melphalan

Melphalan (*Alkeran*) is an amino acid derivative of mechlorethamine that possesses the same general spectrum of antitumor activity as do the other nitrogen mustards. However, the bioavailability of the oral preparation is quite variable (25–90%) from one patient to another.

The major indications for melphalan are in the palliative therapy of multiple myeloma and cancers of the breast or ovary. Because it does not produce alopecia, melphalan is occasionally substituted for cyclophosphamide in the CMF regimen for breast cancer.

Melphalan produces less nausea and vomiting than does cyclophosphamide; however, its bone marrow suppression tends to be more prolonged and affects both white cells and platelets. Peak suppression of blood counts occurs 14 to 21 days after a 5-day course of drug therapy; recovery is generally complete within 3 to 5 weeks.

Chlorambucil

Chlorambucil (*Leukeran*) is an aromatic nitrogen mustard that is intermediate in chemical reactivity between mechlorethamine and melphalan. Its mechanisms of action and range of antitumor activity are similar to theirs. It is well absorbed orally, but detailed information concerning its metabolic fate in humans is lacking.

Chlorambucil is used primarily as daily palliative therapy for chronic lymphocytic leukemia, Waldenström's macroglobulinemia, myeloma, and other lymphomas.

Bone marrow toxicity is the major side effect of chlorambucil. Nausea is uncommon or mild, and hair loss does not occur. Chlorambucil shares the immunosuppressive, teratogenic, and carcinogenic properties of the nitrogen mustards.

Nitrosoureas
Carmustine, Lomustine, and Semustine

The nitrosoureas are alkylating agents that are highly lipid soluble and share similar pharmacological and clinical properties. Carmustine (BCNU), lomustine (CCNU), and semustine (methyl-CCNU) are chemically unstable, forming highly reactive decomposition products. The chemical half-life of these drugs in plasma is only 5 to 15 minutes. Their marked lipid solubility facilitates distribution into the brain and cerebrospinal fluid (CSF).

The chloroethyl moiety of these nitrosoureas is capable of alkylating nucleic acids and proteins and producing single-strand breaks and interstrand cross-linkage of DNA. *Both alkylation and carbamoylation* contribute to the therapeutic and toxic effects of the nitrosoureas. These agents can kill cells in *all* phases of the cell cycle.

Oral absorption of lomustine and semustine is complete, but degradation and metabolism are so rapid that the parent drug cannot be detected after oral administration. Although the plasma half-lives of the parent drugs are only a few minutes, degradation products with antitumor activity may persist for longer periods.

Carmustine and lomustine can produce remissions that last from 3 to 6 months in 40 to 50% of patients with primary brain tumors. Both drugs also are used as secondary treatment of Hodgkin's disease and in experimental combination chemotherapy for various types of lung cancer. Other tumors in which remission rates of 10 to 30% have been obtained are non-Hodgkin's lymphomas, multiple myeloma, melanoma, renal cell carcinoma, and colorectal cancer.

The nitrosoureas produce severe nausea and vomiting in most patients 4 to 6 hours after administration. The major site of dose-limiting toxicity is the bone marrow; leukopenia and thrombocytopenia occur after 4 to 5 weeks. Less frequent side effects include alopecia, stomatitis, and mild abnormalities of liver function. Pulmonary toxicity, manifested by cough, dyspnea, and interstitial fibrosis, is becoming increasingly recognized as a complication of long-term nitrosourea treatment. As alkylating agents, these drugs are potentially mutagenic, teratogenic, and carcinogenic.

Streptozocin

Streptozocin (*Zanosar*), a water-soluble nitrosourea produced by the fungus *Streptomyces achromogenes*, acts through methylation of nucleic acids and proteins. In addition, it produces rapid and severe depletion of the pyridine nucleotides nicotinamide adenine dinucleotide (NAD) and its reduced form (NADH) in liver and pancreatic islets.

Streptozocin is not well absorbed from the gastrointestinal tract and must be administered intravenously or intraarterially. In preclinical studies, the plasma half-life was 5 to 10 minutes.

Streptozocin produces remission in 50 to 60% of patients with islet cell carcinomas of the pancreas. It is also useful in malignant carcinoid tumors.

Almost all patients have nausea and vomiting. The major toxicity is *renal tubular damage*, which may be severe in 5 to 10% of patients taking streptozocin. Treatment of metastatic insulinomas may result in the release of insulin from the tumor and subsequent hypoglycemic coma. Less severe toxicities include diarrhea, anemia, and mild alterations in glucose tolerance or liver function tests.

Alkyl Sulfonates
Busulfan

Busulfan (*Myleran*) is a bifunctional methanesulfonic ester that forms intrastrand cross-linkages with DNA. The drug is well absorbed after oral administration and has a plasma half-life of less than 5 minutes. Metabolites and degradation products are excreted primarily in the urine.

Busulfan is used in the palliative treatment of chronic granulocytic leukemia. Daily oral therapy results in decreased peripheral white blood cells and improved symptoms in almost all patients during the chronic phase of the disease. Excessive uric acid production from rapid tumor cell lysis should be prevented by coadministration of allopurinol.

At usual therapeutic dosages, busulfan is selectively toxic to granulocyte precursors rather than lymphocytes. Thrombocytopenia and anemia and less commonly, nausea, alopecia, mucositis, and sterility also may occur. Unusual side effects of busulfan include gynecomastia, a general increase in skin pigmentation, and interstitial pulmonary fibrosis.

Ethylenimines
Thiotepa

Although thiotepa is chemically less reactive than the nitrogen mustards, it is thought to act by similar mechanisms. Its oral absorption is erratic. After intravenous injection, the plasma half-life is less than 2 hours. Urinary excretion accounts for 60 to 80% of eliminated drug.

Thiotepa has antitumor activity against ovarian and breast cancers and lymphomas. However, it has been largely supplanted by cyclophosphamide and other nitrogen mustards for treatment of these diseases. It is used by direct instillation into the bladder for multifocal local bladder carcinoma.

Nausea and myelosuppression are the major toxicities of thiotepa. It is not a local vesicant and has been safely injected intramuscularly and even intrathecally.

Triazenes
Dacarbazine

Dacarbazine (*DTIC-Dome*) is activated by photodecomposition and by enzymatic *N*-demethylation. Eventual formation of a methyl carbonium ion results in methylation of DNA and RNA and inhibition of nucleic acid and protein synthesis. *As with other alkylating agents, cells in all phases of the cell cycle are susceptible to dacarbazine.*

The plasma half-life of dacarbazine is biphasic, with a distribution phase of 19 minutes and an elimination phase of 5 hours. The drug is not appreciably protein bound, and it does not enter the central nervous system

(CNS). Urinary excretion of unchanged drug is by renal tubular secretion. Dacarbazine metabolism and decomposition is complex.

Dacarbazine is the most active agent used in metastatic melanoma, producing a 20% remission rate. It is also combined with doxorubicin and other agents in the treatment of various sarcomas and Hodgkin's disease.

Dacarbazine may cause severe nausea and vomiting. Leukopenia and thrombocytopenia occur 2 weeks after treatment, with recovery by 3 to 4 weeks. Less common is a flulike syndrome of fever, myalgias, and malaise. Alopecia and transient abnormalities in renal and hepatic function also have been reported.

ANTIMETABOLITES

Folate Antagonists

In general, antimetabolites used in cancer chemotherapy are drugs that are *structurally related to naturally occurring compounds,* such as vitamins, amino acids, and nucleotides. These drugs can compete for binding sites on enzymes or can themselves become incorporated into DNA or RNA and thus interfere with cell growth and proliferation. The antimetabolites in clinical use include the folic acid analogue methotrexate, the pyrimidines (fluorouracil and cytarabine), and the purines (thioguanine, mercaptopurine, fludarabine, pentostatin, and cladribine).

Methotrexate

Methotrexate competitively inhibits the binding of folic acid to the enzyme dihydrofolate reductase. This enzyme catalyzes the formation of tetrahydrofolate, as follows:

$$\text{Folic acid} \xrightarrow{\text{dihydrofolate reductase}} \text{tetrahydrofolate}$$
$$\text{(FH}_2) \qquad\qquad\qquad \text{(FH}_4)$$

Tetrahydrofolate is in turn converted to N^5,N^{10}-methylenetetrahydrofolate, which is an essential cofactor for the synthesis of thymidylate, purines, methionine, and glycine. The major mechanism by which methotrexate brings about cell death appears to be inhibition of DNA synthesis through a blockage of the biosynthesis of thymidylate and purines.

Cells in S-phase are most sensitive to the cytotoxic effects of methotrexate. RNA and protein synthesis also may be inhibited to some extent and may delay progression through the cell cycle, particularly from G_1 to S.

Resistance

Mammalian cells have several mechanisms of resistance to methotrexate. These include an increase in in-tracellular dihydrofolate reductase levels, appearance of altered forms of dihydrofolate reductase with decreased affinity for methotrexate, and a decrease in methotrexate transport into cells (see Chapter 55). The relative importance of each of these mechanisms of resistance in various human tumors is not known.

Cellular uptake of the drug is by carrier-mediated active transport. Drug resistance due to decreased transport can be overcome by greatly increasing extracellular methotrexate concentration, which provides a rationale for high-dose methotrexate therapy. Since bone marrow and gastrointestinal cells do not have impaired folate methotrexate transport, these normal cells can be selectively rescued with reduced folate, bypassing the block of dihydrofolate reductase. Leucovorin (citrovorum factor, folinic acid, 5-formyltetrahydrofolate) is the agent commonly used for rescue.

Absorption, Metabolism, and Excretion

Methotrexate is well absorbed orally and at usual dosages is 50% bound to plasma proteins. The plasma decay that follows an intravenous injection is triphasic, with a distribution phase, an initial elimination phase, and a prolonged elimination phase. The last phase is thought to reflect slow release of methotrexate from tissues. The major routes of drug excretion are glomerular filtration and active renal tubular secretion.

The formation of polyglutamic acid conjugates of methotrexate has been observed in tumor cells and in the liver and may be an important determinant of cytotoxicity. These methotrexate polyglutamates are retained in the cell and are also potent inhibitors of dihydrofolate reductase.

Clinical Uses

Methotrexate is part of curative combination chemotherapy for acute lymphoblastic leukemias, Burkitt's lymphoma, and trophoblastic choriocarcinoma. It is also useful in adjuvant therapy of breast carcinoma; in the palliation of metastatic breast, head, neck, cervical, and lung carcinomas; and in mycosis fungoides.

High-dose methotrexate administration with leucovorin rescue has produced remissions in 30% of patients with metastatic osteogenic sarcoma.

Methotrexate is one of the few anticancer drugs that can be safely administered intrathecally for the treatment of meningeal metastases. Its routine use as prophylactic intrathecal chemotherapy in acute lymphoblastic leukemia has greatly reduced the incidence of recurrences in the CNS and has contributed to the cure rate in this disease. Daily oral doses of methotrexate are used for severe cases of the nonneoplastic skin disease psoriasis (see Chapter 41), and methotrexate has been used as an immunosuppressive agent in severe rheumatoid arthritis.

Adverse Effects

Myelosuppression is the major dose-limiting toxicity associated with methotrexate therapy. Gastrointestinal toxicity may appear in the form of ulcerative mucositis and diarrhea. Nausea, alopecia, and dermatitis are common with high-dose methotrexate. The greatest danger of high-dose therapy is renal toxicity due to precipitation of the drug in the renal tubules, and the drug should not be used in patients with renal impairment. Intrathecal administration may produce neurological toxicity ranging from mild arachnoiditis to severe and progressive myelopathy or encephalopathy. Chronic low-dose methotrexate therapy, as used for psoriasis, may result in cirrhosis of the liver. Occasionally methotrexate produces an acute, potentially lethal lung toxicity that is thought to be allergic or hypersensitivity pneumonitis. Additionally, methotrexate is a potent teratogen and abortifacient.

Drug Interactions

Salicylates, probenecid, and sulfonamides inhibit the renal tubular secretion of methotrexate and may displace it from plasma proteins. Asparaginase inhibits protein synthesis and may protect cells from methotrexate cytotoxicity by delaying progression from G_1-phase to S-phase. Methotrexate may either enhance or inhibit the action of fluorouracil, depending on its sequence of administration.

Gemcitabine

Gemcitabine (*Gemzar*), an antimetabolite, undergoes metabolic activation to difluorodeoxycytidine triphosphate, which interferes with DNA synthesis and repair. It is the single most active agent for the treatment of metastatic pancreatic cancer, and it is used as a first-line treatment for both pancreatic and small cell lung cancer. It is administered by intravenous infusion. The dose-limiting toxicity is bone marrow suppression.

Purine Analogues
Thioguanine (6-Thioguanine)

Thioguanine is an analogue of the natural purine guanine in which a hydroxyl group has been replaced by a sulfhydryl group in the 6-position. Two major mechanisms of cytotoxicity have been proposed for 6-thioguanine: (1) incorporation of the thio nucleotide analogue into DNA or RNA and (2) feedback inhibition of purine nucleotide synthesis. Both of these actions require initial activation of the drug by the enzyme hypoxanthine guanine–phosphoribosyltransferase (HGPRTase), as follows:

$$\text{6-Thioguanine} \xrightarrow{\text{HGPRTase}} \text{6-thioguanosine-5-}$$
$$\text{(6-TG)} \qquad\qquad \text{monophosphate (6-TGMP)}$$

The product of this reaction, 6-TGMP, can eventually be converted to deoxy-6-thioguanosine-triphosphate (dTGTP), which has been shown to be incorporated into DNA. *Resistance* of human leukemia cells to thioguanine has been correlated with decreased activity of HGPRTase and to increased inactivation of the thio nucleotides by alkaline phosphatase.

Thioguanine is slowly absorbed after oral administration; parent drug levels are barely detectable, and peak levels of metabolites occur only after 6 to 8 hours. Total urinary excretion of metabolites in the first 24 hours is 24 to 46% of the administered dose.

Thioguanine is used primarily as part of a combined induction of chemotherapy in acute myelogenous leukemia.

Myelosuppression, with leukopenia and thrombocytopenia appearing 7 to 10 days after treatment, and mild nausea are the most common adverse effects. Liver toxicity with jaundice has been reported in some patients but appears to be less common than with mercaptopurine.

Mercaptopurine (6-Mercaptopurine)

Mercaptopurine (*Purinethol*) is an analogue of hypoxanthine and was one of the first agents shown to be active against acute leukemias. It is now used as part of maintenance therapy in acute lymphoblastic leukemia. Mercaptopurine must be activated to a nucleotide by the enzyme HGPRTase. This metabolite is capable of inhibiting the synthesis of the normal purines adenine and guanine at the initial aminotransferase step and inhibiting the conversion of inosinic acid to the nucleotides adenylate and guanylate at several steps. Some mercaptopurine is also incorporated into DNA in the form of thioguanine. The relative significance of these mechanisms to the antitumor action of mercaptopurine is not clear.

Resistance to mercaptopurine may be a result of decreased drug activation by HGPRTase or increased inactivation by alkaline phosphatase.

The plasma half-life of an intravenous bolus injection of mercaptopurine is 21 minutes in children and 47 minutes in adults. After oral administration, peak plasma levels are attained within 2 hours. The drug is 20% bound to plasma proteins and does not enter the CSF. Xanthine oxidase is the primary enzyme involved in the metabolic inactivation of mercaptopurine.

Mercaptopurine is used in the maintenance therapy of acute lymphoblastic leukemia. It also displays activity against acute and chronic myelogenous leukemias.

The major toxicities of mercaptopurine are myelosuppression, nausea, vomiting, and hepatic toxicity.

Fludarabine

Fludarabine (*Fludara*) is a fluorinated purine analogue of the antiviral agent vidarabine. The active metabolite,

2-fluoro-ara-adenosine triphosphate, inhibits various enzymes involved in DNA synthesis, including DNA polymerase-α, ribonucleotide reductase, and DNA primase. Unlike most antimetabolites, it is toxic to nonproliferating as well as dividing cells, primarily lymphocytes and lymphoid cancer cells.

The drug is highly active in the treatment of chronic lymphocytic leukemia, with approximately 40% of patients achieving remissions after previous therapy with alkylating agents has failed. Activity is also seen in the low-grade lymphomas.

The major side effect is myelosuppression, which contributes to fevers and infections in as many as half of treated patients. Nausea and vomiting are mild. Occasional neurotoxicity has been noted at higher doses, with agitation, confusion, and visual disturbances.

Pentostatin

Pentostatin (*Nipent,* deoxycoformycin) is a purine isolated from fermentation cultures of the microbe *Streptomyces antibioticus.* Its mechanism of action involves inhibition of the enzyme adenosine deaminase, which plays an important role in purine salvage pathways and DNA synthesis. The resulting accumulation of deoxyadenosine triphosphate (dATP) is highly toxic to lymphocytes.

Pentostatin is effective in the therapy of hairy cell leukemia, producing remissions in 80 to 90% of patients and complete remissions in more than 50%. The major toxic effects of the drug include myelosuppression, nausea, and skin rashes.

Cladribine

Cladribine (*Leustatin*) is a synthetic purine nucleoside that is converted to an active cytotoxic metabolite by the enzyme deoxycytidine kinase. Like the other purine antimetabolites, it is relatively selective for both normal and malignant lymphoid cells and kills resting as well as dividing cells by mechanisms that are not completely understood.

The drug is highly active against hairy cell leukemia, producing complete remissions in more than 60% of patients treated with a single 7-day course. Activity has also been noted in other low-grade lymphoid malignancies. The major side effect is myelosuppression.

Pyrimidine Analogues
Cytarabine

Cytarabine (cytosine arabinoside, ara-C, *Cytosar-U*) is an analogue of the pyrimidine nucleosides cytidine and deoxycytidine. It is one of the most active agents available for the treatment of acute myelogenous leukemia. *Cytarabine kills cells in the S-phase of the cycle by competitively inhibiting DNA polymerase.* The drug must

first be activated by pyrimidine nucleoside kinases to the triphosphate nucleotide ara-cytosine triphosphate (ara-CTP). The susceptibility of tumor cells to cytarabine is thought to be a reflection of their ability to activate the drug more rapidly (by kinases) than to inactivate it (by deaminases).

Cytarabine is rapidly metabolized in the liver, kidney, intestinal mucosa, and red blood cells and has a half-life in plasma of only 10 minutes after intravenous bolus injection. The major metabolite, uracil arabinoside (ara-U), can be detected in the blood shortly after cytarabine administration. About 80% of a given dose is excreted in the urine within 24 hours, with less than 10% appearing as cytarabine; the remainder is ara-U. When the drug is given by continuous infusion, cytarabine levels in CSF approach 40% of those in plasma.

Cytarabine is used in the chemotherapy of acute myelogenous leukemia, usually in combination with an anthracycline agent, thioguanine, or both. It is less useful in acute lymphoblastic leukemia and the lymphomas and has no known activity against other tumors. It has been used intrathecally in the treatment of meningeal leukemias and lymphomas as an alternative to methotrexate.

Myelosuppression is a major toxicity, as is severe bone marrow hypoplasia. Nausea and mucositis also may occur. Intrathecal administration occasionally produces arachnoiditis or more severe neurological toxicity.

Fluorouracil

Fluorouracil (5-fluorouracil, 5-fluorouracil, *Efudex, Adrucil*) is a halogenated pyrimidine analogue that must be activated metabolically. The active metabolite that inhibits DNA synthesis is the deoxyribonucleotide 5-fluoro-2′deoxyuridine-S′-phosphate (FdUMP). *5-Fluorouracil is selectively toxic to proliferating rather than non-proliferating cells and is active in both the G_1- and S-phases.* The target enzyme inhibited by 5-fluorouracilfluorouracil is thymidylate synthetase, which catalyzes the following reaction:

$$\text{Uridylate} \xrightarrow{\text{thymidylate synthetase}} \text{thymidylate}$$
$$\text{(dUMP)} \qquad\qquad \text{(dTMP)}$$
$$\text{methylenetetrahydrofolate} \rightarrow \text{dihydrofolate}$$

The carbon-donating cofactor for this reaction is N^5,N^{10} methylenetetrahydrofolate, which is converted to dihydrofolate. The reduced folate cofactor occupies an allosteric site on thymidylate synthetase, which allows for the covalent binding of 5-FdUMP to the active site of the enzyme.

Another action proposed for 5-fluorouracil may involve the incorporation of the nucleotide 5-fluorouridine triphosphate (5-FUTP) into RNA. The cytotoxic role of these "fraudulent" 5-fluorouracil-containing RNAs is not well understood.

Several possible mechanisms of resistance to 5-fluorouracil have been identified, including increased synthesis of the target enzyme, altered affinity of thymidylate synthetase for FdUMP, depletion of enzymes (especially uridine kinase) that activate 5-fluorouracil to nucleotides, an increase in the pool of the normal metabolite deoxyuridylic acid (dUMP), and an increase in the rate of catabolism of 5-fluorouracil.

The drug has been administered orally, but absorption by this route is erratic. The plasma half-life of 5-fluorouracil after intravenous injection is 10 to 20 minutes. It readily enters CSF. Less than 20% of the parent compound is excreted into the urine, the rest being largely metabolized in the liver.

5-Fluorouracil is used in several combination regimens in the treatment of breast cancer. It also has palliative activity in gastrointestinal adenocarcinomas, including those originating in the stomach, pancreas, liver, colon, and rectum. Other tumors in which some antitumor effects have been reported include carcinomas of the ovary, cervix, oropharynx, bladder, and prostate. Topical 5-fluorouracil cream has been useful in the treatment of premalignant keratoses of the skin and superficial basal cell carcinomas, but it should not be used in invasive skin cancer.

Floxuridine (FUDR) is the nucleoside of 5-fluorouracil that is readily converted into 5-fluorouracil in vivo. It has similar pharmacological effects but is preferred to 5-fluorouracil for hepatic arterial infusions because it is more extensively metabolized in the liver than 5-fluorouracil, with less systemic toxicity.

The toxicities of 5-fluorouracil vary with the schedule and mode of administration. Nausea is usually mild if it occurs at all. Myelosuppression is most severe after intravenous bolus administration, with leukopenia and thrombocytopenia appearing 7 to 14 days after an injection. Daily injection or continuous infusion is most likely to produce oral mucositis, pharyngitis, diarrhea, and alopecia. Skin rashes and nail discoloration have been reported, as have photosensitivity and increased skin pigmentation on sun exposure. Neurological toxicity is manifested as acute cerebellar ataxia that may occur within a few days of beginning treatment.

ANTIBIOTICS

Doxorubicin and Daunorubicin

The anthracycline antibiotics are fermentation products of *Streptomyces peucetius*. Daunorubicin (*Cerubidine*) is used to treat acute leukemias, while its structural analogue, doxorubicin (*Adriamycin*) is extensively employed against a broad spectrum of cancers. Although the two drugs have similar pharmacological and toxicological properties, doxorubicin is more potent against most animal and human tumors and will be discussed in greater detail.

Doxorubicin binds tightly to DNA by its ability to *intercalate* between base pairs and therefore is preferentially concentrated in nuclear structures. Intercalation results in steric hindrance, hence production of single-strand breaks in DNA and inhibition of DNA synthesis and DNA-dependent RNA synthesis. The enzyme topoisomerase II is thought to be involved in the generation of DNA strand breaks by the anthracyclines. *Cells in S-phase are most sensitive to doxorubicin,* although cytotoxicity also occurs in other phases of the cell cycle.

In addition to the intercalation mechanism described, the anthracycline ring of doxorubicin can undergo a one-electron reduction to form free radicals and participate in further electron transfer. These highly active substances can then react with tissue macromolecules. This type of interaction suggests an alternative mechanism of cytotoxicity for the anthracyclines. In particular, the cardiac toxicity of anthracyclines may result from the generation of free radicals of oxygen.

Resistance to the anthracyclines usually involves decreased drug accumulation due to *enhanced active efflux* of drug. This form of drug resistance is common among the large, heterocyclic naturally derived anticancer agents. It is termed *multidrug resistance* because of the high degree of cross-resistance among the anthracyclines, vinca alkaloids, dactinomycin, and podophyllotoxins (see Chapter 55).

Doxorubicin is not absorbed orally, and because of its ability to cause tissue necrosis must not be injected intramuscularly or subcutaneously. Distribution studies indicate rapid uptake in all tissues except the CNS. Extensive tissue binding, primarily intranuclear, accounts for the prolonged elimination half-life. The drug is extensively metabolized in the liver to hydroxylated and conjugated metabolites and to aglycones that are primarily excreted in the bile.

Doxorubicin is one of the most effective agents used in the treatment of carcinomas of the breast, ovary, endometrium, bladder, and thyroid and in oat cell cancer of the lung. It is included in several combination regimens for diffuse lymphomas and Hodgkin's disease. Doxorubicin can be used as an alternative to daunorubicin in acute leukemias and is useful in Ewing's sarcoma, osteogenic sarcoma, soft-tissue sarcomas, and neuroblastoma. Some activity has been reported in non–oat cell lung cancer, multiple myeloma, and adenocarcinomas of the stomach, prostate, and testis.

The most important toxicities caused by doxorubicin involve the heart and bone marrow. Acutely, doxorubicin may cause transient cardiac arrhythmias and depression of myocardial function. Doxorubicin may cause radiation recall reactions, with flare-ups of dermatitis, stomatitis, or esophagitis that had been produced previously by radiation therapy. Less severe toxicities include phlebitis and sclerosis of veins used for injection, hyperpigmentation of nail beds and skin creases, and conjunctivitis. Because of its intense red color, doxorubicin will impart a reddish color to the urine for 1 or 2 days after administration.

Idarubicin

Idarubicin (*Idamycin*) differs from its parent compound, daunorubicin, by the absence of the methoxy group in the anthracycline ring structure. Its mechanisms of action and resistance are similar to those of doxorubicin and daunorubicin; however, it is more lipophilic and more potent than these other anthracyclines. Idarubicin undergoes extensive hepatic metabolism and biliary excretion. Adverse reactions of idarubicin are similar to those of its congeners.

Bleomycin

The bleomycins are a group of glycopeptides that are isolated from *Streptomyces verticillus*. The clinical preparation, bleomycin sulfate (*Blenoxane*), is a mixture of several components. Bleomycin binds to DNA, in part through an intercalation mechanism, without markedly altering the secondary structure of the nucleic acid. The drug produces both single- and double-strand scission and fragmentation of DNA. It is thought that the bleomycins, which are avid metal-chelating agents, form a bleomycin–Fe^{++} complex that can donate electrons to molecular oxygen, thus forming the superoxide and hydroxyl free radicals. It is these highly reactive intermediates that attack DNA and produce DNA strand breakage and maximum cytotoxicity in the late G_2 and early M-phases of the cell cycle.

Bleomycin is poorly absorbed orally, but it can be given by various parenteral routes. Its plasma half-life is not affected by renal dysfunction as long as creatinine clearance is greater than 35 mL/minute.

Bleomycin hydrolase, which inactivates bleomycin, is an enzyme that is abundant in liver and kidney but virtually absent in lungs and skin; the latter two organs are the major targets of bleomycin toxicity. It is thought that bleomycin-induced dermal and pulmonary toxicities are related to the persistence of relatively high local concentrations of active drug.

Bleomycin, in combination with cisplatin or etoposide, is important as part of the potentially curative combination chemotherapy of advanced testicular carcinomas. Bleomycin is used in some standard regimens for the treatment of Hodgkin's and non-Hodgkin's lymphomas, and it is useful against squamous cell carcinomas of the head and neck, cervix, and skin.

A potentially fatal lung toxicity occurs in 10 to 20% of patients receiving bleomycin. Patients particularly at risk are those who are over 70 years of age and have had radiation therapy to the chest. Rarely, bleomycin also may cause allergic pneumonitis. Bleomycin skin toxicity is manifested by hyperpigmentation, erythematosus rashes, and thickening of the skin over the dorsum of the hands and at dermal pressure points, such as the elbows. Many patients develop a low-grade transient fever within 24 hours of receiving bleomycin. Less common adverse effects include mucositis, alopecia, headache, nausea, and arteritis of the distal extremities.

Mitomycin

Mitomycin (mitomycin C, *Mitocin-C, Mutamycin*) is an antibiotic that is derived from a species of *Streptomyces*. It is sometimes classified as an alkylating agent because it can covalently bind to and cross-link DNA. Mitomycin is thought to inhibit DNA synthesis through its ability to alkylate double-strand DNA and bring about interstrand cross-linking. There is evidence that enzymatic reduction by a reduced nicotinamide–adenine dinucleotide phosphate (NADPH) dependent reductase is necessary to activate the drug.

The drug is rapidly cleared from serum after intravenous injection but is not distributed to the brain.

Mitomycin has limited palliative effects in carcinomas of the stomach, pancreas, colon, breast, and cervix.

The major toxicity associated with mitomycin therapy is unpredictably long and cumulative myelosuppression that affects both white blood cells and platelets. A syndrome of microangiopathic hemolytic anemia, thrombocytopenia, and renal failure also has been described. Renal, hepatic, and pulmonary toxicity may occur. The drug is teratogenic and carcinogenic, and it can cause local blistering.

Dactinomycin

Dactinomycin (actinomycin D, *Cosmegen*) is one of a family of chromopeptides produced by *Streptomyces*. It is known to bind noncovalently to double-strand DNA by partial intercalation, inhibiting DNA-directed RNA synthesis. The drug is most toxic to proliferating cells, but it is not specific for any one phase of the cell cycle. *Resistance* to dactinomycin is caused by decreased ability of tumor cells to take up and retain the drug, and it is associated with cross-resistance to vinca alkaloids, the anthracyclines, and certain other agents (multidrug resistance).

Dactinomycin is cleared rapidly from plasma, does not enter the brain, is not appreciably metabolized or protein bound, and is gradually excreted in both bile and urine. Virtually no drug is detected in CSF.

Dactinomycin is used in curative combined treatment of Wilms' tumor, Ewing's sarcoma, rhabdomyosarcoma, and gestational choriocarcinoma. It is active in testicular tumors, lymphomas, melanomas, and sarcomas, although its use in most of these malignancies has been supplanted by other agents.

The major side effects of dactinomycin are severe nausea, vomiting, and myelosuppression. Mucositis, diarrhea, alopecia, and radiation recall reactions may occur. The drug is immunosuppressive and carcinogenic.

Plicamycin

Plicamycin (mithramycin, *Mithracin*) is one of the chromomycin group of antibiotics produced by *Streptomyces tanashiensis*. Plicamycin binds to DNA and inhibits transcription. It also inhibits resorption of bone by osteoblasts, thus lowering serum calcium levels. Very little is known about its distribution, metabolism, and excretion. Because of its severe toxicity, plicamycin has limited clinical utility. The major indication for plicamycin therapy is in the treatment of life-threatening hypercalcemia associated with malignancy. Plicamycin also can be used in the palliative therapy of metastatic testicular carcinoma when all other known active drugs have failed.

PLANT-DERIVED PRODUCTS

Three classes of plant-derived drugs, the vinca alkaloids (vincristine, vinblastine, and vinorelbine), the epipodophyllotoxins (etoposide and teniposide), and the taxanes (paclitaxel and taxotere), are used in cancer chemotherapy. These classes differ in their structures and mechanisms of action but share the multidrug resistance mechanism, since they are all substrates for the multidrug transporter P-glycoprotein.

Vinca Alkaloids
Vincristine, Vinblastine, and Vinorelbine

Vincristine (*Oncovin*) and vinblastine (*Velban*) are both produced by the leaves of the periwinkle plant. Despite their structural similarity, there are significant differences between them in regard to clinical usefulness and toxicity.

The vinca alkaloids *bind avidly to tubulin,* a class of proteins that form the mitotic spindle during cell division. The drugs cause cellular arrest in metaphase during mitosis, and cell division cannot be completed. Although the vinca alkaloids usually have been regarded as phase specific in the cell cycle, some mammalian cells are most vulnerable in the late S-phase.

Resistance to vinca alkaloids has been correlated with a decreased rate of drug uptake or an increased drug efflux from these tumor cells. Cross-resistance usually occurs with anthracyclines, dactinomycin, and podophyllotoxins.

Both vincristine and vinblastine are extensively bound to tissues, and only small amounts of the drug are distributed to the brain or CSF. The plasma disappearance of vinblastine and vinorelbine is triphasic. Similar clinical pharmacokinetics have been noted with vincristine and vinorelbine. Biliary excretion is the major route of drug excretion.

Vincristine is an important component of the curative combination chemotherapy for acute lymphoblastic leukemia, Hodgkin's disease (the MOPP regimen), and non-Hodgkin's lymphomas. It is also used in several regimens for pediatric solid tumors, including Wilms' tumor, Ewing's sarcoma, rhabdomyosarcoma, and neuroblastoma; in adult tumors of the breast, lung, and cervix; and in sarcomas. Its relative lack of myelosuppression makes it more attractive than vinblastine for use in combination with myelotoxic drugs. Vinblastine is especially useful in testicular carcinomas and is also active in Hodgkin's disease, other types of lymphomas, breast cancer, and renal cell carcinoma.

Vinorelbine is particularly useful in the treatment of advanced non–small cell lung cancer and can be administered alone or in combination with cisplatin. It is thought to interfere with mitosis in dividing cells through a relatively specific action on mitotic microtubules.

Neurological toxicity is the major dose-limiting toxicity of vincristine, whereas bone marrow toxicity is limiting for vinblastine. Severe neutropenia occurs in approximately half of the patients receiving vinorelbine. Severe leukopenia is the major side effect of vinblastine. These drugs are potent local blistering agents and will produce tissue necrosis if extravasated.

Epipodophyllotoxins
Etoposide

Etoposide (*VePesid*) is a semisynthetic derivative of podophyllotoxin that is produced in the roots of the American mandrake, or May apple. Unlike podophyllotoxin and vinca alkaloids, etoposide does not bind to microtubules. It forms a complex with the enzyme topoisomerase II, which results in a single-strand breakage of DNA. It is most lethal to cells in the S- and G_2-phases of the cell cycle. Drug *resistance* to etoposide is thought to be caused by decreased cellular drug accumulation.

Etoposide is most useful against testicular and ovarian germ cell cancers, lymphomas, small cell lung cancers, and acute myelogenous and lymphoblastic leukemia. Toxicities include mild nausea, alopecia, allergic reaction, phlebitis at the injection site, and bone marrow toxicity.

Teniposide

Teniposide (VM-26, *Vumon*) is closely related to etoposide in structure, mechanisms of action and resistance, and adverse effects. It is more lipophilic and approximately threefold more potent than etoposide. Its major uses have been in pediatric cancers, particularly in acute lymphoblastic leukemias.

Taxanes
Paclitaxel

Paclitaxel (*Taxol*) is a highly complex, organic compound isolated from the bark of the Pacific yew tree. It binds to tubulin dimers and microtubulin filaments, promoting the assembly of filaments and preventing their depolymerization. This increase in the stability of microfilaments results in disruption of mitosis and cytotoxicity and disrupts other normal microtubular functions, such as axonal transport in nerve fibers.

The major mechanism of resistance that has been identified for paclitaxel is transport out of tumor cells, which leads to decreased intracellular drug accumulation. This form of resistance is mediated by the multidrug transporter P-glycoprotein.

Paclitaxel's large volume of distribution indicates significant tissue binding. The drug is extensively metabolized by the liver, and doses must be reduced in patients with abnormal liver function or with extensive liver metastases. Very little of the drug is excreted in the urine.

Paclitaxel is among the most active of all anticancer drugs, with significant efficacy against carcinomas of the breast, ovary, lung, head, and neck. It is combined with cisplatin in the therapy of ovarian and lung carcinomas and with doxorubicin in treating breast cancer.

Myelosuppression is the major side effect of paclitaxel. Alopecia is common, as is reversible dose-related peripheral neuropathy. Most patients have mild numbness and tingling of the fingers and toes beginning a few days after treatment. Mild muscle and joint aching also may begin 2 or 3 days after initiation of therapy. Nausea is usually mild or absent. Severe hypersensitivity reactions may occur. Cardiovascular side effects, consisting of mild hypotension and bradycardia, have been noted in up to 25% of patients.

ENZYMES

L-Asparaginase

The enzyme L-asparaginase (*Elspar*) is derived from the bacteria *Escherichia coli* and *Erwinia carotovora*. It catalyzes the hydrolysis of L-asparagine to aspartic acid and ammonia. L-Glutamine also can undergo hydrolysis by this enzyme, and during therapy, the plasma levels of both amino acid substrates fall to zero. Tumor cells sensitive to L-asparaginase are deficient in the enzyme asparagine synthetase and therefore cannot synthesize asparagine. *Depletion of exogenous asparagine and glutamine inhibits protein synthesis in cells lacking asparagine synthetase,* which leads to inhibition of nucleic acid synthesis and cell death.

The half-life of L-asparaginase in human plasma is 6 to 30 hours. The drug remains primarily in the intravascular space, so its volume of distribution is only slightly greater than that of the plasma. Metabolism and disposition are thought to occur through serum proteases, the reticuloendothelial system, and especially in patients with prior exposure to the drug, binding by antibodies. The drug is not excreted in urine, and very little appears in the CSF.

The major indication for L-asparaginase is in the treatment of acute lymphoblastic leukemia; complete remission rates of 50 to 60% are possible. Lack of cross-resistance and bone marrow toxicity make the enzyme particularly useful in combination chemotherapy. L-Asparaginase also can be used in the treatment of certain types of lymphoma. It has no role in the treatment of nonlymphocytic leukemias or other types of cancer.

Since it is a foreign protein, L-asparaginase may produce hypersensitivity reactions, including urticarial skin rashes and severe anaphylactic reactions. One-third of patients have nausea, anorexia, weight loss, and mild fever. Almost all patients develop elevated serum transaminases and other biochemical indices of hepatic dysfunction. Severe hepatic toxicity occurs in fewer than 5% of cases. Patients receiving L-asparaginase may develop symptoms of CNS toxicity, including drowsiness, confusion, impaired mentation, and even coma. Pancreatitis occurs in 5 to 10% of cases. Hyperglycemia, possibly due to inhibition of insulin synthesis, also may occur. *L-Asparaginase differs from most cytotoxic drugs in its lack of toxicity to bone marrow, gastrointestinal tract, and hair follicles.*

HORMONE DERIVATIVES

Tamoxifen

Tamoxifen (*Nolvadex*) is a synthetic antiestrogen (see Chapter 63) used in the treatment of breast cancer. Normally, estrogens act by binding to a cytoplasmic protein receptor, and the resulting hormone–receptor complex is then translocated into the nucleus, where it induces the synthesis of ribosomal RNA (rRNA) and messenger RNA (mRNA) at specific sites on the DNA of the target cell. *Tamoxifen also avidly binds to estrogen receptors and competes with endogenous estrogens for these critical sites.* The drug–receptor complex has little or no estrogen agonist activity. Tamoxifen directly inhibits growth of human breast cancer cells that contain estrogen receptors but has little effect on cells without such receptors.

Tamoxifen is slowly absorbed, and maximum serum levels are achieved 4 to 7 hours after oral administration.

The drug is concentrated in estrogen target tissues, such as the ovaries, uterus, vaginal epithelium, and breasts. Hydroxylation and glucuronidation of the aromatic rings are the major pathways of metabolism; excretion occurs primarily in the feces.

The presence of estrogen receptors (ER) in biopsies of breast cancers is a good predictor of responsiveness to tamoxifen therapy: 60% of women with ER-positive tumors will have a remission, as opposed to fewer than 10% with ER-negative tumors. Overall, 35 to 40% of women with breast cancer will respond to some degree, with antitumor effects lasting an average of 9 to 12 months. Complete remissions may occur in 10 to 15% of patients and may last several months to a few years. Therapy should be continued for at least 6 weeks to establish efficacy.

Tamoxifen administration is associated with few toxic side effects, most frequently hot flashes (in 10–20% of patients) and occasionally vaginal dryness or discharge. Mild nausea, exacerbation of bone pain, and hypercalcemia may occur.

Estramustine

Estramustine phosphate sodium (*Emcyt*) is a hybrid structure combining estradiol and a nitrogen mustard in a single molecule. The drug has been approved for use in prostatic carcinomas and will produce clinical remissions in one-third of patients who have failed to respond to previous estrogen therapy. The mechanism of action of estramustine is not well defined, but it does not appear to require either alkylation of DNA or the presence of estrogen receptors in tumor cells. Nonetheless, the toxicities of the drug are similar to those of estrogen therapy: breast tenderness and enlargement (gynecomastia), fluid retention, mild nausea, and an increased risk of thrombophlebitis and pulmonary embolism. The drug is not myelosuppressive.

Flutamide

Flutamide (*Eulexin*) is a nonsteroidal antiandrogen (see Chapter 63) compound that competes with testosterone for binding to androgen receptors. The drug is well absorbed on oral administration. It is an active agent in the hormonal therapy of cancer of the prostate and has been shown to complement the pharmacological castration produced by the gonadotropin-releasing hormone (GnRH) agonist leuprolide. Flutamide prevents the stimulation of tumor growth that may occur as a result of the transient increase in testosterone secretion after the initiation of leuprolide therapy. The most common side effects of flutamide are those expected with androgen blockade: hot flashes, loss of libido, and impotence. Mild nausea and diarrhea occur in about 10% of patients.

Buserelin and Leuprolide

Buserelin (*Suprefact*) and leuprolide (*Lupron*) are peptide analogues of the hypothalamic hormone LH-RH (luteinizing hormone–releasing hormone). Chronic exposure of the pituitary to these agents abolishes gonadotropin release and results in markedly decreased estrogen and testosterone production by the gonads. Their major clinical use is in the palliative hormonal therapy of cancer of the prostate.

Leuprolide is a potent LH-RH agonist for the first several days to a few weeks after initiation of therapy, and therefore, it initially stimulates testicular and ovarian steroidogenesis. Because of this initial stimulation of testosterone production, it is recommended that patients with prostatic cancer be treated concurrently with leuprolide and the antiandrogen flutamide (discussed earlier). Leuprolide is generally well tolerated, with hot flashes being the most common side effect.

Somatostatin Analogue

Octreotide acetate (*Sandostatin*) is a synthetic peptide analogue of the hormone somatostatin. Its actions include inhibition of the pituitary secretion of growth hormone and an inhibition of pancreatic islet cell secretion of insulin and glucagon. Unlike somatostatin, which has a plasma half-life of a few minutes, octreotide has a plasma elimination half-life of 1 to 2 hours. Excretion of the drug is primarily renal.

Octreotide is useful in inhibiting the secretion of various autacoids and peptide hormones by metastatic carcinoid tumors (serotonin) and islet cell carcinomas of the pancreas (gastrin, glucagon, insulin, vasoactive intestinal peptide). The diarrhea and flushing associated with the carcinoid syndrome are improved in 70 to 80% of the patients treated with octreotide. Its side effects, which are usually mild, include nausea and pain at the injection site. Mild transient hypoglycemia or hyperglycemia may result from alterations in insulin, glucagon, or growth hormone secretion.

MISCELLANEOUS AGENTS

Hydroxyurea

Hydroxyurea (*Hydrea*) inhibits the enzyme *ribonucleotide reductase* and thus depletes intracellular pools of deoxyribonucleotides, resulting in a specific impairment of DNA synthesis. The drug therefore is an S-phase specific agent whose action results in an accumulation of cells in the late G_1- and early S-phases of the cell cycle.

Hydroxyurea is rapidly absorbed after oral administration, with peak plasma levels achieved approximately 1 to 2 hours after drug administration; its elimination half-life is 2 to 3 hours. The primary route of excretion is renal, with 30 to 40% of a dose excreted unchanged.

Hydroxyurea is used for the rapid lowering of blood granulocyte counts in patients with chronic granulocytic leukemia. The drug also can be used as maintenance therapy for patients with the disease who have become resistant to busulfan. Only a small percentage of patients with other malignancies have had even brief remissions induced by hydroxyurea administration.

Hematological toxicity, with white blood cells affected more than platelets, may occur. Megaloblastosis of the bone marrow also may be observed. Recovery is rapid, generally within 10 to 14 days after discontinuation of the drug. Some skin reactions, including hyperpigmentation and hyperkeratosis, have been reported with chronic treatment.

Procarbazine

Procarbazine (*Matulane*) may autooxidize spontaneously, and during this reaction hydrogen peroxide and hydroxyl free radicals are generated. These highly reactive products may degrade DNA and serve as one mechanism of procarbazine-induced cytotoxicity. Cell toxicity also may be the result of a transmethylation reaction that can occur between the *N*-methyl group of procarbazine and the N7 position of guanine.

Procarbazine is rapidly absorbed after oral administration and has a plasma half-life of only 10 minutes. The drug crosses the blood-brain barrier, reaching levels in CSF equal to those obtained in plasma. Metabolism is extensive and complex. Urinary excretion accounts for 70% of the procarbazine and its metabolites lost during the first 24 hours after drug administration.

When originally tested as a single agent in advanced Hodgkin's disease, procarbazine produced tumor regression responses that were brief, usually lasting only 1 to 3 months. The combination of procarbazine with mechlorethamine, vincristine, and prednisone in the MOPP regimen, however, resulted in an 81% complete remission rate in Hodgkin's disease. Most of these patients are considered cured. Procarbazine is also used in various combination chemotherapy protocols for non-Hodgkin's lymphomas and small cell anaplastic (oat cell) carcinoma of the lung. Limited antitumor effects have been observed against multiple myeloma, melanoma, and non–oat cell lung cancers.

The major side effects associated with procarbazine therapy are nausea and vomiting, leukopenia, and thrombocytopenia. Skin rashes have been reported, as have rare cases of allergic interstitial pneumonia. Procarbazine administration produces a high degree of chromosomal breakage, and the compound is mutagenic, teratogenic, and carcinogenic in experimental systems.

Procarbazine may potentiate the effects of tranquilizers and hypnotics. Hypertensive episodes can result if procarbazine is administered simultaneously with adrenomimetic drugs or with tyramine-containing foods. Rarely, a reaction to alcohol similar to that provoked by disulfiram may occur.

Mitotane

The observation that mitotane (*Lysodren*) could produce adrenocortical necrosis in animals led to its use in the palliation of inoperable adrenocortical adenocarcinomas. A reduction in both tumor size and adrenocortical hormone secretion can be achieved in about half of the patients taking the drug. Because normal adrenocortical cells also are affected, endogenous glucocorticoid production should be monitored and replacement therapy administered when appropriate.

Mitotane is incompletely absorbed from the gastrointestinal tract after oral administration. However, once absorbed, it tends to accumulate in adipose tissue. Mitotane is slowly excreted and will appear in the urine for several years. The major toxicities associated with its use are anorexia, nausea, diarrhea, lethargy, somnolence, dizziness, and dermatitis.

Hexamethylmelamine

Although both DNA and RNA synthesis are inhibited in cells exposed to hexamethylmelamine (*Hexalen*), the molecular mechanisms of these effects are not known.

Hexamethylmelamine is readily absorbed after oral administration, with peak plasma levels achieved after 1 hour. The drug is readily metabolized to form a number of demethylated metabolites. Urinary elimination is the primary route of drug excretion.

Hexamethylmelamine is useful for the treatment of ovarian adenocarcinoma and is frequently combined with cyclophosphamide, cisplatin, and doxorubicin in the treatment of this tumor. It also has some activity against small cell lung cancer.

Nausea and vomiting are the major toxicities associated with hexamethylmelamine administration. Myelosuppression and a peripheral neuropathy also may occur.

Cisplatin

Cisplatin (*Platinol*) is an inorganic coordination complex with a broad range of antitumor activity. It is especially useful in the treatment of testicular and ovarian cancer. It binds to DNA at nucleophilic sites, such as the N7 and O6 of guanine, producing alterations in DNA structure and inhibition of DNA synthesis. Adjacent guanine residues on the same DNA strand are preferentially cross-linked. This platinating activity is analogous to the mode of action of alkylating agents. Cisplatin also binds extensively to proteins. It does not appear to be phase specific in the cell cycle.

Cisplatin shows biphasic plasma decay with a distribution phase half-life of 25 to 49 minutes and an elimination half-life of 2 to 4 days. More than 90% of the drug is bound to plasma proteins, and binding may approach 100% during prolonged infusion. Cisplatin does not cross the blood-brain barrier. Excretion is predominantly renal and is incomplete.

Cisplatin, combined with bleomycin and vinblastine or etoposide, produces cures in most patients with metastatic testicular cancer or germ cell cancer of the ovary. Cisplatin also shows some activity against carcinomas of the head and neck, bladder, cervix, prostate, and lung.

Renal toxicity is the major potential toxicity of cisplatin. Severe nausea and vomiting that often accompany cisplatin administration may necessitate hospitalization. Cisplatin has mild bone marrow toxicity, yielding both leukopenia and thrombocytopenia. Anemia is common and may require transfusions of red blood cells. Anaphylactic allergic reactions have been described. Hearing loss in the high frequencies (4000 Hz) may occur in 10 to 30% of patients. Other reported toxicities include peripheral neuropathies with paresthesias, leg weakness, and tremors. Excessive urinary excretion of magnesium also may occur.

Carboplatin

Carboplatin (*Paraplatin*) is an analogue of cisplatin. Its plasma half-life is 3 to 5 hours, and it has no significant protein binding. Renal excretion is the major route of drug elimination.

Despite its lower chemical reactivity, carboplatin has antitumor activity that is similar to that of cisplatin against ovarian carcinomas, small cell lung cancers, and germ cell cancers of the testis. Most tumors that are resistant to cisplatin are cross-resistant to carboplatin.

The major advantage of carboplatin over cisplatin is a markedly reduced risk of toxicity to the kidneys, peripheral nerves, and hearing; additionally, it produces less nausea and vomiting. It is, however, more myelosuppressive than cisplatin. Other adverse effects include anemia, abnormal liver function tests, and occasional allergic reactions.

Mitoxantrone

Mitoxantrone (*Novantrone*) is a synthetic anthraquinone that is structurally and mechanistically related to the anthracyclines. It intercalates with DNA and produces single-strand DNA breakage. It is cross-resistant with doxorubicin in multidrug-resistant cells and in patients who have failed to respond to doxorubicin therapy.

Mitoxantrone is active against breast carcinomas, leukemias, and lymphomas. Its antitumor efficacy in patients with breast cancer is slightly lower than that of doxorubicin. Its major toxicity is myelosuppression; mucositis and diarrhea also may occur. Mitoxantrone produces less nausea, alopecia, and cardiac toxicity than does doxorubicin.

IMMUNOMODULATING AGENTS

Levamisole

Levamisole (*Ergamisol*) is an antiparasitic drug that has been found to enhance T-cell function and cellular immunity. The drug improves survival of patients with resected colorectal cancers when combined with 5-fluorouracil; the mechanism of this interaction is not known. Levamisole does not have antitumor activity against established or metastatic cancer and has not been found useful in the adjuvant therapy of cancers other than colorectal cancer.

The major adverse effects of levamisole are nausea and anorexia. Skin rashes, itching, flulike symptoms, and fevers also have been observed.

Interferon Alfa-2b

Interferon alfa-2b (*Intron A*) is a recombinant DNA product derived from the interferon alfa-2b gene of human white blood cells. Its mechanism of antitumor action involves binding to a plasma membrane receptor but is otherwise poorly understood. Its serum half-life is 2 to 3 hours after parenteral administration.

Interferon alfa-2b is useful in the treatment of a rare form of chronic leukemia, hairy cell leukemia, in which it produces remissions in 60 to 80% of patients. However, it has minimal antitumor activity in most human cancers. Remissions lasting a few months have been observed in 10 to 20% of patients with lymphomas, multiple myeloma, melanoma, renal cell carcinoma, and ovarian carcinoma.

The adverse effects of interferon alfa-2b include fever and a flulike syndrome of muscle ache, fatigue, headache, anorexia, and nausea. Other less common side effects include leukopenia, diarrhea, dizziness, and skin rash.

Interleukins
Aldesleukin

Aldesleukin (IL-2, *Proleukin*) is a human recombinant interleukin-2 protein. Its antitumor action is thought to include multiple effects on the immune system, such as enhancement of T-lymphocyte cytotoxicity, induction of natural killer cell activity, and induction of interferon-γ production. Aldesleukin has been used alone and in combination with lymphokine activated killer (LAK) cells or tumor-infiltrating lymphocytes (TIL).

The drug produces remissions in 15% of patients with renal cell carcinoma, with median durations of remission of 18 to 24 months.

Several serious toxicities have been observed, with a fatality rate of 5% in the initial studies. The major adverse effect is severe hypotension in as many as 85% of patients, which may lead to myocardial infarctions, pulmonary edema, and strokes. This hypotension is thought to be due to a capillary leak syndrome resulting from extravasation of plasma proteins and fluid into extravascular space and a loss of vascular tone. Patients with significant cardiac, pulmonary, renal, hepatic, or CNS conditions should not receive therapy with aldesleukin. Other adverse reactions include nausea and vomiting, diarrhea, stomatitis, anorexia, altered mental status, fevers, and fatigue.

CELLULAR GROWTH FACTORS

Filgrastim

Filgrastim (*Neupogen*) is a human recombinant granulocyte colony–stimulating factor (rG-CSF) produced using recombinant DNA technology. It acts on precursor hematopoietic cells in the bone marrow by binding to specific receptors that stimulate cellular proliferation and differentiation into neutrophils. It also enhances some neutrophil functions, including phagocytosis and antibody-dependent killing.

Filgrastim is used to accelerate recovery of neutrophils after chemotherapy, both to prevent infections and to shorten the duration of neutropenia in patients in whom infections have developed.

The drug is generally well tolerated, with the major adverse reaction being mild to moderate bone pain secondary to stimulation of bone marrow proliferation.

Sargramostim

Sargramostim (GM-CSF, *Leukine, Prokine*) is a human recombinant granulocyte and macrophage colony–stimulating factor that stimulates the production and potentiates the function of both granulocytes and macrophages from hematopoietic progenitor cells. It is used to accelerate bone marrow repopulation after high-dose chemotherapy, radiation therapy, and bone marrow transplantation. Adverse effects associated with sargramostim use include bone pain (similar to that of filgrastim), fatigue, fevers, skin rash, malaise, and fluid retention.

NEW DRUG THERAPIES FOR CANCER

Imantinib

Imantinib mesylate (*Gleevec*) is a rationally designed inhibitor of the tumor-specific bcr-abl kinase. The Philadelphia chromosome, present in nearly all patients with chronic myelogenous leukemia (CML), is produced by a chromosomal rearrangement linking the bcr and the abl genes. The bcr-able kinase is therefore a unique drug target in leukemic cells, and imantinib selectively and potently inhibits this kinase. Remissions in CML patients are achieved with high frequency and very low toxicity, and this compound may become a front-line agent for treating this cancer. Unfortunately, drug resistance has already been observed in the clinic as a result of mutations in the bcr-abl kinase, and this magic bullet does not appear to be curative for CML patients. Extension of the use of imantinib to other tumor types with overexpression of c-kit kinase or platelet-derived growth factor kinase is undergoing development because of its observed activity against these kinases.

Herceptin

The introduction of herceptin (*Trastuzumab*) into clinical practice for the treatment of breast cancer marks a major advance in the use of monoclonal antibody cancer therapy. Herceptin is a humanized antibody directed against the HER-2 antigen that is overexpressed on the tumor cell surface in approximately 25% of breast cancer patients. HER-2/neu/erbB2 overexpression marks an aggressive estrogen receptor–negative form of breast cancer. Therefore, a therapeutic agent selective for this target is particularly valuable. Herceptin is administered by intravenous infusion and in conjunction with paclitaxel can extend survival in patients with HER-2/neu/erbB2 overexpressing metastatic breast cancer. Herceptin use is associated with infusion- related hypotension, flushing and bronchoconstriction, and skin rash but no bone marrow toxicity. Herceptin appears to sensitize patients to cardiotoxicity, an important concern in patients also receiving doxorubicin.

Iressa

Iressa (ZD1839) is an orally active tyrosine kinase inhibitor selective for the epidermal growth factor (EGF) receptor tyrosine kinase. Iressa is undergoing clinical trials in the treatment of various solid tumors, including head and neck cancer, breast cancer and non-small cell lung cancer. Its antitumor activity is derived from the fact that the EGF receptor and EGF signaling are frequently overactivated in sensitive tumors. The major side effects include diarrhea and skin rash. Bone marrow toxicity has not been a dose-limiting problem.

A summary of the principal clinical uses of most of the drugs mentioned in this chapter can be found in Table 56.2.

TABLE 56.2 Major Clinical Uses of the Anticancer Drugs

Drugs	Therapeutic Uses
Aldesleukin	**Renal cell carcinoma**
L-Asparaginase	Acute lymphocytic leukemia, lymphomas
Bleomycin	Advanced testicular carcinoma; Hodgkin's and non-Hodgkin's lymphomas; squamous cell carcinoma of head, neck, cervix, skin
Buserelin, estramustine, flutamide, leuprolide	Prostatic cancer
Busulfan	Chronic granulocytic leukemia
Carboplatin, cisplatin	Testicular and ovarian cancer
Carmustine, lomustine, semustine	CNS tumors, Hodgkin's disease, lymphomas, melanoma, colorectal and renal cell cancer
Chlorambucil	Chronic lymphocytic leukemia, myeloma, lymphomas
Cladribine, pentostatin	Hairy cell leukemia
Cyclophosphamide	Lymphoma, breast and ovarian cancer, oat cell lung cancer
Cytarabine	Acute myelogenous and acute lymphoblastic leukemia, lymphomas
Dacarbazine	Metastatic melanoma, sarcomas, Hodgkin's disease
Dactinomycin	Wilms' tumor, Ewing's sarcoma, rhabdomyosarcoma, gestational choriocarcinoma, testicular tumors, lymphomas, melanomas
Daunorubicin, doxorubicin, idarubicin	Breast, ovarian, endometrial, bladder, thyroid cancers; oat cell cancer of the lung
Etoposide, teniposide	Testicular, ovarian germ cell cancers, small-cell lung cancer, acute myelogenous and lymphoblastic leukemia
Filgrastim	Promotes recovery of neutrophils after chemotherapy
Fludarabine	Chronic lymphocytic leukemia, low-grade lymphomas
Fluorouracil	Breast, ovarian, cervical, bladder and prostate cancer; gastrointestinal adenocarcinomas
Gemcitabine	Metastatic pancreatic cancer; small cell lung cancer
Gleevec	Leukemia
Herceptin	Breast cancer
Hexamethylmelamine	Ovarian adenocarcinoma, small-cell lung cancer
Hydroxyurea	Chronic myelogenous leukemia
Ifosfamide	Multiple myeloma, breast and ovarian cancer
Interferon alfa-2b	Hairy cell leukemia
Iressa	Head, neck, breast, and lung cancer
Levamisole	Colorectal cancer
Mechlorethamine	Hodgkin's disease
Melphalan	Multiple myeloma, breast and ovarian cancer
Mercaptopurine	Acute lymphoblastic leukemia; acute and chronic myelogenous leukemias
Methotrexate	Acute lymphoblastic leukemia; Burkitt's lymphoma; trophoblastic choriocarcinoma; breast cancer; head, neck, cervical, lung carcinomas
Mitomycin	Stomach, pancreatic, colon, breast, cervical carcinomas
Mitotane	Adrenocortical adenocarcinoma
Mitoxantrone	Breast carcinoma, leukemia, lymphomas
Octreotide	Metastatic carcinoid, islet cell carcinomas
Paclitaxel	Breast, ovarian, lung, head, neck tumors
Plicamycin	Hypercalcemia of malignancy, metastatic testicular carcinoma
Procarbazine	Lymphomas, small cell anaplastic lung cancers
Sargramostim	Stimulates granulocyte and macrophage production after chemotherapy
Streptozocin	Islet cell pancreatic carcinoma, malignant carcinoid tumor
Tamoxifen	Breast cancer
Thioguanine	Acute myelogenous leukemia
Thiotepa	Breast, ovarian cancer, lymphomas
Vincristine, vinblastine, vinorelbine	Acute lymphoblastic leukemia, Hodgkin's disease, pediatric solid tumors (e.g., Wilms', Ewing's), neuroblastoma

Study Questions

1. The nitrogen mustard with the broadest spectrum of antitumor activity in its class is
   (A) Ifosfamide
   (B) Cyclophosphamide
   (C) Mechlorethamine
   (D) Chlorambucil
   (E) Melphalan

2. The first demonstration of the curative potential of chemotherapy in human cancer was the use of which agent in trophoblastic choriocarcinoma in women?
   (A) Chlorambucil
   (B) Thiotepa
   (C) Methotrexate
   (D) Melphalan
   (E) Carmustine

3. Which class of drugs bind avidly to tubulin and cause arrest of cells in metaphase?
   (A) Vinca alkaloids
   (B) Nitrogen mustards
   (C) Alkylating agents
   (D) Antiestrogens
   (E) Antimetabolites

4. You see a patient with breast cancer whose cancer is ER positive. You prescribe tamoxifen. The patient inquires about her chances for remission. What do you tell her?
   (A) You indicate that you do not have a good idea and that only time will tell.
   (B) You indicate that her chances are not too good.
   (C) You indicate that her chances of remission are about 95%.
   (D) You indicate that her chances are somewhat better than 50%.
   (E) You indicate that her chances would be better if her tumor were ER negative.

5. Interferon alfa-2b has been somewhat of a disappointment as an anticancer drug. However, it has proved useful in the treatment of which of the following tumors?
   (A) Oat cell tumors of the lung
   (B) Melanoma
   (C) Wilms' tumor
   (D) ER-positive breast cancer
   (E) Hairy cell leukemia

ANSWERS

1. **B.** Although all of the compounds are nitrogen mustards and have the same basic mechanism of action, differences in the toxicity profile, duration of action, metabolism, and distribution within the body account for the fact that differences in the spectrum of antitumor activity and clinical indications differ for agents within the same class. Ifosfamide also has a broad spectrum of antitumor activity although it is not as broad as that of cyclophosphamide. Mechlorethamine is indicated for use only in Hodgkin's disease. Bone marrow toxicity limits the usefulness of chlorambucil. The effectiveness of melphalan is limited because a substituted phenyl ring in the molecule reduces its reactivity.

2. **C.** The long-term complete remissions of trophoblastic choriocarcinoma in women was the first demonstration of the curative potential of chemotherapy in human cancer. The other choices are all nitrogen mustard compounds. Although carmustine has been shown to produce long-lasting remission in patients with primary brain tumor, the toxicity of nitrogen mustards limits their use. They are usually used in combination with other agents.

3. **A.** The mechanism of action of nitrogen mustards is to form covalent bonds with adjacent guanine residues and inhibit DNA replication and transcription. The nitrogen mustards are also alkylating agents. Antiestrogens inhibit in vitro growth of human breast cancer cells that contain estrogen receptors. Antimetabolites are drugs that are structurally related to naturally occurring compounds, such as vitamins, amino acids, or nucleotides. They can compete for binding sites on enzymes or can become incorporated into DNA or RNA and thus interfere with cell growth and proliferation.

4. **D.** Actually the chances of remission are about 60%. The presence of ER-positive tumors is much more favorable for tamoxifen therapy than if the tumors were ER negative.

5. **E.** The discovery that the endogenous proteins known as interferons were capable of containing viral infections led to the hope that they would have many beneficial results, including anticancer activity. Although they are effective in the treatment of hairy cell leukemia and AIDS-associated Kaposi's sarcoma, they have not been shown to be the panacea that was originally envisioned.

SUPPLEMENTAL READING

Cheson BD, Keating MJ, and Plunkett W (eds.). Nucleoside Analogs in Cancer Therapy. New York: Marcel Dekker, 1997.

Danesi R et al. Pharmacogenetic determinants of anticancer drug activity and toxicity. Trends Pharmacol Sci 2001;22:420–426.

DeVita VT, Hellman S, and Rosenberg SA (eds.). Cancer: Principles and Practice of Oncology (4th ed.). Philadelphia: Lippincott, 1993.

Faroni RE and DeCupis A. The role of polypeptide growth factors in human carcinomas: New targets for a novel pharmacological approach. Pharmacol Rev 2000;52:179–206.

Foye WO (ed.). Cancer Chemotherapeutic Agents. New York: American Chemical Society, 1995.

George DJ. Receptor tyrosine kinases as rational targets for prostate cancer treatment: Platelet-derived growth factor receptor and imatinib mesylate. Urology 2002;60:115–121.

Habib NA. Cancer Gene Therapy: Past Achievements and Future Challenges. New York: Kluwer/Plenum, 2000.

Kirby RS, Christmas TJ, and Brawer MK. Prostate Cancer (2nd ed.). New York: Mosby, 2001.

Suffness M. Taxol: Science and Applications. Boca Raton, FL: CRC, 1995.

Vinorelbine for treatment of advanced non-small cell lung cancer. Med Lett Drugs Ther 1995;37:72–73.

CASE Study   Treatment of Leukemic Meningitis

A 15-year-old girl moves into your neighborhood and makes an appointment to see you. She is being treated for acute lymphoblastic leukemia. She tells you that she has been doing well, but recently she has had frequent severe headaches, and her mother said she has stumbled a couple of times during the past week for no apparent reason. She is being treated with cytarabine. If leukemic meningitis is suspected, what should be done next?

ANSWER: Immediately arrange for an evaluation of the CSF. If the CSF reveals leukemic cells, you can consider administering methotrexate 12 mg intrathecally every day for 4 days. With such a regimen, subsequent evaluations of the CSF often indicate no leukemic cells present. The headaches and balance problems typically disappear. Six months later, most patients show no evidence of leukemia.

57 Immunomodulating Drugs

Leonard J. Sauers

DRUG LIST

Immunopharmacology is the study of the use of pharmacological agents as modulators of immune responses. The principal applications are in the use of *immunosuppressive agents* (i.e., compounds that suppress undesirable immune responses) and *immunostimulating agents* (i.e., drugs, microorganisms, or biological products that enhance or augment immune responses). Three major indications for immunotherapy are in the treatment of autoimmune diseases, primary immunodeficiency diseases, and organ transplantation.

AUTOIMMUNE DISEASES

Cells from the body's immune system can on occasion react against normal endogenous proteins and thereby effect a reaction against certain body tissues. This abnormal immune response is termed *autoimmunity*. Ordinarily, a complex network of feedback loops keeps autoimmune reactions in check. However, under certain circumstances, normal control is lost and the aberrant immune reaction will result in disease.

Myasthenia gravis is an example of an autoimmune disease in which antibodies are produced against the acetylcholine receptors in the neuromuscular junction. The abnormal immune response results in the breakdown of junctional receptors, ultimately rendering patients weak and unable to move voluntary muscles. Rheumatoid arthritis is another autoimmune disease in which antibodies are secreted against a component of an individual's own immune globulins. These antibody–immune globulin conjugates (immune complexes) form precipitates in the joints of affected individuals. Phagocytic cells are in turn attracted to these sites, where they release enzymes that destroy surrounding tissue (inflammation). *Immunosuppressive agents are often employed in debilitating cases of autoimmune disease to curb the production of autoantibodies.*

TABLE 57.1	Some Autoimmune Disorders Treated with Immunosuppressive Therapy

Autoimmune hemolytic anemia
Myasthenia gravis
Cranial arteritis
Idiopathic thrombocytopenic purpura
Membranous glomerulonephritis
Polymyalgia rheumatica
Polymyositis
Psoriatic arthropathies
Rheumatoid arthritis
Systemic lupus erythematosus
Ulcerative colitis
Uveitis
Wegener's granulomatosis

A list of autoimmune diseases for which immunosuppressive therapy is commonly used can be found in Table 57.1.

ORGAN TRANSPLANTATION

Suppression of the immune system is a requirement during organ transplantation because of the propensity of the recipient to reject the foreign tissue by immunological mechanisms. Since transplantation is usually performed in patients with a poor prognosis for survival, the use of immunosuppressive agents has potentially great therapeutic benefit, because it provides the only real hope of continued life for many individuals. Immunosuppression, however, is frequently an adverse reaction when these drugs are used as antineoplastic drugs.

In the past, immunosuppression could be achieved only through the use of *nonspecific* cytotoxic drugs (e.g., cyclophosphamide or azathioprine), which are particularly toxic to rapidly proliferating cells, such as those of the bone marrow, gonadal tissue, and gastrointestinal tract. Consequently, serious side effects, including bone marrow depression, overwhelming infections, and sterility, limited their usefulness as immunosuppressants. The concurrent use of corticosteroids with the immunosuppressants increased the risk of additional toxicity. With the development of the immunosuppressants cyclosporine and tacrolimus it is now possible to avoid much of this toxicity. Because of their relatively low toxicity, these drugs have revolutionized the field of transplantation. It is now possible to successfully transplant tissues to patients not previously considered as candidates for transplantation.

PRIMARY IMMUNODEFICIENCY DISEASES

Primary immunodeficiency diseases (PIDs) are defects of the immune system that are due to genetic abnormalities or some failure in normal embryological development. They are usually apparent at birth or develop shortly thereafter. Approximately 70 PIDs have been described, including those specific for humoral immunity (e.g., X-linked agammaglobulinemia, immune globulin [Ig] A deficiency), cellular immunity (e.g., DiGeorge's syndrome), or both (e.g., severe combined immunodeficiency syndrome).

The treatment of a PID is based on the aspect of the immune system that is lacking. For those with deficiencies in humoral immunity, the only effective treatment available is antibody replacement (e.g., immune globulin) and medical management of infections. For those with deficiencies in cell-mediated immunity, there is no effective pharmacological treatment.

The clinical manifestations of PIDs vary with the aspect of the immune system affected. In general, because of the role of antibodies in protection against bacterial infections, individuals with deficiencies in humoral immunity are particularly prone to infections from *Streptococcus pneumoniae* and *Haemophilus influenzae*. These individuals are also prone to infections of the respiratory, gastrointestinal, and urinary tracts because of the protective role of IgA in secretions.

Individuals with defects in cellular immunity are prone to fungal, protozoal, and viral infections, such as *Candida albicans,* cytomegalovirus, and *Pneumocystis carinii,* since cell-mediated immune responses are the primary defenses against these types of infection. Because of the role of cell-mediated immunity in tumor surveillance, these individuals will also demonstrate an increased incidence of malignancy if they survive long enough.

GENERAL PRINCIPLES OF IMMUNOSUPPRESSIVE THERAPY

Before describing individual drugs, it is important to consider three principles of immunosuppressive therapy. (1) *Primary immune responses are more readily inhibited than are secondary responses.* Therefore, components of the primary phase of the immune response, such as processing, proliferation, and differentiation, will be the most sensitive to drug action. Drugs that are effective in suppressing an immune response in an unsensitized person generally will show much less effect, if any, in a sensitized individual. Once a population of memory cells has been established, immunosuppressive drugs show little effectiveness. (2) *Not all immune responses are equally affected by immunosuppressive drugs.* Cellular and humoral immunity may be affected differentially. Additionally, the different classes of immune globulins in a humoral response may be variably affected. (3) *Beneficial effects other than immunosuppression may result from therapy with these drugs.* In particular, the antiinflammatory properties of certain of these drugs may be valuable because inflammation often accompanies the immune response. If only an inflammatory reaction is present, a true antiinflammatory drug, such as a corticosteroid, that is devoid of the many side effects of immunosuppressive agents should be used.

The focus in the next section is on immunosuppressants that have been shown to be clinically useful. Others that may hold promise in the future are mentioned briefly.

INDIVIDUAL DRUGS USED TO SUPPRESS THE IMMUNE SYSTEM

Cyclosporine

Cyclosporine (*Sandimmune*) is a potent inhibitor of antibody- and cell-mediated immune responses and *is the immunosuppressant of choice for the prevention of transplant rejection.* It also has application in the treatment of autoimmune diseases.

Cyclosporine is a highly stable 11–amino acid cyclic polypeptide. The molecule is very lipophilic and essentially is not soluble in water. It can be administered intravenously, orally, or by injection.

Mechanism of Action

Cyclosporine can bind to the cytosolic protein cytophilin C. This drug–protein complex inhibits calcineurin phosphatase activity, which leads to a decreased synthesis and release of several cytokines, including interleukins IL-2, IL-3, IL-4, interferon-α, and tumor necrosis factor.

Cyclosporine exhibits a high degree of specificity in its actions on T cells without significantly impairing B-cell activity. It can inhibit the T cell–dependent limb of antibody production by lymphocytes by preventing the differentiation of B cells into antibody-secreting plasma cells. Because T cells appear to require IL-2 stimulation for their continuous growth, cyclosporine impairs the proliferative response of T cells to antigens. However, once T cells have been stimulated by antigens to synthesize IL-2, cyclosporine cannot suppress the proliferation of T cells induced by this cytokine.

Absorption, Metabolism, and Excretion

After oral administration, cyclosporine is absorbed slowly and incompletely, with great variation among in-

dividuals. Peak plasma concentrations are reached in 3 to 4 hours, and the plasma half-life is 10 to 27 hours. The drug is extensively metabolized by hepatic mixed-function oxidase enzymes and is excreted principally via the bile into the feces. Metabolism results in inactivation of the immunosuppressive activity. Agents that enhance or inhibit the mixed-function oxidase enzymes will alter the therapeutic response to cyclosporine.

Clinical Uses

Cyclosporine has been approved for use in allogeneic kidney, liver, and heart transplant patients and is under study for use in pancreas, bone marrow, single lung, and heart–lung transplant procedures. It is recommended that corticosteroids, such as prednisone, be used concomitantly, although at half or less of their usual dose. Such combined therapy leads to fewer side effects, a decreased incidence of infectious complications, efficacy of lower doses of cyclosporine, and a better history of patient survival.

Cyclosporine appears to have promise in the treatment of autoimmune diseases. It has a beneficial effect on the course of rheumatoid arthritis, uveitis, insulin-dependent diabetes, systemic lupus erythematosus, and psoriatic arthropathies in some patients. Toxicity is more of a problem in these conditions than during use in transplantation, since higher doses of cyclosporine are often required to suppress autoimmune disorders.

Adverse Effects

Compared with previously available therapy, the adverse effects associated with cyclosporine are much less severe but still worthy of concern. Nephrotoxicity, which can occur in up to 75% of patients, ranges from severe tubular necrosis to chronic interstitial nephropathy. This effect is generally reversible with dosage reduction. Vasoconstriction appears to be an important aspect of cyclosporine-induced nephrotoxicity. Hypertension occurs in 25% of the patients and more frequently in patients with some degree of renal dysfunction; the concomitant use of antihypertensive drugs may prove useful. Hyperglycemia, hyperlipidemia, transient liver dysfunction, and unwanted hair growth are also observed.

Corticosteroids

Corticosteroids, such as prednisone (*Deltasone, Meticorten*) and prednisolone (*Prelone, Delta-Cortef*), have been used alone or in combination with other agents in the treatment of autoimmune disorders and for the prevention of allograft rejection. However, the toxicity associated with their use necessitates prudent administration. Additional information on corticosteroids can be found in Chapter 60.

Although corticosteroids possess immunosuppressive properties, their real value is in controlling the inflammation that can accompany transplantation and autoimmune disorders. Virtually all phases of the inflammatory process are affected by these drugs. Corticosteroid therapy alone is successful in only a limited number of autoimmune diseases, such as idiopathic thrombocytopenia, hemolytic anemia, and polymyalgia rheumatica.

Tacrolimus

Tacrolimus (*Prograf*) is a second-generation immunosuppressive agent that has been approved for use in liver transplantation. Its efficacy for other transplantations is being evaluated. It has properties similar to those of cyclosporine except that weight for weight it is 10 to 100 times more potent. It is a macrolide antibiotic that selectively inhibits transcription of a specific set of lymphokine genes in T lymphocytes (e.g., IL-2, IL-4, and interferon-γ) and binds to cytoplasmic proteins in lymphocytes. Although the binding proteins (cytophilins) for cyclosporine and tacrolimus are different, they share similar functions in that the cytophilins are important for the intracellular folding of proteins. It is speculated that these proteins are important in regulating gene expression in T lymphocytes and that both drugs somehow interfere in this process.

Absorption of tacrolimus from the gastrointestinal (GI) tract is variable. It is extensively metabolized in the liver and excreted in the urine. As with cyclosporine, nephrotoxicity is its principal side effect.

Sirolimus

Sirolimus (*Rapamune*) is structurally related to tacrolimus. It is approved for use as an adjunctive agent in combination with cyclosporine for prevention of acute renal allograft rejection. It blocks IL-2-dependent T-cell proliferation by inhibiting a cytoplasmic serine–threonine kinase. This mechanism of action is different from those of tacrolimus and cyclosporine. This allows sirolimus to augment the immunosuppressive effects of these drugs.

Azathioprine

Azathioprine (*Imuran*) is a cytotoxic agent that preferentially destroys any rapidly dividing cell. Since immunologically competent cells are generally rapidly dividing cells, azathioprine is very effective as an immunosuppressive drug. Unfortunately, any cell that is replicating is a target for this action. This lack of specificity leads to serious side effects.

Azathioprine, in combination with corticosteroids, has historically been used more widely than any other drug in immunosuppressive therapy. It is classified as a purine antimetabolite and is a derivative of 6-mercaptopurine (see Chapter 56).

Mechanism of Action

Azathioprine is a phase-specific drug that is toxic to cells during nucleic acid synthesis. Phase-specific drugs are toxic during a specific phase of the mitotic cycle, usually the S-phase, when DNA synthesis is occurring, as opposed to cycle-specific drugs that kill both cycling and intermitotic cells.

Azathioprine is converted in vivo to thioinosinic acid, which competitively inhibits the synthesis of inosinic acid, the precursor to adenylic acid and guanylic acid. In this way, azathioprine inhibits DNA synthesis and therefore suppresses lymphocyte proliferation. This effectively inhibits both humoral and cell-mediated immune responses.

Absorption, Metabolism, and Excretion

Azathioprine is well absorbed following oral administration, with peak blood levels occurring within 1 to 2 hours. It is rapidly and extensively metabolized to 6-mercaptopurine, which is further converted in the liver and erythrocytes to a variety of metabolites, including 6-thiouric acid. Metabolites are excreted in the urine. The half-life of azathioprine and its metabolites in the blood is about 5 hours.

Clinical Uses

Azathioprine is a relatively powerful antiinflammatory agent. Although its beneficial effect in various conditions is principally attributable to its direct immunosuppressive action, the antiinflammatory properties of the drug play an important role in its overall therapeutic effectiveness.

Azathioprine has been used widely in combination with corticosteroids to inhibit rejection of organ transplants, particularly kidney and liver allografts. However, it is usually reserved for patients who do not respond to cyclosporine plus corticosteroids alone.

Azathioprine also has applications in certain disorders with autoimmune components, most commonly rheumatoid arthritis. It is as effective as cyclophosphamide in the treatment of Wegener's granulomatosis. It has largely been replaced by cyclosporine in immunosuppressive therapy. Relative to other cytotoxic agents, the better oral absorption of azathioprine is the reason for its more widespread clinical use.

Adverse Effects

The therapeutic use of azathioprine has been limited by the number and severity of adverse effects associated with its administration. Bone marrow suppression resulting in leukopenia, thrombocytopenia, or both may occur. GI toxicity may be a problem. It is also mildly hepatotoxic. Because of its immunosuppressive activity, azathioprine therapy can lead to serious infections. It has been shown to be mutagenic in animals and humans and carcinogenic in animals.

Mycophenolate Mofetil

Mycophenolate mofetil (*CellCept*), in conjunction with cyclosporine and corticosteroids, has clinical applications in the prevention of organ rejection in patients receiving allogeneic renal and cardiac transplants. By effectively inhibiting de novo purine synthesis, it can impair the proliferation of both T and B lymphocytes. Following oral administration, mycophenolate mofetil is almost completely absorbed from the GI tract, metabolized in the liver first to the active compound mycophenolic acid, and then further metabolized to an inactive glucuronide.

Early clinical trials indicate that mycophenolate mofetil in conjunction with cyclosporine and corticosteroids is a more effective regimen than azathioprine in preventing the acute rejection of transplanted organs. GI side effects are most common.

Other Cytotoxic Drugs

Although azathioprine is the most popular cytotoxic drug used for immunosuppression, others have been employed. Among these is cyclophosphamide, a cycle-specific agent that acts by cross-linking and alkylating DNA, thereby preventing correct duplication during cell divisions. Methotrexate is a phase-specific agent that acts by inhibiting folate metabolism. It is highly toxic and appears to offer no advantages over azathioprine. Chlorambucil, an alkylating agent, has actions similar to those of cyclophosphamide. In contrast, its adverse effects are fewer in that alopecia and GI intolerance are almost never encountered. See Chapter 56 for further details of these agents.

Antibodies

Antiserum can be raised against lymphocytes or thymocytes by the repeated injection of human cells into an appropriate recipient, usually a horse. The use of such antiserum or the immune globulin fraction derived from it has been used to produce immunosuppression. Although antilymphocytic serum can suppress cellular and often humoral immunity against a variety of tissue graft systems, the responses are variable, particularly from one batch of serum to another.

Antithymocyte Globulin

Antithymocyte globulin (*Atgam*) is purified immune globulin obtained from hyperimmune serum of horses immunized with human thymus lymphocytes. It has been used successfully alone and in combination with azathioprine and corticosteroids to prevent renal allograft rejection. Although it has benefits when administered prophylactically, its use during rejection episodes may be its greatest value.

Antithymocyte globulin binds to circulating T lymphocytes in the blood, which are subsequently removed from the circulation by the reticuloendothelial system. This globulin also reduces the number of T lymphocytes in the thymus-dependent areas of the spleen and lymph nodes.

Since the preparations are raised in heterologous species, reactions against the foreign proteins may lead to serum sickness and nephritis. The concomitant use of corticosteroids may alleviate this response.

Muromonab-(CD3)

Muromonab-(CD3) (*Orthoclone OKT3*) is a mouse monoclonal antibody that is a purified IgG. It is used for the prevention of acute allograft rejection in kidney and hepatic transplants and as prophylaxis in cardiac transplantation. It is also used to deplete T cells in marrow from donors before bone marrow transplantation.

Muromonab-(CD3) alters the cell-mediated immune response by binding to the CD3 (cluster of differentiation antigen, T3) glycoprotein on T lymphocytes. This binding inhibits lymphocyte activation so that affected T cells cannot recognize foreign antigen and cannot participate in rejecting an organ graft. Within minutes of the first muromonab-(CD3) injection, total circulating T cells are rapidly depleted from the blood. They later reappear devoid of CD3 and antigen recognition complexes.

Adverse side effects include fever, pulmonary edema, vomiting, headache, and anaphylaxis. Neutralizing antibodies may develop over time and necessitate adjusting the dosage upward to compensate for the loss of therapeutic activity.

Rho(D) Immune Globulin

An Rh-negative mother can become sensitized to Rh antigen during delivery of an Rh-positive infant. This sensitization may lead to Rh hemolytic disease in future newborns. Rho(D) immune globulin (*RhoGAM*) is a preparation of human IgG that contains a high titer of antibodies against the Rh(D) red cell antigen. Rho(D) immune globulin functions to prevent the mother from becoming sensitized to the Rh antigen by binding to and destroying fetal red blood cells that have entered her blood. It is generally given at 28 weeks of pregnancy and within 72 hours after delivery. Rh incompatibility can be identified with routine blood tests.

INDIVIDUAL DRUGS USED TO STIMULATE THE IMMUNE SYSTEM

A number of disorders can be treated with *immuno-stimulating agents* (also known as biological response modifiers or immunomodulating agents); these drugs enhance the body's immune response. These conditions include immunodeficiency diseases, cancer, some types of viral and fungal infections, and certain autoimmune disorders. The drugs may work on cellular or humoral immune systems or both.

Immunostimulating agents are nonspecific; they cause general stimulation of the immune system. Among the agents capable of general potentiation of the immune system are extracts and derivatives from bacteria, yeast, and fungi. They also include a variety of peptides, cytokines, and synthetic compounds. In most cases, the pharmacology of these agents has not been well described. The most commonly used agents are discussed next.

Bacillus Calmette-Guérin

Bacillus Calmette-Guérin (BCG) is a viable attenuated strain of *Mycobacterium bovis*. Nonviable strains of the bacterium also have been shown to augment the immune response. The smallest active compound derived from BCG thus far has been identified as muramyl dipeptide. The T cell is a principal target for BCG. It also appears to stimulate natural killer cells, which in turn can kill malignant cells. It has been suggested that BCG cross-reacts immunologically with tumor cell antigens.

BCG immunotherapy has been most successful in the treatment of bladder cancers. It is instilled directly into the bladder, where it is held for 2 hours before urination.

The most dangerous complications of BCG therapy are severe hypersensitivity and shock. Chills, fever, malaise, immune complex, and renal disease are among the other side effects. The route of administration influences the nature of the side effects.

Levamisole

Levamisole (*Ergamisol*) was originally developed as an antihelminthic drug (see Chapter 54). It potentiates the stimulatory effects of antigens, mitogens, lymphokines, and chemotactic factors on lymphocytes, granulocytes, and macrophages. It has been shown to increase T cell–mediated immunity.

Levamisole has been used successfully in treating chronic infections. It also has been approved for use in combination with fluorouracil in the treatment of colorectal cancer.

Immune Globulin

Immune globulin is isolated from pooled human plasma either from donors in the general population or from hyperimmunized donors. It is used principally in the treatment of certain immune deficiencies. Standard immune globulin solutions contain a distribution of all subclasses, with antibody titers for most major bacterial, viral, and fungal pathogens.

Immune globulin, given intramuscularly or intravenously, is recommended in the treatment of primary humoral immunodeficiency, congenital agammaglobulinemias, common variable immunodeficiency, severe combined immunodeficiency, idiopathic thrombocytopenic purpura, and autoimmune hemolytic anemia. There are six licensed preparations of immune globulin.

The principal side effects are possible anaphylactoid reactions and severe hypotension.

Thymic Factors

Thymic factors are naturally occurring substances that promote T-lymphocyte differentiation and differentiation of early stem cells into prothymocytes. Each of the available preparations (e.g., thymic humoral factor, thymosin fraction 5, and thymodulin) are mixtures of several polypeptides isolated from a calf thymus extract.

By promoting the formation of T lymphocytes, thymic factors are used to enhance T-lymphocytic functions. Thymic factors have been used with some success in clinical trials in patients with severe combined immunodeficiency, DiGeorge's or Nezelof's syndrome, and viral disorders. Studies with thymodulin show promise in treating symptoms in asthmatics and patients with allergic rhinitis. The primary consideration in the use of thymic factors for immunodeficiency states is the presence of T-lymphocyte precursors.

Few major side effects have been reported, especially with purer forms produced by genetic engineering. Crude thymic preparations have produced allergic side effects in some patients.

Cytokines

An exciting application of immunomodulating therapy is in the use of cytokines (*lymphokines, monokines*). As mentioned earlier in this chapter, immune cell function is regulated by cytokines produced by leukocytes or other supporting cells. With the advent of genetic engineering, cytokines can be produced in pure form and in large quantities.

Interleukin-2

IL-2 (*Proleukin*) is a cytokine that promotes the proliferation, differentiation, and recruitment of T and B lymphocytes, natural killer cells, and thymocytes. Human recombinant IL-2 is designated as rIL-2. rIL-2 binds to IL-2 receptors on responsive cells and induces proliferation and differentiation of T helper cells and T cytotoxic cells. It also can induce B-lymphocyte proliferation, activate macrophage activity, and augment the cytotoxicity of natural killer cells.

rIL-2 is administered systemically as an immunostimulating agent in patients with AIDS and to augment specific antitumor immunity. Patients with renal cell carcinoma or melanoma have been effectively treated with rIL-2 in combination with adoptive transfer immunotherapy. The latter refers to the injection of the patient's own cytokine-activated killer cells or tumor-infiltrating lymphocytes after they reside in tissue culture for several weeks in the presence of rIL-2.

Systemic administration of rIL-2 causes fever, nausea, vomiting, fatigue, and malaise. Other adverse affects include flushing, diarrhea, chills, rash, edema, symptomatic hypotension, and certain renal abnormalities. These tend to occur at increased dosage levels and are attenuated by reducing the dosage.

Myeloid Colony–Stimulating Factors

Recombinant granulocyte-macrophage colony–stimulating factor (GM-CSF) (*Sargramostim*) and granulocyte stimulating factor (G-CSF) (*Filgrastim*) are cytokines, or growth factors, that support the survival, clonal expansion, and differentiation of hematopoietic cells. These factors are normally produced in the body by monocytes, fibroblasts, and endothelial cells. GM-CSF induces bone marrow progenitor cells belonging to the granulocyte or macrophage lineage to divide and differentiate into mature cells. G-CSF induces the maturation of granulocyte progenitor cells.

In general these recombinant cytokines are indicated for acceleration of the recovery of circulating white blood cells in patients who have depressed hematopoiesis, as a result of either chemotherapy or congential disorders of hematopoiesis. A list of indications for the use of GM-CSF and G-CSF is provided in Table 57.2.

Results of several phase 1 and phase 2 clinical trials suggest that these cytokines are well tolerated. Adverse effects are those commonly observed following the administration of molecules produced by biotechnological

TABLE 57.2	Clinical Indications for the Use of Myeloid Colony–Stimulating Factors
G-CSF, GM-CSF	Autologous and allogenic bone marrow transplant
	HIV infections
	Primer for stem cell collection
	Acute myeloid leukemia
GM-CSF	Aplastic anemia
	Myelodysplasia
G-CSF	Congenital neutropenia
	Chemotherapy-induced neutropenia
	Cyclic neutropenia

means. They include diarrhea, asthenia, rash, malaise, fever, headache, bone pain, chills, and myalgia. Many of these effects can be ameliorated by the administration of analgesics and antipyretics.

Other Cytokines

Human recombinant interferon-α(rIFN-α) and rIL-1 also show promise as immunostimulators, principally as adjuvants in the treatment of viral and malignant disorders.

rIFN-α is produced by leukocytes and inhibits viral DNA and RNA replication. At lower doses, it can stimulate macrophages, T lymphocytes, and natural killer cell activity.

rIL-1 is produced by macrophages in the host and is necessary for activation and development of immune cells. Intravenous administration of rIL-1 is associated with the general augmentation of immune responses.

rIL-6 is a protein that stimulates lymphocyte and megakaryocyte proliferation. It is in clinical trials in patients with refractory cancer and myelodysplastic syndrome. Trials also are ongoing with rIL-3, a multipotent factor that stimulates the growth of monocytes, erythrocytes, neutrophils, and megakaryocytes.

Study QUESTIONS

1. An Rh-negative mother gives birth to an Rh-positive baby. This is the mother's first child. Is immunotherapy necessary?
   (A) Yes. The mother should receive Rho(D) immune globulin to prevent hemolytic anemia in future neonates.
   (B) Yes. The mother's immune system reacted against the baby's T cells. Thymosin should be given to augment the baby's cellular immunity.
   (C) Yes. The mother's immune system reacted against the baby's B cells. Fetal interferon-γ should be given to augment the baby's humoral immunity.
   (D) No. Immunotherapy is not necessary, since this is the first child.
   (E) No. Immunotherapy would only have been necessary if the mother were Rh positive and baby Rh negative.

2. Cytotoxic agents such as azathioprine are effective immunosuppressants because they
   (A) Bind to and inactivate circulating immunocomplexes
   (B) Specifically inhibit IL-2 gene transcription
   (C) Prevent the clonal expansion of T and B cells by inhibiting purine synthesis
   (D) Induce the synthesis of antiidiotype antibodies
   (E) Alkylate and cross-link DNA, preventing blastogenesis

3. Interleukin-2 can be beneficial in the treatment of AIDS because it can
   (A) Attach to the HIV virus, making it more susceptible to phagocytosis
   (B) Bind to IL-2 receptors on responsive immune cells and stimulate the production of T helper and T cytotoxic cells.
   (C) Cross-link antibodies on mast cell surfaces leading to degranulation.
   (D) Activate the complement cascade by binding to the C5a fragment.
   (E) Inhibit T suppressor cell activity and thereby stimulating the immune response

4. A 4-year-old boy has significantly reduced levels of IgA, IgM, IgD and IgE in his blood. Testing demonstrates that he did not develop the appropriate antibody titer following standard childhood vaccinations. The most probable cause of these deficiencies is
   (A) Deficiency in macrophage function that is preventing the proper presentation of antigens to T cells
   (B) Lack of a specific component of the complement cascade
   (C) Alcohol abuse by the mother during pregnancy
   (D) A primary immunodeficiency disease that is blocking the maturation of B cells into plasma cells
   (E) An autoimmune disease targeted at basophil surface receptors

5. Which of the following best describes the side effects of cyclosporine therapy?
   (A) Leukopenia, hypotension, hemolytic anemia
   (B) Nephrotoxicity, neurotoxicity, hirsutism
   (C) Thrombocytopenia, hypokalemia
   (D) Hemorrhagic cystitis, hypoglycemia
   (E) Increase circulating immune complexes, cardiac arrhythmia

ANSWERS

1. **A.** An Rh-negative mother can develop antibodies against the Rh antigen if she is exposed to the blood of an Rh-positive baby during pregnancy or birth. If no therapy is given, hemolytic anemia can occur in future Rh-positive babies. Rho(D) immune globulin contains antibodies against the Rh antigen. Administered to the mother, it will destroy any red blood cells from the baby that entered her blood, preventing the mother from developing an immune response to the Rh antigen.

2. **C.** Azathioprine is a phase-specific cytotoxic agent that functions by inhibiting purine synthesis. The other answers are wrong because azathioprine is nonspecific, is not an alkylating agent, has no effect on immune complexes, and does not induce antibody synthesis.

3. **B.** IL-2 stimulates the immune system by binding to the IL-2 receptors on responsive immune cells, causing differentiation and proliferation of T helper and T cytotoxic cells. It has no direct effect on the HIV virus, complement. or basophils.

4. **D.** The boy has significantly reduced serum antibody levels and a reduced ability to mount an antibody response to childhood vaccinations. The most probably cause is a primary immunodeficiency disease affecting humoral immunity.

5. **B.** The primary side effect of cyclosporine therapy is nephrotoxicity, occurring in up to 75% of cases. Unwanted hair growth and neurotoxicity are also commonly noted. The other answers are wrong because cyclosporine therapy is associated with hypertension, hyperkalemia, and hyperglycemia. There are no references to cyclosporine having cardiac or immune complex effects or causing hemorrhagic cystitis.

SUPPLEMENTAL READING

Campistol JM and Grinyo JM. Exploring treatment options in renal transplantation: The problems of chronic allograft dysfunction and drug-related nephrotoxicity. Transplantation 2001;71:SS42–SS51.

Gorantla VS et al. Immunosuppressive agents in transplantation: Mechanisms of action and current anti-rejection strategies. Microsurgery 2000;20:420–429.

Graham RM. Cyclosporine: Mechanism of action and toxicity. Cleveland Clin I Med 1994;61:308–313.

Kupiec-Weglinski JW. New Immunosuppressive Modalities and Anti-rejection Approaches in Organ Transplantation. Boca Raton, FL: CRC, 1994.

Nakamura T and Matsumoto K. Growth Factors: Cell Growth, Morphogenesis, and Transformation. Boca Raton, FL: CRC, 1994.

Nicola NA (ed.). Guidebook to Cytokines and Their Receptors. New York: Oxford University Press, 1995.

Yin EZ, Frush DP, Donnelly LF, and Buckley RH. Primary immunodeficiency disorders in pediatric patients: Clinical features and imaging findings. Am J Roentgenol 2001;176:1541–1552.

CASE **Study** **Adverse Reactions to Transplantation**

Four weeks after receiving a bone marrow transplant, Mary Smith developed jaundice and a skin rash on her hands, feet, and face. She also had occasional episodes of vomiting and diarrhea. Clinical chemistry results showed her serum liver enzymes (LDH, ALT) and bilirubin level to be elevated. What is the most likely cause of Mary's symptoms and what is the best therapy?

ANSWER: Ms. Smith has an acute graft-versus-host (GVH) reaction. Such reactions usually occur when immunologically competent cells are introduced into an immunocompromised host. When they develop, it is usually within 100 days following transplant. In choosing tissues and organs for transplantation, the HLA antigens of donors and patients are matched as closely as possible to decrease the risk of rejection. However many minor antigenic markers that can cause immunological incompatibility differ between individuals. In this case, T lymphocytes from the donor's bone marrow are attacking her skin, liver, stomach, and intestines. Patients with GVH reactions are already receiving cyclosporine or other immunosuppressive therapy. When a GVH reaction is diagnosed, treatment with corticosteroids, such as prednisone and prednisolone, is usually added.

58 | Gene Therapy

John S. Lazo and Jennifer Rubin Grandis

Most drugs used today are designed to treat symptoms rather than cure the underlying disease. Notable exceptions include cytotoxic chemotherapeutic agents, as described in Chapter 56, and agents that restore or modulate hormone function, as outlined in Chapter 57. However, increased understanding of the molecular and genetic etiology of diseases may permit permanent modification of organ function by drug-oriented methods. The first disease-associated gene, β-globin, was cloned over 25 years ago. It is now theoretically possible to isolate, sequence, and analyze genes causally associated with many heritable and acquired human diseases, including cystic fibrosis, Duchenne's muscular dystrophy, and Gaucher's disease. Moreover, with the complete sequencing of the human genome, many of the estimated 100,000 human genes may become candidates for genetic manipulations. Thus, it is now possible to propose molecular pharmacological and genetic approaches to therapy. Many of these approaches fall under the general rubric of *gene therapy*.

Germ cell gene therapy will require considerable discussion about ethical issues and extensive information before it can be applied to humans, but somatic cell gene therapy in humans is now being extensively explored. During the past 5 years in the United States alone, more than 500 human gene therapy clinical trials aimed at treating conditions ranging from inherited disorders such as cystic fibrosis to cancer and AIDS, have been approved by the Office of Biotechnology Activities (OBA, formerly the Recombinant DNA Advisory Committee) of the National Institutes of Health. Nearly 3500 patients have been enrolled in these studies (Fig. 58.1).

With few exceptions, gene therapy was considered safe if not particularly effective until the death of an 18-year-old man in 1999, the first fatal outcome for a pa-

tient in a phase I gene therapy protocol. This death has stimulated a substantial review of the oversight mechanisms in human gene transfer research. One of the first successes of gene therapy was reported in 2000, when three infants with a fatal form of severe combined immunodeficiency syndrome (SCID) received ex vivo gene therapy with a recombinant mouse leukemia viral vector encoding the γC receptor gene. After 10 months, γC transgene expression in T- and NK cells was detected and T-, B-, and NK-cell counts and function were comparable to those of age-matched controls.

Although numerous obstacles must be overcome before gene therapy will be routinely employed, a rigorous approach to investigating the safety and efficacy of gene transfer will ensure that clinical strategies employing genetic manipulation are rationally incorporated into the therapeutic armamentarium.

GENE THERAPY: DEFINITION AND GOALS

The broadest definition of human gene therapy includes the in vivo (direct administration of the gene therapy formulation) and ex vivo (transfection of cells in tissue culture by gene therapy followed by administration of the transfected material into the patient) transfer of defined genetic material to cells of patients. Principles of gene therapy include transfer of one or more transgenes to prevent a disease, prevent an adverse consequence of a disease, or facilitate recovery from the consequence. Although most of the controversy and excitement have centered on the transfer of functional genes, the therapeutic potential of genes that abrogate aberrant function (e.g. antisense and ribonucleic acid–based strate-

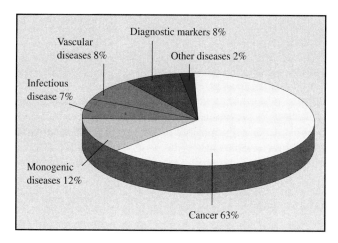

FIGURE 58.1
Proposed uses or targets of human gene therapy trials. During the past 5 years in the United States more than 500 human gene therapy clinical trials have been approved by the Office of Biotechnology Activities of the National Institutes of Health.

gies) should also be considered. Two fundamental approaches underlie the basis of gene therapy. In the first, genetic material is introduced into cells to alter the cellular phenotype but not the genotype. This is typified by the transfer of unintegrated DNA, antisense oligomers, and ribozymes. In this regard, gene therapy has many of the attributes and problems of conventional endocrine or antimicrobial therapy with respect to efficiency of targeting and the duration of effect. A second approach seeks permanent alteration of the genotype of the cell, leading to a modified phenotype that prevents or alters a disease state. In this setting, gene therapy will permanently modify organ function.

Theoretically, mutated or nonfunctional genes could be excised and replaced, and new genes with desired functions could be permanently inserted into the genome. Stable integration of an antisense DNA might also be desirable in some circumstances. Because of the technical difficulties associated with the delivery of nucleic acid–based products selectively to specific target cells in vivo, more experimental information is available for ex vivo human gene therapy.

ANTISENSE

The antisense approach is use of nucleic acids to reduce the expression of a specific target gene. As shown in Figure 58.2, a small piece of DNA, an oligodeoxynucleotide that is in the reverse orientation (antisense) to a portion of a target messenger RNA (mRNA) species, is introduced into a cell and a DNA–RNA duplex is formed by complementary Watson-Crick base pairing. Cessation of protein synthesis then may result from the rapid

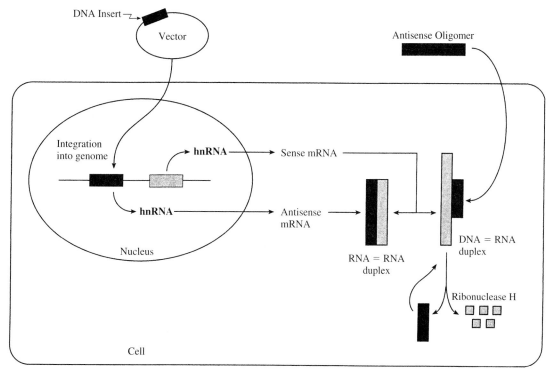

FIGURE 58.2
Translation arrest or nuclease digestion by exogenously applied antisense oligonucleotides or by antisense mRNA produced from DNA delivered by a plasmid. Heterogeneous nuclear RNA is hnRNA.

degradation of the mRNA species due to activation of ribonuclease H or disruption of translation. Cells and organisms protect themselves against foreign DNA and RNA by producing nucleases that degrade phosphodiester bonds in oligodeoxynucleotides. Chemical modification of the phosphodiester moiety can produce nuclease-resistant oligomers. In the two most common chemical analogues, the backbone phosphate is replaced either with a methyl group to form a methyl phosphonate or with a sulfur group to form a phosphorothioate (Fig. 58.3). These modifications grant extra stability to the oligonucleotides, allowing for a longer half-life in vivo.

The antisense RNA can also be generated within cells after delivery via a plasmid or attenuated virus containing a suitable promoter that controls expression of the antisense strand using methods of gene insertion described later (Fig. 58.2). In addition to the strict antisense strategies, several related approaches have been considered. Catalytic RNA, catalytic DNA, or ribozymes capable of degrading complementary mRNA may decrease translation of targeted sequences. Oligomers designed to interact with genes directly via Hoogsteen hydrogen binding in a triplex formation have been suggested as a means of disrupting transcrip-

tion (Fig. 58.4). Transcription factor decoys that are duplexes designed to bind to a particular transcription factor and prevent its normal function are another approach examined in the context of NFκB blockade. These strategies, like antisense itself, do not require integration into the genome, and thus they share the pharmacological problems of absorption, distribution, metabolism, and elimination of any traditional drug not based on nucleic acid.

GENE EXCISION AND REPLACEMENT

Diseases at a genetic level can result from several causes, including (1) mutation in a gene, (2) loss of expression of a gene, (3) elevated expression of a gene, or (4) expression of a pathogenic viral or foreign gene. In each case, gene replacement or excision therapy might be desirable. Theoretically, the disease gene could be replaced through a homologous recombination event. Depending on the design of the replacement gene, it also would be possible to engineer stop codons or nonsense sequences into the internal domains of a gene to ensure loss of protein production. Excision of an entire

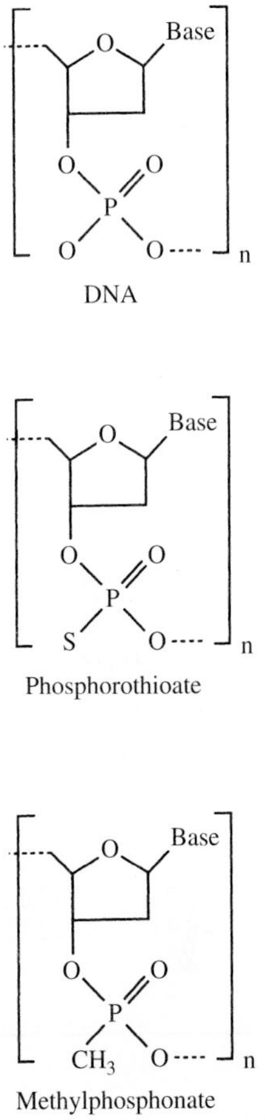

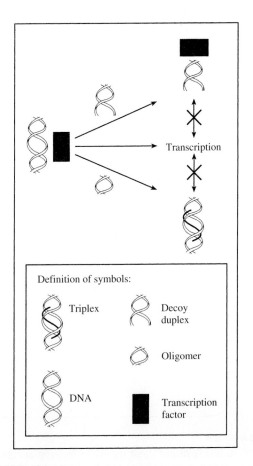

FIGURE 58.3

Chemical structures of oligodeoxynucleotides and the analogues used in gene therapy.

FIGURE 58.4

Theoretical mechanism of transcription disruption by oligomers.

gene also is feasible. This strategy, however, requires extremely efficient and specific homologous recombination events in the target cell population. Such strategies have allowed for the development of knockout animals, but to date have not been practical for human somatic cell gene therapy. Ongoing investigations are exploring the feasibility of inducible vectors, use of the cre-lox system, or cell type specific promoters to optimize gene expression in target cells.

GENE ADDITION

A more practical approach has been to permit the introduced genes to integrate into the genome in a site-nonspecific manner. The newly added gene could then function to provide a missing or mutated gene product (Fig. 58.5A). *This is the approach of most current gene therapy protocols and is exemplified by the development of clinical trials for adenosine deaminase (ADA) defi-*

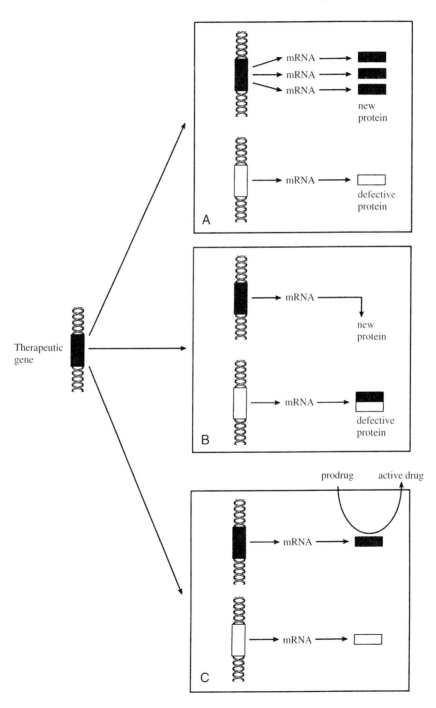

FIGURE 58.5

Possible mechanisms by which inserted therapeutic genes may alter cellular function. **A.** Gene addition with return to a normal phenotype. **B.** Dominant-negative or phenotype deletion. **C.** Gene addition to a unique phenotype, such as an enzyme that activates a prodrug.

ciency, which is an example of inherited SCID. ADA is a reasonable target for these reasons: (1) It is an autosomal recessive disorder in which a defect in a single gene produces absence of or diminished ADA activity with fatal combined immunodeficiency. (2) ADA expression is characteristic of a normal maintenance gene with considerable variation in the normal ADA levels, suggesting that stringent regulation of expression is unnecessary. (3) A significant level of expression is not required to correct the phenotype. (4) Ex vivo gene transfer studies can be conducted. (5) Replacement of ADA may reduce the production of toxic DNA metabolites and thus provide a growth advantage for transfected cells.

For ethical reasons, children enrolled in these clinical trials have also received standard therapy of enzyme infusions, so the results of these studies have been difficult to interpret and are controversial. Nevertheless, there is some evidence that the ex vivo gene transfer approach may evoke a biological response relevant to the treatment of ADA deficiency. Such interpretations have stimulated efforts to use the ex vivo strategy for other monogenic disorders, such as familial hypercholesterolemia, hemophilia B, and Gaucher's disease.

Alternatively, the introduced gene could generate a protein that acts to block or suppress the function of another undesirable protein in a dominant-negative manner (Fig. 58.5*B*). Last, the introduced gene could result in the production of an entirely new and unique protein that provides the recipient cell with a desirable phenotype (Fig. 58.5*C*). In theory, an enzyme required for the metabolic activation of a prodrug could be expressed, leading to the desired pharmacological activity near the genetically altered cell. This approach is used in cancer gene therapy in which tumor cells are transfected with a gene encoding for an enzyme such as thymidine kinase in the presence of systemic administration of a nontoxic prodrug. The transfected enzyme in the tumor cells converts the prodrug, such as ganciclovir, to an active cytotoxic compound. Theoretically, such an approach selectively kills tumor cells and is nontoxic to untransfected cells. Clinical trials to assess the safety and efficacy of enzyme–prodrug cancer therapy are under way.

DELIVERY SYSTEMS

In many cell types it is feasible to deliver nucleic acids and genes by a variety of methods when the cells are grown in tissue culture (Table 58.1). Nonetheless, some cells, such as pneumocytes and neurons, are not readily isolated from humans and do not grow well in vitro. Furthermore, for many diseases it is essential to alter the phenotype of a significant proportion of the total cell population, making ex vivo gene therapy of limited use.

There is general agreement that no ideal delivery system is available for in vivo gene therapy. Direct or intratumoral injection of plasmid DNA or antisense oligomers without a viral vector has been attempted. Expression of genes using traditional nonviral vectors has been low compared to viral strategies. Nonetheless, recent breakthroughs in nonviral delivery systems, including the gene gun, electroporation and naked DNA, suggest that nonviral gene therapy can achieve local expression of therapeutic genes at levels equivalent to those of viral vectors.

Although the mechanism remains undetermined, the injection of naked DNA into skeletal muscle has demonstrated relatively high transfection efficiency. In this setting, DNA is precipitated onto the surface of microscopic metal beads (e.g., gold) and the microprojectiles are accelerated and penetrate intact tissue to several cell layers.

TABLE 58.1   Vectors Approved for Human Use by the U. S. Office of Biotechnology Activities

Vector	Advantages	Disadvantages
Nonviral		
Liposomes	No replication risk, nonimmunogenic, useful for plasmids or viruses	Limited efficiency
Naked or particle-mediated DNA	No replication risk	Moderate efficiency, nonspecific cell targeting
Viral		
Retrovirus	Efficient transfer, manufacturing easy, most commonly used	Small DNA capacity (9 kb), random DNA insertion, targets only dividing cells, replication risk
Adenovirus	Infects nonproliferating cells, noninte-grating	Immunogenic, small DNA capacity (7.5 kb), replication risk, repeated injections required for long-term expression
Adeno-associated virus	Low immunogenicity, targets nonproliferating cells, may have discrete genome insertion sites	Difficult to manufacture, low titer
Herpesvirus	Targets central nervous system, low immunogenicity	Difficult to manufacture, host toxicity

In preclinical trials, efficiency remains low, but expression has been noted to last for several weeks, and there has been no significant inflammatory response.

Some investigators have used electrical current (*electroporation*) to improve DNA (or drug) entry into tumor cells with some preliminary success. Liposomes are attractive vehicles for gene delivery, since they can carry plasmid, antisense, or viral DNA. Compared with viral approaches, however, liposomes remain relatively inefficient at facilitating gene transfer, although their safety profile remains more desirable. Some of the attributes and limitations of the nonviral methods are listed in Table 58.1.

Because viruses can efficiently integrate into the genome, many clinical trials are exploring the use of *replication-defective recombinant viral vectors* and delivery systems. Retroviruses contain their genetic information as a double-strand DNA genome that is transcribed, and the single-strand proviral DNA product is stably integrated into the host genome. Recombinant DNA technology has been used to remove deleterious viral genes involved in replication, and the resulting vector is replication defective, nonpathogenic, and unable to produce infectious particles. Ideally, with a retroviral vector, only a single administration should be required because the gene should be permanently retained and expressed. No clinical evidence of mutagenesis has emerged from the clinical trials performed to date, but the number of patients treated and the time of exposure has been limited.

Adenoviral vectors have also been used in human trials. These vectors enter cells by either an adenovirus fiber–specific receptor or a surface integrin receptor. They efficiently transfer genes in nonreplicating and replicating cells. Nonetheless, immunological responses to viruses have been noted with adenoviral vectors. *Replication-selective adenovirus vectors* have been introduced to optimize infection of target cells and minimize infection of normal cells. Over 200 cancer patients have been treated to date in more than 10 clinical trials with little evidence of toxicity reported. Replication, however, has generally been transient (<10 days), with limited efficacy observed when the gene therapy was administered as a single agent. More encouraging antitumor effects have been observed when the gene therapy was combined with cytotoxic chemotherapy. Further modifications are likely to be required before there can be general application of adenoviral vectors for cancer therapy.

DISEASE APPLICATION AND FUTURE DIRECTIONS

Antisense clinical trials, most with phosphorothioates, have been directed toward blocking viral production in patients with AIDS or genital warts, disrupting the func-

tionality of protooncogenes in cancer, blocking immune cell activity after kidney transplantation, treating rheumatoid arthritis, or influencing autoimmune diseases. Studies to date have not reported marked clinical efficacy, which might be due to protein binding and poor entry into cells. Additional chemical modifications and possibly the use of carriers, such as liposomes, may improve drug delivery and utility.

A proportion of the human gene therapy trials approved by the OBA seek to correct a single-gene defect, such as adenosine deaminase deficiency, glucocerebrosidase deficiency in Gaucher's disease, or the mutated chloride transport gene in cystic fibrosis. The major difficulties limiting success have been immunogenicity associated with the vector delivery system, low transfection efficiency, and transient transgene expression.

Most human gene therapy trials are designed to express a new gene product that facilitates the correction of a disease process, such as cancer. Almost half of the current gene therapy–based protocols in the United States are aimed at boosting the immune response to tumor antigens. Thus, there are attempts to express the lymphokine interleukin-2 in tumor cells to stimulate a natural immune response against the producing tumor cell and its malignant neighbors. In other types of studies, malignant cells infected with a vector that encodes a tumor suppressor gene, p53, lead to growth arrest, apoptosis or enhanced sensitivity to cytotoxic agents. Others have used vectors encoding the herpesvirus protein thymidine kinase that target cells for killing when exposed to the antiviral prodrug ganciclovir; this is known as *suicide gene therapy*. Similarly, attempts are being made to produce HIV-infected cells that express thymidine kinase or other enzymes that activate the nontoxic prodrugs to cytotoxic compounds. Disruption of viral functions with decoy molecules that compete with, sequester, or cleave products produced by HIV also is being examined.

Most of these trials have been early phase I or II studies that are designed to evaluate safety rather than efficacy of the gene therapy formulation. Results of ongoing and pending phase III studies will more precisely place the role of gene therapy in a clinical context. Although the feasibility of human gene transfer has been demonstrated in the completed clinical trials, there has been a paucity of evidence to support the efficacy and reliability of gene transfer approaches. Future gene therapy studies will capitalize on preclinical efforts to improve cellular targeting, gene transfer efficiency, and sustained expression. Regulation of the expression of the introduced transgene would be desirable, and use of cell type–specific promoters, such as the actin or surfactant promoter, or drug-controlled promoters, such as the tetracycline promoter, are being examined in preclinical models.

Study QUESTIONS

1. Severe combined immunodeficiency (SCID) syndromes are excellent models for gene therapy because of the genetic basis of these disorders and significant advances in the technology to transfer therapeutic genes into hematopoietic precursor cells. For all these reasons, which of the following syndromes represents an ideal candidate for gene therapy?
   (A) B-cell deficiency
   (B) DiGeorge's syndrome
   (C) γC Deficiency
   (D) Adenine deaminase deficiency
   (E) T-cell deficiency

2. All of the following are desirable characteristics in the design of a gene therapy vector EXCEPT
   (A) Ability to produce at high titer on a commercial scale
   (B) Ability to transfect both dividing and nondividing cells
   (C) Ability to produce site-specific integration into the chromosome of the target cell
   (D) Ability to limit size of genetic material it can deliver
   (E) Ability to deliver only certain cell types

3. A patient with ornithine transcarbamylase (OTC) deficiency is being treated in a gene therapy clinical trial. The gene therapy approach for this disease is primarily designed to
   (A) Replace the enzyme ornithine transcarbamylase
   (B) Decrease the accumulation of ammonia
   (C) Eliminate the need for a modified diet
   (D) Target a protooncogene
   (E) Enhance the immune system

4. A 25-year-old hemophiliac is interested in receiving gene therapy. He should contemplate all of the following approaches EXCEPT
   (A) Intravenous infusion of a retroviral vector expressing the B-domain-deleted factor VIII
   (B) Ex vivo transfection of autologous fibroblasts transfected with a plasmid encoding B-domain-deleted factor VIII
   (C) Intravenous adenoviral-mediated delivery of factor VIII
   (D) Adeno-associated virus (AAV) vector delivered to skeletal muscle
   (E) Retroviral vector expressing B-domain deleted factor VIII transfected into dermal fibroblasts that are then reimplanted

5. A patient with advanced inoperable squamous cell carcinoma of the head and neck receives a replication-selective adenovirus on a gene therapy clinical trial. The rationale for the use of this treatment:

(A) Deletion of viral genes will reduce toxicity of the viral vector to normal cells.
(B) Deletion of a p53 inhibitory protein will be selective for tumors that have lost p53 function.
(C) Deletion of a key regulatory sequence will allow for induction of the therapeutic gene in tumor cells.
(D) Results of preclinical studies suggest that only tumor cells are affected by this treatment.
(E) Clinical results support that only patients with p53 mutations in their tumors respond to the treatment.

ANSWERS

1. **C.** SCID-X1 (γC deficiency) is an optimal model for gene therapy because there is little γC gene transcription regulation; γC expression is ubiquitous and constitutive among different hematopoietic lineages; and γC exerts no autonomous function.

2. **D.** The vector should have no size limit to the genetic material it can deliver. The coding sequence of a therapeutic gene can vary from several hundred base pairs to more than 10,000 base pairs. In addition, the requirement for appropriate regulatory sequences may be required for efficient transduction and expression of the therapeutic DNA. The ability to produce a high titer on a commercial scale is essential to carry out large-scale tests. It is necessary to be able to transfer genes in nonreplicating and replicating cells. It is also important to optimize delivery to target cells and minimize delivery to normal cells.

3. **A.** OTC is a metabolic enzyme required to break down ammonia. Total lack of this enzyme leads to death shortly after birth owing to a buildup of ammonia. The partial presence of OTC also leads to accumulation of ammonia, which can be controlled by drugs and dietary intake. The genetic cause of this disease, its morbidity, and the need for rapid production of OTC by adenoviral vectors may extend the life span of OTC-deficient newborns to allow for drug treatment and dietary manipulation. Jesse Gelsinger, the 18-year-old patient who was the first patient to die on a phase I gene therapy trial, had OTC deficiency.

4. **C.** Systemic administration of adenoviral vectors has not been used in the treatment of hemophilia because of the transient gene expression and immunogenic consequences of adenoviral delivery. All of the other approaches are under investigation or have been published in the literature on treatment of hemophilia.

5. B. dl1520 (Onyx-015) was the first adenovirus developed with deletion of a gene encoding a p53-inhibitory protein, E1B-55kD, theoretically making it selective for tumor cells that have lost p53 function. Controversial data demonstrate that the mechanism of selectivity is more complex than originally thought. In addition, clinical results have demonstrated responses in patients whose tumors did not have mutant p53.

SUPPLEMENTAL READING

Huber BE and Lazo JS. (eds.). Gene therapy for neoplastic diseases. Ann N Y Acad Sci 1994;716;1–351.

Fischer A et al. Gene therapy for human severe combined immunodeficiencies. Immunity 2001;15:1–4.

Somia N and Verma IM. Gene therapy: Trials and tribulations. Nature Rev Genet 2000;1:91–99.

Friedman T, Noguchi P, and Mickelson C. The evolution of public review and oversight mechanisms in human gene transfer research: Joint roles of the FDA and NIH. Curr Opin Biotechnol 2001;12:304–307.

Mannucci PM and Tuddenham EGD. The hemophilias: From royal genes to gene therapy. N Engl J Med 2001;344:1773–1784.

Kirn D. Clinical research results with dl1520 (Onyz-015), a replication-selective adenovirus for the treatment of cancer: What have we learned? Gene Therapy 2001;8:89–98.

McCormick F. Cancer gene therapy: Fringe or cutting edge? Nature Rev Cancer 2001;1:130–141.

CASE Study   Cystic Fibrosis and Gene Therapy

Kris Allen was diagnosed with cystic fibrosis (CF) shortly after birth. Genetic analysis revealed that he had the most common form of dysfunction of the CF transmembrane conductance regulator gene (CFTR) leading to faulty processing and protein trafficking. His therapy to date has consisted of palliative treatments, such as daily physiotherapy to improve chest and lung function, pancreatic enzyme replacement, and a high calorie diet. Conventional treatment of his recurrent pulmonary disease is less and less effective, and he is interested in gene therapy. What would be a logical strategy for this patient?

Answer: Aerosol delivery of the CFTR gene. Both viruses and liposome–DNA complexes are capable of successful CFTR gene transfer to the nasal and airway epithelia of patients with CF. In fact, gene transfer to the airways is one of the few areas where liposome–DNA complexes match the expression obtained using viral vectors without the viruses' inflammatory side effects. Current trials are aimed at optimizing gene delivery with reduced toxicity to produce sustained correction of the epithelial transport defect.

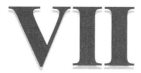

DRUGS AFFECTING
THE ENDOCRINE SYSTEM

59

Hypothalamic and Pituitary Gland Hormones

Priscilla S. Dannies

 DRUG LIST

GENERIC NAME	PAGE	GENERIC NAME	PAGE
Desmopressin	682	Oxytocin	683
Gonadotropin	681	Prolactin	679
Goserelin	682	Somatrem	679
Leuprolide	682	Somatropin	679
Octreotide	681	Vasopressin	682

The hormones of the pituitary gland participate in the control of reproductive function, body growth, and cellular metabolism; deficiency or overproduction of these hormones disrupts this control. Clinical use of protein hormones in the past was limited because preparations had to come from glands or urine. The ability to prepare at least some of these hormones in large quantities by recombinant DNA techniques and the development of more stable analogues that can be injected in a depot form permit increased and more effective use of these hormones.

ANTERIOR PITUITARY HORMONES

Six major hormones are secreted by the adenohypophysis, or anterior pituitary gland (Fig. 59.1). Cells in the anterior pituitary gland also secrete small amounts of a variety of other proteins, including renin, angiotensinogen, sulfated proteins, fibroblast growth factor, and other mitogenic factors. The physiological significance of these other secretory products is not known, but they may participate in autocrine regulation of the gland.

The secretion of anterior pituitary hormones is controlled in part by hypothalamic regulatory factors that are stored in the hypothalamus and are released into the adenohypophyseal portal vasculature. Hypothalamic regulatory factors so far identified are peptides with the exception of dopamine. Secretion of anterior pituitary hormones is also controlled by factors produced more distally that circulate in the blood. Predominant control of hormone production may be relatively simple, as with thyroid-stimulating hormone (TSH), the production of which is primarily stimulated by thyrotropin-releasing hormone (TRH) and inhibited by thyroid hormones, or it may be complex, as with prolactin, the production of which is affected by many neurotransmitters and hormones.

All anterior pituitary hormones are released into the bloodstream in a pulsatile manner; the secretion of many also varies with time of day or physiological conditions, such as exercise or sleep. At least part of the pulsatility of anterior hormone secretion is caused by pulsatile secretion of hypothalamic regulatory hormones. Understanding the rhythms that control hormone secretion has led to better uses of hormones in therapy.

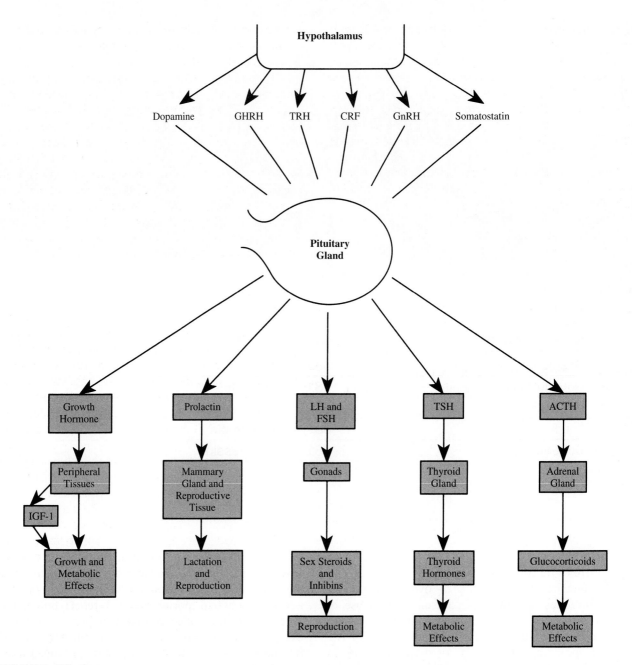

FIGURE 59.1

Hormones of the hypothalamus and the anterior pituitary gland. Hormones released from the hypothalamus are one of the major means of controlling secretion from the anterior pituitary gland. GHRH, growth hormone releasing hormone; TRH, thyrotropin releasing hormone; CRF, corticotropin releasing hormone; GnRH, gonadotropin releasing hormone; LH, luteinizing hormone; FSH, follicle-stimulating hormone; TSH, thyroid-stimulating hormone; ACTH, adrenocorticotropic hormone; IGF-1, insulinlike growth factor 1.

Growth Hormone

Growth hormone, or somatotropin, is a protein that stimulates linear body growth in children and regulates cellular metabolism in both adults and children. Growth hormone stimulates lipolysis, enhances production of free fatty acids, elevates blood glucose, and promotes positive nitrogen balance. Many of its anabolic actions are mediated by enhanced production of an insulinlike growth factor (IGF-1), a protein produced in many tissues in response to growth hormone.

The episodic release of growth hormone is the most pronounced among the pituitary hormones. Serum levels between bursts of release are usually low (<5 ng/mL) and increase more than 10-fold when release is elevated. The marked variation in serum levels is in part the result of strong controls in opposite directions by the hypothalamic hormones, growth hormone–releasing hormone (GHRH), and somatostatin. Circulating factors, such as IGF-1 and ghrelin, a peptide produced in large amounts in neuroendocrine cells of the stomach, also affect growth hormone secretion. Growth hormone is released during sleep, with maximum release occurring an hour after the onset of sleep. Growth hormone is also released after exercise, by hypoglycemia, and in response to arginine and levodopa.

Growth Hormone Deficiency

Growth hormone deficiency in children results in short stature and in adults increases fat mass and reduces muscle mass, energy, and bone density. Measurements of serum growth hormone levels are used for diagnosis of deficiency, but random measurements are not useful, because normal episodic release results in large variations in growth hormone levels. Growth hormone deficiency is most convincingly demonstrated by lack of response to provocative stimuli, such as administration of insulin, levodopa, or arginine. Recently a combination of GHRH and ghrelin have been used and have given large responses in normal subjects. Deficiencies are corrected by giving human growth hormone. Growth hormone is also sometimes given to individuals who are not growth hormone–deficient; it is used to increase the height of girls with Turner's syndrome and in certain conditions to counteract the wasting that may occur in AIDS.

In the past human growth hormone was prepared from human pituitary glands, but this source was discontinued after people who had received treatment contracted Creutzfeldt-Jakob disease. Now two forms of recombinant human growth hormone are available: somatropin (*Humatrope* and others), which has the same amino acid sequence as pituitary-derived growth hormone, and somatrem (*Protropin*), which has an *N*-terminal methionine that the pituitary form does not. Subcutaneous injections each evening, which mimic the natural surge that occurs at the start of sleep, are the usual regimen. Stimulation of growth in children is most effective when treatment begins early.

Growth Hormone Excess

Acromegaly results from chronic secretion of excess growth hormone, usually as a result of pituitary adenoma. Long bones will not grow in adults because the epiphyses are closed, but bones of the extremities (hands, feet, jaw, and nose) will enlarge. The skin and soft tissues thicken, and the viscera enlarge. Excessive growth hormone secretion is demonstrated by elevated serum levels of growth hormone after glucose administration, since glucose is less effective in inhibiting

growth hormone secretion in acromegalics than it is in normal subjects. In addition, serum IGF-1 levels are elevated in acromegalics.

The primary treatment of acromegaly is surgery. Pharmacotherapy is used when surgical treatment is not successful. Two dopamine agonists (see Chapter 31), bromocriptine and cabergoline, are sometimes effective; they are taken orally. Although dopamine stimulates growth hormone release in normal individuals, it inhibits growth hormone release in up to 50% of acromegalics. The somatostatin analogue octreotide is usually more effective, and now that a long-acting form is available that requires only monthly injections, it is the preferred treatment. Another possible growth hormone antagonist, pegvisomant, is being investigated.

Prolactin

Human prolactin is similar in structure to human growth hormone, and both are good lactogens. In women, prolactin acts with other hormones on the mammary gland during pregnancy to develop lactation and after birth to maintain it. Hyperprolactinemia causes impotence in men and amenorrhea and infertility in women. Chronically elevated levels of circulating prolactin are associated with suppression of 17-β-estradiol and testosterone production in the ovaries and testes.

Prolactin serum levels increase during pregnancy and breast-feeding, at least immediately after the birth. In both men and women, prolactin increases after sleep starts, continues to increase during the night, and increases markedly during stress. Prolactin release is episodic during the day. More than 20 hormones and neurotransmitters affect prolactin production, but the dominant physiological control is primarily negative, mediated by dopamine from the hypothalamus. Dopaminergic agonists inhibit prolactin release and antagonists, such as the antipsychotic drugs, increase release.

There is no known therapeutic use for prolactin, but serum levels are measured to diagnose hyperprolactinemia. The normal range of serum prolactin is 1 to 20 ng/mL. Elevated prolactin levels (>100 ng/mL) in the absence of stimulatory factors, such as antipsychotic drugs, are an indication of pituitary adenoma. Approximately one-third of women who need treatment for infertility have high serum prolactin levels. Galactorrhea, or inappropriate lactation, is sometimes associated with high prolactin levels. Hyperprolactinemia has been traditionally treated by the dopaminergic agonist bromocriptine (*Parodel*). The doses, usually 5 mg/day, are lower than those used to treat Parkinson's disease, and therefore, the side effects, nausea and postural hypotension, are less likely to cause problems. More recently, however, the more potent, long-lasting dopaminergic agonist cabergoline (*Dostinex*) has been found to be at least as effective and has a lower incidence of side effects.

Thyroid-Stimulating Hormone

TSH, or thyrotropin, is a glycosylated protein of two subunits, α and β. TSH stimulates the thyroid gland to produce thyroid hormones. Deficiencies are treated by giving thyroxine itself rather than TSH, but TSH is available for diagnostic purposes to differentiate between pituitary and thyroid gland failure as causes of hypothyroidism (see Chapter 65).

Gonadotropins

Follicle-stimulating hormone (FSH), luteinizing hormone (LH), and human chorionic gonadotropin (hCG) are glycoproteins that are similar in structure to TSH. Glycosylation is not identical among the different hormones, and the type of glycosylation influences the half-life of the hormones. A sulfated *N*-acetylgalactosamine attached to LH but not FSH causes LH to be more rapidly metabolized; the half-life of LH is 30 minutes and that of FSH is 8 hours.

LH and FSH are pituitary hormones secreted in pulsatile fashion approximately every 2 hours. In women before menopause, this pattern is superimposed on much larger changes that occur during the normal menstrual cycle. FSH is released in substantial amounts during the follicular phase of the menstrual cycle and is required for proper development of ovarian follicles and for estrogen synthesis from granulosa cells of the ovary. Most LH secretion occurs in an abrupt burst just before ovulation. LH is required for progesterone synthesis in luteal cells and androgen synthesis in thecal cells of the ovary. FSH stimulates spermatogenesis and synthesis of androgen-binding protein in Sertoli cells of the testes. LH stimulates testosterone production from Leydig cells. Production of LH and FSH is controlled by gonadotropin-releasing hormone (GnRH) from the hypothalamus and by feedback control from target organs through steroids and multiple forms of a protein, inhibin.

Injections of these hormones are used to treat infertility in women and men. Traditional sources of gonadotropins are from human urine. Human menopausal gonadotropins (menotropins, *Humegon, Pergonal*) are isolated from urine of postmenopausal women and contain both FSH and LH. Purified preparations of FSH from the same source are also available (urofollitropin, *Fertinex, Fertinorm HP*). During early pregnancy, trophoblasts of the placenta produce hCG in large amounts. LH and hCG bind to the same gonadal receptors, but hCG is more stable and can be isolated from urine of pregnant women, so hGH preparations (*Pregnyl, Profasi*) are used to mimic the burst of LH secretion before ovulation. Recombinant preparations of FSH are also available (follitropin, *Gonal F, Follistim*).

Gonadotropins are used to treat infertility in women with potentially functional ovaries who have not responded to other treatments. The therapy is designed to simulate the normal menstrual cycle as far as is practical. A common protocol is daily injections of menotropins for 9 to 12 days, until estradiol levels are equal to that in a normal woman, followed by a single dose of hCG to induce ovulation. Two problems with this treatment are risks of ovarian hyperstimulation and of multiple births. Ovarian hyperstimulation is characterized by sudden ovarian enlargement associated with an increase in vascular permeability and rapid accumulation of fluid in peritoneal, pleural, and pericardial cavities. To prevent such occurrences, ovarian development is monitored during treatment by ultrasound techniques and by measurements of serum levels of estradiol.

Purified FSH is used to prepare follicles for in vitro fertilization because LH activity in menotropins may cause premature ovulation. Purified FSH is also used to treat infertility in women with polycystic ovarian disease; in this disease LH and androgen production may already be elevated.

Gonadotropins are used to induce spermatogenesis in hypogonadotropic hypogonadal men; a lengthy treatment is required to obtain mature sperm. For several weeks hCG is injected to increase testosterone levels, followed by injections of menotropins for several months. Prepubertal cryptorchidism can be treated by injections of hCG for up to several months.

Adrenocorticotropic Hormone

Adrenocorticotropic hormone (ACTH), or corticotropin, a peptide of 39 amino acids, is first synthesized as a larger precursor from which ACTH is derived by proteolytic cleavage. ACTH stimulates production of glucocorticoids from the adrenal cortex (see Chapter 60). Release of ACTH depends on diurnal rhythms with serum levels highest in the early morning. Secretion of this peptide also increases under stress. It is easier and less expensive to treat patients having adrenocortical insufficiency with glucocorticoid replacement therapy than it is to use ACTH. Therefore, use of ACTH (*Acthar*) is restricted to diagnosis; a shorter 24–amino acid analogue (*Cosyntropin*) is also used. Intravenous administration of ACTH should result in peak plasma levels of glucocorticoids within 30 to 60 minutes if the adrenal gland is functional. Prolonged administration of ACTH in a repository form, however, may be necessary to stimulate steroid production, because ACTH has long-term trophic effects on adrenal cells in addition to the rapid stimulation of steroid production. If the cause of steroid deficiency is at the level of the pituitary gland, ACTH should eventually stimulate steroid production.

HYPOTHALAMIC REGULATORY HORMONES

Five peptides isolated from the hypothalamus regulate release of one or more pituitary hormones. In addition, dopamine released from the hypothalamus inhibits prolactin production.

Somatostatin

Somatostatin (or somatotropin release–inhibiting factor [SRIF]) occurs primarily as a 14–amino acid peptide, although a 28–amino acid form also exists. As with the other hypothalamic peptides, it is formed by proteolytic cleavage of a larger precursor. Somatostatin, originally isolated from the hypothalamus, is also in many other locations, including the cerebral cortex, brainstem, spinal cord, gut, urinary system, and skin. Somatostatin inhibits the secretion of many substances in addition to growth hormone (Table 59.1).

Somatostatin has a very brief half-life in serum and is not useful clinically. An 8–amino acid analogue with 2 D-amino acids substituted for the naturally occurring L-amino acids is more stable, and monthly injections of a depot form of this analogue (octreotide, *Sandostatin LAR*) have several uses. Long-acting octreotide is used to treat acromegaly, as described earlier. It is also used to counteract unpleasant effects caused by overproduction of secreted bioactive substances produced by neuroendocrine tumors, including hyperinsulinemia from insulinomas and secretions from carcinoid tumors that cause severe diarrhea. Octreotide may also control severe diarrhea associated with AIDS that has not responded to other treatments.

Transient side effects, gastrointestinal discomfort and decreased glucose tolerance, usually last only a few weeks after initiation of therapy. The most significant side effect associated with prolonged use of octreotide is formation of gallstones resulting from reduced bile flow.

Thyrotropin-Releasing Hormone

Thyrotropin-releasing hormone, or protirelin, consists of three amino acids. TRH (*Relefact TRH*) is used for tests to distinguish primary from secondary hypothyroidism (see Chapter 65).

Gonadotropin-Releasing Hormone

GnRH (gonadorelin, luteinizing hormone–releasing hormone) is a decapeptide that stimulates production of LH and FSH. It is released in bursts from the hypothalamus at regular intervals, about every 2 hours, although in women the interval may lengthen in the luteal end of the menstrual cycle. The pituitary gland responds to these regular pulses by producing LH and FSH. The pattern of LH and FSH in cycling women, including the large burst of LH release before ovulation, can be stimulated by regular administration of GnRH pulses. The large burst of LH from the pituitary gland appears to be induced by feedback through estradiol and other products of the gonads that change the response of the pituitary gland to the GnRH pulses rather than by large changes in the amounts of GnRH secreted. The stimulatory response to GnRH depends on pulsatile administration and the timing of the pulses. Continual administration of GnRH does not have the same effects as pulsatile administration; although production of LH and FSH is stimulated initially, it is suppressed within a few days. Part of this desensitization to GnRH is caused by a decrease in the number of pituitary receptors for GnRH; additional postreceptor mechanisms are also important in this complete suppression.

GnRH itself has a short half-life, 7 minutes, if given intravenously. Structural variations of the decapeptide have resulted in more stable analogues with higher affinity for the GnRH receptor; a common modification is to substitute a D-amino acid for the sixth amino acid, glycine, in GnRH.

Gonadotropin Stimulation

When stimulation of gonadotropin production is needed, the pituitary gland is usually capable of responding to appropriately administered GnRH, even in cases of hypogonadotropic hypogonadism, when LH and FSH levels are always low. Therefore, GnRH therapy can be substituted for gonadotropin therapy by administering GnRH (*Lutrepulse*) pulses intravenously via an indwelling pump. GnRH itself is used, since the short half-life is important to prevent accumulation between pulses. The advantage of this procedure compared with intramuscular injections of gonadotropins

---

TABLE 59.1 Effects of Somatostatin

Inhibition of secretion of
  Growth hormone
  Thyroid-stimulating hormone
  Prolactin
  ACTH
  Insulin
  Glucagon
  Pancreatic polypeptide
  Gastrin
  Cholecystokinin
  Secretin
  Vasoactive intestinal peptide
  Exocrine pancreas secretion
Inhibition of bile flow
Inhibition of mesenteric blood flow
Decreased gastrointestinal motility

for treating infertility is that normal levels of LH and FSH should be maintained because of feedback from the gonads. This should reduce the risk of ovarian hyperstimulation and multiple births, since the procedure should not result in inappropriately high levels of gonadotropins (Table 59.2).

Gonadotropin Suppression

Stable potent derivatives of GnRH include leuprolide (*Lupron*) and goserelin (*Zoladex*). Because these agonists are long acting, they suppress gonadotropin production after an initial stimulation. In some uses, the initial stimulation of gonadotropin is undesirable; a newer GnRH antagonist, ganirelix (*Antagon*) inhibits gonadotropin production without the stimulation and may ultimately replace the long-acting agonists. These compounds are formulated so they can be injected monthly or even less frequently.

In men, androgens stimulate growth of prostatic cancer; therefore, a reduction in androgen actions is used for palliative treatment (see Chapter 63). Estrogen use increases mortality in men primarily as a result of cardiovascular complications, and castration is not popular. Therefore, treatment with GnRH analogues to suppress gonadotropin release is favored. When long-acting agonists are given, signs and symptoms of prostatic cancer may increase shortly after initiation of therapy because of the initial stimulation of the pituitary gland. These analogues are also used to suppress puberty in young children with central precocious puberty.

In women, GnRH agonists are sometimes given along with FSH when stimulating follicles in fertility treatments; this addition prevents premature ovulation caused by the release of pituitary LH. Uterine leiomyomas and endometriosis regress when gonadotropin secretion is decreased. GnRH analogues relieve these conditions, but the relief usually lasts only as long as the analogue is administered, and the condition generally returns within a few months after therapy ceases. The main side effects are a result of estradiol deprivation and include hot flashes (sudden intense surface temperature elevation and sweating), dry skin and vagina; long-term use may decrease bone density. The addition of estrogen and progesterone can reduce the adverse effects while maintaining gonadotropin suppression. However, there is a continuing need to address the recent cancer risk cautions issued for short-term versus long-term use of estrogen–progesterone combinations as hormonal replacement therapy.

Corticotropin-Releasing Hormone

Corticotropin-releasing hormone consists of 41 amino acids; it stimulates ACTH release. It is used for investigational purposes.

HORMONES OF THE POSTERIOR PITUITARY GLAND

Antidiuretic hormone (ADH) and oxytocin are synthesized in the supraoptic and paraventricular nuclei in the brain and are transported in secretory granules through axons to the posterior lobe. These hormones are cyclic peptides of eight amino acids. Each is synthesized as a larger precursor, which is processed into the hormone plus a protein that binds the hormone, called neurophysin. ADH and oxytocin have different amino acids at positions 3 and 8.

Antidiuretic Hormone

ADH (vasopressin) is released primarily in response to increases in plasma osmolarity or decreases in blood volume. It produces its antidiuretic activity in the kidney, causing the cortical and medullary parts of the collecting duct to become more permeable to water, thereby increasing water reabsorption, reducing serum osmolarity, and increasing its volume. It produces this effect by binding to a subset of vasopressin receptors (Table 59.3) called V_2 that have relatively high affinity for the hormone. ADH also has actions at sites other than the kidney. V_2 receptors also mediate an increase in circulating levels of two proteins involved in blood coagulation: factor VIII and von Willebrand's factor. At higher concentrations, ADH interacts with V_1 receptors to cause a general constriction of most blood vessels. It also interacts with V_3 (or V_{1b}) receptors to increase ACTH release, although the major control of ACTH release occurs through corticotropin-releasing hormone.

ADH itself is available for injections (*Pitressin*) but has a half-life of about 15 minutes. Desmopressin (*DDAVP*) is an analogue without an amino group at the first amino acid and with D-arginine instead of L-arginine. This analogue is more stable and has very little pressor activity. Desmopressin can be given subcutaneously or nasally, and the effects last for 12 hours.

	Dose and	
Drug	**regimen**	**Effect**
Agonist	Low, pulsatile	Pituitary and gonadal stimulation
Agonist	High, constant	Initial pituitary and gonadal stimulation followed by suppression within 2 weeks
Antagonist	Constant	Pituitary and gonadal suppression

TABLE 59.2 **Biological Actions of GnRH Agonists and Antagonists**

TABLE 59.3 Actions of ADH

Receptor type	Response
V_1	Pressor
V_2	Antidiuretic
	Hemostatic
V_3	ACTH release

Because it is stable, desmopressin is preferred for treatments especially if pressor effects are not desired. The primary indication for therapy is central diabetes insipidus, a disorder that results when ADH secretion is reduced and that is characterized by polydipsia, polyuria, and dehydration. Desmopressin is also used to reduce primary nocturnal enuresis, or bedwetting, in children. It is useful in people with mild hemophilia A or with some types of von Willebrand's disease, in which von Willebrand's factor is present at low levels. In these cases, desmopressin is given when excessive bleeding occurs or before surgery to help reduce bleeding indirectly by increasing the amounts of coagulation factors.

A possible adverse effect of desmopressin is water intoxication if too much is taken.

ADH antagonists, including nonpeptide analogues that may be taken orally, have been developed with specificity for each of the receptor types. In the future, those that block V_1 receptors may be useful in treating hypertension, and those that block V_2 receptors may be useful in any condition of excessive water retention or hyponatremia, for which so far there is no satisfactory therapeutic treatment.

Oxytocin

Oxytocin (*Pitocin, Syntocinon*) causes milk release (letdown) by stimulating contraction of the myoepithelial cells of the milk ducts in lactating mammary glands; this forces milk from the alveoli of the breast. Oxytocin release is stimulated by suckling and by auditory and visual stimuli, such as a baby's cry. Oxytocin is available as a nasal spray, which is used as an aid to lactation when milk ejection is impaired.

Oxytocin also stimulates contraction of uterine smooth muscle in late phases of pregnancy. See Chapter 62 for a full discussion of the use of oxytocin in labor and delivery.

Study QUESTIONS

1. A patient with severe diarrhea as a result of a carcinoid tumor is a candidate for which of the following treatments?
   (A) Pulsatile administration of GnRH
   (B) Nasal administration of desmopressin
   (C) Depot injections of octreotide
   (D) Oral administration of bromocriptine
2. The actions of ADH include all of the following EXCEPT
   (A) Stimulation of ACTH release
   (B) Stimulation of bile secretion
   (C) Constriction of most blood vessels
   (D) Stimulation of coagulation factor VIII production
   (E) Production of concentrated urine
3. A patient with endometriosis who is being treated with leuprolide has hot flashes and dry skin and vagina. What additional treatment would relieve these unpleasant effects?
   (A) Estrogen and progesterone
   (B) Ganirelix
   (C) Testosterone
   (D) Bromocriptine
4. A 30-year-old woman has secondary amenorrhea and serum prolactin levels of 75 ng/mL. She has vis-

ited a fertility clinic to attempt to become pregnant. What treatment should be given?
   (A) Clomiphene
   (B) Ganirelix
   (C) Cabergoline
   (D) Estradiol
5. Growth hormone deficiency in children must be determined by measuring hormone levels after giving an agent that stimulates release because
   (A) Normal growth hormone secretion in children is too low to be measured by current assays
   (B) Growth hormone secretion occurs only during sleep
   (C) Growth hormone secretion is episodic
   (D) A different form of growth hormone is secreted after stimulation

ANSWERS

1. **C.** Carcinoid tumors arise from neuroendocrine cells of the gut and secrete serotonin and gastrointestinal hormones, which activate the gastrointestinal tract and result in diarrhea. Most of these tumors have receptors for somatostatin, which inhibit secretion when activated, resulting in reduced activity of the gut. Octreotide is a stable analogue of

somatostatin that is effective in treating carcinoid-induced diarrhea and that may slow tumor growth. The long-acting form requires only monthly injections to maintain effective levels. GnRH, desmopressin, and bromocriptine will not inhibit secretion from these neuroendocrine tumors.

2. **B.** ADH has many actions through three receptors but does not affect bile secretion. It stimulates ACTH release, although the predominant control occurs through corticotropin-releasing hormone. It has pressor activity by causing smooth muscles cells of most blood vessels to constrict. It stimulates production of coagulation factor VIII and von Willebrand's factor, and it increases the permeability of the collecting duct in the kidney to water, resulting in urine that has high osmolarity and low volume.

3. **A.** Endometriosis is growth of the endometrium beyond the uterine cavity. Leuprolide is a GnRH analogue that suppresses LH and FSH when present continuously, resulting in endometrial atrophy and low estrogen levels, causing hot flashes and skin dryness; long-term use may also reduce bone density. Low-dose estrogen and progesterone replacement therapy relieves the side effects caused by reduced estrogen levels, usually without stimulating endometrial growth. However, the recent warning of relative cancer risk of estrogen–progesterone combinations as short-term versus long-term hormonal replacement therapy must be carefully considered. Ganirelix, testosterone, and bromocriptine would not relieve the side effects.

4. **C.** High prolactin levels may cause amenorrhea and infertility through mechanisms not understood. Prolactin levels in normal women are less than 20 ng/mL. The primary control of prolactin is through inhibition of secretion by dopamine from the hypothalamus. Cabergoline is a stable dopamine agonist that reduces prolactin secretion. Clomiphene, an estrogen antagonist, is used to stimulate LH and FSH release to enhance fertility but should not be used until it has been determined whether reducing pro-lactin levels alone is sufficient to cause fertility. Ganirelix and estradiol are not useful in treating infertility.

5. **C.** Growth hormone secretion is episodic, and a single measurement without stimulation may give a false impression of growth hormone levels that are too low (<5 ng/mL). Growth hormone release occurs not only immediately after sleep but also after eating and after exercise. A 20-kilodalton form of growth hormone is secreted with the normal 22-kilodalton form, but the former is present in about one-fifth the amount. Both forms have biological activity and are secreted basally and after stimulation of growth hormone release.

SUPPLEMENTAL READING

Conn PM and Crowley WF. Gonadotropin-releasing hormone and its analogs. Annu Rev Med 1995;45:391.

deVos A, Ultsch M, and Kossiakoff AA. Human growth hormone and extracellular domain of its receptor: Crystal structure of the complex. Science 1992;255:306.

Grinspoon S and Gelato M. The rational use of growth hormone in HIV-infected patients. J Clin Endocrinol Metab 2001; 86: 3478 (editorial).

Oberg K. Established clinical uses of octreotide and lanreotide in oncology. Chemotherapy 2001;45(Suppl 2):40–53.

Olive DL and Pritts EA. Treatment of endometriosis. N Engl J Med 2001;345:266.

Taplin ME and Ho SH. Clinical Review 134: The endocrinology of prostate cancer. J Clin Endocrinol Metab 2001;86:3467.

Thibonnier M, Coles P, Thibonnier A, and Shoham M. The basic and clinical pharmacology of nonpeptide vasopressin receptor antagonists. Ann Rev Pharmacol Toxicol 2001;41:175–202.

Utiger RD. Treatment of acromegaly. N Engl J Med 2000;342:1210.

CASE Study Changes in Body Size

A 53-year-old man visits his physician because he is bothered by headaches, which are becoming more intense and more frequent, so that he has one most of the time. The physician notices that the man's hands, feet, nose, and jaw are large and his voice is hoarse. The physician learns by questioning that the man has needed to purchase a larger wedding ring and larger shoes several times in the past 7 years. In a photograph of the man taken 10 years earlier, the nose and jaws are not large. The physician suspects acromegaly and finds after tests that the patient's serum growth hormone levels are elevated after oral glucose administration. A pituitary macroadenoma 1.1 cm in diameter is detected by magnetic resonance imaging. If surgery does not result in normal growth hormone levels, what treatment should be used?

ANSWER: Excessive growth hormone secretion in adults causes acromegaly, which is slow in onset but eventually results in growth of soft tissue and bones of the hands, feet, and parts of the face. Growth of nasopharyngeal soft tissue may result in hoarseness. Growth hormone is secreted episodically, so normal people may have briefly elevated levels of serum growth hormone through the day. In normal subjects but not acromegalics, oral glucose suppresses these spikes of growth hormone secretion. Surgical removal of the macroadenoma should help the headaches, but it returns serum growth hormone levels to normal only in 50% of cases. In patients whose levels are still elevated, treatment with long-acting somatostatin analogues, which inhibit growth hormone secretion, are the treatment of choice. Octreotide is available in a long-acting form that may be given biweekly to monthly. The dopamine agonists bromocriptine and cabergoline work in some acromegalic patients but are in general less effective than the somatostatin analogue.

60 Adrenocortical Hormones and Drugs Affecting the Adrenal Cortex

Ronald P. Rubin

 DRUG LIST

GENERIC NAME	PAGE	GENERIC NAME	PAGE
Aminoglutethimide	700	Hydrocortisone	692
Beclomethasone	692	Ketoconazole	700
Betamethasone	692	Metyrapone	699
Clobetasol	692	Mifepristone (RU 486)	701
Corticotropin	699	Mitotane	700
Cosyntropin	699	Prednisolone	692
Dexamethasone	701	Triamcinolone	692

The steroidal nature of adrenocortical hormones was established in 1937, when Reichstein synthesized desoxycorticosterone. Eventually it was clearly established that the adrenal cortex elaborated a number of hormones and that these compounds differed in their amount of inherent metabolic (glucocorticoid) and electrolyte regulating (mineralocorticoid) activity. The actions of these hormones extend to almost every cell in the body. In humans, hydrocortisone (cortisol) is the main carbohydrate-regulating steroid, and aldosterone is the main electrolyte-regulating steroid.

STEROID PHYSIOLOGY

Anatomy of the Adrenal Cortex

The mammalian adrenal cortex is divided into three concentric zones: the zona glomerulosa, zona fasciculata, and zona reticularis. The zona glomerulosa produces hormones, such as aldosterone, that are responsible for regulating salt and water metabolism; the zona fasciculata produces glucocorticoids; and the zona reticularis produces adrenal androgens. While secretion by the two inner zones is controlled by pituitary adrenocorticotropic hormone (corticotrophin, ACTH), aldosterone produced by the zona glomerulosa is principally controlled by the renin–angiotensin system. Desoxycorticosterone, a mineralocorticoid produced in the zona fasciculata, is under corticotrophin control.

Steroid Biosynthesis

Although the adrenal cortex is primarily involved in the synthesis and secretion of corticosteroids, it is also capable of producing and secreting such steroid intermediates as progesterone, androgens, and estrogens. The adrenal gland synthesizes steroids from cholesterol, which is derived from plasma lipoproteins via the low- and high-density lipoprotein pathways. Additionally, cholesterol is enzymatically released extramitochondrially from cholesterol esters catalyzed by a cholesterol ester hydrolase. The corticotrophin-dependent stimulation of cholesterol ester hydrolase activity provides an additional source of cholesterol for steroidogenesis.

Cholesterol is transported into the mitochondria of steroidogenic tissue, where side chain cleavage is carried out. In common with other mixed-function oxidase systems, the cholesterol side chain cleavage requires reduced nicotinamide-adenine dinucleotide phosphate

(NADPH), oxygen, and a specific cytochrome P450. *The rate-limiting step in steroid biosynthesis is the conversion of cholesterol to pregnenolone* (Fig. 60.1).

Pregnenolone leaves the mitochondria to become the obligatory precursor of corticosteroids and adrenal androgens. The biosynthetic pathway next branches into two separate routes. One route passes through progesterone and corticosterone to aldosterone, and the other

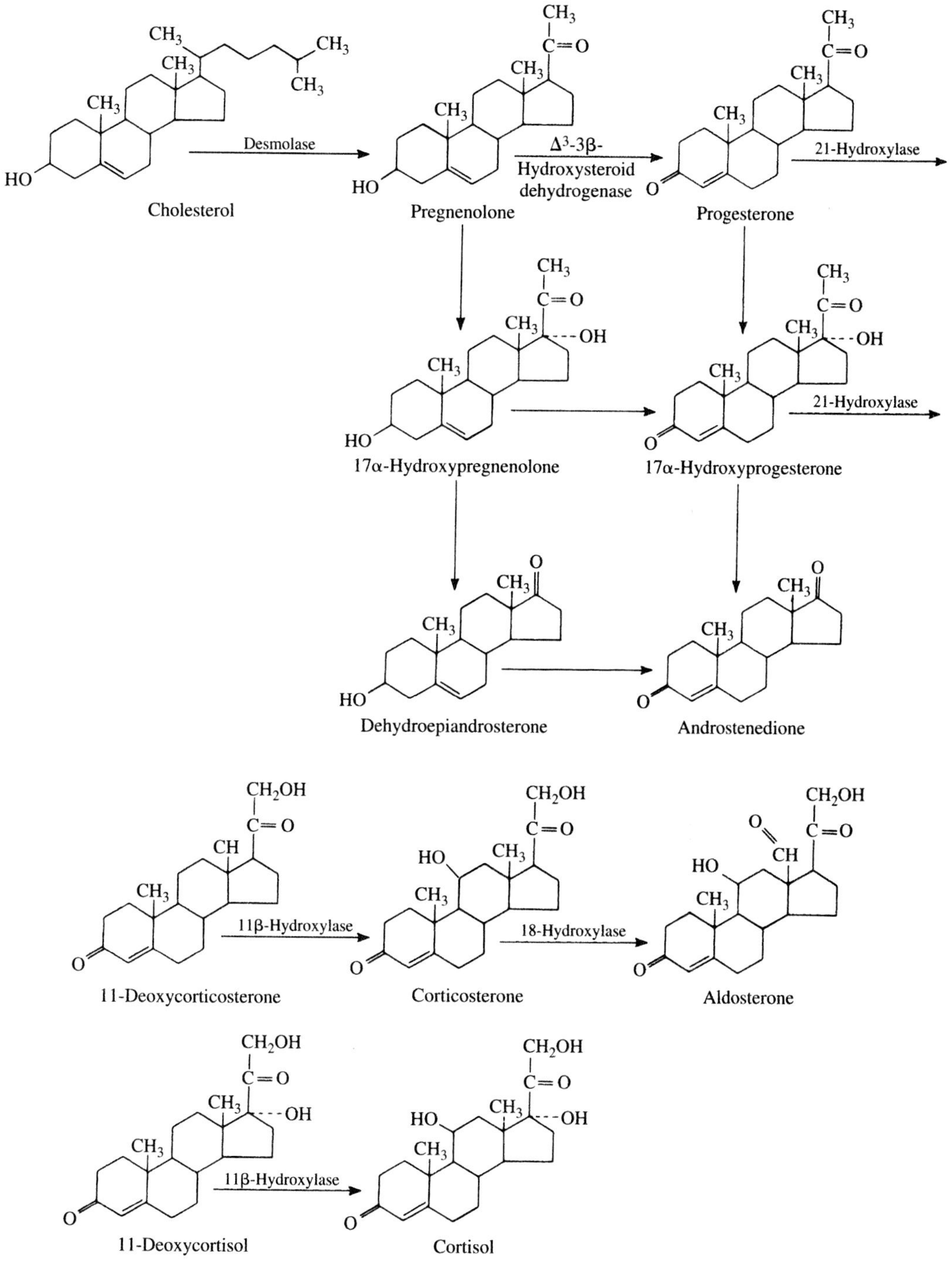

FIGURE 60.1
Metabolic pathways of corticosteroid biosynthesis.

proceeds from 17α-hydroxyprogesterone and 1-deoxy-cortisol to yield cortisol. Thus, steroid intermediates are converted to steroid end products by sequential 17-, 21-, and 11-hydroxylation reactions. 11-β-Hydroxylation is essential for glucocorticoid and mineralocorticoid activity of a steroid. The steroid hydroxylase system has the characteristics of a mixed-function oxidase, since two substrates, steroid and NADPH, are oxidized. All hydroxylases seem to be associated with a specific cytochrome P450.

The 17- and 21-hydroxylase enzymes are associated with microsomes, whereas the 11-β-hydroxylase has a mitochondrial origin. Since the last-named enzyme is not detectable in other steroid-producing tissues, the term 11-oxygenated steroids is considered synonymous with adrenal steroids. Aldosterone synthesis involves an essential 18-hydroxylation step catalyzed by $P450_{c18}$ with corticosterone as the precursor; this reaction also takes place within the mitochondria.

Steroid Transport in Blood

Glucocorticoids secreted into the systemic circulation are reversibly bound to a specific α-globulin known as *transcortin* or *corticosteroid-binding globulin*. This binding system has a high affinity and low capacity for corticosteroids, which contrasts with the low-affinity binding of these compounds to plasma albumin. Approximately 80% of the normal cortisol content in human plasma (12 μg/dL) is bound to corticosteroid-binding globulin, while 10% is bound to serum albumin; the remaining 10% is the biologically active unbound hormone.

Transcortin acts as a reservoir from which a constant supply of unbound cortisol may be provided to target cells. In addition, when serum albumin levels are low, less circulating cortisol becomes bound, which yields a greater physiological effect. Not only does protein binding control the amount of biologically active cortisol available, but it also reduces the rate at which steroids are cleared from the blood and thus limits steroid suppression of corticotrophin release from the pituitary gland.

The binding affinity of human transcortin is not limited to corticoids. Progesterone and the synthetic glucocorticoid prednisone also can bind to this macromolecule. High estrogen states (pregnancy, estrogen administration, use of oral contraceptives) greatly increase circulating transcortin levels. Thyroxine also stimulates transcortin formation, while androgen administration will decrease transcortin levels and the amount of bound glucocorticoids.

Steroid Metabolism

Most of the cortisol circulating in the blood is metabolized before its excretion. The metabolism of adrenal steroids occurs primarily in the liver, and when metabolic processes are altered, as occurs in liver disease, the half-life of cortisol may increase from 100 minutes to 7 hours.

Two major steps are involved in the metabolism of cortisol. The first is reduction of double bonds and introduction of a hydroxyl group in the A ring to form tetrahydric derivatives; this pathway accounts for 20 to 30% of the cortisol excreted. The glucocorticoid-metabolizing microsomal enzymes 11β-hydroxysteroid dehydrogenases (11β-HSD) play a crucial role in determining the availability of glucocorticoids. 11 β-HSD-1 acts as a reductase, regenerating active glucocorticoids, whereas 11β-HSD-2 acts as a dehydrogenase, converting cortisol to its inactive 11-keto derivative (cortisone). By inactivating glucocorticoids, 11β-HSD-2 protects the mineralocorticoid receptor from occupation by glucocorticoids, thereby endowing specificity to the aldosterone regulatory effects despite the predominance of glucocorticoids in the circulation. By contrast, congenital deficiency of 11β-HSD-2 results in inappropriate activation of the mineralocorticoid receptor by cortisol, leading to hypertension and hypokalemia. The second step in the metabolism of cortisol is a glucuronic acid or sulfate conjugation to form more soluble derivatives that are poorly bound to plasma proteins and readily pass into the urine. Adrenal androgens also are excreted, primarily as sulfates; they constitute about two-thirds of the total urinary 17-ketosteroids excreted. In the male, the other third is contributed by gonadal secretions. Knowledge of corticosteroid metabolism is important to the clinician, since alterations in adrenocortical function can be determined by measuring the amounts of 17-hydroxycorticosteroids. However, radioimmunoassay of urinary free cortisol (and plasma cortisol) is supplanting measurements of urinary metabolites.

Since the metabolism of steroid hormones occurs in part through the action of the hepatic oxidative drug-metabolizing enzymes, concomitant administration of anticonvulsant drugs (e.g., phenytoin and carbamazepine), which are potent inducers of glucocorticoid metabolism, will augment the elimination of methylprednisolone severalfold. Also, since steroids such as prednisone lack glucocorticoid activity until converted to prednisolone by hepatic enzymes, patients with liver disease should be treated with prednisolone rather than prednisone.

ACTIONS OF THE CORTICOSTEROIDS

The pharmacological actions of steroids are generally an extension of their physiological effects. Adrenal corticosteroids exert effects on almost every organ in the body. In normal physiological concentrations, they are essential for homeostasis, for coping with stress, and for the very maintenance of life.

The designation "glucocorticoid activity" is arbitrary, since naturally occurring glucocorticoids, such as cortisol, also possess mineralocorticoid activity, and the principal mineralocorticoid, aldosterone, when administered in very high doses, has glucocorticoid activity. Moreover, hydrocortisone, as well as certain synthetic glucocorticoids, such as prednisone and dexamethasone, binds to mineralocorticoid receptors. However, the distinction between these two groups serves a useful purpose when dissociation of the basic actions becomes crucial for optimizing steroids' therapeutic efficiency.

Carbohydrate, Protein, and Fat Metabolism

The glucocorticoids increase blood glucose and liver glycogen levels by stimulating gluconeogenesis. The source of this augmented carbohydrate production is protein, and the protein catabolic actions of the glucocorticoids result in a negative nitrogen balance. The inhibition of protein synthesis by glucocorticoids brings about a transfer of amino acids from muscle and bone to liver, where amino acids are converted to glucose.

Supraphysiological concentrations of glucocorticoids will induce the synthesis of specific proteins in various tissues. For instance, glucocorticoids stimulate the synthesis of enzymes involved in glucose and amino acid metabolism, including glucose 6-phosphatase and tyrosine transaminase. The relation of this action of glucocorticoids to their overall effects on general metabolic processes remains obscure, although the latency of their therapeutic actions (several hours) is consistent with the fact that steroids regulate RNA and protein synthesis.

Glucocorticoids not only break down protein but also stimulate the catabolism of lipids in adipose tissue and enhance the actions of other lipolytic agents. This occurrence results in an increase in plasma free fatty acids and an enhanced tendency to ketosis. The mechanism of this lipolytic action is unknown. The net effect of the biochemical changes induced by the glucocorticoids is antagonism of the actions of insulin. These biochemical events promote hyperglycemia and glycosuria, which are similar to the diabetic state.

Electrolyte and Water Metabolism

Another major function of the adrenal cortex is the regulation of water and electrolyte metabolism. The principal mineralocorticoid, aldosterone, can increase the rate of sodium reabsorption and potassium excretion severalfold. This will occur physiologically in response to sodium or volume depletion or both. The primary site of this effect is the distal tubule (see Chapter 21). The steroid-binding specificity of mineralocorticoid and glucocorticoid receptors overlaps in the distal cortical cells and collecting tubules, so that glucocorticoids may mediate mineralocorticoid-like effects. Glucocorticoids also decrease the intestinal transport of calcium by antagonizing the action of 1,25-dihydroxyvitamin D_3 and promote calcium excretion by the kidney (see Chapter 66).

Cardiovascular Function

Glucocorticoids directly stimulate cardiac output and potentiate the responses of vascular smooth muscle to the pressor effects of catecholamines and other vasoconstrictor agents. Such actions on vascular smooth muscle may be secondary to effects mediated through the central nervous system or on circulating volume. However, the presence of steroid receptors on vascular smooth muscle suggests a direct effect on vasomotor activity. *Thus, corticosteroids appear to play an important role in the regulation of blood pressure by modulating vascular smooth muscle tone, by having a direct action on the heart, and through stimulating renal mineralocorticoid and glucocorticoid receptors.* The resulting hypertension may predispose patients to coronary heart disease if a prolonged course of rigorous glucocorticoid therapy is employed.

Immune and Defense Mechanisms

The inflammatory response is a highly complex process that involves a number of cell types of the reticuloendothelial system and a number of chemical mediators, including prostaglandins, leukotrienes, kinins, and biogenic amines (See Chapter 36). The inhibitory effects of glucocorticoids on various aspects of the inflammatory and immunological responses constitute the basis for their therapeutic efficacy. All steps of the inflammatory process are blocked: there is a diminution in heat, erythema, swelling, and tenderness. Both the early components (edema, fibrin deposition, neutrophil migration, and phagocytosis) and late components (collagen synthesis and deposition) may be retarded.

Glucocorticoids promote apoptosis and reduce survival, differentiation, and proliferation of a variety of inflammatory cells, including T lymphocytes and macrophages. These effects are mediated by changes in the production and activity of inflammatory cytokines, such as interleukin (IL) 6 and IL-β, tumor necrosis factor-α, and interferon-γ. Many of the antiinflammatory actions of glucocorticoids are mediated by cross-talk between the activated glucocorticoid receptor and transcription factors, such as the proinflammatory nuclear factor-κ-B (NF-κB) and activator protein (AP) 1. These transcription factors, which promote the expression of a number of inflammatory genes, are potential targets for antiinflammatory therapy as observed in asthma, for example.

A prominent histological feature of glucocorticoid action on the late-phase response to bronchial inhalation challenge with antigen is inhibition of the influx of polymorphonuclear leukocytes, eosinophils, basophils, mononuclear cells, and lymphocytes into tissues (Fig. 60.2). The ability of glucocorticoids to alter reticuloendothelial cell traffic, which is a prominent antiinflammatory action of glucocorticoids, is regulated by adhesion molecules. Glucocorticoids reduce the expression of adhesion molecules through the inhibition of proinflam-

Late phase—untreated

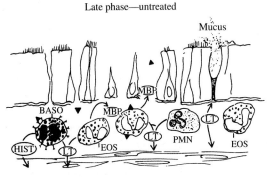

1. Inflammatory cell infiltrate
2. Bronchoconstriction
3. Hypersecretion of mucus
4. Epithelial permeability
5. Epithelial destruction
6. Edema

Late phase—steroid-treated

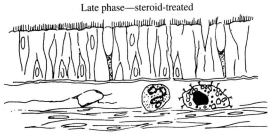

1. No inflammatory cell infiltrate
2. No Bronchoconstriction
3. No Hypersecretion of mucus
4. No Epithelial permeability
5. No Epithelial destruction
6. No Edema
7. Reduced arachidonate metabolites
8. Increased β-adrenergic tone

FIGURE 60.2

Model of steroid action on the late-phase response to bronchial inhalation challenge with antigen. Steroid therapy (*bottom*) prevents the inflammatory cell infiltrate and concomitant sequelae usually observed in response to the antigen challenge (*top*). BASO, basophils; EOS, eosinophils; PMN, polymorphonuclear leukocytes; HIST, histamine; LT, leukotrienes; MBP, major basic protein. (Reprinted with permission from Schleimer RP. The mechanisms of antiinflammatory steroid action in allergic disease. Annu Rev Pharmacol Toxicol 1985;25:400. Copyright 1985 by Annual Reviews Inc.)

matory cytokines and by direct inhibitory effects on the expression of adhesion molecules. Chemotactic cytokines, such as IL-8, which attract immune cells to the inflammatory site, are also inhibited by glucocorticoids. In addition to their ability to inhibit the adherence of inflammatory cells, particularly neutrophils, to the vascular endothelium, steroids are vasoconstrictors. This action would further impede inflammatory cell migration into tissues.

As mentioned previously, glucocorticoids promote apoptosis and reduce survival, differentiation, and proliferation of a number of inflammatory cells. While there is an increase in the number of polymorphonuclear leukocytes in the circulation, corticosteroids cause the involution and atrophy of all lymphoid tissue and decrease the number of circulating lymphocytes. The striking lymphocytopenia is caused in large part by an inhibition of lymphocyte proliferation, although diminished growth with preferential accumulation of cells in the G_1-phase of the cell cycle is followed by cell death. These effects are mainly mediated by alterations in cytokine production and action.

Another important aspect of the inflammatory cascade is arachidonic acid metabolism, leading to the synthesis of the proinflammatory prostaglandins and leukotrienes. Through the formation of lipocortin, an inhibitor of phospholipase A_2, glucocorticoids depress the release of arachidonic acid from phospholipids and hence the production of arachidonic acid metabolites.

Other Endocrine Organs

Since the synthesis and release of cortisol are regulated by pituitary corticotrophin, removal of the pituitary gland results in decreased function and eventual atrophy of the zona fasciculata and zona reticularis. Infusion of supraphysiological concentrations of cortisol will suppress corticotrophin secretion from the pituitary and will markedly decrease circulating corticotrophin levels. This occurrence implies a negative feedback control for corticotrophin and corticosteroid release (Fig. 60.3).

In addition to the humoral control of corticotrophin release, direct nervous control is mediated through the median eminence of the hypothalamus (Fig. 60.3). Nerve terminals in the median eminence store and release various hormones and neurotransmitters, including corticotropin-releasing factor (CRF), which is under the control of higher neural centers. During stress, CRF is released into the pituitary portal system to stimulate corticotrophin release. Activation of the hypothalamic–pituitary system also accounts for the diurnal, or circadian, nature of cortisol secretion; plasma cortisol concentrations reach a maximum between 6 and 8 A.M. and then slowly decrease through the afternoon and evening. Human and animal studies suggest the existence of an early (fast) and more prolonged (delayed,

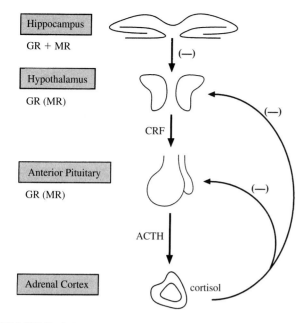

FIGURE 60.3

The role of the hypothalamic–pituitary axis in the regulation of adrenocortical hormone synthesis and release. The major physiological stimulus for the synthesis and release of glucocorticoids is corticotropin (ACTH) secreted from the anterior pituitary gland. ACTH secretion is regulated by corticotropin-releasing factor (CRF) from the paraventricular region of the hypothalamus. The release of CRF in turn is controlled by glucocorticoid levels and by input from the hippocampus. Both endogenous and exogenous glucocorticoids feed back negatively to regulate the secretion of ACTH and CRF. Glucocorticoid and mineralocorticoid receptors (GR and MR) in the hippocampus also negatively modulate CRF synthesis and release.

>2 hours) feedback of corticotrophin suppression. Both inhibitory systems are operative at the hypothalamic and pituitary levels. The hippocampus also highly expresses glucocorticoid and mineralocorticoid receptors, which when activated, decrease the synthesis and release of CRF. This results in a decrease in basal and corticotrophin-induced cortisol secretion (Fig. 60.3).

Corticosteroids also affect adrenomedullary function by increasing epinephrine production; the mechanism is exertion of a stimulatory action on two of the enzymes that regulate catecholamine synthesis, tyrosine hydroxylase, the rate-limiting enzyme, and phenylethanolamine N-methyltransferase, which catalyzes the conversion of norepinephrine to epinephrine. Steroids also influence the metabolism of circulating catecholamines by inhibiting their uptake from the circulation by nonneuronal tissues (i.e., extraneuronal uptake; see Chapter 9). This effect of corticoids may explain their permissive action in potentiating the hemodynamic effects of circulating catecholamines.

Finally, steroids can exert suppressive actions on certain endocrine systems. Glucocorticoids inhibit thyroid-stimulating hormone pulsatility and the nocturnal surge of this hormone by depressing thyrotropin-releasing hormone secretion at the hypothalamic level. In addition to hypercortisolism being associated with insulin resistance, glucocorticoids are inhibitors of linear growth and skeletal maturation in humans. A pivotal component of this inhibition is the depression of growth hormone secretion. The anticalcemic effect of the glucocorticoids, which is associated with an amplification of the actions of parathyroid hormone, also may retard bone growth. The inhibitory action of high levels of glucocorticoids on reproductive function is probably because of attenuation of luteinizing hormone secretion and direct action on the reproductive organs.

GENERAL PHARMACOLOGY OF CORTICOSTEROIDS

Structure-Activity Relationships
Natural Corticosteroids

Within the basic structure of the steroid molecule (Fig. 60.4), a 4,5 double bond and a 3-ketone group are needed for typical steroid activity. A hydroxyl group on C11 is needed for glucocorticoid activity (corticosterone) but is not required for sodium-retaining activity (desoxycorticosterone). The addition of a hydroxyl group on C17, which converts corticosterone to cortisol, also increases glucocorticoid activity.

Synthetic Corticosteroids

The ultimate aim in altering the steroid molecule is to decrease sodium-retaining activity and to increase anti-inflammatory glucocorticoid activity.

Ring A

The addition of a double bond at the 1,2 position of cortisol or cortisone yields prednisone or prednisolone, respectively, and increases the ratio of carbohydrate to

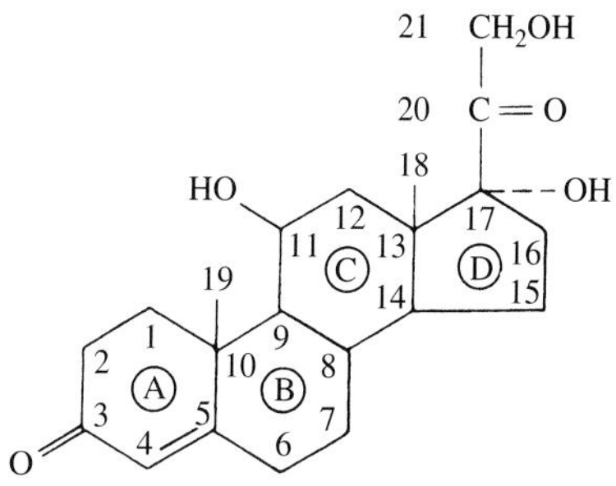

FIGURE 60.4
Basic corticosteroid nucleus.

sodium-retaining potency. Prednisone is inactive and must be converted to prednisolone in the liver by reduction at the 11-keto position.

Ring B

The inclusion of an α-methyl group in position 6 of prednisolone will yield 6-α-methylprednisolone, a compound with slightly greater glucocorticoid potency. This small structural modification greatly diminishes the binding of methylprednisolone to transcortin.

Ring C

The addition of a fluoride group on the 9 position of cortisol to give 9-α-fluorocortisol will greatly increase all biological activity.

Ring D

Hydroxylation or methylation at the 16 position of α-fluoroprednisolone to give triamcinolone, dexamethasone, or betamethasone increases antiinflammatory potency and drastically diminishes sodium-retaining activity.

The relative antiinflammatory potency of each of the synthetic analogues is compared with cortisol in Table 60.1 and is roughly correlated with its biological half-life. Hydrocortisone is considered a short-acting steroid; triamcinolone and prednisolone, intermediate-acting; and betamethasone and dexamethasone, long-acting. Thus, prednisone 5 mg, dexamethasone 0.75 mg, and hydrocortisone 20 mg should possess equal glucocorticoid potency.

The synthetic analogues (except 9-α-fluorocortisol) share an advantage over hydrocortisone in that sodium retention is not as marked at equipotent antiinflammatory doses. However, all of the other undesirable side effects of supraphysiological concentrations of hydrocortisone have been observed with the synthetic analogues.

Steroid Preparations

Glucocorticoids are available in a wide range of preparations, so that they can be administered parenterally, orally, topically, or by inhalation. Obviously the oral route is preferred for prolonged therapy. However, parenteral administration is required in certain circumstances. Intramuscular injection of a water-soluble ester (phosphate or succinate) formed by esterification of the C21 steroid alcohol produces peak plasma steroid levels within 1 hour. Such preparations are useful in emergencies. By contrast, acetate and tertiary butylacetate esters must be injected locally as suspensions and are slowly absorbed from the injection site, which prolongs their effectiveness to approximately 8 hours.

Topical preparations usually contain relatively insoluble steroids, such as clobetasol propionate, triamcinolone acetonide, or triamcinolone diacetate. Side effects of this mode of drug application are usually milder and more transient than those seen after systemically administered steroids. However, potent topical corticosteroids, such as clobetasol propionate (*Temovate*), can suppress adrenal function when used in large amounts for a long time, especially when the skin surface is denuded or when occlusive dressings are employed. Since the high potency topical preparations carry a higher risk of local side effects, their use should be held in reserve.

Inhaled glucocorticoid preparations, such as beclomethasone dipropionate and betamethasone valerate, provide an effective alternative to systemic steroids in the treatment of chronic asthma, with lesser side effects than oral or parenteral glucocorticoids (see Chapter 39). In fact, inhaled glucocorticoids have become a mainstay of asthma therapy. Inhalation delivers the agent directly to the target site in relatively low doses, with the potential for more frequent administration. Moreover, inhaled glucocorticoids are metabolized in the lung before they are absorbed, which reduces their systemic effects. However, even modest doses of

---

TABLE 60.1   General Classification of Glucocorticoids

Steroid	Carbohydrate Potency[a] (mg)	Antiinflammatory Potency	Sodium-retaining Potency	Biological Half-life (hr)
Cortisol	20.0	1	1.00	8–12
Prednisolone (Δ^1-cortisone)	5.0	4	0.50	12–36
6-α-Methylprednisolone	4.0	5	0.50	12–36
9-α-Fluorocortisol	0.1	10	125.00	12–36
Triamcinolone (9-α-fluoro-16-hydroxyprednisolone)	4.0	5	0.10	12–36
Betamethasone (9-α-16-β-methylprednisolone)	0.6	25	0.05	36–54
Dexamethasone (9-α-fluoro-16-α-methylprednisolone)	1.0	30	0.05	36–54

[a]Carbohydrate action of glucocorticoids is defined as the stimulation of glucose formation, diminution of its use, and promotion of its storage as glycogen.

inhaled steroid can have a measurable effect on the hypothalamic–pituitary axis, although the clinical effects may be marginal. There is also a close association in adults between the heavy use of inhaled glucocorticoids and the risk of posterior subcapsular cataract. Since the dose–response curve to inhaled glucocorticoids is relatively flat, the use of steroid-sparing agents (long-acting inhaled β-adrenergic agonists, low-dose theophylline, or antileukotrienes) is recommended instead of increasing the dose of glucocorticoid. This strategy will also limit the severity of hypothalamic–pituitary–adrenal depression and other side effects.

ADVERSE EFFECTS

General Considerations

Short-term glucocorticoid therapy of life-threatening diseases, such as status asthmaticus, provides dramatic improvement with few complications. However, when administered in pharmacological doses for long periods, steroids generally produce serious toxic effects that are extensions of their pharmacological actions. No route or preparation is free from the diverse side effects (Table 60.2), although individuals receiving comparable doses of glucocorticoids exhibit variations in side effects.

Glucocorticoids are cautiously employed in various disease states, such as rheumatoid arthritis, although they still should be regarded as adjunctive rather than primary treatment in the overall management scheme. The toxic effects of steroids are severe enough that a number of factors must be considered when their prolonged use is contemplated.

The first point is that treatment with steroids is generally palliative rather than curative, and only in a very few diseases, such as leukemia and nephrotic syndrome, do corticosteroids alter prognosis. One must also consider which is worse, the disease to be treated or possible induced hypercortisolism. The patient's age can be an important factor, since such adverse effects as hypertension are more apt to occur in old and infirm individuals, especially in those with underlying cardiovascular disease. Glucocorticoids should be used with caution during pregnancy. If steroids are to be employed, prednisone or prednisolone should be used, since they cross the placenta poorly.

Once steroid therapy is decided upon, the lowest possible dose that can provide the desired therapeutic effect should be employed. Relationships of dosage, duration, and host responses are essential elements in determining adverse effects. Increasing attention is being given to the use of lower doses of glucocorticoids in combination with other drugs that can have a synergistic effect on a given disease. Moreover, the lowered dose levels of steroid will minimize the side effects.

TABLE 60.2 Complications of Glucocorticoid Therapy

Hematological and immuno-logical	Central nervous system
Leukocytosis	Insomnia
Lymphopenia	Depression
Eosinopenia	Nervousness
Altered inflammatory response	Psychosis
Gastrointestinal	Fluid and electrolyte
Peptic ulceration	Na^+ retention
Fatty liver	K^+ loss
Pancreatitis	Negative Ca^{++} balance
Nausea, vomiting	Hypertension
Metabolic	Endocrinological
Hyperglycemia	Suppression of HPA axis[a]
Protein wasting	Antagonisms with insulin, parathyroid, thyroid
Hyperlipidemia	Skin
Obesity	Thinning of skin
Musculoskeletal	Striae purpurae
Myopathy	Ecchymoses
Growth failure	Acne
Osteopenia	Hirsutism
Ocular	General
Posterior subcapsular cataracts	Cushingoid features
Increased intraocular pressure	Truncal obesity
	Withdrawal syndrome

[a]Hypothalamic-pituitary-adrenocortical axis.

Osteoporosis

The most damaging and therapeutically limiting adverse effect of long-term glucocorticoid therapy is impairment of bone formation. This effect is associated with a decrease in serum levels of osteocalcin, a marker of osteoblastic function. In fact, *glucocorticoid administration is the most common cause of drug-induced osteoporosis.* Most patients receiving chronic steroid therapy develop osteoporosis, particularly during the first year of therapy, and more than 50% will have a bone fracture. Trabecular bone is particularly affected.

Systemic glucocorticoid therapy increases the probability of osteoporosis even with dosages sufficiently low so as not to affect the hypothalamic–pituitary–adrenal axis. By enhancing bone resorption and decreasing bone formation, glucocorticoids decrease bone mass and increase the risk of fractures. The overall effects appear to be due to direct actions of glucocorticoids on osteoblasts and to indirect effects, such as impaired Ca^{++} absorption and a compensatory increase in parathyroid hormone secretion. Inhibition of bone growth is a well-known side effect of long-term systemic glucocorticoid therapy in children with bronchial asthma, even in those receiving alternate-day therapy. Glucocorticoids can also augment bone loss, decreasing testosterone levels in men and estrogen levels in women by direct effects on the gonads and inhibition of gonadotropin release. Thus, patients taking glucocorticoids can also develop hypogonadism. It is recommended that all patients who receive long-term glucocorticoid treatment should have measurements of bone density, gonadal steroids, vitamin D, and 24-hour urinary Ca^{++}. Deficiencies in either testosterone or estradiol increase bone loss and should be corrected if possible. Bisphosphonates (etidronate, alendronate, or risedronate) and calcitonin, which inhibit bone resorption, have become increasingly popular for treating osteoporosis.

The Infectious Process

Steroids can alter host–parasite interactions, suppress fever, decrease inflammation, and change the usual character of the symptoms produced by most infectious organisms. There is a heightened susceptibility to serious bacterial, viral, and fungal infections. Local infections may reactivate and spread, and infections acquired during the course of therapy may become more severe and even more difficult to recognize. By interfering with fibroblast proliferation and collagen synthesis, glucocorticoids cause dehiscence of surgical incisions, increase risk of wound infection, and delay healing of open wounds. This untoward effect of steroids may make it mandatory to administer antibiotics with the steroids, especially when there is a history of a chronic infectious process (e.g., tuberculosis). On the other hand, individuals with normal defenses who are treated with low to moderate doses of glucocorticoids are not at great risk of infection. While the incidence of infections has probably decreased with the increased use of inhaled steroids and combination therapy, inhaled steroids carry an increase in the incidence of oral candidiasis that can be reduced by using proper doses. Nevertheless, glucocorticoids are used to treat herpes zoster, bacterial meningitis, and skin infections.

Effects on Gastric Mucosa

Steroid administration was once thought to lead to the formation of peptic ulcers, with hemorrhage or perforation or reactivation of a healed ulcer. It is now realized that this effect is principally observed in patients who have received concomitant nonsteroidal antiinflammatory treatment. Since there is a minimal increase in the incidence of ulcers in patients receiving glucocorticoid treatment alone, prophylactic antiulcer regimens are usually not necessary.

Hyperglycemic Action

In about one-fourth to one-third of the patients receiving prolonged steroid therapy, the hyperglycemic effects of glucocorticoids lead to decreased glucose tolerance, decreased responsiveness to insulin, and even glycosuria. Ketoacidosis occurs very rarely. Pharmacological concentrations of steroids may precipitate frank diabetes in individuals who cannot produce the necessary additional insulin. Mild hyperglycemia can often be managed with oral hypoglycemic agents. The effects of glucocorticoids on hyperglycemia are usually reversed within 48 hours following discontinuation of steroid therapy. If glucocorticoid therapy is continued for an extended period, the alterations of glucose metabolism and the resulting hyperinsulinemia may lead to enhanced cardiovascular risk.

Ophthalmic Effects

Glucocorticoids induce cataract formation, particularly in patients with rheumatoid arthritis. An increase in intraocular pressure related to a decreased outflow of aqueous humor is also a frequent side effect of periocular, topical, or systemic administration. Induction of ocular hypertension, which occurs in about 35% of the general population after glucocorticoid administration, depends on the specific drug, the dose, the frequency of administration, and the glucocorticoid responsiveness of the patient.

Central Nervous System Effects

Treatment with steroids may initially evoke euphoria. This reaction can be a consequence of the salutary effects of the steroids on the inflammatory process or a direct effect on the psyche. The expression of the unpredictable and often profound effects exerted by steroids on mental processes generally reflects the personality of the individual. Psychiatric side effects induced by glucocorticoids may include mania, depression, or mood disturbances. Restlessness and early-morning insomnia may be forerunners of severe psychotic reactions. In such situations, cessation of treatment might be considered, especially in patients with a history of personality disorders. In addition, patients may become psychically dependent on steroids as a result of their euphoric effect, and withdrawal of the treatment may precipitate an emotional crisis, with suicide or psychosis as a consequence. Patients with Cushing's syndrome may also exhibit mood changes, which are reversed by effective treatment of the hypercortisolism.

The hippocampus is a principal neural target for glucocorticoids. It contains high concentrations of glucocorticoid and mineralocorticoid receptors and has marked sensitivity to these hormones.

Fluid and Electrolyte Disturbances

The normal subject may retain sodium and water during steroid therapy, although the synthetic steroid analogues represent a lesser risk in this regard. Prednisolone produces some edema in doses greater than 30 mg; triamcinolone and dexamethasone are much less liable to elicit this effect. Glucocorticoids may also produce an increase in potassium excretion. Muscle weakness and wasting of skeletal muscle mass frequently accompany this potassium-depleting action. The expansion of the extracellular fluid volume produced by steroids is secondary to sodium and water retention. However, the presence of specific steroid receptors in vascular smooth muscle suggests that glucocorticoids are also more directly involved in the regulation of blood pressure. The major adverse effects of glucocorticoids on the cardiovascular system include dyslipidemia and hypertension, which may predispose patients to coronary artery disease. A separate entity, steroid myopathy, is also improved by decreasing steroid dosage.

Pseudorheumatism

In certain patients, whose large dosages of corticosteroids for rheumatoid arthritis are gradually diminished, new symptoms develop that may be mistaken for a flare-up of the joint disease. These can include emotional lability, fever, muscle aches, and general fatigue. It is tempting to increase the dosage of steroid in this situation, but continued maintenance at the lower dosage with a subsequent gradual decrease in the dose usually improves symptoms.

Additional Effects

Other side effects include acne, striae, truncal obesity, deposition of fat in the cheeks (moon face) and upper part of the back (buffalo hump), and dysmenorrhea. Topical administration may produce local skin atrophy. In patients with AIDS who are treated with glucocorticoids, Kaposi's sarcoma becomes activated or progresses more rapidly.

Iatrogenic Adrenal Insufficiency

In addition to the dangers associated with long-term use of corticosteroids in supraphysiological concentrations, withdrawal of steroid therapy presents problems. The suppression of the hypothalamic–pituitary axis observed with modest doses and short courses of glucocorticoid therapy is usually readily reversible. However, steroid therapy with modest to high doses for 2 weeks or longer will depress hypothalamic and pituitary activity and result in a decrease in endogenous adrenal steroid secretion and eventual adrenal atrophy. These patients have a limited ability to respond to stress and an enhanced probability that shock will develop. Long-acting steroids, such as dexamethasone and betamethasone, suppress the hypothalamic–pituitary axis more than do other steroids. The functional state of the hypothalamic–pituitary axis can be evaluated by tests involving basal plasma cortisol determinations, low and high doses of cosyntropin (peptide fragment of corticotrophin), insulin hypoglycemia, metyrapone, and corticotrophin-releasing hormone.

Glucocorticoids are not withdrawn abruptly but are tapered. The doses are altered so that the condition being treated will not flare up and recovery of the hypothalamic–pituitary axis will be facilitated. Tapering the dose may reduce the potential for the development of Addison-like symptoms associated with steroid withdrawal. Alternate-day therapy will relieve the clinical manifestations of the inflammatory diseases while allowing a day for reactivation of endogenous corticosteroid output, thereby causing less severe and less sustained hypothalamic–pituitary suppression. This is feasible with doses of shorter-acting corticosteroids, such as prednisolone. The usual daily dose is doubled and is given in the early morning to simulate the natural circadian variation that occurs in endogenous corticosteroid secretion. The benefits of alternate-day therapy are seen only when steroids are used for a long period and are particularly useful for tapering the dose of glucocorticoid.

Although not always predictable, the degree to which a given corticosteroid will suppress pituitary activity is related to the route of administration, the size of the dose, and the length of treatment. The parenteral route causes the greatest suppression, followed by the oral route, and finally topical application. Hypothalamic–pituitary suppression also may result if large doses of a steroid aerosol spray are used to treat bronchial asthma. Patients given high concentrations of steroids for long periods and subsequently exposed to undue stress (e.g., severe infection, surgery) face the danger of adrenal crisis. These patients must be given supplemental steroids to compensate for their lack of adrenal reserve and to sustain them during the crisis.

Acute adrenal insufficiency will, of course, occur from an abrupt cessation of steroid therapy. The causation of fever, myalgia, arthralgia, and malaise may be difficult to distinguish from reactivation of rheumatic disease. Steroid treatment should be reduced gradually over several months to avoid this potentially serious problem. Also, continued suppression may be avoided by administering daily physiological replacement doses (5 mg prednisone) until adrenal function is restored. Although tapering of dose may not facilitate recovery of the hypothalamic–pituitary–adrenal axis, it may reduce the possibility of adrenal insufficiency. This is important, since severe hypotension caused by adrenal insufficiency may evoke a medical emergency. Adrenal insufficiency should always be considered in patients who are being withdrawn from prolonged glucocorticoid therapy unless metyrapone or insulin hypoglycemia tests are performed to exclude this possibility.

An additional problem associated with glucocorticoid therapy is that certain side effects can be caused by the diseases for which glucocorticoids are administered. Thus, osteoporosis can be a sequela of rheumatoid arthritis, and the physician is left to determine whether the untoward effect is iatrogenic or is merely a sign of the disease being treated. In addition to these problems, the physician must also be aware of the patient's natural reluctance to reduce the dose of steroid because of its salutary effects, both on the inflammatory process and on the psyche. Thus, the problems associated with withdrawal from long-term steroid therapy in rheumatoid arthritis are additional reasons steroid treatment should be initiated only after rest, physiotherapy, and nonsteroidal antiinflammatory drugs or after methotrexate, gold, and D-penicillamine have been used.

THERAPEUTIC USES OF STEROID HORMONES

Replacement Therapy

Adrenal insufficiency may result from hypofunction of the adrenal cortex (primary adrenal insufficiency, Addison's disease) or from a malfunctioning of the hypothalamic–pituitary system (secondary adrenal insufficiency). In treating primary adrenal insufficiency, one should administer sufficient cortisol to diminish hyperpigmentation and abolish postural hypotension; these are the cardinal signs of Addison's disease.

Although patients may require varying amounts of replacement steroid, 20 to 30 mg/day of cortisol supplemented with the mineralocorticoid 9-α-fluorocortisol (0.1 mg/day) is generally adequate. A doubling of the cortisol dose may be required during minor stresses or infections. In patients who require high-dose supplementation, prednisone can be substituted for cortisol to avoid fluid retention.

In the treatment of secondary adrenocortical insufficiency, lower doses of cortisol are generally effective, and fluid and electrolyte disturbances do not have to be considered, since patients with deficient corticotrophin secretion generally do not have abnormal function of the zona glomerulosa. Since cortisol replacement therapy is required for life, adequate assessment of patients is critical to avoid the serious long-term consequences of excessive or insufficient treatment. In many cases, the doses of glucocorticoid used in replacement therapy are probably too high. Patients should ideally be administered three or more doses daily. To limit the risk of osteoporosis, replacement therapy should be carefully assessed on an individual basis and overtreatment avoided.

Inflammatory States

Since glucocorticoids possess a wide range of effects on virtually every phase and component of the inflammatory and immune responses, they have assumed a major role in the treatment of a wide spectrum of diseases with an inflammatory or immune-mediated component. Rheumatoid arthritis is the original condition for which antiinflammatory steroids were used, and they remain a mainstay of therapy. Intraarticular glucocorticoid injections have proven to be efficacious, particularly in children. However, the detrimental effects of glucocorticoids on growth are significant for children with active arthritis. Although steroids offer symptomatic relief from this disorder by abolishing the swelling, redness, pain, and effusions, they do not cure. Progressive deterioration of joint structures continues, and the disease process may be exacerbated after steroid therapy is terminated (see Chapter 36).

Based on the concept that asthma is an inflammatory disease that leads to airway obstruction, inhaled glucocorticoids are the first-line treatment for moderate to severe asthma. Inhaled preparations are particularly effective when used to prevent recurrent attacks. This therapy is often combined with an inhaled bronchodilator such as a β-adrenergic agonist. The use of β-adrenergic agonists or theophylline enables use of a lower dose of glucocorticoid, especially in patients relatively resistant to therapy (see Chapter 39).

Steroids are used in other collagen diseases, such as lupus erythematosus; in hypersensitivity or allergic states, such as nephrotic syndrome, ulcerative colitis, and Crohn's disease; in granulomatous disease, such as sarcoid; and in a wide range of dermatological and ophthalmological conditions. Glucocorticoids may also be used at lower doses in combination with other drugs for the treatment of vasculitis, lupus nephritis, and amyloidosis. Steroids are valuable in the prevention and treatment of organ transplant rejection and in the improvement of muscle function in polymyositis.

Corticosteroids are the mainstay of therapy for inflammatory demyelinating polyneuropathies. In Guillain-Barré syndrome glucocorticoids reduce the inflammatory attack and improve final outcome, while in chronic inflammatory demyelinating polyneuropathy glucocorticoids suppress the immune reaction but may not retard the progression of the disease. Glucocorticoids also exert a facilitatory action on neuromuscular transmission that may contribute to their efficacy in certain neuromuscular disorders. The fact that acetylcholine receptor antibodies are responsible for the neuromuscular transmission defect in myasthenia gravis has provided a rationale for exploiting the immunosuppressive effects of glucocorticoids (see Chapter 28).

Although infections are generally thought to be particularly frequent and possibly severe in patients treated with steroids, they have been used as short-term adjunctive therapy to reduce the severe symptoms associated with such bacterial infections as acute *H. influenzae* and miliary tuberculosis and in viral infections, such as hepatitis and infectious mononucleosis.

Glucocorticoids are also used in the treatment of a number of HIV-related disorders, including *Pneumocystis carinii* pneumonia, demyelinating peripheral neuropathies, tuberculous meningitis, and nephropathy. Glucocorticoids are used as adjunctive therapy in Pneumo cystitis carinii pneumonia to decrease the inflammatory response and allow time for antimicrobial agents to exert their effects. In patients who are immunocompromised because of HIV infection, adjunctive steroids may be less beneficial in promoting survival.

Leukemia

Steroids are important components in the treatment of hematopoietic malignancies. Their efficacy in chronic lymphocytic leukemia and multiple myeloma stems from their lympholytic effects to reduce cell proliferation, promote cell cycle arrest, and induce cell death by apoptosis. A complication of chronic lymphocytic leukemia, that is, autoimmune hemolytic anemia, also responds favorably to steroids. However, the development of resistance may limit the effectiveness of steroid therapy.

Shock

Prompt intensive treatment with corticosteroids may be lifesaving when an excessive inflammatory reaction has resulted in septic shock. A massive infusion of corticosteroids can restore cardiac output and reverse hypotension by sensitizing the response of adrenoceptors in the heart and blood vessels to the stimulating action of catecholamines. This protective role of steroids may be due to a direct effect on vascular smooth muscle. The combination of glucocorticoids and dopamine therapy preserves renal blood flow during shock.

Congenital Adrenal Hyperplasia

Congenital enzymatic defects in the adrenal biosynthetic pathways lead to diminished cortisol and aldosterone production and release. In these conditions, corticotrophin secretion is increased, and adrenal hyperplasia occurs, accompanied by enhanced secretion of steroid intermediates, especially adrenal androgens. More than 90% of cases of congenital adrenal hyperplasia are due to 21-hydroxylase deficiency, which is created by mutations in the CYP21 gene encoding the en-

zyme. Overproduction of androgens causes virilization, accelerated growth, and early epiphysial fusion. Treatment of this condition requires administration of glucocorticoid in amounts adequate to suppress adrenal androgen secretion but insufficient to compromise bone growth and mineralization. Approximately 75% of patients have concomitant mineralocorticoid deficiency and therefore cannot synthesize sufficient aldosterone to maintain sodium balance. These patients may develop potentially fatal salt-wasting if not treated.

PROPOSED MECHANISM OF STEROID ACTION

While certain properties of glucocorticoid action are a result of direct posttranscriptional effects, most are a consequence of effects on gene expression. Steroids transported by transcortin enter the target cell by diffusion and then form a complex with its cytosolic receptor protein. Glucocorticoids bind to cytoplasmic glucocorticoid receptors containing two subunits of the heat shock protein that belong to the 90-kDa family. The heat shock protein dissociates, allowing rapid nuclear translocation of the receptor–steroid complex. Within the nucleus, the glucocorticoid receptor induces gene transcription by binding to specific sequences on DNA called glucocorticoid response elements in the promoter–enhancer regions of responsive genes (Fig. 60.5). In certain cases, the glucocorticoid receptor can interact with nuclear factor-κB and AP-1 to inhibit gene expression activated by these proinflammatory transcription factors. Because their side effects are thought to be a consequence of gene induction, glucocorticoids that can repress inflammatory genes without inducing gene transcription are in development.

The pivotal role that the glucocorticoid receptor plays in hormone action is illustrated by the fact that the magnitude of induction of a regulatable gene and cellular responsiveness are directly proportional to the number of occupied receptors. A decrease in glucocorticoid receptor number (down-regulation) produced by protein degradation may be responsible for the increase in steroid resistance observed clinically. Down-regulation of glucocorticoid receptors also is a potential mechanism for terminating glucocorticoid-dependent responses and for curtailing excessive cell stimulation when circulating levels of steroids are high. The effectiveness of glucocorticoids will also be compromised by the concomitant administration of other drugs that enhance the clearance of glucocorticoids (ephedrine, phenytoin, rifampin). Glucocorticoids, which bind to mineralocorticoid receptors in the kidney to regulate salt balance, are inactivated by 11-β-hydroxysteroid reductase so that they do not elicit mineralocorticoid

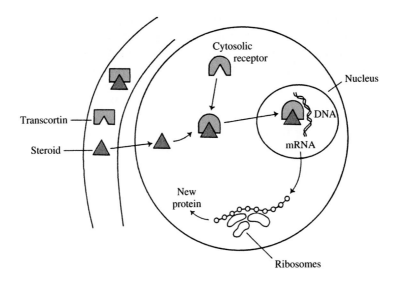

FIGURE 60.5
Mechanism of action of glucocorticoids.

actions in this tissue. However, in other tissues gluco-corticoids may exert their actions through mineralocor-ticoid receptors. Several actions of glucocorticoids that are too rapid to be explained by actions on transcription are mediated by effects on membrane receptors.

Because glucocorticoids regulate gene expression and protein synthesis, there is generally a lag of several hours before their effects are manifest. Moreover, the duration of various responses can endure after steroid levels fall. This may account for the fact that side effects elicited by steroids can be minimized by alternate-day therapy.

Metabolites of arachidonic acid, including prosta-glandins (PG), thromboxanes, and leukotrienes, are considered strong candidates as mediators of the in-flammatory process. Steroids may exert a primary effect at the inflammatory site by inducing the synthesis of a group of proteins called lipocortins. These proteins sup-press the activation of phospholipase A_2, thereby de-creasing the release of arachidonic acid and the produc-tion of proinflammatory eicosanoids (Fig. 60.6).

Another possible glucocorticoid-sensitive step is the PG endoperoxide H synthase (or cyclooxygenase) (COX) mediated conversion of arachidonate to PG en-doperoxides (Fig. 60-6). The endoperoxides (PGG and PGH) are the precursors of PGE_2, thromboxane A2 (TBXA2), and PGI_2, (prostacyclin). PG endoperoxide H synthase has two isoforms: one is constitutively ex-pressed (PGHS-1, or COX-1), and another is induced by growth factors, cytokines, and endotoxins (PGHS-2, or COX-2). One component of the antiinflammatory ac-tion of glucocorticoids appears to involve the suppres-sion of PGHS-2 induction in inflammatory cells by

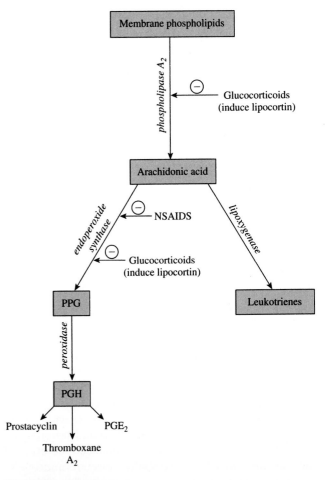

FIGURE 60.6
Possible site or sites of action of glucocorticoids on prostanoid production.

proinflammatory stimuli. Inhibition of the production and effects of inflammatory cytokines (IL-6 and IL-β) by the transcription factors nuclear factor-κB and AP-1 may also contribute to the antiinflammatory effects of glucocorticoids.

DRUGS USED IN THE DIAGNOSIS OR TREATMENT OF ADRENOCORTICAL ABNORMALITIES

Corticotropin

Corticotropin (*ACTH, Acthar, Cortrophin Gel*) is an open-chain polypeptide that consists of 39 amino acid residues, the first 24 of which are essential for its biological activity. The remainder of the amino acids are also clinically important, since they may be involved in stimulating antibody formation and causing allergic reactions. This is true especially when corticotropin of animal origin is injected into humans. Commercially available corticotropin is prepared from animal pituitary glands.

Absorption, Metabolism, Excretion

Corticotropin is rapidly inactivated by gastrointestinal proteolytic enzymes and therefore must be administered parenterally. It is rapidly removed from the circulation ($T_{1/2}$, 15 minutes) and is probably inactivated in body tissues, since no intact compound is found in the urine.

Clinical Uses

The rationale for using corticotropin instead of pharmacological concentrations of glucocorticoids stems from the fact that corticotropin provides enhanced amounts of all endogenously secreted adrenocortical hormones, including androgens. However, obvious disadvantages are associated with the use of this polypeptide: (1) It must be given daily parenterally. (2) It is quite expensive. (3) It is antigenic and thus can produce resistance and hypersensitivity reactions. Corticotropin is used as a diagnostic tool for the identification of primary adrenal insufficiency or as a method for evaluating the hypothalamic–pituitary–adrenal axis before surgery in patients previously treated with glucocorticoids.

Adverse Effects

Aside from hypersensitivity and allergic reactions, corticotropin administration has been associated with electrolyte disturbances and masculinization in women.

Cosyntropin

Cosyntropin (*Cortrosyn*) is a polypeptide that consists solely of the first 24 amino acids of corticotropin. It ap-

pears to offer an advantage over the naturally occurring hormone in that it has a longer duration of action and lacks the antigenic portion of corticotropin. Although the short cosyntropin test is recognized as a valid screening test to assess adrenocortical insufficiency, the overnight metyrapone test or insulin hypoglycemia test may prove more sensitive.

Metyrapone
Mechanism of Action

Metyrapone (*Metopirone*) produces its primary pharmacological effect by inhibiting 11-β-hydroxylase, thereby causing diminished production and release of cortisol. The resulting reduction in the negative feedback of cortisol on the hypothalamus and pituitary causes an increase in corticotrophin release and in the secretion of precursor 11-deoxysteroids.

Clinical Uses

Metyrapone is used in the differential diagnosis of both adrenocortical insufficiency and Cushing's syndrome (hypercortisolism). The drug tests the functional competence of the hypothalamic–pituitary axis when the adrenals are able to respond to corticotrophin; that is, when primary adrenal insufficiency has been ruled out.

After metyrapone administration, a patient with a disease of pituitary origin cannot achieve a compensatory increase in the urinary excretion of 17-hydroxycorticosteroids or 11-deoxysteroids. Moreover, if pituitary corticotrophin is suppressed by an autonomously secreting adrenal carcinoma, there will be no increase in response to metyrapone. On the other hand, if pituitary corticotrophin secretion is maintained, as occurs in adrenal hyperplasia, the inhibition of corticoid synthesis produced by metyrapone will stimulate corticotrophin secretion and the release of metabolites of precursor urinary steroids, which can be measured as 17-hydroxycorticosteroids. Metyrapone is now used less frequently in the differential diagnosis of Cushing's syndrome because of the ability to measure plasma corticotrophin directly.

The steroid-inhibiting properties of metyrapone have also been used in the treatment of Cushing's syndrome, and it remains one of the more effective drugs used to treat this syndrome. However, the compensatory rise in corticotrophin levels in response to falling cortisol levels tends to maintain adrenal activity. This requires that glucocorticoids be administered concomitantly to suppress hypothalamic–pituitary activity. Although metyrapone interferes with 11β- and 18-hydroxylation reactions and thereby inhibits aldosterone synthesis, it may not cause mineralocorticoid deficiency because of the compensatory increased production of 11-desoxycorticosterone.

Adverse Effects

Side effects associated with the use of metyrapone include gastrointestinal distress, dizziness, headache, sedation, and allergic rash. The drug should not be used in cases of adrenocortical insufficiency or when hypersensitivity reactions can be expected. When administered to pregnant women during the second or third trimesters, the drug may impair steroid biosynthesis in the fetus. Because metyrapone is relatively nontoxic, it is used in combination therapy with the more toxic aminoglutethimide to reduce its dosage.

Aminoglutethimide

Aminoglutethimide (*Cytadren*) is a competitive inhibitor of desmolase, the enzyme that catalyzes the conversion of cholesterol to pregnenolone; it also inhibits 11-hydroxylase activity. This drug also reduces estrogen production by inhibiting the aromatase enzyme complex in peripheral (skin, muscle, fat) and steroid target tissues.

Such a medical adrenalectomy is an efficacious treatment for metastatic breast and prostate cancer, since it diminishes the levels of circulating sex hormones. Glucocorticoids are administered concomitantly to suppress enhanced corticotrophin release. Cortisol is preferable to dexamethasone in this situation because aminoglutethimide markedly enhances the hepatic microsomal metabolism of dexamethasone. Hepatic enzyme induction may be responsible for the development of tolerance to the side effects of aminoglutethimide, such as ataxia, lethargy, dizziness, and rashes.

Aminoglutethimide is suitable for use in Cushing's syndrome that results from adrenal carcinoma and in congenital adrenal hyperplasia, in which it protects the patient from excessive secretion of endogenous androgens. The drug is not curative, and relapse occurs when treatment is terminated. Since aminoglutethimide therapy is frequently associated with mineralocorticoid deficiency, mineralocorticoid supplements may be needed. Aminoglutethimide and metyrapone are frequently used in combination at lower doses of both drugs as an adjunct to radiation or surgical therapy.

Mitotane

Mitotane (*Lysodren*) produces selective atrophy of the zona fasciculata and zona reticularis, which results in a decrease in the secretion of 17-hydroxycorticosteroids. Direct inhibition of cholesterol side-chain cleavage and 11β/18-hydroxylase activities has also been demonstrated. Mitotane is capable of inducing remission of Cushing's disease, but only after several weeks of therapy and at the price of severe gastrointestinal distress. Moreover, more than half of patients relapse following cessation of therapy. Other side effects include lethargy, mental confusion, skin rashes, and altered hepatic function. Being a lipid-soluble substance, mitotane remains stored in body tissues for extended periods. This may account for the marked patient-to-patient variability in its therapeutic and/or toxic effects.

Mitotane is the drug of choice for the treatment of primary adrenal carcinoma when surgery or radiation therapy is not feasible (see Chapter 56). Its effectiveness in curtailing adrenal activity is due to an action on adrenocortical mitochondria to impair cytochrome P450 steps in steroid biosynthesis. Mitotane requires metabolic transformation to exert its therapeutic action, and the differential ability of tumors to metabolize the drug may determine its clinical effectiveness. It is advised to measure serum mitotane levels and urinary free cortisol excretion to ensure adequate therapeutic concentrations. Mitotane increases circulating cholesterol by inhibiting cytochrome P450–mediated reactions and therefore contributes to the cardiovascular events that are a significant cause of mortality in untreated Cushing's syndrome.

Mitotane, being closely related to the organochlorine insecticides, shares its inductive effects on the liver microsomal drug-metabolizing enzyme system, and its use may therefore alter the requirement for concomitantly administered drugs that are also metabolized by this pathway.

Ketoconazole

Ketoconazole (*Nizoral*), an orally effective broad-spectrum antifungal agent (see Chapter 52), blocks hydroxylating enzyme systems by interacting with cytochrome P450 at the heme iron site to inhibit steroid and/or androgen synthesis in adrenals, gonads, liver, and kidney. The most sensitive site of action appears to be the C17-20 lyase reaction involved in the formation of sex steroids. This explains the greater suppressibility of testosterone production than with cortisol. Cholesterol side-chain cleavage and 11β/18-hydroxylase are secondary sites of inhibition.

Ketoconazole can be used as palliative treatment for Cushing's syndrome in patients undergoing surgery or receiving pituitary radiation and in those for whom more definitive treatment is still contemplated. Because surgical treatment is not always well tolerated by elderly patients, ketoconazole 200 to 1,000 mg/day can be a valuable alternative for the control of hypercortisolism. Common side effects include pruritus, liver dysfunction, and gastrointestinal symptoms.

Because of its effectiveness in blocking C17-20 lyase activities, ketoconazole does not enhance existing hirsutism associated with metyrapone. On the other hand, the antiandrogenic effects of ketoconazole may prove disconcerting to male patients.

Mifepristone (RU 486)

Mifepristone is a progesterone receptor antagonist that has a high affinity for glucocorticoid receptors and little agonist effect. This drug has recently been approved for use in the United States for the treatment of hypercortisolism. At high doses, mifepristone blocks negative feedback of the hypothalamic–pituitary axis, thereby increasing endogenous corticotrophin and cortisol levels. Because mifepristone exerts its effects at the receptor level and not by altering glucocorticoid production, elevated serum cortisol and corticotrophin levels may not accurately reflect the effectiveness of the therapeutic regimen. Mifepristone does not inhibit cortisol binding to the mineralocorticoid receptor, so that the resulting corticotrophin disinhibition may cause potassium depletion. Thus, administration of a mineralocorticoid receptor antagonist such as spironolactone may be indicated with mifepristone. Hypoadrenalism, nausea, and drowsiness have been reported during prolonged administration of mifepristone.

Dexamethasone

Cushing's disease is defined as hypercortisolism due to chronic overproduction of corticotrophin by a corticotroph adenoma. Cortisol's lack of suppressibility during the administration of low doses of dexamethasone but suppressibility during high-dose dexamethasone is the key diagnostic finding in 99% of the patients with Cushing's disease. This contrasts with the lack of glucocorticoid suppressibility typically found in patients with corticotrophin-independent hypercortisolism (Cushing's syndrome). A judicious selection of the available tests may be necessary to obtain an accurate diagnosis in patients with Cushing's syndrome.

Study QUESTIONS

1. During the period of withdrawal from extended glucocorticoid therapy
   (A) Prompt recovery of the hypothalamic–pituitary–adrenal axis results in restoration of endogenous corticotrophin release.
   (B) The patient may be eager to further reduce the dose of glucocorticoid.
   (C) The physician should rapidly reduce glucocorticoid therapy to physiological doses.
   (D) Patients should not require an increment in steroid therapy during increased stress (e.g., severe infection).
   (E) The appearance of fever and malaise attributed to steroid withdrawal may be difficult to distinguish from reactivation of rheumatic disease.
2. Which one of the following enzymes is required for cortisol biosynthesis?
   (A) 21-hydroxylase
   (B) 17,20 lyase
   (C) Cyclooxygenase
   (D) 11-β-hydroxysteroid dehydrogenase-2
   (E) 18-hydroxylase
3. The primary goal of glucocorticoid treatment in rheumatic arthritis is
   (A) Suppression of inflammation and improvement in functional capacity
   (B) Eradication of all symptoms
   (C) Reversal of the degenerative process
   (D) Development of a sense of well-being in the patient
   (E) Prevention of suppression of the hypothalamic–pituitary–adrenal axis

4. The addition of a fluoride group on ring C of cortisol to give 9-α-fluorocortisol
   (A) Will shorten its half-life
   (B) Will increase both glucocorticoid and mineralocorticoid activity
   (C) Shares an advantage over cortisol in that sodium retention is not as marked at equipotent inflammatory doses
   (D) Will not cause suppression of the hypothalamic–pituitary–adrenal axis when applied topically.
   (E) Provides a steroid widely used in the treatment of rheumatoid arthritis
5. Dexamethasone
   (A) Is adequate replacement therapy in an adrenalectomized patient
   (B) Has a half-life equivalent to that of cortisol
   (C) Produces salt retention in therapeutic doses
   (D) Possesses most of the undesirable side effects of cortisol
   (E) Has antiinflammatory potency equivalent to that of cortisol
6. Which answer is most appropriate for the action of ketoconazole?
   (A) It has a single major action that is confined to the adrenal cortex.
   (B) It provides long term treatment for Cushing's disease.
   (C) It has an action on the adrenal cortex that is irreversible.
   (D) Its action may be associated with liver dysfunction.
   (E) It preferentially blocks cortisol synthesis as opposed to testosterone production.

ANSWERS

1. **E.** Recovery from prolonged steroid therapy is slow, and the withdrawal may be unpleasant. The patient may be reluctant to reduce the dose of steroid because of its salutary effects on the psyche. Tapering the dose of steroid is important in steroid withdrawal; however, the patient may temporarily require a dose increase during periods of heightened stress.

2. **A.** 17,20 lyase is required for androgen synthesis, cyclooxygenase for prostaglandin production, 11-β-hydroxysteroid dehydrogenase-2 acts as a reductase-converting cortisol to its inactive 11-keto derivative cortisone, whereas 18-hydroxylase is required for aldosterone production.

3. **A.** Glucocorticoid treatment of rheumatoid arthritis does not eradicate all symptoms, nor does it reverse the degenerative process. Suppression of the hypothalamic–pituitary–adrenal axis is an unwanted side effect of glucocorticoid therapy. While development of a sense of well-being may be attributed to the relief of symptoms, it is not the primary basis for employing the potent glucocorticoids.

4. **B.** The addition of a fluoride group to ring C of cortisol to give 9-α-fluorocortisol greatly increases and prolongs all biological activity. The result is an agent with potent glucocorticoid and mineralocorticoid activity, making it inappropriate to use in rheumatoid arthritis. Because of its potency and extended action, fluorocortisol will have a greater tendency to depress the hypothalamic–pituitary axis than cortisol, even when applied topically.

5. **D.** Dexamethasone is a fluorinated glucocorticoid that is more potent and longer acting than cortisol. While devoid of salt-retaining activity in therapeutic doses, this glucocorticoid does possess most of the adverse effects observed with cortisol. Because it lacks mineralocorticoid activity, dexamethasone is not used in replacement therapy.

6. **D.** In addition to its ability to block steroid biosynthesis, ketoconazole is frequently used as an antifungal agent. Its action is readily reversible and is used principally for interim management of Cushing's disease prior to surgery or radiotherapy. Ketoconazole preferentially blocks the C17,20 lyase reaction that is involved in the synthesis of sex steroids.

SUPPLEMENTAL READING

Adcock IM. Molecular mechanisms of glucocorticoid actions. Pulmon Pharmacol Therap 2000;13:115–126.

Barnes PJ. Efficacy of inhaled corticosteroids in asthma. J Allergy Clin Immunol 1998;102:531–538.

Baxter JD. Advances in glucocorticoid therapy. Adv Intern Med 2000;45:317–349.

Boushey HA. Effects of inhaled corticosteroids on the consequences of asthma. J Allergy Clin Immunol 1998;102:S5–S16.

Compston JE. Management of bone disease in patients on long term glucocorticoid therapy. Gut 1999;44:770–772.

DaSilva JA and Bijlsma JW. Optimizing glucocorticoid therapy in rheumatoid arthritis. Rheumatol Dis Clin North Am 2000;26:859–880.

Hasinski S. Assessment of adrenal glucocorticoid function. Which tests are appropriate for screening? Postgrad Med 1988;104:61–64.

Manelli F and Giustina A. Glucocorticoid-induced osteoporosis. Trends Endocrinol Met 2000;11:79–85.

Sholter DE and Armstrong PW. Adverse effects of corticosteroids on the cardiovascular system. Can J Cardiol 2000;16:505–511.

Sonino N and Boscaro M. Medical therapy for Cushing's disease. Endocrinol Metab Clin North Am 1999;28:211–222.

CASE Study Diagnosis and Treatment of Cushing's Disease

Julie Singer is a 55-year-old white woman who was admitted to the emergency department in acute distress. A previous physical examination showed hypertension and diabetes mellitus type 2. The patient's present medications include enalapril 40 mg, nifedipine 60 mg, and 100 U insulin. A physical examination revealed prominent ankle edema, a palpable spleen, and hepatomegaly. Chest radiography revealed diffuse cardiac enlargement and left ventricular hypertrophy. Based upon the history and clinical findings, what is your diagnosis and what treatment do you recommend?

ANSWER: This study describes the clinical features of Cushing's disease (pituitary-dependent hypercortisolism), the tests for its diagnosis, and its treatment. The combination of hypertension, congestive heart failure, and hyperglycemia (blood glucose 220 mg/dL) suggest hypercortisolism (Cushing's syndrome). This tentative diagnosis was supported by a low-dose (1 mg) dexamethasone overnight suppression test demonstrating unsuppressed serum cortisol (1409 nM). It was further substantiated by elevated corticotrophin (85 pM) and suppression of serum cortisol (598 nM) by high-dose (10 mg) dex-

amethasone. Inferior petrosal sinus sampling provided a final confirmation of the diagnosis. The patient was prescribed metyrapone 2 g/day and aminoglutethimide 500 mg/day. Hyponatremia and hyperkalemia required the concomitant administration of a mineralocorticoid, fludrocortisone acetate 0.1 mg/day. With this treatment regimen, the patient's overall appearance and the clinical findings began to improve slowly. Blood pressure became better controlled, congestive failure showed improvement, insulin resistance diminished, and bone density improved. Corticotrophin levels eventually fell (from 18.5 to 8 ng/L) and serum cortisol became normally responsive to exogenous corticotrophin (rising from 407 to 1089 nM). After 6 months, the combination of metyrapone and aminoglutethimide was tapered and terminated, and radiation therapy was initiated. This study illustrates the important principle that clinical acumen and judicious use of drugs in diagnosis and treatment can lead to the dramatic reversal of the metabolic and cardiovascular abnormalities in a patient with severe Cushing's syndrome.

61 | Estrogens, Progestins, and Specific Estrogen Receptor Modulators (SERMs)

Jeannine S. Strobl

 DRUG LIST

GENERIC NAME	PAGE	GENERIC NAME	PAGE
Estrogens		Norgestrel	708
Estradiol	705	Mifepristone (anti-progestin)	709
Estropipate	710	**SERMs**	
Estrone	705	Clomiphene	707
Ethinyl estradiol	707	Faslodex	707
Mestranol	707	Raloxifene	707
Progestins		Tamoxifen	707
Medroxyprogesterone acetate	707	**Nonsteroidal Aromatase Inhibitors**	
Megestrol	707	Anastrozole	711
Norethindrone	707	Letrozole	711

NATURAL ESTROGENS AND PROGESTINS

Biologically important natural estrogens and progestins include estradiol, estrone, estriol, and progesterone. *Estradiol-17β is the most potent estrogen that is found naturally in women.* Estrone is one-tenth as biologically active as estradiol, and estriol is the weakest of the three. Estriol is synthesized by the placenta and is excreted at high levels in the urine of pregnant women. Progesterone is the most important naturally occurring progestin.

The ovary is the major site of estrogen and progestin biosynthesis in nonpregnant premenopausal women. In pregnant women, the fetoplacental unit is the major source of estrogens and progestins. Peripheral sites of estrogen synthesis include the liver, kidney, brain, adipose tissue, skeletal muscle, and testes. Progesterone is secreted in small amounts by the testes and adrenal gland. The combined estrogen and progestin production by all of these peripheral sites amounts to 10% or less of ovarian synthesis in normal premenopausal women. In postmenopausal women, ovarian steroid synthesis declines and peripheral estrogen biosynthesis accounts for all estrogen produced, both in postmenopausal women and in males.

The naturally occurring estrogens and progestins are not orally active because they are rapidly metabolically inactivated. The major site of estrogen and progestin metabolism is the liver. Both are subject to first-pass metabolism. Metabolites are also formed in the gastrointestinal tract, brain, skin, and other steroid target tissues. Estrogens and progestins are primarily excreted in the urine. Estrone, estradiol, 2-methoxyestrone, and their respective glucuronide or sulfate conjugates are the most abundant estrogen urinary metabolites. Progesterone is excreted as pregnanediol or as a pregnanediol conjugate. A small fraction (10% or less) of the estrogen metabolites enter the bile, where they may undergo enterohepatic recirculation before elimination.

Plasma proteins bind estrogens and modulate estrogenic activity. More than 90% of estradiol in the bloodstream is protein bound, with sex hormone–binding globulin (SHBG) being the major serum estrogen-binding moiety. Estrogens that are bound to SHBG are biologically inactive because of their high binding affinity, while estrogens that are bound loosely to serum albumin are available for entry into tissues and are therefore biologically active. Progesterone in plasma is 89% protein bound. Progesterone binds with a relatively high affinity to the serum protein corticosteroid-binding globulin and also to albumin.

MECHANISMS OF ACTION

Estrogens and progestins exert their effects in target tissues by a combination of cellular mechanisms. High-affinity estrogen and progestin receptors are found in target tissues. There are two forms of the estrogen receptor, ER-α and ER-β, and two forms of the progesterone receptor, PR-α and PR-β. Receptor binding by estrogens and progestins can activate a classic pathway of steroid hormone gene transcription. Gene activation is mediated by the ability of steroid hormone receptor complexes to recruit nuclear coactivator proteins to the transcription complex. Gene repression occurs in a ligand-dependent fashion by the recruitment of nuclear corepressor proteins to the transcription complex. This latter effect is an important mechanism of action of estrogen antagonism. Activation of steroid hormone receptors by their cognate ligands proceeds through receptor phosphorylation events. It is well established that estrogen and progesterone receptor activation also takes place in a ligand-independent fashion. As a result of cross-talk among cell signaling pathways, ER and PR are activated by phosphorylation events triggered by such diverse stimuli as epidermal growth factor, insulinlike growth factor, protein kinase A, and protein kinase C.

An additional mode of estrogen and progesterone action is classified as nongenomic effects. Nongenomic mechanisms for steroid hormone action are attributed to responses to estrogens and progestins that occur in a very short time (seconds to several minutes) such that they are difficult to explain by transcriptional activation. The role of the ER and PR receptors in these responses is incompletely understood. One important example of a nongenomic estrogen action that is mediated by ER-α is the rapid stimulation of endothelial nitric oxide synthase (eNOS). This enzyme produces nitric oxide. Nitric oxide has vasodilatory activity, and activation of eNOS may be an important mediator of the cardioprotective effects of estrogens.

Estradiol can augment target tissue responses to progesterone by inducing an increase in the concentration of progesterone receptors. Progesterone, on the other hand, appears to limit tissue responses to estrogen by decreasing the concentration of ERs.

ACTIONS OF ESTROGENS AND PROGESTINS IN FEMALES

The Menstrual Cycle

Secretion of gonadotropin-releasing hormone (GnRH) from the hypothalamus stimulates the release of follicle-stimulating hormone (FSH) and luteinizing hormone (LH) from the anterior pituitary. FSH and LH regulate the production of estrogen and progesterone by the ovary. Ovarian estrogen and progesterone secretion proceed in a cyclical manner. It is this cyclical release of estrogen and progesterone that determines the regular hormonal changes in the uterus, vagina, and cervix associated with the menstrual cycle. Cyclical changes in blood levels of estrogen and progesterone, together with FSH and LH, modulate the development of ova, ovulation, and the corpus luteum in the ovary.

During the first, or *follicular*, phase of the menstrual cycle, estradiol blood levels rise slowly and then fall quite rapidly. Estradiol blood levels peak around midcycle (days 12–14). The midcycle estrogen peak is thought to be important in triggering a midcycle surge of LH and FSH secretion. Estrogens have a biphasic effect on LH and FSH release, with high levels of estrogen at midcycle triggering LH and FSH release; subsequently they suppress LH and FSH secretion. This suppression is mediated by inhibition of GnRH release from the hypothalamus.

The *luteal* phase of the menstrual cycle follows the LH and FSH surge (days 14–28). The brief elevation of the LH level stimulates production of the ovarian corpus luteum. The high levels of estradiol and the FSH surge at midcycle inhibit estradiol biosynthesis by the ovarian granulosa cells. As a consequence, during the luteal phase, estrogen production is reduced and androgens produced by the ovarian thecal cells accumulate. Androgens, together with low levels of FSH, stimulate the production of progesterone by the granulosa cells in the corpus luteum. The menstrual cycle ends about 14 days later with the regression of the corpus luteum and a concomitant fall in estrogen and progesterone production. The triggering mechanism for this regression may involve both estrogens and prostaglandins. In the event that pregnancy occurs, human chorionic gonadotropin secretion by the embryo maintains the corpus luteum through stimulation of progesterone and estrogen synthesis.

Control of Pregnancy
Ovulation

During the follicular phase of the menstrual cycle, one or more follicles are prepared for ovulation. FSH and estrogens are the most important hormones for this developmental process. Complete follicular maturation cannot occur in the absence of LH. Rupture of a mature follicle follows the midcycle peak of LH and FSH by about 24 hours. In humans, usually one mature ovum is released per cycle. During the luteal phase of the menstrual cycle and under the influence of LH, the ovarian granulosa cells of the corpus luteum become vacuolated and accumulate a yellow pigment called *lutein*.

Implantation

The lining of the uterus, that is, the endometrium, is critical for implantation of the fertilized ovum. The endometrium consists of a layer of epithelial cells overlying a layer of vascularized stromal cells. Under the influence of estrogen and progesterone, the endometrium undergoes cyclical changes that prepare it for the implantation of a fertilized ovum. The follicular phase of the menstrual cycle also may be called the *proliferative phase* when referring to changes that occur in the uterus. Estrogens induce endometrial cell division and growth.

During the luteal phase, when the uterus is exposed to high concentrations of progesterone and moderate estradiol levels, the mitotic activity in the endometrial cells is suppressed. The action of progesterone on the endometrium converts it from a proliferative state to a secretory state. The epithelial cell structure assumes a more glandular appearance. Vascularization of the stroma increases, and some stromal cells begin to look like the decidual cells of early pregnancy. Estrogens and progesterone are key hormones in the maintenance of pregnancy. Estriol is produced in high concentrations by the placenta in pregnant women.

Cervical mucus is secreted by the endocervical glands and is regulated by estrogens and progestins. Under the influence of high levels of estrogen or progesterone, the physicochemical composition of cervical mucus may reduce sperm motility and provide a barrier to fertilization.

When implantation of the ovum does not occur, estrogen and progesterone levels fall and menstrual bleeding ensues. The endometrial lining, but for a single layer of epithelial cells, is shed.

Growth and Development

Estrogens cause the growth of the uterus, fallopian tubes, and vagina. Stimulation of proliferation of the vaginal epithelium is checked by the cyclical exposure to progesterone during the luteal phase in the mature female. Estrogens also are responsible for the expression of female secondary sex characteristics during puberty. These include breast enlargement, the distribution of body hair, body contours as determined by subcutaneous fat deposition, and skin texture. During development, estrogens stimulate proliferation of the ductal epithelial cells in breast tissue. Progesterone mediates lobuloalveolar development at the ends of these mammary ducts. In women, cyclical changes in the breast cell proliferation occur during the menstrual cycle, with the highest levels of proliferation occurring during the luteal phase, when circulating levels of both estrogen and progesterone are high. This has led to the idea that progesterone, as well as estrogens, exerts mitotic effects in adult human breast tissue. The effects of estrogens and progesterone on breast development are most noticeable during puberty and pregnancy.

Estrogens can stimulate the release of growth hormone and exert a positive effect on nitrogen balance. These effects contribute to the growth spurt during puberty. Closure of the bone epiphyses signaling the end of long bone growth is also estrogen mediated.

Bone remodeling occurs throughout adult life. Osteoblasts are the bone cells that are responsible for increasing bone mass. Bone loss occurs through the activity of other bone cells, called osteoclasts. Normal bone remodeling takes place when there is a balance between osteoblast and osteoclast activities. Estrogens maintain bone mass by inhibiting bone resorption by the osteoclasts. Estrogens inhibit the production of cytokines by peripheral blood cells and the osteoblasts that stimulate osteoclast activity. In postmenopausal women, declining estrogen levels give rise to a net increase in osteoclast activity and loss of bone mass resulting in the serious condition osteoporosis. Also, progestins antagonize loss of bone.

Other Actions of Estrogens and Progestins

The high levels of estrogens and progesterone associated with pregnancy may alter liver function and glucose metabolism. High circulating levels of estrogen can cause mild glucose intolerance. Estrogens increase the synthesis of many liver proteins, including transferrin, SHBG, corticosteroid-binding globulin, thyroid-binding globulin, and proteins involved in blood clotting.

Estrogens lower serum cholesterol levels by stimulating the formation of high-density lipoproteins and reducing low-density lipoproteins. Reductions in serum albumin and antithrombin III synthesis can occur in the presence of elevated female sex steroids.

In males, estrogens stimulate the growth of the stromal cells in the accessory sex organs.

SYNTHETIC AGENTS ACTING VIA ESTROGEN AND PROGESTERONE RECEPTORS

Long-acting semisynthetic estrogens and progestins contain esterified lipophilic substituents. Esterification of steroids prolongs their release from depot injection sites. Medroxyprogesterone acetate (*Amen, Cyctin, Provera, Depo-Provera*) is a widely used long-acting synthetic progestin.

Synthetic steroid hormones retain the common steroid nucleus, but they may contain novel substituents that affect their pharmacological activity. The two most widely used synthetic steroid estrogens are ethinyl estradiol (*Estinyl*) and mestranol, found in oral contraceptives. Synthetic steroids containing an ethinyl substitution are metabolized more slowly. Thus, *these synthetic steroid hormones have better oral absorption properties and extended biological half-lives than the natural estrogens.*

Approximately 50% of a dose of mestranol is demethylated to form ethinyl estradiol. Ethinyl estradiol also can be deethinylated. Subsequently, the metabolism of these two synthetic estrogens proceeds by means of the same pathways as the natural steroid hormones. The principal metabolites of mestranol and ethinyl estradiol are hydroxylated derivatives that are conjugated with either glucuronic acid or sulfate. The synthetic steroid estrogens, in contrast to the natural estrogens, are excreted primarily in the feces.

One chemical class of synthetic progestins is derived from testosterone and is referred to as the 19-nortestosterones. These compounds have progestational activity yet retain some androgenic activity. Norethindrone (*Micronor, Nor-QD*) and norethindrone acetate (*Aygestin*) are two synthetic progestins derived by the addition of an ethinyl group at the C17 position of 19-nortestosterone. There is little difference between the pharmacological activity of norethindrone and norethindrone acetate because in humans the acetate group is very readily cleaved to yield norethindrone. Norethindrone is metabolized by hydroxylation and conjugation, just as are the natural progestins. The majority of the 19-nortestosterone metabolites are conjugates that are excreted in the urine.

A second chemical class of synthetic progestins contains the pregnane nucleus structure of progesterone along with some additional substitutions. Alkyl chain additions to the C17 position increase the biological half-life of these compounds. Modifications at positions C6 and C7 increase their progestational activity. Examples of these synthetic progestins include medroxyprogesterone and megestrol acetate (*Megace*). These compounds are metabolized in the same manner as progesterone and are excreted in the urine.

SELECTIVE ESTROGEN RECEPTOR MODULATORS (SERMs)

Selective ER modulators (SERMs) are nonhormonal pharmacological agents that bind to ERs. A characteristic feature of the SERMs is that a given agent will act as an estrogen agonist in one or more tissues and as an estrogen antagonist in one or more other estrogen target organs. Tamoxifen citrate (*Nolvadex*), clomiphene citrate (*Clomid, Serophene*) and raloxifene (*Evista*) are examples of nonsteroidal SERMs. The best studied SERM is tamoxifen citrate, a drug formerly characterized as an antiestrogen.

Tamoxifen is a partial estrogen agonist in breast and thus is used as a treatment and chemopreventative for breast cancer. Tamoxifen is a full agonist in bone and endometrium, and prolonged use of tamoxifen leads to a fourfold to fivefold increase in the incidence of endometrial cancer. See Chapter 56 for a detailed discussion of the use of tamoxifen in breast cancer.

Raloxifene (*Evista*) is a new SERM approved for use in the treatment and prevention of osteoporosis because it has estrogenic activity in bone. Raloxifene is an estrogen antagonist in both breast and endometrial tissues. The estrogenlike properties of raloxifene result in the maintenance of a favorable serum lipid profile (decreased low-density lipoprotein levels with no change in either high-density lipoproteins or triglycerides). Raloxifene is 95% bound to plasma proteins. Absorption of raloxifene is impaired by cholestyramine.

Tamoxifen, clomiphene, and raloxifene are orally active. The primary route of excretion of all three drugs is in the feces. The undesirable effects common to all three of these SERMs are increased frequency of hot flashes and increased risk of thromboembolism. Both effects are attributable to their estrogenic activity.

Faslodex (*Fulvestrant*) is a SERM with no known agonist activity on the ER. It is administered as a monthly injection. In phase III clinical trials faslodex showed good activity against advanced breast cancer.

CLINICAL USES

The chief therapeutic uses of estrogens and progestins are as oral contraceptives and hormone replacement therapy. Progestins and SERMs are also important agents in the treatment of osteoporosis, breast cancer, endometrial cancer, and infertility.

Oral Contraception

Oral contraceptives are among the most effective forms of birth control (Table 61.1). The most widely used type of oral contraceptive in the United States today is the *combination* preparation, that is, a combination of estrogen and progestin (Table 61.2). Users take a tablet daily that contains both an estrogen and a progestin for 20 to 21 days of the menstrual cycle and then nothing or a placebo for the remainder of the cycle or the next 7 to 8 days. Withdrawal bleeding occurs 2 to 3 days after discontinuation of this regimen. Combination preparations vary in the dose of synthetic estrogen and progestin they contain. The use of sequential and triphasic oral contraceptives minimizes the overall dose of hormone delivered. These preparations are designed to more closely simulate estrogen-to-progestin ratios that occur physiologically during the menstrual cycle. *Ethinyl estradiol and mestranol are the only two estrogen constituents used for oral contraception in the United States.* The use of ethinyl estradiol is favored. Mestranol is inactive until it is metabolized to ethinyl estradiol.

Several progestins are used in combination products. Norgestrel (*Ovrette*) is a mixture of active and inactive enantiomers; levonorgestrel (*Norplant*) is the active enantiomer. Levonorgestrel and norethindrone are the most potent synthetic progestins in oral contraceptive preparations.

Inhibition of ovulation is the primary mechanism of the contraceptive action of sequential and combination birth control preparations. Ovulation is prevented by the suppression of the midcycle surge of FSH and LH. Estrogens are most active in inhibiting FSH release, but at high enough doses, they also inhibit LH release. In low-dose combination products, the progestin causes LH suppression. The progestin component is also important in causing withdrawal bleeding at the end of the cycle.

Combination oral contraceptive drugs having the lowest effective concentration of both estrogen and progestin should be prescribed. These preparations are known as low-dose oral contraceptive agents. Adverse effects of both estrogen and progestin are minimized with the use of these agents.

Clinical experience with the low-dose combination drugs indicates that the estrogen-to-progestin ratio is critical in achieving maximum contraceptive activity. In certain combinations (*Ortho-Novum 7/7/7, Tri-Norinyl, Tri-Levlen, Triphasil*), the estrogen-to-progestin ratio is varied in three phases over the initial 21 days by changing the progestin content of the tablets. An example of the estrogen and progestin doses found in this type of oral contraceptive is shown in Table 61.3.

Progestin-only oral contraceptive formulations consist of a low dose of either norethindrone or norgestrel

---

TABLE 61.1   Pregnancy Rates vs. Contraceptive Method

Method	Pregnancies (%)[a]
Male sterilization	0.15
Norplant System	0.20
Female sterilization	0.40
Oral contraceptives	3.00
Intrauterine device	3.00
Condom	12.00
Diaphragm or sponge	18-28
Spermicide	21.00
None	85.00

[a]Accidental pregnancy rate during a 1-year period.
Data from Trussell J and Kost K. *Stud Fam Plann* 1987:18:237.

TABLE 61.2   Some Oral Contraceptive Preparations Available in the Untied States, with Estrogen–Progestin Content

Estrogen	Progestin	Trade name
Ethinyl estradiol (20 μg)	Norethindrone acetate (1 mg)	Loestrin
Ethinyl estradiol (30 μg)	Norgestrel (300 μg)	Lo-Ovral
Ethinyl estradiol (30 μg)	Levonorgestrel (150 μg)	Nordette, Levlen
Ethinyl estradiol (35 μg)	Norethindrone (0.5 mg)	Brevicon, Modicon
Ethinyl estradiol (50 μg)	Norgestrel (0.5 mg)	Ovral
Ethinyl estradiol (50 μg)	Ethynodiol diacetate (1 mg)	Demulen
Mestranol (50 μg)	Norethindrone (1 mg)	Ortho-Novum, Norinyl, Norethin
None	Norethindrone (0.35 mg)	Micronor, Nor-QD
None	Norgestrel (0.075 mg)	Ovrette

TABLE 61.3   Estrogen and Progestin Composition of Tri-Levlen 28, a Triphasic Oral Contraceptive

	Estrogen	Progestin	Days
Phase I	Ethinyl estradiol (30 μg)	Levonorgestrel (50 μg)	1–6
Phase II	Ethinyl estradiol (40 μg)	Levonorgestrel (75 μg)	7–11
Phase III	Ethinyl estradiol (30 μg)	Levonorgestrel (125 μg)	12–21
Blank tablets	0	0	22–28

(Table 61.2). Because of an increased incidence of certain side effects and slightly decreased contraceptive activity, progestin-only oral contraceptives are not extensively used. The undesirable side effects associated with progestin-only contraceptives are irregular bleeding episodes, headache, weight gain, and mood changes. Progestin-only contraceptive *devices* are used. The *Norplant System* for contraception consists of a series of levonorgestrel-filled pliable plastic tubes that are implanted subcutaneously on the inside of the upper arm by a physician. While one set of six tubes can remain effective for up to 5 years, the contraceptive effects are readily reversible with removal of the implant. Adverse effects are similar to those seen with other progestin-only contraceptives; however, accidental pregnancy is less frequent.

Mirena is a relatively new intrauterine contraceptive device that releases levonorgestrel into the uterine cavity for 5 years. Use of this contraceptive device is associated with fewer systemic progestin side effects and is at least as effective as *Norplant.*

Abortifacients and Emergency Contraceptives

Progesterone is a hormone required for the maintenance of pregnancy. Termination of early pregnancy is effected using the steroidal antiprogestin drug, mifepristone (RU486), which acts by blocking progestin binding to the progesterone receptor. A single oral dose of RU486 followed by a single dose of a prostaglandin (*Misoprostol*) 48 hours later is 90 to 95% effective in terminating pregnancy. The side effects are generally mild except for heavy bleeding. Severe cardiovascular complications have occurred and may be due to the prostaglandin component of this treatment. The use of RU486 is therefore contraindicated in women at risk for cardiovascular disease, including smokers and women over 35 years of age.

High-dose estrogen and high-dose progestin are effective in emergency contraception when given immediately following unprotected coitus. *Plan B* is an emergency contraceptive kit consisting of two tablets of the progestin levonorgestrel (0.75 mg). The first tablet must be taken as soon as possible but no later than 3 days after coitus, and the second tablet is taken 72 hours later. This regimen is more effective and better tolerated than the *Preven* emergency contraceptive kit, an estrogen–progestin combination (two tablets of 50 μg ethinyl estradiol and two tablets of 0.25 mg of levonorgestrel). The high doses of estrogen in the *Preven* regimen are associated with severe nausea and vomiting.

Hormone Replacement Therapy

The beginning of menopause is marked by the last menstrual cycle. This is the result of declining ovarian func-

tion and reduced synthesis of estrogens and progesterone. Estrogen production in postmenopausal women is usually only about 10% of that in premenopausal women. Almost no progesterone is synthesized in postmenopausal women. Hormone replacement therapy (HRT) generally refers to the administration of estrogen–progestin combinations. Estrogen replacement therapy (ERT) consists of the use of an estrogen alone, usually in the form of conjugated equine estrogens or an estrogen transdermal patch.

The four most common symptoms associated with menopause are vasomotor disorders, or hot flashes; urogenital atrophy; osteoporosis; and psychological disturbances. A varying proportion of women may have one or more of these symptoms.

Osteoporosis

One in four postmenopausal women have osteoporosis. *Osteoporosis, a decrease in bone mass, constitutes the most serious effect of menopause.* It has been estimated that following cessation of ovarian function, the loss of bone mass proceeds at a rate of 2 to 5% per year. As a result of osteoporosis, as many as 50% of women develop spinal compression fractures by age 75, and 20% will have hip fractures by age 90.

Estrogen replacement therapy can prevent bone loss and actually increase bone density in postmenopausal women. *Estrogen treatment is the most effective therapy for osteoporosis* and significantly reduces the incidence of bone fractures in postmenopausal women. The usual dose of estrogen prescribed is 0.625 mg/day of conjugated equine estrogens (*Premarin*). Alternatively, a transdermal estrogen patch can be used.

Endometrial cancer is not a concern in women who have undergone hysterectomy. However, in women with an intact uterus, there is a risk of endometrial cancer with ERT. A preliminary endometrial biopsy should be performed before instituting therapy to rule out endometrial hyperplasia or cancer, and biopsies should be repeated at 6- to 12-month intervals in women receiving ERT. When endometrial cancer is a concern, patients should consider HRT. Estrogens should be given in an intermittent fashion followed by at least 7 to 10 days of treatment with a progestin alone. Oral norgestimate, norethindrone acetate, and medroxyprogesterone acetate are progestins given to postmenopausal women receiving estrogens to control endometrial proliferation.

Alternatives to steroid hormone therapy for osteoporosis include raloxifene, bisphosphonates, sodium fluoride, vitamin D and calcium supplementation, calcitonin, and parathyroid hormone. Tamoxifen has estrogenic effects on bone and delays bone loss in postmenopausal women. However as a result of estrogenic activity in the uterus, long-term tamoxifen administration has been associated with an increased risk of endometrial cancer. Raloxifene has estrogenic activity on bone but antiestrogenic activity in uterus and breast tissue. Raloxifene is a SERM that was specifically approved for the prevention and treatment of osteoporosis.

Cardiovascular Actions

Declining estrogen levels associated with menopause are correlated with an increased risk of cardiovascular related deaths in women. The protective effects of estrogens on the lipid profile are well recognized. There is a relationship between elevated levels of cholesterol, triglycerides, very low density lipoproteins, low-density lipoproteins, and coronary artery disease; in contrast, the elevation of high-density lipoproteins appears to be related to a reduced incidence of cardiovascular effects. The hormonal effects produced by estrogen and progestin therapy vary with the dosage, duration, route of administration, and particular preparation. In general, estrogenic compounds lower levels of "bad cholesterol" (low-density lipoproteins), while progestins raise low-density lipoproteins and triglycerides.

The use of HRT for mitigation of cardiovascular disease is not supported by the most recent clinical studies. The use of estrogen–progestin combinations in postmenopausal women was associated with a slight increase in coronary artery disease and a threefold elevation in thromboembolic episodes.

Conjugated equine estrogens (*Premarin*) are the most commonly used estrogens in the treatment of menopause-associated vasomotor symptoms and osteoporosis. *Premarin* is a mixture of estrogen sulfates, including estrone, equilin, and 17-β-dihydroequilin. The sulfate derivatives are orally active and are cleaved within the body to yield the active, unconjugated estrogen.

Premphase is an estrogen–progestin combination that introduces a cyclic progestin component. *Premphase* packets consist of a 2-week regimen of daily 0.625-mg conjugated equine estrogens followed by a 2-week period of a combination of conjugated equine estrogens and daily medroxyprogesterone. Esterified estrogens, primarily sodium estrone sulfate (*Estratab*), and estropipate (*Ogen*) are also used. Several transdermal patches deliver estradiol continuously. These products differ in their dose of estradiol: *Climara*, 0.025 mg/day; *Estraderm*, 0.05 mg/day; and *Vivelle*, 0.0375 mg/day.

Vasomotor Symptoms

Vasomotor disorders (hot flashes) are common, affecting 70 to 80% of postmenopausal women. The cause of the vasomotor changes appears to be associated with the release of LH after normal female estrogen levels have fallen. These symptoms occur with variable frequency but generally disappear without treatment within 2 to 3 years of onset. Estrogen or progestin therapy is often effective in suppressing vasomotor symptoms. Short-term estrogen therapy (2 years) for these symptoms is recommended and is not associated with increased cancer risk. Continuous therapy is usually not required.

Urogenital Atrophy

The tissues of the distal vagina and urethra are of similar embryonic origin, and both are sensitive to the trophic action of estrogens. Postmenopausal atrophy of these tissues may result in painful sexual intercourse, dysuria, and frequent genitourinary infections. Unlike the vasomotor complaints, these symptoms seldom improve if untreated. Treatment with a combination of minimally effective dosages of an estrogen and a progestin is recommended. Estrogen can be administered orally or in a topical preparation with equivalent efficacy. Progestins are given orally.

Replacement Therapy in Premenopausal Women

Oophorectomy causes many of the symptoms seen in menopause. The onset and intensity of vasomotor symptoms and osteoporosis, however, may be more severe than in women proceeding into the more gradual age-associated process of menopause. The regimens for estrogen–progestin replacement therapy in oophorectomized patients are comparable to those recommended for postmenopausal women.

Several genetic conditions lead to a failure of ovarian development. These genetic alterations lead to a failure in the synthesis of normal amounts of estrogen or progesterone, so that female secondary sex characteristics do not appear at puberty. Only with estrogen treatment is there stimulation of the growth of the genitalia, breast enlargement, and development of female body contours and distribution of body hair. Some increases in body height also occur with estrogen therapy, but this is more marked after androgen treatment. Replacement estrogens can be administered using a transdermal patch formulation or micronized estradiol (*Estrace, Gynodiol*).

Central Nervous System Effects

Insomnia and fatigue in many postmenopausal women may be related to reduced estrogen levels; there is a correlation between the incidence of waking episodes and low levels of estrogen. Estrogen replacement therapy may be used to treat severe cases.

There is considerable interest in the role of estrogen hormone replacement therapy as a cognitive enhancer in postmenopausal women. Although there is some evidence for improved cognitive abilities in postmenopausal women receiving estrogen replacement therapy, the effects reported thus far are modest.

Infertility

Anovulation, often related to altered ratios of estrogen to progestin, can be treated with a variety of agents, including estrogen–progestin replacement, clomiphene citrate, bromocriptine, FSH, LH, human chorionic gonadotropin, and GnRH. Clomiphene citrate (*Clomid, Serophene*) and bromocriptine (*Parlodel*) are the two most widely used agents.

Induction of Ovulation

Anovulation can be due to an insufficient release of LH and FSH during the mid phase of the menstrual cycle. Induction of ovulation by clomiphene citrate is the result of stimulation of FSH and LH release. The mechanism of this action is probably related to the *estrogen antagonist* properties of clomiphene citrate. Although estrogens generally exert a negative-feedback inhibition on FSH and LH secretion by means of a suppression of GnRH from the hypothalamus, clomiphene exerts its action by stimulating secretion of these hormones. Antagonism of this feedback system results in a surge of FSH and LH secretion, hence ovulation.

Patients with normal or elevated estrogen levels and normal pituitary and hypothalamic function respond most frequently to treatment with clomiphene citrate. In this group, the ovulation rate following clomiphene citrate may be 80%. Clomiphene citrate is administered on a cyclic schedule. First, menstrual bleeding is induced; next drug is given orally for 5 days at 50 mg/day. Ovulation is expected 5 to 11 days after the dose of clomiphene citrate. Pregnancy rates approach 50 to 80% after six such treatment cycles, with most pregnancies occurring during the first three treatment cycles. Clomiphene is also used in conjunction with gonadotropins to induce ovulation for in vitro fertilization.

CANCER

Certain tissues of the female reproductive tract, which are subject to the trophic action of hormones, exhibit a high frequency of neoplasia. Cancer of the breast, the second most common form of cancer in American women, and the rarer endometrial cancer in women, are often responsive to treatments with estrogens or progestins. The toxicity of these hormonal treatments compared with standard cancer chemotherapy is low.

Breast Cancer

Early breast cancer is usually treated by surgery and local irradiation. Hormonal therapy is reserved for patients with advanced metastatic breast cancer. Breast cancer occurs in both premenopausal and postmeno- pausal women. Approximately one-third of patients have a complete or partial remission with a mean duration of 9 to 12 months after hormonal therapy. Hormonal therapy of advanced breast cancer is not curative, but extended control of disease is possible by the use of different hormonal therapies sequentially.

Estrogen receptor–positive breast cancer in premenopausal and postmenopausal women responds equally to tamoxifen therapy (see Chapter 58). In addition, daily tamoxifen administration for 5 years is a successful therapy for the prevention of breast cancer in the contralateral breast in women who have already had one episode of breast cancer.

Progestins have been used with some success in the treatment of breast cancer, and the response rate is approximately the same as with tamoxifen. Most clinical experience has been obtained using oral megestrol acetate.

The successful response of breast cancers to tamoxifen or progestin treatment depends on the presence of high-affinity receptors for estrogen, progesterone, or both. Fewer than 10% of mammary tumors that lack detectable ER levels will respond to hormonal therapies. *Determination of hormone receptor levels in tumor samples is highly recommended before selecting a therapy.*

Although estrone is a weak estrogen, breast tissue metabolizes estrone and estrone sulfate to estradiol, providing a trophic signal for tumor growth. *The newest drug introduced for the hormonal control of breast cancer is letrozole (Femara).* It is a nonsteroidal aromatase inhibitor that dramatically reduces serum levels of estradiol, estrone, and estrone sulfate in postmenopausal women by blocking the conversion of adrenal androgens, androstenedione, and testosterone to estrone and estradiol. The duration of remission in breast cancer patients treated with letrozole exceeds that of tamoxifen, and the drug can be used even in tumors that have developed resistance to tamoxifen. Letrozole is orally active and is excreted primarily in the urine. The incidence of side effects is rare. It does not change serum corticosteroid, aldosterone, or thyroid hormone levels. Anastrozole (*Arimidex*) is another promising third-generation aromatase inhibitor.

Endometrial Cancer

Progesterone administration induces remissions in approximately one-third of patients with metastatic endometrial cancer. The mean duration of response is 27 months. Almost 60% of endometrial adenocarcinomas contain progesterone receptors. Preliminary data show a correlation between progesterone receptor status and response rates in this disease. The mechanism of the effect of progesterone on endometrial cancer is not known.

OTHER USES

Other clinical uses of estrogens and progestins include the treatment of dysfunctional uterine bleeding, dysmenorrhea, endometriosis, and rarely, metastatic prostate cancer.

Breast Cancer

Administration of estrogen alone or estrogen–progestin combinations multiplies by 1.2 to 1.8 the relative risk of breast cancer in postmenopausal women. The risk is slightly greater in women taking estrogen–progestin (conjugated equine estrogens plus medroxyprogesterone acetate) compared with women taking estrogen alone (conjugated equine estrogens). In addition, the risk is greater for lean women (low body mass index) with either therapy. Thus, the ability of progestins to protect the endometrium from cancer risk is not observed in breast tissue. Oral contraceptive use in younger women does not seem to be associated with an increased breast cancer risk.

Ovarian Cancer

Oral contraceptive use lessens the incidence of ovarian cancer.

Hepatic Cancer

Hepatocellular carcinoma and benign hepatomas are rare complications of oral contraceptive and tamoxifen use.

Cardiovascular Complications

Estrogen replacement therapy is associated with an increased risk of thromboembolic disease, and alternative therapies for osteoporosis and cardiovascular protection are recommended for individuals with prior thromboembolic episodes. The problems generally are more severe and/or more frequent when either of the synthetic estrogens, ethinyl estradiol or mestranol, is used. These preparations alter liver function more significantly than do the natural estrogens, such as the sulfate conjugates or esterified estrogens. Alterations in the synthesis of specific liver proteins, such as coagulation factors and fibrinogen, are implicated in the formation of thromboembolisms. Conjugated estrogens, tamoxifen, clomiphene and raloxifene also increase the frequency of thromboembolic disease.

Current estimates are that oral contraceptive use doubles to triples the overall risk of thromboembolic disease. The increased use in recent years of oral contraceptives with lower estrogen content probably contributes to the decreased risk. However, the risk is greater in women who smoke, who are over age 35, or who are diabetic.

Mild hypertension and fluid retention frequently occur in oral contraceptive users. Systolic blood pressure is elevated 5 to 6 mm Hg; diastolic blood pressure increases are on the order of 1 to 2 mm Hg. Hypertension is not commonly a problem in postmenopausal women receiving conjugated estrogens.

Migraine Headaches

A 0.5% incidence of migraines has been reported among users of oral contraceptives. Migraine headaches may be a warning signal for an oncoming stroke, and immediate discontinuation of oral contraceptive use is recommended.

Teratogenesis

Diethylstilbestrol (DES) was once given to prevent spontaneous abortion, but it no longer has such a medical indication. There is a 0.01 to 0.1% incidence of a rare vaginal and cervical clear cell adenocarcinoma among the daughters of mothers who received DES during their first trimester of pregnancy. An increased cancer incidence in male offspring of mothers who had received DES has also been noted.

Progestins may be teratogenic during the first trimester of pregnancy. Therefore, if pregnancy is suspected, oral contraceptive use should not be initiated or use should be stopped promptly.

Fertility

There is some delay in the return of fertility after discontinuation of oral contraceptive use. Gonadotropin profiles should be normal 3 months after combination oral contraceptive use is stopped. The incidence of prolonged amenorrhea extending beyond 6 months is 2 to 3%. This reaction is especially a problem with the use of progestin-only minipills.

Breast Feeding

The use of oral contraceptives may interfere with lactation. In addition, the hormones may be present in the mother's milk, hence be taken in by the nursing child. If breast feeding is planned, the use of oral contraceptives should be discontinued until after weaning.

Gallbladder Disease

There is a 2.5-fold increased incidence of gallbladder disease in postmenopausal women receiving estrogens. This occurrence may be related to changes in plasma lipid metabolism.

Glucose Tolerance

Estrogen usage is associated with a mild decrease in glucose tolerance. Estrogens do not cause diabetes, but their concurrent use in the diabetic patient may necessitate adjustment in insulin dosage.

ADVERSE EFFECTS

Common side effects associated with estrogen use include nausea, weight gain, and edema. Progestin use is associated with weight gain and mild depression. Tolerance to these effects usually develops over several months.

Low-dose estrogen combination oral contraceptives result in irregular midcycle bleeding episodes in some patients. High-progestin preparations, especially the progestin-only minipill, can cause irregular bleeding and prolonged amenorrhea.

Endometrial hyperplasia frequently develops in premenopausal and postmenopausal women receiving estrogens alone. This reaction is generally regarded to be a premalignant state, because individuals reported to have endometrial hyperplasia later have a higher than normal incidence of endometrial carcinoma. *Administration of estrogens only is associated with a 1.7- to 15-fold increased risk of endometrial carcinoma.* The relative risk rises with increased dosage and duration of estrogen use. Women receiving progestins 10 days per month during estrogen therapy generally do not develop endometrial carcinoma. Women taking combination oral contraceptives have slightly less risk of developing endometrial carcinoma than nonusers. This may be related to the constant exposure of the endometrium to both progestin and estrogen.

Adverse Reactions to SERMs

Ovarian enlargement is the most common side effect of clomiphene use. The occurrence of multiple births following ovulation induction with clomiphene is 4 to 9%; 90% of these multiple births are twins. Since clomiphene is teratogenic, therapy should be discontinued if there is a chance that conception has occurred. Rarely, irreversible ocular toxicities have been reported with clomiphene use.

Nausea, vomiting, and hot flashes may accompany tamoxifen administration. Tamoxifen may cause a transient flare of tumor growth and increased pain due to bone metastases. These reactions are thought to be due to an initial estrogenic action of this drug. Mild or tran-

sient depression of platelet counts often occurs in patients receiving tamoxifen. At very high doses, generally no longer used in cancer treatment, ocular toxicity has been reported. There is a slight risk of hepatocellular carcinoma in humans receiving long-term (5 years) tamoxifen therapy as well as a slightly (0.4%) elevated incidence of endometrial cancer.

Raloxifene and clomiphene use is associated with an increased frequency of vasomotor disturbances (hot flashes) and thromboembolism formation.

CONTRAINDICATIONS AND DRUG INTERACTIONS

Some of the contraindications to the use of estrogens, progestins, and estrogen–progestin combinations are presented in Table 61.4.

Certain concomitantly administered drugs may interfere with the effectiveness of the oral contraceptives or lead to an increased incidence of breakthrough bleeding. These include rifampin, isoniazid, ampicillin, neomycin, penicillin V, chloramphenicol, sulfonamides, nitrofurantoin, phenytoin, barbiturates, primidone, analgesics, and phenothiazines.

The oral contraceptives also may decrease the effectiveness of anticoagulants, anticonvulsants, tricyclic antidepressants, guanethidine, and hypoglycemic agents. The causes of such drug interactions include alterations in hepatic microsomal drug-metabolizing enzymes, competition for binding sites on plasma proteins, and enhanced excretion.

Raloxifene absorption is inhibited by cholestyramine.

TABLE 61.4 Contraindications for Drug Use

Formulation	
Estrogens	Breast or endometrial cancer or vaginal bleeding of unknown origin
	Pregnancy
	Hepatic dysfunction or liver cancer
	Preexisting cardiovascular disease
Progestins	Pregnancy
	Depression
Oral contraceptives	Pregnancy
	Smokers over age 35
Antiestrogens	Pregnancy
	Endometrial cancer

Study Questions

1. Raloxifene is a SERM. A characteristic of SERMs is that they
   (A) Act as estrogen agonists at all ERs
   (B) Antagonize estrogens at all ERs
   (C) Act as agonists at some and antagonists at other ERs

2. The most widely used type of oral contraceptive in the United States is
   (A) Estrogen only
   (B) Progestin only
   (C) Combination of estrogen and progestin

3. Osteoporosis is the most serious effect of menopause. All of the following statements about osteoporosis are true EXCEPT
   (A) Estrogen is an effective treatment.
   (B) If endometrial cancer is a concern, a combination of estrogen and progestin should be considered.
   (C) Vitamin D and calcium supplementation are alternatives to steroid hormone therapy.
   (D) Bisphosphonates are ineffective in prevention of osteoporosis.
   (E) Calcitonin is a useful alternative agent.

4. Breast cancer is the second most common cancer in women. All of the following statements concerning breast cancer at true EXCEPT
   (A) Hormonal therapy is reserved for patients with advanced metastases.
   (B) Estrogen treatment is an acceptable form of hormonal therapy.
   (C) Progestin treatment is an accepted form of hormonal therapy.
   (D) Tamoxifen is an accepted form of nonhormonal therapy.

5. The mechanism of action of the compound RU486 is to
   (A) Block estrogen binding to ERs
   (B) Block progestin binding to progesterone receptors
   (C) Act as an estrogen agonist
   (D) Act as a progesterone agonist

ANSWERS

1. **C.** Raloxifene is a recently approved SERM. It is a partial estrogen agonist in breast tissue but was initially characterized as an antiestrogen. It, like the best-studied SERM, tamoxifen, has estrogen agonist properties in some tissues and estrogen antagonism properties in others.

2. **C.** Although progestin-only oral contraceptive formulations are available, the combination of estrogen and progestin is considered the safest and most desirable type.

3. **D.** The bisphosphonates are a useful alternative therapy to steroid hormones. Estrogen treatment is effective, but in some patients the risks outweigh the benefits.

4. **B.** Estrogen therapy is contraindicated in the presence of breast cancer. Normal breast growth is stimulated by estrogens, and estrogen administration is therefore contraindicated. Hormonal therapy is normally reserved for patients with advanced metastases. Surgery and local irradiation are the preferred therapy for early breast cancer. Progestin treatment and tamoxifen therapy are both accepted forms of therapy. Both are more effective in treatment of cancers with high-affinity receptors for estrogen, progesterone, or both.

5. **B.** RU 486 acts as a competitive progesterone antagonist and blocks progesterone binding at its receptors. It has no activity at estrogenic receptors.

SUPPLEMENTAL READING

Choice of Contraceptives. Med Lett 1995;37:9–12.

McClung B and McClung M. Pharmacologic therapy for the treatment and prevention of osteoporosis. Nursing Clin North Am 2001;36:433–440.

Schairer C et al. Menopausal estrogen and estrogen-progestin replacement therapy and breast cancer risk. JAMA 2000;283:485–491.

Willett WC, Colditz G, and Stampfer M. Postmenopausal estrogens: Opposed, unopposed, or none of the above. JAMA 2000;283:534–535.

CASE Study   Use of Hormones in Menopause

Joan Jenkins is a 56-year-old woman who comes to your office complaining of hot flashes, increased irritability, and inability to concentrate on day-to-day tasks. She indicates that she is undergoing menopause but that she does not want to take any hormones because her mother had breast cancer and she was afraid that this would increase her risk. She says the symptoms are almost unbearable. What do you advise?

ANSWER: You should try to allay her fears but point out that she is correct in being concerned. Tell her that there is an increased risk of breast cancer after estrogen or estrogen–progestin combination therapy but that the risk is relatively small. Inform her that her severe symptoms will be relatively short-lived and suggest trying hormone replacement therapy for a short time to see if the condition is greatly improved. The use of estrogen replacement for short periods (up to 2 years) is not associated with an increased incidence of breast cancer. You should also point out that osteoporosis is the most serious menopausal symptom and that there are alternatives to hormone therapy in preventing the decrease in bone mass associated with menopause. She should be encouraged to take calcium and vitamin D supplementation immediately. She should be scheduled for baseline determination of her bone density so that any evidence of loss of bone mass can be ascertained.

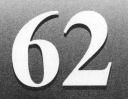

62 Uterine Stimulants and Relaxants

Leo R. Brancazio and Robert E. Stitzel

 DRUG LIST

GENERIC NAME	PAGE	GENERIC NAME	PAGE
Atosiban	721	Magnesium sulfate	720
Carboprost tromethamine	719	Methylergonovine	718
Dinoprostone	719	Misoprostol	719
Ergonovine	718	Oxytocin	718
Hydroxyprogesterone	721	Nifedipine	721
Indomethacin	721	Terbutaline	720

The physiological processes involved in *parturition* (i.e., labor, delivery, and birth) require a complex interplay of hormonal action, neuronal activity, and uterine smooth muscle contraction. During the first two trimesters of pregnancy, the uterus remains in a relatively quiescent state, demonstrating little or no contraction of the myometrium. This inactivity is largely the result of the inhibitory action of high circulating levels of progesterone on the uterine musculature (see Chapter 63). During the final trimester, however, uterine smooth muscle becomes increasingly excitable, such that mild muscle contractions are seen (Braxton-Hicks contractions); these gradually increase in both strength and frequency, occasionally to the extent that they may even be thought to signal the onset of labor, a phenomenon termed *false labor.* Parturition requires in part the integration of processes that involve cervical canal dilation and uterine smooth muscle contractions that are strong enough to expel the fetus.

Other physiological events must occur at the end of pregnancy to facilitate birth. The cervix begins to soften (*cervical ripening*) as a direct result of connective tissue dissociation; this process may involve the actions of the peptide hormone *relaxin,* which is produced both in the corpus luteum and in the placenta. Relaxin also aids in the dissociation of the connective tissue between the pelvic bones, a process that also aids in the facilitation of birth. At the true onset of labor, coordinated, rhythmic contractions of the uterus begin, and as labor progresses, the myometrial contractions increase in intensity and strength. These contractions force the fetus against the cervix, further dilating the cervix. Once the cervix has dilated sufficiently, the uterine contractions push the fetus through the birth canal.

A variety of endocrine hormones play a role in initiating the changes in uterine contractility, especially during the final trimester. It is probable that the concentration of receptors responsive to the hypothalamic peptide hormone *oxytocin* (see Chapter 59) increases in the uterine musculature in response to the increasing levels of estrogen during pregnancy. Although circulating blood levels of oxytocin do not change markedly throughout pregnancy, it is likely that the augmented number of oxytocin receptors in the uterus makes the muscle increasingly responsive to plasma oxytocin. There also is speculation that the uterus itself may be capable of synthesizing oxytocin. If such a synthesis does indeed occur, much higher local concentrations of the peptide will be found than would be predicted strictly on the basis of circulating amounts of the hormone. Increases in the number of myometrial α-adrenergic and angiotensin receptors also will increase the sensitivity of these muscle cells to contractile stimuli. Finally, the possibility of fetal factors playing a role in the initiation of parturition should be considered.

Although, like other smooth muscle, the myometrium is capable of contraction at any time, it is generally quiescent throughout most of pregnancy. As pregnancy progresses, spontaneous repetitive action potentials can be seen, but muscle tension will develop only once these action potentials become synchronized electrical discharges. Contractions do become evident, however, several weeks before labor begins. The contractions of the myometrium progressively increase during the onset of labor, in part through the action of a positive neuroendocrine feedback system that involves both synthesis and release of oxytocin and prostaglandins. The stretching of the softened cervix induced by increasing fetal pressure results in local receptor stimulation and the initiating of a spinal reflex that eventually results in the release of oxytocin from the posterior pituitary. This additional oxytocin will further promote uterine contractions.

Release of oxytocin at this stage of parturition promotes prostaglandin production, particularly of the E and F series, within the decidua; these prostaglandins are powerful myometrial stimulants and thus further enhance uterine contractions. The prostaglandin concentration in maternal serum and amniotic fluid increases with the progression of labor.

Many of the biochemical and molecular events that are responsible for uterine smooth muscle contraction are the same as those that control other smooth muscle tissues (Fig. 62.1). Once uterine smooth muscle sensitivity has been augmented, actin and myosin must interact for contraction to occur. This interaction depends on the phosphorylation of the contractile proteins by the enzyme *myosin light chain kinase* (MLCK). This enzyme requires Ca^{++} and is active only when associated with calmodulin. *Activation of the entire muscle contraction*

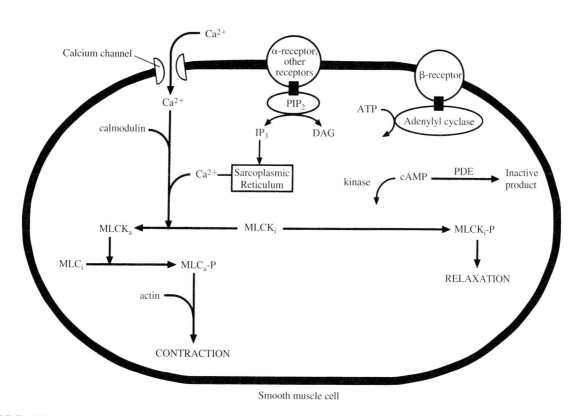

FIGURE 62.1

Major biochemical events of smooth (uterine) muscle contraction and relaxation. Calcium (Ca^{++}) binds to calmodulin and initiates a series of biochemical reactions that ultimately lead to muscle contraction. $MLCK_i$, myosin light chain kinase (inactivated); $MLCK_a$, myosin light chain kinase (activated); MLC_i, inactive myosin light chain; MLC_a-P, phosphorylated active myosin light chain; $MLCK_i$-P, phosphorylated MLCK; PDE, phosphodiesterase; PIP_2, phosphatidylinositol; IP_3, inositol triphosphate; DAG, diacylglycerol.

process involves the receptor binding of estrogen, oxytocin, α_1-adrenergic agonists, and prostaglandins (PGE$_1$ and PGE$_2$). A decrease in the progesterone–estrogen ratio in the myometrium is also an important factor in the timing and initiation of labor; this altered ratio may involve increased fetal estrogen production, particularly in the latter weeks of pregnancy. *Cytokines produced by the fetus* are also thought to be responsible for stimulating uterine contraction.

Uterine relaxation is mediated in part through inhibition of MLCK. This inhibition results from the phosphorylation of MLCK that follows the stimulation of myometrial β-adrenoceptors; relaxation involves the activity of a cyclic adenosine monophosphate (cAMP) mediated protein kinase, accumulation of Ca^{++} in the sarcoplasmic reticulum, and a decrease in cytoplasmic Ca^{++}. Other circulating substances that favor quiescence of uterine smooth muscle include progesterone, which increases throughout pregnancy, and possibly prostacyclin. Progesterone's action probably involves hyperpolarization of the muscle cell membrane, reduction of impulse conduction in muscle cells, and increased calcium binding to the sarcoplasmic reticulum.

Drugs and hormones used clinically to enhance uterine contractions are primarily employed either to induce or to augment contractions during labor and delivery. They have particular value in limiting an extended pregnancy, preventing the early rupture of membranes, or aiding placental insufficiency. Many of these compounds also are useful in limiting postpartum hemorrhage. *The primary use of uterine relaxants (tocolytic agents) is in the prevention of premature labor.* These drugs act either directly to suppress myometrial smooth muscle contraction or indirectly to inhibit synthesis or release of the prostaglandins and/or other endogenous uterine stimulants.

UTERINE STIMULANTS

Oxytocin

Oxytocin (*Pitocin, Syntocinon*) is a cyclic 8–amino acid peptide that is synthesized in the paraventricular nucleus of the hypothalamus and transported within hypothalamic neurons (in association with neurophysin) to the posterior pituitary for storage. Its mechanism of action involves the direct stimulation of oxytocin receptors found on the myometrial cells. Oxytocin circulates unbound in the plasma, where it has a half-life of approximately 15 minutes. It is primarily inactivated in the kidneys and liver.

Oxytocin is generally considered to be the drug of choice for inducing labor at term. In combination with amniotomy, oxytocin is highly successful in inducing and augmenting labor. When given oxytocin, approximately 80% of patients with documented labor disorders progress into labor and deliver vaginally. It has also been used following incomplete abortion after 20 weeks of gestation (although use of prostaglandins may be preferred in this instance), and it may be used after full-term delivery to prevent or control uterine hemorrhage. Oxytocin in high doses is used to induce abortion. An oxytocin challenge test (an assessment of the fetal heart rate in response to oxytocin-induced contractions) can be performed in certain high-risk (e.g., those with hypertension, diabetes, preeclampsia) obstetrical patients as a measure of fetal well-being.

Inappropriate use of oxytocin can lead to uterine rupture, anaphylactoid and other allergic reactions, and possibly maternal death. Prolonged stimulation of uterine contractions can result in the following fetal adverse reactions: persistent uteroplacental insufficiency, sinus bradycardia, premature ventricular contractions, other arrhythmias, and fetal death. Prolonged use of oxytocin can lead to water intoxication secondary to the antidiuretic hormone–like effects of oxytocin. Maternal and fetal cardiovascular parameters should be monitored during oxytocin administration.

Oxytocin may be given by intravenous infusion (e.g., labor induction), intramuscular injection (e.g., control of postpartum bleeding), or as a nasal spray (e.g., to promote milk ejection).

Ergonovine Maleate and Methylergonovine Maleate

Ergonovine (*Ergotrate*) and methylergonovine (*Methergine*) are compounds obtained either directly or semisynthetically from ergot, a fungus that grows on rye and other grains. These compounds stimulate uterine smooth muscle directly, thereby increasing muscular tone and enhancing the rate and force of rhythmical contractions. Ergonovine also stimulates cervical contractions. These drugs are capable of inducing a sustained tetanic contraction, which can shorten the final stage of labor and aid in the reduction of postpartum blood loss. Both are commonly used for the routine expulsion of the placenta after delivery and in postpartum and postabortal atony and hemorrhage.

Both drugs are partial agonists at α-adrenergic receptors and at some serotonin and dopamine receptors; they also can inhibit the release of endothelial-derived relaxation factor. They may induce arterial vasoconstriction and have minor actions on the central nervous system. Their α-adrenergic blocking activity is relatively weak compared with those of other ergot alkaloids.

Absorption is rapid and largely complete after oral administration, and onset of action occurs in 5 to 15 minutes and lasts about 3 hours. Both ergonovine and methylergonovine can be given intramuscularly or intravenously, although intravenous administration can be associated with transient but severe hypertension. These compounds undergo hepatic metabolism, with elimination primarily by renal excretion of metabolites. They also can be found in breast milk, and therefore, neither drug should be administered longer than necessary, since prolonged use can lead to ergot poisoning (ergotism), including gangrene, in the nursing infant.

Adverse reactions associated with their administration include hypertension, headache, and possible seizures. Nausea, vomiting, chest pains, difficulties in breathing, and leg cramps also have been reported. These alkaloids should not be used in cases of threatened spontaneous abortion or in patients with known allergies to the drugs. Contraindications generally include angina pectoris, myocardial infarction, pregnancy, and a history of a cerebrovascular accident, transient ischemic attack, or hypertension.

Dinoprostone, Carboprost Tromethamine, and Misoprostol

Dinoprostone (*Prostin E₂*) is a naturally occurring prostaglandin E_2 found in mammalian tissues, human seminal plasma, and menstrual fluid (see Chapter 36). Carboprost tromethamine (*Hemabate, Prostin/15M*) is a synthetic analogue of the naturally occurring prostaglandin $PGF_{2\alpha}$. Both drugs stimulate uterine smooth muscle contractions and can be used to induce abortion during gestation weeks 12 to 20. Abortion was successful in 96% of the cases in which these agents were used, with complete passage of fetal products occurring more than 75% of the time without surgical intervention. The mean time to abortion after drug administration was 16 hours. The prostaglandins are more effective stimulants of uterine contraction through the second trimester of pregnancy than is oxytocin. Inhibition of endogenous prostaglandin synthesis with a nonsteroidal antiinflammatory agent, such as aspirin or ibuprofen, can increase the length of gestation, prolong spontaneous labor, or interrupt premature labor.

Dinoprostone is slowly absorbed from the amniotic fluid into the systemic circulation. It and its metabolites readily cross the placenta and can concentrate in the fetal liver. Dinoprostone is primarily metabolized in the maternal lungs and liver and has a half-life in plasma and amniotic fluid of less than 1 minute and 3 to 6 hours, respectively. Carboprost also is metabolized in maternal lung and liver but somewhat more slowly than dinoprostone. It is primarily eliminated by renal excretion of its metabolites, with small amounts appearing in the feces.

Because dinoprostone produces cervical ripening along with stimulation of the uterus, it has been used as an alternative to oxytocin for the induction of labor. Preparations of dinoprostone can be placed in either the cervix or the posterior fornix. *Prepidil* is a formulation and delivery system of dinoprostone that delivers a dose of 0.5 mg into the cervix, while *Cervidil* consists of the drug embedded in a plastic matrix. The matrix is designed to deliver a dose of 0.3 mg per hour for 12 hours.

Carboprost has been used successfully to control postpartum bleeding that was secondary to loss of uterine tone and where the myometrium was unresponsive to oxytocin, ergonovine, or methylergonovine. Given intramuscularly, carboprost causes an almost immediate and sustained uterine contraction. Clinical experience has shown that the use of this agent has saved many women from operative interventions (including hysterectomy) to control postpartum hemorrhage.

Misoprostol (*Cytotec*) is a prostaglandin E_1 analogue that is being evaluated as a cervical ripening agent. It also is used in the treatment and prevention of peptic ulcer disease (see Chapter 40). Clinical trials show that misoprostol is an effective agent for both cervical ripening and labor induction. It appears to be as effective as dinoprostone and is much less expensive.

While adverse reactions are common following the use of abortion-inducing doses of the prostaglandins, most are not serious. Gastrointestinal disturbances include nausea, vomiting, and diarrhea. Transient fever, retained placental fragments, excessive bleeding, decreased diastolic blood pressure, and headache also have been noted. These drugs should be used with caution in patients with asthma, cervicitis, vaginitis, hypertension or hypotension, anemia, jaundice, diabetes, or epilepsy. They should not be used in patients with acute pelvic inflammatory disease, drug hypersensitivity, or an active renal, hepatic, or cardiovascular disorder. Since prostaglandins are potentially carcinogenic, if pregnancy is not effectively terminated following their use, another method should be used. The prostaglandins are not generally used concomitantly with oxytocin because of the possibility of uterine rupture.

UTERINE RELAXANTS

Many risk factors are associated with the triggering of premature labor, that is, labor that begins before the end of week 37 of gestation. These include maternal smoking or drug abuse, lack of prenatal care, multiple gestation, placental abnormalities, infection of the fetal membranes, cervical incompetence, and previous preterm birth. Although most episodes are of unknown origin, premature labor can develop spontaneously or may follow early rupture of fetal membranes, perhaps as a result of a genetically associated abnormality.

Uterine relaxants (*tocolytic drugs*) are administered where prolonged intrauterine life would greatly benefit the fetus or would permit additional time to allow treatment with drugs such as corticosteroids, which promote the production of fetal lung surfactant. Tocolytics are also used when temporary uterine relaxation is desirable (e.g., intrauterine fetal resuscitation). While hydration, bed rest, and sedation have been used to inhibit uterine contractions, tocolytics are more likely to inhibit labor early in gestation, especially before labor is far advanced. Agents used in this regard include magnesium sulfate, alcohol, prostaglandin inhibitors, calcium channel blockers, hydroxyprogesterone, and β_2-adrenergic agonists.

All tocolytic agents are powerful drugs that must be used with extreme care, since pulmonary edema, myocardial infarction, respiratory arrest, cardiac arrest, and death can occur during tocolytic therapy. Newborns of mothers given tocolytics have had respiratory depression, intraventricular hemorrhage, and necrotizing enterocolitis. Absolute contraindications to tocolysis include acute fetal distress (except during intrauterine resuscitation), chorioamnionitis, eclampsia or severe preeclampsia, fetal demise (of a singleton pregnancy), fetal maturity, and maternal hemodynamic instability.

Ethanol

Intravenous use of *ethanol*, while once widely employed to inhibit premature labor, is now of historical interest only. *Ethanol inhibits oxytocin release from the pituitary* and thus indirectly decreases myometrial contractility. Today, β_2-adrenomimetics and magnesium sulfate have replaced ethanol for parenteral tocolysis.

β_2-Adrenoceptor Agonists

Although β_2-adrenoceptor agonists (see Chapter 10) are the most commonly used tocolytic agents in the United States, they are not completely successful in treating preterm labor. Prophylactic administration of these agents to patients at high risk for preterm labor is not always effective. There is, however, clear evidence that β_2-agonists can arrest preterm labor for at least 48 to 72 hours. The efficacy of these drugs beyond this time frame is in dispute. Even a short delay in delivery can be desirable, however, in that at very early preterm gestations (24–28 weeks) a 2-day delay in delivery may mean a 10 to 15% increase in probability of survival for the newborn. Furthermore, such a delay allows for corticosteroid administration to the mother, which has been shown to decrease the incidence and severity of respiratory distress syndrome of the newborn, decrease the incidence of neonatal intraventricular hemorrhage, and improve survival in the premature newborn. Tocolysis also allows for the transport of the mother to a tertiary center where delivery of the preterm infant often results in its improved survival.

These drugs act by binding to β_2-adrenoceptors on myometrial cell membranes and activating adenylyl cyclase. This in turn increases levels of cAMP in the cell (Fig. 62.1), activating cAMP-dependent protein kinase, hence decreasing intracellular calcium concentrations and reducing the effect of calcium on muscle contraction.

β_2-Adrenergic drugs have many side effects. These result both from their residual β_1 activity and from their ability to stimulate β_2-receptors elsewhere in the body (see Chapter 2). The side effects include palpitations, tremor, nausea, vomiting, nervousness, anxiety, chest pain, shortness of breath, hyperglycemia, hypokalemia, and hypotension. Serious complications of drug therapy are pulmonary edema, cardiac insufficiency, arrhythmias, myocardial ischemia, and maternal death.

Terbutaline

Terbutaline (*Brethine, Bricanyl*) is a relatively specific β_2-adrenoceptor agonist (see Chapters 10 and 39). Terbutaline can prevent premature labor, especially in individuals who are more than 20 weeks into gestation and have no indication of ruptured fetal membranes or in whom labor is not far advanced. Its effectiveness in premature labor after 33 weeks of gestation is much less clear. Terbutaline can decrease the frequency, intensity, and duration of uterine contractions through its ability to directly stimulate β_2-adrenoceptors. While it appears to be especially selective for β_2-receptor activation, terbutaline does have some β_1 activity as well.

Terbutaline should be initially used only in an appropriate hospital setting where any obstetric complications can be readily addressed. After initial administration, it can be used in the outpatient setting. Concomitant use of β_2-adrenergic agonists and corticosteroids have additional diabetic effects and may rarely lead to pulmonary edema. The combination of β_2-adrenergic agonists and magnesium sulfate can cause cardiac disturbances, while coadministration of terbutaline with other sympathomimetics can lead to the potentiation of the actions of the latter drugs.

Terbutaline is frequently used in the management of premature labor, although it has not been marketed for such use. Its effectiveness, side effects, precautions, and contraindications are similar to those of all β_2-adrenergic agonists. Terbutaline can cause tachycardia, hypotension, hyperglycemia, and hypokalemia. It can be given orally in addition to subcutaneous or intravenous administration.

Magnesium Sulfate

Magnesium sulfate prevents convulsions in preeclampsia and directly uncouples excitation–contraction in myometrial cells through inhibition of cellular action potentials. Furthermore, magnesium sulfate decreases calcium uptake by competing for its binding sites, activating adenylyl cyclase (thereby reducing intracellular calcium), and stimulating calcium-dependent adenosine triphosphatase (ATPase), which promotes calcium uptake by the sarcoplasmic reticulum. Magnesium is filtered by the glomerulus, so patients with low glomerular filtration will have low magnesium clearance. Although the compound does have some cardiac side effects, magnesium sulfate may be preferred over β-adrenergic agents in patients with heart disease, diabetes, hypertension, or hyperthyroidism.

There is much debate as to the efficacy of magnesium sulfate. For effective inhibition of uterine activity, enough must be given to maintain a blood plasma level of at least 5.5 mEq/L. Even at this level, tocolysis may be hard to achieve.

Magnesium toxicity can be life threatening. Patients given magnesium lose patellar reflexes at plasma levels greater than 8 to 10 mEq/L. Respiratory depression can occur at levels greater than 10 to 12 mEq/L, with respiratory paralysis and arrest soon after (e.g., at levels greater than 12–15 mEq/L). Higher levels cause cardiac arrest. Toxicity can be avoided by following urine output and checking patellar reflexes in patients receiving magnesium. Other side effects include sweating, warmth, flushing, dry mouth, nausea, vomiting, dizziness, nystagmus, headache, palpitations, pulmonary edema, maternal tetany, profound muscular paralysis, profound hypotension, and neonatal depression.

Other Agents

Since certain prostaglandins are known to play a role in stimulating uterine contractions during normal labor, it is logical that inhibitors of prostaglandin synthesis have been used to delay preterm labor. Indomethacin (*Indocin*) has been the principal agent for this use. Indomethacin is given orally or rectally for 24 or 48 hours to delay premature labor. A potential worry concerning the use of indomethacin is premature closure of the fetal ductus arteriosus induced by its ability to inhibit prostaglandin synthesis. The fetal ductus is more sensitive to indomethacin beyond 32 weeks of gestation. Indomethacin use also can decrease amniotic fluid volume and cause oligohydramnios through its ability to decrease fetal urinary output. Long-term use of maternal indomethacin is associated with primary pulmonary hypertension and an increased incidence of intraventricular hemorrhage in the newborn.

The calcium channel blocking agent nifedipine (*Procardia;* see Chapter 19), is one of the more recent drugs examined as a tocolytic agent. It acts by impairing the entry of Ca^{++} into myometrial cells via voltage-dependent channels and thereby inhibits contractility. Although preliminary results appear promising, more studies are needed before its usefulness can be fully assessed.

Hydroxyprogesterone has been used prophylactically for the 12th to 37th week of pregnancy, particularly in women who are in the high-risk category for premature delivery (e.g., those with a history of premature delivery or spontaneous abortion). A concern relating to teratogenic potential has limited its use. Hydroxyprogesterone as a tocolytic agent requires further evaluation before its routine prophylactic administration can be recommended.

With the increasing evidence that oxytocin is important in human labor, investigators are studying oxytocin antagonists for the treatment of preterm labor. *Atosiban* is an analogue of oxytocin that is modified at positions 1, 2, 4, and 8. It is a competitive inhibitor of oxytocin binding. Early studies have demonstrated that this drug does decrease and stop uterine contractions. Atosiban is not available for use in the United States.

Study QUESTIONS

1. Which of the following is the drug of choice for inducing labor?
   (A) Oxytocin
   (B) Misoprostol
   (C) Methyl ergonovine
   (D) Dinoprostone
   (E) Carboprost tromethamine
2. Adverse reactions to the prostaglandin analogue carboprost tromethamine include all of the following EXCEPT
   (A) Diarrhea
   (B) Fever
   (C) Water intoxication
   (D) Nausea
   (E) Dyspnea

3. Carboprost is used primarily to
   (A) Induce labor
   (B) Control postpartum bleeding
   (C) Antagonize effects of dinoprostone
   (D) Inhibit premature labor
   (E) Close the fetal ductus arteriosus
4. All of the following are properties of magnesium sulfate that may be related to its ability to relax uterine smooth muscle EXCEPT
   (A) Uncoupling excitation–contraction in myometrial cells through inhibition of cellular action potentials
   (B) Decreasing calcium uptake by competing for binding sites
   (C) Activating adenylate cyclase

(D) Stimulating calcium-dependent ATPase
(E) Antagonizing prostaglandin action

5. Which of the following is a special concern for the use of indomethacin for inducing labor (tocolysis)?
(A) Fetal cardiac arrest
(B) Fetal gastrointestinal bleeding
(C) Fetal hematuria
(D) Closure of the fetal ductus arteriosis
(E) Fetal muscular paralysis

ANSWERS

1. **A.** Oxytocin is considered the drug of choice for inducing labor. All other methods of labor induction are compared to oxytocin to establish their efficacy. Data demonstrate that oxytocin is highly effective in inducing, establishing, and augmenting labor. Oxytocin is not as effective for labor induction when a woman has a cervix that is not favorable for labor. Another agent, such as misoprostol or dinoprostone, may be better for women with unfavorable cervices. Both misoprostol and dinoprostone are prostaglandin analogues. They cause changes in the substance of the cervix and uterine contraction. Although all agents used for labor induction carry the risk of uterine hyperstimulation, prostaglandins are more likely to cause hyperstimulation in women with favorable cervices. Furthermore, the current formulations of prostaglandins do not allow for tight control of blood levels and rapid clearance of medication if hyperstimulation occurs. Methyl ergonovine is an α-agonist that causes direct smooth muscle contraction. Carboprost tromethamine is a methylated analogue of prostaglandin $F_{2\alpha}$. It is highly potent in causing prolonged uterine contraction. Both medications are used for the control of uterine bleeding after delivery by causing tetanic uterine contractions. These medications are contraindicated for labor induction in women with live fetuses. Both medications can be used in facilitating medical abortions.

2. **C.** Carboprost tromethamine is methylated at the 15 position. This methylation causes the analogue to be 10 to 15 times more potent then the natural prostaglandin. Smooth muscles that are especially sensitive to prostaglandin $F_{2\alpha}$ are uterine, gastrointestinal, and bronchial. The uterine sensitivity allows for the therapeutic efficacy. The gastrointestinal sensitivity causes the diarrhea and nausea. Prostaglandins are involved in the pyretic response, and thus a side effect of their use may be fever. Oxytocin has antidiuretic hormone qualities, and with prolonged use may cause water intoxication.

3. **B.** Clinical evidence has shown that the use of this agent has saved many women from surgery by controlling postpartum hemorrhage. It can also induce labor but is not the drug of choice. It will induce

rather than inhibit premature labor. A prostaglandin antagonist would be useful to produce closure of the fetal ductus arteriosus.

4. **E.** Magnesium has no known effect on prostaglandins. The mechanism of action by which magnesium sulfate causes smooth muscle contraction is complex and poorly understood. Magnesium sulfate uncouples excitation–contraction in myometrial cells through inhibition of cellular action potentials. Furthermore, magnesium sulfate decreases calcium uptake by competing for binding sites, activating adenylate cyclase (reducing intracellular calcium), and stimulating calcium-dependent ATPase, which promotes calcium uptake by sarcoplasmic reticulum.

5. **D.** Indomethacin is a potent prostaglandin synthesis inhibitor. Patency of the ductus arteriosis depends on the formation of prostaglandins. Closure of the ductus arteriosis can lead to fetal heart failure and death. Also, fetal closure can lead to neonatal pulmonary hypertension. Neonatologists use indomethacin for the treatment of neonatal patent ductus arteriosis, thus often obviating neonatal heart surgery. Prostaglandin synthesis inhibitors are associated with bleeding. Although bleeding is well documented in children and adults, the use of indomethacin has not been shown to cause hematuria or gastrointestinal bleeding in the fetus. There is some evidence, however, that maternal use of indomethacin may increase the risk of neonatal intraventricular hemorrhage. Neither muscular paralysis nor cardiac arrest has been demonstrated in the fetus with maternal use of indomethacin.

SUPPLEMENTAL READING

Challis JR et al. Prostaglandins and mechanisms of preterm birth. Reproduction 2002;81:633–641.

Cox SM, Sherman M, and Leveno KJ. Randomized investigation of magnesium sulfate for prevention of preterm birth. Am J Obstet Gynecol 1990;163:797–801.

Diddy GA 3rd. Postpartum hemorrhage: New management options. Clin Obstet Gynecol 2002;45:330–344.

Goldberg AB, Greenberg MB, and Darney PD. Misoprostol and pregnancy. N Engl J Med 2001;344:38–47.

Gyetvai K, Hannah ME, Hodnett ED, and Ohlsson A. Tocolytics for preterm labor: A systematic review. Obstet Gynecol 1999;94:869–77.

Rodts-Palenik S and Morrison JC. Tocolysis: An update for the practitioner. Obstet Gynecol Surv 2002;1:127–131.

Winkler M and Rath W. A risk-benefit assessment of oxytocics in obstetric practice. Drug Safety 1999;20:323–345.

CASE Study   Is Labor Induction Justified?

A 25-year-old woman is 2 weeks beyond her estimated date of delivery. She reports no pain, no labor contractions, no vaginal bleeding, no leaking fluid from her vagina, and no vaginal discharge. She reports that her fetus is moving. On further history, you find that the patient reports no other complaints, and her medical, surgical, social, and family histories are all negative. The physical examination you perform produces normal findings. Notably, her uterine fundal size measurement is 40 cm. Her pelvic examination reveals that her cervix is 3 cm dilated, 50% effaced, soft in consistency, and midposition in the vagina. The fetal station is presenting at 0. You find no evidence of ruptured membranes. Uterine monitoring shows no contractions. You and the patient decide that labor induction would be safe and appropriate. What would be a good course of action?

ANSWER: In this case, the decision to induce labor is appropriate. In caring for patients, physicians must decide who are appropriate patients for labor induction. The median length of human pregnancy is 40 weeks (when using the woman's menstrual period to date the pregnancy). Pregnancy is considered to be full-term from the 37 0/7 weeks to 41 6/7 weeks.

Patients who are pregnant 2 or more weeks beyond their due date are classified as having postterm or postdate pregnancy. These prolonged pregnancies carry the increased risk of fetal death (2 to 6 times as high as for women who are at 40 weeks' gestation). Women who are postterm have a higher risk of cesarean section, trauma from delivery, prolonged bleeding after delivery, and prolonged hospitalization. Newborns who are born postterm have an increased risk of being pathologically large (macrosomia), birth trauma, intolerance to labor, meconium staining, meconium aspiration, and possible subsequent hypoxia or anoxia brain injury. With all these concerns, labor induction may be safer than continuing the pregnancy.

Oxytocin is the drug of choice for inducing labor. In appropriate patients, it nearly always leads to safe vaginal delivery. Patients whose cervix is favorable for labor are good candidates for oxytocin. Obstetricians traditionally use a scoring system to rate the cervix (Bishop EH. Pelvic Scoring for Elective Induction. Obstet Gynecol 1964;24: 266–268). The following table defines the scoring system. Scores of ≥6 are considered favorable. Our patient has a score of 8.

Score	Dilation (cm)	Effacement (%)	Station	Cervical Consistency	Cervical Position
0	Closed	0–30	−3	Firm	Posterior
1	1–2	40–50	−2	Medium	Midposition
2	3–4	60–70	−1,0	Soft	Anterior
3	≥5	≥80	≥+1	–	–

63

Androgens, Antiandrogens, and Anabolic Steroids

Frank L. Schwartz and Roman J. Miller

 DRUG LIST

GENERIC NAME	PAGE	GENERIC NAME	PAGE
Androgens		Stanozolol	731
Danazol	730	**Antiandrogens**	
Methyltestosterone	730	Cyproterone acetate	732
Testosterone	724	Finasteride	732
Anabolic agents		Flutamide	732
Methandrostenolone	731	Ketoconazole	732
Nandrolone	730	Leuprolide Acetate	732
Oxandrolone	730	Spironolactone	732
Oxymetholone	731		

Androgens are steroid hormones that are secreted primarily by the testis, and *testosterone* is the principal androgen secreted. Its primary function is to regulate the differentiation and secretory function of male sex accessory organs. Androgens also possess protein anabolic activity that is manifested in skeletal muscle, bone, and kidneys. As a class, androgens are reasonably safe drugs, having limited and relatively predictable side effects.

CHEMISTRY AND BIOSYNTHESIS

The basic structure of all steroid hormones is similar (see Chapter 60, Fig. 60.4). The addition of a *hydrogen atom at position 5* and an *angular methyl group at positions 18 and 19* establishes the basic chemical framework for androgenic activity.

CHARACTERIZATION OF PLASMA ANDROGENS

In males, *testosterone* is the principal circulating androgen, and the testes are the principal source. Although the adrenals are capable of androgen synthesis, less than 10% of the circulating androgens in men are produced in the adrenals. Testosterone is synthesized by Leydig cells of the testes at the rate of about 8 mg/24 hours, providing a plasma concentration of 0.5 to 0.6 µg/dL. In females, the ovaries contribute approximately one-third of the total androgens synthesized, while the adrenals contribute the rest.

Androstenedione, dehydroepiandrosterone (DHEA), and *dehydroepiandrosterone sulfate* (DHEA-S) are other mildly androgenic compounds of secondary importance in males and females. The gonads and the adrenal cortex are capable of secreting androstenedione and DHEA, while DHEA-S is secreted primarily by the adrenal.

Concentrations of plasma testosterone and other androgens vary throughout the day in both sexes; whether such variation is simply random or fits a repeatable diurnal pattern is a matter of debate. Compared with the diurnal variation seen with cortisol, plasma testosterone concentrations are reasonably constant. Plasma androgen concentrations also vary greatly in women through the menstrual cycle, with peak levels seen in the luteal phase.

SEX HORMONE–BINDING PROTEINS

Circulating testosterone is reversibly bound to two major plasma proteins, *albumin* and *gamma globulin*. Binding to albumin is a relatively nonspecific low-affinity and high-capacity association. In contrast, binding to the specific γ-globulin fraction, called *sex hormone–binding globulin (SHBG)*, is a high-affinity steroid-specific interaction. Under physiological conditions, 98% of testosterone is protein bound, 40% to albumin and 58% to SHBG. Thus, 2% or less of circulating testosterone is unbound or free. *Free testosterone reflects the amount that is biologically active and available for interaction with peripheral target cells.*

SHBG levels are known to be influenced by a variety of clinical conditions. In females, the high estrogen levels of pregnancy or the use of oral contraceptives result in increased SHBG concentrations. In males, elevated levels of SHBG are seen most commonly in individuals with liver cirrhosis or during normal aging. Elevated SHBG levels are also seen in hyperthyroidism and hypogonadism. All of these conditions are associated with elevated estrogen levels, which result in increased hepatic SHBG synthesis. SHBG levels are suppressed by androgen replacement or chronic glucocorticoid therapy. Elevations of SHBG do not necessarily result in a fall in free testosterone levels. *When assessing the androgenic status of an individual, whether male or female, it is necessary to measure both total and free testosterone plasma levels.*

Plasma testosterone levels also exhibit age-associated changes. The levels of the hormone are very low throughout childhood and until early adolescence, when increasing testicular steroidogenesis precedes the onset of puberty in boys. Levels peak in the early 20s, and beginning at about age 30, testicular production of testosterone begins to decline. Urinary 17-ketosteroid excretion declines slowly as a result of a concomitant decrease in the metabolic clearance rate of testosterone. Therefore, there is a relatively constant serum testosterone concentration that often does not decline significantly until after age 70. After the fifth decade, free testosterone levels do decrease as a result of increased SHBG levels. In females, testosterone levels also decline with age; however, at menopause the decline in female hormones is so much greater that many postmenopausal women have higher androgen to estrogen ratios, resulting frequently in significant hirsutism.

STEROIDOGENESIS

The main steroidogenic components of the testis are the interstitial cells of Leydig found between the seminiferous tubules. The principal secretory product of Leydig cells, testosterone, is not stored to any significant degree within these cells. Biochemical studies of Leydig cell steroidogenic function have shown that *testosterone synthesis begins with acetate derived either from glucose or products of lipid metabolism.* Acetate is converted to cholesterol through numerous reactions in or on the smooth endoplasmic reticulum. Cholesterol, once formed, is stored in lipid droplets in an esterified form. The cholesterol required for steroidogenesis is transferred into the mitochondria, where the side chain is cleaved by enzymes on the inner membranes to form pregnenolone. *This reaction is the rate-limiting step in testosterone biosynthesis and is the step stimulated by luteinizing hormone (LH).* Pregnenolone is then returned to the cytoplasm, where it serves as the principal precursor of testosterone.

Testosterone synthesis from pregnenolone can occur along two distinct metabolic pathways (Fig. 63.1). The names given to these two routes of metabolism refer to the position in the steroid molecule where an unsaturated bond is maintained. Thus, in the delta-4 pathway an unsaturated position is between C4 and C5 of ring A, whereas in the delta-5 pathway, the unsaturated position is between C5 and C6 of ring B. *In the human testis, the delta-5 pathway is the predominant (but not exclusive) one used for the biosynthesis of testosterone.*

Sertoli cells, in the seminiferous tubule wall, are known to be important in spermatogenesis, in part through their synthesis of an *androgen-binding protein (ABP)*. ABP, when secreted into the lumen of the seminiferous tubules, selectively binds testosterone of Leydig cell origin and serves as a hormone reservoir and transport protein for the androgen.

REGULATION OF PLASMA TESTOSTERONE

The regulation of plasma testosterone is accomplished through a dynamic feedback interaction among the hypothalamus, pituitary, and testis (Fig. 63.2). The hypothalamus synthesizes and releases gonadotropin releasing hormone (GnRH) into the hypothalamic–hypophyseal portal system. Pulsatile release of GnRH stimulates the release of the pituitary gonadotropins LH and follicle-stimulating hormone (FSH). LH and FSH then reach the

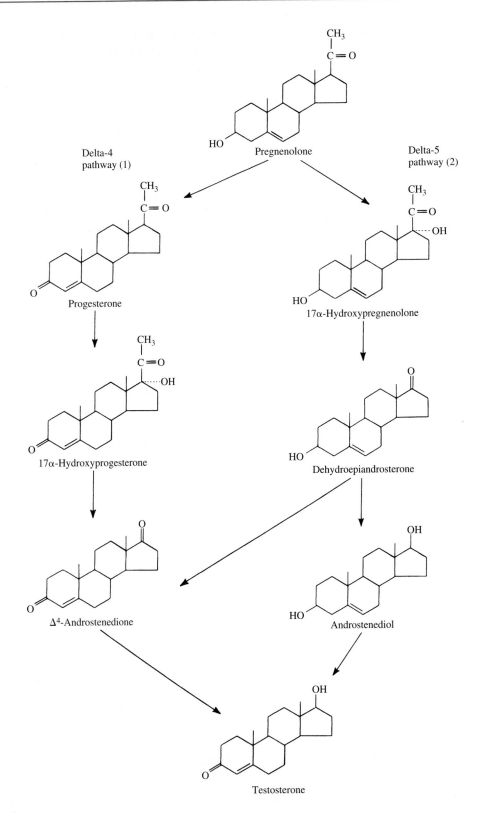

FIGURE 63.1

Synthetic pathways of testosterone. *1.* Andrenostenedione pathway (delta-4).
2. Dehydroepiandrosterone pathway (delta-5).

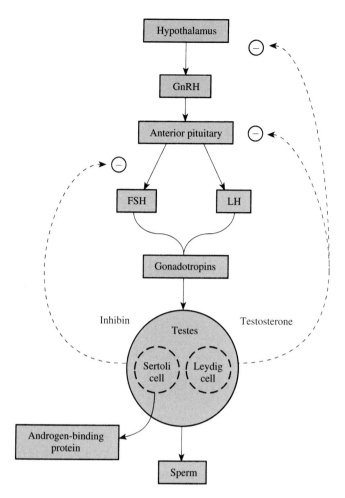

FIGURE 63.2

Hormonal interrelationships between the hypothalamus, anterior pituitary, and testes. *Solid arrows,* Excitatory effects; *dashed arrows,* inhibitory effects. GnRH, gonadotropin-releasing hormone; FSH, follicle-stimulating hormone; LH, luteinizing hormone. (Modified with permission from Fox SI. Human Physiology (3rd ed.). Copyright 1990 Wm. C. Brown, Dubuque, IA. All rights reserved.)

testes, where they regulate testosterone synthesis and spermatogenesis, respectively. The resultant increases in serum testosterone levels exert a negative feedback at both the hypothalamic and the pituitary levels.

The hypothalamus releases GnRH in a pulsatile manner. The pulse frequency is sex specific, with males exhibiting a 120-minute frequency and females exhibiting a 60- to 90-minute frequency. The pulsating levels of GnRH from the pituitary modulate LH and FSH release. Androgens and estrogens can modulate gonadotropin release at both the hypothalamus and pituitary levels. In this regard, the gonadal steroids modulate GnRH pulse frequency and amplitude at the hypothalamus level while simultaneously modifying pituitary responses to GnRH by influencing GnRH receptor levels in the pituitary. Increases in GnRH recep-

tor levels with a resultant increased sensitivity to GnRH is termed up-regulation, while a decrease in GnRH receptors is termed down-regulation. In the hypothalamus, the negative feedback of testosterone involves both the conversion to dihydrotestosterone (DHT) and aromatization into estradiol.

A separate protein hormone produced primarily in the testis, called *inhibin,* also affects the secretion of FSH. Inhibin has been isolated primarily from testicular extracts but also may be found in the antral fluid of ovarian follicles in females. Inhibin decreases the release of FSH from the pituitary but does not affect hypothalamic production of GnRH.

The catabolism of plasma testosterone and other androgens occurs primarily in the liver (Fig. 63.3), where they are conjugated into water-soluble compounds that are excreted by the kidney as the urinary 17-ketosteroids.

MECHANISM OF ACTION

Given the wide spectrum of androgen actions, it is reasonable to expect the intracellular processes mediating these diverse effects to vary among target tissues. The currently accepted hypothesis of androgen action in male sex accessory organs is depicted in Fig. 63.4. Testosterone diffuses from the blood across the plasma membrane of the sex accessory organ cell, where it is rapidly metabolized to DHT and androstanediol. *In many sex accessory organs, DHT, rather than testosterone, is the primary intracellular androgen* and is more potent than testosterone. Once formed, DHT preferentially binds to a receptor protein in the nucleus. This DHT–receptor complex is subsequently activated and binds to proteins on the nuclear matrix. Following this interaction, RNA synthesis results in enhanced protein synthesis and cellular metabolism. If sufficient androgen stimulation occurs, DNA synthesis and cellular division begin.

Non-sex accessory tissues also are targets for the protein anabolic actions of androgens. These tissues possess lower levels of endogenous hormone, minimal 5α-reductase activity, and lower concentrations of specific androgen receptors. The protein anabolic actions are probably mediated by an interaction with the androgen receptor.

PHARMACOLOGICAL ACTIONS

Androgens produce both virilizing and protein anabolic actions (Table 63.1). The virilizing actions of testosterone include irreversible effects that occur during embryogenesis, that is, those that induce differentiation of the central nervous system and male reproductive tracts, and the *excitatory actions* at puberty that are

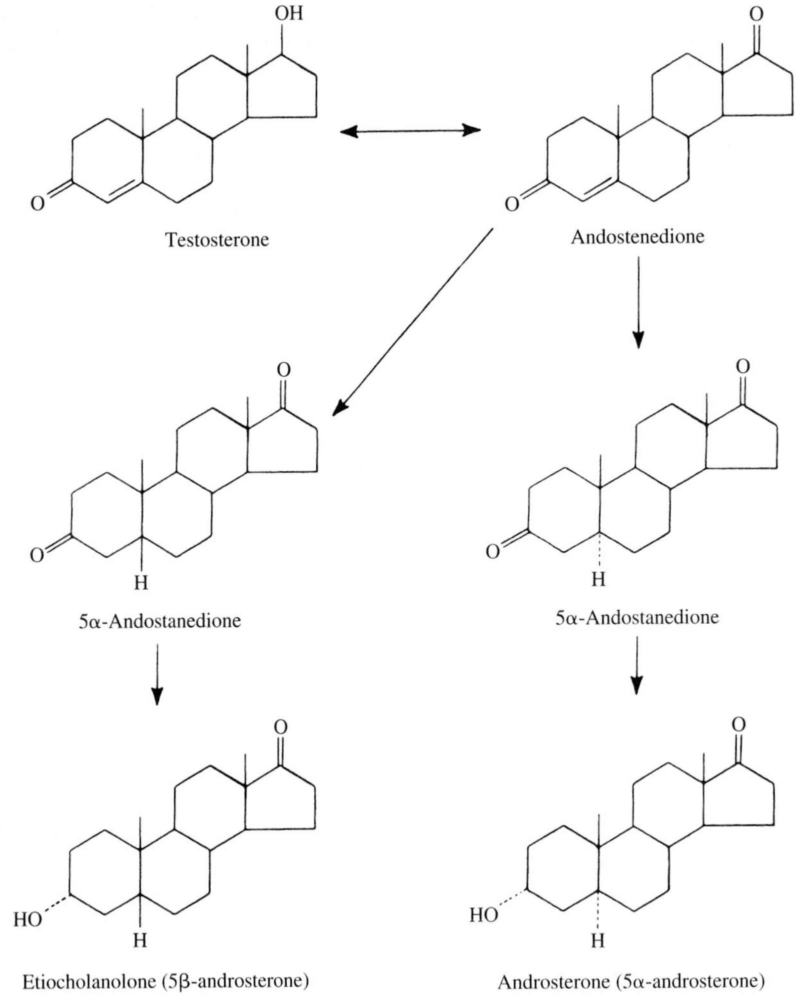

FIGURE 63.3
Primary pathways for testosterone catabolism.

responsible for secondary sexual development. In addition to the effects on male reproductive function, androgens influence a number of other systems, many of which are associated with masculinity. These actions include the growth of male-pattern facial, pubic, and body hair, the lower vocal pitch resulting from a thickening and lengthening of the vocal cords, and a significant (30%) increase in the rate of long bone growth. Androgens also terminate long bone growth by inducing closure of the epiphyses. The degree of virilization and timing of puberty also affect peak bone density and risk of osteoporosis in males.

The protein anabolic actions of androgens on bone and skeletal muscle are responsible for the larger stature of males than females. Androgens induce some degree of anabolism in other tissues, including bone marrow, liver, kidney, and heart. They also have several other actions, not necessarily associated with maleness, such as lymphoid tissue regression during puberty.

CLINICAL USES

The primary therapeutic use of androgens is as replacement therapy in testicular deficiency (Table 63.2), a condition in which induction and maintenance of male secondary sex characteristics are desired. Although re-

TABLE 63.1   **Pharmacological Actions of Androgens**

Virilizing effects
  Gonadotropin regulation
  Spermatogenesis
  Sexual dysfunction
  Sexual restoration and development
Protein anabolic effects
  Increased bone density
  Increased muscle mass
  Increased red blood cell mass

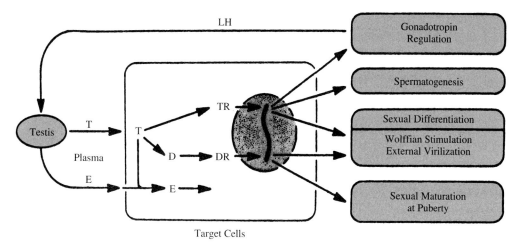

FIGURE 63.4

Mechanism of action of androgens. T, testosterone; D, dihydrotestosterone; E, estradiol; R, receptor protein; LH, luteinizing hormone. (Reprinted with permission from Wilson JD. Androgen abuse by athletes. Endocr Rev 1988;9:181. Copyright 1988 by The Endocrine Society.)

placement therapy is the primary use of androgen administration, these hormones also are used and abused for their protein anabolic effects.

Hypogonadism

Testicular failure may occur before puberty and present as delayed puberty and the eunuchoid phenotype, or after puberty, with the development of infertility, impotence, or decreased libido in otherwise fully virilized males. The source of hypogonadism can be testicular, as occurs in *primary hypogonadism,* or it may result from abnormalities of the hypothalamic–pituitary axis, as in *secondary hypogonadism.*

Prepuberal Hypogonadism

Prepuberal hypogonadism is often unsuspected until a delay in male sexual development is noticed at the time

TABLE 63.2	Androgenic Steroids Used Primarily for Androgen Replacement
Agent (trade name)	
Testosterone *(Oreton, Neo-Hombreol F, Testoderm, Androderm)*	
Testosterone propionate *(Neo-Hombreol, Oreton Propionate, others)*	
Testosterone enanthate *(Delatestryl,* others)	
Testosterone cypionate *(DEPO-Testosterone,* others)	
Methyltestosterone *(Metandren, Neo-Hombreol* [M], others)	
Fluoxymesterone *(Halotestin)*	

of puberty. The eunuchoid phenotype is caused by absent or deficient androgenic induction of the undifferentiated embryonic bipotential tissue into fully developed male sex accessory organs. Causes of this condition include deficient testicular steroidogenesis (both congenital and acquired), target organ androgen insensitivity syndromes (receptor defects, 5α-reductase deficiency), deficient pituitary LH and FSH secretion, or deficient hypothalamic GnRH production. Androgen replacement therapy is effective only when the end organs are sensitive to androgens, so certain forms of pseudohermaphroditism are unresponsive to androgen replacement.

The compounds most effective in bringing about masculinization are the long-acting enanthate, cypionate, or propionate esters of testosterone; these preparations require intramuscular injection. Recently effective cutaneous forms of androgens have become available and may be equally effective. Owing to inconsistent drug absorption, oral androgen preparations do not result in full sexual development in prepuberal hypogonadotropic males.

Postpuberal Hypogonadism

Postpuberal hypogonadism is also classified as either primary hypogonadism or secondary hypogonadism. Primary hypogonadism occurs after puberty as the result of surgical castration or testicular destruction (e.g., through orchitis, radiation) and is associated with elevated levels of LH and FSH. Secondary hypogonadism is usually associated with hypopituitarism from destruction or infiltration of the hypothalamus or pituitary by infarction, tumoral replacement, or surgical removal.

Thus, these individuals have inappropriately low LH and FSH levels that do not respond to GnRH stimulation. Androgen replacement in these individuals usually restores secondary male sexual characteristics, such as libido and potency.

Aging and Impotence

Aging in men is associated with decreased testicular function that results in reduced testicular steroidogenesis, decreased free plasma testosterone levels, decreased 17-ketosteroid excretion, and increased gonadotropin levels. Decreased testicular function has been implicated as a cause of reduced libido, muscle mass, muscle strength, and bone density in elderly men. However, these observations are so variable that a causal relationship between lowered androgen levels has not been firmly established. *Androgen replacement in elderly men has not been demonstrated to be beneficial unless there is true androgen deficiency.* In addition, it is wise to avoid the indiscriminate use of androgens in this age group because of the high incidence of prostate neoplasms (benign and malignant). Androgen administration in replacement doses has proved to be moderately successful in increasing libido and sexual performance in men who have true testicular failure.

Anemia

Androgens stimulate erythrocytosis and are effective in the treatment of certain anemias that are secondary to endocrine hypofunction or myeloid hypoplasia. In high dosages, these compounds in the past were used in the treatment of several forms of anemia. However recombinant erythropoietin has replaced the androgens as a more effective treatment of most forms of anemia.

Therapeutic Use of Androgens in Women

Because of the antagonistic action of androgens in many estrogen-sensitive tissues, it would seem logical that androgens might be effective therapeutic agents in clinical situations of estrogen excess or in the presence of estrogen-dependent neoplasms. However, the *virilizing side effects of these compounds have limited their clinical use.* Selective protein anabolic forms of androgens have been used in certain clinical situations.

Endometriosis

Endometriosis is abnormal growth of endometrial tissue in the peritoneal cavity. Women with this disorder have dysmenorrhea, dyspareunia, chronic pelvic pain, and infertility. Danazol (*Danocrine*) is a 2,3-isoxazol derivative of 17α-ethynyl testosterone (ethisterone) that has weak virilizing and protein anabolic properties. It is effective in endometriosis through its negative feedback inhibition of LH and FSH release, which in turn results in decreased ovarian steroidogenesis and regression of endometriomas. Because of the virilizing side effects of danazol, causing acne and hirsutism, its use in endometriosis has been largely supplanted by the use of GnRH analogues. Danazol is also approved for use in fibrocystic breast disease and hereditary angioneurotic edema.

Female Hypogonadism

Female hypogonadism, especially prepuberal, may be an indication for androgen therapy. Androgens are necessary for normal pubic hair induction and long bone growth in both sexes. In prepuberal females with hypopituitarism in whom all other hormonal deficiencies (estrogen, progesterone, thyroid, adrenal, and growth hormone) have been corrected, normal sexual development and long bone growth are not complete without androgen hormone replacement. Estrogen administration during adolescence is necessary for the development of the breast, the gynecoid pelvis, and other female characteristics. However, maximal long bone growth and development of axillary and pubic hair will not occur without small amounts of androgen replacement. The use of *methyltestosterone* (*Android*) and *diethylstilbestrol* in combination has been demonstrated to be very effective in inducing complete secondary sexual development in these females. Finally, low doses of androgens have been used to facilitate impaired libido in postmenopausal women when combined with estrogen replacement therapy.

Use of Androgens as Protein Anabolic Agents

Anabolic activities of testosterone, such as increases in amino acid incorporation into protein and in RNA polymerase activity, have been demonstrated in skeletal muscle. Apart from the direct anabolic effects in specific tissue, androgens antagonize the protein catabolic action of glucocorticoids. The androgen compounds with the greatest ratio of protein anabolic effects to virilizing effects are the *19-nortestosterone derivatives.* Compounds that are used clinically (Table 63.3) include nandrolone phenpropionate (*Durabolin*), nandrolone decanoate

TABLE 63.3 Clinical Uses of Protein Anabolic Steroids

Protein catabolic states (burns, malnutrition, maintenance)
Short stature
Anemia
Endometriosis
Breast cancer
Osteoporosis

(*Deca-Durabolin*), methandrostenolone (*Dianabol*), oxymetholone (*Anadrol, Adroyd*), stanozolol (*Winstrol*), and oxandrolone (*Anavar*).

The protein anabolic compounds are most commonly used to stimulate appetite and muscle mass in persons with advanced malignancy or other conditions characterized by advanced malnutrition. These compounds are also often abused by athletes who are trying to build muscle mass. Athletes often take multiple compounds at the same time (stacking) or sequentially to try to maximize their anabolic effects. This type of use is not based on scientific data but rather on hyperbole often spread by individuals with no medical or scientific background. Athletes who use these compounds in this way are unaware of the potential adverse effects or do not care.

ADVERSE EFFECTS

As a class, the androgens are relatively safe and nontoxic. However, in inappropriate doses or for inappropriate reasons, their use can result in significant toxicity.

Toxicity in Men

The administration of androgens to sexually mature hypogonadal men is associated with few untoward effects. However, prepuberal or hypogonadal males never exposed to testosterone show enhanced sensitivity to administered androgens, and many do not like the effects. Testosterone administration can cause irritability, agitation, or aggressive behavior. Androgen administration to normal males inhibits the release of the pituitary gonadotropins FSH, LH, and as a consequence, endogenous testicular production of testosterone is reduced. Spermatogenesis is also reduced, and if administration is continued, azoospermia and infertility may result. Peripheral aromatization of androgens to estrogens can cause gynecomastia. Cessation of exogenous androgen treatment in normal males usually results in restoration of normal sperm levels over a 6-month period. Finally, androgen replacement therapy in elderly men should be monitored closely. Men at this age are at risk for developing prostatic neoplasms (benign and malignant), and use of androgens in this setting is contraindicated because of the likelihood of stimulating growth of these tumors.

Toxicity in Women

Although masculinization is a desired action of androgens in the treatment of men with testicular deficiencies, these effects can be quite distressing to women. The degree of virilization in women will vary with the dosage, duration of therapy, and particular androgen preparation used. In women receiving high doses of androgen for any reason, facial hair growth may progress to total body hair growth, baldness may develop, breasts may shrink, and the voice may deepen. In addition, clitoral hypertrophy, uterine atrophy, and menstrual irregularities may develop. Although some of the symptoms are reversible and disappear upon cessation of therapy, several effects—baldness, growth of facial hair, clitoral enlargement, and deepening of the voice—are commonly irreversible. Steroids taken by women during pregnancy may cause pseudohermaphroditism in the genetically female fetus and may even cause its death.

Toxicity in Either Sex

Androgen administration to male or female adults, especially at high dosages, results in *erythrocytosis* and *polycythemia,* fluid retention, and it may produce or exacerbate edema. This can be serious when associated with congestive heart failure, cirrhosis of the liver, or nephrotic syndrome. Since androgens stimulate the activity of sebaceous glands, oily skin and acne are found in some individuals who are receiving androgen therapy. A change in cholesterol levels can result from androgen therapy, such as *decreased levels of high-density lipoprotein cholesterol and increased levels of low-density lipoprotein cholesterol*. This change in the distribution of cholesterol may contribute to increased risk of atherosclerosis and coronary artery disease, especially in athletes who are exposed for long periods to high levels of anabolic steroids.

Oral androgen preparations that have the 17-methyl substitution on the steroid molecule are associated with the development of liver disorders, including hyperbilirubinemia, and elevated liver function tests. As many as 80% of individuals who take these compounds have been shown to develop liver problems. Although these changes are usually reversed if steroid treatment is discontinued, use of the oral preparations is also associated with the development of *benign liver tumors* and a rare liver disorder involving the development of blood-filled sacs (*peliosis hepatis*). Finally, worsening of *sleep apnea* and precipitation of *superior sagittal sinus thrombosis*—seizures, facial palsy, hemiplegia, stupor, and coma—have been associated with androgen therapy.

ANTIANDROGENS

By definition, antiandrogens are substances that prevent or depress the action of male hormones in their target organs. Potential sites of action include gonadotropin suppression, inhibition of androgen synthesis, and androgen receptor blockade. Compounds that affect each of these sites are available. Potential clinical uses of antiandrogens include suppression of androgen excess and treatment of androgen-dependent tumors.

Extreme clinical examples of androgen excess include central precocious puberty, the adrenogenital syndromes, and androgen-secreting adrenal, ovarian, or testicular tumors. Less severe problems include idiopathic hirsutism, premenstrual syndrome, and severe cystic acne.

Inhibitors of Androgen Biosynthesis

Ketoconazole (*Nizoral*) is a broad-spectrum antifungal agent (see Chapter 52) that in very high doses inhibits several steps in the biosynthesis of both adrenal and gonadal steroids. While the normal antifungal dose is 200 mg/day, testosterone biosynthesis in both the adrenal and testis is completely abolished by doses of 800 to 1,600 mg/day. This drug is used most commonly for large virilizing adrenal tumors that cannot be surgically removed.

Androgen Receptor Antagonists

Spironolactone (*Aldactone*) is a compound originally developed as a mineralocorticoid antagonist and is used as a diuretic and antihypertensive agent (see Chapter 21). However, at high doses spironolactone binds to the androgen receptor. In clinical practice it is a weak androgen antagonist used to treat hirsutism in women by blocking testosterone binding to androgen receptors in hair follicles. Use of spironolactone in women for the treatment of hirsutism or male pattern baldness can result in elevated serum potassium levels; these levels should be checked within 1 month of starting the medication.

Flutamide (*Eulexin*) is a nonsteroidal androgen receptor antagonist that inhibits androgen binding to its nuclear receptor. It is effective in inducing prostatic regression and is approved for the treatment of prostatic carcinoma. For maximum clinical effectiveness it has to be used in combination with a GnRH antagonist (e.g., leuprolide acetate) that inhibits androgen production. Flutamide may eventually be used for the treatment of hirsutism and male pattern baldness in women if a topical preparation is developed.

Cyproterone acetate is a progestational antiandrogen that blocks androgen receptor binding and suppresses androgen-sensitive tissues. It is available in a topical form in Europe for the treatment of hirsutism.

5α-Reductase Inhibitors

Finasteride (*Proscar*) is a 5α-reductase inhibitor that blocks the conversion of testosterone to DHT in target tissues. Since DHT is the major intracellular androgen in the prostate, finasteride is effective in suppressing DHT stimulation of prostatic growth and secretory function without markedly affecting libido. It is approved for the treatment of benign prostatic hyperplasia. Although there is usually some regression in the size of the prostate gland following administration of finasteride, clinical response may take 6 to 12 months. If the obstructive symptoms are severe, there is often not enough time to allow this compound to work. The principal adverse effects of finasteride are impotence, decreased libido, and decreased volume of ejaculate. The compound is generally well tolerated in men.

Gonadotropin-Releasing Hormone Analogues

GnRH analogues (see Chapter 59) can induce chemical castration by suppressing the pulsatile release of LH and FSH, hence inhibiting testicular steroidogenesis. Administration of these compounds reduces circulating testosterone levels. These compounds are inhaled, injected subcutaneously, or implanted subcutaneously. They are used in males in the treatment of precocious puberty and carcinoma of the prostate.

PREPARATIONS

Androgens come in oral, injectable, implantable, and topical preparations. Because of the toxicity of the oral preparations and the inconvenience of the injectable forms, the transdermal gels have been a major clinical advance for treatment of hypogonadal males.

Study QUESTIONS

1. The serum level of testosterone in males from adolescence through the fifth decade of life is a primarily a consequence of
   (A) A relatively constant level of testicular testosterone production
   (B) A significant decline in testosterone production

   (C) A decline in the metabolic clearance rate of testosterone
   (D) An increase in the metabolic clearance rate of testosterone
   (E) A sharp drop in urinary 17-ketosteroid levels

2. Which of the following is mostly likely to be found in a male who lacks functional 5α-reductase?

(A) Depressed serum levels of testosterone

(B) Elevated serum levels of dihydrotestosterone

(C) Highly depressed protein anabolic activity in skeletal muscle, bone, and kidney

(D) Elevated serum levels of testosterone with subnormal prostatic function

(E) Decreased binding of testosterone to sex hormone–binding globulin in the serum

3. The formation of what as a principal precursor of testosterone is considered the biosynthetic rate-limiting step?

(A) Pregnenolone

(B) Cholesterol

(C) Androstenediol

(D) Estrogen

(E) Progesterone

4. Normal skeletal muscle cells

(A) Typically lack androgen receptors and thus are not affected by high concentrations of testosterone

(B) Respond more readily to dihydrotestosterone than to testosterone

(C) Have higher levels of 5α-reductase than do prostatic tissue cells

(D) Use the androgen receptor to enhance protein anabolic activity

(E) Produce testosterone in response to FSH stimuli

5. Upon examination, a 68-year-old married man was found to have a greatly enlarged prostate. Which one of the following drugs is most likely to suppress prostatic growth without affecting libido?

(A) Spironolactone

(B) Finasteride

(C) Ketoconazole

(D) Flutamide

(E) Stanozolol

ANSWERS

1. **C.** In adolescent males, testicular testosterone production dramatically rises from prepuberal levels and then declines into adulthood. However, with advancing adulthood there is a drop in the metabolic clearance rate of testosterone, increasing the length of time that testosterone remains in the serum. Evidence of a relatively constant level of serum testosterone is seen in the relative constant levels of urinary 17-ketosteroids, a metabolite of testosterone, from the second to the fifth decade of life.

2. **D.** The enzyme 5α-reductase catalyzes the formation of dihydrotestosterone from testosterone. In normal accessory sex gland tissues, such as the prostate, most of the direct androgen effect is due to dihydrotestosterone rather than testosterone. Thus when 5α-reductase is lacking, serum levels of testosterone may be normal or even slightly elevated with a hypotrophied prostate gland.

3. **A.** In the Leydig cell the rate-limiting step in testosterone synthesis is the enzymatic cleavage of side chains from cholesterol to form pregnenolone.

4. **D.** Skeletal muscle cells use the androgen receptor to bind testosterone that promotes the anabolic effect of this hormone.

5. **B.** Finasteride is a 5α-reductase inhibitor, which essentially makes dihydrotestosterone unavailable to the prostate but does not reduce serum testosterone levels. The decreased prostatic levels of dihydrotestosterone frequently result in a size regression of the prostate, while the relatively normal testosterone levels minimize a depressed libido. Flutamide and spironolactone exhibit antiandrogen effects by competing for the androgen receptor; ketoconazole inhibits testosterone synthesis; and stanozolol is an oral anabolic androgen preparation.

SUPPLEMENTAL READING

Finkelstein JW et al. Estrogen or testosterone increase self-reported aggressive behaviors in hypogonadal adolescents. J Clin Endocrinol Metab 1997;82:2433–2438.

Griffin JE. Male reproductive function. In Griffin JE and Ojeda SR (eds.). Textbook of Endocrine Physiology. New York: Oxford University, 1992:169–188.

Hall PF. Testicular steroid synthesis: organization and regulation. In Knobil F and Neill JD (eds.). The Physiology of Reproduction. Vol. 1. New York: Raven, 1994:1335.

Luke MC and Coffey DS. The male sex accessory tissues: structure, androgen action, and physiology. In Knobil F and Neill JD (eds.). The Physiology of Reproduction. Vol. 1. New York: Raven, 1994:1435.

Parker MG (ed.). Nuclear Hormone Receptors. New York: Academic, 1991.

Strauss RH and Yesalis CE. Anabolic steroids in the athlete. Annu Rev Med 1991;42:449–457.

Snyder PJ et al. Effects of testosterone replacement in hypogonadal men. J Clin Endocrinol Metab 2000;85:2670–2677.

CASE **Study**   Athletics and Anabolic Steroids

Ron Diggs is a 15-year-old white cross-country runner who comes to your office requesting help in gaining muscle strength and endurance. He is a good athlete who would like to get a college scholarship and thinks that if he can increase his muscle strength, he will get better and win a scholarship. He knows of some other athletes who are using anabolic steroids and requests your help. What would you do?

ANSWER: The use and abuse of anabolic steroids by athletes and body builders of either sex to increase strength and muscle mass is widespread. Surveys indicate that in the United States 6% of high school athletes, 20% of college athletes, and more than 50% of professional athletes in certain sports use or abuse anabolic steroids at some time. Use of these compounds does result in increased muscle mass, strength, and endurance. However, much of this benefit is now thought to be due as much to en-hanced training effort as it is to the protein anabolic effects of the androgens. Individuals who take these compounds typically use 100 to 200 times the normal dose and will cycle or stack multiple anabolic compounds together in an effort to enhance the biological effect.

Common endocrine side effects of these compounds include virilization in women, suppression of endogenous gonadotropins, hypogonadism (amenorrhea in women, impotency in men), and severe psychological disturbances (depression, mania, steroid rage). Other physiological side effects are hepatotoxicity, suppression of high-density lipoprotein cholesterol, increased cardiovascular risk, insulin resistance, and decreased thyroid hormone production. It would be malpractice and unlawful to consider such treatment for this person. However, it is important to educate him about the risk–benefit ratio and reason for not using them.

64

Drugs Used in the Treatment of Erectile Dysfunction

John A. Thomas and Michael J. Thomas

 DRUG LIST

GENERIC NAME	PAGE	GENERIC NAME	PAGE
Alprostadil	737	Papaverine	738
Apomorphine	737	Phentolamine	738
Calcitonin gene-related peptide	739	Sildenafil	738
Forskolin	739	Testosterone	738
Linsidomine	739	Trazodone	739
Minoxidil	739	Vardenifil	736
Naltrexone	739	Yohimbine	739
Nitroglycerin	739		

The term impotence has been used to indicate the inability of the male to attain and maintain erection of the penis sufficient to permit satisfactory sexual intercourse. Erectile dysfunction (ED) is the preferred term. ED is a common problem, especially among older men. Perhaps a more precise term for ED is that used to signify inability of the man to achieve an erect penis as part of the multifaceted process of male sexual function. Overall, the process encompasses a variety of physical aspects with significant psychological and behavioral components.

In the United States approximately 10 million men have ED. While erectile function may not be the most important indicator of sexual satisfaction, ED may contribute to mental stress that affects interactions with family and associates. While many advances have occurred in the diagnosis and treatment of ED, other aspects remain poorly understood by the general population and even health care professionals. ED is frequently assumed to be a physiological event associated with aging, but that is not entirely accurate.

The incidence of ED can be as high as 50% in men aged 40 to 70, with the percentage increasing with age. Other risk factors associated with ED include chronic illnesses, medications, cigarette smoking, heavy alcohol consumption, sedentary patterns, and obesity. ED can be due to vasculogenic, neurogenic, hormonal, and/or psychogenic factors. It can also be due to changes in the nitric acid–cyclic guanosine monophosphate (cGMP) biochemical pathway.

Most cases of secondary ED are related to arteriosclerosis. ED is also associated with hypertension, antihypertensive therapy, and diabetes mellitus, particularly in the older diabetic. Other chronic diseases, such as psychogenic disorders and Peyronie's disease, may be associated with ED.

Several therapeutic agents, especially those that affect neurotransmitter activity (both agonist and antagonist) are often associated with ED. Many such reports have been anecdotal, although 25% of ED may be drug-related. Several classes of drugs have been associated with ED (Table 64.1). The mechanism or mechanisms of

TABLE 64.1	Drugs That May Cause Erectile Dysfunction
Therapeutic Class	**Drug or Drug Class**
Antihypertensives	Thiazide diuretics, β-blockers, clonidine, methyldopa
Antidepressants	SSRIs, MAOIs
Antipsychotics	Phenothiazines, thioxanthenes
Antianxiety agents	Benzodiazepines
Hormones	Estrogens, antiandrogens
Miscellaneous	Alcohol, metoclopramide, opioids

SSRI, selective serotonin reuptake inhibitor; MAOI, monoamine oxidase inhibitor.

drug-induced ED may be neural, endocrine, or idiopathic. ED seems to be most frequently associated with antihypertensive medications, particularly β-blockers and thiazide diuretics. Estrogen therapy (see Chapter 61) and the use of antiandrogens (see Chapter 63) can lead to changes in the endocrine system resulting in ED. Paradoxically, selective serotonin reuptake inhibitors (SSRIs) can be associated with ED while also being useful be for the treatment of premature ejaculation.

Erection involves a coordinated action of the autonomic nervous system, and certain drugs may interfere with either the sympathetic division (e.g., α_1- receptors) or the parasympathetic division (e.g., noncholinergic neurotransmitters).

PHYSIOLOGY OF PENILE ERECTION

The physiology of penile erection involves an interplay of anatomical, hemodynamic, neurophysiological, and sex hormone interaction. Penile erection is the result of a complex interaction between the central nervous system and other local factors. This physical event also can be influenced by psychological factors.

The penis is mainly supplied by the internal pudendal artery, and three major sets of veins, superficial, intermediate, and deep veins, drain it. Drug-induced changes in neurotransmitter action can affect local blood flow. Vascular supply, intrinsic smooth muscles of the penis, and adjacent striated muscles are controlled by nerves arising from the thoracolumbar sympathetic, the lumbosacral parasympathetic, and the lumbosacral somatic systems. The pudendal nerve is the major somatic pathway innervating the male genitalia.

In addition to the integrated participation of the peripheral nerves, central neural pathways are involved in the process. These central mechanisms interact during normal sexual activity and require complex coordination between the autonomic nervous system and the somatic outflow at the level of the spinal cord.

5-Hydroxytryptamine (5-HT), dopamine, and norepinephrine play important roles as central neurotransmitters in the process of erection. Still other substances or hormones, such as endorphins, oxytocin, vasopressin, adrenocorticotropic hormone (ACTH) and related peptides, and prolactin, appear to participate in the complex and coordinated process of penile erection. Central nonadrenergic neurons also may influence male sexual behavior.

Nitric oxide (NO) released during nonadrenergic, noncholinergic (NANC) neurotransmission and from the vascular endothelium is most likely the major neurotransmitter mediating penile erection. NO is a mediator of relaxation of the corpus cavernosum in response to NANC neurotransmission. An endothelium-derived relaxing factor (EDRF) in the peripheral vasculature also can induce relaxation of vascular smooth muscles. NO functions as EDRF in many blood vessels, and its release from the endothelial cell relaxes vascular smooth muscle by activating soluble guanylate cyclase, thereby increasing the production of the intracellular messenger cGMP.

The role of NO in the physiology of male sexual function establishes its importance as the principal modulator of penile erection. An increase in cGMP activates specific protein kinases, which in turn phosphorylate certain proteins, activate ion channels, and through intermediary biochemical events lead to reduction in cytosolic calcium and relaxation of smooth muscles. Following an erection or the return to a flaccid state, cGMP is hydrolyzed to GMP by phosphodiesterase type 5 (PD-5). Although other types of phosphodiesterases are present in the corpus cavernosum, they do not appear to play a significant physiological role in erection.

Certain drugs (e.g., sildenafil, vardenafil, and cialis) exert their pharmacological actions by inhibiting the breakdown of cGMP. Sildenafil (*Viagra*) is a selective inhibitor of PD-5, an enzyme that inactivates cGMP. Vardenifil (*Levitra*) is a particularly effective inhibitor of PD-5. It has a shorter onset of action and can be used in smaller doses than sildenafil. Other drugs used in the treatment of ED exert their effects through other biochemical pathways, both central and peripheral.

INDIVIDUAL AGENTS

The pharmacological agents useful in this disorder may be grouped under five broad categories of treatment (Table 64.2). Such a classification system takes into account the mode of drug action, the route of administration, and the means by which target organ selectivity is achieved.

Oral medication for treatment of ED is relatively new. Earlier measures often employed the intracaver-

TABLE 64.2 **Classification by Mode of Action for Treatments of Erectile Dysfunction**

Class	Name	Definition
I	Central initiator	Compounds that have the main site of action in the CNS to activate neural events that result in coordinated signaling that results in the initiation of a penile erection (e.g. apomorphine)
II	Peripheral initiator	Compounds that have the main site of action in the periphery to activate events that result in a penile erection (e.g. PGE_1)
III	Central conditioner	Compounds that act mainly to improve the internal milieu of the CNS so that penile erection is enabled or enhanced, they do not on their own initiate an erection (e.g. trazodone)
IV	Peripheral conditioner (local or systemic)	Compounds that act mainly to improve the local or systemic internal milieu so that penile erection is enabled or enhanced (e.g. sildenafil)
V	Other	Other ways of promoting penile rigidity including devices and surgery (e.g. prostheses)

Reprinted with permission from Heaton JP, Adams MA, and Morales A. A therapeutic taxonomy of treatment for erectile dysfunction: An evolutional imperative. *Int J Impot Res* 1997;9:115–121. Dept of Urology, Queen's University, Kingston, Ontario.

nosal injection of a vasoactive agent or a systemic mode of drug administration. Local injections or dermal applications were frequently required for satisfactory pharmacological actions upon the vascular smooth muscles of the penis. Compounds with relatively short duration of action were found to be less than satisfactory in maintaining penile erections.

Combinations of drugs have sometimes been used to take advantage of the differing onset and duration of action of the individual compounds. A rapid onset of action and a sufficient duration are important characteristics of drugs used in the treatment of ED. Vasoactive agents that are orally effective have been available for about 20 years, but sildenafil and apomorphine (buccal) have significantly improved upon the therapeutic efficacy of orally active agents.

Alprostadil

Alprostadil (prostaglandin E_1 [PGE_1]; *Edex, Topiglan*) exerts a number of effects, including systemic vasodilation, inhibition of platelet aggregation, and stimulation of intestinal motility. PGE_1 relaxes isolated smooth muscle cells contracted by norepinephrine. It has become widely used in the treatment of ED. Alprostadil binds with PGE receptors and results in a cyclic adenosine monophosphate (cAMP) mediated smooth muscle relaxation. Little is known about the pharmacokinetics of PGE_1, but it is believed that as much as 80% is metabolized in one pass through the lungs. Such rapid degradation probably accounts for its lack of significant cardiovascular side effects when administered intracavernosally. PGE_1 can also be metabolized in the penis.

PGE_1 is not orally effective. Its therapeutic success depends on its being injected intracavernosally or administered transurethrally or intraurethrally. PGE_1 has

also been used in combination with other agents, such as papaverine. The injection does not appear to produce any long-term side effects on penile smooth muscle. Transurethral therapy with alprostadil, such as MUSE (alprostadil urethral suppository or *m*edicated *u*rethral *s*ystem for *e*rection) is also an effective therapeutic technique, and there may be a role for this form of administration in selected patients with ED. The intracavernosal injection of alprostadil (e.g., alprostadil alfadex; *Edex, Viridal*) is safe and effective in patients with ED when sildenafil is ineffective. Both of these delivery systems have been used in the treatment of ED. MUSE can also be used in conjunction with a penile constrictor device (e.g., *ACTIS*).

Apomorphine

Apomorphine (*Uprima*) is a short-acting central and peripheral dopamine receptor agonist that can elicit male sexual responses. Dopamine appears to have an important role in normal erectile function. Apomorphine is a D_1-like, D_2-like dopamine receptor agonist. Apomorphine is not a new drug, and it has been used with limited success in ameliorating the symptoms of Parkinson's disease and to induce emesis. It is not orally active except for a special buccal formulation, but it can be given parenterally, usually subcutaneously. Apomorphine is rapidly cleared from the kidney because of its high lipid solubility, its large volume of distribution, and its rapid metabolism.

Aside from sildenafil, apomorphine is one of the few orally active (buccal route) pharmacological agents used in the treatment of ED. Apomorphine stimulates penile erection in both normal men and in men who are impotent. Apomorphine can be the drug of choice in patients with coexisting benign prostatic hyperplasia (BPH), coronary artery disease, and hypertension.

When formulated into a controlled release sublingual capsule, apomorphine becomes a very effective orally active drug representative of a new class of centrally acting drugs useful in the treatment of ED. It has a narrow range (2 to 6 mg) of effective doses for its erectogenic actions, with the higher doses being more effective in inducing erections. Apomorphine can cause nausea, emesis, drowsiness, and dizziness.

Androgens: Testosterone

Androgen deficiency can lead to decreases in nocturnal erections and libido. Hypogonadism is associated with impotence, yet erection in response to visual stimulation is preserved in men with hypogonadism, suggesting that androgens are not essential for erection. Although androgens can enhance male sexual function, testosterone therapy for the treatment of ED should be discouraged unless the cause is clearly related to hypogonadism. Androgen therapy in normal men may enhance sexual behavior but is without significant effect upon erectile function.

Usefulness of oral methyltestosterone is limited in men with hypogonadal impotence. Improvement following transdermal testosterone may require several months of therapy. Androgen replacement regimens for treating male hypogonadism include long-acting intramuscular injections (e.g., testosterone enanate, testosterone cypionate) and oral preparations (e.g. methyltestosterone, fluoxymesterone). Transdermal patches (*Testoderm*, *Androderm*) and topical testosterone gel (*Androgel*) are also available. Transdermal testosterone also may improve sexual function and psychological well-being in women who have undergone oophorectomy and hysterectomy. Transdermal delivery systems can provide a more constant serum testosterone level than do intramuscular injections, but they are more expensive.

Papaverine

Papaverine (*Pavabid*) is a nonspecific phosphodiesterase inhibitor that increases cAMP and cGMP levels in penile erectile tissue. Papaverine is particularly known as a smooth muscle relaxant and vasodilator. Its principal pharmacological action is as a nonspecific vasodilator of smooth muscles of the arterioles and capillaries. Various vascular beds and smooth muscle respond differently to papaverine administration both in intensity and duration. Papaverine decreases the resistance to arterial inflow and increases the resistance to venous outflow.

Papaverine is highly effective in men with psychogenic and neurogenic ED but less effective in men with vasculogenic ED. Papaverine–phentolamine combinations have been used in self-injection procedures. Papaverine doses may range from 15 to 60 mg. Papa-

verine treatment in patients with severe arterial or venous incompetence is usually unsuccessful, but autoinjections using low doses sufficient to achieve an erection are safe and efficient.

Major side effects associated with papaverine therapy include priapism, corporeal fibrosis, and occasional increases in serum aminotransferases. Intracorporeal scarring may be related to the low pH of the vehicle that is necessary to solubilize papaverine. Attempts to buffer papaverine to render it more suitable for intracavernosal injection have not been entirely satisfactory, and such delivery may still lead to intracorporeal scarring.

Phentolamine

Human erectile tissue has a population of membrane receptors that are predominantly of the α-adrenoceptor subtype. Phentolamine (*Vasomax*) is a nonselective α-adrenoceptor blocking agent (see Chapter 11), and like other such agents, it has been used to treat ED. Nonselective adrenoceptor antagonists may provoke a reflex that increases both sympathetic outflow and the release of norepinephrine.

Phentolamine has been used orally and intracavernosally in the treatment of ED. Following oral administration, phentolamine has a plasma half-life of about 30 minutes and a duration of action of 2 to 4 hours. An intracavernosal injection of phentolamine results in the drug reaching maximum serum levels in about 20 to 30 minutes. It is rapidly metabolized.

Phentolamine has been used in combination with papaverine, chlorpromazine, and vasoactive peptides in the treatment of ED.

Side effects of phentolamine are dose related. It may cause orthostatic hypotension, reflex tachycardia, cardiac arrhythmias, and rarely, myocardial infarction. Phentolamine also may reduce sperm motility in vitro.

Other α-adrenoceptor receptor antagonists include yohimbine, phenoxybenzamine, and thymoxamine. Yohimbine is an α_2-adrenoceptor antagonist, and thymoxamine is a competitive and relatively selective blocking agent for α_1- adrenoceptors. Phenoxybenzamine blocks both α_1- and α_2-adrenoreceptors, although it has a greater affinity for the α_1-subtype. All three of these α-receptor blocking drugs can induce penile erection, but their effects are generally less consistent and less effective than those of phentolamine. Yohimbine is only moderately effective in treating patients with organic impotence, and side effects may include postural hypotension, heart palpitations, fine tremors, and cavernosal fibrosis, especially following intracavernosal injections.

Sildenafil

Sildenafil (*Viagra*) was developed more than 10 years ago as an antihypertensive and antianginal drug. It proved ineffective in these applications but was shown to affect the smooth muscles of the penis.

Sildenafil is a selective inhibitor of cGMP-specific PD-5 and therefore inhibits the degradation of cGMP. PD-5, the predominant type in the corpus cavernosum, also is present in other tissues (e.g., lungs, platelets, and eye). The selective inhibition of this enzyme facilitates the release of nitric oxide and smooth muscle relaxation of the corpus cavernosa. Sildenafil enhances erection by augmenting nitric oxide–mediated relaxation pathways. It has been suggested that sildenafil's mechanism of action is due to cross-talk between cGMP- and cAMP-dependent transduction pathways within the cavernous muscles.

Sildenafil is readily absorbed after oral administration and reaches peak plasma levels after about an hour. It undergoes hepatic metabolism and has a terminal half-life of about 4 hours. An initial dose of 50 mg is taken about an hour prior to sexual activity to induce penile erection.

Orally administered sildenafil is an effective and well-tolerated treatment for men with ED, including those with diabetes mellitus. It has also been used for so-called salvage therapy in men who do not respond to intracorporeal injections of other agents.

Headache is a common side effect, as are flushing and rhinitis. More serious side effects include definite or suspected myocardial infarctions and cardiac arrest.

Trazodone

Trazodone (*Apothecon*) is also classified as an antidepressant agent. It is a selective serotonin reuptake inhibitor (SSRI), partial agonist at postsynaptic 5-HT$_{1A}$ receptors, and exhibits α-adrenoceptor blocking actions.

Trazodone may cause priapism and enhance libido, and it prolongs nocturnal erections. This drug has been used both orally and by intracavernosal injection. It can be used alone or in combination with yohimbine. Overall, trazodone has not been as effective in treating ED as other available agents. However, it may be an option for selected patients, particularly those with performance anxiety or low libido.

Other Agents

Many other drugs and herbals exhibit varying degrees of potency with respect to penile erection. Some have undergone limited clinical trials, while others are associated with anecdotal reports. Generally, these agents are not particularly effective and are not widely used among mainstream therapeutic options for ED.

Linsidomine (SIN-1) is an active metabolite of the antianginal drug molsidomine. Its mechanism of action upon the corpus cavernosum involves the release of ni-

tric oxide. Injected intracavernosally it can produce penile erections, but its clinical usefulness has not been fully established.

Nitroglycerin (also isosorbide nitrate) relaxes isolated strips of human corpus cavernosum. Its mechanism involves the stimulation of guanylate cyclase. Clinically, nitroglycerin has been of limited use in the treatment of ED.

Minoxidil, an antihypertensive agent, produces arteriolar vasodilation by an unknown mechanism. In limited clinical studies, minoxidil increases penile rigidity and has been used in the long-term treatment of organic impotence.

Naltrexone, an orally active opioid receptor antagonist, restores erectile function in some patients with idiopathic ED.

Calcitonin gene–related peptide (CGRP) induces a dose-related increase in penile arterial inflow, cavernous smooth muscle relaxation, cavernous outflow occlusion, and an erectile response. CGRP plus PGE$_1$ may be an alternative to penile implants in selected patients.

Forskolin, an herbal, relaxes smooth muscle. Injected intracavernosally, forskolin has been of limited use in the treatment of vasculogenic impotence.

Other herbal remedies or so-called natural products purportedly can enhance male sexual activity. Some may contain yohimbine. Natural prosexual agents of herbal origin include *Epidemicum sagthatum, Tribulas terrestris,* and *Murira puama.* Their use in folk medicine in China and other countries is likely due to their sexual stimulating properties and their aphrodisiac effects. *Ginkgo biloba* extract also has been used in the therapy of ED and sexual dysfunction.

Drug Interactions

Orally active agents used in the treatment of ED are more affected by aging and disease processes than are those injected intracavernosally. In addition, alterations in hepatic metabolism and/or renal clearance in the elderly man (see Chapter 6) influence the frequency of appearance of adverse reactions between several coadministered drugs in the treatment of ED. For example, the concomitant use of sildenafil and nitroglycerin is contraindicated by cardiovascular complications. Also, the use of testosterone in the presence of androgen-dependent tumors may promote tumor growth.

Sildenafil has other minor adverse effects, such as headache, nasal congestion, and flushing. There are no clinically significant drug interactions between sildenafil and apomorphine. Apomorphine, like sildenafil, is orally active. However, unlike sildenafil, it exerts its action through the central nervous system. Apomorphine can produce dizziness, nausea, pallor, and hypotension, and in the presence of ethanol, it purportedly increases the incidence of these side effects. Such a synergy caused by ethanol and apomorphine coadministration is not unique and would likely be present with other agents that induce mild hypotension.

The concomitant intake of grapefruit juice increases the concentration of many drugs (e.g., testosterone, sildenafil) in humans. Such actions appear to be mediated mainly by the suppression of the cytochrome P450 enzyme CYP3A4 in the small intestine. The resultant diminished first-pass metabolism and increased bioavailability can lead to increased drug levels in the blood. Because sildenafil is metabolized by CYP3A and to a lesser extent by CYP2C9, grapefruit juice can reduce the clearance of this drug. Other drugs can either increase or decrease serum levels of sildenafil. Administration of cimetidine, erythromycin, or ritonavir can lead to increases in serum concentrations of sildenafil, while rifampin diminishes blood levels of sildenafil.

Therapy with phentolamine may result in reflex tachycardia, arrhythmias, and hypotension; the latter effect can be exacerbated by other vasodilatory drugs and by the simultaneous ingestion of ethanol. The pharmacological actions of trazodone can be reduced by paroxetine and possibly other SSRIs.

Study QUESTIONS

1. Sildenafil's mechanism of action can best be described as
    (A) Selective inhibitor of phosphodiesterase type 5
    (B) Selective serotonin uptake inhibitor
    (C) Nonselective inhibitor of phosphodiesterase
    (D) β-Adrenoceptor blocking agent
2. Apomorphine
    (A) Has dopamine receptor antagonist properties
    (B) Efficacy depends upon a special buccal formulation
    (C) Actions are mediated only centrally
    (D) Action is contraindicated in patients with BPH
3. All of the following agents possess erectogenic properties EXCEPT
    (A) Papaverine
    (B) Phentolamine
    (C) Trazodone
    (D) Alcohol
4. All of the following classes of agents may produce erectile dysfunction EXCEPT
    (A) β-Adrenoceptor blocking agents
    (B) Oral hypoglycemic agents
    (C) Phenothiazines
    (D) Thiazide diuretics
    (E) α-Adrenoceptor blocking agents
5. Testosterone therapy may be indicated for the treatment of erectile dysfunction in which of the following situations?
    (A) Aged patient
    (B) Hypogonadism
    (C) Alcoholism
    (D) Depression

ANSWERS

1. **A.** The principal action of sildenafil is selective inhibition of the enzyme phosphodiesterase type 5. This is the enzyme that inactivates cGMP. Sildenafil does not appear to inhibit other forms of the enzyme. Sildenafil has no actions on either serotonin receptors or β-adrenoceptors.
2. **B.** Apomorphine is an older drug with dopamine receptor agonist properties. It acts both centrally and peripherally. It is not contraindicated in cases of BPH but rather may be the drug of choice in this instance.
3. **D.** Heavy use of alcohol is associated with impotence. The other choices are agents that possess erectogenic properties.
4. **E.** The first four choices all are associated with erectile dysfunction. Although α-adrenoceptor blocking agents are not approved for the treatment of erectile dysfunction, they have been shown to have some effectiveness.
5. **B.** The only time testosterone is indicated for the treatment of erectile dysfunction is if the cause is clearly related to hypogonadism. In other situations, the adverse effects related to testosterone and its limited effectiveness preclude its use.

SUPPLEMENTAL READING

Andersson KE. Pharmacology of erectile function and dysfunction. Urol Clin North Am 2001;28:233–248.
Keene LC and Davies PH. Drug-related erectile dysfunction. Adverse Drug React Toxicol Rev 1999;18:5–24.
Lue T. Erectile dysfunction. N Engl J Med 2000;348:1802–1813.
Melman A and Gingell JC. The epidemiology and pathophysiology of erectile dysfunction. J Urol 1999;161:5–11.
Padma-Nathan H and Giuliano F. Oral drug therapy for erectile dysfunction. Urol Clin North Am 2001;28:321–334.

CASE Study   Diabetes and Erectile Dysfunction

A 48-year-old white man went to the local urology clinic with the chief complaint of sexual incompatibility associated with failure to attain an erection. He states that he has a family history of diabetes mellitus but is not receiving any insulin or oral hypoglycemic drugs. He is married and has fathered two children, aged 12 and 15. Blood chemistries and hormone levels are as follows: total insulin (free and bound), 15 microunits/mL; T_4 (thyroxine), 10 μg/dL; testosterone (total), 200 ng/dL; fasting blood glucose, 210 mg/dL; dihydrotestosterone, 10 ng/dL. Based on this medical history and the hormone levels, what treatment would you initiate?

ANSWER: This patient has possible diabetes mellitus with hypogonadism. Both testosterone and DHT levels lower than normal suggests hypogonadism. Whether or not there is a vasculogenic problem from the diabetes mellitus cannot be determined. The blood glucose is elevated, and a workup for diabetes may be pursued (blood insulin is normal). Initial therapy is administration of testosterone.

65 Thyroid and Antithyroid Drugs

John Connors

DRUG LIST

GENERIC NAME	PAGE	GENERIC NAME	PAGE
Iocetamic acid	751	Methylthiouracil	750
Iodine	743	Potassium perchlorate	751
Iopanoic acid	751	Propylthiouracil	750
Levothyroxine sodium	748	Sodium ipodate	751
Liothyronine sodium	748	Thyroglobulin	748
Liotrix	748	Thyroid USP	748
Lithium carbonate	752	Tyropanoic acid	751

Three hormones, thyroxine (3,5,3′,5′-tetraiodothyronine, or T_4), triiodothyronine (3,5,3′-triiodothyronine, or T_3), and calcitonin (see Chapter 66) are secreted by the thyroid gland. The hormones T_4 and T_3 are iodine-containing amino acid derivatives and are unique in that they have no discrete target tissue. Every tissue in the body is affected in some way by thyroid hormones, and almost all cells appear to require constant optimal amounts for normal operation.

Thyroid hormones exert a wide variety of physiological actions through genomic and nongenomic mechanisms and influence the metabolism of proteins, carbohydrates, and lipids; cell morphology; membrane transport; ion homeostasis; oxygen consumption; heat production; and so on. Relatively constant circulating concentrations of T_4 and T_3 are required for normal growth and development and the proper functioning of the neural, reproductive, cardiovascular, gastrointestinal, and hematopoietic systems. Unlike most other hormones, whose circulating concentrations vary widely in response to external and internal stimuli, the circulating concentrations of thyroid hormones are usually held relatively constant over time.

In health, two negative feedback control systems operate to maintain circulating thyroid hormone levels. The first, the *hypothalamic–pituitary-thyroid axis* (HPTA), acts to regulate the concentration of thyroid hormones in the blood by controlling their synthesis and secretion by the thyroid gland. The second negative feedback control system is the *thyroid autoregulatory system*. It is intrinsic to the thyroid gland and acts to ensure that an adequate supply of iodide is extracted from the blood and made available for thyroid hormone synthesis despite variations in dietary iodine intake.

Worldwide, the most common thyroid disorder is hypothyroidism resulting from dietary iodine deficiency. In iodine-replete areas of the world, most thyroid disorders are the result of autoimmune disease. The symptoms manifested in hypothyroid and hyperthyroid states are largely independent of any underlying disorder of the thyroid gland itself; they are a function of the degree of hormone deficiency or excess.

A second dietary trace element, selenium, is also essential for normal thyroid hormone metabolism. Selenium in the form of selenocysteine is a required component for three enzymes that remove iodide from thyroid hormones. Deiodination is the major metabolic pathway by which T_4 and T_3 are cleared from the system. After secretion by the thyroid gland, T_4 may be deiodinated to yield either T_3 or the physiologically inactive reverse T_3 (3,3',5'-triiodothyronine, or rT_3). T_3 and rT_3 are further deiodinated to form less active metabolites. Selenium, like iodine, is deficient in many areas of the world.

BIOSYNTHESIS, STORAGE, SECRETION, AND METABOLISM OF THYROID HORMONES

Thyroid epithelial cells synthesize and secrete T_4 and T_3 and make up the functional units of thyroid glandular tissue, the thyroid follicles. Thyroid follicles are hollow vesicles formed by a single layer of epithelial cells that are filled with *colloid*. T_4, T_3, and iodine are stored in the follicular colloid. T_4 and T_3 are derived from tyrosyl residues of the protein *thyroglobulin* (Tg). Thyroid follicular cells synthesize and secrete Tg into the follicular lumen. Thyroid follicular cells also remove iodide (I^-) from the blood and concentrate it within the follicular lumen. Within the follicles, some of the tyrosyl residues of Tg are iodinated, and a few specific pairs of iodotyrosyl residues may be coupled to form T_4 and T_3. Thus, T_4, T_3, and iodine (in the form of iodinated tyrosyl residues) are found within the peptide structure of the Tg that is stored in the follicular lumen.

The secretion of T_4 and T_3 requires the uptake of follicular contents across the follicular cell apical membrane, the enzymatic release of T_4 and T_3 from peptide linkage within Tg, and the transport of T_4 and T_3 across the follicular cell basal membrane to the blood. Several of the steps in synthesis and secretion of T_4 and T_3 may be compromised by iodine deficiency or disease and can be blocked selectively by a variety of chemicals and drugs.

Requirement for Iodine

A normal rate of thyroid hormone synthesis depends on an adequate dietary intake of iodine. Iodine is naturally present in water and soil, although some soils contain very low amounts. As a result, seafood is a more reliable source of iodine than crop plants. Approximately 1.6 billion people in more than 100 countries live in areas where natural sources of dietary iodine intake are marginal or insufficient. A minimum of 60 μg of elemental iodine is required each day for thyroid hormone synthesis, and at least 100 μg/day is required to eliminate thyroid follicular cell hyperplasia and thyroid enlargement (i.e., iodine deficiency goiter).

Subsequent to the ingestion of iodine in various forms, I^- is absorbed by the small intestine and enters the blood. Two competing pathways are involved in the clearance of I^- from the blood: renal filtration into urine and thyroidal uptake. The renal clearance rate for I^- (30–50 mL/minute) varies only with the glomerular filtration rate. However, the thyroidal I^- clearance rate is autoregulated to maintain an absolute thyroidal I^- uptake rate of approximately 100 μg I^- each day. To accomplish this, the thyroidal I^- clearance rate may vary (3 to 100 mL/minute) depending on the concentration of I^- in the blood.

Iodide Transport by Follicular Cells and Iodine Trapping Within Follicles

The thyroid follicular cells transport I^- across the cell and secrete the precursor protein, Tg, into the follicular lumen. In addition, these cells contain an apical membrane–bound enzyme, thyroperoxidase (TPO), and the enzymatic machinery to produce hydrogen peroxide (H_2O_2). In the presence of H_2O_2, TPO catalyzes the incorporation of I^- into tyrosyl residues of Tg to form monoiodotyrosine (MIT) and diiodotyrosine (DIT) and the coupling of these iodotyrosyl residues to form T_4 and T_3.

Thyroid follicular cells actively transport iodide into the cell against both a concentration gradient and a negative potential (Fig. 65.1). At the basal (blood side) follicular cell membrane, an iodide pump actively transports

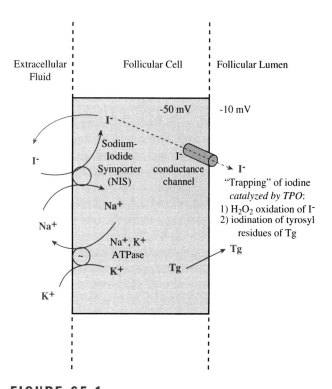

FIGURE 65.1

Concentration of iodine within the thyroid follicular cell and follicular lumen.

I⁻ from the extracellular fluid (pertechnetate) into the cytoplasm and concentrates I⁻ within the follicular cell. The I⁻ concentration gradient between the thyroid gland and the blood normally ranges from 25 to 100 and is referred to as the thyroid–plasma or thyroid–serum ratio. During periods of active stimulation, the concentration of I⁻ within the follicle may be as high as 250 times that of the blood. On the luminal side of the apical membrane, the I⁻ is rapidly oxidized in the presence of H_2O_2 and TPO and incorporated into the tyrosyl residues in newly formed Tg to form MIT or DIT.

The thyroidal mechanism used for concentrating I⁻ may also concentrate other monovalent anions, including pertechnetate, perchlorate, and thiocyanate, within the follicular lumen. However, none of these anions become incorporated into Tg, although they may act as a competitive inhibitor of I⁻ transport. The ability of the thyroid gland to concentrate radioactive pertechnetate makes it a useful agent for thyroid imaging, since it is concentrated by the thyroid cells without further metabolism. The perchlorate and thiocyanate discharge tests make use of the ability of these anions to inhibit I⁻ transport to test for defects in the incorporation of I⁻ into Tg.

Coupling of Iodotyrosines to Form Iodothyronines

The final step in thyroid hormone synthesis is the coupling of two *iodotyrosines* within a single peptide chain of Tg to form the *iodothyronine* T_4 or T_3. Both the coupling of two DITs to form T_4 and the coupling of a MIT with a DIT to form T_3 are catalyzed by the enzyme TPO.

Storage of Thyroid Hormones and Iodine in Colloid

T_4, T_3, MIT, and DIT are stored outside the cell in the follicular colloid in peptide linkage within the Tg molecules. In normal humans on an iodine-sufficient diet, Tg makes up approximately 30% of the mass of the thyroid gland and represents a 2- to 3-month supply of hormone. The total amount of iodine contained as T_4, T_3, MIT, and DIT within Tg varies with the dietary iodine intake.

Secretion of Thyroid Hormones

The secretion of T_4 and T_3 is a relatively complex process because T_4 and T_3 are stored in the peptide structure of Tg within the follicular lumen and therefore are separated from the pertechnetate and the capillary endothelium by the thyroid follicular cells.

Endocytosis

The first step in the release of thyroid hormones from the thyroid gland is through *endocytosis* of colloid from the follicular lumen into the follicle cells. This may occur by macropinocytosis or micropinocytosis. Both processes are stimulated by TSH and result in the uptake of macropinocytotic or micropinocytotic vesicles that are limited by a single membrane and are filled with colloid inclusions. These endocytotic vesicles migrate from the follicular cell apical membrane toward the basal membrane. Within a few minutes of their formation, the colloid-containing endocytotic vesicles become surrounded by lysosomes containing glycoside hydrolases and proteases. The lysosomes eventually fuse with the endocytotic vesicles to form lysoendosomes. Within the lysoendosomes, Tg is hydrolyzed to yield peptide fragments, iodoamino acids (MIT and DIT), iodothyronines (T_4 and T_3), and other free amino acids. Once released from Tg, T_4 and T_3 rapidly diffuse across the basal plasma membrane into the pertechnetate and eventually into the circulation. During thyroidal secretion, only T_4, T_3 and a small amount of I⁻ normally reach the circulation; no Tg, MIT, or DIT escapes.

The T_4 and T_3 that are released from the thyroid gland are firmly but reversibly bound to several plasma proteins. More than 99% of the circulating thyroid hormone is protein bound, with only the free hormone available to enter cells (Table 65.1). The amount of T_4 or T_3 entering the cells and the ultimate physiological response are directly related to the plasma concentrations of free T_4 and free T_3. It is the concentrations of free T_4 and T_3 in the plasma that are regulated by the HPTA (Fig. 65.2) rather than the total (i.e., free plus protein-bound) plasma T_4 and T_3 concentrations.

Thyroxine-binding globulin is the least abundant of the three major transport proteins. Nevertheless, it carries about 70% of the circulating T_4 and T_3 by virtue of its high affinity for the two hormones. *Transthyretin*, formerly known as thyroxine-binding prealbumin, binds only about 10 to 15% of the hormones. *Albumin*, a protein that has a binding affinity for a multitude of small molecules, has an even lower affinity for T_4 and T_3 than

TABLE 65.1 Approximate Values for Thyroid Hormone Plasma Concentrations and Various Kinetic Parameters

	T_4	T_3
Plasma concentration		
Total	7.77 mg/dL	0.14 mg/dL
Free	1.554 ng/dL	0.389 ng/dL
Total hormone in free form	0.02%	0.3%
Plasma half-life	6.7 days	0.75 days
Volume of distribution	10 L	40 L
Metabolic clearance rate	1.1 L/day	24 L/day
Total production rate	85.47 mg/day	33.6 mg/day
From thyroid secretion	100%	20%

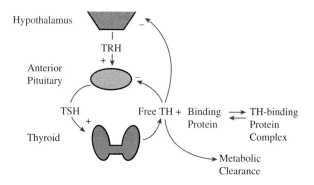

FIGURE 65.2
The hypothalamic–pituitary–thyroid axis.

transthyretin, but the high plasma albumin concentration results in the binding of about 15 to 20% of the circulating thyroid hormones. Like T_4 and T_3 bound to transthyretin, the hormones may dissociate rapidly from albumin to generate free T_4 and free T_3. Circulating T_4 and T_3 are also bound by high-density lipoproteins (HDL). Plasma HDL may carry about 3% of the T_4 and 6% of the T_3. The physiological significance of this HDL binding is uncertain, but it may play a role in targeting thyroid hormone delivery to specific tissues.

The thyroid hormone transport proteins are not essential for hormone action. Rather, they participate in the maintenance of a steady supply of free hormone to tissues. Because of the presence of the binding proteins in the plasma, the size of the circulating thyroid hormone pool is quite large, and both T_4 and T_3 have very long half-lives in humans (Table 65.1). The total amount of thyroid hormone bound to plasma proteins is about three times that secreted and degraded in the course of a single day. Three functions can be postulated for the thyroid hormone transport proteins: (1) extrathyroidal storage of hormone, (2) a buffering action, such that effects of acute changes in rates of thyroid gland secretion or hormone metabolic clearance on plasma concentrations of free thyroid hormones are minimized, and (3) a hormone-releasing function that allows the very small free hormone pool to be continuously replenished and made available to cells as intracellular hormone is metabolized. Thus, the large pools of protein-bound T_4 and T_3 in the blood act to stabilize plasma free T_4 and free T_3 concentrations and consequently the intracellular concentrations of T_4 and T_3 and thyroid hormone receptor (TR) occupancy.

Cellular Uptake and Intracellular Binding of T_3 to Nuclear Thyroid Hormone Receptors

Free T_4 and T_3 can enter cells by carrier-mediated facilitated diffusion or active transport. After gaining access to the cell interior, T_4 may undergo 5′-monodeiodination to yield T_3. The T_3 thus mixes with T_3 entering the

cell from the plasma and binds to nuclear TRs. The specific 5′-monodeiodinase enzyme and the level of activity vary from tissue to tissue, as does the contribution of plasma T_4 to nuclear TR-bound T_3.

Thyroid Hormone Activation and Inactivation by Selenodeiodinases

In humans, the major pathway in the metabolism of the thyroid hormones consists of the removal of iodine or deiodination. Three deiodinase isoenzymes, encoded on three distinct genes, catalyze the reductive deiodination. All three enzymes contain the rare amino acid selenocysteine. The essential trace element selenium therefore plays an important role in thyroid hormone economy.

The most important pathway for the metabolism of T_4 is monodeiodination. The removal of an iodide from the outer ring of T_4 yields T_3. Since the affinity of nuclear TRs is much higher for T_3 than T_4, outer ring monodeiodination of T_4 to yield T_3 produces a more active metabolite. Conversely, removal of an iodide from the inner ring of T_4 yields an inactive metabolite, rT_3. Both T_3 and rT_3 may undergo subsequent deiodinations to yield totally deiodinated thyronine (T_0).

Up to 80% of the circulating T_3 originates from deiodination of T_4. This is due mainly to a deiodinase (D1) activity in the liver, where most of the T_3 formed is exported into the circulation. Monodeiodination of T_4 to yield T_3 is catalyzed by another deiodinase (D2). It appears that D2 catalyzes T_3 from T_4 for local cellular demands independent of circulating T_3. The third enzyme involved in the reductive deiodination of T_4, T_3, and other iodothyronines is D3. The sole action of this enzyme is the removal of iodide from the inner ring of iodothyronines.

The three deiodinases have differing tissue distributions, substrate preferences, and K_m values. This arrangement allows for control of thyroid hormone action at the cellular level. The source and quantity of T_3

TABLE 65.2	**TSH-Stimulated Events at the Thyroid Gland**
Cyclic AMP– Mediated Events	**Phospholipase C–Mediated Events**
Sodium iodide symporter activity	H_2O_2 generation
Thyroglobulin synthesis	I^- conductance of the apical membrane
Thyroperoxidase synthesis	
Hormone synthesis	
Endocytosis and hydrolysis of colloid	
Hormone secretion	
Type 1 deiodinase activity	
Hypertrophy	

bound to nuclear TRs may vary among tissues depending on the distributions and relative activities of D1, D2, and D3.

MECHANISMS OF ACTION OF THYROID HORMONES

Thyroid hormone mechanisms of action can be classified into two types: (1) genomic or nuclear and (2) nongenomic, including effects at the plasma membrane and mitochondria. Genomic effects involve modification of gene transcription, are mediated only by T_3, and require at least several hours to detect. Nongenomic actions are generally rapid in onset and occur in response to T_4 and some T_4 metabolites (e.g., rT_3, T_3, and T_2).

Genomic Actions of Thyroid Hormones

Thyroid hormone receptors are members of a superfamily of nuclear receptors that includes receptors for estrogen, glucocorticoid, mineralocorticoid, retinoic acid, 9-cis-retinoic acid (retinoid X), and vitamin D. Similar to the mechanism of action of lipophilic steroid hormones, the lipophilic T_3 binds to a protein receptor to form a complex and the hormone–receptor complex binds to an appropriate hormone response element on DNA to alter the transcription of specific genes. The current view of the mechanism of thyroid hormone action differs from that for steroid hormones, however, in three major ways: (1) There are apparently no cytosolic receptors for thyroid hormones. (2) The nuclear TRs can bind to DNA nucleotide sequences in the regulatory region of thyroid hormone–responsive genes in the absence of thyroid hormone binding. (3) In the absence of T_3 binding, TR bound to these specific areas of DNA may repress or promote the transcription of the associated thyroid hormone-responsive gene.

Nongenomic Actions of Thyroid Hormone

The nongenomic actions of thyroid hormone are increasingly recognized as physiologically significant. Nongenomic actions may be observed within minutes of stimulation and respond to a range of thyroid hormone metabolites (T_4, T_3, rT_3, T_2). The magnitude of nongenomic actions is usually only a few fold in contrast to the multifold genomic actions. The nongenomic actions (Table 65.2) may involve interactions with components of the cellular signal transduction pathways, such as cyclic adenosine monophosphate (cAMP), phosphatidyl inositol, and protein kinases. Examples include effects on cellular respiration, cell morphology, vascular tone, and ion homeostasis. Possible nongenomic targets of thyroid hormone include the plasma membrane, cy-toskeleton, sarcoplasmic reticulum, mitochondria, and contractile elements of vascular smooth muscle.

PHYSIOLOGICAL EFFECTS OF THYROID HORMONES

There is no discrete target tissue for thyroid hormones; virtually every cell in the body is affected by thyroid hormones in some way. These hormones are intimately involved in the maintenance of normal function in virtually every cell type, including cellular responsiveness to other hormones, to the availability of metabolic substrates, to growth factors, and so on. Thyroid dysfunction can produce dramatic changes in the metabolism of proteins, carbohydrates, and lipids at the cellular level that can have repercussions for the operation of the cardiovascular, gastrointestinal, musculoskeletal, reproductive, and nervous systems. Some of the clinical manifestations of thyroid dysfunction are presented next in the discussions of hypothyroid and hyperthyroid states.

HYPOTHYROID STATES

Hypothyroidism refers to the exposure of body tissues to a subnormal amount of thyroid hormone. This can result from a defect anywhere in the HPTA. As a consequence of the lack of thyroid hormone, a wide variety of physiological and clinical disturbances involving virtually every organ system may result.

Primary hypothyroidism results from an inability of the thyroid gland itself to produce and secrete sufficient quantities of T_4 and T_3 and accounts for most cases of hypothyroidism. In iodine-sufficient areas of the world, the most common cause of primary hypothyroidism is *chronic autoimmune thyroiditis* (Hashimoto's thyroiditis). Other causes of primary hypothyroidism include spontaneous degeneration of glandular tissue (idiopathic hypothyroidism), thyroid ablation with radioactive iodine uptake (^{131}I), and total or subtotal surgical thyroidectomy. Primary hypothyroidism is accompanied by an elevation in pituitary TSH secretion and circulating TSH levels. An enlargement of the thyroid, or goiter, usually develops with increasing duration of the primary hypothyroidism.

Biosynthetic defects in thyroid hormonogenesis may also result in an inability of the thyroid gland to produce sufficient hormone and may be due to inherited enzymatic deficiencies or the ingestion of natural or therapeutically administered antithyroid agents. An example in the latter category is lithium, widely used to treat psychiatric disorders and associated with the development of hypothyroidism and goiter. It is concentrated by the thyroid, where it inhibits thyroidal I⁻ uptake, incorporation of I⁻ into Tg, coupling of iodotyrosine, and, eventually, thyroid hormone secretion.

Secondary hypothyroidism, or pituitary hypothyroidism, is the consequence of impaired thyroid-stimulating hormone (TSH) secretion and is less common than primary hypothyroidism. It may result from any of the causes of hypopituitarism (e.g., pituitary tumor, postpartum pituitary necrosis, trauma). Patients with secondary hypothyroidism exhibit undetectable or inappropriately low serum TSH concentrations. In secondary hypothyroidism, a normal thyroid gland lacks the normal level of TSH stimulation necessary to synthesize and secrete thyroid hormones. Such patients usually also have impaired secretion of TSH in response to exogenous thyrotropin-releasing hormone (TRH) administration.

Tertiary hypothyroidism, or hypothalamic hypothyroidism, results from impaired TRH stimulation of pituitary TSH. This may be due to a disorder that damages the hypothalamus or interferes with hypothalamic–pituitary portal blood flow, thereby preventing delivery of TRH to the pituitary. Tumors, trauma, radiation therapy, or infiltrative disease of the hypothalamus can cause such damage. This relatively rare form of hypothyroidism is also characterized by inappropriately low levels of serum TSH.

Clinical Manifestations of Hypothyroidism

During the perinatal period, there is an absolute requirement for thyroid hormone for the development and maturation of the nervous and musculoskeletal systems. In the perinatal nervous system, thyroid hormone plays a critical role in normal growth of the cerebral and cerebellar cortices, the proliferation of axons, the branching of dendrites, synaptogenesis, myelination, cell migration, and so on.

Thyroid hormone also plays a major role in the maturation of bone. A deficiency of thyroid hormone in early life leads to both delay in and abnormal development of epiphyseal centers of ossification (epiphyseal dysgenesis). Hypothyroidism-induced impairment of linear growth can lead to dwarfism in which the limbs are disproportionately short in relation to the trunk with the apparent bone age retarded in relation to chronological age.

The hallmarks of infantile hypothyroidism (e.g., retardation of mental development and growth) become manifest only in later infancy and are largely irreversible. Consequently, early recognition and initiation of replacement therapy are crucial. In the absence of thyroid hormone therapy, the symptoms of infantile hypothyroidism include feeding problems, failure to thrive, constipation, a hoarse cry, and somnolence. In succeeding months, especially in severe cases, protuberance of the abdomen, dry skin, poor growth of hair and nails, delayed eruption of the deciduous teeth, and delay in reaching the normal milestones of development (e.g., holding up the head, sitting, walking, and talking) become evident.

In adults, the signs and symptoms of hypothyroidism include somnolence, slow mentation, dryness and loss of hair, increased fluid in body cavities (e.g., the pericardial sac), low metabolic rate, tendency to gain weight, hyperlipidemia, subnormal temperature, cold intolerance, bradycardia, reduced systolic and increased diastolic pulse pressure, hoarseness, muscle weakness, slow return of muscle to the neutral position after a tendon jerk, constipation, menstrual abnormalities, infertility, and sometimes myxedema (hard edema of subcutaneous tissue with increased content of proteoglycans in the fluid). A goiter (i.e., enlargement of the thyroid gland) may be present.

Juvenile or adult patients with primary hypothyroidism (as indicated by low serum free T_4 and high serum TSH concentrations) are usually treated with thyroxine with the aim of relieving symptoms and reducing the serum TSH concentration into the normal reference range. If the primary hypothyroidism is the result of iodine deficiency, then gradually increasing dietary iodine supplementation may also be instituted in addition to the thyroxine replacement therapy. Iodine supplementation alone may lead to the development of acute hyperthyroidism.

Patients with secondary or tertiary hypothyroidism are also usually treated with thyroxine, but the serum TSH concentration is not a reliable guide to therapy. The efficacy of thyroid hormone replacement in these patients must be assessed clinically and by measurement of the serum T_4 concentration.

The most extreme manifestation of untreated hypothyroidism is *myxedema coma,* which even if detected early and appropriately treated, carries a mortality rate of 30 to 60%. Myxedema coma is a misnomer. Most patients exhibit neither the myxedema nor coma. Patients with myxedema coma usually have longstanding hypothyroidism with the classic symptoms of hypothyroidism. Decompensation into myxedema coma may occur when the homeostatic mechanisms of the severely hypothyroid patient are subject to a stressful precipitating event (e.g., infection, trauma, some medications, stroke, surgery). The principal manifestation of myxedema coma is a deterioration of mental status (apathy, confusion, psychosis, but rarely coma). Other common clinical features include hypothermia, diastolic hypertension (early), hypotension (late), hypoventilation, hypoglycemia, and hyponatremia. If myxedema coma is suspected, the patient is usually admitted to an intensive care unit for pulmonary and cardiovascular support and treated with intravenous T_4 (or sometimes T_3). Until coexisting adrenal insufficiency is ruled out, hydrocortisone should also be administered.

DRUGS USED IN THE TREATMENT OF HYPOTHYROIDISM

Levothyroxine Sodium

Levothyroxine sodium (*Levothroid, Synthroid, Levoxine*) is the sodium salt of the naturally occurring levorotatory isomer of T_4. It is the preparation of choice for maintenance of plasma T_4 and T_3 concentrations for thyroid hormone replacement therapy in hypothyroid patients. It is absorbed intact from the gastrointestinal tract, and its long half-life allows for convenient once-daily administration. Since much of the T_4 is deiodinated to T_3, it is usually unnecessary to use more expensive preparations containing both T_4 and T_3. The aim is to establish euthyroidism with measured serum concentrations of T_4, T_3, and TSH within the normal range.

The TSH-suppressive effects of exogenous T_4 also prove useful in removing the stimulatory effects of TSH on the thyroid gland in the management of simple nonendemic goiter, chronic thyroiditis, and TSH-dependent thyroid carcinoma.

Liothyronine Sodium

Liothyronine sodium (*Cytomel*) is the sodium salt of the naturally occurring levorotatory isomer of T_3. Liothyronine is generally not used for maintenance thyroid hormone replacement therapy because of its short plasma half-life and duration of action. The use of T_3 alone is recommended only in special situations, such as in the initial therapy of myxedema and myxedema coma and the short-term suppression of TSH in patients undergoing surgery for thyroid cancer. The use of T_3 alone may also be useful in patients with the rare condition of 5'-deiodinase deficiency who cannot convert T_4 to T_3.

Liotrix

Liotrix (*Euthroid, Thyrolar*) is a 4:1 mixture of levothyroxine sodium and liothyronine sodium. Like levothyroxine, liotrix is used for thyroid hormone replacement therapy in hypothyroid patients. Although the idea of combining T_4 and T_3 in replacement therapy so as to mimic the normal ratio secreted by the thyroid gland is not new, it does not appear that liotrix offers any therapeutic advantage over levothyroxine alone.

Thyroid USP and Thyroglobulin

Thyroid USP (*Thyrar, Thyroid Strong, S-P-T*) is derived from dried and defatted thyroid glands of domestic an-imals (bovine, ovine, or porcine), while Tg (*Proloid*) is a partially purified extract of frozen porcine thyroid glands. Although used extensively in the past, these preparations are rarely used today.

The total thyroid hormone content of thyroid glands and the ratio of T_3 to T_4 vary somewhat from one species to another. Thyroid USP preparations are therefore standardized on the basis of their iodine content. Much of the iodine in these preparations is in the metabolically inactive form of iodotyrosines. Thus, a given preparation may satisfy the USP iodine assay requirements and yet contain low amounts of T_4 and T_3. *Thyrar* (a beef extract) and *Armour Thyroid* tablets (a pork extract) are evaluated by additional biological assays to ensure consistent potency from one batch to another.

The production of *Proloid*, which is a partially purified frozen porcine Tg preparation, is an attempt to avoid the variability in desiccated thyroid preparations. It is also assayed and standardized for biological potency. Thyroglobulin is slightly more expensive and offers no particular therapeutic advantage over Thyroid USP. These two preparations have a higher ratio of T_3 to T_4 than that found in human thyroid secretion, so supraphysiological levels of T_3 may occur in the immediate postabsorptive period because of the rapid release of T_3 from ingested Tg, its immediate absorption, and the relatively long period (1 day) required for T_3 to equilibrate in its volume of distribution.

ADVERSE EFFECTS OF TREATMENT WITH THYROID HORMONE

The most common adverse effects (i.e., symptoms of hyperthyroidism) are the result of a drug overdose; they include cardiac palpitation and arrhythmias, tachycardia, weight loss, tremor, headache, insomnia, and heat intolerance. Symptoms subside if medication is withheld for several days.

In patients with longstanding hypothyroidism and those with ischemic heart disease, rapid correction of hypothyroidism may precipitate angina, cardiac arrhythmias, or other adverse effects. For these patients, replacement therapy should be started at low initial doses, followed by slow titration to full replacement as tolerated over several months. If hypothyroidism and some degree of adrenal insufficiency coexist, an appropriate adjustment of the corticosteroid replacement must be initiated prior to thyroid hormone replacement therapy. This prevents acute adrenocortical insufficiency that could otherwise arise from a thyroid hormone–induced increase in the metabolic clearance rate of adrenocortical hormones.

DRUG INTERACTIONS

Administration of sympathomimetic agents and thyroid hormone to patients with coronary artery disease may increase the risk of coronary insufficiency. Since thyroid hormones increase the catabolism of vitamin K–dependent clotting factors, the effects of coumarin anticoagulants may be enhanced. During concomitant therapy, the dosage of the anticoagulant may have to be reduced. Conversely, initiation of thyroid hormone therapy in patients with diabetes mellitus may increase the requirement for insulin or oral hypoglycemic agents. Similarly, a larger dose of cardiac glycosides (e.g., digitoxin, digoxin) may be required in digitalized patients.

THYROTOXICOSIS

Thyrotoxicosis is any condition in which the body tissues are exposed to supraphysiological concentrations of thyroid hormones. This designation is preferred to the term *hyperthyroidism* to describe this disorder because its origin may not result from excessive thyroid gland secretion. Thyrotoxicosis factitia arises from the ingestion of excessive quantities of thyroid hormone rather than from overactivity of the thyroid gland. The term hyperthyroidism is reserved for disorders that result from overproduction of hormone by the thyroid itself. This distinction is important because only conditions caused by hyperthyroidism respond to treatment with agents that decrease iodine uptake, thyroid hormone production, and the release of thyroid hormone, and only these conditions may require permanent radioactive or surgical ablation of the gland.

The manifestations of hyperthyroidism depend on the severity of the disease, the age of the patient, the presence or absence of extrathyroidal manifestations, and the specific disorder producing the thyrotoxicosis. Of the various types of hyperthyroidism, only two are common: Graves' disease and toxic multinodular goiter. Less common causes include toxic adenoma and postpartum thyroiditis, among others.

Graves' disease, the most common type of hyperthyroidism, is an autoimmune disease that is characterized by the presence of TSH receptor–stimulating antibodies (TSAB) that bind to the TSH receptors (TSHR) on thyroid follicular cells. These TSABs mimic TSH in stimulating growth of the thyroid gland (diffuse goiter) and by causing an increase in synthesis and secretion of T_4 and T_3. In these patients, serum concentrations of T_4, T_3, and TSAB are elevated, while TSH levels are suppressed. Additional symptoms of Graves' disease may include infiltrative ophthalmopathy (*exophthalmos*) and occasionally infiltrative dermopathy. Both of these are also thought to result from an autoimmune process.

In older patients *toxic multinodular goiter* typically presents as longstanding asymptomatic multinodular goiters. Functional autonomy of the nodules develops over time by an unknown mechanism and causes the disease to move from the nontoxic to the toxic phase. The onset of hyperthyroidism is gradual, and the symptoms are usually milder than those of Graves' disease.

Toxic adenoma (Plummer's disease) is less common and is caused by one or more autonomous adenomas of the thyroid gland. These autonomously secreting tumors occur in an intrinsically normal thyroid gland and result from point mutations in the TSHRs on thyroid follicular cells. These point mutations lead to constitutive activation of the TSHR in the absence of TSH. Tumor growth is progressive over many years, and with growth, a progressively larger share of thyroid hormone secretion is assumed by the adenoma; TSH secretion is inhibited, while the remainder of the gland is unstimulated and may atrophy. Continued autonomous growth results in excessive secretion of T_4 and T_3 and thyrotoxicosis.

Clinical Manifestations of Thyrotoxicosis

The signs and symptoms of thyrotoxicosis, regardless of the cause, may include the following: increased basal metabolic rate, heat intolerance, tachycardia, widened pulse pressure, cardiac arrhythmias, skeletal muscle weakness, muscle wasting, tremor, hyperreflexia, emotional instability, nervousness, insomnia, change in menstrual pattern, frequent bowel movements (occasionally diarrhea), and weight loss despite an increased appetite. In addition, very frequent manifestations of all forms of thyrotoxicosis, irrespective of the underlying cause, are retraction of the upper eyelid (evident as the presence of a rim of sclera between the lid and the limbus) and lid lag. These ocular manifestations appear to be due largely to increased adrenergic stimulation and are ameliorated by adrenergic antagonists and reversed promptly upon successful treatment of the thyrotoxicosis. These eye signs do not indicate Graves' infiltrative ophthalmopathy and are not accompanied by protrusion of the eyes.

In Graves' disease, the autoimmune processes mediate the enlargement of the thyroid gland, the infiltrative ophthalmopathy with exophthalmos, and the dermopathy and thereby distinguish Graves' disease from other causes of thyrotoxicosis.

Thyrotoxic Crisis, or Thyroid Storm

Thyrotoxic crisis, thyroid storm, or accelerated hyperthyroidism is an extreme accentuation of thyrotoxicosis. Although uncommon, this serious complication of hyperthyroidism usually occurs in association with Grave's disease and occasionally with toxic multinodular goiter.

If unrecognized, it is invariably fatal. Thyroid storm is usually abrupt in onset and occurs in patients whose preexisting thyrotoxicosis has been treated incompletely or not at all. Thyrotoxic crisis may be related to cytokine release and an acute immunological disturbance caused by a precipitating condition, such as trauma, surgery, diabetic ketoacidosis, toxemia of pregnancy, or parturition. Although the serum thyroid hormone levels may not be appreciably greater than those in uncomplicated thyrotoxicosis, the clinical picture is severe hypermetabolism with fever, profuse sweating, tachycardia, arrhythmias, and so on. Pulmonary edema or congestive heart failure may also develop. With progression of the disorder, apathy, stupor, and coma may supervene, and hypotension can develop. There are no foolproof criteria by which severe thyrotoxicosis complicated by some other serious disease can be distinguished from thyrotoxic crisis induced by that disease. In any event, the differentiation between these alternatives is of no great significance because treatment of the two is the same, directed at systemic support and amelioration of the thyrotoxicosis.

DRUGS USED IN THE TREATMENT OF HYPERTHYROIDISM

Treatment of hyperthyroidism is directed at reducing the excessive synthesis and secretion of thyroid hormones. This may be accomplished by inhibiting thyroidal synthesis and secretion with antithyroid drugs, by reducing the amount of functional thyroid tissue, or by both. Unfortunately, only a small proportion of patients treated with antithyroid drugs obtain long-term remission of their hyperthyroidism. Ablative therapy is often necessary. Since many of the signs and symptoms of hyperthyroidism reflect increased cellular sensitivity to adrenergic stimulation, a β-adrenergic antagonist is often used adjunctively. Propranolol (Inderal), the most widely used β-adrenoceptor blocker, is effective in ameliorating many of the manifestations of thyrotoxicosis. It may reduce thyrotoxicosis-induced tachycardia, palpitations, tremor, sweating, heat intolerance, and anxiety, which are largely mediated through the adrenergic nervous system. Propranolol may also impair the conversion of T_4 to T_3. The use of propranolol is contraindicated in thyrotoxic patients with asthma or chronic obstructive pulmonary disease because it impairs bronchodilation. It is also contraindicated in patients with heart block and those with congestive heart failure, unless severe tachycardia is a contributory factor.

Thionamides

Thionamides are the primary drugs used to decrease thyroid hormone production. They do not inhibit secretion of stored thyroid hormone, and therefore, when they are used alone, their clinical effects are not appar-

ent until the preexisting intrathyroidal store of thyroid hormone is depleted. This may take several weeks. Propylthiouracil and methylthiouracil (methimazole; Tapazole) are the most commonly used preparations in the United States.

Thionamide drugs interfere with peroxidase-catalyzed reactions. In the thyroid gland, they inhibit the activity of the enzyme TPO, which is required for the intrathyroidal oxidation of I^-, the incorporation of I^- into Tg, and the coupling of iodotyrosyl residues to form thyroid hormones. Thus, these drugs inhibit thyroid hormone synthesis and with time, also secretion. Propylthiouracil, but not methimazole, also inhibits D1, which deiodinates T_4 to T_3. Because of this additional action, propylthiouracil is often used to provide a rapid alleviation of severe thyrotoxicosis.

In patients with autoimmune thyroid disease, thionamide drugs may also exert an immunosuppressive effect. As the drug is concentrated in thyroid follicular cells, the expression of thyroid antigen and the release of prostaglandins and cytokines are decreased. Subsequently, the autoimmune response is impaired. Thionamides also inhibit the generation of oxygen radicals in T cells, B cells, and particularly the antigen-presenting cells within the thyroid gland. Thus, thionamides may cause a decline in thyroid autoantibody titers, although the clinical importance of immunosuppression is unclear.

Thionamide drugs are well absorbed from the gastrointestinal tract. Although they have short plasma half-lives (propylthiouracil 1.5 hours; methimazole 6 hours), they accumulate in the thyroid gland, and a single daily dose may exert effects for greater than 24 hours. Thionamides undergo hepatic conjugation to form glucuronides and are excreted in the bile and urine. Nevertheless, few glucuronide conjugates are found in the feces because they are absorbed from the gastrointestinal tract.

The thionamide drugs are used in the management of hyperthyroidism and thyrotoxic crisis and in the preparation of patients for surgical subtotal thyroidectomy. Although the use of thionamides alone may restore euthyroidism, it is difficult to adjust the dosage in some patients. This has led to the development of block-and-replace regimens in which a full blocking dose of thionamide plus a levothyroxine supplement is prescribed. Although thionamides may be used to treat hyperthyroidism during pregnancy, they should be given in minimally effective doses to avoid inducing infantile hypothyroidism and thyroid enlargement in the developing fetus.

If given in excessive amounts over a long period, thionamides may cause hypothyroidism and enlargement of the thyroid gland. The most serious adverse effects are granulocytopenia and agranulocytosis, which occur in about 0.5% of patients and usually within 3 months of starting therapy. The most frequently observed adverse effect is rash. Arthralgia, myalgia, cholestatic jaundice, lymphadenopathy, drug fever, psychosis, and a lupuslike syndrome have also been reported.

Iodine and Iodine-Containing Agents
Iodides

The effects of iodide on the thyroid gland are complex. When administered in pharmacological amounts, potassium iodide (KI) causes a transient inhibition of the uptake and incorporation of I^- into Tg (Wolff-Chaikoff effect). In addition, high doses of KI also inhibit the secretion of thyroid hormone and thyroid blood flow. These effects make KI an ideal agent for treating severe thyrotoxicosis or thyroid crisis when a rapid decrease in plasma T_4 and T_3 is desirable. As the thyroid gland escapes from Wolff-Chaikoff effect, I^- accumulates within the gland and hormone synthesis resumes. With continued treatment with KI alone, the inhibition of thyroid secretion may also diminish. Hypersecretion of thyroid hormone and thyrotoxicosis may return at the previous or a more severe intensity. For this reason, iodide alone is not used for the management of hyperthyroidism. Nevertheless, KI has long been used in combination with propylthiouracil in the management of thyrotoxic crisis to rapidly inhibit thyroid hormone secretion. Iodide plus a thionamide has also been used in the immediate preoperative preparation of patients about to undergo total or subtotal surgical thyroidectomy.

The ability of KI to block the thyroidal uptake of I^- and its incorporation into Tg would prove useful in the event of an accident at a nuclear power plant. In such an event, large quantities of radionuclides, including isotopes of radioiodine, could be released into the atmosphere. Administration of KI (*Thyro-Block*) to inhibit the uptake and incorporation of radioiodine would be the most effective means of limiting the potential damage to the thyroid gland.

Adverse reactions to iodine can be divided into intrathyroidal and extrathyroidal reactions. Among the intrathyroidal reactions is iodine-induced thyrotoxicosis (Jod-Basedow's phenomenon), which may occur in patients with nontoxic nodular goiter given low doses (<25 mg/day) of potassium or sodium iodide. At higher doses (50–500 mg/day), iodide goiter or hypothyroidism or both may develop, but this usually requires long exposure. Extrathyroidal adverse reactions to iodine are relatively rare and generally not serious. These include rash, which may be acneiform; drug fever; sialadenitis (inflammation of the salivary glands); conjunctivitis and rhinitis; vasculitis; and a leukemoid eosinophilic granulocytosis.

Oral Cholecystographic Agents

The iodine-containing oral cholecystographic contrast agents (OCAs) include sodium ipodate (*Oragrafin*),

iopanoic acid (*Telepaque*), tyropanoic acid (*Bilopaque*), and iocetamic acid (*Cholebrine*). They all inhibit D1 and D2. These actions make OCAs useful as adjunctive therapy with other antithyroid drugs by promoting a rapid fall in the plasma T_3 concentration of the seriously thyrotoxic patient.

In addition, the metabolism of OCAs results in the release of large amounts of I^- into the circulation. As described for KI, I^- released from OCAs may have effects at the thyroid gland and if used alone to treat hyperthyroidism, OCAs carry the same potential to induce increased secretion of thyroid hormone and exacerbation of thyrotoxicosis. When an OCA is used in the treatment of hyperthyroidism, large doses of antithyroid agents are usually administered concomitantly. However, the combination of OCAs and antithyroid drugs may cause resistance to the antithyroid drugs with time, presumably because of the elevation in intrathyroidal I^- content. Thus, it is recommended that the use of OCAs be reserved for short-term treatment of patients with severe thyrotoxicosis and significant comorbidity (e.g., myocardial infarction, sepsis, stroke) for rapid control of plasma T_3 concentrations.

When the OCAs are used for these purposes, they are administered at much lower doses than when used for cholecystography. At the higher doses, the major adverse effects of these compounds are acute renal failure, thrombocytopenia, and athrombocytosis; possible minor adverse reactions include diarrhea, nausea, vomiting, and dysuria.

Radioiodine

Millicurie amounts of ^{131}I (*Iodotope I-131*) are used for thyroid ablation in the management of hyperthyroidism. ^{131}I is taken up and trapped in the same manner as I^-. The ablative effect is exerted primarily through β-particle emissions, which destroy thyroid tissue. The major disadvantage associated with this therapy is the development of hypothyroidism after thyroid ablation. Microcurie amounts of radioiodine also are used for the diagnostic evaluation of thyroid function.

Potassium Perchlorate

The perchlorate ion of potassium perchlorate, $KClO_4$, is a competitive inhibitor of thyroidal I^- transport via the Sodium Iodide Symporter (NIS). This drug can cause fatal aplastic anemia and gastric ulcers and is now rarely used. If administered with careful supervision, in limited low doses and for only brief periods, serious toxic effects can be avoided. The compound is especially effective in treating iodine-induced hyperthyroidism, which may occur, for example, in patients treated with the antiarrhythmic compound amiodarone. Perchlorate ion can also be used in a diagnostic test of I^- incorporation into Tg, the so-called perchlorate discharge test.

Lithium Carbonate

Lithium inhibits thyroidal incorporation of I^- into Tg, as well as the secretion of thyroid hormones, but it does not inhibit the activity of the $Na^+–I^-$ symporter or the accumulation of I^- within the thyroid. Lithium offers no particular advantage over drugs of the thionamide class but may be employed for temporary control of thyrotoxicosis in patients who are allergic to both thionamides and iodide.

Drug Interactions

As the plasma levels of T_4 and T_3 fall after the administration of antithyroid drugs, the catabolism of vitamin K–dependent clotting factors decreases, thus reducing the effectiveness of coumarin anticoagulants. During concomitant therapy, the dosage of the anticoagulant may have to be increased. Conversely, the use of antithyroid therapy in patients with diabetes mellitus may decrease the patient's requirement for insulin or oral hypoglycemic agents. Similarly, patients receiving cardiac glycosides, such as digitoxin, may require a smaller dose.

Lithium carbonate, administered for affective and bipolar disorders, may enhance the effects of antithyroid drugs. Potassium iodide, used as an expectorant, is a major ingredient in many cough medications. Iodide derived from this source may enhance the effects of antithyroid drugs and lead to iodine-induced hypothyroidism. Iodine in topical antiseptics and radiological contrast agents may act in a similar manner.

Study QUESTIONS

1. All of the following are common adverse effects associated with drug overdose of thyroid hormone replacement therapy EXCEPT
   (A) Cardiac palpitation
   (B) Arrhythmias,
   (C) Tachycardia
   (D) Weight gain
   (E) Heat intolerance.

2. An adequate dietary intake of iodine is essential to prevent hypothyroidism. In many areas of the world, dietary iodine intake is insufficient and must be supplemented. There is another element in which a dietary intake may be insufficient that is also associated with thyroid hormone metabolism. This element is
   (A) Calcium
   (B) Selenium
   (C) Fluorine
   (D) Sodium
   (E) Potassium

3. What is the primary reason for administering β-adrenergic receptor blocking drugs as adjunct therapy in the treatment of thyrotoxicosis?
   (A) They reduce the elevated thyroid hormone levels.
   (B) Many of the effects of elevated thyroid hormones result from an increase in number of β-adrenoceptors.
   (C) They elevate the levels of prostaglandins through indirect mechanism.
   (D) The effects of elevated thyroid hormones are directly antagonized by β-adrenoceptor agonists.

4. What is the basic mechanism of action of thiocyanate in inhibiting iodide uptake by the thyroid gland?

   (A) Thiocyanate inhibits the binding of iodide to thyroid hormone receptors.
   (B) Thiocyanate becomes incorporated into Tg.
   (C) Thiocyanate competitively inhibits iodide uptake by the thyroid follicular cells.
   (D) Thiocyanate inhibits iodide uptake by a noncompetitive mechanism.
   (E) Thiocyanate causes an increase in the transcription of RNA polymerase.

5. The following statements regarding the mechanism of action of thionamide drugs in the treatment of hyperthyroidism are true EXCEPT
   (A) The clinical effects are apparent soon after administration.
   (B) The compounds inhibit the action of the enzyme TPO.
   (C) The drugs inhibit thyroid hormone synthesis.
   (D) These drugs do not inhibit secretion of preexisting stored thyroid hormone.

ANSWERS

1. **D.** The cardiac effects (A, B, and C) are symptoms of hyperthyroidism, as is E. Instead of weight gain, a loss in body weight would be expected.

2. **B.** Selenium in the form of selenocysteine is required for three enzymes that remove iodide from thyroid hormones. There are no significant areas in which dietary intake of sodium or potassium are problems. Fluorine deficiency is not associated with thyroid hormone metabolism.

3. **B.** The symptoms of thyrotoxicosis are largely mediated through the adrenergic nervous system, and β-adrenoceptor blockers may ameliorate some of

the manifestations of the disorder. They have no effect on thyroid hormone levels or on prostaglandins. The effects are directly antagonized by antagonists rather than agonists.

4. **C.** Thiocyanate and other monovalent anions, such as perchlorate, inhibit iodide uptake by acting as competitive inhibitors of iodide uptake by the thyroid follicular cells. This is the only relevant action of these anions in this situation.

5. **A.** The clinical effects are not apparent until the preexisting intrathyroidal stores of thyroid hormone are depleted. This may take several weeks. This class of drugs do inhibit the action of the enzyme TPO and thus inhibit thyroid hormone synthesis. They do not inhibit secretion of preexisting stored thyroid hormone.

SUPPLEMENTAL READING

Burman KD and Wartofsky L. Iodine effects on the thyroid gland: Biochemical and clinical aspects. Rev Endocr Metab Disord 2000;1(1-2):19–25.

Daniels GH. Clinical review 120. Amiodarone-induced thyrotoxicosis. J Clin Endocrinol Metab 2001;86(1): 3–8.

Fatourechi V. Medical treatment of Graves' ophthalmopathy. Ophthalmol Clin North Am 2000;13: 683–691.

Freitas JE. Therapeutic options in the management of toxic and nontoxic nodular goiter. Semin Nucl Med 2000;30(2): 88–97.

Girling JC. Thyroid disease in pregnancy. Hosp Med 2000;61:834–840.

Graves PN and Davies TF. New insights into the thyroid-stimulating hormone receptor: The major antigen in Graves's disease. Endocrinol Metab Clin North Am 2000;29:267–286.

Heuston WJ. Treatment of hypothyroidism. Am Fam Physician 2001;64:1717–1724.

Taurog A. Hormone synthesis: Thyroid iodine metabolism. In Braverman LE and Utiger RD (eds.). Werner and Ingbar's The Thyroid (8th ed.). New York: Lippincott Williams & Wilkins, 2000:61–84.

CASE Study   Hypothyroxinemia in a 36-year-old Woman with an Enlarged Thyroid Gland

Sara Gwynn, aged 38, complains to her family physician of weight gain, constipation, and lethargy. Significant findings upon physical examination include the following: At 5 feet, 4 inches and 169 lb, she is moderately overweight. Blood pressure is 152/92; pulse, 59; neck is full, with an enlarged (1.5 to 2 times normal) thyroid gland; deep tendon reflexes display delayed relaxation.

Significant Results of Laboratory Studies

Test	Sara Gwynn	Normal Range
Total serum T_4	2.7 mg/dL	5.0–12.0 mg/dL
T_3 resin uptake	20%	25–35%
Serum TSH	87.5 mU/L	0.3–5.0 mU/L

Weight gain, constipation, and lethargy can all be symptoms of hypothyroidism. In addition, mild hypertension, goiter, and delayed relaxation of deep tendon reflexes are among the common physical findings of hypothyroidism. What are your interpretations of the clinical findings and what treatment would you suggest?

ANSWER: The results of the laboratory tests confirm the hypothyroxinemia (i.e., low serum total T_4 concentration). The calculated free thyroxine index (total serum T_4 concentration $\times T_3$ resin uptake) of 0.54 is below normal (1.25–4.2), indicating that the reduced total serum T_4 concentration is not due to a decrease in the concentration of serum thyroid hormone–binding proteins. The accompanying elevation in the serum TSH concentration indicates that Mrs. Gwynn's hypothyroxinemia is due to thyroid gland failure (i.e., primary hypothyroidism). The responsiveness of her thyroid gland to TSH is subnormal, resulting in subnormal thyroid hormone synthesis and secretion. Autoimmune thyroiditis (Hashimoto's thyroiditis) is the most common cause of this condition.

Treatment is thyroid hormone replacement. The goal of the therapy is to relieve the symptoms of hypothyroidism by normalizing the levels of circulating thyroid hormones. In addition to the amelioration of symptoms, the clinical effectiveness of the thyroid hormone replacement may be monitored by periodically measuring the serum TSH concentration. The lowest dose of thyroid hormone that is needed to normalize the serum TSH concentration is usually the appropriate dose. Most or all of the symptoms of hypothyroidism should improve with appropriate thyroid hormone replacement, but this may require weeks or months of therapy.

66

Parathyroid Hormone, Calcitonin, Vitamin D, and Other Compounds Related to Mineral Metabolism

Frank L. Schwartz

 DRUG LIST

GENERIC NAME	PAGE	GENERIC NAME	PAGE
Alendronate	760	Pamidronate	760
Calcitonin	756	Parathyroid hormone	760
Calcitriol	760	Plicamycin	759
Cholecalciferol	757	Risedronate	760
Dihydrotachysterol	757	Tiludronate	760
Ergocalciferol	757	Zoledronic acid	760
Etidronate	760		

The principal hormones involved in calcium metabolism and bone remodeling are *parathyroid hormone* (PTH), *calcitonin,* and *vitamin D* (D$_3$). Other hormones, such as the thyroid hormones, growth hormone, androgens, estrogens, and the glucocorticoids also influence mineral homeostasis and bone metabolism. The three primary target tissues for these hormones are bone, kidney, and intestine. These three hormones and their target tissues maintain serum calcium levels, extracellular calcium levels, and bone integrity.

CALCIUM HOMEOSTASIS

Calcium is the principal extracellular electrolyte regulated by PTH, calcitonin, and D$_3$. *Extracellular calcium* is a critical component of signal transduction across the plasma membrane, which regulates a wide spectrum of physiological events including muscle contraction, secretion of neurotransmitters and hormones, and the ac-

tion of growth factors, cytokines, and protein hormones. *Intracellular calcium* is an important cofactor in many enzymatic reactions. Plasma calcium exists in three forms: *ionized* (50%), *protein bound* (46%), and *complexed* to organic ions (4%). Total plasma calcium concentration is normally tightly maintained within the range of 4.5 to 5.7 mEq/L, primarily by the actions of PTH and D$_3$, which regulate bone resorption and calcium absorption from the intestine and kidney. The calcium-lowering actions of calcitonin may regulate postprandial plasma calcium deposition into bone and prevent hypercalcemia.

The regulation of serum calcium concentration is a complex process that requires the coordinated responses of these three hormones and their target tissues. The model shown in Figure 66.1 consists of three wings depicting overlapping feedback loops that represent the interrelationship between *bone* (wing 1), *intestine* (wing 2), and *kidney* (wing 3) in modulating calcium homeostasis. The left side of the model (A loops) de-

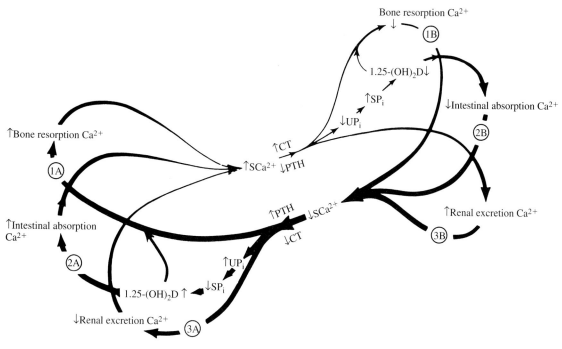

FIGURE 66.1

The butterfly model of calcium homeostasis. The model consists of three overlapping control loops (negative feedback) that interlock and relate to one another through the level of blood concentrations of ionic calcium, parathyroid hormone (PTH), and calcitonin (CT). The loops are numbered 1, 2, and 3; the limbs of the three loops describing physiological events that increase blood concentrations of calcium are designated A (left), and the limbs that describe events that decrease blood concentrations of calcium are designated B (right). UP_i, urinary phosphate; SP_i, serum phosphate; SCa^{++}, serum calcium. (Reprinted with permission from Arnaud CD. Calcium homeostasis: Regulatory elements and their integration. Fed Proc 1987;37:2557.)

scribes events that increase blood calcium in response to *hypocalcemia*, whereas the right side (B loops) describes events that decrease blood calcium in response to *hypercalcemia*.

Hypocalcemia directly increases PTH synthesis and release and inhibits calcitonin release. PTH in turn restores plasma calcium by initially stimulating transport of free or labile calcium from bone into the blood. PTH also increases renal 1,25-dihydroxycholecalciferol $(1,25\text{-}(OH)_2D_3)$ production, which is the most active form of D_3. $1,25\text{-}(OH)_2D_3$ induces enterocyte differentiation in the intestine, which in turn results in increased absorption of calcium. Finally, during long periods of hypocalcemia, PTH can mobilize more stable calcium deep in the hydroxyapatite of bone by activating deep osteoclasts.

Hypercalcemia, in contrast, results in calcitonin synthesis and release, while PTH release and formation of $1,25\text{-}(OH)_2D_2$ are inhibited. Calcitonin inhibits bone resorption directly by reducing osteocyte activity. Calcitonin also induces an initial phosphate diuresis, followed by increased renal calcium, sodium, and phosphate excretion.

PARATHYROID HORMONE

PTH is secreted from the parathyroid glands in response to a low plasma concentration of ionized (free) calcium. PTH immediately causes the transfer of labile calcium stores from bone into the bloodstream. PTH increases rates of dietary calcium absorption by the intestine indirectly via the vitamin D_3 system activation of enterocyte activity. Within the kidney, PTH directly stimulates calcium reabsorption and a phosphate diuresis.

Chemistry

PTH is a single-chain polypeptide composed of 84 amino acid residues that is devoid of disulfide bonds and has a molecular weight of 9500. Biological activity of the human hormone resides primarily in the amino terminal end of the protein (i.e., amino acids 1–34). This portion of PTH has full biological activity both in vivo and in vitro. Synthetic fragments of the 1-34 portion of the PTH molecule have been synthesized. A paraneoplastic hormone, *PTH related peptide (PTHrP)* has been identified, isolated, and synthesized. PTHrP is structurally homologous to the amino terminal portion of PTH and interacts with the PTH receptor in bone and kidney. This hormone is responsible for hypercalcemia in certain forms of malignancy. It has been used as a therapeutic agent in osteoporosis in some clinical trials.

Synthesis and Secretion

Plasma calcium concentration is the principal factor regulating PTH synthesis and release. The increase in PTH synthesis and secretion induced by hypocalcemia is believed to be mediated through activation of parathyroid gland adenylyl cyclase and a subsequent increase in intracellular cyclic adenosine monophosphate (cAMP).

Formation of PTH begins with the synthesis of several precursor molecules. *PreproPTH* is the initial peptide that is synthesized within the parathyroid gland, and it serves as a precursor to both proPTH and PTH. PreproPTH is formed within the rough endoplasmic reticulum, transported into the cisternal space, and then cleaved to form proPTH. The proPTH polypeptide is transported into the cisternal space, where another proteolytic cleavage occurs, forming PTH.

PTH in Target Tissues

PTH has two levels of action in bone. First, in response to acute decreases in serum calcium, PTH stimulates surface osteocytes to increase the outward flux of calcium ion from bone to rapidly restore serum calcium. Thus, during brief periods of hypocalcemia, PTH release results in mobilization of calcium from labile areas of bone that lie adjacent to osteoclasts. This effect is not associated with any significant increase in plasma phosphate or bone resorption. Second, PTH induces transformation of osteoprogenitor cells into osteoclasts, which increase bone formation. Thus, PTH has anabolic action on bone formation at physiological levels, and it is this action that allows it to be used pharmacologically to treat osteoporosis. However, in conditions that result in chronic calcium deficiency or prolonged hypocalcemia (e.g., renal osteodystrophy, vitamin D deficiency, or malabsorption syndromes), PTH mobilizes deep osteocytes in perilacunar bone and can result in significant bone resorption and eventual osteopenia as it attempts to maintain normal concentrations of ionic or free plasma calcium.

In the kidney, PTH stimulates the conversion of 25-$(OH)D_3$ into $1,25$-$(OH)_2D_3$. Intrarenal $1,25$-$(OH)_2 D_3$ causes an amplification of the PTH-induced calcium reabsorption and phosphate diuresis. $1,25$-$(OH)_2D_3$ enhances PTH action in bone also. Once again, *PTH does not directly affect intestinal calcium absorption*, but it does so indirectly through induction of $1,25$-$(OH)_2 D_3$ synthesis and enhanced enterocyte absorption.

CALCITONIN

Calcitonin release is normally stimulated by rising serum calcium levels and suppressed by hypocalcemia. The major physiological effects of calcitonin are inhibition of bone resorption and deposition of postabsorptive calcium into bone following a meal, which prevents postprandial hypercalcemia.

Chemistry

Calcitonin is a single-chain polypeptide composed of 32 amino acid residues having a molecular weight of approximately 3600. A cysteine disulfide bridge at the 1-7 position of the amino terminal end of the peptide is essential for biological activity; however, the entire amino acid sequence is required for optimal activity.

Synthesis and Secretion

The regulation of calcitonin synthesis and release from the parafollicular C cells of the thyroid gland is calcium dependent. *Rising serum calcium is the principal stimulus responsible for calcitonin synthesis and release.* Other hormones, such as glucagon, gastrin, and serotonin, also stimulate calcitonin release. Calcitonin has been isolated in tissues other than the parafollicular C cells (parathyroid, pancreas, thymus, adrenal), but it is not known whether this material is biologically active.

Secretagogues, such as gastrin and pancreozymin, may contribute significantly to the regulation of endogenous calcitonin. In fact, it has been postulated that gastrin-induced calcitonin release following meals may help regulate the postprandial calcium deposition in bone.

A calcitonin precursor has been identified within the thyroid parafollicular C cells. It is thought to function in a manner analogous to that of proPTH to facilitate intracellular transport and secretion of the hormone. The metabolic degradation of calcitonin appears to occur in both the liver and kidney.

Although blood calcitonin levels are normally low, excessive levels have been found in association with medullary carcinoma of the thyroid and more rarely carcinoid tumors of the bronchus and stomach. Serum calcitonin levels are used to screen and monitor patients who have or are suspected of having medullary carcinoma of the thyroid.

Mechanism of Action

Calcitonin interacts with specific plasma membrane receptors within target organs to initiate biological effects. This interaction has been directly linked to the generation of cAMP via adenylyl cyclase activation.

VITAMIN D₃ (CHOLECALCIFEROL)

Vitamin D_3, through its active metabolite, $1,25-(OH)_2D_3$, also plays an important role in maintaining calcium homeostasis by enhancing intestinal calcium absorption, PTH-induced mobilization of calcium from bone, and calcium reabsorption in the kidney.

Synthesis and Activation

The primary supply of vitamin D_3 in humans is not obtained from the diet but rather is derived from the ultraviolet photoconversion of 7-dehydrocholesterol to vitamin D_3 in skin. Thus, vitamin D_3 synthesis varies with the seasons. D_3 is a prohormone and requires further metabolic conversion to exert biological activity in its target organs (Fig. 66.2). The liver and the kidney are the major sites of metabolic activation of this endogenous sterol hormone. The initial transformation of D_3 occurs in the liver and is catalyzed by the enzyme 25-OH-D_3-hydroxylase

to form $25-(OH)D_3$; this is the primary circulating form of D_3. Circulating $25-(OH)D_3$ is then converted by the kidney to the most active form of D_3, $1,25-(OH)_2D_3$, by the 1-(OH)-D_3-hydroxylase enzyme. Blood concentrations of $1,25-(OH)_2D_3$ are approximately one five-hundredth of those of $25-(OH)D_3$. $1,25-(OH)_2D_3$ is converted to the metabolite $24R,25-(OH)_2D_3$, which is capable of suppressing parathyroid secretion.

In addition to the endogenous metabolites, some exogenous sterols possess biological activity similar to that of D_3. *Ergocalciferol* (vitamin D_2) is derived from the plant sterol ergosterol and may act as a substrate for both the 25-hydroxylase and the 1-hydroxylase enzyme systems of the liver and kidney to form $25-(OH)D_2$ and $1,25-(OH)_2D_2$, respectively. *Ergocalciferol* (vitamin D_2) is the form used in commercial vitamins and supplemented dairy products. *Dihydrotachysterol,* another sterol that is used as a therapeutic agent, also functions as a substrate for the hydroxylase enzymes in the liver and kidney.

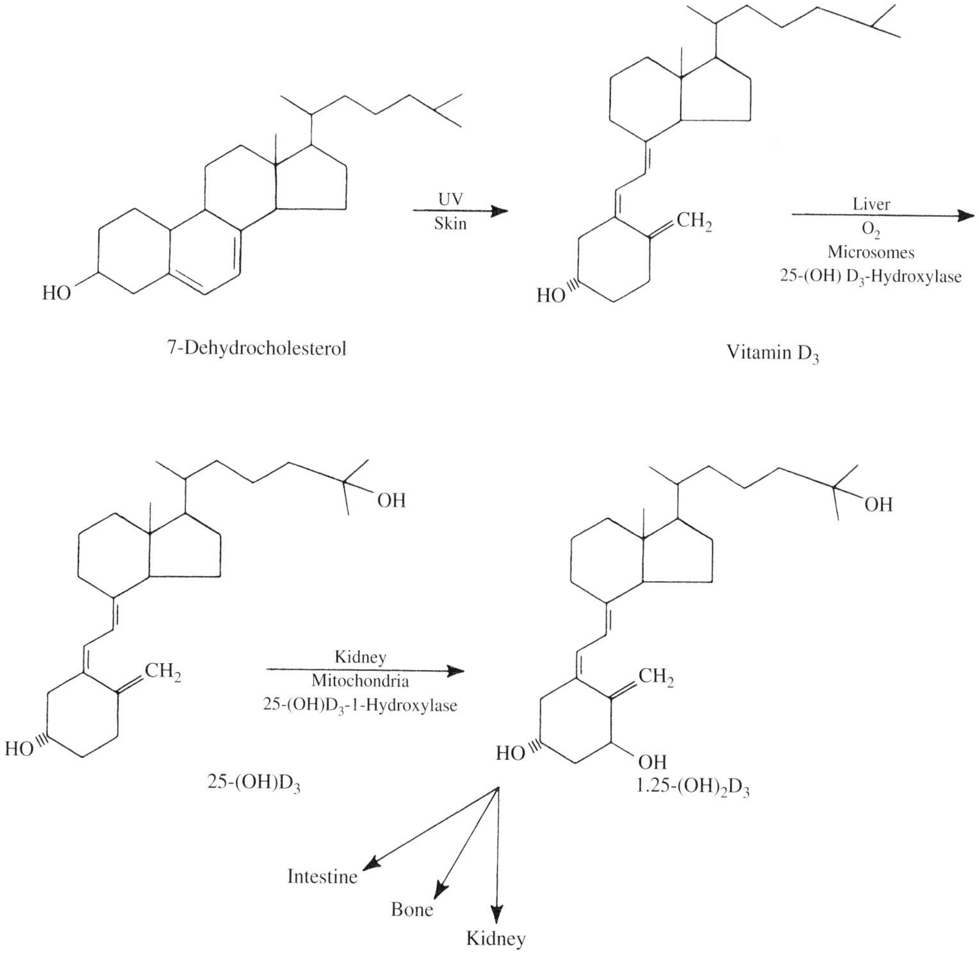

FIGURE 66.2
Functional metabolism of vitamin D, including its biosynthesis by photolysis reaction in skin. (Reprinted with permission from DeLuca HF. Vitamin D metabolism and function. Arch Intern Med 1987;138:836.)

Mechanism of Action

1, 25-(OH)$_2$D$_3$ exerts its influence within target tissues through high-affinity sterol-specific intracellular receptor proteins. The D$_3$ receptor, similar to steroid receptor systems, translocates the hormone from the cell cytoplasm to the nucleus, where biological response is initiated via transcription and translation (Fig. 66.3).

BISPHOSPHONATES

The bisphosphonates are synthetic organic compounds that are incorporated directly into the hydroxyapatite of bone and then inhibit osteoclastic bone resorption. This antiresorptive action makes them useful in the pharmacological treatment of hypercalcemia, osteoporosis, and Paget's disease.

Chemistry

The bisphosphonates have a common structure, P-C-P, which is similar to the structure of the native pyrophosphate P-O-P found in bone hydroxyapatite. The different compounds in clinical use vary by the attachments to the R component of the native molecule.

Mechanism of Action

The bisphosphonates inhibit osteoclastic resorption of bone by binding to the hydroxyapatite crystals of bone. When osteoclasts first attach to bone in the active resorptive sites, the bisphosphonates are released from that bone. The release of these compounds locally prevents further osteoclastic attachment to those resorptive surfaces. The bisphosphonates also may inhibit resorption by inducing apoptosis of osteoclasts and by inhibiting release of interleukins and other compounds involved in bone resorption. The net result of actions of these compounds is inhibition of bone osteoclastic resorption. This action allows new bone formation to catch up in the remodeling process and can result in a net gain in bone density.

CLINICAL USES OF PARATHYROID HORMONE, CALCITONIN, VITAMIN D, AND BISPHOSPHONATES

These hormones and drugs are used most commonly for disorders of calcium and bone metabolism rather than to correct specific hormone deficiencies. For example, the use of PTH replacement in hypoparathyroidism in the past was not practical because of the difficulty in ob-

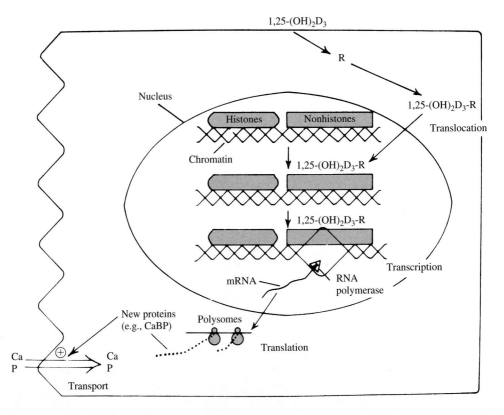

FIGURE 66.3

Proposed molecular mechanism of action of 1,25-(OH)$_2$D$_3$ in an intestinal mucosa cell. R, receptor protein; CaBP, calcium-binding protein. (From Haussler MR and McCain TA. Basic and clinical concepts related to vitamin D metabolism and action. I. N Engl J Med 1977;297:974.)

taining purified hormone and the fact that it is injected subcutaneously. With the recent ability to produce large quantities of recombinant PTH (rPTH), its use will be more common, especially for severe osteoporosis.

Hypercalcemia of Malignancy

Hypercalcemia is a common clinical condition that can accompany a variety of other medical conditions, such as sarcoidosis, vitamin D toxicity, hyperparathyroidism, and malignancy. When calcium levels are exceptionally high, adjunctive measures for the control of plasma calcium levels are necessary, as this is a medical emergency. Various modalities in combination are used to treat this condition; intravenous hydration with normal saline and the use of loop diuretics (e.g., furosemide) to induce calcium diuresis are the most important supportive measures.

The *bisphosphonates are the most effective compounds available to treat hypercalcemia of malignancy.* Pamidronate (*Aredia*) and zoledronic acid (*Zometa*) can be infused intravenously and are the most effective compounds available for rapid reduction of serum calcium levels.

Calcitonin is also effective in reducing serum calcium levels in life-threatening hypercalcemia; however, it is not as rapid or as effective as the bisphosphonates. Subcutaneous administration of salmon (*Calcimar*) or human (*Cibacalcin*) calcitonin reduces serum calcium levels within 3 to 5 days in 75 to 90% of malignant hypercalcemias.

Plicamycin (*Mithracin*), an inhibitor of RNA synthesis in osteoclasts, reduces serum calcium levels when infused over 4 to 6 hours every 3 to 4 days. Plicamycin's effects are slower than those of the bisphosphonates; the drug is a bone marrow suppressant that can complicate clinical management if the patient is already receiving chemotherapy for the malignancy.

Osteoporosis

Postmenopausal osteoporosis is the most common form of osteoporosis. In perimenopausal women, the greatest amount of bone density is lost during the first 5 years after onset of menopause. Women going through menopause at a particularly early age are especially at risk for developing osteoporosis, and they should take some prophylactic regimen at the onset of menopause. Previously, estrogen replacement therapy (ERT), along with calcium supplementation and D_3, were the standard of care. However, the benefits of ERT, including increased bone density, decreased risk of colon cancer, and decreased vaginal atrophy, must be weighed against the slightly increased risk of breast cancer, endometrial cancer, stroke, and deep vein thrombosis. While unopposed estrogen may slightly increase the incidence of

endometrial cancer, appropriate combinations with a progestin negate such risk. Other compounds are available for the prevention of osteoporosis. These include the selective estrogen receptor modulators (See Chapter 61), the bisphosphonates, and nasally administered calcitonin. For example, the bisphosphonates are now indicated for prophylaxis of osteoporosis when individuals are going to be treated with glucocorticoids or the gonadotropin antagonists.

Once bone loss is sufficient to result in a compression fracture, pharmacological therapy is much less effective. However, even after fractures have occurred, the use of the bisphosphonates and rPTH has been shown to increase bone densities and reduce the rate of subsequent fractures. Nasal calcitonin (200 units daily) is effective in promoting fracture healing and also exhibits an analgesic effect by reducing pain in persons with acute lumbar compression fractures. *Whatever compound is used for prophylaxis or treatment of osteoporosis, calcium and D_3 supplementation are required for maximum benefit.*

Drug-Induced Osteopenia

Chronic administration of many drugs, especially anticonvulsant medications, glucocorticoids, and GnRH agonists, are known to produce osteopenia and osteoporosis. The anticonvulsants inhibit formation of active D_3; chronic glucocorticoid therapy increases bone turnover by altering osteoblast differentiation and inhibiting collagen synthesis; and the GnRH agonists induce chemical hypogonadism.

Clinical trials have demonstrated that the use of the bisphosphonates, nasal calcitonin, or human rPTH combined with calcium and vitamin D supplementation is effective in preventing drug-induced osteoporosis. Thus, individuals receiving over the long term any medication that can induce osteomalacia should also take one of these compounds and have periodic bone density determinations.

Renal Osteodystrophy

Patients with chronic renal failure develop hyperphosphatemia, hypocalcemia, secondary hyperparathyroidism, and severe metabolic bone disease. The secondary hyperparathyroidism is thought to be due to hyperphosphatemia and decreased $1,25\text{-}(OH)_2$ formation. Oral or intravenous $1,25\text{-}(OH)_2 D_3$ (calcitriol) therapy along with oral phosphate-binding agents and calcium supplementation is effective in reducing the effects of renal osteodystrophy.

Paget's Disease

Paget's disease is an uncommon disorder of bone characterized by mixed lytic and sclerotic bone changes.

These individuals have areas of increased bone resorption and other areas of abnormal new bone formation. The abnormal bone formation can result in pain, deformity, and fracture of affected bones. The bisphosphonates and calcitonin are most commonly used in the treatment of this disease. Long-term continuous use of bisphosphonates can be associated with the induction of osteomalacia through a direct impairment of new bone formation. Therefore, the bisphosphonates are given in a cyclic pattern to treat Paget's disease.

ADVERSE EFFECTS

With the exception of the possible development of a hypervitaminosis associated with high-dose administration of vitamin D_2 or D_3, the compounds discussed in this chapter are relatively safe. Allergic reactions to the injection of calcitonin and PTH have occurred and chronic use of some bisphosphonates has been associated with the development of osteomalacia. The principal side effects of intravenous bisphosphonates are mild and include low-grade fever and transient increases in serum creatinine and phosphate levels. Oral bisphosphonates are poorly absorbed and can cause esophageal and gastric ulceration. They should be taken on an empty stomach; the individual must remain upright for 30 minutes after ingestion.

Human Parathyroid Hormone

Human rPTH (1-34) has been produced by recombinant technologies, is now approved, and will soon be available for the treatment of osteoporosis. It is given subcutaneously, 25 µg/day cyclically for 12 to 18 months, to increase bone density in individuals with a history of fractures, severe osteopenia, or osteoporosis. PTHrP (1-36) has also been synthesized and is in early clinical trials.

Calcitonin

Calcitonin (*Miacalcin, Miacalcin Nasal Spray*) is a synthetic 32–amino acid polypeptide that is identical to salmon calcitonin. Salmon calcitonin is more potent than human calcitonin because of its higher affinity for the human calcitonin receptor and its slower metabolic clearance. Administration is by subcutaneous or intramuscular injection or by nasal spray. The absorption of the nasal form is slower than that of the parenteral routes.

Vitamin D Compounds

Vitamin D comes in many formulations, including multivitamin preparations, fish liver oils with or without vitamin A, combinations with calcium salts, and vitamin D preparations alone. Most forms of vitamin D contain either cholecalciferol (D_3) or ergocalciferol (D_2).

Cholecalciferol is pure vitamin D_3 derived from the ultraviolet conversion of 7-dehydrocholesterol to cholecalciferol. *Ergocalciferol (vitamin D_2)* is a sterol derived from yeast and fungal ergosterol. *Calcitriol* [*Rocaltrol*, $1,25\text{-}(OH)_2D_3$] is the metabolically active vitamin D_3 compound. *Dihydrotachysterol* is a synthetic compound that may act somewhat more quickly than either vitamin D_2 or D_3.

Bisphosphonates

Multiple bisphosphonates compounds are available for both oral and intravenous use. Some [alendronate (*Fosamax*) and etidronate (*Didronel*)] are used for osteoporosis, others [etidronate, tirludronate (*Skelid*), risedronate (*Actonel*)] for Paget's disease, and yet others [pamidronate (*Aredia*), zoledronic acid] for the hypercalcemia of malignancy.

Study QUESTIONS

1. Why are elderly individuals more likely to be vitamin D deficient than young adults? All of the choices are true EXCEPT
   (A) They spend less time outdoors exposed to the sun, which is important in the synthesis of vitamin D.
   (B) Their appetite and intake of essential nutrients is diminished because of chronic medical conditions associated with aging.
   (C) The formation of the active form of vitamin D is diminished by chronic liver and renal conditions.

   (D) The vitamin D receptor has less affinity for D_3 with aging.
2. A 48-year-old white man is noted to have osteopenia on a routine LS spine film while being evaluated for back pain. His bone density reveals osteoporosis of both his hip and LS spine. All of the choices are possible EXCEPT
   (A) He has been taking gabapentin (*Neurontin*) for the past 2 years for a seizure disorder.
   (B) He has Crohn's disease and has had to take prednisone off and on since age 16.

(C) He has had multiple calcium kidney stones over the past few years and has been on a low-calcium diet.

(D) He had glomerulonephritis at age 24 and developed chronic renal failure but received a kidney transplant 10 years ago.

(E) He drinks 2 to 3 glasses of wine each day at dinner.

3. An 85-year-old black man is noted to have sclerosis of the sacroiliac joint on routine films for back pain. The radiologist suggests that this might indicate Paget's disease. Workup for this condition reveals minimal involvement of the pelvis and LS spine. How would you treat this patient?

(A) Reassure the patient and tell him that unless his symptoms become much worse, there will be no specific treatment.

(B) Begin calcitonin nasal spray to prevent further bone resorption and help with the pain.

(C) Use tiludronate in 18-month cycles to prevent progression of the disease to other parts of the body.

4. A 36-year-old white woman is noted to have a 1.5-cm nodule in the right lower lobe of her thyroid on routine examination. Her thyroid functions are normal and a ^{123}I uptake and scan of the thyroid produce normal findings. Her serum calcium levels were determined to be 14 mg/dL (normal levels 9 to 10.3 mg/dL). What is the most likely diagnosis?

(A) Hyperparathyroidism; serum calcium, PTH level, and ultrasound of the thyroid should be obtained.

(B) This may be a lymph node, not associated with any thyroid disease.

(C) She may have medullary carcinoma of the thyroid. Therefore, serum calcitonin, ret-Pro-Oncogene determination, and ultrasound of the thyroid should be obtained.

(D) This may be a thyroid carcinoma that is anterior in the thyroid and therefore not picked up by the ^{123}I scan. She should have thyroglobulin level measurement and ultrasound of the thyroid.

ANSWERS

1. **D.** There is no evidence that affinity for D_3 with its receptor is altered during aging. Aging is associated with vitamin D deficiency for several reasons. It is important for the elderly to receive vitamin D supplementation to prevent osteoporosis and the other problems associated with hypocalcemia. If they have chronic liver or renal conditions, use of one of the specific metabolites should be used, such as calcitriol.

2. **E.** There is no good evidence that moderate amounts of alcohol contribute to osteoporosis. All

of the other listed conditions can contribute to osteoporosis. Antiseizure medications interfere with activation of vitamin D; glucocorticoids stimulate bone resorption of calcium; renal loss of calcium can result in secondary hyperparathyroidism; and organ transplantation is associated with osteoporosis because of the glucocorticoids and other immunosuppressive medications used. Individuals chronically taking these medications should take a bisphosphonate for prophylaxis. In patients prone to form kidney stones, a low dose of a thiazide diuretic will often block the renal loss of calcium and prevent osteoporosis and further stone formation.

3. **A.** Paget's disease is often asymptomatic and picked up on plain bone films. Patients with Paget's disease should have their serum calcium level determined to make sure that they are not hypercalcemic from excessive bone resorption, their serum alkaline phosphatase measured as a marker of new bone formation, a bone scan to determine whether other bones are involved, and a 24-hour urinary hydroxyproline measurement to assess bone resorption. The patient who has minimal involvement and is biochemically normal does not need pharmacological therapy. No studies indicate that early treatment slows progression in individuals with the more severe form of this disorder.

4. **A.** Although all of the conditions can present as an asymptomatic nodule in the thyroid, the marked hypercalcemia in this patient makes hyperparathyroidism the probable diagnosis. Carcinomas of the thyroid are common, and outcomes are improved with early diagnosis. Medullary carcinoma and hyperparathyroidism caused by hyperplasia may be inherited and are associated with the multiple endocrine neoplasia syndromes.

SUPPLEMENTAL READING

Eastell R. Treatment of postmenopausal osteoporosis. N Engl J Med 1998;338:736–746.

Fleich H. Bisphosphonates: mechanisms of action. Endocrinol Rev 1998;19:80–100.

Neer RM et al. Effect of parathyroid hormone (1-34) on fractures and bone mineral density in postmenopausal women with osteoporosis. N Engl J Med 2001;344:1434–1441.

Nelson HD et al. Postmenopausal hormone replacement therapy: Scientific review. JAMA 2002;288:872–881.

Plotkin H et al. Dissociation of bone formation from resorption during two-week treatment with PTHrP (1-36) in humans: Potential anabolic therapy for osteoporosis. J Clin Endocrinol Metab 1998;83:2786–2791.

CASE Study   Hypercalcemia

Alan Aldrich is a 67-year-old white man who goes to the emergency department with lethargy, increased thirst, and increased urination for 3 days. His family states that he has been somewhat confused for the past day and is not eating or drinking as much as he should. He has a history of chronic bronchitis, a 60–pack year history of smoking, and has lost 12 lb over the past month. Physical examination reveals an arousable thin elderly white man in no acute distress. Blood pressure is 110/60; pulse is 88; respiration rate is 22; temperature is 100.3°F (37.9°C). Chest radiography reveals chronic obstructive pulmonary disease with a questionable subpleural mass on the right. His initial blood chemistry revealed serum Ca^{++}, 13.8 mg/dL; alkaline phosphatase, 489; and elevated liver functions. What is the likely cause of his condition, and how would you treat it?

ANSWER: The cause of hypercalcemia most likely is malignancy. However, he may have longstanding hyperparathyroidism or milk alkali syndrome from the ingestion of large amounts of calcium carbonate to treat indigestion. He should be examined for each of these causes, but in the interim, this is a medical emergency and you have to treat empirically. The proper initial treatment is rehydration with 0.9% normal saline, use of a loop diuretic such as furosemide, and treatment with one of the intravenous preparations of a bisphosphonate, alendronate or zolindronic acid. Serum Ca^{++} is usually restored within 24 to 48 hours with this regimen. Retreatment with a bisphosphonate is often required if the patient has widespread bone metastasis. Once his serum Ca^{++} level is normalized, the diagnostic workup can be completed to determine the cause of the hypercalcemia.

67

Insulin and Oral Drugs for Diabetes Mellitus

Michael J. Thomas and John A. Thomas

DRUG LIST

GENERIC NAME	PAGE	GENERIC NAME	PAGE
Acarbose	775	Metformin	773
Acetohexamide	772	Miglitol	775
Chlorpropamide	772	Nateglinide	773
Glargine	769	Pioglitazone	774
Glimeperide	773	Repaglinide	773
Glipizide	773	Rosiglitazone	774
Glyburide	773	Tolazamide	772
Lispro	769	Tolbutamide	772

GLUCOSE HOMEOSTASIS

Carbohydrates, particularly glucose, are an important source of fuel for living organisms. Glucose is a major energy source for all cells, and some tissues (e.g., brain) need a continuous delivery of glucose. Maintenance of serum glucose concentrations within a normal physiological range, critical to the maintenance of normal fuel use, is primarily accomplished by two pancreatic hormones, insulin and glucagon. Derangements of glucagon or insulin regulation can result in hyperglycemia or hypoglycemia, respectively.

Glucose penetrates most tissues slowly unless insulin is present to facilitate its uptake; however, central nervous system (CNS) cells, capillary endothelial cells, gastrointestinal epithelial cells, pancreatic cells, and renal medullary cells are freely permeable to glucose.

The endocrine portion of the pancreas, called the *islets of Langerhans,* consists of cordlike groups of cells arranged along pancreatic capillary channels. Two major types of secretory cells exist within the islets: α-cells, which produce glucagon; and β-cells, which produce insulin. Other cell types are also present in the islets, including the δ-cells, which secrete somatostatin, and PP cells, which produce pancreatic polypeptide. These pancreatic cells monitor changes in the availability of small calorigenic molecules, namely glucose, and to a lesser extent amino acids, ketone bodies, and fatty acids. Pancreatic β-cells appropriately alter their rates of insulin secretion in response to fluctuations in the levels of these calorigenic molecules, with *glucose playing the dominant role in regulation of insulin secretion.* Pancreatic α-cells secrete glucagon in response to increases in amino acid and fatty acid levels; however, glucose inhibits glucagon secretion. If blood glucose levels fall (e.g., during hypoglycemia or fasting), glucagon secretion is augmented, providing a counterregulatory hormonal response that stimulates

763

gluconeogenesis in the liver and other tissues to avoid hypoglycemia.

Blood glucose concentrations are strictly maintained within homeostatic limits by a variety of biochemical and physiological control mechanisms. Circulating glucose levels are determined by the balance among absorption, storage, production, and use (metabolic rate). *Glucagon* and *insulin* are the two most important hormones that maintain glucose homeostasis when blood concentrations are perturbed.

INSULIN

More than a century has passed since von Mering and Minkowski first demonstrated that pancreatectomized dogs exhibited signs and symptoms characteristic of diabetes mellitus. Shortly thereafter, Banting and Best used pancreatic extracts to reverse these symptoms in dia-

betic patients, thus providing a basis for establishing a cause-and-effect relationship between insulin deficiency and diabetes. Insulin was subsequently isolated, crystallized, and eventually synthesized in the laboratory. Insulin replacement therapy has been widely used in the clinical management of diabetes mellitus for more than 70 years. In 1982, recombinant DNA (rDNA) derived *human insulin* was first produced and is now widely used instead of insulin derived from beef or pork. More recently, insulin analogues have been produced that modulate the activity and rate of insulin action.

Chemistry

Insulin is a relatively simple protein consisting of 51 amino acids arranged as two polypeptide chains, an α-chain and β-chain, connected by disulfide bonds; the latter are necessary to maintain tertiary structure and biological activity (Fig 67.1). Although the amino acid

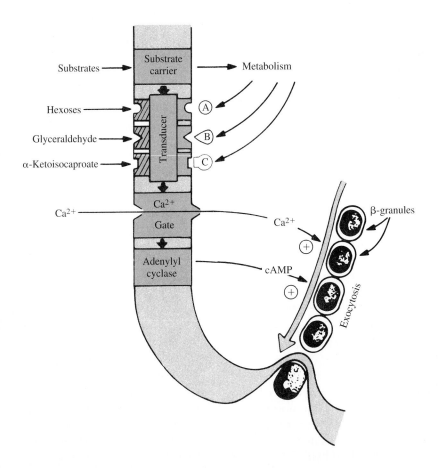

FIGURE 67.1

Hypothetical mechanisms in pancreatic islet cells. The cell membrane of the islet cell contains five coupled systems: (1) the substrate carriers; (2) a receptor–transducer complex with receptors for hexoses (primary glucose), glyceraldehyde, and αketo-isocaproate on the outside and sites for various metabolites and cofactors (e.g., A, B, C) on the inside of the membrane; (3) a Ca^{++} entry; (4) an adenylyl cyclase system; and (5) secretory complex composed of microtubules and secretory granules involved in exocytosis driven by Ca^{++} and cyclic adenosine monophosphate (cAMP). (Reprinted with permission from Matschinsky FM et al. Metabolism of pancreatic islets and regulation of insulin and glucagon secretion. In DeGroot LJ et al. (eds.). Endocrinology. Vol. 2. New York: Grune & Stratton, 1979.)

sequence and composition of animal insulins may differ slightly from those of human insulin, their biological actions are similar. Alteration of specific amino acid residues within the insulin molecule yields novel derivatives that vary in their pharmacokinetics and binding affinity for the insulin receptor. Some insulin analogues display mitogenic properties in addition to their metabolic effects.

Biosynthesis and Secretion

The insulin molecule is initially translated in pancreatic β-cells as a large single-chain polypeptide called *preproinsulin*, then further processed to *proinsulin* by specific endopeptidases and packaged into storage granules prior to release. Proinsulin has little inherent biological activity and must be converted to insulin by the action of specific proteases in the Golgi apparatus; this enzyme action results in the formation of insulin and C (*connecting*) *peptide*. C-peptide facilitates the correct folding of the α- and β-chains of insulin and maintains the alignment of the disulfide bridges in insulin before cleavage of the C-peptide from insulin. Both insulin and C-peptide are stored in the pancreatic β-cell granules, and both are liberated during insulin secretion. Though it is unclear whether C-peptide has any function after it enters the circulation, it is sometimes measured as an indicator of endogenous insulin production.

The specific stimulus for insulin release involves fluctuations in the serum glucose levels and to a much lesser extent levels of other substrates. Glucose enters the pancreatic β-cell via glucose transporter isoform (GLUT) 4 glucose transporters, is quickly phosphorylated to glucose-6-phosphate, and triggers an intracellular influx of calcium ions that promotes fusion of the insulin-containing secretory granules with the cell membrane (*exocytosis*).

Insulin is continuously secreted at a low basal level during fasting, but a postprandial rise in serum glucose or amino acid levels can augment blood levels of insulin severalfold. Other nutrients (e.g., arginine, leucine) and several hormones (e.g., glucagon, growth hormone, secretin, gastrin cholecystokinin, pancreozymin, adrenocorticotropin) modulate insulin release. The autonomic nervous system also participates in the regulation of the rate of insulin secretion, with the islets of Langerhans receiving both cholinergic and adrenergic innervation. Insulin secretion is enhanced by vagal (cholinergic) and diminished by sympathetic (adrenergic) stimulation.

Glucose-induced stimulation of insulin release from cells is biphasic. The initial rapid rise in insulin that follows a rise in glucose is termed the first phase of insulin release and is thought to reflect the release of the presynthesized insulin in the storage granules; a more delayed and prolonged rise in insulin secretion follows. This second phase of insulin secretion is due to an upregulation of insulin expression and production. The first phase of insulin secretion is often blunted in diabetes.

Biochemical and Pharmacological Actions of Insulin

The biochemical actions of insulin are complex and involve many steps to integrate carbohydrate, protein, and lipid metabolism for the maintenance of fuel homeostasis. In addition to its effects on stimulating glucose uptake by tissues, insulin has five major physiological effects on fuel homeostasis. It can (1) diminish hepatic glycogenolysis by inhibiting glycogen phosphorylase; (2) promote hepatic glucose storage into glycogen by stimulating glycogen synthetase; (3) inhibit hepatic gluconeogenesis (i.e., convert noncarbohydrate substrates like amino acids into glucose); (4) inhibit lipolysis by inhibiting hormone-sensitive lipase activity, thereby decreasing plasma free fatty acid and glycerol levels; and (5) promote the active transport of amino acids into cells for incorporation into protein, thereby producing a net positive nitrogen balance.

The biological actions of insulin are initiated following a reversible binding of the hormone to a high-affinity specific insulin receptor on the cell membrane surface (Fig. 67.2). The insulin receptor is a heterotetrameric tyrosine kinase receptor composed of two α- and two β-subunits. Insulin binds to the α-subunit on the extracellular surface of the cell and activates tyrosine kinase activity in the intracellular portion of the β-subunit. This results in the autophosphorylation of the adjacent insulin β-receptor subunit and the phosphorylation of tyrosine residues on cytoplasmic proteins, termed the insulin receptor substrate (IRS) 1 and 2. IRS phosphorylation provides a docking site for other intracellular signaling proteins. The regulatory subunit of phosphatidyl inositol 3 (PI-3) kinase (p85) becomes activated and dimerizes with its catalytic subunit (p110), and this complex mobilizes the translocation of glucose transporters to the cell membrane surface, which promotes hexose transport. Other downstream signaling pathways include activation of p70-S6 kinase, protein kinase B (both via PI-3 kinase), and Grb2 activation of the Ras-Raf-MAP kinase pathway, which controls glycogen synthesis and cell growth. The hormone–receptor complex may then be internalized by endocytosis, which results in degradation of insulin and recycling of the receptor to the cell membrane surface.

Absorption, Metabolism, and Excretion

Insulin is usually administered subcutaneously. Depending on the type of insulin being administered, the rate of insulin absorption can be modulated by al-

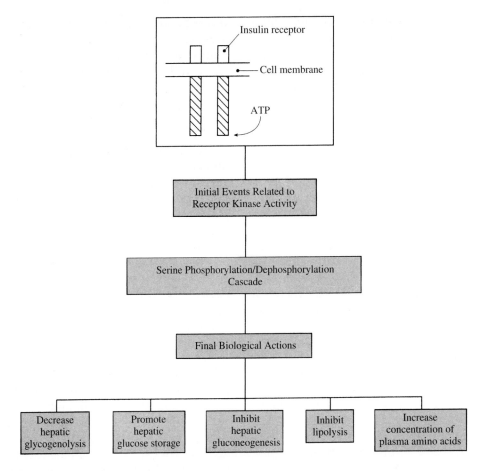

FIGURE 67.2

Levels of insulin action. Insulin acts in stages, with the initial events related to receptor tyrosine kinase activity. The second stage is a cascade of serine phosphorylation and dephosphorylation reactions involving the enzyme MAP (mitogen-activated protein–microtubule-associated protein kinase). The final stage includes the glucose transport molecules themselves, enzymes for glycogen and lipid synthesis, and proteins involved in the hormone's action on gene expression and cell growth.

tering the polymerization of the insulin molecule (e.g., monomers, dimers, or hexamers). Intramuscular injections of insulin are used less often because absorption is more rapid. Being a polypeptide hormone, insulin is readily inactivated if administered orally. In emergencies, such as severe diabetic ketoacidosis, insulin can be given intravenously. Clinical studies are examining the efficacy and safety of inhaled insulin, which may be promising for some patients.

Once insulin enters the circulation, its plasma half-life is less than 10 minutes. Hepatic insulinases destroy approximately 50% of circulating insulin, with the remainder degraded by circulating proteases. Therefore, only a relatively small amount of the total endogenous insulin secreted ever reaches the peripheral tissues. Although a number of tissues accumulate small amounts of insulin, *the liver and kidney are the principal sites of hormone uptake and degradation.* Insulin metabolism is accomplished both through the actions of an insulin-

specific protease found in the cytosol of many tissues and by the reductive cleavage of the insulin disulfide bonds by glutathione–insulin transhydrogenase. In the kidney, insulin that undergoes glomerular filtration is almost completely reabsorbed and metabolized within the proximal convoluted tubules of the nephron.

DIABETES MELLITUS

Diabetes mellitus affects approximately 5 to 8% of the population. A large number of individuals are asymptomatic and do not know they have the disease. The recent rise in obesity in the United States accounts for much of the observed and anticipated rise in cases of diabetes mellitus in this country. Although insulin treatment has greatly increased the life expectancy of the diabetic patient, diabetes remains the third leading cause of death by disease, the second leading cause of blindness, and the second leading cause of renal failure.

Diabetes mellitus is a heterogeneous group of disorders characterized by abnormalities in carbohydrate, protein, and lipid metabolism. The central disturbance in diabetes mellitus is an abnormality in insulin production or action or both, although other factors can be involved. Hyperglycemia is a common end point for all types of diabetes mellitus and is the parameter that is measured to evaluate and manage the efficacy of diabetes therapy.

Diabetes mellitus has been traditionally classified into *insulin-dependent* diabetes mellitus (IDDM), also known as type I (formerly called juvenile-onset diabetes mellitus), and *non–insulin-dependent* diabetes mellitus (NIDDM), also known as type II (formerly referred to as adult-onset diabetes mellitus). There are clearly varying degrees of overlap, and though it is often important to know whether a particular individual possesses relative insulin deficiency or relative insulin resistance or both, some of the more salient differences between IDDM and NIDDM are summarized in Table 67.1.

The pathogenesis of type I diabetes is autoimmune destruction of the cells of the pancreas. The factor or factors that trigger this autoimmune response are unknown. Predisposing factors appear to include certain major histocompatibility complex haplotypes and autoantibodies to various islet cell antigens. The progression of the autoimmune response is characterized by lymphocytic infiltration and destruction of the pancreatic cells resulting in insulin deficiency. Type I diabetes mellitus constitutes about 10% of cases of diabetes mellitus.

The other type of diabetes mellitus, type II, is far more common. In contrast, type II is not an autoimmune process and may or may not be insulin dependent; that is, a diabetic state that is most effectively managed by insulin therapy. Frequently, NIDDM is used interchange-

ably with type II diabetes mellitus, and efforts are being made to avoid the term adult onset, since many adolescents (and occasionally children) are developing NIDDM. Because the incidence of diabetes is high in families of persons with NIDDM, a strong genetic predisposition is suspected. However, NIDDM is most likely a polygenic disease, involving multiple genetic predispositions to the development of the diabetic state.

The three major metabolic abnormalities that contribute to hyperglycemia in NIDDM are defective glucose-induced insulin secretion, increased hepatic glucose output, and inability of insulin to stimulate glucose uptake in peripheral target tissues. These abnormalities also involve the cellular glucose transport in cells, liver, adipose tissue, and skeletal muscle, and they may be the result of alterations in GLUTs. Another essential problem in NIDDM may be reduced sensitivity of fat and muscle cells to the effects of insulin (i.e., *insulin resistance*). Consequently, in early stages of NIDDM, the pancreas may produce normal or even excessive amounts of insulin and only become impaired at insulin production at a later stage of the disease. Recently, a hormone produced in adipose tissue, *resistin,* has been identified and is postulated to cause many of the derangements that ultimately result in insulin resistance.

Several putative sites of insulin resistance have been identified in humans, including a defective binding of insulin to a receptor and a blunting of insulin signal transduction. Conditions associated with elevated insulin levels (*hyperinsulinism*), such as obesity, may be the result of *down-regulation* in the number of insulin receptors, effectively resulting in a state of insulin resistance. Conversely, decreases in insulin levels (e.g., diabetes) may lead to an *up-regulation* of the receptors, which may shift the insulin dose–response curve to the left; that is, less insulin would be required to produce a given biological effect. The extent to which receptor regulation actually participates in adjustments to changing physiological conditions has not been definitively established.

TABLE 67.1 Features of Type I and Type II Diabetes Mellitus

Characteristic	Type I	Type II
Onset (age)	Usually <30	Usually >40
Type of onset	Abrupt	Gradual
Nutritional status	Often thin	Often obese
Clinical symptoms	Polydipsia, polyuria, polyphagia	Often asymptomatic
Ketosis	Present	Usually absent
Endogenous insulin	Absent	Variable
Insulin therapy	Required	Sometimes
Oral hypoglycemics	Usually not effective	Often effective
Diet	Mandatory with insulin	Mandatory with or without drugs

Insulin resistance also has been associated with a number of hormonal and metabolic states, including Cushing's syndrome (excessive corticosteroids), acromegaly (excessive growth hormone), and gestational diabetes. Physiological or psychological stress also can contribute to insulin resistance. *Gestational diabetes mellitus* is a condition that develops during the second trimester of pregnancy; the cause may be rises in human placental lactogen and other hormones that contribute to insulin resistance. This condition usually resolves during the postpartum period. Another relatively common form of insulin resistance is often seen in women with *polycystic ovarian syndrome,* a disorder that is associated with hyperandrogenism, hirsutism, menstrual irregularities, obesity, and infertility.

METABOLIC DISTURBANCES AND COMPLICATIONS OF THE DIABETIC STATE

There are only two major sources of blood glucose: *exogenous,* or the ingestion of dietary carbohydrate, and *endogenous,* which is contributed by hepatic and renal gluconeogenesis and hepatic glycogenolysis. *Diabetes mellitus is a metabolic disorder in which carbohydrate metabolism is reduced while that of proteins and lipids is increased.* In diabetics, exogenous and endogenous glucose is not used effectively, and it accumulates in the blood (*hyperglycemia*). As blood glucose levels increase, the amount of glucose filtered by the glomeruli eventually exceeds the reabsorption capacity (T_m, transport maximum) of the proximal tubule cells, and glucose appears in the urine (*glucosuria*). Protein catabolism and the rate of nitrogen excretion are increased when blood insulin falls to low levels; stimulation of hepatic gluconeogenesis converts amino acids to glucose. The catabolism of lipids and fatty acids is also accelerated in the absence of insulin, leading to the formation of *ketone bodies,* such as acetoacetic acid, β-hydroxybutyric acid, and acetone. Renal losses of glucose, nitrogenous substances, and ketone bodies promote osmotic diuresis that can result in dehydration, electrolyte abnormalities, and acid–base disturbances. *Diabetic ketoacidosis* is the end result of insulin deficiency in uncontrolled type I diabetes.

Type II diabetics are less prone to develop ketone bodies or diabetic ketoacidosis but may develop *hyperosmolar coma,* a condition characterized by severe hyperglycemia and dehydration. Both diabetic ketoacidosis and hyperosmolar coma are medical emergencies that require prompt insulin administration and intravenous fluids.

Diabetes mellitus is associated with many complications that are increased in the setting of poor glycemic control. Diabetes mellitus can cause microvascular complications (e.g., retinopathy, nephropathy, and neuropathy) and macrovascular complications (e.g., atherosclerotic cardiovascular disease), associated with diabetic dyslipidemia (usually elevated triglycerides and low-density lipoprotein cholesterol). Recent clinical trials have demonstrated that the risk of developing chronic complications of diabetes is reduced by achieving good glycemic control. This can be accomplished by a combination of diet, exercise, and rational pharmacological therapy directly targeted to optimize diabetes management.

CLINICAL MANAGEMENT OF DIABETES

Diet is the cornerstone of the management of diabetes, regardless of the severity of the symptoms or the type of diabetes. Exercise is also an important component in managing diabetes, particularly in obese individuals with NIDDM who may have a component of insulin resistance as a consequence of obesity. Treatment regimens that have proved effective include a calorie-restricted diet in combination with exogenous insulin or oral hypoglycemic drugs. However, since diet, exercise, and oral hypoglycemic drugs (Table 67.2), often because of noncompliance by the patient, will not always achieve the clinical objectives of controlling the symptoms of diabetes, insulin remains universally important in therapeutic management. The administration of insulin is required for the treatment of type I (IDDM) and in cases of type II (NIDDM) that are refractory to management with oral hypoglycemic drugs.

Because the spectrum of patients with diabetes extends from the totally asymptomatic individual to one with life-threatening ketoacidosis, *therapeutic management must be highly individualized.* An important objective is to maintain a glucose level as close to normal as possible without producing frequent hypoglycemia or overly restricting the patient's lifestyle. Many diabetics aim to achieve an average blood glucose below 150 (hemoglobin A1c < 7%). Unstable or ketoacidosis-prone diabetics are difficult to maintain with a single dose of either intermediate- or long-acting insulin; they usually require multiple injections of combinations of short-, intermediate-, and/or long-acting insulin preparations.

Insulin Preparations

Commercially available insulins differ in their onset of action, maximal activity, and duration of action (Table 67.3). They can be classified as *rapid acting* (0–5 hours), *short acting* (0–8 hours), *intermediate acting* (2 to 16 hours), and *long acting* (4 to 36 hours). Human insulin (e.g. *Humulin, Novolin*) produced by rDNA technology is now widely available and has largely supplanted in-

TABLE 67.2 Antidiabetic Drugs

Augment Insulin Supply	Enhance Insulin Action	Delay Carbohydrate Absorption
Sulfonylureas	Biguanides	α-Glucosidase inhibitors
Meglitinides	Thiazolidine-	
Insulins	diones	

sulins derived from beef and pork. Some insulins have been modified through genetic engineering to produce insulin analogues, derivatives that possess novel pharmacokinetic properties (lispro, insulin aspart, and insulin glargine). The duration of action can vary with factors such as injection volume, injection site, and blood flow at the site of administration.

Rapid-acting insulin analogues (lispro, insulin aspart [*Humalog, Novolog*]) have been engineered to contain amino acid modifications that promote rapid entry into the circulation from subcutaneous tissue. They begin to exert their effects as early as 5 to 10 minutes after administration. Lispro insulin, the first insulin analogue to be approved in Europe and the United States, is produced by switching the positions of lysine-proline amino acid residues 28 and 29 of the carboxy terminus of the β-chain. Lispro insulin displays very similar actions to insulin and has a similar affinity for the insulin receptor, but it cannot form stable hexamers or dimers in subcutaneous tissue, which promotes its rapid uptake and absorption.

Insulin aspart is absorbed nearly twice as fast as regular insulin. In addition to binding to the insulin receptor, insulin aspart also binds to the insulinlike growth factor (IGF-1) receptor, which shares structural homology with the insulin receptor. However, at physiological and pharmacological levels, the metabolic effects of insulin aspart predominate. Both lispro insulin and insulin aspart have relatively fast onsets and short

half-lives, making them ideal for controlling the upward glycemic excursions that occur immediately after meals in diabetics.

Short-acting or *regular* insulins (*Humulin R, Novolin R*) take 30 minutes to begin to exert their effect but have a longer duration of action than does either lispro insulin or insulin aspart. Typically, regular insulin is administered several minutes before a meal; it has a more gradual onset of action and is designed to control postprandial hyperglycemia. Regular insulin is primarily used to supplement intermediate- and long-acting insulin preparations; however, it is also the preparation of choice for glucose management during surgery, trauma, shock, or diabetic ketoacidosis. Regular insulin can be given intravenously when emergency diabetes management is required (e.g., diabetes ketoacidosis). Prompt insulin zinc suspension (*Semilente*) is also a fast-acting form of insulin, but unlike regular insulin, it should be mixed only with *Lente* or *Ultralente* insulin preparations. Rapid-acting and short-acting insulins are often administered two to three times a day or more. These insulins are also employed in sliding scale insulin regimens, which supplement a person's glucose control based on blood glucose monitoring equipment.

Intermediate-acting preparations (e.g., isophane insulin suspension [*NPH* insulin] or insulin zinc suspension [*Lente* insulin]) have a more delayed onset of action, but they act longer. Conjugation of the insulin molecule with either *zinc* or *protamine* or both will convert the normally rapidly absorbed parenterally administered insulin to a preparation with a longer duration of action. Isophane insulin suspension (*Neutral protamine Hagedorn, NPH*) has a rate of absorption that has been slowed by complexing insulin with protamine, a polyvalent cation. Both NPH and *Lente* insulin are used to control diabetes in a variety of situations except during emergencies (e.g., diabetic ketoacidosis). Intermediate-acting insulin preparations are usually given once or twice a day.

TABLE 67.3 Pharmacokinetic Properties of Insulin Formulations and Analogues

Drug	Onset	Peak	Duration
Short Acting			
Lispro (Humalog)	10–20 min	1–2 hr	2–4 hr
Insulin Aspart (Novolog)	10–20 min	1 hr	3–5 hr
Regular	30–60 min	2–3 hr	5–7 hr
Prompt Insulin Zn Suspension (Semi-Lente)	30–60 min	2–3 hr	5–7 hr
Intermediate Acting			
Isophane Insulin Suspension (NPH)	1–2 hr	5–7 hr	13–18 hr
Insulin Zn Suspension (Lente)	1–3 hr	4–8 hr	13–20 hr
Long Acting			
Extended Zn Suspension (Ultralente)	2–4 hr	8–14 hr	18–36 hr
Insulin Glargine (Lantus)	2–hr	None	up to 24 hr

Protamine zinc and extended insulin zinc suspension (*Ultralente*) are often referred to as *long-acting* insulin preparations. These insulins have more protamine and zinc in the mixture than is found in isophane insulin suspension. Insulin zinc suspension, extended (*Ultralente Insulin*), is quite similar to the protamine zinc insulin suspension except that it does not contain protamine. Both of these long-acting insulins have an approximate duration of action of 36 hours.

Insulin glargine (*Lantus*) is a long-acting insulin analogue that does not use zinc or protamine to modulate insulin solubility. The introduction of two positive arginine residues at the carboxy terminus of the β-chain shifts the isoelectric point of the peptide from 5.4 to 6.7, thus creating a molecule that is soluble at pH 4 but less soluble at neutral (physiological) pH (in subcutaneous tissue). A second modification of insulin, glargine, involves the substitution of a charge-neutral glycine for a negatively charged asparagine at the amino terminal end of the α-chain; this prevents deamidation and dimerization and enhances stability at physiological pH. Injection of insulin glargine forms microprecipitates in subcutaneous tissue as the pH is raised from 4 to physiological. A steady, sustained release of insulin from the site of injection mimics the basal secretion of insulin from the pancreas. Absorption of insulin glargine commences within a few hours of injection, and there is usually little or no peak or trough in the levels of insulin glargine as it dissolves from its site of injection. Because it is necessary to maintain its acidic pH prior to injection, insulin glargine must not be mixed with any other form of insulin during injection.

Adverse Reactions to Insulin Therapy

The most common side effect associated with insulin therapy is *hypoglycemia,* which may result in such CNS symptoms as tremors, lethargy, hunger, confusion, motor and sensory deficits, seizures, and unconsciousness. Adrenergic manifestations include anxiety, palpitations, tachycardia, and diaphoresis. In many cases, diabetics are aware that hypoglycemia is developing, and prompt administration of oral carbohydrates (e.g., fruit juice or glucose tablets) can restore normoglycemia. In more severe cases (e.g., unconsciousness, seizures), intravenous glucose or intramuscular glucagon is required to reverse the hypoglycemia.

Another frequent side effect of insulin therapy is weight gain. Some is due to increased caloric storage of glucose by insulin, and some is due to renal sodium retention resulting in fluid retention and edema. These effects can synergize with oral agents that are often coadministered with insulin, particularly sulfonylureas and thiazolidinediones.

Other complications arising from insulin therapy are uncommon. Sometimes, diabetics treated with exogenous insulin develop insulin-binding immunoglobulins, although the clinical significance of these antibodies remains unclear. Allergic reactions due to the use of animal-derived insulins has subsided since the use of recombinant DNA-derived human insulin became widespread. Over time, repeated subcutaneous injections of insulin can cause local lipodystrophy (lipohypertrophy or lipoatrophy), which may alter the pharmacokinetics of insulin absorption from this site. Also, hypokalemia can follow acute insulin administration, an effect that is due to the stimulation of Na^+–K^+–ATPase (adenosine triphosphatase) with its resultant redistribution of K^+ to the intracellular compartment. This property of insulin is sometimes used in the emergency treatment of *hyperkalemia.*

Insulin Regimens

The rational design of insulin regimens involves estimates and consideration of the patient's diet, lifestyle, level of physical activity, and type of diabetes. A thin, active type I diabetic will have very different insulin requirements from those of a sedentary, obese type II diabetic. Hence, it is not possible to provide a cookbook approach for designing all diabetes regimens. There is usually less insulin resistance in type I diabetics, and it is possible to estimate metabolic needs of insulin based on the type I diabetic patient's weight (typically 0.5 to 1 units/kg/day). Other considerations, such as work schedule and mealtimes, are important in determining the way the insulin is divided proportionally to cover short-range and long-range glycemic control. Although there is quite a bit of variation, most diabetics have about half to two-thirds of their insulin as a long-acting preparation, and the rest is usually delivered as a rapid- or short-acting insulin.

Some insulin preparations are combinations of NPH and *regular* insulin packaged in premixed ratios of 70:30 or 50:50 of NPH and *regular* insulin (*70/30 Humulin, 70/30 Novolin, 50/50 Humulin*). A similar combination product is 75/25 insulin, which contains 75% protamine lispro and 25% lispro insulin. Insulin zinc suspension (*Lente* insulin) is an intermediate-acting mixture of prompt insulin zinc suspension (30%) and extended insulin zinc suspension (70%). While these combination products may be convenient for some patients and can improve compliance, they are not ideal regimens for most diabetics, who may achieve better control by separately mixing their rapid- or short-acting insulin with an intermediate- or long-acting insulin to arrive at a ratio that is better suited to manage their diabetes.

Insulin pumps are small, portable devices worn externally that deliver a continuous supply of insulin subcutaneously through a hypodermic needle. The pumps provide a basal rate of insulin between meals and can be manually adjusted to facilitate glycemic control at mealtimes. Rapid and short-acting insulins are typically used in insulin pumps. Pumps are usually worn 2 to 3 days before the tubing and needle are changed.

ORAL AGENTS FOR TREATING DIABETES MELLITUS

Although insulin has the disadvantage of having to be injected, it is without question the most uniformly effective treatment of diabetes mellitus. Some milder forms of diabetes mellitus that do not respond to diet management or weight loss and exercise can be treated with oral hypoglycemic agents. The success of oral hypoglycemic drug therapy is usually based on a restoration of normal blood glucose levels and the absence of glycosuria. Traditionally, the term *oral hypoglycemic* was used interchangeably with sulfonylureas, but more recently the development of several new drugs has broadened this designation to include all oral medications for diabetes. Because these drugs do not have to be injected, oral agents enhance compliance in type II diabetics. These classes of drugs are not generally used in type I diabetes. The pharmacokinetic profile of oral agents for diabetes is depicted in Table 67.4.

Sulfonylureas

Sulfonylureas are the most widely prescribed drugs in the treatment of type II diabetes mellitus. The initial sulfonylureas were introduced nearly 50 years ago and were derivatives of the antibacterial sulfonamides. Although their structural similarities to the sulfonamide antibacterial agents are readily apparent, the sulfonylureas possess no antibacterial activity.

Mechanism of Action

The primary mechanism of action of the sulfonylureas is *direct stimulation of insulin release from the pancreatic β-cells.* In the presence of viable pancreatic β-cells, sulfonylureas enhance the release of endogenous insulin, thereby reducing blood glucose levels. At higher doses, these drugs also decrease hepatic glucose production, and the second-generation sulfonylureas may possess additional extrapancreatic effects that increase insulin sensitivity, though the clinical significance of these pharmacological effects is unclear. These mechanisms are summarized in Table 67.3.

The sulfonylureas are *ineffective* for the management of type I and severe type II diabetes mellitus, since the number of viable β-cells in these forms of diabetes is small. Severely obese diabetics often respond poorly to the sulfonylureas, possibly because of the insulin resistance that often accompanies obesity.

The Sulfonylurea Receptor

The sulfonylurea receptor was identified as an adenosine triphosphate (ATP) sensitive potassium (K_{ATP}) channel that is present on the β-cell membrane surface. Closure of these K_{ATP} channels causes β-cell membrane

TABLE 67.4 Pharmacokinetic Properties of Oral Hypoglycemic Drugs

Drug	Half-Life (hr)	Duration of Action (hr)	Activity of Metabolites
Sulfonylureas			
First generation			
Acetohexamide	0.8–2.4	12–18	+
Chlorpropamide	24–48	60	+
Tolazamide	4–7	12–24	+
Tolbutamide	3–28	6–12	−
Second generation			
Glyburide	2–4	16–24	±
Glipizide	1–5	12–24 (XL > 24)	−
Glimeperide	5–9	>24	+
Meglitinides			
Repaglinide	1	4–6	−
Nateglinide	1–2	4	−
Biguanides			
Metformin	4–8	18–24	−
α-Glucosidase inhibitors			
Acarbose	2	4–6	±
Miglitol	2	4–6	−
Thiazolidinediones			
Pioglitazone	26–30	days	−
Rosiglitazone	4	days	−

depolarization and triggers the opening of voltage-dependent calcium channels. The influx of calcium into the β-cell triggers insulin granule fusion to the β-cell membrane and insulin release. The intracellular levels of ATP and adenosine diphosphate (ADP) modulate the activity of the K_{ATP} channel, depending on the availability of glucose.

The activity of the K_{ATP} channels is modulated by the direct binding of sulfonylureas to a specific subunit of the K_{ATP} channel called SUR1. SUR1 is a member of the K^+ inwardly rectifying (Kir) 6.0 subfamily of proteins and can bind nucleotides and sulfonylureas with high affinity. Four SUR1 subunits form a complex with four subunits from the Kir 6.2 subfamily and create the pore for K^+ permeation in the pancreatic β-cell. Sulfonylurea binding to SUR1 directly promotes the closure of these K_{ATP} channels, lowering the threshold for glucose-dependent insulin release. Diazoxide (a direct vasodilator discussed in Chapter 20) also binds to SUR1 but keeps the K_{ATP} channels open, raising the threshold for glucose-stimulated insulin secretion and sometimes causing hyperglycemia in patients.

Absorption, Metabolism, and Excretion

Sulfonylureas are readily absorbed from the gastrointestinal tract following oral administration but undergo varying degrees and rates of metabolism in the liver and/or kidney; some metabolites possess intrinsic hypoglycemic activity. Thus, the biological half-lives of the sulfonylureas vary greatly, and a comparison of the drug half-life with the observed duration of action does not always show a good correlation. Sulfonylureas and their metabolites are excreted either renally or in the feces.

Clinical Uses

Sulfonylureas are generally effective in individuals with mild to moderate type II diabetes. The chance for successful glycemic control with sulfonylureas is poor in diabetic patients requiring more than 40 units of insulin per day. When beginning therapy with one of these drugs, a low to intermediate dose is given initially and then gradually increased until the dosage results in normoglycemia. Once the maximum recommended dosage for a particular sulfonylurea is reached, further increasing the dose will not improve glycemic control.

Adverse Effects and Drug Interactions

The most common adverse effect associated with sulfonylurea administration is hypoglycemia, which may be provoked by inadequate calorie intake (e.g., skipping a meal), or increased caloric needs (e.g., increased physical activity). Collectively, sulfonylureas also tend to cause weight gain, which is undesirable in individuals who already are obese. Some of this weight can be due to fluid retention and edema. Less common adverse reactions include muscular weakness, ataxia, dizziness, mental confusion, skin rash, photosensitivity, blood dyscrasias, and cholestatic jaundice. Occasionally, persons who display drug sensitivities to sulfa-containing antibiotics show a cross-reactivity to the sulfonylureas. In this situation, a nonsulfonylurea insulin secretagogue can be used (if desired), such as repaglinide or nateglinide (discussed later). Sulfonylureas are not used in gestational diabetes, which is generally managed by a combination of intensive diet control and insulin.

Since diabetic patients with renal or hepatic disease are particularly vulnerable to hypoglycemia, the sulfonylurea compounds should be avoided in these individuals. A decrease in alcohol tolerance also has been observed in some patients taking sulfonylurea compounds. Since sulfonylureas are highly bound to plasma proteins and are extensively metabolized by microsomal enzymes, coadministration of drugs capable of displacing them from their protein binding sites or inhibiting their metabolism (e.g., sulfonamide antibacterials, propranolol, salicylates, phenylbutazone, chloramphenicol, probenecid, and alcohol) also may potentiate hypoglycemia.

First-Generation Sulfonylureas

The first-generation sulfonylureas are not frequently used in the modern management of diabetes mellitus because of their relatively low specificity of action, delay in time of onset, occasional long duration of action, and a variety of side effects. They also tend to have more adverse drug interactions than the second-generation sulfonylureas. They are occasionally used in patients who have achieved previous adequate control with these agents.

Acetohexamide (*Dymelor*) is the only sulfonylurea with uricosuric activity, an action that may be of benefit in diabetic patients who also have gout.

Chlorpropamide (*Diabinese*) has a relatively slow onset of action, with its maximal hypoglycemic potential often not reached for 1 or 2 weeks. Similarly, several weeks may be required to eliminate the drug after discontinuation of therapy. This drug can cause flushing, particularly when taken with alcohol, and can also cause hyponatremia. This effect has been employed to treat some patients who have partial central diabetes insipidus, an unrelated condition due to a pituitary ADH deficiency.

Tolazamide (*Tolinase*) is an orally effective hypoglycemic drug that causes less water retention than do the other compounds in this class.

Tolbutamide (*Orinase*) is a relatively short-acting compound that may be useful in patients who are prone to hypoglycemia.

Second-Generation Sulfonylureas

The second-generation sulfonylureas display a higher specificity and affinity for the sulfonylurea receptor and more predictable pharmacokinetics in terms of time of onset and duration of action, and they have fewer side effects. Second-generation sulfonylureas may also exert mild diuretic effects on the kidney and are highly protein bound, primarily through nonionic binding (in contrast to the ionic binding observed with the first-generation compounds).

Glyburide (*DiaBeta, Micronase, Glynase*), also known as glibenclamide, is approximately 150 times as potent as tolbutamide on a molar basis and twice as potent as glipizide (discussed later). Glyburide is completely metabolized in the liver to two weakly active metabolites before excretion in the urine. Its average duration of action is 24 hours.

Glipizide (*Glucotrol*) is similar to glyburide, but it is metabolized by the liver to two inactive metabolites; these metabolites and glipizide are renally excreted.

Glimepiride (*Amaryl*) is metabolized to at least one active metabolite. It is quickly absorbed from the gastrointestinal tract within an hour of oral administration and excreted in the urine and feces. Its half-life varies from 5 to 9 hours depending on the frequency of multiple dosing.

Meglitinides

Though structurally unrelated to sulfonylureas, the meglitinide class of hypoglycemic drugs bind to the same K_{ATP} channel as do the sulfonylureas, but it is unclear whether they bind to the same SUR1 subunit within the K_{ATP} complex. As a class, the meglitinides are incapable of stimulating insulin secretion in nutrient-starved β-cells, but in the presence of glucose, they demonstrate hypoglycemic effects by augmenting the release of insulin. Consequently, meglitinides seem relatively unlikely to cause fasting hypoglycemia.

Repaglinide (*Prandin*), a member of the meglitinide class, is approved for monotherapy or in combination with metformin. Repaglinide is taken before each meal, three times a day, and is rapidly absorbed; it is metabolized by the liver and has a half life of an hour. Insulin levels transiently rise postprandially after repaglinide administration but generally return to baseline by the next meal. Although repaglinide does not appear to offer any advantage over the sulfonylureas, it may be helpful in patients with a known allergy to sulfa drugs. Hypoglycemia is the most common side effect.

Nateglinide (*Starlix*), a newer drug in the meglitinide class, is a phenylalanine derivative that also works by binding to a specific site on the K^+–ATP–sensitive channel on the surface of β-cells. Nateglinide binds with a higher affinity than does repaglinide and has a faster onset of action and a shorter duration of action. Like repaglinide, it is approved for both monotherapy and in combination with metformin. Nateglinide is taken three times a day before meals and achieves peak plasma levels within an hour. Nateglinide administration results in plasma insulin levels that peak within 2 hours; they return to baseline by 4 hours. Nateglinide is metabolized by the liver and excreted by the kidney. The main side effect of nateglinide is hypoglycemia, though its effects on fasting insulin levels is not substantially reduced.

Biguanides

Biguanides are a group of oral hypoglycemic agents that are chemically and pharmacologically distinct from the sulfonylureas. One biguanide, phenformin, was briefly used in the United States more than 30 years ago but was withdrawn from the market because it produced severe lactic acidosis in some patients. Metformin (*Glucophage*) was used in Europe for many years before it was approved for use in the United States in 1995. Metformin is the only approved biguanide for the treatment of patients with NIDDM that are refractory to dietary management alone. Metformin does not affect insulin secretion but requires the presence of insulin to be effective. The exact mechanism of metformin's action is not clear, but it does decrease hepatic glucose production and increase peripheral glucose uptake. When used as monotherapy, metformin rarely causes hypoglycemia.

Metformin works best in patients with significant hyperglycemia and is often considered first-line therapy in the treatment of mild to moderate type II overweight diabetics who demonstrate insulin resistance. The United Kingdom Prospective Diabetes Study demonstrated a marked reduction in cardiovascular comorbidities and diabetic complications in metformin-treated individuals. Metformin has also been used to treat hirsutism in individuals with polycystic ovarian syndrome and may enhance fertility in these women, perhaps by decreasing androgen levels and enhancing insulin sensitivity.

Adverse gastrointestinal symptoms (nausea, vomiting, anorexia, metallic taste, abdominal discomfort, and diarrhea) occur in up to 20% of individuals taking metformin; this can be minimized by starting at a low dose and slowly titrating the dose upward *with food*. Like phenformin, metformin can cause lactic acidosis, but its occurrence is rare except when renal failure, hypoxemia, or severe congestive heart failure is present or when coadministered with alcohol. Metformin is also contraindicated in persons with hepatic dysfunction, but it appears to be safe for use in the hepatic steatosis that often occurs with fatty infiltration of the liver in poorly controlled type II diabetics.

Two relatively new formulations of metformin are available. *Glucovance* is a combination of metformin and glyburide that may be helpful for diabetics who require both a sulfonylurea and metformin, and *Glucophage XR* is an extended-release product of metformin that may be better tolerated in some patients who are prone to gastrointestinal side effects. Metformin is usually given two to three times a day at mealtimes.

Thiazolidinediones

Thiazolidinediones (sometimes termed glitazones) are a novel class of drugs that were initially identified for their insulin-sensitizing properties. They all act to decrease insulin resistance and enhance insulin action in target tissues. Thiazolidinediones activate the nuclear peroxisome proliferator–activated receptor (PPAR) γ, a nuclear orphan receptor that is predominantly expressed in adipose tissue and to a lesser extent in muscle, liver, and other tissues. The endogenous ligand for the PPAR-γ receptor is postulated to be prostaglandin J2, and it appears to work by heterodimerizing with other nuclear receptors to modulate the expression of insulin-sensitive genes.

Thiazolidinediones are readily absorbed from the gastrointestinal tract following oral administration and are rapidly metabolized by the liver. Plasma elimination half-life is 2 to 3 hours for rosiglitazone (*Avandia*) and slightly longer for pioglitazone (*Actos*). About two-thirds of conjugated metabolites appear in the urine and the remainder in the feces. The biological effect of these drugs takes several weeks to develop, although patients may see some benefit within a few days to a week. Generally, however, the insulin-sensitizing action of the thiazolidinediones takes a while to develop. For that reason, upward adjustments in dosage are made gradually to avoid hypoglycemia.

The patient who would benefit the most from a thiazolidinedione is a type II diabetic with a substantial amount of insulin resistance (e.g., one who does not respond to other oral therapies or who requires excessive amounts of insulin [>100 units/day]). Improvements in diabetic control are variable, ranging from a 1% reduction in hemoglobin A1c when used as monotherapy to greater reductions (>2% reduction in hemoglobin A1c) when used in combinations with other agents, such as sulfonylureas or metformin.

Rosiglitazone is approved for use as monotherapy and in conjunction with metformin, though it is sometimes combined with a sulfonylurea or insulin. It is usually taken once or twice a day with or without food. Rosiglitazone may cause a modest increase in low-density lipoprotein and triglyceride concentrations, but it is unclear whether this effect has any clinical significance or persists in the long term.

Pioglitazone is approved for use as monotherapy and in conjunction with metformin, sulfonylureas, and insulin. It is taken once a day with or without food. Though pioglitazone may also cause a small increase in low-density lipoprotein concentrations, there is usually a modest decrease in triglyceride levels, but it unclear whether this has any clinical significance or persists in the long term.

The original prototype of this class of drugs, troglitazone (*Rezulin*), was taken off the U.S. market in 2000 because of increasing concerns about idiosyncratic hepatic toxicity that resulted in several deaths worldwide. Consequently, frequent monitoring of liver transaminases is recommended for rosiglitazone and pioglitazone, and these drugs should be stopped if transaminases rise to more than two to three times the upper limit of normal. To date, rosiglitazone and pioglitazone seem to be associated with far fewer incidents of hepatic toxicity.

Thiazolidinediones commonly cause edema that can be quite severe, sometimes requiring cessation of the drug, but mild cases of lower extremity edema can be treated with a low dose of a diuretic. There is often a modest amount of weight gain that is independent of water-retaining effects. In laboratory animals, thiazolidinediones at high doses are associated with ultrastructural histopathological changes in cardiac tissue; therefore, thiazolidinedione use is contraindicated in patients with significant heart failure. Thiazolidinediones can also cause mild anemia. Safety in pregnancy is not established.

Hypoglycemia is rare with thiazolidinedione monotherapy; however, these drugs may potentiate the hypoglycemic effects of concurrent sulfonylurea or insulin therapy. If a thiazolidinedione is to be added to a diabetic's regimen, the sulfonylurea or insulin dosage should be decreased to compensate for any enhanced insulin sensitivity. Occasionally a small portion of insulin-treated type II diabetics may be capable of coming off their insulin altogether, depending on their responsiveness to thiazolidinedione action.

α-Glucosidase Inhibitors

The α-glucosidase inhibitors primarily act to decrease postprandial hyperglycemia by *slowing the rate* at which carbohydrates are absorbed from the gastrointestinal tract. They act by competitively inhibiting α-glucosidases, a group of enzymes in the intestinal brush border epithelial cells that includes glycoamylase, sucrase, maltase, and dextranase. The prolongation of the intestinal absorption of carbohydrates results in a blunted insulin response, keeping postprandial hyperglycemia under control. To be effective, α-glucosidase inhibitors must be taken before or with meals. Theoretically, the α-glucosidase inhibitors are most beneficial in patients with mild to moderate diabetes whose diet is more than 50% carbohydrates. α-Glucosidase inhibitors are not approved for used in type I diabetes.

Acarbose (*Precose*) is an oligosaccharide derivative that has a higher affinity for the α-glucosidase enzymes than do other dietary oligosaccharides. Systemic absorption of acarbose is very low (~2%), with most being broken down in the intestine to several metabolites. About half of the orally administered acarbose is excreted unchanged in the feces, while the remainder, some of which is systemically absorbed, is renally excreted. Acarbose may be associated with hepatotoxicity in rare instances.

Miglitol (*Glyset*) is another α-glucosidase inhibitor, but in contrast to acarbose, miglitol is systemically absorbed prior to its activity in the small intestine. It also appears to inhibit the enzymes sucrase and maltase to a greater extent than does acarbose. It does not undergo metabolism and is renally excreted unchanged.

Gastrointestinal disturbances (loose stools, flatulence, and abdominal cramping) are the most frequently observed side effects of the α-glucosidase inhibitors. These effects can be minimized by starting patients on a low dose and then slowly advancing the dose as tolerance develops; curtailment of carbohydrate consumption also can alleviate these effects. Patients should be counseled that these side effects will occur and that tolerance should develop; otherwise, compliance will be low and about one-third of patients will stop their medication. Unlike the sulfonylureas, insulin, and the thiazolidinediones, α-glucosidase inhibitors do not cause weight gain. Insulin levels do not change in the presence of α-glucosidase inhibitors, so fasting hypoglycemia does not occur when α-glucosidase inhibitors are used as monotherapy. Although the α-glucosidase inhibitors may be used as monotherapy, they are usually used in combination with metformin, sulfonylureas, or insulin. Under the best circumstances, α-glucosidase inhibitors can be expected to promote a 0.5 to 1% reduction in a patient's hemoglobin A1c. Leaving aside their gastrointestinal side effects, α-glucosidase inhibitors appear to be relatively safe.

Study QUESTIONS

1. The main reason metformin should not be used in patients with renal failure is that
   (A) It increases the risk of lactic acidosis.
   (B) It increases the risk of ketoacidosis.
   (C) It causes development of congestive heart failure.
   (D) It causes hepatic necrosis.
   (E) It causes hypoglycemia.

2. All of the following statements are true EXCEPT
   (A) Lispro insulin displays a similar affinity and action with the insulin receptor.
   (B) Lispro insulin has a slower onset of action than glargine insulin.
   (C) Premixed 70/30 insulin is composed of 70% NPH and 30% regular insulin.
   (D) Glucagon is a hormone that counteracts many of the metabolic effects of insulin.
   (E) Glargine insulin has a longer duration of action than lispro insulin.

3. Hypoglycemia is rarely seen with these drugs when used as monotherapy EXCEPT:
   (A) Metformin
   (B) Rosiglitazone
   (C) Miglitol
   (D) Glyburide
   (E) A, B, and C

4. All of the following are true statements about the thiazolidinediones EXCEPT

   (A) Thiazolidinediones may be hepatotoxic in some individuals.
   (B) Thiazolidinediones increase the number of insulin receptors on the cell membrane surface.
   (C) Thiazolidinediones bind a nuclear receptor in tissue termed PPAR-γ, which augments the expression of insulin-regulated genes.
   (D) Thiazolidinediones take many days to weeks to begin exerting a blood glucose–lowering effect in diabetics.
   (E) The most common side effects of thiazolidinediones are weight gain and edema.

ANSWERS

1. **A.** Metformin causes lactic acidosis in patients with renal failure and severe congestive heart failure. It does not increase the risk of ketoacidosis and showed a reduction in cardiovascular comorbidities in a large study. It is contraindicated in patients with severe liver disease but does not cause hepatic necrosis. When used as monotherapy, metformin rarely causes hypoglycemia.

2. **B.** Lispro insulin was engineered to have a rapid onset of action. Lispro insulin displays a similar affinity and action with the insulin receptor as regular insulin. Premixed 70/30 insulin is composed of a 70:30 ratio of NPH to regular insulin. Glucagon has opposite effects to many of those of insulin.

Glargine insulin has substituent groups that prevent deamidation and dimerization and that enhance its stability at physiological pH.

3. **D.** One of the most important therapeutic objectives is to maintain normal glucose levels without producing frequent hypoglycemia. The main class of hypoglycemic drugs that have a propensity to cause hypoglycemia are the sulfonylureas, of which glyburide is one. This is not a problem with the other choices.

4. **B.** The thiazolidinediones decrease insulin resistance and enhance insulin action in target tissues. The original prototype drug of this class was removed from the market because of hepatotoxicity. These compounds activate the PPAR-γ-receptor. Although patients may see some benefit within a few days, a clinically significant effect generally takes weeks. The most common side effects are edema and weight gain that is independent of the weight gain seen in edema.

SUPPLEMENTAL READING

Ashcroft SJ. The beta-cell K(ATP) channel. J Membr Biol 2001;176:187–206.

Bailey CJ. Insulin resistance and antidiabetic drugs. Biochem Pharmacol 1999;58:1511–1520.

Holleman F and Hoekstra JBL. Insulin Lispro. N Engl J Med 1997;337:176–183.

Kahn CR et al. Unraveling the mechanism of action of thiazolidinediones. J Clin Invest 2000;106:1305–1307.

Miki TK et al. The structure and function of the ATP-sensitive K+ channel in insulin-secreting pancreatic beta-cells. J Molec Endocrinol 1999;22:113–123.

Mudaliar S and Henry RR. New oral therapies for type 2 diabetes mellitus: The glitazones or insulin sensitizers. Annu Rev Med 2001;52:239–257.

Virkamaki A et al. Protein–protein interaction in insulin signaling and the molecular mechanisms of insulin resistance. J Clin Invest 1999;103:931–943.

CASE Study   Insulin Regimens

George Smith is taking insulin for the first time. His physician prescribes 20 units NPH and 5 units regular insulin at breakfast, and 10 units NPH and 5 units regular insulin at dinner. After a few days, Mr. Smith begins to notice this approximate pattern in his blood sugar measurements:

8 A.M. (fasting), about 110; noon (before lunch), about 120; 5 P.M. (before dinner), about 55; bedtime, about 115.

When his blood sugar is about 55, he feels shaky and sweaty, but this goes away if he has something to eat. Which of the following changes would you recommend to his regimen?

Decrease his morning regular insulin
Decrease his morning NPH insulin
Stop evening insulin and add a sulfonylurea at bedtime

Have him eat a larger lunch
Move his evening NPH insulin from supper time to bedtime

ANSWER: Mr. Smith should decrease his morning NPH insulin. Since on awakening his fasting glucose is in the normal range and after taking his morning regular insulin his blood glucose remains in the normal range, there is no need to adjust either his morning regular insulin or his bedtime NPH insulin. Regular insulin is short-acting and would not result in a 5 P.M. low glucose level. The longer-acting NPH insulin given in the morning would continue to lower glucose for the rest of the morning and afternoon, in this case resulting in excessive blood glucose at dinner time.

68 | Vitamins

Suzanne Barone

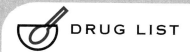

DRUG LIST

GENERIC NAME	PAGE	GENERIC NAME	PAGE
Biotin	780	Pyridoxine	780
Cyanocobalamin	780	Retinol	778
Folic acid	780	Riboflavin	779
Nicotinic acid	780	Thiamine	779
Pantothenic acid	780		

Vitamins are a group of unrelated chemical substances that are essential in small amounts for the regulation of normal metabolism, growth, and function of the human body. Not all of the vitamins can be synthesized in the body, and therefore, some vitamins must be obtained from an external source, such as a proper well-balanced diet or dietary supplements.

Vitamins become a pharmacological concern when there is an imbalance in the body's vitamin supply. Deficiency diseases can result from insufficient vitamin ingestion, irregular absorption, or impaired metabolic use of these nutrients. The ingestion or administration of excessive quantities of vitamins, also known as hypervitaminosis, may result in toxicity.

This chapter focuses on the pharmacological and toxicological properties of vitamins.

DIETARY REFERENCE STANDARDS

The Food and Nutrition Board of the Institute of Medicine (IOM) has been developing reference standards for vitamins and other nutrients called Dietary Reference Intakes (DRIs). In the past, the recommended dietary allowances (RDAs), which are the levels of intake of essential nutrients that are considered to be adequate to meet the known nutritional needs of practically all healthy persons, were the primary reference value for vitamins and other nutrients. The DRIs also include other reference values, such as the estimated average requirement (EAR) and the adequate intake (AI). The RDA, EAR, and AI reference standards define nutritional intake adequacy. Since these recommendations are given for healthy populations in general and not for individuals, special problems, such as premature birth, inherited metabolic disorders, infections, chronic disease, and use of medications, are not covered by the requirements. Separate RDAs have been developed for pregnant and lactating women. Vitamin supplementation may be required by patients with special conditions and for those who do not consume an appropriate diet.

A varied diet containing a wide range of foodstuffs provides adequate intake of vitamins for most people, and supplementing these amounts will have no beneficial effect and may result in the toxicity associated with hypervitaminosis. The DRI also includes the tolerable upper intake level (UL) of vitamins. The UL is defined as the highest level of intake of a nutrient that will not pose a risk of adverse health effects to most individuals in the general population. The UL is an important reference standard, especially with the current promotion and wide availability of vitamin preparations. A table of the DRIs for vitamins is available on the IOM's web site at http://www.nationalacademies.org/IOM/IOMHome.nsf/Pages/Ongoing+Studies#FNB.

DEFICIENCY DISEASES

Medical personnel who work in affluent areas are unlikely to see large numbers of people with vitamin deficiency diseases. However, certain groups of the population are particularly at risk, such as low-income families and chronically ill patients. The classic symptoms of any vitamin deficiency disease as observed in laboratory animals are often blurred in humans. The clinical picture is often complicated by deficiencies of other vitamins, minerals, calories, and protein and by infections and parasite infestations, which usually accompany longstanding malnutrition. Biochemical, physiological, and behavioral changes can occur in the marginal deficiency state without or before the appearance of more specific symptoms. Since the nonspecificity of these changes makes them difficult to detail, this section focuses on the symptoms associated with individual vitamin deficiency diseases.

VITAMIN TOXICITY

Toxic effects have been observed when large dosages of some vitamins are ingested. Generally the water-soluble vitamins are less toxic, since excess quantities are usually excreted in the urine. Excessive amounts of fat-soluble vitamins, however, are stored in the body, which makes toxic levels of these vitamins easier to obtain.

PHYSIOLOGICAL FUNCTION AND DIETARY SOURCES

Vitamins are usually classified as either fat soluble (vitamins A, D, E, and K) or water soluble (vitamins B and C). The fat-soluble vitamins are generally metabolized slowly and are stored in the liver. In contrast, the water-soluble vitamins are rapidly metabolized and are readily excreted in the urine.

Fat-Soluble Vitamins
Vitamin A

Vitamin A, or retinol, is essential for the proper maintenance of the functional and structural integrity of epithelial cells, and it plays a major role in epithelial differentiation. Bone development and growth in children have also been linked to adequate vitamin A intake. Vitamin A, when reduced to the aldehyde 11-*cis*-retinal, combines with opsin to produce the visual pigment rhodopsin. This pigment is present in the rods of the retina and is partly responsible for the process of dark adaptation.

Principal dietary sources of vitamin A are milk fat (cheese and butter) and eggs. Since it is stored in the liver, inclusion of liver in the diet also provides vitamin A. A plant pigment, carotene, is a precursor for vitamin A and is present in highly pigmented vegetables, such as carrots, rutabaga, and red cabbage.

An early sign of hypovitaminosis A is night blindness. This condition is related to the role of vitamin A as the prosthetic group of the visual pigment rhodopsin. The night blindness may progress to *xerophthalmia* (dryness and ulceration of the cornea) and blindness. Other symptoms of vitamin A deficiency include cessation of growth and skin changes due to hyperkeratosis.

Since vitamin A is a fat-soluble vitamin, any disease that results in fat malabsorption and impaired liver storage brings with it the risk of vitamin A deficiency; these conditions include biliary tract disease, pancreatic disease, sprue, and hepatic cirrhosis. One group at great risk are children from low-income families, who are likely to lack fresh vegetables (carotene) and dairy products (vitamin A) in the diet.

Acute hypervitaminosis A results in drowsiness, headache, vomiting, papilledema, and a bulging fontanel in infants. The symptoms of chronic toxicity include scaly skin, hair loss, brittle nails, and hepatosplenomegaly. Anorexia, irritability, and swelling of the bones have been seen in children. Retardation of growth also may occur. Liver toxicity has been associated with excessive vitamin A intake. Vitamin A is teratogenic in large amounts, and supplements should not be given during a normal pregnancy. The IOM has reported the UL of vitamin A to be 3,000 µg/day.

Vitamin D

Vitamin D is the collective term for a group of compounds formed by the action of ultraviolet irradiation on sterols. Cholecalciferol (vitamin D_3) and calciferol (vitamin D_2) are formed by irradiation of the provitamins 7-dehydrocholesterol and ergosterol, respectively. The conversion to vitamin D_3 occurs in the skin. The liver is the principal storage site for vitamin D, and it is here that the vitamin is hydroxylated to form 25-hydroxyvitamin D. Additional hydroxylation to form 1,25-dihydroxyvitamin D occurs in the kidney in response to the need for calcium and phosphate. A discussion of the role of vitamin D in calcium homeostasis is provided in Chapter 66.

The principal disorder associated with inadequate vitamin D intake is rickets. The low blood calcium and phosphate levels that occur during vitamin D deficiency stimulate parathyroid hormone secretion to restore calcium levels (see Chapter 66). In children, this deficiency leads to the formation of soft bones that become deformed easily; in adults, osteomalacia results from the removal of calcium from the bone. Vitamin D deficiency may occur in patients with metabolic disorders, such as hypoparathyroidism and renal osteodystrophy. The requirement for vitamin D is slightly higher in members of darker-pigmented races, since melanin interferes with the irradiation that produces vitamin D_3 in the skin. People with limited exposure to the sun may need to supplement vitamin D intake.

The hypercalcemia resulting from *hypervitaminosis D* is responsible for toxic symptoms such as muscle weakness, bone pain, anorexia, ectopic calcification, hypertension, and cardiac arrhythmias. Toxicity in infants can result in mental and physical retardation, renal failure, and death.

Vitamin E

Vitamin E is a potent antioxidant that is capable of protecting polyunsaturated fatty acids from oxidative breakdown. This vitamin also functions to enhance vitamin A use. Although several other physiological actions have been suggested, to date no unifying concept exists to explain these actions. Vitamin E (α-tocopherol) is found in a variety of foodstuffs, the richest sources being plant oils, including wheat germ and rice, and the lipids of green leaves.

Deficiency of vitamin E is characterized by low serum tocopherol levels and a positive hydrogen peroxide hemolysis test. This deficiency is believed to occur in patients with biliary, pancreatic, or intestinal disease that is characterized by excessive steatorrhea. Premature infants with a high intake of fatty acids exhibit a deficiency syndrome characterized by edema, anemia, and low tocopherol levels. This condition is reversed by giving vitamin E.

Prolonged administration of *large dosages of vitamin E* may result in muscle weakness, fatigue, headache, and nausea. This toxicity can be reversed by discontinuing the large-dose supplementation.

Vitamin K

Vitamin K activity is associated with several quinones, including phylloquinone (vitamin K_1), menadione (vitamin K_3), and a variety of menaquinones (vitamin K_2). These quinones promote the synthesis of proteins that are involved in the coagulation of blood. These proteins include prothrombin, factor VII (proconvertin), factor IX (plasma thromboplastin), and factor X (Stuart factor). A detailed discussion of blood coagulation is found in Chapter 22. The vitamin K quinones are obtained from three major sources. Vitamin K is present in vari-

ous plants, especially green vegetables. The menaquinones that possess vitamin K_2 activity are synthesized by bacteria, particularly gram-positive organisms; the bacteria in the gut of animals produce useful quantities of this vitamin. Vitamin K_3 is a chemically synthesized quinone that possesses the same activity as vitamin K_1.

Vitamin K deficiency results in increased bleeding time. This hypoprothrombinemia may lead to hemorrhage from the gastrointestinal tract, urinary tract, and nasal mucosa. In normal, healthy adults, deficiency is rare. The two groups at greatest risk are newborn infants and patients receiving anticoagulant therapy; hypoprothrombinemia preexists in these two groups. Any disease that causes the malabsorption of fats may lead to deficiency. Inhibition of the growth of intestinal bacteria from extended antibiotic therapy will result in decreased vitamin K synthesis and possible deficiency.

Toxicity of vitamin K has not been well defined. Jaundice may occur in a newborn if large dosages of vitamin K are given to the mother before birth. Although kernicterus may result, this can be prevented by using vitamin K.

Water-Soluble Vitamins
The B Vitamins

The B vitamin group is made up of substances that tend to occur together in foods and are given the collective name vitamin B complex. The vitamins of the B group usually have to be converted to an active form, and most of them play a vital role in intracellular metabolism (Table 68.1). The B vitamins are obtained from both meat and vegetable products, except for vitamin B_{12}, which occurs only in animal products. The richest source of the B vitamin group is seeds, including the germ of wheat or of rice.

The deficiency diseases associated with the lack of the individual B vitamins are briefly described next.

Severe *thiamine (vitamin B_1) deficiency* results in beriberi. The symptoms can include growth retardation, muscular weakness, apathy, edema, and heart failure. Neurological symptoms, such as personality changes and mental deterioration, also may be present in severe cases. Because of the role played by thiamine in metabolic processes in all cells, a mild deficiency may occur when energy needs are increased. Since thiamine is widely distributed in food, beriberi is rare except in communities existing on a single staple cereal food. The disease does occur with some frequency in alcoholics, whose poor diet may lead to an inadequate daily intake of thiamine.

Riboflavin (vitamin B_2) deficiency results in local seborrheic dermatitis that may be limited to the face and scrotum. Other symptoms of ariboflavinosis include angular stomatitis, cheilitis, and glossitis. Specific ocular

TABLE 68.1 The B Vitamins

Vitamin	Active Form	Role
Thiamine (B_1)	Thiamine pyrophosphate	Carbohydrate metabolism
Riboflavin (B_2)	Flavin adenine dinucleotide; flavin mononucleotide	Carbohydrate metabolism
Nicotinic acid (niacin)	Nicotinamide adenine dinucleotide	Dehydrogenation of proteins in cellular respiration
Pyridoxine (B_6)	Pyridoxal phosphate Pyridoxamine phosphate	Amino acid transformations
Pantothenic acid	Coenzyme A	Transfer of acetyl groups
Cyanocobalamin (B_{12})	—	Nucleic acid synthesis
Biotin	—	Fatty acid synthesis
Folic acid (folacin)	Pteroylglutamic acid-containing coenzymes	Nucleic acid synthesis, protein metabolism

signs include vascularization of the cornea and keratitis. This deficiency usually occurs in association with deficiency of other B complex vitamins.

Niacin or *nicotinic acid deficiency* produces the symptoms of pellagra. The clinical picture progresses from an initial phase of general malaise to symptoms including photosensitivity, sore and swollen tongue, gastritis, and diarrhea. Neurological disturbances, depression, and apathy also may occur. Both niacin and the amino acid tryptophan can be converted to diphosphopyridine nucleotide and triphosphopyridine nucleotide. These reactions require the presence of thiamine, riboflavin, and pyridoxine. Therefore, treatment of the symptoms of pellagra should include, in addition to B complex vitamin supplementation, an intake of dietary proteins to provide adequate amounts of tryptophan.

Pyridoxine (vitamin B_6) deficiency symptoms are generally expressed as alterations in the skin, blood, and central nervous system. Symptoms include sensory neuritis, mental depression, and convulsions. Hypochromic, sideroblastic anemia also may result. Since pyridoxine is required for the conversion of tryptophan to diphosphopyridine and triphosphopyridine nucleotides, pellagralike symptoms can occur with vitamin B_6 deficiency. This deficiency is found most often in conjunction with other B complex deficiencies.

The symptoms of *pantothenic acid deficiency* have not been clinically described. Since pantothenic acid is a ubiquitous vitamin, isolated deficiency is unlikely. However, marginal deficiency may exist in persons with general malnutrition.

Severe *cyanocobalamin (vitamin B_{12}) deficiency* results in pernicious anemia that is characterized by megaloblastic anemia and neuropathies. The symptoms of this deficiency can be masked by high intake of folate. Vitamin B_{12} is recycled by an effective enterohepatic circulation and thus has a very long half-life. Absorption of vitamin B_{12} from the gastrointestinal tract requires the presence of gastric intrinsic factor. This factor binds to the vitamin, forming a complex that can now be absorbed in the terminal ileum. Lack of this factor results in pernicious anemia. Following a gastrectomy, patients must be given vitamin B_{12} parenterally. There is no way to determine how many people have undiagnosed vitamin B_{12} deficiency. Since Vitamin B_{12} is found in almost all animal products, dietary deficiencies are rare except in some vegan vegetarians who consume no animal products and need to get their vitamin B_{12} from a supplement. However, marginal nutritional levels of Vitamin B_{12} have been observed in elderly persons, demented patients, AIDS patients, and patients with malignant diseases.

Biotin deficiency is characterized by anorexia, nausea, vomiting, glossitis, depression, and dry, scaly dermatitis. Biotin deficiency occurs when *avidin,* a biotin-binding glycoprotein, is present. Avidin, which is found in raw egg whites, binds the biotin, making it nutritionally unavailable.

Folic acid deficiency symptoms include megaloblastic anemia, glossitis, diarrhea, and weight loss. The requirement for this vitamin increases during pregnancy and lactation.

The effects of most *vitamin B overdoses* have not been documented, although large dosages of pyridoxine have been reported to cause peripheral neuropathies. Ataxia and numbness of the hands and feet and impairment of the senses of pain, touch, and temperature may result. Excessive niacin intake may result in flushing, pruritus, and gastrointestinal disturbances. These symptoms are due to niacin's ability to cause the release of histamine. Large dosages of niacin can result in hepatic toxicity.

Vitamin C

Vitamin C (ascorbic acid) is essential for the maintenance of the ground substance that binds cells together and for the formation and maintenance of collagen. The exact biochemical role it plays in these functions is not known, but it may be related to its ability to act as an oxidation–reduction system.

Vitamin C is found in fresh fruit and vegetables. It is very water soluble, is readily destroyed by heat, especially in an alkaline medium, and is rapidly oxidized in air. Fruit and vegetables that have been stored in air, cut or bruised, washed, or cooked may have lost much of their vitamin C content.

The deficiency disease associated with a lack of ascorbic acid is called scurvy. Early symptoms include malaise and follicular hyperkeratosis. Capillary fragility results in hemorrhages, particularly of the gums. Abnormal bone and tooth development can occur in growing children. The body's requirement for vitamin C increases during periods of stress, such as pregnancy and lactation.

Megavitamin intake of vitamin C may result in diarrhea due to intestinal irritation. Since ascorbic acid is partially metabolized and excreted as oxalate, renal oxalate stones may form in some patients.

THERAPEUTIC USES

All of the vitamins are used as specific treatments for their respective deficiency diseases. The dosages required will vary depending on the severity of the disease and the vitamin. Vitamins have also been used like drugs to "treat" diseases. However, unlike drug products, vitamins are not reviewed by the U. S. Food and Drug Administration before formulations appear on the market. Vitamins are considered to be dietary supplements under the Dietary Supplement Health and Education Act (DSHEA). Vitamins and other dietary supplements are not permitted to be marketed as a treatment or cure for a specific disease or condition unless the vitamin is approved as a drug for that purpose. However, under DSHEA, supplement manufacturers may make health claims, such as the link between a food substance and a disease or health-related condition. This may make it difficult for patients to assess the need for vitamin supplementation.

Legitimate clinical research is being conducted with vitamins in many areas including heart disease, ophthalmological disease, neurocognitive function, and dermatological diseases. It is important for physicians to be aware of scientific information that either supports or refutes a role for vitamins in the maintenance of health or in the avoidance of disease.

Cancer

Vitamin A can suppress many chemically induced tumors in the laboratory. Epidemiological evidence suggests that foods rich in carotenes or vitamin A are associated with a lower risk of cancer. However, the use of vitamin A supplementation is not advised because of the toxicities produced by large amounts of this vitamin.

The antioxidant properties of vitamins C and E can inhibit the formation of some carcinogens. The antioxidant vitamins have been studied as cancer chemopreventive agents for many cancer types, including gastrointestinal and ovarian cancers. However, data are not sufficient to draw conclusions about the vitamins' effects on human cancers.

Coronary Heart Disease

The role of the antioxidant properties of vitamins C, E, and β-carotene in the prevention of cardiovascular disease has been the focus of several recent studies. Antioxidants reduce the oxidation of low-density lipoproteins, which may play a role in the prevention of atherosclerosis. However, an inverse relationship between the intake or plasma levels of these vitamins and the incidence of coronary heart disease has been found in only a few epidemiological studies. One study showed that antioxidants lowered the level of high-density lipoprotein 2 and interfered with the effects of lipid-altering therapies given at the same time. While many groups recommend a varied diet rich in fruits and vegetables for the prevention of coronary artery disease, empirical data do not exist to recommend antioxidant supplementation for the prevention of coronary disease.

Niacin has been used clinically to lower serum cholesterol levels (see Chapter 23). It is used as adjunctive therapy in patients with hyperlipidemia. It is one of the drugs of first choice for patients who do not respond adequately to diet and weight loss.

Miscellaneous Uses

Vitamin A and its retinoid analogues have gained popularity in the treatment of acne and other dermatological diseases (see Chapter 41).

Vitamin K supplements are given to neonates until normal intestinal bacteria that are capable of producing the vitamin develop.

Folic acid supplements are given to pregnant women to decrease the risk of neural tube defects such as spina bifida. Prenatal vitamin preparations that contain higher concentrations of folic acid must be dispensed under a health care worker's guidance because high folate intakes can mask the symptoms of pernicious anemia.

A study of the vitamins in neurocognitive diseases such as Alzheimer's disease have not provided sufficient evidence to demonstrate that vitamins play a role in the prevention of these diseases.

Clinical trials have also been conducted to study the effect of the antioxidants on the progression of age-related macular degeneration (AMD) and vision loss. The Age-Related Eye Disease Study Research Group recommends supplements of zinc and antioxidants for adults at risk for developing AMD. However, the group cautions about unknown long-term effects of high-dose supplementation.

VITAMIN–DRUG INTERACTIONS

Drug interactions and the adverse effects that can result are a special concern. Although vitamins are not always thought of as being drugs, these nutrients can interact with drugs and result in a variety of effects. Vitamin–drug interactions can produce either a decrease or an increase in the effectiveness of the drug; conversely, the intake of drugs can affect the disposition of vitamins in the body. Many drugs, such as some laxatives and cholestyramine, can produce vitamin malabsorption or fecal nutritional loss, resulting in drug-induced nutrient depletion and hypovitaminosis. Both fat-soluble and water-soluble vitamins can be affected by drug intake.

Vitamin A

Vitamin A absorption from the small intestine requires dietary fat and pancreatic lipase to break down retinyl esters and bile salts to promote the uptake of retinol and carotene. Drugs, such as mineral oil, neomycin and cholestyramine, that can modify lipid absorption from the gastrointestinal tract can impair vitamin A absorption. The use of oral contraceptives can significantly increase plasma vitamin A levels.

Since alcohol dehydrogenase is required for the conversion of retinol to retinal, excessive and prolonged ethanol ingestion can impair the physiological function of vitamin A. The decreased conversion of retinol to retinal results from competitive use of the enzyme by ethanol. Night blindness may result, since the visual cycle is a retinol-dependent physiological process.

Vitamin D

Laxatives and agents that bind bile salts inhibit the gastrointestinal absorption of vitamin D. The glucocorticoids in high dosages may interfere with the hepatic metabolism of vitamin D. Prolonged administration of hepatic microsomal enzyme inducers, such as phenobarbital, phenytoin, primidone and glutethimide, can lead to an accelerated degradation of vitamin D_3 to form inactive metabolites. The synthesis of vitamin D_3 can be impaired by physical and chemical barriers to ultraviolet light (e.g., sunscreens).

Vitamin K

The most common group of drugs that produce vitamin K deficiency are the coumarin anticoagulants. The hypoprothrombinemic effects of dicumarol can be overcome by administration of vitamin K.

Vitamin C

Oral contraceptives decrease the plasma levels of ascorbic acid. Aspirin also decreases tissue levels of vitamin C. The renal excretion of acidic and basic drugs may be altered when they are coadministered with large doses of vitamin C.

Vitamin B Complex

Many drugs interact with folate to affect its absorption, antagonize its biochemical activity, or increase its loss from the body. These drugs include ethanol, phenytoin, and oral contraceptives. Salicylates can compete with folic acid for plasma protein binding. Methotrexate, a cytotoxic agent, is a folate antagonist that inhibits the biosynthesis of this coenzyme.

Many drug classes have been shown either to act as vitamin B_6 antagonists or to increase vitamin B_6 turnover. Alcohol decreases the production of pyridoxal phosphate, the coenzyme formed from vitamin B_6. Hydrazines, such as isoniazid, act as coenzyme inhibitors. Cycloserine, an antitubercular drug, and penicillamine, a chelating agent, inactivate the coenzyme. Steroid hormones, such as those in oral contraceptive preparations, compete with the coenzyme. Pyridoxine can decrease the efficacy of levodopa, an antiparkinsonian drug, by stimulating the decarboxylation of dopa to dopamine in peripheral tissues. Phenobarbital and phenytoin serum levels may be decreased following pyridoxine supplementation.

Four groups of drugs have been shown to affect the absorption of vitamin B_{12}. These include the oral hypoglycemic biguanides, colchicine, ethanol, and aminosalicylic acid.

Drug-induced niacin deficiency has resulted from the use of isonicotinic acid hydrazide, which interferes with the conversion of niacin from tryptophan. Administration of ethanol or the antimetabolites 6-mercaptopurine and 5-fluorouracil also may lead to niacin deficiency. The uricosuric effects of sulfinpyrazone and probenecid may be inhibited by nicotinic acid.

Drugs that increase intestinal motility or induce diarrhea may decrease riboflavin absorption. Hyperthyroidism and the administration of thyroxine also reduce riboflavin absorption.

Alcoholics may have both decreased intake and decreased absorption of thiamine. Liver disease can prevent the formation of the active coenzyme.

ANEMIA

Anemia occurs when the hemoglobin concentration of blood is reduced below normal levels. This condition may result from chronic blood loss, abnormal hemolysis, or nutritional deficiency. Many therapeutic agents can induce this change in hemoglobin as an unwanted side effect.

Different classifications of anemia are based in part on the pathophysiological factor inducing the decreased hemoglobin concentration. Anemias due to cell hypoproliferation include aplastic anemia and iron deficiency anemia. Hemolytic anemia results from excessive destruction of red blood cells. Megaloblastic anemia, sideroblastic anemia, and iron deficiency anemia result from an abnormality in the maturation of red blood cells.

Iron Deficiency Anemia

Iron is a constituent of hemoglobin, and iron deficiency will lead to a decrease in hemoglobin synthesis. Since iron is conserved by the body, deficiency usually results from acute or chronic loss of blood or insufficient iron intake during physiological stress. Infants, children, and premenopausal women require more iron than do men because of the increased demand that occurs during growth, pregnancy, and loss of blood during menstruation. In tropical climates, bleeding due to an infestation by the hookworm parasite is a common cause of iron deficiency.

The symptoms of iron deficiency anemia include fatigue, weakness, shortness of breath, and soreness of the tongue. Therapeutic iron supplementation is used to treat this type of anemia. Oral administration of ferrous salts (generic ferrous sulfate, *Feosol, Slo Fe*) is preferred, but parenteral iron (iron dextran, *InfeD*) can be given if oral therapy fails. Toxic reactions occur more frequently after parenteral iron administration. Gastrointestinal disturbances are common following oral dosages.

Antacids may decrease the gastrointestinal absorption of iron. Iron may chelate or decrease the gastrointestinal absorption of drugs like levodopa and tetracycline.

Megaloblastic Anemia

Megaloblastic anemia is characterized by the appearance of large cells in the bone marrow and blood due to defective maturation of hematopoietic cells. Folic acid or vitamin B_{12} deficiency will result in this type of anemia. Malabsorption, impaired use, chronic infections, and drugs can lead to folic acid or vitamin B_{12} deficiency.

Folic acid or folate salts (*Folvite*) are administered to correct folate-deficient megaloblastic anemia. Vitamin B_{12}–deficient patients receive cyanocobalamin supplements. Dosage is very important, since patients with severe megaloblastic anemia may develop hypokalemia and die suddenly if treated intensively with vitamin B_{12}. Vitamin B_{12} deficiency due to a lack of gastric intrinsic factor results in pernicious anemia. This type of megaloblastic anemia causes neurological damage if it is not treated. Treatment of Vitamin B_{12}–deficient megaloblastic anemia with folic acid may improve the symptoms; however, neurological damage may still occur if vitamin B_{12} intake is not supplemented. Parenteral injections of vitamin B_{12} must be given.

Sideroblastic Anemia

Sideroblastic anemia is characterized by excessive iron in the cells that cannot be incorporated into porphyrin to form heme. Although it is rare, the most common cause of sideroblastic anemia is alcoholism and pyridoxine deficiency. Pyridoxine is required for the formation of pyridoxal phosphate, a coenzyme in porphyrin synthesis.

Study Questions

1. A patient with pancreatic disease complains of difficulty driving at night because of vision problems. Ulceration of the cornea is detected on ophthalmic examination. Which of the following should be recommended?
   (A) Supplementation with vitamin B complex
   (B) Supplementation with vitamin A
   (C) Decreased intake of vitamin A
   (D) Supplementation of diet with more red meat
   (E) Decreased vitamin C intake

2. A patient comes into the clinic for a pregnancy test. It is positive. Which of the following should be recommended?
   (A) A multivitamin without iron
   (B) A multivitamin with iron
   (C) A diet rich in carrots
   (D) No vitamin supplement
   (E) A vitamin A supplement

3. Capillary fragility, malaise, and abnormal bone and tooth development describe a deficiency of which vitamin?
   (A) Vitamin A
   (B) Vitamin B_6
   (C) Vitamin C
   (D) Riboflavin
   (E) Vitamin E

4. Which vitamin can mask the symptoms of pernicious anemia by alleviating the anemia but not preventing the neurological damage?
   (A) Vitamin B_{12}
   (B) Niacin
   (C) Folic acid

(D) Vitamin C

(E) Vitamin D

5. An epileptic patient who is taking phenytoin and lamotrigine to control her seizures is in the first month of pregnancy and definitely wants to have the baby. What vitamin supplement would be essential?

(A) Vitamin B$_6$

(B) Vitamin D

(C) Vitamin C

(D) Niacin

(E) Folic Acid

ANSWERS

1. **B.** Supplement with vitamin A. Vitamin A deficiency symptoms include night blindness that can lead to corneal ulceration. This deficiency can occur in patients with impaired liver storage or fat malabsorption. Dairy products, such as milk, are a good source of vitamin A. β-Carotene, a vitamin A precursor, is found in pigmented vegetables, such as carrots. When a deficiency is diagnosed, it is appropriate to treat the patient with a supplement rather than to rely on increased consumption of vitamin A–rich foods. A patient with pancreatic disease and malabsorption syndrome will need parenteral supplementation.

2. **B.** Pregnancy increases the need for vitamins and iron in general. Folic acid has been shown to decrease the risk of neural tube defects, such as spina bifida. It is important to assess the nutritional status of the patient to determine whether higher levels of folic acid are needed. Vitamin A is a teratogen and should not be given in high doses during pregnancy.

3. **C.** Early symptoms of vitamin C deficiency, or scurvy, include malaise. Hemorrhages, especially of the gums, may result from capillary fragility.

4. **C.** The only effective treatment of pernicious anemia is supplementation of vitamin B$_{12}$. It is important to determine whether megaloblastic anemia is from a deficiency of folic acid or vitamin B$_{12}$. Treatment of vitamin B$_{12}$–deficient anemia with folic acid may result in neurological damage if vitamin B$_{12}$ is not adequately supplemented.

5. **E.** Folic acid supplements should be given to all pregnant women. In addition, phenytoin use is associated with lowered folate levels.

SUPPLEMENTAL READING

AREDS Report No. 8. A randomized, placebo-controlled, clinical trial of high-dose supplementation with vitamins C and E, beta carotene, and zinc for age-related macular degeneration and vision loss. Arch Ophthalmol 2001;119:1417.

Combs GF. The Vitamins: Fundamental Aspects in Nutrition and Health (2nd ed.). San Diego: Academic, 1998.

Fleming A. The role of folate in the prevention of neural tube defects: Human and animal studies. Nutr Rev 2001;58:S13.

Gaytan RJ and Prisant LM. Oral nutritional supplements and heart disease: A review. Am J Ther 2001;8:255.

Institute of Medicine. Dietary Reference Intakes for Thiamin, Riboflavin, Niacin, Vitamin B$_6$, Folate, Vitamin B$_{12}$, Pantothenic Acid, Biotin, and Choline. Washington: National Academy, 1998.

Rosenberg IH. B Vitamins, homocysteine, and neurocognitive function. Nutr Rev 2001;59:S69.

Sarubin A. The Health Professional's Guide to Popular Dietary Supplements. Chicago: American Dietetic Association, 2000.

Willett WC and Stampfer MJ. What vitamins should I be taking, doctor? N Engl J Med 2001;345:1819.

C A S E **Study**   Vitamin Deficiency and Alcoholism

A patient has muscular weakness, apathy, and edema in both legs. You schedule a series of tests, including a cardiac stress test. The results of the stress test suggest that the patient is in moderate congestive heart failure. The patient suffered a personal loss last year with the death of a son. Soon after his son's death he began drinking heavily. You suspect that the drinking is responsible for his present condition. Give an analysis of this clinical picture.

Answer: The symptoms resemble those you remember from medical school for beriberi, but you fail to see the connection. Then a light clicks on. If the patient were consuming most of his calories as alcohol, he may have a nutritional deficiency, a beriberi-like syndrome, as a result of insufficient intake of thiamine. You prescribe a daily vitamin tablet and admonish the patient to cut back on alcohol intake. At the next appointment, the edema is much better and the cardiac stress tests results are normal. He has joined Alcoholics Anonymous and indicates that he is doing better.

69 | Herbal Medicine

Gregory Juckett

 DRUG LIST

Herbal therapies have become an integral part of the American health care scene. Since 1991, public use of herbal products has increased quite markedly, with over $5 billion spent annually. This does not include the many (up to 25%) pharmaceutical products used in conventional practice that originally were, and in some cases still are, derived from plants (Table 69.1). The perennial appeal of herbs may stem from their "natural" origin, giving them the reputation of being somehow safer and better tolerated than prescription drugs. In addition, they are available without prescription, often at much lower cost. For much of the world's population, herbal treatments remain the first and sometimes the only available treatment. Proponents of herbal therapy also state that the multiple compounds found in most herbal preparations have the advantage of acting *synergistically;* that is, they act in concert to produce a more enhanced effect than would a single isolated component. An example is St. John's wort (*Hypericum perfoliatum*), which contains not only hypericin, the ingredient it is usually standardized for, but also hyperforin and a variety of other compounds. It is now believed that these other ingredients, far from be-ing extraneous, contribute significantly to the herb's effectiveness.

The study of natural product medicines is termed *pharmacognosy,* which includes the study of herbal medicine. The resurgence of herbal medicine use has once again made pharmacognosy extremely relevant to the medical curriculum.

HERBAL MEDICINE TRADITIONS

The popular *western herbalism* discussed in this chapter is one of many philosophical systems of herbal treatment. It is also sometimes described as *eclectic,* since it has drawn on many other traditions, including the native American and Chinese. *Chinese traditional medicine, Ayurvedic* (Indian), and *Tibetan* traditions use complex herbal recipes and nutrition to achieve "balance" in the ill patient. Although these practices are most commonly found in ethnic populations, they are also becoming popular in some western complementary and alternative circles.

Homeopathic treatments frequently bear herbal names and are often confused with allopathic herbal

TABLE 69.1 Plant-Derived Medicines

Active Ingredients	Botanical Source
Aspirin (acetylsalicylic acid)	Willow bark (salicylic acid)
Atropine	Belladonna nightshade
Capsaicin	Pepper plant
Colchicine	Autumn crocus
Digitalis	Foxglove
Morphine	Opium poppy
Pilocarpine	Jaborandi tree
Podophyllin	Mayapple root
Quinine	Cinchona bark
Reserpine	Indian snake root
Taxol	Pacific yew tree bark
Vincristine, vinblastine	Madagascar periwinkle

TABLE 69.2 Herbal Formulations

Formulation	Means of Preparation
Infusion	Near-boiling water poured on herb for 5–10 minutes
Tea (tisane)	Infusion of aromatic herbs
Decoction	Simmer herb for 15 minutes, then strain
Maceration	Steep herb in room-temperature water
Tincture	Steep herb in ethyl alcohol and water
Fluid extract	1 part herb to 1 part ethyl alcohol
Glycerin extract	Steep herb in glycerin–water mix
Juice	Juice expressed by crushing herb
Inhalation	Breathe in vapor from heated herb mix
Oil	Steep herb in olive or other plant oil
Ointment	Herb salve made with lanolin or beeswax
Lozenge	Herb preparation that dissolves in the mouth
Powder	Dried powdered herb
Tablet	Compressed herb material in pill form
Capsule	Encapsulated herbal material
Syrup	Concentrated sugar solution to preserve infusion
Compress	Cloth soaked in herbal solution
Poultice	Application of moist herbal paste

preparations. The difference is that homeopathic remedies are serially diluted and shaken until they may lack any molecule of the original herb ingredient. Therefore, there is no risk of pharmacological toxicity from a homeopathic preparation. *Bach's Flower Remedies* are a homeopathic variation in which flower essences are created by floating flowers in sunlit water. These essences are usually intended as remedies for emotional and spiritual rather than specific physical complaints.

Aromatherapy uses a variety of fragrant plant oils to treat mood or physical problems either topically (as an adjunct to massage) or through inhalation. Some of these oils are quite potent, and if not used in proper dilution, they may cause skin irritation or contact allergy. Toxic ingestions are also possible.

Herbs from these traditions often are administered in a confusing array of preparations (Table 69.2). In the U. S. market, tablet and capsule formulations are the most popular, while overseas, *teas* or *infusions* of herbs are the most widely used. *Tinctures* consist of an herb steeped in a mix of alcohol and water, and *extracts* consist of one part herb to one part ethyl alcohol. The alcohol content can be a concern, particularly with children. Some of these products have been withdrawn by the U. S. Food and Drug Administration (FDA) for this reason but may still be available outside the United States.

POTENTIAL CONCERNS

Detractors of herbal medicine use have legitimate concerns about dosage variability, possible toxicity and adulteration, herb–drug interactions, and above all, lack of FDA regulation. Far from being intrinsically harmless, many pharmacologically active plant alkaloids and other compounds are natural defensive poisons; their very effectiveness may be an unanticipated consequence of their adaptive toxicity to grazing animals and

insects. Thus, herbal products like digitalis, while quite "natural," may also be dangerous or even fatal in overdose. Other herbs may not be superior to better-researched pharmaceuticals, or they may delay the use of more effective therapy. While herbal research has understandably lagged far behind that of patented medications, a surprising number of clinical trials exist, although some of them are fraught with methodological problems and much of the data is foreign and therefore not readily accessible to U. S. physicians. There is also the frustrating problem of interpreting conflicting research results; it is possible to assemble impressive arrays of studies both supporting and questioning the effectiveness of a particular herbal product. These conflicting findings may result from flawed study design, the use of differing preparations, or different study end points. Unfortunately, despite the recent increase in herb research, significant gaps in knowledge remain. An additional concern is that few if any available studies have been conducted on pregnant women or children.

Some herbal preparations, particularly some unbranded Asian imports, have been found to contain inactive fillers or *adulterants*. In one assessment, 24% of imported herbs were found to contain ingredients not on the label. These included specific medications (aspirin, caffeine, diuretics, and even benzodiazepines), not to mention heavy metals, such as lead. Some Asian formulations may also contain animal components. Therefore, it is advisable to buy only products that list the following information: botanical name or names, parts used, expiration date, batch or lot number, and the manufacturer's name and address.

Of special concern today are the possible *herb–drug interactions* with which patients and their health care providers must be familiar. Some herbs, such as ginkgo, garlic, ginger, chamomile, horse chestnut, and feverfew, can prolong bleeding time and should be avoided with coumadin and antiplatelet regimens. It is also necessary that they be stopped 2 weeks prior to surgery. Other herbs, including kava, St. John's wort, and valerian, also must be discontinued prior to surgery because they can unpredictably alter the effects of common anesthetics. *Panax* ginseng may cause blood pressure fluctuations, and some herbs, notably St. John's wort, may lower the blood levels of many coadministered medications. For this reason, it is critical for consumers and their health care providers to maintain an open dialogue about herb use; the use of over-the-counter herbs and supplements should be inquired about when obtaining a medical history. Patients are frequently reluctant to discuss their herb use either because they fear disapproval or because of the all too often correct perception that the provider is not knowledgeable enough to warrant giving the information. *Blanket condemnation of herb use often has the counterproductive effect of terminating any further communication between physician and patient.*

REGULATORY ISSUES

The explosion in popularity of herbs dates to the *Dietary Supplement Health and Education Act of 1994 (DSHEA)*, in which the FDA recognized herbal preparations as dietary supplements outside of its direct regulatory control. The act was a compromise between the FDA and manufacturing lobbies brought about in large measure by increased public demand for herbal products. Instead of FDA regulation, these products now fall under the far less stringent Current Good Manufacturing Practice for Human Foods. Unlike prescription pharmaceuticals, which must be proved safe and effective before being marketed, supplements do not have to be either safe or effective as long as they avoid therapeutic claims on the label. Neither are they policed in regard to delivering accurate doses, although some consumer-oriented organizations, such as *Consumer Lab* (www.ConsumerLab.com), are starting to hold manufacturers more accountable through random testing and reporting of their results. Supplements are permitted to have *"structure–function"* statements on their label stating only the product's supposed physiological function. For instance, an Echinacea product label might read "supports immune function" but may not claim to prevent or abort the common cold. The FDA recommended in 1999 an improved dietary supplement labeling system with a supplement facts panel that is be-

TABLE 69.3 Potentially Toxic Herbs

Herbal Preparation	Type of Toxicity
Aristolochia	Nephrotoxicity
Bloodroot	General toxicity
Chaparral tea	Liver toxicity
Coltsfoot tea	Possible carcinogen, liver toxicity
Comfrey tea	Liver toxicity
Ephedra (ma huang)	Arrhythmias, stroke, elevated blood pressure
Lobelia	Nervous system toxicity, respiratory paralysis
Pennyroyal	CNS stimulation
Sassafras (safrole) tea	Carcinogen
Yohimbe	CNS stimulation, psychosis

ing gradually adopted by the industry. Future legislation may further tighten the quite lax U. S. regulatory environment. Unsafe herbs (Table 69.3) also will be increasingly restricted.

The European system differs from that of the United States in that the manufacture of the more pharmacologically active herbs is for the most part regulated and is much more widely accepted by the medical community. Many health care providers routinely prescribe herbal treatments either alongside or in place of more conventional medications. The German government's *Commission E* publishes a set of herbal monographs that not only officially sets the standard for that country but has also become a widely respected clinical reference throughout the world.

HERBAL PREPARATIONS

Echinacea

The purple coneflower *Echinacea purpura,* and its close relatives, *E. angustifolia* and *E. pallida,* are the source of the herb Echinacea, which is widely popular as a nonspecific immune stimulant. These perennials are native to the prairies of North America and are now widely grown garden ornamentals. The root and aerial parts of the plant are the portions used, and the preparation's potency can be verified by the transient tingling sensation produced when it is tasted. Echinacea contains alkamides, caffeic acid esters (echinacoside, cichoric acid, caftaric acid), polysaccharides (heteroxylan), and an essential oil. Some echinacea products are standardized for their *echinacoside* content. In the past, adulteration with American feverfew (*Parthenium integrifolium*) was common. Echinacea is now sold either by itself or in combination with golden seal or zinc for the treatment of colds and influenza.

Mechanism of Action

Echinacea extracts appear to stimulate the number and activity of immune cells (i.e., increasing physiological levels of tumor necrosis factor and other cytokines) and to increase leukocyte mobility and phagocytosis. The extracts also have antiviral and antiinflammatory properties and inhibit bacterial hyaluronidase.

Indications

There are numerous studies on echinacea in the literature, many of which indicate either an in vitro immune stimulation or a significant clinical reduction in the severity and duration of upper respiratory viral symptoms, especially when taken early in the onset of symptoms. Despite several of these meta-analyses concluding that echinacea is an effective immunomodulator of acute infection, there is still controversy as to the extent of its clinical effectiveness. A number of trials now clearly indicate that echinacea is unlikely to be effective in the prevention of colds, even if it may slightly shorten their course.

In vitro antiinflammatory effects have been documented, and the herb has a long history of being used externally for wound healing, psoriasis, and the reduction of skin irritation. Although there are a few small positive studies, the available evidence is not yet conclusive in regard to clinical use.

Adverse Reactions, Contraindications, and Interactions

Echinacea appears to be a very safe herb, producing only minor gastrointestinal (GI) side effects and an occasional allergic reaction, usually in atopic patients already sensitized to other members of the Compositae plant family. Anaphylaxis has occurred rarely. Use in HIV is discouraged because of the concern that long-term therapy may eventually suppress the immune system.

It is recommended that echinacea not be taken by anyone for more than 8 continuous weeks, and most clinical use is under 2 weeks' duration. Echinacea has not yet been shown to be safe in pregnant or breastfeeding women and small children. No specific herb–drug interactions are reported, but for theoretical reasons those taking immunosuppressant drugs should avoid echinacea.

Dose

Usually echinacea is given as a capsule, but it is also available as an alcohol-based tincture. The use of echinacea tea is less desirable, since not all of the components are water soluble. Unfortunately, there are significant differences in the potency of commercially available supplies, depending on the plant species and the part and age of the plant used.

Conclusion

While it is still controversial, there is some evidence that echinacea stimulates the immune system and may mitigate some of the symptoms of viral infection. However, it does not appear to be helpful in *preventing* viral infections, and long-term use should be avoided.

Feverfew

Feverfew (*Tanacetum parthenium*) is a common European composite herb with daisylike white flowers now widely naturalized in the United States. While its name (a corrupted version of the Latin *febrifugia*) indicates a long history in herb lore, feverfew's current popularity is due to its use in the prevention and treatment of migraines. Feverfew has also been used for rheumatoid arthritis and numerous other conditions with far less substantiation. The leaves contain sesquiterpene lactones, including *parthenolide*, which is thought to be the most active and important ingredient. Feverfew preparations are frequently standardized for parthenolide content, which can vary substantially depending on time of harvest (levels drop after seeds form) and other factors. Most studies have used feverfew standardized to 0.6 to 0.7% parthenolide; the value of leaves containing less than 0.2% parthenolide is questionable.

Mechanism of Action

Parthenolide inhibits serotonin release, an action that is thought to be a likely source of its effectiveness in migraine. Extracts have also been shown to reduce the production of prostaglandins (another possible mechanism) and leukotrienes. Interestingly, *melatonin* has been identified in feverfew, a possibly significant observation, since chronic migraines have been associated with low melatonin levels.

Indications

At least three studies have demonstrated that feverfew (dried leaf, not extract) can reduce the frequency and severity of migraine headaches, although one study failed to find any significant difference from placebo. Prophylaxis appears to be more effective than acute treatment. There is also a consensus that feverfew is probably less effective than conventional migraine prophylaxis, although it may have a role as a second-line option. Although feverfew has also been used for rheumatism, it has never been verified to be effective in clinical trials.

Adverse Reactions, Contraindications, and Interactions

Although feverfew appears generally safe in nonpregnant adults, the use of fresh leaves has caused *mouth irritation* and even ulceration. This is far less likely to occur when the herb is encapsulated. *Allergic reactions* (contact dermatitis) have occurred with topical use in sensitized individuals, and ingestion may also produce allergic reactions in people with preexisting allergies to members of the Compositae family. Feverfew has caused contractions in term pregnancy and has been implicated in cattle abortions and so should be avoided in pregnancy and lactation. A *feverfew withdrawal syndrome* consisting of joint pain and muscle stiffness may occur following abrupt discontinuation. Theoretically, because of its antiprostaglandin effects, feverfew should not be coadministered with *anticoagulants* or *antiplatelet drugs*.

Dosage

For migraine prophylaxis: 50 to 125 mg per day with food, preferably in capsule form to prevent mouth irritation.

Conclusion

Feverfew may be considered as an *alternative migraine prophylaxis* regimen in patients failing to respond to conventional therapy. It has not been shown to be effective for rheumatoid arthritis. There is insufficient evidence to support its use in other conditions.

Garlic

Garlic (*Allium sativum*) is an ancient culinary and medicinal herb related to the onion and reputed to have many health benefits. Today it is popularly used to lower cholesterol and blood pressure and is even reputed to reduce the risk of cancer. It is also taken for its antimicrobial effects. The active ingredient, *allicin,* is the source of garlic's famous odor, and many sulfur-containing garlic constituents are derived from it. Odorless *alliin,* found in the garlic bulb, is converted to allicin by the enzyme *allinase,* which is released by chopping or cutting. Aged or cooked garlic has less odor but also much less active allicin.

Mechanism of Action

Garlic clearly has *antithrombotic* properties. Ajoene (an allicin metabolite) and methyl allyl trisulfide inhibit platelet aggregation. Garlic may promote *vasodilation* by relaxing smooth muscle, and it may *reduce low-density lipoprotein (LDL) oxidation.*

Indications

Some studies support garlic having a modest but significant effect on lowering total cholesterol, LDL cholesterol, and triglycerides and raising high-density lipoprotein (HDL) cholesterol. More recent studies have found no significant effect, even though similar preparations and doses were used. Therefore, the effectiveness of garlic for this indication remains unresolved. Likewise,

some *blood pressure* studies have shown a modest reduction in diastolic more than systolic blood pressures, while others have not.

The antifungal effect of allicin in fresh garlic extract has been demonstrated against cryptococcal meningitis and a variety of yeasts and fungi. However, this effectiveness appears diminished in commercial preparations. Fresh but not aged garlic also appears to have activity against *Escherichia coli, Staphylococcus aureus,* and a variety of bacteria and viruses. Topical use also appears to be effective, albeit with occasional local irritation being produced. The high oral dosages of fresh garlic required for *antimicrobial* treatment may make clinical use less feasible due to odor and side effects. Garlic has been shown to reduce cancer susceptibility in mice, but epidemiological studies in human colorectal and other cancers are mixed.

For lipid reduction, garlic is used at 600 to 900 mg daily, usually divided into three doses, or 4 g fresh garlic or 8 ml of garlic oil daily.

Adverse Reactions, Contraindications, Interactions

Garlic can cause heartburn, nausea, and loose stools at high doses, especially in those unaccustomed to it. Its most characteristic and troublesome side effect, however, is persisting *breath odor,* which no amount of tooth brushing will eradicate. Allicin and its odoriferous metabolic products are actually released into the lung alveoli and exhaled.

Allergic contact dermatitis and even burns from prolonged skin contact with the cloves have been reported. Systemic allergy with bronchospasm or hives from ingestion occurs rarely. There is some concern that chronic high doses may lead to decreased hemoglobin production.

Garlic should be avoided in gastroesophageal reflux disease and peptic ulcer disease. High doses should be avoided in pregnancy. Garlic does pass into breast milk but so far has not been shown to be harmful. Cases of botulism have been reported from chopped garlic or garlic oil left out for long periods at room temperature. Administration of garlic with anticoagulant and antiplatelet drugs should be avoided because of the risk of bleeding.

Conclusion

Fresh garlic may have some cardiovascular benefits, but it is unclear whether it lowers blood lipids or blood pressure as much as originally thought. Aged preparations and cooked garlic are likely to be less effective despite being better tolerated.

Ginkgo Biloba Leaf Extract

Ginkgo, or maidenhair tree (*Ginkgo biloba*), is thought to be the most ancient of living tree species, and it is now also one of the top selling herbs in Europe and the United States because of its reputed ability to improve cognitive function. *Ginkgo leaf extract* is prepared from ginkgo leaf by a complex process that removes toxic *ginkgolic acid*. This reduces the risk of allergic reactions to the leaves if they are consumed directly. Ginkgo leaf extract contains *24% flavone glycosides* (including the antioxidant *rutin,* which improves capillary fragility) and *6% terpene lactones.*

Mechanism of Action

Ginkgo leaf extract appears to act primarily as a mild *cerebral vasodilator* that increases cerebral blood flow and reduces blood viscosity. *Ginkgolides* inhibit platelet activating factor, and this may improve microcirculatory blood flow in atherosclerotic disease with slightly increased risk of bleeding. There appears to be an antioxidant effect that may be neuroprotective. Although some studies suggested a monoamine oxidase inhibitor (MAOI) effect, this is considered to have questionable clinical relevance.

Indications

Ginkgo leaf extract is most popular for cognitive disorders, including memory loss, dementia, and cerebrovascular insufficiency. A number of well-designed clinical trials have shown modest benefit in Alzheimer's disease, with ginkgo extract appearing as effective as second-generation cholinesterase inhibitors. At least one large (214 patient) study, however, failed to show a memory improvement in dementia patients. Studies are now under way to see whether ginkgo use will protect against development of Alzheimer's disease.

Intermittent claudication appears to benefit from ginkgo therapy: many studies demonstrate improved walking distance and decreased pain. One meta-analysis of eight studies documented statistically significant improvement but questioned its clinical relevance. In some studies, the high doses (240 mg) appeared more effective.

Vertigo and *tinnitus* are difficult to treat conditions for which ginkgo is frequently recommended. At least two trials support the use of gingko extract for vertigo, but the evidence for tinnitus remains inconclusive.

Other suggested uses include sexual dysfunction secondary to selective serotonin reuptake inhibitors (SSRIs), macular degeneration, premenstrual syndrome, and the prevention of acute mountain sickness at high altitude. Some of these uses are supported only by a single study.

Adverse reactions, Contraindications, and Interactions

Allergic reactions are a significant concern with unprocessed ginkgo leaf (ginkgolic acid) but are much less likely to occur with the leaf extract. The malodorous ginkgo fruit cross-reacts with poison ivy (urushiol) and may cause an identical contact dermatitis.

Children eating large numbers (>50) of the uncooked ginkgo kernels have had seizures, and consequently there is some concern about using high doses of ginkgo in seizure patients. However, most patients tolerate gingko extract very well, with only occasional GI upset or headache being reported, and the product is considered safe for healthy nonpregnant adults.

Bleeding complications are an infrequent but serious concern, with subdural hematomas, subarachnoid hemorrhages, hyphema (bleeding of the iris), and surgical bleeding occasionally reported. Stopping ginkgo administration prior to surgery and the avoidance of its use with anticoagulant drugs and perhaps with aspirin is recommended. Use of ginkgo extract should be *avoided in pregnant women and children,* since at least one study showed in a ginkgo preparation small amounts of colchicine, a compound that can block cellular division and cause abortion; however, it is unclear whether this is a problem in all ginkgo preparations.

Ginkgo may reduce the effectiveness of *thiazide diuretics* for blood pressure control and at least theoretically should be avoided with MAOIs. There is also a suggestion that ginkgo may decrease male and female fertility, and it should be avoided in those trying to conceive.

Dose

For cognitive function, total daily doses of 120 to 240 mg divided into 2 or 3 doses of ginkgo leaf extract are recommended. For intermittent claudication, 240 mg a day would be preferable.

Conclusion

The preponderance of evidence indicates that ginkgo is an effective mild cerebral and perhaps general vasodilator that may mitigate cognitive decline in the elderly. Its effect on memory in younger adults is less clear; although some studies show a benefit, others do not. Ginkgo should be avoided with anticoagulants and used with caution with antiplatelet medication. Although ginkgo's effectiveness in intermittent claudication, vertigo, SSRI-induced sexual dysfunction, acute mountain sickness, and other indications may not yet be well enough established for widespread clinical use, this ancient herb may still play a role in 21st-century medicine.

Ginseng

Panax ginseng describes the root from two species of plants, *Asian* ginseng (*Panax ginseng*) and *American* ginseng (*Panax quinquefolius*), popularly used for improving stamina and providing a sense of well-being. The terms red and white ginseng refer to how the root is processed, not the species of origin. *Red* ginseng roots are steam-cured prior to drying, while *white* ginseng is bleached and dried. Panax ginsengs contain triterpenoid saponins called *ginsenosides* (also called *panaxosides*), of which up to 18 types are recognized as having differing and sometimes opposing pharmacological properties.

Siberian ginseng (*Eleutherococcus senticosus*) should not be confused with Panax ginseng. Although it belongs to the same plant family (Araliaceae), it is a much larger, more abundant, and consequently less expensive plant. Like Panax ginseng, however, it is used as a tonic and adaptogen, a nonmedical term meaning that it helps the body adapt to stress in a variety of ways. Siberian ginseng does contain saponins (*eleutherosides*) but no ginsenosides. To date, in spite of its popularity, there is little conclusive evidence of clinical efficacy.

Mechanism of Action

Ginsenosides are thought to be the active principles in Panax ginseng root. The various subtypes can have opposing pharmacological actions: Rg1 stimulates the central nervous system (CNS) and elevates blood pressure, while Rb1 does just the opposite. Somehow these multiple ginsenoside constituents are thought to act in concert to provide increased stamina. In addition, these compounds have antiplatelet aggregation effects and antioxidant properties, and they may stimulate the immune system.

Indications

Despite the long popularity of ginseng and its evident mild stimulatory effect, there is less conclusive evidence for its clinical effectiveness than for many of the other herbs discussed in this chapter. In regard to improving cognitive function, most studies have failed to prove a consistent benefit. A recent investigation of ginseng's effect on physical stamina found that an 8-week course of therapy failed to improve aerobic *work capacity*. Ginseng has been studied as a diabetic agent, with reduced hemoglobin A1c levels and improved glucose control being documented in a small trial. Although there is some intriguing work with ginseng as a cancer preventive, there is not enough evidence to suggest its clinical use at this time.

Adverse Reactions, Contraindications, and Interactions

Ginseng is generally considered safe for nonpregnant healthy adults; however, at sufficient doses, ginseng may elevate blood pressure and cause insomnia, palpitations, nervousness, and tremor in susceptible individuals. These effects are increased if caffeine or other stimulants are taken concurrently. Both Panax and Siberian ginsengs should definitely be avoided in any patient with poorly controlled hypertension. Dizziness, headache, diarrhea, and nausea have also been reported. A controversial *ginseng abuse syndrome* consisting of tremor, elevated blood pressure, insomnia, and anxiety may also occur.

Diabetic patients have had hypoglycemia on ginseng, so sugars must be monitored, and insulin or other hypoglycemic medication dosages may have to be reduced. The use of ginseng with anticoagulants (e.g., warfarin) and antiplatelet drugs is to be avoided because of the theoretical risk of increased bleeding. Also, coadministration of ginseng with digoxin and MAOIs should be avoided.

Dose

Capsules of powdered root (100, 250, and 500 mg) are available, and doses range from *200 to 600 mg per day*. Ginseng may also be taken as a tea or extract. A *3-month maximum* treatment course followed by a 2-week break between courses has been recommended. A major concern is that many commercial preparations do not contain the quantity of herb stated on the label. In one assessment of 54 tested ginseng products, 60% showed subtherapeutic amounts of active ingredients, and 25% showed no evidence of any ginseng at all.

Conclusion

Ginseng has been popular for more than 2000 years as a tonic for improved stamina and sense of well-being, particularly in the elderly. Although subjective quality of life reports substantiate this tradition, objective evidence of improved cognitive function and physical stamina remains incomplete or lacking. Further studies of standardized ginseng preparations will be necessary to clarify its use in fatigue and diabetes.

Kava

Kava-kava (*Piper methysticum*) is a South Pacific island shrub the rhizome or root of which was used in the past as a ceremonial beverage and that today is popular as an *anxiolytic*. Historically, women prepared the kava by pounding and then chewing it. After being allowed to ferment in bowls, the kava was drunk by male islanders to mark a special event. The herb would induce a pleasant euphoric tranquility and contribute to the group's social cohesion. The active ingredients are thought to be *kavapyrones* (also known as kavalactones), a family of related synergistically active compounds that include *kawain* and *methysticin*.

Mechanism of Action

The exact mechanism of action is unclear, but it is thought that kavapyrones may act in the amygdala, producing a tranquilizing and muscle relaxant effect.

Despite inducing mild sedation and euphoria, there is usually no cognitive or memory impairment at typical doses. Chewing the root results in a *local anesthetic* effect with temporary numbness. High doses may cause gait impairment, dilated pupils, and eventually impaired motor performance.

Indications

Kava may be effective for the short-term treatment of anxiety. A number of small trials have shown extracts, standardized to 70% kavapyrones, to be significantly and consistently more effective than placebo. Additional studies suggest that kava acts centrally as a *muscle relaxant* and likely has *neuroprotective* and nonopioid *analgesic* properties.

Adverse Reactions, Contraindications, and Interactions

Although kava was considered relatively safe until recently, GI upset, headache, allergic skin reactions, elevated liver function tests, and rare extrapyramidal reactions may occur. It should be avoided in patients with known liver disease. Slowed reflexes and diminished judgment may occur at high doses. Heavy chronic use may produce a psychological (rather than physiological) *habituation* and a pellagralike skin condition known as *kava dermatitis* characterized by reddened eyes and dry flaking skin with a yellow discoloration; flavokawains A and B are yellow pigments isolated from kava and are likely causative. Despite the resemblance to pellagra, niacin does not reverse this condition.

Heavy kava users have also been observed to lose weight and have low plasma protein levels and low platelet and lymphocyte counts. Pulmonary hypertension and shortness of breath have rarely occurred. Kava should be avoided in pregnant women and children, since the consequences of use are unknown. A recent cause for concern is an uncommon idiosyncratic liver toxicity associated with kava use; in some cases, this has been severe enough to warrant liver transplantation. It is unclear whether kava alone is to blame, but the safety of this herb is under review. Several European countries, where this problem was first reported, have either suspended sales or are acting to make kava a prescription drug.

Kava should not be used with alcohol, benzodiazepines, barbiturates or other sedatives because of their additive effects. In one case, coma resulted from mixing alprazolam and kava. Patients have complained that kava, while relaxing the body, may be less effective for mental anxiety with obsessive or racing thoughts than are the benzodiazepines.

Dosage

Kava preparations are frequently *standardized to 30 to 70% kavapyrones*. Doses of *100 mg (70% kavapyrones) three times daily* are often used for anxiety. Kava is sometimes drunk as a tea (2–4 g of root placed in 150 mL of hot water followed by straining). Treatment may take several weeks to be fully effective, but should be *limited to no more than 3 months* of drug administration.

Conclusion

Kava appears to act somewhat like an *herbal tranquilizer* to produce a calm, relaxed state, often with mild euphoria. At recommended doses it has little effect on cognitive performance. Although it is safe for most adults, prolonged or excessive use may create psychological dependency and health problems.

Milk Thistle

Milk thistle (*Silybum [Carduus] marianus*) is a spiny European plant with white-veined leaves and milky sap, the seed of which is used to treat liver disease. Milk thistle *seed extract* is used orally in the treatment of *alcoholic and other cirrhoses* and in Europe intravenously for its *hepatoprotective effect in Amanita and other mushroom poisonings*. It is grown in this country primarily as a "*liver cleanser*" and is reputed to protect this organ from a wide array of toxins. Milk thistle seed contains the active principle *silymarin*, a complex of flavonolignan compounds including silibinin (silybin), silidianin, and silychristin.

Mechanism of Action

Silymarin is thought to protect the liver by *preventing the entry of toxins* into the hepatocyte and by stimulating *nucleolar polymerase A,* which, in turn, increases protein synthesis and liver regeneration. Silymarin undergoes enterohepatic circulation, increasing its concentration in hepatocytes. It is also an *antioxidant* in its own right and is considered to have some cytoprotective effect against carcinogens.

Indications

Alcoholic cirrhosis has been improved (faster return of liver enzymes to baseline) in at least three trials, although one multicenter Spanish study failed to demonstrate any change in the clinical course. There is no evidence to support the use of milk thistle to increase alcohol tolerance, although it is certainly being used for this purpose. The effectiveness of silymarin for *viral hepatitis* is not clear, although several trials demonstrated enough benefit to encourage further studies.

Intravenous silymarin has been demonstrated to lower mortality from *Amanita mushroom poisonings,* but this formulation is available only in Europe. Animal studies have demonstrated hepatic protection against alcohol, acetaminophen, and mushroom toxins and protection against hepatic fibrosis with bile duct occlusion. There is also evidence of silybin protecting against cis-platin-induced *nephrotoxicity* in rats. It is not yet clear whether milk thistle extract offers any renal protection to humans.

Adverse Reactions, Contraindications, and Interactions

Milk thistle appears to be remarkably safe, with *loose stools* due to increased bile solubility and occasional *allergic reactions* being the common side effects. It has not been evaluated in children or in pregnant women. There are no known serious drug or herb interactions.

Dosage

Dry extract capsules standardized to *70% silymarin* (*calculated as silibinin*) are administered at 200 to 400 mg/day or 12 to 15 g of dried seed per day. Teas are not recommended, since silymarin is not water soluble.

Conclusion

Milk thistle has shown promise in improving liver function parameters in various hepatotoxic situations, such as alcoholic cirrhosis and mushroom poisoning. It is still unclear whether it will offer protection against viral hepatitis and various nephrotoxic agents.

Saw Palmetto

Saw palmetto (*Serenoa repens*) is a dwarf American palm native to the extreme southeastern United States. A lipidosterolic extract of its berries contains fatty acids (especially lauric acid), phytosterols, monocylglycerides, and polysaccharides. Fatty acids constitute more than 80% of the extract and are thought to be the most clinically effective component. It is widely used to treat *benign prostatic hypertrophy* (*BPH*). The berries themselves are less well absorbed than the extract and are therefore believed to be less effective.

Mechanism of Action

Saw palmetto extract can *inhibit the enzyme 5-α-reductase in vitro.* This enzyme converts testosterone into *dihydrotestosterone* (*DHT*), which in turn contributes to prostatic enlargement. Saw palmetto also appears to have an *antiinflammatory effect* and can reduce *DHT binding* to prostatic androgen receptors (*antiandrogenic effect*). Despite its proposed 5-α-reductase mechanism,

saw palmetto has not consistently lowered serum testosterone, DHT, or *prostate-specific antigen* (*PSA*) levels, so it is likely that other mechanisms exist. While several earlier studies did indicate lowered PSA levels, more recent research has not supported these findings. It appears that saw palmetto does not shrink the total prostate either, although it may reduce the size of the transition zone or inner prostatic epithelium.

Indication

Numerous (but not all) trials have indicated improvement in *BPH symptom scores* compared to placebo with 1 to 3 months of therapy. Saw palmetto extract appears to be equally effective as finasteride (see Chapter 63) but is less effective than α_1-adrenoceptor antagonists. No information appears to be available on the use of saw palmetto in the prevention of hair loss.

Adverse Reactions, Contraindications, and Interactions

Headache and GI symptoms are the most frequently reported side effects. It is possible to reduce GI side effects, such as nausea, abdominal discomfort, and diarrhea, by taking the extract with food. Theoretically, decreased libido or erectile dysfunction could also occur. Because of saw palmetto's possible hormonal effects (and lack of indications for use), pregnant and nursing women should avoid it. It is important to rule out prostate cancer in those taking saw palmetto for BPH, since the symptoms are similar. The effect of saw palmetto on prostatic cancer would likely be beneficial but not curative. No drug interactions have been reported.

Dose

For BPH, 320 mg of the lipidosterolic extract by mouth daily in two divided doses with food is usually recommended. It must be taken for a *minimum of 3 months* and perhaps indefinitely. The dried berries and tea are not recommended, since the fatty acids responsible for clinical effect would be largely lost.

Conclusion

Saw palmetto extract is a fairly well tolerated, safe alternative to finasteride for *long-term treatment of BPH,* although α_1-adrenoceptor blocking agents undoubtedly afford more rapid symptom relief.

St. John's Wort

St. John's wort (*Hypericum perforatum*) is a yellow-flowered perennial European herb that has become widely naturalized in the United States. Its name is derived from the Old English word for plant, *wort,* and from the fact that it often starts blooming around June 24, St. John's day. Although St. John's wort has traditionally been used for wound healing, insomnia, rheumatism, and depression, it is most popular today for the treatment of mild to moderate depression.

The leafy parts of the herb contain naphthodianthrones (e.g., *hypericin*), flavonoids (e.g., *quercetin*), and phloroglucinols (e.g., *hyperforin*). Although this herb is now commonly *standardized for its hypericin content,* it appears that its other constituents may also be just as pharmacologically active.

Mechanism of Action

Just how St. John's wort treats depression is not clearly understood. It is possible that this herb's various components may work synergistically rather than through a single active substance, mimicking the action of traditional antidepressants. High concentrations can affect in vitro *serotonin reuptake,* but it is unclear whether this would occur in a patient taking standard oral doses. The hyperforin constituent may possess serotonin reuptake inhibitor activity, and it also inhibits synaptic uptake of γ amino butyric acid (GABA) and L-glutamate. Earlier studies demonstrated some monoamine oxidase inhibition, but this action now seems unlikely to be clinically relevant. Flavonoid components and hypericin also may weakly inhibit catechol-*O*-methyl-transferase (COMT). *Melatonin,* surprisingly, has also been identified in St. John's wort and may play a role in its sleep-enhancing and antidepressant effects.

Indications

St. John's wort is very popular as a physician-prescribed antidepressant in Europe and is widely used for this purpose—usually without medical guidance—in the United States. A meta-analysis of 23 studies concluded that St. John's wort was more effective than placebo in treating mild to moderate depression and was as effective as imipramine and standard antidepressants. It was also better tolerated than the antidepressants to which it was compared. A recent meta-analysis, however, *failed to find St. John's wort effective for severe depression.*

Adverse Reactions, Contraindications, and Interactions

St. John's wort is usually well tolerated, but insomnia, dizziness, fatigue, restlessness, GI upset, constipation, dry mouth, and allergy are reported as possible side effects. Hypomania has also been reported in several cases, and rarely, photosensitivity can be a problem following high doses; hypericin seems to be the component responsible for the photosensitivity. Sun-induced neu-

ropathy has also been described, and it is possible that hypericin may also increase the risk of cataracts with prolonged use. While a prior allergy to the herb is the main contraindication, St. John's wort should also be avoided in pregnant and breast-feeding women (it may increase uterine tone) and in children until its safety is further established.

A major emerging concern in St. John's wort use is the numerous clinically significant herb–drug interactions that have been reported. St. John's wort appears to be a major inducer of the cytochrome *P450 3A4 (CYP3A4) enzyme system* in the liver. This first came to light following acute heart transplant rejection in a person taking *cyclosporin* and St. John's wort. The cyclosporin levels remained subtherapeutic until St. John's wort was discontinued. A similar phenomenon was noted with AIDS patients taking *protease inhibitors* and *nonnucleoside reverse transcriptase inhibitors (NNRTIs).* Concomitant use of St. John's wort reduced the effectiveness of these medicines as well. Since then, St. John's wort has been shown to reduce plasma levels of *digoxin, warfarin, theophylline,* and *oral contraceptives.* Breakthrough bleeding has been observed in young women taking this herb, and patients starting oral contraceptives should be counseled to use backup contraception if they take St. John's wort or antibiotics. St. John's wort can adversely affect many other common medications, including *nonsedating antihistamines, antifungals, chemotherapeutic agents,* and *calcium channel blockers.*

SSRIs should not be taken with St. John's wort because of the risk of the onset of a *serotonin syndrome* characterized by nausea, tremor, and weakness. Alcohol also should be avoided. St. John's wort can increase *opioid*-induced sleep.

Dose

St. John's wort is commonly used at 300 mg of extract (standardized to 0.3% hypericin) three times daily for 6 weeks or longer. Short-term treatment is usually ineffective.

Conclusion

St. John's wort is probably effective for mild to moderate but not severe depression. Although well tolerated in most patients, a major concern is its numerous herb–drug interactions mediated by its induction of the cytochrome P450 enzyme system.

Soy and Other Phytoestrogens

Soybeans (*Glycine max*) are protein-rich legumes widely grown around the world as a food crop. They are the major dietary source of *isoflavones,* which are broken down in the intestine into the phytoestrogens *genis-*

tein and *daidzein.* It is believed that the lower risk of breast cancer, cardiovascular disease, and osteoporosis in Asian women is partly due to their high soy diet, since these benefits are lost when they adopt Western dietary habits. Flaxseed, from flax (*Linum usitatissimum*), is the source of another type of phytoestrogen, *lignan,* as well as linolenic acid and omega-3 fatty acids. Red clover (*Trifolium pratense*) contains *isoflavones* as well as *coumarin* and produces effects somewhat similar to those of diethylstilbestrol. The negative effect of red clover on sheep fertility threatened the economy in New Zealand at one time.

Perhaps the most marketed herbal phytoestrogen is black cohosh, or black snakeroot (*Cimicifuga racemosa*), a tall woodland perennial with white torchlike flowers native to eastern North America. The rhizome contains *triterpene glycosides* and many other ingredients that appear to have phytoestrogenic effects. Other traditional herbs sometimes promoted as phytoestrogens, such as dong quai (*Angelica sinensis*), have little medical evidence to support their use.

Mechanism of Action

Soy isoflavones appear to act as *selective estrogen receptor modulators* in that they can occupy and block the β-estrogen receptor. In premenopausal women with normal estrogen levels, soy therefore would have an overall antiestrogen (estrogen blocking) effect, whereas in postmenopausal women lacking estrogen, a weak estrogenic effect would be observed. Soy may also increase the excretion of bile acids and lower cholesterol.

The mechanism of black cohosh's phytoestrogen effect is unclear, although it may also inhibit estradiol binding to estrogen receptors. It does not appear to contain isoflavones like soy, and there are conflicting findings on its estrogenic activity. Early reports of luteinizing hormone suppression have been contradicted by more recent research showing no change in gonadotropins or estradiol. There appears to be no stimulatory effect on estrogen receptor–positive breast cancer cells.

Indications

Soy is possibly effective in reducing menopausal symptoms, such as hot flashes, although it is much less effective than estrogens for this purpose. Higher isoflavone doses than are typically achieved in the U. S. diet are necessary to protect against osteoporosis. High isoflavone soy protein intake outperformed lower isoflavone supplements in this regard. *Ipriflavone,* a semisynthetic isoflavone, is effective in the treatment and prevention of osteoporosis and is used for this purpose in Europe and Japan. In the United States, the FDA has approved the use of soy in conjunction with a low-fat diet for cholesterol reduction. There also is evidence that diets high in soy protein re-

duce the likelihood of prostate cancer. There is much less evidence available regarding the effectiveness of red clover and flaxseed; however, they too appear to hold some promise for menopausal symptoms, lipid reduction, and prostate cancer.

Black cohosh (*Remifemin* preparation) appears modestly effective in menopausal symptom relief, according to several German studies of up to 6 months' duration; however, more research is necessary before it can be recommended as an estrogen alternative. Black cohosh is less effective than estrogen for symptom reduction and is not known to have any effect against osteoporosis.

Adverse Reactions, Contraindications, and Interactions

While soy is generally considered safe, it may induce *nausea, bloating,* and *allergic reactions* (itchy rashes or even asthma if inhaled as dust) in some people. One study suggested that high midlife soy (tofu) consumption may be associated with *cognitive decline* in later life. However, educational and social differences between the high- and low-tofu groups may also account for some of these findings. Research findings in regard to the safety of soy in breast cancer patients conflict, with an in vitro study suggesting possible stimulation of estrogen-dependent breast cell cultures.

Black cohosh may cause nausea, vomiting, hypotension, and even miscarriage. It is absolutely contraindicated in pregnancy. Red clover contains coumarins and should therefore be avoided with anticoagulants. Diets high in red clover isoflavones have reduced livestock fertility and theoretically could do the same in humans. *Flaxseed may cause nausea, diarrhea, and flatulence.* Cyanogenic nitrates in flax (especially in immature seed pods) have produced toxic reactions.

Dose

Soy protein doses of 20 to 60 g daily are used to reduce hot flashes and to lower elevated cholesterol. Higher doses of isoflavones (2.25 mg/g soy protein) or more than 60 g soy protein may help prevent osteoporosis.

Black cohosh root doses vary widely, with up to 2000 mg/day of root being taken several times daily. *Remifemin* is the best-studied brand, and tablets containing 40 mg of black cohosh extract with 1 mg of triterpenes are given as one or two tablets twice daily.

Conclusions

Soy appears to have weak estrogenic activity when taken after menopause but may block the effects of more potent estrogens (thereby reducing breast cancer risk) when used before menopause. It can reduce menopausal symptoms but is less effective than estrogen in this regard. Although long-term high soy diets may help prevent osteoporosis, it is likely that most U. S. women will not consume enough to be adequate for osteoporosis treatment. Semisynthetic or concentrated isoflavone preparations may play a role in the future.

Black cohosh may reduce menopausal symptoms, and it appears safe and well tolerated for at least a 6-month period. It lacks the other proven benefits of estrogen, however. There is less information to recommend red clover and flaxseed, although they remain widely used for this purpose.

A listing of other popular herbs and their proposed actions is given in Table 69.4.

TABLE 69.4 Other Popular Herbs and Their Chief Indications

Herb	Principal Indication
Aloe vera	Topical use for burns and skin irritation
Bearberry (*Uva ursi*)	Urinary tract infections
Bilberry	Visual and circulatory problems
Boldo	Digestive disorders
Butcher's broom (Ruscus)	Vein disorders
Cascara sagrada	Laxative
Cat's-claw	Inflammatory conditions (little evidence)
Chamomile	Digestive disorders, antispasmodic
Chaste tree	Menstrual disorders
Dong quai (*Angelica sinensis*)	Gynecological disorders (little evidence)
Evening Primrose	Eczema, mastalgia
Ginger	Motion sickness, Antiemetic
Golden seal	Anti-infective (toxic at higher doses)
Gotu kola (Indian pennywort)	Mental fatigue
Green tea	Antioxidant (cancer and heart disease prevention)
Hawthorn	Mild heart failure, BP reduction
Horse chestnut seed	Varicose veins
Licorice	Demulcent, peptic ulcer (high doses elevate BP)
Mistletoe	Anticancer agent (scant evidence, potential toxicity)
Pau d'arco	Multiple chronic conditions (scant evidence)
Senna	Laxative
Skullcap	Immune system support
Slippery elm	Demulcent, coughs
Tea tree oil (Melaleuca)	Skin infections
Turmeric	Antioxidant, antiinflammatory
Valerian	Sleep disorders
Wild yam (Dioscorea)	Menopause symptoms; does not supply progesterone

Study Questions

1. Which herb is most frequently used to treat migraine headache?
   (A) Kava
   (B) Hawthorn
   (C) Feverfew
   (D) Ginseng
   (E) Garlic

2. Which herb is most frequently used to treat benign prostatic hyperplasia?
   (A) Green tea
   (B) Bilberry
   (C) Cayenne
   (D) Ginseng
   (E) Saw palmetto

3. Which herb is most frequently used to treat anxiety?
   (A) Garlic
   (B) Saw palmetto
   (C) Ginkgo
   (D) Kava
   (E) Echinacea

4. Select the herb most frequently used to treat fatigue.
   (A) Ginseng
   (B) Uva ursi
   (C) Horse chestnut
   (D) Evening primrose
   (E) Golden seal

5. Your 80-year-old patient complains of forgetfulness and frequent ringing in his ears (tinnitus) and vertigo. He has seen an ear, nose, and throat specialist, but his examination produced normal findings, and he was told that the problem would probably wax and wane in severity. An extensive neurological evaluation and head computed tomography scan also produced normal findings. What herb might be beneficial for his condition?
   (A) Garlic
   (B) Peppermint
   (C) Ginkgo
   (D) Ginger
   (E) Valerian

6. Before giving permission for the patient in question 5 to take this herb, you forgot to ask about his other medications. Which one of the following drugs could present a problem if taken concomitantly?
   (A) Coumadin
   (B) Propranolol
   (C) Lisinopril
   (D) Acetaminophen
   (E) Amlodipine

7. Which one of the following statements is true regarding St. John's wort?
   (A) It may produce photosensitivity at low doses.
   (B) It may induce the cytochrome P450 system.
   (C) It may be unsafe when high tyramine foods are ingested.
   (D) It may increase the levels of many commonly prescribed medications.

8. Which one of the following statements is true of the Chinese herb ma huang (*Ephedra sinensis*)?
   (A) *Ephedra* has been associated with increased risk of hypertension and tachycardia but not stroke.
   (B) The FDA recommends that it be taken for no more than 1 month.
   (C) The FDA recommends that ephedra alkaloids be limited to no more than 8 mg per dose.
   (D) Ephedra is dangerous at any dose and has no legitimate role in herbal medicine.

ANSWERS

1. **C.** Feverfew has several studies supporting its effectiveness as a prophylactic agent for migraine headache. Kava is best known for its antianxiety effects, hawthorn for its use in congestive heart failure, and ginseng as a tonic to increase energy levels. Garlic is used for a variety of conditions, including hyperlipidemia and hypertension.

2. **E.** Saw palmetto reduces the symptoms of prostatic obstruction with long-term use and appears to be as effective as finasteride. Green tea is recommended as an antioxidant and for its reputed cardiovascular benefits. Bilberry is used for improving night vision, while cayenne pepper is applied topically as a coun-

terirritant for neuralgia. Ginseng is commonly used to boost energy and stamina.

3. **D.** Kava is often recommended for anxiety, and it appears significantly more effective than placebo for this condition. Garlic is used for cardiovascular benefits, saw palmetto for prostatic hypertrophy, and ginkgo as a cerebral vasodilator. Echinacea is considered an immunomodulating herb with potential benefit in viral illnesses.

4. **A.** Ginseng is used to increase energy levels and induce a general sense of physical and mental well-being. Bearberry or uva ursi is a natural treatment for urinary tract infections, whereas golden seal is taken as a general anti-infective. Horse chestnut is used in the management of varicosities. Evening primrose oil (linoleic acid) is commonly thought of as a treatment for either eczema or mastalgia.

5. **C.** Ginkgo would be the most likely herbal treatment to benefit this patient, since it would improve cerebrovascular blood flow and cognitive function. Vertigo and tinnitus may also respond, although there is more evidence for the former. Garlic is traditionally used for cardiovascular benefits (lipid, blood pressure reduction), but it would be unlikely to produce immediate results. Peppermint is used as an antispasmodic in irritable bowel syndrome, while ginger tea is a common carminative (gas reducer) and motion sickness treatment. Valerian is useful as a sedative.

6. **A.** Coumadin, taken in conjunction with ginkgo, could increase the risk of bleeding. Ginkgo has an antiplatelet effect, which has produced bleeding complications in this clinical setting. The other medications listed are not known to have this problem. Acetaminophen, unlike aspirin, does not have an antiplatelet effect.

7. **B.** St. John's wort significantly induces the cytochrome P450 system. St. John's wort has numerous herb–drug interactions thought to be caused by this mechanism, which speeds the elimination of many medications and results in subtherapeutic (not higher) drug levels. Photosensitivity may be associated with high doses but is unlikely to be caused by average or low doses of this herb. St. John's wort does interact with selective serotonin reuptake inhibitors and MAO inhibitors. However, it is not thought necessary to avoid tyramine while taking St. John's wort because it is no longer thought to have clinically significant MAO activity.

8. **C.** The FDA now recommends that for safety reasons, ephedra should be limited to 8 mg or less per single dose and that a total daily dose of 24 mg not be exceeded. These are much lower than past dosage recommendations. The new recommendations also suggest a 1-week (not 1 month) limitation of treatment. Stroke is certainly a possible complication.

Despite many concerns about unsupervised use of ephedra, it may still have a useful role when used in healthy patients at proper doses.

SUPPLEMENTAL READING

Blumenthal M, Goldberg A, and Brinckmann J. (eds.). Herbal Medicine: Expanded Commission E Monographs. Newton, MA: Integrative Medicine Communications, 2000.

Cupp MJ. (ed.). Toxicology and Clinical Pharmacology of Herbal Products. Totowa, NJ: Humana, 2000.

Fetrow CW and Avila JR (eds.). Professional's Handbook of Complementary and Alternative Medicines. Springhouse, PA: Springhouse, 1999.

Jellin JM et al. Pharmacist's Letter/Prescriber's Letter Natural Medicines Comprehensive Database (3rd ed.). Stockton, CA: Therapeutic Research Faculty, 2000.

C A S E   Study   Ma Huang and Athletic Performance

A 20-year-old student athlete went to a university health service with supraventricular tachycardia (heart rate above 200), dizziness, weakness, nausea, tremor, and diaphoresis. He denied any history of heart arrhythmias, and medical history was unremarkable save for penicillin allergy. Family history was negative for heart disease. The patient said he took no medications except creatine for weight lifting. His alcohol intake was limited to up to a six-pack of beer on weekends and he denied both smoking and drug abuse. On further questioning, the patient reluctantly admitted drinking an orange-flavored beverage that had been spiked with ma huang (*Ephedra sinica*) to enhance his performance prior to a weightlifting session that afternoon. The symptoms began shortly afterward. He had used this preparation before without becoming ill, but this time he had added an extra scoop "for good measure." The patient was transferred to the emergency department and observed closely until his tachycardia resolved. Explain the causes of the patient's symptoms.

ANSWER: The active ingredient of ma huang is ephedra, an alkaloid whose derivatives (ephedrine, pseudoephedrine) are ingredients in FDA-approved over-the-counter cold and allergy medicines. Although effective and safe at correct dosages in healthy patients, the intake of ephedra compounds became controversial after their widespread use as a stimulant and appetite suppressant ("herbal fen-phen") caused a spate of adverse reactions (>800) along with several fatalities. The FDA has recommended that total ephedra alkaloids in herbal preparations be limited to no more than 8 mg per dose and that no more than 24 mg per 24 hours (rather than previous recommendations) be taken. Therapy should also be limited to only 1 week. Excessive dosages have caused insomnia, nervousness, headaches, tremor, hypertension, seizures, heart attack, stroke, and death. However, in vulnerable patients, life-threatening adverse reactions have occurred with doses as small as 4 to 20 mg/day.

The correct diagnosis was somewhat delayed in this case by the patient's understandable reluctance to confess to ma huang supplementation. Although up to one-third of U. S. patients may be using herbs, few ever inform their health care providers. Frequently patients are reluctant to discuss the use of unauthorized therapies (stimulants, anabolic steroids, illicit drugs, and herbs), especially if they fear a disapproving reaction on the part of their health care provider. This extends to a wide variety of other behaviors as well and can place both the patient and the physician in difficult or dangerous situations. Fortunately, it is possible to counsel patients about the dangers of an herb or drug without condemning them personally. Providers should create a comfortable environment for the patient to share vital information without fear of reprisal or loss of confidentiality. A blanket off-the-cuff rejection of anything the patient values (sexual issues, herbs, dietary supplements) may result in loss of rapport, with the patient likely continuing the behavior in a clandestine manner. The best way to encourage patients to discuss their use of herbs is to ask them about herb use while taking a medical history. Most patients are glad for the opportunity to discuss their herb use once they realize they won't face condemnation.

Patients with cardiovascular disease (including hypertension), diabetes (risk of hyperglycemia), pregnancy (uterine contractions), prostatism, and anxiety disorders are among those who should not take ma huang at any dose. Drug–herb interactions occur with MAOIs (hypertensive crisis), phenothiazines (tachycardia, hypotension), β-blockers (hypertension) and theophylline (increased CNS effects). Of course, caffeine and other stimulants have an additive effect.

CASE Study   Phytoestrogens and Menopause

A 55-year-old postmenopausal patient returns to the clinic 6 months after being prescribed *Premarin* and *Provera* for hot flashes, vaginal dryness, insomnia, and mood swings. She took hormone replacement therapy (HRT) for 2 months and had significant relief of symptoms. Even so, she noted breast tenderness on this regimen that worried her despite her recent negative mammogram report. When she read in an article that long-term estrogen (>5 years) might increase her risk of breast cancer by up to 30%, she abruptly stopped therapy. Despite the return of her earlier symptoms, she adamantly refused further HRT even when informed again of its effectiveness for osteoporosis. However, she was very interested in pursuing dietary therapy with phytoestrogens, since this is what several women in her church group are doing.

This patient asks how much soy and what type of soy products she must eat to get relief. She questions whether soy phytoestrogens will do "all of the good things and none of the bad," as she has been told. She asks about the safety and effectiveness of other phytoestrogens and about any other "natural" estrogen alternatives to conjugated equine estrogens.

ANSWER: In spite of the many benefits of HRT, about 80% of prescriptions for it are never filled or are discontinued. Many physicians are frustrated when they discover their patients have stopped therapy without their input, more often than not because of fear of breast cancer. Other commonly cited side effects include weight gain, bloating, and spotting. It appears that the tide of public and possibly even scientific opinion may be turning against estrogen therapy. The Heart and Estrogen/Progesterone Replacement Study trial has demonstrated a possible increase in cardiac events in the first 2 years of therapy, although subsequent cardiac risk appears to decline. Overall there was no benefit in reducing risk of death from chronic heart disease in women at risk. Other trials, including the Nurse's Health Trial, suggest that HRT can be associated with a significant (up to 30%) increase in breast cancer after 5 or more years of use, and more than 10 years of HRT has been associated with increased mortality from ovarian cancer. Finally, the recent National Institute of Health trial demonstrating increased breast cancer and cardiovascular risk associated with HRT has altered professional practice as well as public perception of estrogen's risk.

Phytoestrogen dietary therapy has become increasingly attractive to women in the present climate of care. These substances are not estrogens at all, but they bind to estrogen receptors and may act like selective estrogen receptor modulators. Many plant sources of phytoestrogens were found, including soybeans, other legumes, and flaxseed. Soybeans are among the best sources of the isoflavones genistein and daidzein. Soy may now be consumed in a variety of ways: fresh, frozen, dried, roasted (soy nuts), tofu (soybean curd), tempeh (fermented soybeans and grains), soy milk, soy flour, miso (fermented soy paste), and textured vegetable protein. Some soy products may have lost their isoflavone content in processing: soy cheese, soy oil, and tofu yogurt. Flaxseed contains another type of phytoestrogen, lignans, as well as omega-3 fatty acids. About 1 tablespoon of flaxseed could be considered equivalent to one serving (50 g) of soy, and flaxseed may be an alternative for those who dislike tofu.

Although there is some controversy about how much soy must be consumed to benefit from its phytoestrogen effect, it is believed that two servings per day will modestly reduce menopausal symptoms and the risk of breast cancer. More than three servings may reduce cholesterol. Although it has yet to be proved that dietary soy will stop osteoporosis, a synthetic isoflavone, ipriflavone, has been used in Japan and Europe to treat osteoporosis. Large doses of soy (6–8 servings per day) are believed by some to help this condition as well.

Phytoestrogens appear to reduce the risk of breast cancer, because their estrogenic effect is actually quite weak (one two-hundredth of estradiol) and yet by occupying estrogen receptors, they protect the breasts from more potent estrogens. In an estrogen-deficient postmenopausal patient, they provide a modest estrogenic effect, while in an estrogen-rich environment they actually protect the breasts from estrogen stimulation. Soy may also block tyrosine kinase, an enzyme necessary for the growth of cancer cells.

Allergies to soy may be a concern for some patients, and there may be a cross-reaction with peanut allergy. Bloating and gas occur, especially in those unaccustomed to soy products.

Some women are rejecting conjugated equine estrogens in favor of preparations containing lower-potency estriol, a weak human estrogen produced in pregnancy and thought to be more protective of the

CASE Study   Phytoestrogens and Menopause—cont'd

breast. *Tri-Est,* a human estrogen formulation comprised of 80% estriol, 10% estradiol, and 10% estrone (the latter two to increase potency) and *Bi-est,* composed of 80% estriol and 20% estradiol (some converted to estrone) may be ordered at compounding pharmacies. Usual doses of both are 2.5 to 5 mg per day. Many other women elect to take phytoestrogenic herbs rather than soy isoflavone dietary supplements. These less well studied herbs include black cohosh (*Remifemin*) and red clover (*Promensil*). The Chinese herb dong quai has not yet been shown to be effective for menopausal symptoms in clinical trials.

It is not yet clear what the ideal postmenopausal regimen is, but certainly the risks of estrogen replacement are becoming more of a concern to physicians and their patients. Phytoestrogens appear to be relatively safe for the breast, but there are legitimate concerns that they will fail to protect women from osteoporosis. In addition, their safety for women with a history of breast cancer is still quite controversial. Although the epidemiological evidence indicates a protective effect against breast cancer, some in vitro studies on soy isoflavones suggest a possible stimulatory effect on estrogen-dependent breast cancer cells. It makes sense to tailor regimens to bone density studies and assessment of breast cancer risk.

INDEX

Page numbers in italics denote figures; those
followed by a t denote tables.

Mivacurium, 342–343
Modafinil, 351
Moexipril, 212
Monoamine oxidase (MAO), 90, 91
  adrenomimetic drugs and, 98
  inhibitors, 386t, 391–393
Monobactam, 532t
Monobactams, 534
Monobenzone, 495
Monoiodotyrosine (MIT), 743, 744
Montelukast, asthma and, 465, 466t
Moraxella catarrhalis, quinolones and, 519
Moricizine, 170t, 175–176
  electrophysiological effects of, 171t
Morphine, 4, *317*, 317
  abuse of, 409
    consequences, 408t
  adverse reactions, 321
  botanical source of, 786t
  breast milk, 45t
  enterohepatic recirculation, 44t
  renal tubular secretion, 42t
  uses of, 320–321
Multidrug resistance gene (MDR gene), 27
Multiple dosing, *52*, 53
Muromonab (CD3), 661
Muscarine, 121–122
Muscarinic blocking drugs, 134
  absorption, metabolism, excretion, 136
  clinical uses, 136–138
  mechanism of action, 134–135
  pharmacological actions of, 135–136, 135t
  poisoning, 138–139, 138t
Muscarinic receptors, ganglionic blocking
    agents and, 142, 142t
Muscle relaxants, toxicity of, 138t
Muscle tremor, antiasthmatics and, 462
Muscular dystrophy, 666
Muscular system
  catecholamines and, 102–103
  histamine and, 452
  neuromuscular transmission (*see* neuro-
    muscular transmission)
  pulmonary smooth muscle, innervation of,
    87
Mutagenesis, 65
Myasthenia gravis, 341, 657, 658t
  case study, 347
  cholinesterase inhibitors and, 129–130
Mycobacterium avium-intracellulare, clin-
    damycin and, 548
Mycophenolate mofetil (MMF), 493, 661
Mycoplasma
  chloramphenicol and, 546
  macrolides and, 548
  tetracyclines and, 544
Mydriatics, toxicity of, 138t
Myeloid colony-stimulating factors, 663, 663t
Myocardial excitation-contraction coupling,
    152, *153*
Myocardial oxygen supply, 197t
Myosin light chain kinase, *717*, 717–718
Myxedema coma, 747–748

Nabumetone, 428t, 431
N-acetylcysteine, 66t
N-acetyltransferases, 37–38, *38*
Nadolol, 170t
  angina and, 202, 202t
  characteristics of, 113t, 114
Nafcillin, 529–530, 529t
Naftifine, 492t
Naked DNA, as a vector, 670t
Nalbuphine, *317*, 326
  abuse of, consequences, 408t

Nalidixic acid, 519
Nalmefene, *317*, 327
Naloxone, 66t, *317*, 326–327
Naltrexone, *317*, 327
  erectile dysfunction and, 739
Nandrolone, 730
  abuse of, consequences, 408t
Naproxen, 315, 428t, 430
Narcolepsy, psychomotor stimulants and,
    350–351
Nateglinide, 771t, 773
National Formulary, 6
Natriuretic peptides, 215
Natural penicillins, 528–529, 529t
Nausea
  chemotherapy and, case study, 637
Nedocromil, 455
  asthma and, 466–467, 466t
Nefazodone, 388t, 389
  half-life, 386t
Neisseria gonorrhoeae, quinolones and, 519
Neisseria meningitis, chloramphenicol and,
    547
Nelfinavir, 591t, 592
Nematodes, drugs for, 621–625, 622t
Neomycin, 491t, 539t
  case study, 543
  gut flora and, 540
Neostigmine, 126
  renal tubular secretion, 42t
Nephrotic syndrome, diuretics and, 248,
    252–253
Nephrotoxicity, *64*, 64–65
Nervous system
  adrenal medulla, 87
  angiotensins and, 210
  autonomic
    ganglia, 84
    vs. somatic, 83–84, *84*
  autonomic effector cells, receptors, 92–94,
    93t
  blood-brain barrier, 30–31, 287–288, *288*
  catecholamines and, 103
  corticosteroids and, 694
  histamine and, 452
  hormone replacement therapy and, 710
  intercranial pressure, diuretics and, 252
  medulla, opioids and, 319
  meningitis, aminoglycosides and, 540
  muscarinic blocking drugs and, 135t, 136
  nerve impulse transmission, 87–88, *88*, *89*
    neurochemical transmission, 88
      acetylcholine, *88*, 89
      norepinephrine, *89*, *90*, 90–92, *91*
  neurons
    adrenergic, 85
    defined, 83
    noradrenergic, 85
    postganglionic, *84*, 84–85
    preganglionic, *84*, 84–85
  neuroscience, 281–282, *282*
  neurotransmitters, 282–284
    amino acid, *284*, 284–285, *285*, 285t
    autonomic, 85
    peptides, 285–287, 286t
  nicotine and, 144
  organization and functions, 83
  parasympathetic, *84*, 85
    organs innervated by, 85–87
  somatic, *84*
  stimulants, 348–349, 349t
  sympathetic, *84*
    organs innervated by, 85–87
Netilmicin, 539t
Neurokinin A, 286t

Neurokinin B, 286t
Neuroleptic malignant syndrome, 402
Neuromuscular blockade, reversal of, 130
Neuromuscular transmission
  acetylcholine depression, 340–341
  acetylcholine enhancement, 340
  agents affecting, 338, *339*, 340
  antispasticity agents, 344–345, 345t
  blocking agents, 341–344
Neuronal uptake, 90
Neurons (*see* nervous system)
Neuropeptide Y, 286t
Neurotensin, 286t
Neurotoxicity, *64*, 65
Neurotoxins, 341
Neurotransmission, ganglionic, *144*
Neurotransmitters, autonomic, 85
Nevirapine, 589t, 590
  enzyme induction, 37t
New Drug Application (NDA), 6
Newborn
  drugs and, case study, 290
N-hexane, *64*
Niacin, 780, 780t
Niclosamide, 622t, 625
Nicotine, 143
  abuse of, 411
    consequences, 408t
  breast milk, 45t
  CYP isoforms and, 35t
  pharmacological actions of, 144
  smoking cessation, case study, 147
Nicotinic acid, 272–273, 273t
  drug interactions, 275t
Nicotinic receptor, 10–11, 143
  ganglionic, blockade of, 143–144
  muscarinic blocking drugs and, 136
Nifedipine, 197, 220t
  adverse reactions, 222t
  induced vasodilation, case study, 224
  pharmacokinetics of, 222t
Nifurtimox, 607t, 610–611
Nikethamide, 349t
Nitrates
  chronic (congestive) heart failure and, 155
  as a food additive, 67t
  organic, angina and, *197*, 197–200, *198*, 200t
Nitric oxide, 215–216, 426
Nitrites
  antidote for, 66t
  as a food additive, 67t
Nitrofurans, 521–522
Nitrofurantoin, *64*, 521
Nitrofurazone, 521–522
Nitrogen dioxide, *64*, 66
Nitrogen mustards, 639t, 640–641
Nitroglycerin
  angina and, 197, 200t
  erectile dysfunction and, 739
Nitrosoureas, 639t, 641–642
Nitrous oxide, 292t, 298–300, 300t, 305
  partition coefficient of, 301t
Nocardia, sulfonamides and, 517
Noncompetitive antagonism, 18, *18*
Nonhalogenated inhalational anesthetics,
    305
Non-Hodgkin's disease, cure rates for, 631t
Non-insulin-dependent diabetes mellitus
    (NIDDM), 767
Nonionic bisphenols, 502, 503t, 504
Nonlinear pharmacokinetics, *53*, 53
Nonmaleficence, principle of, 73–74
Nonnucleoside reverse transcriptase in-
    hibitors (NNRTIs), 585, 588–590, 589t
Nonopioid analgesics (*see* analgesics)